Neuromuscular Case Studies

SECOND EDITION

Neuromuscular Case Studies

Tulio E. Bertorini, MD, FAAN, FACP

Director, Mid-South MDA and ALS Clinics
Professor of Neurology
Director, Clinical Neurophysiology Fellowship
University of Tennessee Health Sciences Center
Semmes Murphey Clinic
Memphis, Tennessee

ELSEVIER

Elsevier
1600 John F. Kennedy Blvd.
Ste 1800
Philadelphia, PA 19103-2899

NEUROMUSCULAR CASE STUDIES, SECOND EDITION ISBN: 978-0-323-87400-7

Content Strategist: Mary Hegeler
Senior Content Development Specialist: Shilpa Kumar
Publishing Services Manager: Shereen Jameel
Project Manager: Nandhini Thanga Alagu
Design Direction: Amy L. Buxton

Printed in India

Last digit is the print number: 9 8 7 6 5 4 3 2 1

*To my wife, Emma; my son Tulio and his girlfriend, Stacey;
my daughter Paola and her husband, Jay; my son Francisco and his wife, Paulinha;
and my grandchildren Nicolas, Rafael, and Gabrela.*

To the memory of my parents, Nicolas and Enriqueta.

PREFACE

In the first edition of this book we presented cases as diagnostic exercises using clinical evaluations and electrophysiological and histological tests. Since then, more than a decade has passed, during which time we've seen an increase in the use of genetic testing in diagnosis, sometimes avoiding the need to do electrophysiology or histology in myopathies. These, however, are still relevant, particularly in some other disorders. Also, immunology with specific antibody tests has increased our yield to achieve a proper diagnosis.

Several cases included in this edition were evaluated in the past and included histology that could have been avoided if the patients were seen currently and had genetic testing for diagnosis. We have included these cases, however, for their educational relevance in demonstrating their histological characteristics.

Most importantly, we now have many treatments that were not available when the first edition of this book was published; these include new immune and genetic treatments (such as antisense oligonucleotides) and gene replacement, which have revolutionized care. We include several new cases and have expanded old ones emphasizing their treatments, some of which have been newly recognized.

We hope that this new edition provides not only diagnostic exercises but a guidance to treatment as well. This book is not intended to be comprehensive; for more in-depth exploration of the subject, we encourage our readers to refer to larger treatises available in the literature.

ACKNOWLEDGMENTS

I would like to thank Cindy Burchfield and Ginger Lindsey very much for their excellent secretarial help.

The superb histological work and photography by Joseph Null are very much appreciated.

I also want to thank Jason Peck for the professional artwork.

I am grateful to my nursing personnel at Semmes-Murphey Clinic: Teig Wetzel MSN, RN, Samantha Hulsey, MA, and Mary K Norris PA; and to the EMG Clinic Director, Rhonda Walker R.EEG.T, R.NCS.T, and technicians Lori Maynard R.EEG.T, R.NCS.T, Karrie Krone R.EEG.T, R.NCS.T; and also our new technician, Christine Nguyen. They all do great work.

I also want to thank The University of Tennessee Department of Neurology and the Semmes-Murphey Clinic for their support.

Lastly, I appreciate the editorial assistance of Shilpa Kumar, Mary Hegeler and Nandhini Thanga Alagu at Elsevier.

Sincerely yours,
Tulio

CONTENTS

Introduction

1

Neuromuscular Anatomy and Function

Neuromuscular disorders are those that affect the anterior horn (motor neuron diseases, such as amyotrophic lateral sclerosis [ALS]), roots (radiculopathies), plexuses (plexopathies), or peripheral nerves (polyneuropathy, mononeuropathy). These also include diseases of the neuromuscular junction (e.g., myasthenia gravis) and muscle fibers (myopathies) (Fig. 1-1). Several of these disorders could involve other regions of the nervous system such as the spinal cord and its pathways or other organs in the body. The following is a review of the basic anatomy and physiology of muscle and nerve that is of importance in understanding these disorders.

The performance of movements requires the interaction of neuronal systems of the cerebral cortex and the motor neurons of the brainstem and anterior horns of the spinal cord. The fine modulation of these movements is regulated by several pathways that include the proprioceptive input for feedback, the interaction of the cortical neurons, limbic system, brainstem, and interneuronal systems.[1]

The feedback is regulated by the interaction of receptors in *muscle spindles* and *deep tendon organs*. The muscle spindle has intrafusal muscle fibers that when stretched activate their *1 alpha nerve fibers* that stimulate motor neurons of agonist muscles to contract. They also activate *inhibitory* neurons that go to motor neurons of antagonist muscles. The sensitivity of the spindles varies with their length, which is determined by the contraction of its *intrafusal* fibers that are innervated by *gamma* motor neurons. Another regulatory mechanism is the input of the deep tendon organs through their *1b afferent axons* that are activated upon changes in muscle tension, causing the inhibition of agonist motor neurons, while facilitating antagonist muscles to contract.

The **motor unit** is the final pathway of the motor system. This is formed by the motor neurons of the spinal cord or brainstem, their myelinated axons, and the muscle fibers innervated by that neuron, which are intermixed with fibers from other motor units. The physiologic and biochemical characteristics of muscle fibers of a motor unit are determined by the rate of firing of their motor neurons.[2]

There are two major types of muscle fibers, depending on their speed of contraction, their biochemical characteristics, and, thus, their histochemical staining, and all muscle fibers of a motor unit are of the same type. *Type I* fibers correspond to the red or dark meat in animals. *Type II* muscle fibers correspond to white meat (Table 1-1). The characteristics of these fibers could be changed by cross-innervation from nerves of one type of muscle to the other or by prolonged stimulation of their axons at different rates. Type I muscle fibers are slow-contracting and stain pale with ATPase using alkaline pH, and dark with oxidative stains.[1,2] These fibers also have subtypes that can be recognized by special histochemical stains, such as nonspecific esterase and menadione-mediated alpha glycerophosphate dehydrogenase.[3]

Type II fibers stain dark with ATPase at alkaline pH and have two major subtypes. Type IIA fibers are fast-contracting, nonfatigable fibers that stain dark with alkaline ATPase and pale at acid pH of 4.6 and 4.3. Their function depends mainly on aerobic metabolism. The type IIB fibers stain intermediate with ATPase at pH 4.6 (Fig. 1-2). These are fast-contracting, fast-fatiguing fibers that depend mainly on glycolytic, anaerobic metabolism.[2]

In humans, muscle fibers of both fiber types and subtypes are intermixed with fibers of other motor units. They appear in muscle histology in an almost checkerboard pattern, as seen in Fig. 1-2, with a predominance of one or the other in some muscles. The deltoid, for example, has mainly type I fibers, and the quadriceps has mainly type II.

Peripheral nerves carry axons from motor neurons and sensory afferents from the Golgi tendon organs and spindles. They also contain large myelinated fibers that carry proprioceptive sensation. Nerves also have unmyelinated and small myelinated axons that carry touch, pain, and temperature sensations. Their cell bodies are located in the dorsal root ganglia; peripheral nerves also have autonomic fibers with myelinated presynaptic and unmyelinated postsynaptic axons (Table 1-2).

ANATOMY OF THE CRANIAL AND PERIPHERAL NERVES

Human striated muscles are innervated by nerves that originate in the brainstem and spinal cord.[4–7] These are summarized here. Motor cranial nerves include those to the *extraocular* muscles such as the **oculomotor**, **abducens**, and **trochlear** nerves; and the **V cranial** or **trigeminal** nerve that innervates muscles of mastication and provides sensation to the face. The **facial** or **VII cranial nerve** innervates muscles of facial expression, as well as the lacrimal and salivary glands, provides sensation and taste to the anterior part of the tongue, and relays sensation of the tympanic membrane, external auditory canal, and a small area of the skin behind the ear. The **hypoglossal** nerve supplies muscles of the tongue, while the **glossopharyngeal**, **vagal**, and **cranial accessory** nerves innervate the laryngeal muscles.

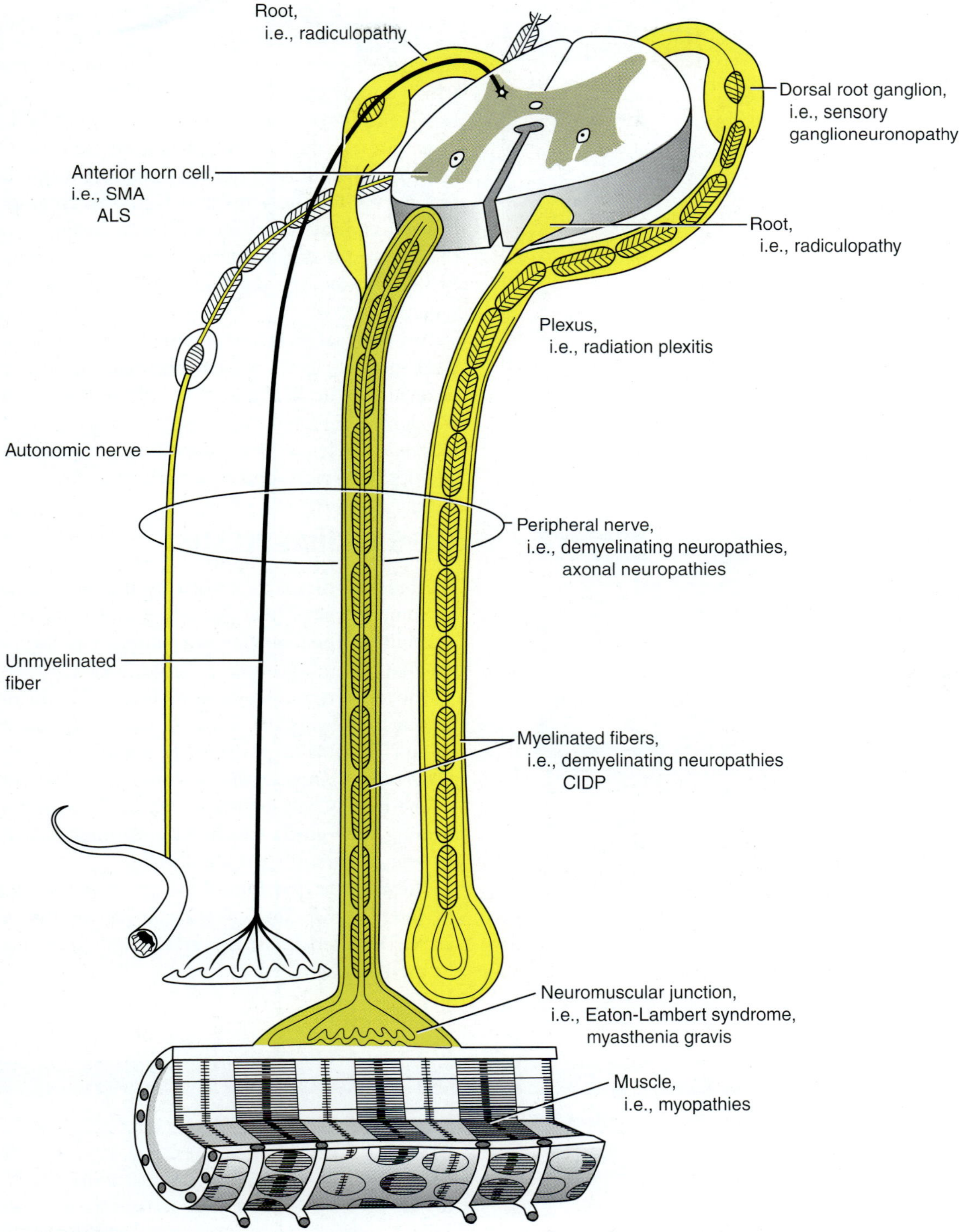

FIG 1-1 The anatomic elements of the peripheral nervous system and related neurologic disorders. (Reprinted with permission from Bertorini TE. Overview and classification of neuromuscular disorders. In: Bertorini TE, ed. *Clinical Evaluation and Diagnostic Tests for Neuromuscular Disorders.* Boston, MA: Butterworth-Heinemann; 2002.)

The **glossopharyngeal** nerve also relays taste sensation of the posterior tongue. The **spinal accessory** nerve supplies the *sternocleidomastoid* and upper portion of the *trapezius* muscles. The *sternocleidomastoid* also receives innervation from C2 and C3 roots, while innervation of the upper *trapezius* also comes from C3 and C4 roots.

The ***anterior roots*** of the spinal cord carry motor axons from the anterior horn, and the **posterior roots** are composed of sensory axons, the cell bodies of which are in the posterior root ganglia. Both are formed by rootlets that exit or enter the cord. They then join to form the **spinal nerves** that exit the spinal canal.

TABLE 1-1 Major Skeletal Muscle Fiber Types

	Type I	Type II
Contraction time	Slow (tonic)	Fast (twitch)
Oxidative enzyme content (i.e., NADH-TR*)	High	Low
Capillary supply	Rich	Poor
Myofibrillar adenosine triphosphatase (pH 9.4)	Low	High
Myofibrillar adenosine triphosphatase (pH 4.3)	High	Low
Glycolytic activity	Low	High
Lipid content	High	Low

**NADH-TR*, Nicotinamide adenine dinucleotide-tetrazolium reductase.
Reprinted from Bertorini TE, ed. *Clinical Evaluation and Diagnostic Tests for Neuromuscular Disorders*. Boston, MA: Butterworth-Heinemann; 2002:600.

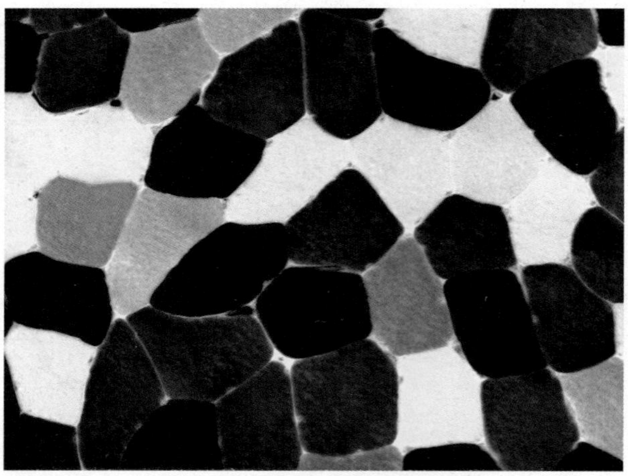

FIG 1-2 Muscle biopsy stained with ATPase at a pH of 4.6. Notice the dark type I fibers, pale type IIA fibers, and intermediate type IIB fibers (×200).

There are 31 pairs of spinal nerves: 8 cervical, 12 thoracic, 5 lumbar, 5 sacral, and 1 coccygeal (Fig. 1-3). After exiting the cord, these branch into two divisions: the ***posterior rami***, which supply the posterior area of the skin in the neck and trunk and paraspinal muscles, and the ***anterior rami***, which innervate the skin of the anterior lateral aspect of the trunk and form the different plexuses that give origin to the peripheral nerves for the arms and legs. The anterior rami of the **thoracic spinal** nerves form the intercostal nerves, supplying the *intercostal* and *abdominal* muscles, and provide sensation to these areas. The dermatomal distribution of the body is seen in Fig. 1-4.

The **cervical plexus** is formed of the anterior rami of the cervical roots *C1* to *C4*, which innervate the anterior and lateral flexors of the neck, and form the **phrenic** nerve from *C3* to *C5*, which innervates the *diaphragm*. The *trapezius* and *sternocleidomastoid* muscles receive innervation from the **accessory** nerve and upper cervical roots, as described earlier.

THE BRACHIAL PLEXUS

The brachial plexus is formed by the anterior rami of *C5* to *T1* spinal nerves which give origin to the nerves of the upper extremities. The following is a summary of the anatomy of the brachial plexus (Fig. 1-5):

The roots from *C5* to *C6* combine to form the ***upper trunk*** in the brachial plexus, the *C7* roots form the ***middle trunk***, and the *C8* and *T1* roots form the ***lower trunk***. The three trunks have ***posterior*** and ***anterior divisions*** that form the **cords**.

The **trunks** pass by the region of the supraclavicular fossa forming their **cords** which travel through the thoracic outlet between the first rib and the clavicle.

The ***anterior divisions*** of the upper and ***middle trunk*** form the ***lateral cord*** which gives origin to the **musculocutaneous** nerve. The ***lateral cord*** also gives origin to the outer branch of the **median** nerve.

TABLE 1-2 Nerve Fiber Classification

Sensory and Motor Fibers	Sensory Fibers	Diameter (μm)	Velocity (m/s)	Function
A-α	Ia	10–20	0–120	Motor: alpha motor neurons Sensory: muscle spindle afferents
A-α	Ib	10–20	50–120	Sensory: Golgi tendon organs, touch, pressure
A-β	II	4–12	25–70	Motor: motoneurons to intra/extrafusal muscle fibers Sensory: secondary muscle spindle afferents, touch, pressure, vibration
A-γ		2–8	10–50	Motor: small gamma motoneurons to intrafusal muscle fibers
A-σ	III	1–5	3–30	Sensory: small touch, pain, temperature fibers
B		1–3	3–15	Small unmyelinated preganglionic autonomic fibers
C	IV	<1	<2	All postganglionic autonomic fibers, pain, and temperature fibers

Modified with permission from Dumitru D, Gitter AJ. Nerve and muscle anatomy and physiology. In: Dumitru D, Amato AA, Zwarts MJ, eds. *Electrodiagnostic Medicine*. 2nd ed. Philadelphia, PA: Hanley & Belfus: 2002:17.

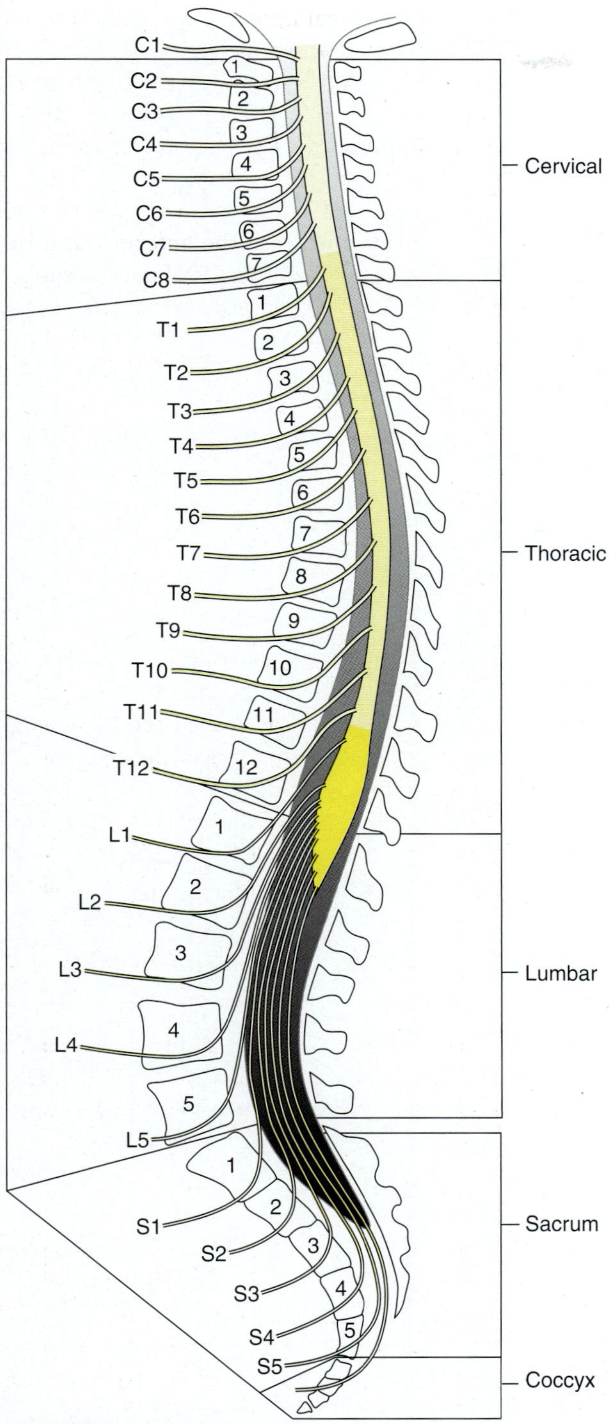

FIG 1-3 The spinal roots and their nerves.

The ***posterior cord*** is formed by the union of the three ***posterior* divisions** and gives off the **subscapular**, **thoracodorsal**, and **axillary** nerves, then proceeds to form the **radial** nerve.

The **anterior division** of the ***lower trunk*** forms the ***medial cord*** that gives origin to the ***ulnar*** nerve, the **medial branch** of the ***median*** nerve, and the ***medial antebrachial cutaneous*** *sensory* nerve of the forearm.

The ***dorsal scapular*** nerve originates *directly* from the C4 and C5 roots and innervates the rhomboids and a portion of the *levator scapulae*. The rhomboid is innervated only by fibers from the C5 root. The ***long thoracic*** nerve also originates *directly* from C5 to C7 roots to supply the *serratus anterior* muscle. It is important to study the rhomboids and *serratus anterior* muscles electromyographically in suspected cervical radiculopathies, particularly for the diagnosis in those without evidence of denervation in paraspinal muscles, because the serratus and the rhomboid muscles are affected in radiculopathies, but not in brachial plexopathies.

Nerves of the Brachial Plexus

The **suprascapular** nerve arises from the *C5* to *C6* roots through the upper trunk supplying the *supraspinatus* and the *infraspinatus* muscles.

The **subscapular** nerve from C5 to C6 roots innervates the *teres major* muscle. The **anterior thoracic** nerve from the C5 to C8 roots innervates the *pectoralis major* and *minor*, and the **thoracodorsal** nerve from C6 to C8 roots innervates the *latissimus dorsi* muscle.

The ***axillary*** nerve is formed by fibers of the C5 to C6 roots which go through the posterior cord of the plexus and innervate the *deltoid* and *teres minor* muscles, as well as part of the skin of the lateral shoulder.

The ***musculocutaneous*** nerve originates in the lateral cord from fibers of the C5 to C6 roots and innervates the *biceps*, *brachialis*, and *coracobrachialis* muscles as well. Its sensory branch, the ***lateral antebrachial cutaneous* nerve**, innervates the lateral aspect of the forearm.

The ***radial*** nerve is formed of axons from C5 to C8 roots going through the posterior cord and innervates the *triceps* and the *anconeus* muscles in the arm; then, after passing the spiral groove of the humerus, it gives off a sensory branch, the ***posterior antebrachial cutaneous*** nerve which innervates the skin of the lateral and the dorsal forearm. After the groove, the nerve supplies the *brachioradialis* and the *extensor carpi radialis longus*. After entering the forearm, the **radial** nerve divides into the motor ***posterior interosseus*** nerve and its sensory branch, the **superficial radial** nerve, which innervates the skin of the lateral aspect of the dorsum of the hand. The **posterior interosseus** nerve innervates the *supinator, extensor carpi radialis brevis, abductor pollicis longus, extensor carpi ulnaris, extensor digitorum communis, extensor pollicis longus* and *brevis, extensor digiti minimi*, and *extensor indicis*.

The ***median*** nerve originates from axons of the *C6* to *T1* roots that travel through the lateral and medial cords of the brachial plexus. The nerve supplies the *flexor carpi radialis, pronator teres, palmaris longus*, and *flexor digitorum superficialis*. Before entering the carpal tunnel, the nerve gives off a sensory branch that innervates the skin of the thenar eminence. The nerve then passes through the carpal tunnel and supplies the *lumbricals I and II* and forms the **recurrent thenar** nerve that innervates the *abductor pollicis brevis*, the *opponens pollicis*, and the *flexor pollicis*. The latter is also partially innervated by the **ulnar** nerve.

In the forearm the median nerve also gives rise to a purely motor branch, the **anterior interosseus** nerve, which innervates the *pronator quadratus, flexor pollicis longus*, and *flexor digitorum profundus* I and II.

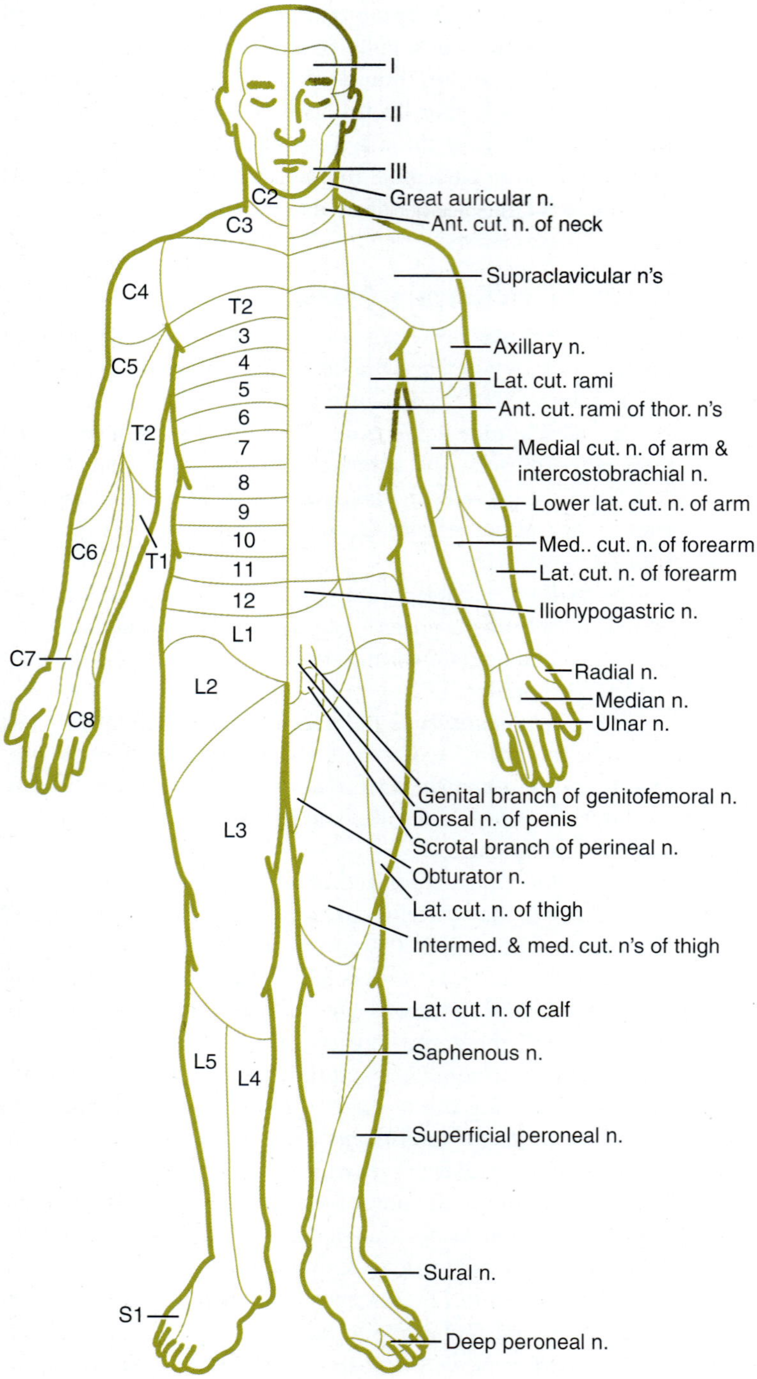

FIG 1-4 **A**, The dermatomes of the body, anterior view.

Continued

The sensory axons of the distal **median nerve** innervate the skin of the lateral aspect of the palm, the dorsal surface of the terminal phalanges, and the volar surface of the first three digits and the middle of the fourth digit. The axons innervating the skin of the thumb come from the *C6* roots and part of *C7;* the index and the middle fingers, from the C7 root.

The most common anomalous cross-innervations in the arm are crossovers between the **median** and **ulnar** nerves. Their fibers, which originate from the median nerve, travel with the ulnar nerve to innervate muscles that are normally innervated by the **ulnar** nerve.

The ***ulnar*** nerve originates from the *C8* and *T1* roots through the medial cord of the plexus and travels in the arm next to the brachial artery and the **median** nerve. After entering the forearm, it supplies the *flexor carpi ulnaris* and *flexor digitorum profundus III* and *IV*, then also gives rise to the ***dorsal cutaneous branch***, which innervates the skin of the medial dorsal aspect of the hand. It then passes the medial aspect of the wrist, then the hand, and gives origin to its ***superficial branch*** supplying the *palmaris brevis* muscle and the skin of the medial aspect of the hand, the hypothenar eminence, and the fifth digit and half of the fourth digit. The ***motor branch*** innervates the muscles of the

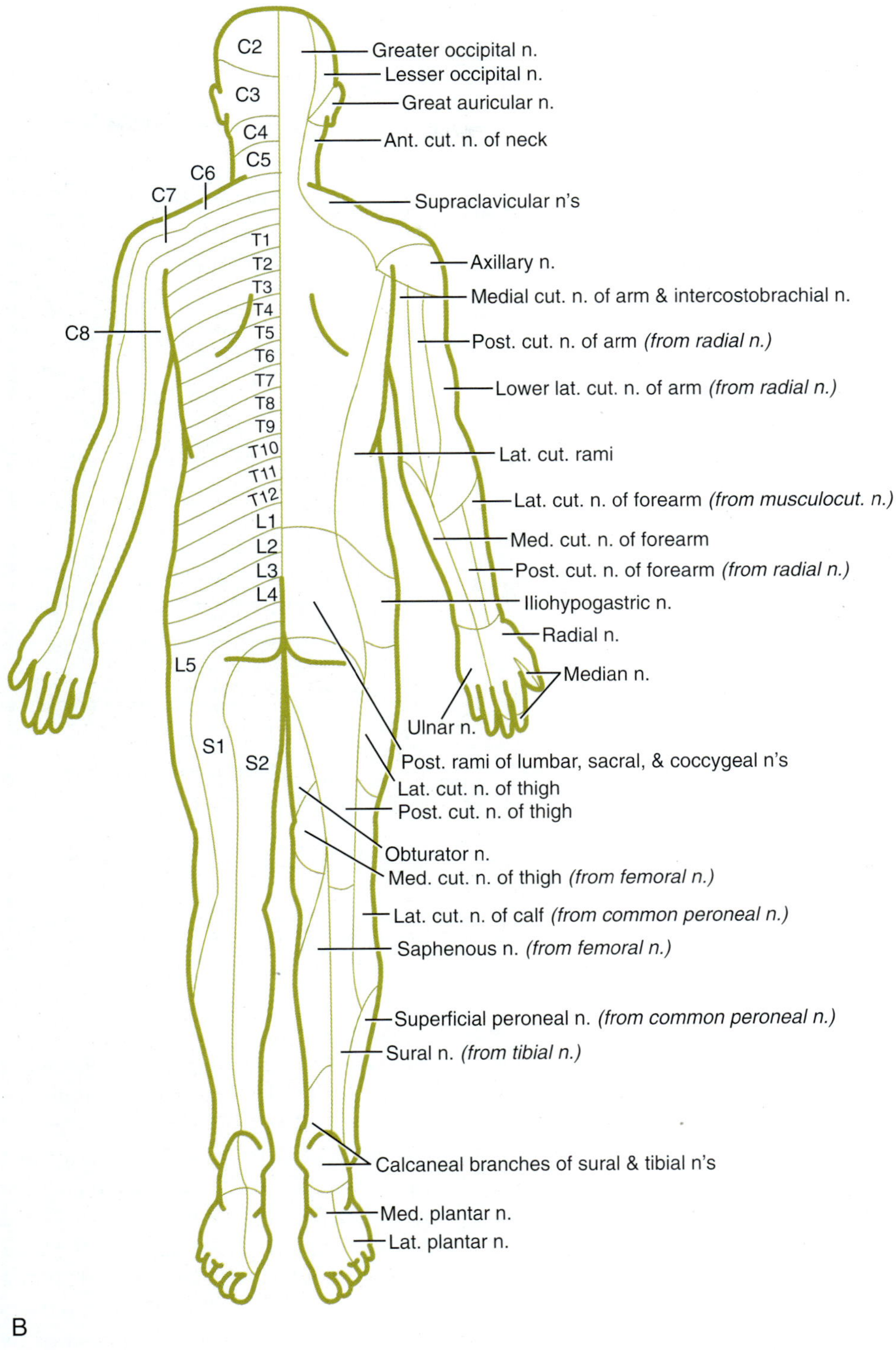

FIG 1-4, cont'd B, The dermatomes of the body, posterior view. (Reprinted with permission from Bertorini TE. Clinical evaluation and clinical laboratory tests. In: Bertorini TE, ed. *Clinical Evaluation and Diagnostic Tests for Neuromuscular Disorders*. Boston, MA: Butterworth-Heinemann; 2002.)

hypothenar eminence and then innervates the dorsal *interossei* and *lumbricals III* and *IV*, the three *volar interossei*, and half of the *flexor pollicis brevis*.

The ***median antebrachial cutaneous*** nerve originates *directly* from the medial cord (from the lower trunk) and supplies the skin over the medial aspect of the forearm. This nerve is important in electrodiagnosis, because it could be affected in plexopathies, helping to differentiate them from ulnar neuropathies and C8–T1 radiculopathies, in which it is not involved.

THE LUMBOSACRAL PLEXUS

The spinal cord ends in the conus medullaris, and the roots of the lower segments form the cauda equina, which gives origin to the **lumbosacral plexus** (Fig. 1-6). The **anterior rami** of the *L1* to *L3* roots and part of the L4 root form the ***lumbar plexus***, which travels within the *psoas muscle*, giving origin to the following: distal branches to the *quadratus lumborum* and branches to the *psoas*; the ***iliohypogastric*** nerve, which

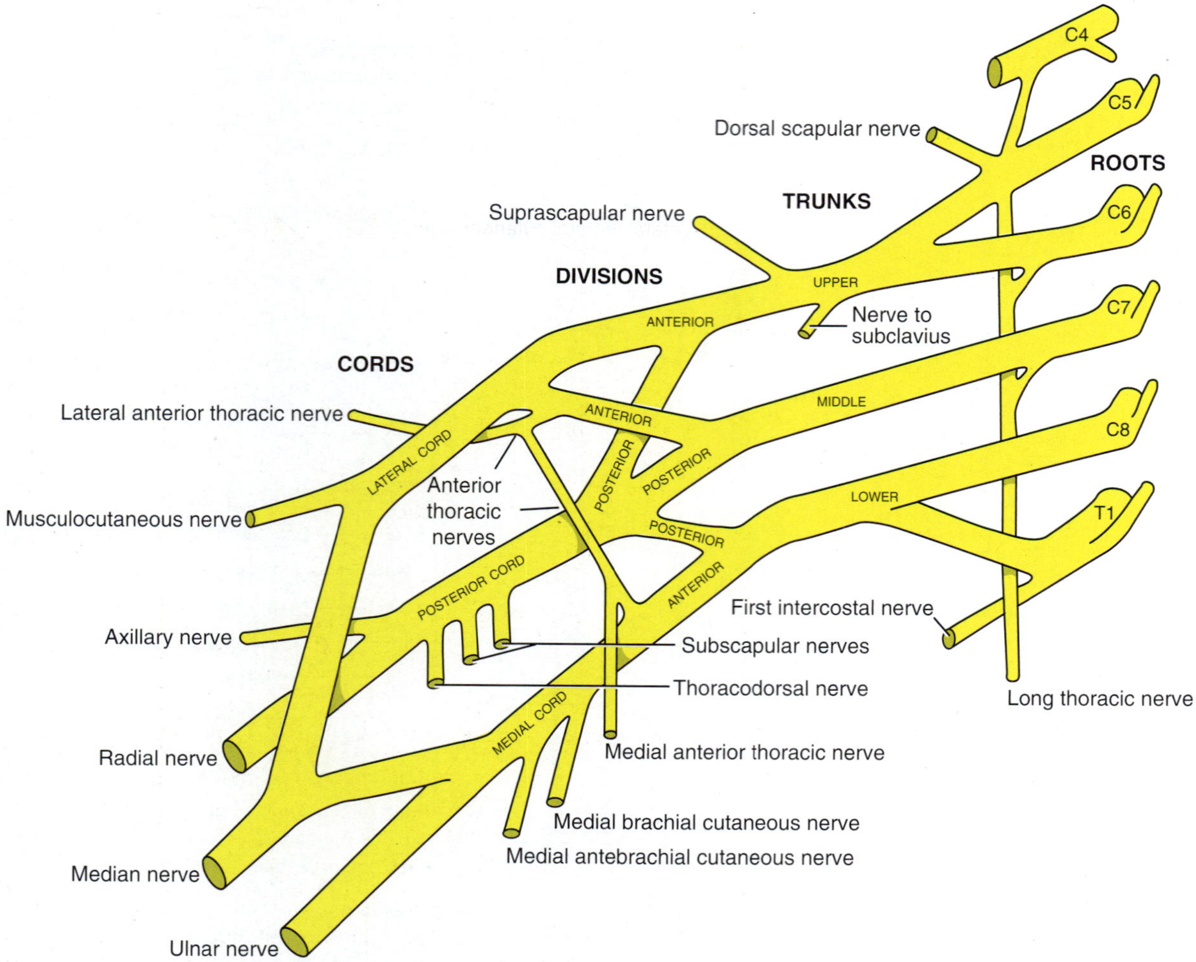

FIG 1-5 The brachial plexus and its nerves. (Reprinted with permission from Bertorini TE. Clinical evaluation and clinical laboratory tests. In: Bertorini TE, ed. *Clinical Evaluation and Diagnostic Tests for Neuromuscular Disorders*. Boston, MA: Butterworth-Heinemann; 2002.)

originates from the L1 root and innervates the skin of the upper buttocks and the hypogastric region; the ***ilioinguinal*** nerve, which arises from *L1* to *L2* roots and innervates the skin of the medial thigh, the root of the penis, part of the scrotum and labia majora, and *internal oblique* and *transversalis* muscles; the ***genitofemoral*** nerve from *L1* to *L2* roots, which forms the ***lumboinguinal*** nerve that supplies the skin of the femoral triangle; and the **external spermatic** nerve, which innervates the *cremasteric* muscle and the skin of the inner area of the upper thigh, scrotum, and labia.

The **anterior divisions** from the L2 to L4 roots give origin to the ***obturator*** **nerve**, which innervates the *adductor muscles* (the *adductor magnus* is also partially innervated by the **sciatic** nerve) and the skin of the medial and upper thigh.

The ***lateral femoral cutaneous*** nerve originates from the **posterior division** of the plexus from fibers of *L2* to *L3* roots and supplies the skin of the lateral thigh.

The ***femoral*** nerve originates from **posterior divisions** of the *L2* to *L4* roots to innervate the *psoas* and *iliacus*, then exits the pelvis under the inguinal ligament, and innervates the *pectineus*, *sartorius*, and *quadriceps muscles*. Its **sensory branches** supply the skin of the anterior thigh and the medial calf. The ***saphenous*** nerve is a sensory branch of the femoral nerve; it originates from the L2 and L4 roots and supplies the skin of the medial aspect of the knee, the medial leg, and medial side of the foot.

The ***sacral plexus*** originates from the *L5* to *S3* roots in front of the sacroiliac joint and the piriformis, giving off the **superior *gluteal*** nerve from the L4 to S1 roots, the ***inferior gluteal*** nerve from the L5 to S2 roots, and a branch to the *piriformis* muscle, all from the posterior divisions. Other posterior division fibers form the **posterior femoral cutaneous** and **perforating cutaneous** nerves. Fibers from the **anterior divisions** innervate the *obturator internus, superior gemellus, quadratus femoris*, and *inferior gemellus*. Branches from S2 to S5 **anterior primary rami** form the **pelvic nerves** such as the **pudendal** nerve, **pelvic splanchnic**, and branches to the *levator ani, coccygeus*, and *external anal sphincter* muscles.

The **superior gluteal** nerve innervates the *gluteus medius* and *minimus* and the *tensor fascia latae*. The **inferior gluteal** nerve innervates the *gluteus maximus*.

The ***sciatic*** nerve is formed by anterior and posterior divisions of the L4 to S2 roots and consists of the ***peroneal portion***, which originates from the ***posterior divisions*** of the plexus, and

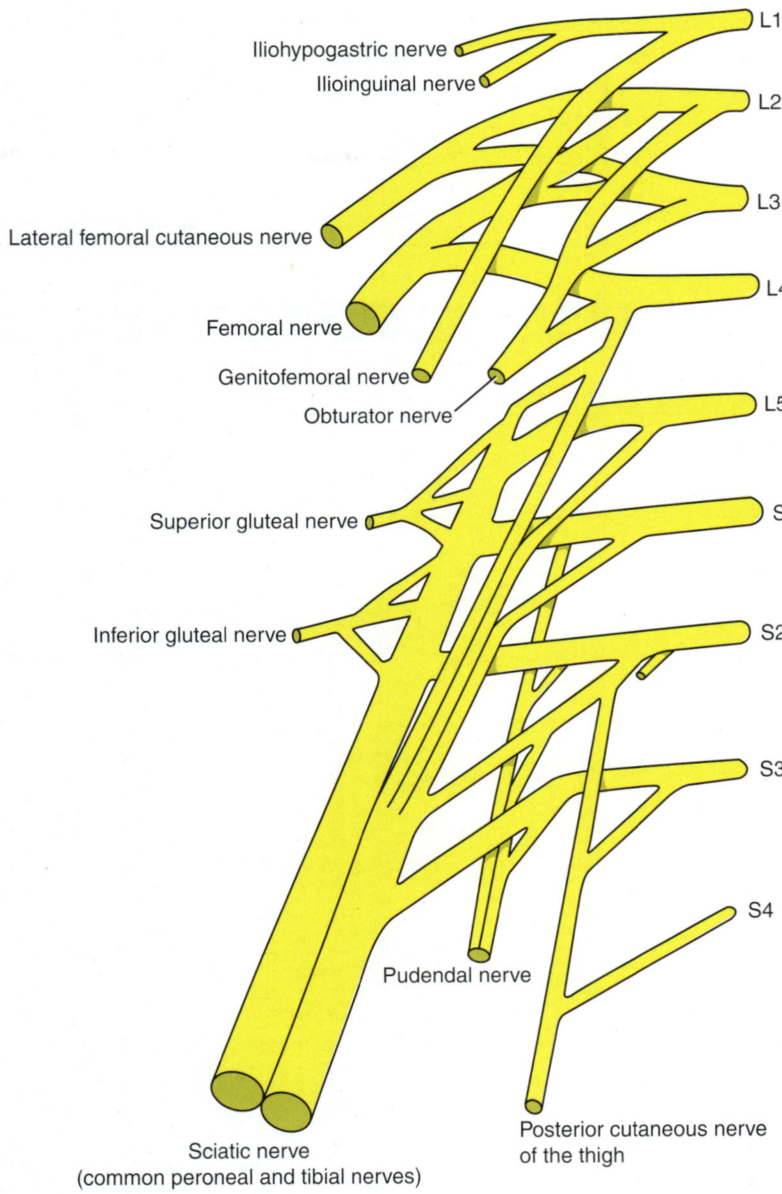

FIG 1-6 The lumbosacral plexus and its nerves. (Reprinted with permission from Bertorini TE. Clinical evaluation and clinical laboratory tests. In: Bertorini TE, ed. *Clinical Evaluation and Diagnostic Tests for Neuromuscular Disorders*. Boston, MA: Butterworth-Heinemann; 2002.)

the ***tibial portion***, formed from the ***anterior divisions***. The ***tibial portion*** innervates the skin of the outer thigh and the *hamstring* muscles, except for the short head of the *biceps*, which is innervated by the **peroneal portion**. The *adductor magnus* is also partially innervated by the **obturator** nerve.

The ***peroneal*** and ***tibial*** portions of the **sciatic** nerve separate to form the **tibial** and **common peroneal** nerves in the posterior aspect of the thigh.

The ***common peroneal*** nerve originates at the popliteal fossa from the **lateral *popliteal*** nerve of the peroneal portion of the ***sciatic***, originating from axons of the *L4* to *S1* roots. The nerve travels around the fibular head and gives a ***sensory branch*** to the patella, then divides into the ***superficial*** and ***deep peroneal*** nerves. The **superficial peroneal** innervates the *peroneus longus* and *brevis*, and its **sensory branch** innervates the anterior lateral aspect of the lower half of the leg and the dorsum of the foot and toes. The ***deep peroneal*** nerve innervates the *tibialis anterior, extensor hallucis longus, peroneus tertius*, and *extensor digitorum brevis* and supplies the small area of the skin between the first and second toes.

The ***tibial*** nerve originates at the popliteal fossa from the **medial popliteal** nerve of the **sciatic** and innervates the *gastrocnemius* and *soleus* muscles, the *tibialis posterior*, the *flexor digitorum longus*, and the *flexor hallucis longus*. It then passes through the tarsal tunnel and into the foot, providing a sensory branch, the **calcaneal** nerve, and divides into the ***medial plantar*** and ***lateral plantar*** nerves. The ***medial plantar*** innervates the *adductor hallucis*, the *flexor digitorum brevis*, and the *flexor hallucis brevis*, and provides sensation to the skin of the medial anterior two-thirds of the sole of the foot and the plantar skin of the first three toes and part of the fourth toe. The **lateral plantar** innervates the *abductor digiti minimi, flexor digiti minimi, adductor hallucis, quadratus plantae*, and *interossei* muscles and supplies the skin of the fifth toe and the lateral aspect of the fourth toe.

The ***sural*** nerve originates below at the popliteal space and is formed purely of sensory axons from the ***peroneal communicating*** branch of the **common peroneal** nerve and the **medial *sural cutaneous*** branch of the **tibial** nerve. The **sural** supplies the skin of the posterolateral area of the distal leg and the lateral foot; its axons come mainly from the *S1* root but also from the *L5* and *S2* roots.

Table 1-3 lists limbs, muscles, and their innervation; the anatomy of individual nerves and their muscles is discussed in various cases in this book.

TABLE 1-3 Muscles of the Extremities and Their Innervation

Muscles, Innervation	Nerve	Cord/Division	Trunk	Roots[a]	Activation
Upper Extremity					
Shoulder Joint					
Trapezius	Spinal accessory	Not from brachial plexus	Not from brachial plexus	**C3, C4** (some branches)	Elevate shoulder
Rhomboids	Dorsal scapular	Directly from roots	Directly from roots	**C4, C5**	Retract scapulae
Levator scapulae	Dorsal scapular + twigs from C3, C4	Directly from roots	Directly from roots	C3, C4, **C5**	Elevate scapulae
Serratus anterior	Long thoracic	Directly from roots	Directly from roots	C5, **C6**,[b] **C7**[b]	Push forward against resistance
Pectoralis major clavicular	Lateral pectoral	Lateral	Upper	**C5, C6**,[b] (C7)[c]	Adduction of the shoulder
Sternal	Medial pectoral	Medial	Lower	**C7, C8**,[b] (T1)[c,d,e]	Extend and rotate the shoulder
Pectoralis minor	Lateral and medial pectoralis	Lateral and medial	Upper, middle, and lower	C6, **C7**,[b] C8	Depress scapula
Supraspinatus and infraspinatus	Suprascapular		Upper	(C4),[c] **C5**, C6	Abduct arm and extend
Latissimus dorsi	Thoracodorsal	Posterior	Upper, middle, and lower	**C6**,[b] **C7**, C8	Internally rotate, adduct, and extend arm
Teres major	Subscapular	Posterior	Upper	C5, **C6**,[b] (C7)[e,f]	Abduct, internally rotate arm
Teres minor	Axillary	Posterior	Upper	(C4),[e] **C5**,[b] C6	Abduct, flex, and extend arm (posterior deltoid)
Deltoid	Axillary	Posterior	Upper	(C4), **C5**, C6	Abduct for and extend the arm
Arm					
Biceps	Musculocutaneous	Lateral	Upper	C5, **C6**[b]	Flex supinated forearm
Brachialis	Musculocutaneous	Lateral	Upper	C5, **C6**,[b] (C7)[c]	Flex supinated forearm
Coracobrachialis	Musculocutaneous	Lateral	Upper and middle	(C5),[c] **C6**,[b] C7	Forward elevation of arm with elbow flexed
Triceps	Radial	Posterior	Middle and lower	C6, **C7, C8**[b]	Extend forearm
Brachioradialis	Radial	Posterior	Upper	C5, **C6**, (C7)[e]	Flex forearm at semipronation
Extensor carpi radialis longus	Radial	Posterior	Upper and middle	C5, **C6**, (C7)[c,e,f]	Extend and abduct hand at wrist
Anconeus	Radial	Posterior	Middle and lower	(C5),[c] **C7, C8**, (T1)[e]	Extend elbow
Supinator	Posterior interosseous	Posterior	Upper	C5,[d,e,f] **C6**,[b] C7	Supinate forearm with elbow extended
Extensor carpi ulnaris	Posterior interosseous	Posterior	Upper, middle, and lower	(C6)[c,d,f] **C7, C8**[b]	Extend and adduct hand at wrist
Extensor digitorum communis	Posterior interosseous	Posterior	Middle and lower	(C6),[c,f] **C7**, C8	Extension of metacarpophalangeal joints
Abductor pollicis longus	Posterior interosseous	Posterior	Middle and lower	(C6),[c,f] **C7, C8**[b]	Abduct thumb at carpometacarpal joint
Extensor pollicis longus	Posterior interosseous	Posterior	Middle and lower	C7, C8[b]	Extend thumb at interphalangeal joint
Extensor pollicis brevis	Posterior interosseous	Posterior	Middle and lower	(C6),[c,f] **C7, C8**[b]	Extend thumb at metacarpophalangeal joint

TABLE 1-3 Muscles of the Extremities and Their Innervation—cont'd

Muscles, Innervation	Nerve	Cord/Division	Trunk	Roots[a]	Activation
Extensor indicis proprius	Posterior interosseous	Posterior	Middle and lower	C7, **C8**[b]	Extend index finger with flexion of others
Pronator teres	Median	Lateral	Upper and middle	C6, **C7**[b]	Pronate forearm
Flexor carpi radialis	Median	Lateral and medial	Upper, middle, and lower	C6, **C7**[b]	Flex and abduct hand at wrist
Flexor digitorum superficialis	Median	Lateral and medial	Middle and lower	C7, **C8**,[b] T1	Flex fingers at proximal interphalangeal joint
Palmaris longus	Median	Lateral and medial	Middle and lower	**C7, C8**,[b] T1	Cup palm of hand
Pronator quadratus	Anterior interosseous	Lateral and medial	Middle and lower	C7, **C8**,[b] T1	Pronate forearm
Flexor digitorum profundus	Anterior interosseous	Medial and lateral	Middle and lower	C7, **C8**, (T1)[c,e,f]	Flex distal phalanx of index finger, third finger
Flexor pollicis longus	Anterior interosseous	Lateral and medial	Middle and lower	**C7**, C8, (T1)[c,e,f]	Flex distal phalanx of thumb
Flexor carpi ulnaris	Ulnar	Medial	Lower	C7, **C8**, T1	Flex and adduct hand at wrist
Flexor digitorum profundus III and IV	Ulnar	Medial	Lower	C7, **C8**, (T1)[c,d,e,f]	Flex distal interphalangeal joint
Hand					
Abductor pollicis brevis	Median	Medial	Lower	**C8**,[b] **T1**	Abduct thumb at right angle to palm
Flexor pollicis brevis	Median	Medial	Lower	**C8**,[b] **T1**	Flex thumb at metacarpophalangeal (S) joint
Opponens pollicis	Median	Medial	Lower	**C8**,[b] **T1**	Touch base of little finger with thumb
Lumbricals I and II	Median	Medial	Lower	C8, **T1**	Extend finger at proximal interphalangeal joint
Abductor digiti minimi	Ulnar	Medial	Lower	**C8, T1**	Abduct little finger
Flexor digiti minimi	Ulnar	Medial	Lower	C8, **T1**	Flex little finger at metacarpophalangeal joint
Opponens digiti minimi	Ulnar	Medial	Lower	C8, **T1**	Oppose little finger to thumb
Adductor pollicis	Ulnar	Medial	Lower	C8, **T1**	Adduct thumb at right angle to palm
Flexor pollicis brevis	Ulnar	Medial	Lower	**C8**,[b] T1	Flex thumb at metacarpophalangeal joint
Palmar interossei	Ulnar	Medial	Lower	C8, **T1**[b]	Adduct fingers
Dorsal interossei	Ulnar	Medial	Lower	C8, **T1**	Adduct fingers
Lumbricals III and IV	Ulnar	Medial	Lower	C8, **T1**[b]	Extend finger at proximal interphalangeal joint
Lower Extremity					
Hip and Thigh					
Iliopsoas	Femoral to psoas major, minor	Posterior	Lumbar	**L1, L2, L3**,[b] L4	Flexion of thigh
Quadriceps femoris	Femoral	Posterior	Lumbar	L2, **L3, L4**	Extension of leg on the thigh
Pectineus	Femoral	Posterior	Lumbar	**L2**,[b] L3, L4	Adduct thigh
Sartorius	Femoral	Posterior	Lumbar	**L2, L3**, L4	Flexion, abduction of hip; flexion of knee
Adductor longus and brevis	Obturator	Anterior	Lumbar	**L2, L3**, L4	Adduction of thigh
Adductor magnus	Obturator; also from sciatic	Anterior	Lumbar	L2, **L3, L4**[b]	Adduction of thigh
Gracilis	Obturator	Anterior	Lumbar	**L2**,[b] L3, L4	Adduct thigh and flex knee
Gluteus medius and minimus	Superior gluteal	Posterior	Sacral	**L4, L5**, S1	Adduct thigh

Continued

TABLE 1-3 Muscles of the Extremities and Their Innervation—cont'd

Muscles, Innervation	Nerve	Cord/Division	Trunk	Roots[a]	Activation
Tensor fasciae latae	Superior gluteal	Posterior	Sacral	**L4, L5**, S1	Flexion and internal rotation of thigh
Gluteus maximus	Inferior gluteal	Posterior	Sacral	**L5, S1, S2**[b]	Extend at the hip
Piriformis	Nerve to piriformis	Posterior	Sacral	(L5),[e] **S1**[b], S2	Externally rotate thigh
Adductor magnus	Sciatic, also from obturator	Anterior	Sacral	L2, L3, L4	Adduction of thigh
Obturator internus and gemellus superior	Obturator internus	Anterior	Sacral	L5, **S1**,[b] S2	Externally rotate thigh with extended leg
Inferior gemellus	Quadratus femoris	Anterior	Sacral	L4, **L5, S1**, S2	Externally rotate thigh with extended leg
Quadratus femoris	Quadratus femoris	Anterior	Sacral	L4, **L5, S1**	Externally rotate thigh
Semitendinosus	Sciatic (tibial portion)	Anterior	Sacral	**L5**,[b] **S1**, S2	Flexion of knee
Semimembranosus	Sciatic (tibial portion)	Anterior	Sacral	(L4),[f] **L5**,[b] **S1**, S2	Flexion of knee
Biceps (long head)	Sciatic (tibial portion)	Anterior	Sacral	L5, **S1**, (S2)[e]	Flexion of knee
Biceps (short head)	Sciatic (common peroneal portion)	Posterior	Sacral	**L5, S1**, S2	Flexion of knee
Leg					
Gastrocnemius and soleus	Tibial	Anterior	Sacral	**S1**,[b] **S2**[b]	Plantar flexion and inversion of foot
Tibialis posterior	Tibial	Anterior	Sacral	L4, **L5**, (S1)[c,d,f]	Plantar flexion and inversion of foot
Flexor digitorum longus	Tibial	Anterior	Sacral	L5, **S1, S2**, (S3)[e]	Flexion of toes
Flexor hallucis longus	Tibial	Anterior	Sacral	L5, S1, **S2**,[b] (S3)[e]	Flex big toe
Popliteus	Tibial	Anterior	Sacral	(L4),[c,e] **L5**, S1	Flex and internally rotate tibia
Tibialis anterior	Deep peroneal	Posterior	Sacral	**L4**, L5, (S1)[c,f]	Dorsiflexion of foot
Extensor hallucis longus	Deep peroneal	Posterior	Sacral	(L4),[c,f] **L5**, S1	Dorsiflexion of distal phalanx of big toe
Extensor digitorum longus	Deep peroneal	Posterior	Sacral	(L4),[c,f] **L5**, S1	Dorsiflexion of toes
Peroneus tertius	Deep peroneal	Posterior	Sacral	**L5**, S1	Dorsiflexion and eversion of foot
Peroneus longus	Superficial peroneal	Posterior	Sacral	**L5**,[b] **S1**,[b] (S2)[d,e]	Eversion of foot
Peroneus brevis	Superficial peroneal	Posterior	Sacral	**L5**,[b] **S1**,[b] (S2)[d,e]	Eversion of foot
Abductor hallucis	Medial plantar	Anterior	Sacral	(L5),[c,f] S1, S2, **S3**[b]	Plantar flexion abduction of first toe
Flexor digitorum brevis	Medial plantar	Anterior	Sacral	(L5),[c,f] S1, S2, **S3**[b]	Flex middle phalanges of toes II–V
Flexor hallucis brevis	Medial plantar	Anterior	Sacral	(L5),[f] S1, S2, **S3**[b]	Flex metatarsophalangeal joint of big toe
Flexor digiti minimi	Lateral plantar	Anterior	Sacral	S1, S2, **S3**[b]	Flex metatarsophalangeal joint of little toe
Abductor digiti quinti	Lateral plantar	Anterior	Sacral	S1, S2, **S3**[b]	Adduct little toe
Adductor hallucis	Lateral plantar	Anterior	Sacral	(L5),[f] S1, S2, **S3**[b]	Adduct big toe
Interossei	Lateral plantar	Anterior	Sacral	S1, S2, **S3**[b]	Spread toes
Quadratus plantae	Lateral plantar	Anterior	Sacral	S1, S2, **S3**[b]	Flex toes
Extensor digitorum brevis	Deep peroneal	Posterior	Sacral	**L5, S1**, (S2)[e]	Dorsiflexion of proximal phalanges of toes

[a]Boldface in the roots column indicates principal nerve roots, according to Medical Research Council of the United Kingdom. *Aids to the Examination of the Peripheral Nervous System*. London: Bailliere Tindall; 1986.
[b]Indicates principal nerve roots as per Williams PL, Warwick R, Dyson M, Bannister LH. *Gray's Anatomy*. Edinburgh: Churchill Livingstone; 1989.
[c]As per Goodgold J. *Anatomical Correlates of Clinical Electromyography*. Baltimore, MD: Williams & Wilkins; 1974.
[d]As per Delagi EF, Iazzetti J, Perotto A, Marrison A. *Anatomic Guide for the Electromyographer*. Springfield, IL: Charles C. Thomas; 1980.
[e]As per Williams PL, Warwick R, Dyson M, Bannister LH. *Gray's Anatomy*. Edinburgh: Churchill Livingstone; 1989.
[f]As per Haerer AF. *DeJongs the neurologic examination*. Philadelphia, PA: Lippincott-Raven; 1992.
Footnotes e–f indicate discrepancies and their references. *C*, Cervical; *D*, deep; *L*, lumbar; *S*, superficial; *T*, thoracic.

STRUCTURE OF THE PERIPHERAL NERVES

The principal components of nerve are the epineurium, the perineurium, and the endoneurium (Figs. 1-7 and 1-8).

The *epineurium* surrounds the entire fascicle and makes up one-half of the cross-sectional area of a nerve. This structure consists of connective tissue, capillaries, arterioles, and veins; it also contains fibroblasts, mast cells, and occasional lymphocytes.

The sural nerve, which is frequently used for histologic studies, has approximately 6–15 fascicles but may have up to 20. The *perineurium* is the connective tissue layer surrounding each individual fascicle. It has a network of collagen fibers in longitudinal and oblique orientations. These are formed primarily of type III collagen.

Small arterioles and venules are found in the epineurial and perineurial areas and are recognized on biopsies by their lack of elastic laminae. Vessels can sometimes be seen in the perineurial septum.

The *endoneurium* is the region of the nerve fascicle internal to the perineurium; it is formed mainly of connective tissue, axons, and Schwann cells. In this area collagen fibers run longitudinally to the axons and are packed more closely in the area immediately adjacent to the perineurium. *Schwann cells* surround both myelinated and unmyelinated axons, and each myelinated axon is associated with only one Schwann cell that provides its myelin (see Fig. 1-8). Several unmyelinated axons are contained within the cytoplasm of one Schwann cell. A *Schwann cell profile*, surrounded by the same basal lamina and

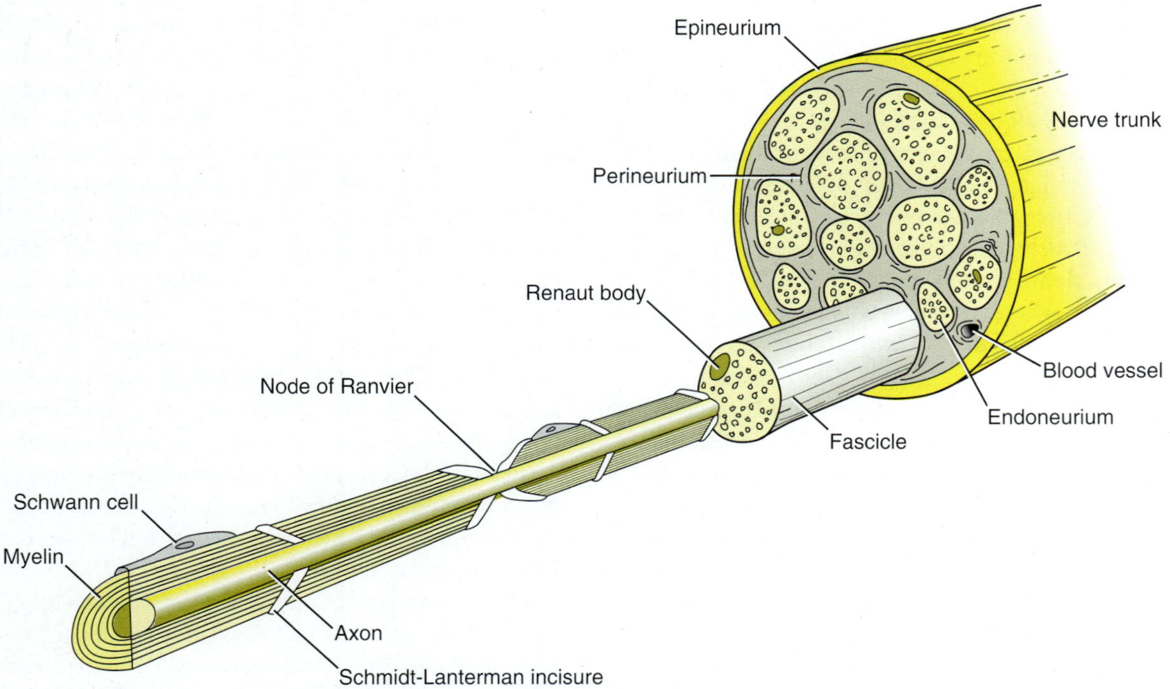

FIG 1-7 The peripheral nerve and its components. (Reprinted with permission from Bertorini TE, Horner LH. Histology and histochemistry of muscle and nerve. In: Bertorini TE, ed. *Clinical Evaluation and Diagnostic Tests for Neuromuscular Disorders*. Boston, MA: Butterworth-Heinemann; 2002.)

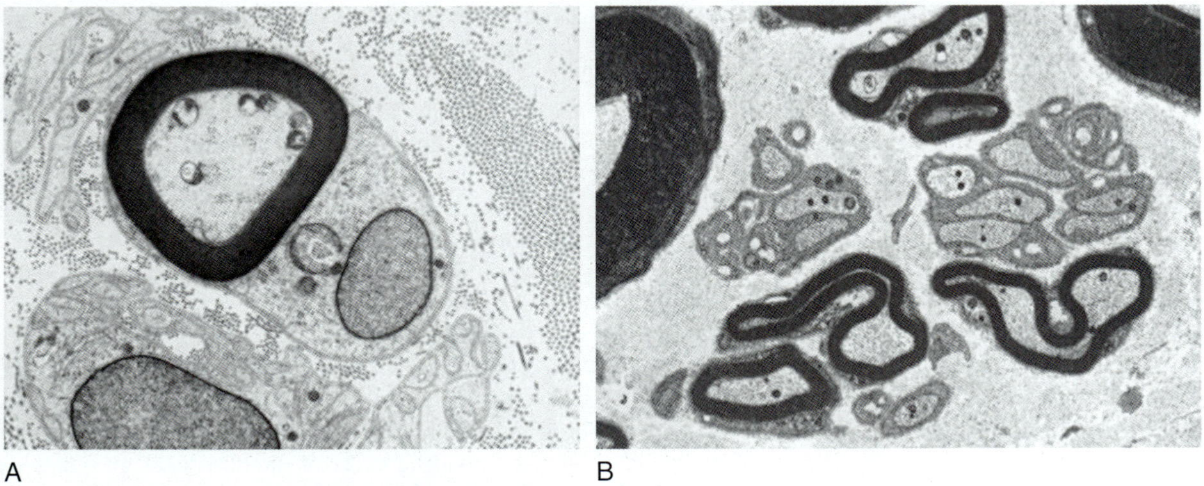

FIG 1-8 A, Myelinated axon and its Schwann cell (×9000). **B**, Several small myelinated and unmyelinated

usually containing one to four unmyelinated axons, is called a *Schwann cell subunit*, or *Remak* fibers.[8]

Capillaries and small venules, fibroblasts, pericytes, vascular endothelial cells, and smooth muscle and mast cells can also be seen in the endoneurium.

The Axons

Nerve fibers within fascicles consist of large and small myelinated and unmyelinated fibers.

The normal sural nerve contains up to 9400 evenly distributed myelinated fibers with a density of 5200–8000 fibers per mm; this varies with age. The number of unmyelinated fibers varies from 18,000 to 42,000 fibers per fascicle.[9]

The axons contain neurofilaments that run parallel longitudinally to form a cytoskeleton. They are approximately 10 nm in diameter and are evenly distributed, with a density of 100–300 fibers per mm. Axonal microtubules have 2.5 nm of external diameter and are 100–800 nm in length. Other elements of the axon are the mitochondria, various membrane-bound structures, vesicles, and glycogen granules of approximately 30 μm. An *internode* is the area of the axon that is myelinated by one Schwann cell; it has a length of 1800 μm in large axons.

The area where two adjacent internodes meet is called the *node of Ranvier*. This region of the axon contains no myelin, and at this point, the membrane-bound organelles and microtubules are compact, whereas the neurofilaments are not significantly changed. The *perinodal segment* describes the area close to either side of the node.

Myelin is a multilayer, laminated structure composed of layers of biochemically modified Schwann cell membranes. Seventy-one percent of dehydrated myelin is lipid and 29% is protein. There are normally 80–160 myelin lamellae in each large myelinated nerve fiber.[8,9]

Peripheral nerves contain important proteins whose alterations are associated with various hereditary neuropathies and are antigenic in autoimmune neuropathies. These include, among others, PMP22, protein 2 and zero, the gap protein connexin, myelin-associated glycoprotein, gangliosides, glycolipids, and ion channels.

THE STRUCTURE OF MUSCLES

The human body has more than 430 striate muscles that produce movement of joints, stabilize the body's position, power breathing, and produce heat. Some striate muscles also form the voluntary sphincters. Striate muscles are surrounded by connective tissue, called the ***epimysium***. The ***perimysium*** separates muscle fascicles which contain up to 150 muscle fibers. The ***endomysium*** is a fine network of collagen around each *myofiber* (Fig. 1-9).

The ***epimysium*** tapers at its distal ends; it blends with and forms intermuscular tissue sheets to give origin to tendons. These tendons are strong and dense formations of connective tissue that connect both ends of the muscles to the periosteum of bone or other muscles. All layers of connective tissue contribute fibers to form the tendons. The *myotendinous junctions* are the areas where muscle and connective tissue join. In these areas the muscle fibers are small and have an increased number of internalized nuclei and increased nonspecific esterase staining histologically.

Medium-sized arterioles and vessels are located between muscle fascicles, whereas small capillaries are parallel and between muscle fibers. The muscle spindles appear as encapsulated formations that contain the small intrafusal muscle fibers.

Myofibers are polygonal in shape and normally have a diameter of approximately 40–80 μm in men and 30–70 μm in women. Individual fibers have a ***sarcolemma***, or muscle membrane. The cytoplasm of muscle is called ***sarcoplasm***.[8]

The fibers are composed of myofibrils that are irregular polygons of approximately 1 μm in diameter in transverse sections on electromicroscopy (EM) (Fig. 1-10). Each myofibril consists of a bundle of myofilaments, the thick filaments of myosin and the thin filaments of actin. On EM the myofilaments are arranged in segments called ***sarcomeres***, which are repeated throughout the length of the fiber, giving the muscle its striated appearance. The *sarcomere* is the region between two *Z lines* with a span of approximately 3 μm. Within the sarcomere there is a dark, central *anisotropic (A) band* that contains the myosin filaments in a regular and parallel arrangement. At the end of the A band, the thick and thin filaments lie side-by-side (zone of overlap). In the middle of the A band there is a dark line called the *M line*, which forms cross-bridges of these filaments; it is formed by supporting proteins. The M line is surrounded by a paler *H zone* that is limited by the termination of the thin filaments and is, therefore, composed of only thick filaments (see Fig. 1-10A). This zone changes in size during muscle contractions. The *pale I (isotropic) band* is situated on either side of the *A band* and consists of parallel thin filaments composed mainly of *actin*, but also of *troponin* and *tropomyosin*. This represents the area where thin filaments lie between two sarcomeres with the Z line in the center.

The cytoskeleton of muscle fiber is held together by filamentous proteins and microtubules. These include the microtubular protein *tubulin*, and the microfilament proteins *severin, fragmin, gelsolin, profilin, dyscoilin*, and *a-actinin*, likely located in the Z line area. Proteins of the Z lines include *betactinin, vimentin, FATZ, myotilin, nebulin, plectin, myopaladin, myopodin, nestin, paranemin, synemin, syncoilin, tropomodulin, alpha filamin*, and *Zasp/cypher* and also paranemin and *desmin*, which surround the *Z line*.[10] Accumulation of desmin is associated with a form of myopathy and cardiomyopathy. *Telethonin* is another sarcomeric protein localized in the Z band; its deficiency causes limb-girdle muscular dystrophy (LGMD) 2G. In LGMD 2A, there is a deficiency of the cytosolic protease *calpain-3*, which interacts with *titin*. *Myomesin* is situated in the *M line* and skelemin is located in its periphery. Other proteins of the *M line* include *M protein* and *MM creatine kinase (CK); MyB-C* and *MyBP-H* are located in the *A band*.[8,10]

Proteins of the elastic filaments include *nebulin and titin* (or *connectin*). *Titin*, located adjacent to thick filaments, links thick myosin with the *Z band* and binds with *telethonin*, a protein important in the assembly of the sarcomere. Mutations of the titin gene cause Welander distal muscular dystrophy. A deficiency of myotilin, a protein similar to titin that binds

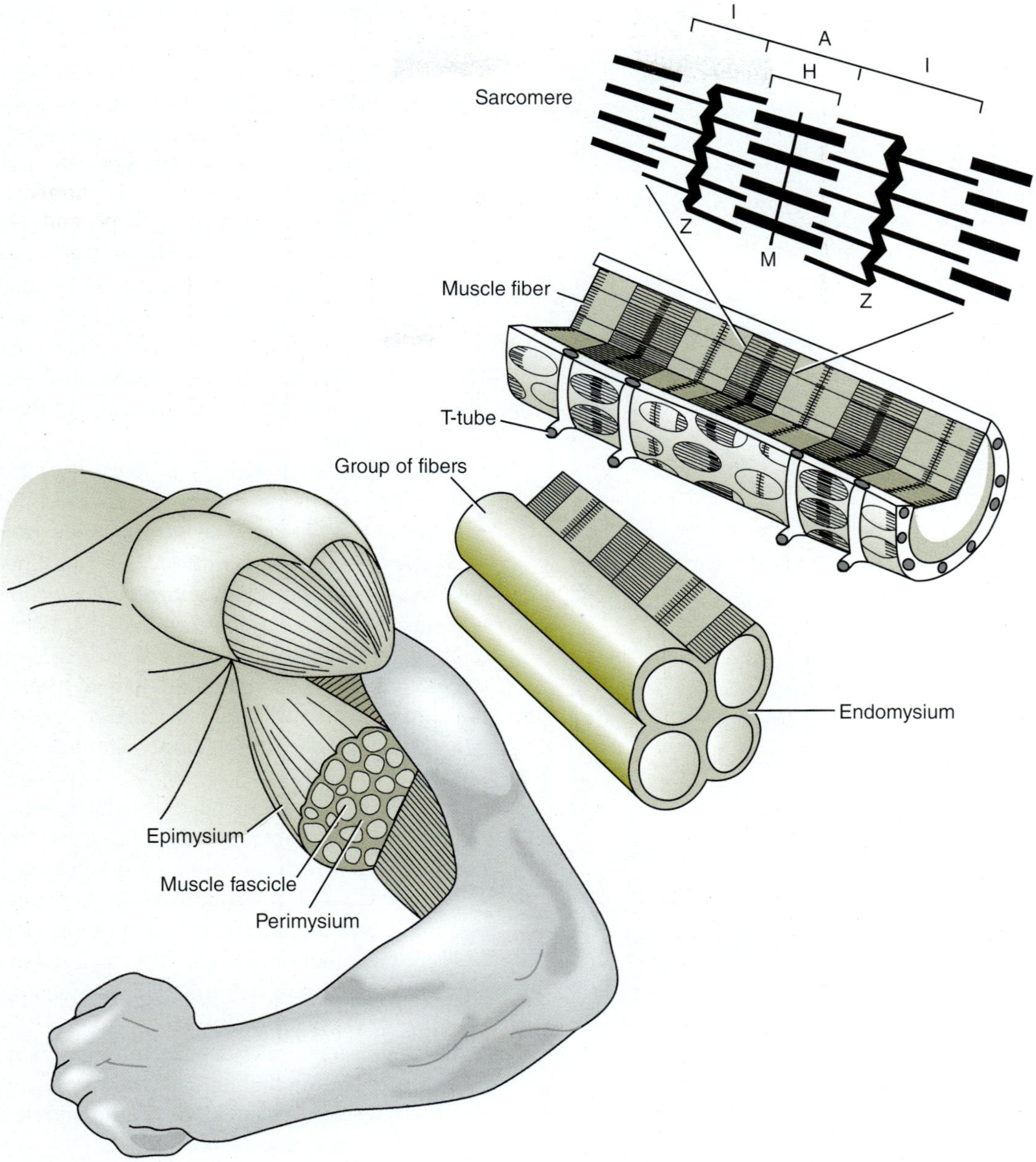

FIG 1-9 Muscle, myofibers, and myofilaments. (Reprinted with permission from Bertorini TE, Horner LH. Histology and histochemistry of muscle and nerve. In: Bertorini TE, ed. *Clinical Evaluation and Diagnostic Tests for Neuromuscular Disorders*. Boston, MA: Butterworth-Heinemann; 2002.)

alpha-actinin to the Z line, causes LGMD 1A. Proteins of the plasma membrane include *vinculin*, which binds actin filaments: *spectrin; ankyrin;* and *dystrophin*, which is absent or deficient in Duchenne's and Becker's muscular dystrophies. Dystrophin is linked to a glycoprotein complex that includes the *sarcoglycans*. Deficiencies of the different sarcoglycans are associated with various forms of LGMD. Dystrophin is also linked to the *dystroglycans, sarcospan, syntrophins*, and *dystrobrevin* (Fig. 1-11).

Other membrane proteins include aquaporins affixin and *dysferlin*, which is deficient in Miyoshi myopathy and in LGMD 2B. *Caveolin* forms membrane invaginations, or *caveolae*, and mutations of *caveolin-3* have been reported in LGMD 1C.

Laminin together with *collagen IV, nidogen*, and *perlecan* form the backbone structure of the basement membrane, which also includes *fibronectin proteoglycans* and *cadherins. Laminin alpha 2* (merosin) links the sarcolemma with the extracellular matrix by binding to *dystroglycan*, which in turn binds dystrophin. *Laminin alpha 2* is deficient in the most frequent form of congenital muscular dystrophy, whereas extracellular collagen VI mutations cause Bethlem myopathy.

The protein *fukutin* has homology to the fringelike enzymes that modify glycosides and glycoproteins. Its deficiency apparently causes a translational defect of alpha *dystroglycans*. These are affected in the Fukuyama type of muscular dystrophy. A homologous protein, "*Fukutin*-related protein," is located in

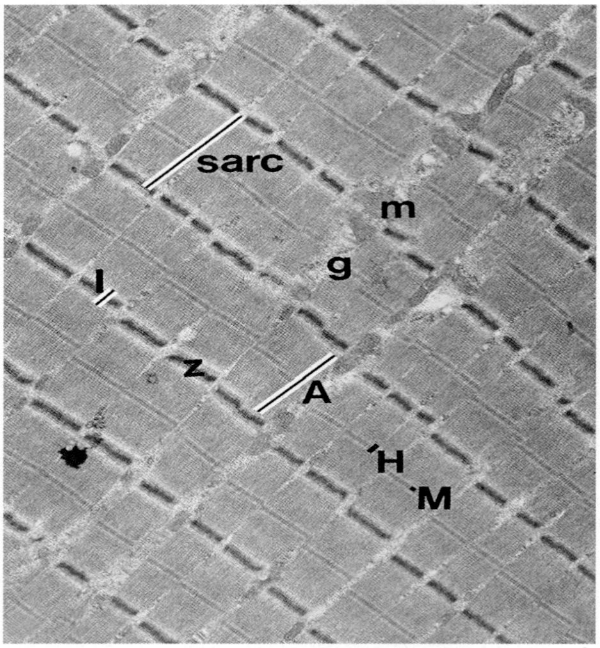

A

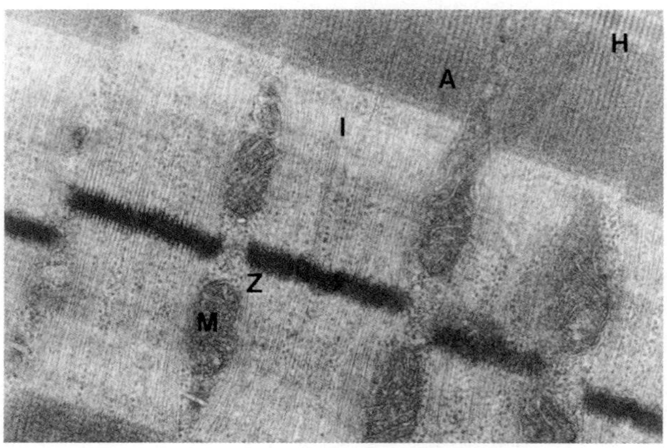

B

FIG 1-10 A, The different components of the sarcomere: sarc= sarcomere, M=M Line, m=mitochondria, g=glycogen, z=Z Line, H=H zone, A=A band (electromicroscopy, ×7000). **B**, Electromicroscopy of muscle at high magnification: A=A band, I=I band, H=H zone, Z=Z Line, M=mitochondria (×58,680).

the Golgi apparatus. It also has a role in glycosylation, mutations of the gene that expresses this protein and causes LGMD 2I. Other proteins of the Golgi apparatus include POMGnT1 and LARGE.

The *integrins* are proteins that also serve as receptors for *laminin*, and mutations of *integrin alpha 7* have been reported as being associated with a form of congenital myopathy.

The contractile proteins include *troponin, tropomyosin, actin*, and *myosin*. The latter is predominantly damaged in the critical illness myopathy. The protein *tropomodulin* caps the heads of the thin filaments.

The *nuclei* of muscle fibers are located beneath the sarcolemma, and the ***satellite cell*** lies between the basal lamina and the **sarcolemma**. The satellite cells have denser nuclei and divide to form myotubules during the process of regeneration. In adults, approximately 4% of peripheral nuclei are from satellite cells.

Nuclear membrane proteins may also be associated with neuromuscular disorders. For example, mutations of the gene for *emerin* and *lamin A/C* are associated with the X-linked and autosomal dominant forms of Emery–Dreifuss muscular dystrophy, respectively.

The ***mitochondria*** are located in the sarcoplasm adjacent to I bands or beneath the sarcolemma. They are ovoid in shape, have a diameter of 0.1 nm, and are more abundant in type I muscle fibers. Aberrations in shape and an increased number of mitochondria can be observed in mitochondrial myopathies. Fatty acids incorporate in the mitochondria for beta-oxidation. The mitochondria also contain enzymes of the Krebs cycle and respiratory chain.

The ***T-tubular* system** is a network of tubes continuous with muscle membrane invaginations that connect throughout the muscle fibers. The ***sarcoplasmic reticulum*** consists of a series of sacs between the A band and the I band. At this level the **sarcoplasmic reticulum *cisterna*** comes in proximity with the T-tubular system, forming what is known as a ***triad***. In these locations, the voltage-activated calcium channels and the calcium-release channels are joined. Important proteins in the sarcoplasmic reticulum include, among others, *calsequestrin, triadin, DMPK, POMT1, seleno protein N. calmodulin*, and *sarcolipin*.

Other constituents of muscle include fine granules of glycogen, which are more abundant in type II fibers; vacuoles of neutral lipids, which are found predominantly in type I fibers; microtubules; and ribosomes. Golgi complexes, granules of lipofuscin, and other elements form in muscle fibers. Enzymes of energy metabolism located in the cytosol and mitochondria are fundamental to muscle function, and their deficiencies cause various metabolic myopathies.

Neuromuscular junctions and intramuscular nerves can also be observed in muscle biopsies. They are identified on EM by the characteristic invaginations on the muscle membrane that surround the associated axon.

THE NEUROMUSCULAR JUNCTION

The neuromuscular junction, or motor endplate,[11] is the area of contact between the motor axon and muscle fibers (Fig. 1-12). Normally there is one endplate per muscle fiber, and it is situated in the middle of the fiber. Occasional muscle fibers have two endplates, and this is particularly common in the extraocular muscles. In the nerve terminal of the neuromuscular junction, the motor axon loses its myelin sheath and is covered only by Schwann cell processes.[12] The axon then terminates in small synaptic boutons.

The ***axonal terminal*** is located in a *groove* in the surface of the myofiber. It is separated from the muscle membrane by spaces of the *primary and secondary synaptic clefts*, facing the *postsynaptic folds* of the fibers.

The axonal terminal contains synaptic vessels, mitochondria, supportive proteins, microtubules, glycogen and filaments, and endoplasmic reticulum.

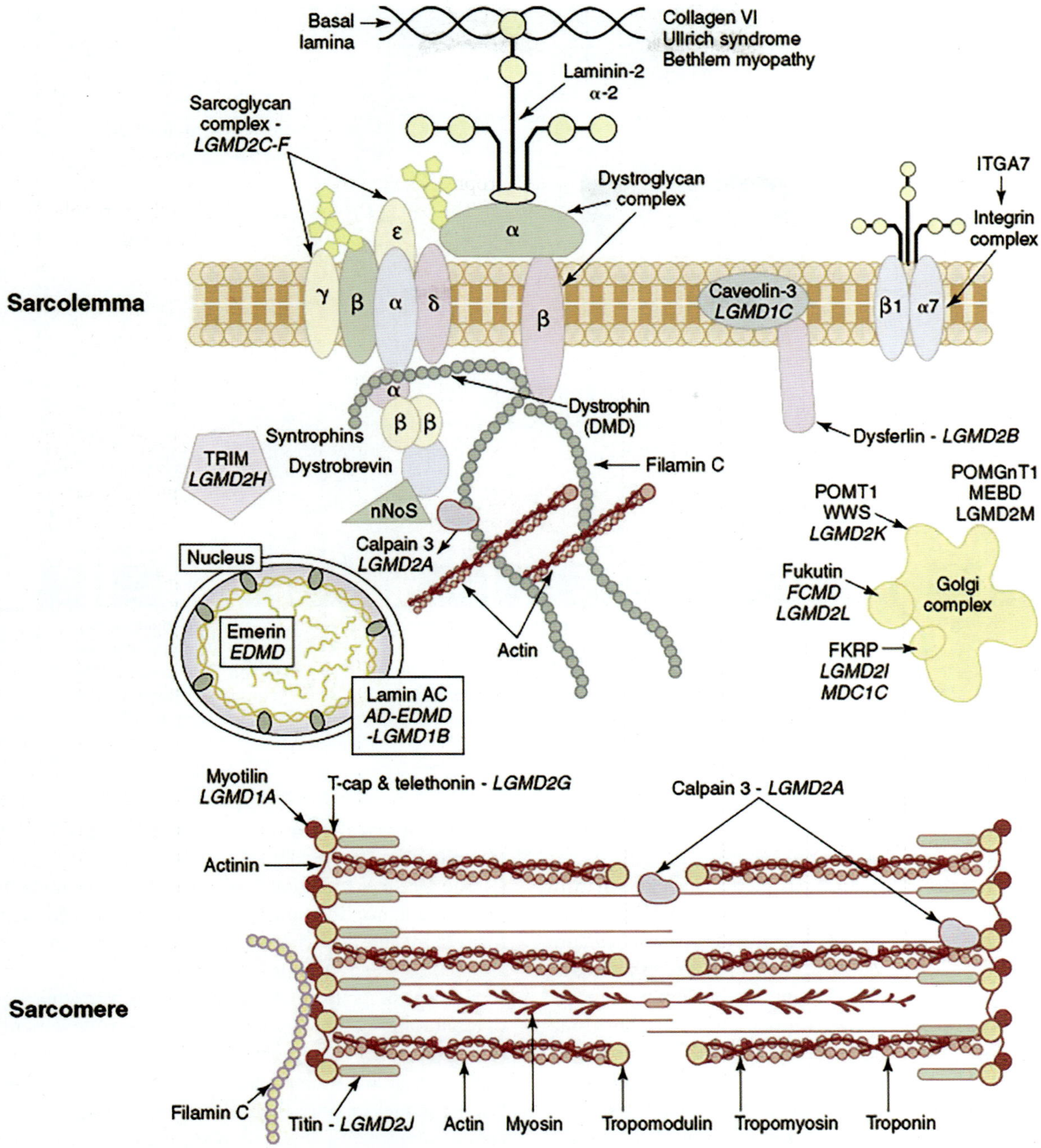

FIG 1-11 Different proteins of sarcolemma and other areas of the muscle fiber associated with muscular dystrophy. *EDMD*, Emery–Dreifuss muscular dystrophy; *FCMD*, Fukuyama congenital muscular dystrophy; *FKRP*, fukutin-related protein; *ITGA7*, integrin, alpha7; *LGMD*, limb-girdle muscular dystrophy; *LGMD2M*, limb-girdle muscular dystrophy 2M; *MEBD*, muscle-eye-brain disease; *nNOS*, neuronal nitric oxide synthase; *POMGnT1*, protein O–linked mannose β1,2-N-acetylglucosaminyltransferase; *POMT*, protein O–mannosyltransferase; *TRIM*, tripartite motif; *WWS*, Walker–Warburg syndrome. (From Bertorini TE. *Neuromuscular Disorders: Treatment and Management*. 2nd ed. Amsterdam: Elsevier; 2022. Copyright 2022 by Elsevier.)

Acetylcholine (ACh) receptors are located at the top of the secondary postsynaptic folds, where they are anchored to the dystrophin-related protein complex through rapsyn, and the Erb B tyrosine kinases. The receptors are connected to the cytoskeleton by their attachment with utropin and the sarcoglycans and dystroglycans. The trough area of the folds contains numerous voltage-sensitive sodium channels that are anchored to the membrane by *ankyrin, syntrophin*, and *spectrin*. Among the proteins in the gap areas are the laminins, agrin, neuregulin, collagen, and Nac beta-x.[11] The enzyme *ACh esterase* lies deep in the secondary clefts of the basement membrane.

The receptor is a ligand-gated pentameric transmembrane protein surrounding a central ionic channel. Adult muscle has five different receptor *subunits:* two *alpha*, one *beta*, one *epsilon*, and one *delta*. Each subunit contains four hydrophobic areas. The binding sites of the receptors are located in the extracellular space of the alpha subunits. In myasthenia gravis antibodies bind epitopes formed by the alpha subunits in an area called the *main immunogenic region*.

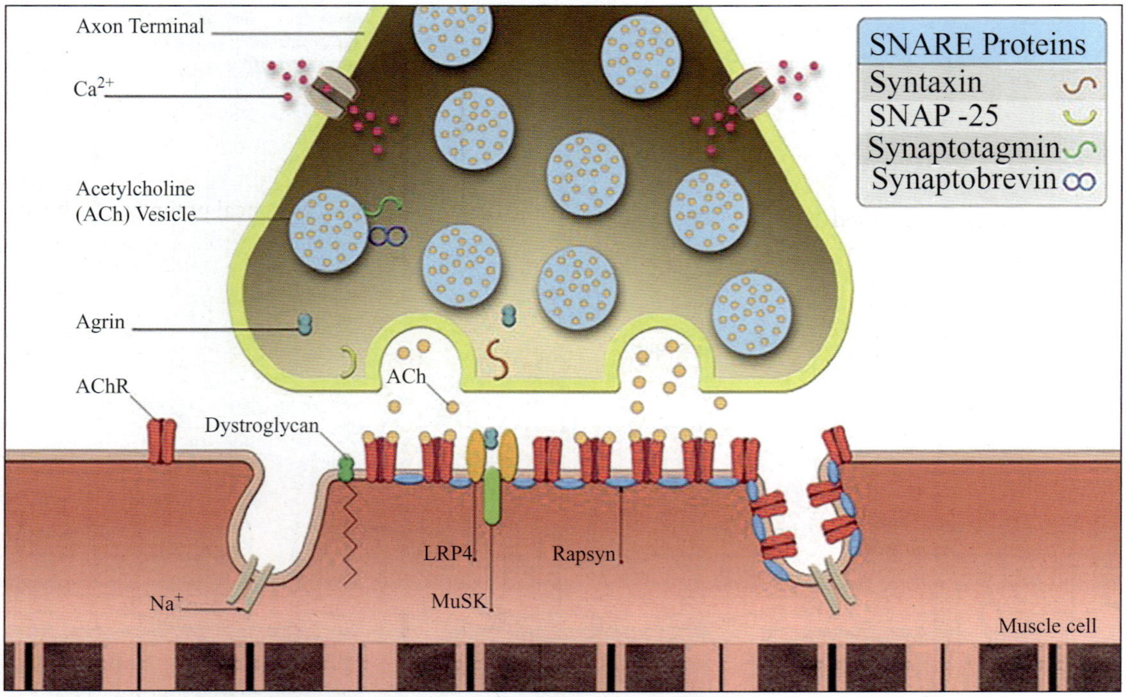

FIG 1-12 Cartoon showing the various components of the neuromuscular junction. Axonal depolarization causes an opening of the voltage-gated calcium channel and influx of calcium triggers the fusion of vesicles with the presynaptic membrane and releases stored acetylcholine into the synaptic cleft. This initiates the binding of acetylcholine to the receptor in the postsynaptic membrane, for which there is an opening with influx of the anions. This opens the sodium channels producing an endplate potential that triggers the muscle action potential. Other various proteins of the neuromuscular junction are also shown.

The neuromuscular junction contains several other proteins such as dystrophin-related phosphoprotein, nitric acid-synthetase, and dystrobrevin. Some proteins, such as synapsin I, synaptotagmin, neurexin, synaptophysin, αSNAP-25, ACh transporter, Rab 3a, raphilin, RIM, syntaxin, and the calcium and potassium channels, are located in the nerve terminal of the junction. Synaptobrevin, syntaxin, and SNAP-25 act as receptors for synaptic vesicle-associated protein αSNAP; this group of proteins is called the soluble N-ethymaleimide-sensitive factor attachment protein receptor complex. Agrin is synthesized in the motor neurons, deposits in the basal lamina of the junctions, and contributes to endplate stabilization. This protein stimulates the tyrosine kinase (MuSK), which promotes the aggregation of receptors during development. This and other proteins such as LRP4 (lipoprotein receptor release protein 4), down-streaming kinase (DOK-7), and rapsyn are required for postsynaptic function and differentiation. Genetic defects and antibodies against some of these proteins can cause disorders of neuromuscular transmission.[13,14]

PHYSIOLOGY

The Membrane and the Action Potentials

To understand the mechanisms of generation of the action potential and its propagation, the origin of the **resting membrane** potential is briefly summarized here.

The plasma membrane maintains not only the integrity of cells but also the concentration gradients and the electrical charge differences of ions across the cells. It also controls nutrition and waste disposal.

The plasma membrane is formed by *carbohydrates, proteins*, and *lipids*. The lipid bilayer of the outer cell membrane is formed by *phospholipids, glycolipids*, and *cholesterol* molecules situated between this bilayer.[15]

Because of its structure, the membrane prevents the crossing of large water-soluble molecules, and their movement requires transmembrane *transport proteins*. These include *channel proteins* that are situated across the bilayer and have a water-filled channel or pore that allows the passage of ions. Others are *carrier proteins*, which bind substances to allow their transport by undergoing conformational changes. Liposoluble molecules pass directly through the membrane.

Ion channels allow the selective entrance of ions.[14] Some of these are open when the membrane is at rest, allowing the entrance and exit of ions according to concentration and electric gradients. These are called *"leak" channels*. Other channels open and close from the action of voltage-gated mechanisms and are thus *voltage-gated channels*. The gate is a protein situated in the membrane whose conformational changes allow the opening of the channel. *Ligand-gated* pores are opened by chemical transmitters, such as ACh, at the neuromuscular junction, while *voltage-gated* channels open after changes in the membrane voltage.[15]

Finally, the movement of some ions against the concentration gradient is maintained by transport mechanisms with the consumption of energy *(the Na–K ATPase pump)*.

The Membrane Potential

Excitable cells have an electrical potential across their membranes, which is approximately 60–90 mV negative inside depending on the cells. This potential is called the *resting membrane potential* or transmembrane potential. In the axon this is called the *resting axonal potential.*

The resting potential is maintained by the concentration and the electrical gradient of ions. The *concentration gradient* causes the ions to try to equilibrate their content across both sides of the membrane (Fig. 1-13). For example, the intracellular space has a high concentration of potassium ions and negative-charged organic ions. Because potassium concentration is higher within the cell, this ion tends to move toward the extracellular space. This causes a loss of positive charges inside the cell, creating an *electrical gradient*, thus the movement of potassium caused by its concentration gradient is balanced by the electrical force generated by electrical charges opposing the efflux. The magnitude of the transmembrane voltage is the *equilibrium potential* for potassium. The membrane potential of nerves depends not only on the permeability of the potassium "leak" channels but also on that of other ions such as sodium and chloride.

The *resting nerve potential* is about −70 mV intracellularly. At this potential, potassium is close to its equilibrium voltage, but sodium is 100 mV from its equilibrium potential. (Potassium is in equilibrium, because there are more potassium than sodium channels.) This creates a strong electrical gradient, in addition to the Na concentration gradient (as more sodium is present outside the cell), both favoring sodium to move *into* the cell. This flow equilibrates the charges in potassium flow, and thus exiting positive potassium balances the influx of positive-charged sodium.

To compensate for the charges created by the ionic flow, and to maintain the equilibrium potential of the membrane, there is a movement of these ions *against* their concentration gradient that requires the consumption of energy from adenosine triphosphate (ATP). This is provided by the *sodium–potassium ATPase pump* (Fig. 1-14).

Chloride ions do not use active transport. The concentration of chloride depends on the resting membrane potential, and its ions cross the membrane according to the concentration gradient, and its electrical potential. Chloride is more concentrated on the outside of the cells, and there is no chloride flux at rest.

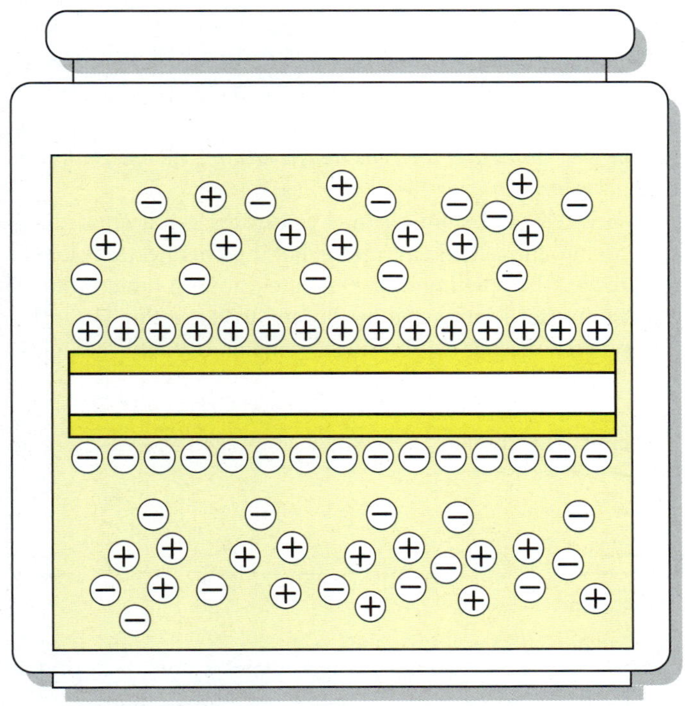

FIG 1-13 The location of ions in a semipermeable membrane. The negative and positive ions accumulate at each border of the membrane and cross according to their concentration and electrical gradient.

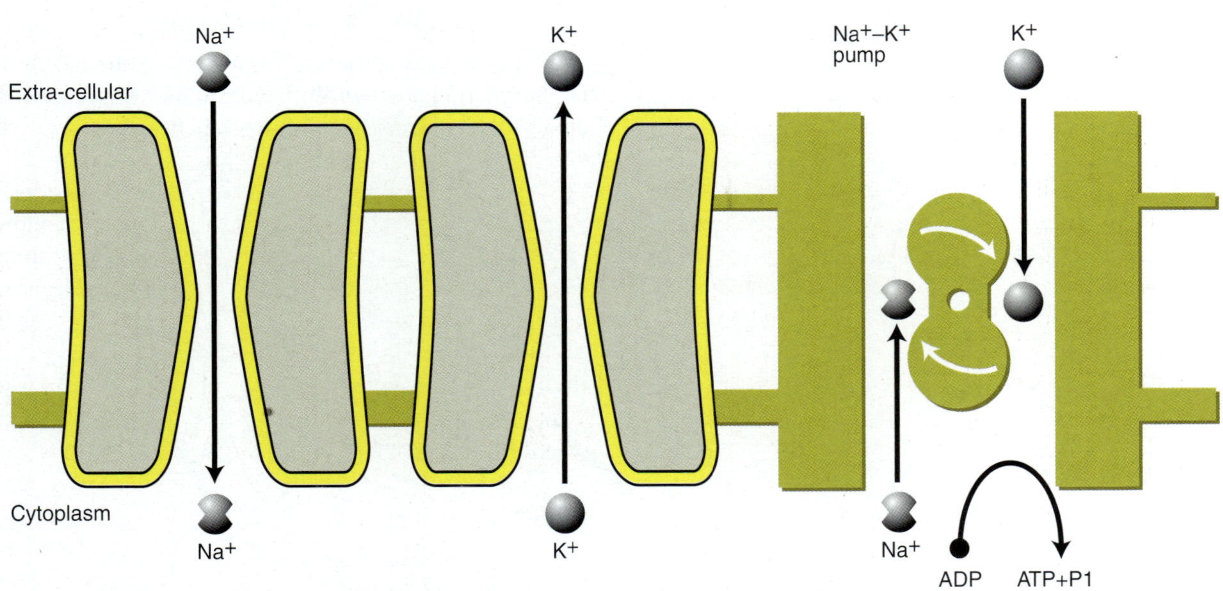

FIG 1-14 The movement of ions producing the resting membrane potential, and the Na–K ATPase pump.

The Action Potential

The action potential is generated by depolarization of the cell due to an increased conductance, causing a rapid reversal of ionic flow, with an inward-directed flow of sodium. This is followed by repolarization from the outward-directed potassium current, both through their *voltage-gated* channels. (These are presented in a simplified diagram in Fig. 1-15.) This depolarizes the membrane to a voltage of approximately 20–40 mV.[16]

While the potassium channel gate can be either opened (activated) or closed (inactivated), the sodium channel has two gates, *its* ***activation*** *and* ***deactivation*** *gates. At rest the activation gate is closed, and the inactivation gate is open. During depolarization a rapid opening of the activation gate allows sodium to flow through the channel. The* ***inactivation*** *gate then closes, and the channel enters its inactivated state. During repolarization, first, the* ***activation*** *gate closes and then the* ***deactivation*** *gate opens and the channel returns to its resting state* (Fig. 1-16).

When the potassium channel senses the rapid entrance of sodium into the cell, its gate opens, but this channel takes longer to activate. The opening of the channel causes a rapid influx of potassium that returns the membrane to its resting potential. The potassium channel, however, remains open for a slightly longer period than required to achieve the resting potential, causing the membrane to become *hyperpolarized* and therefore more negative. The membrane then slowly returns to baseline by the flow of potassium and sodium through their *leak* channels.

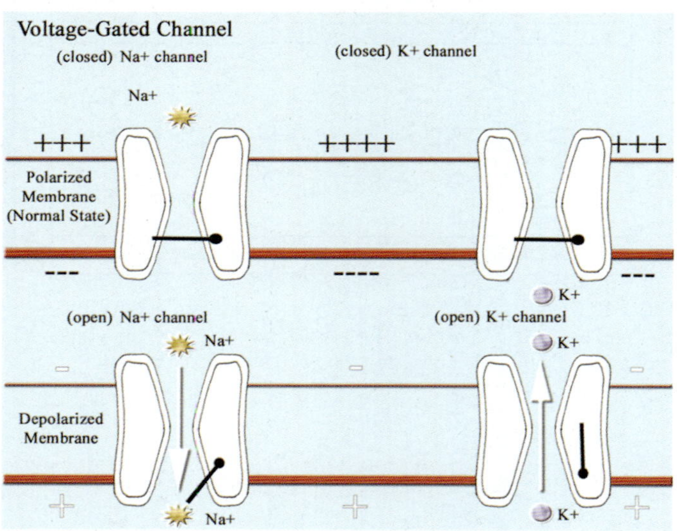

FIG 1-15 Changes of the membrane and the voltage-gated ions at rest and during depolarization.

The period of time in which the sodium channel is inactivated, because its inactivation channel does not open, and the cell cannot be depolarized again, is called the *absolute refractory period.* The *relative refractory period* is the period of time in which the membrane requires a stronger stimulus to be activated.

The action potential propagates longitudinally as the membrane depolarizes in both directions *(a current).* The propagation results in increased membrane capacitance, opening other neighboring voltage-gated sodium channels and depolarizing adjacent segments (Fig. 1-17). The voltage charges can be recorded by electrodes, which detect the propagation of the electrical potential, and the recorded potential is biphasic. Extracellular recordings generate a triphasic potential (except at the neuromuscular or myotendinous junctions); the triphasic potential is produced by the effects of *volume conduction.*

In *myelinated fibers,* myelin contains the lipid sphingomyelin that covers a segment of the axon. This is an isolator of electrical currents and, thus, isolates the axon in the myelinated area or internode. The axon is not covered at the node of Ranvier where ionic changes occur.[17]

The distance separating the nodes reduces the amount of current needed to cause a membrane capacitance change. This causes depolarization to occur *only* in the nonisolated node of Ranvier, and the propagation of the impulse is *not continuous,* as it is in unmyelinated axons, but jumps from node to node *(saltatory conduction)* (see Fig. 1-17). Increased myelin thickness reduces the membrane capacitance of myelinated segments, increasing conduction velocity.[18]

In demyelination there is slowing of conduction and conduction block, whereas remyelination produces shorter internodes, causing a slowing of conduction as the electrical currents have to jump through more, and smaller, segments.

The Neuromuscular Transmission

The neuromuscular transmitter ACh is synthesized in the axon by the reaction of acetyl CoA and choline. This reaction is mediated by the enzyme *choline acetyltransferase.*[19]

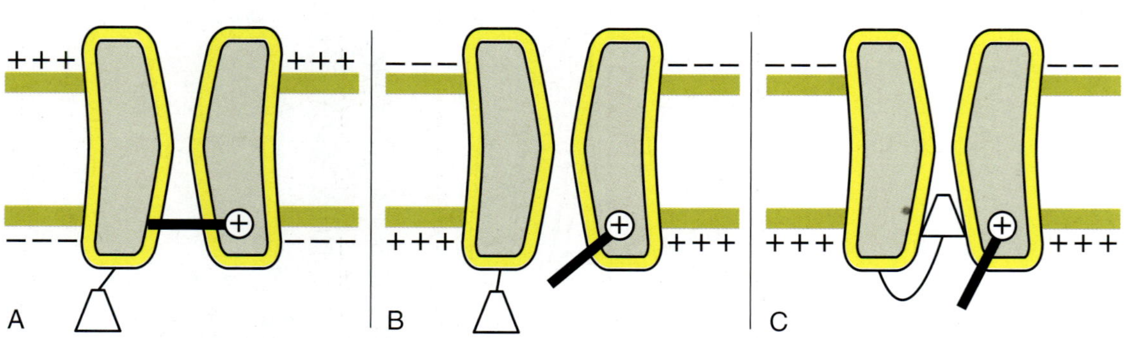

FIG 1-16 The activation and deactivation gates of the sodium channels during depolarization and repolarization. **A**, At rest, the activation gate is closed (bar) and the inactivation gate is open. **B**, During depolarization the activation gate is open. **C**, The inactivation gate closes and the channel is "inactivated."

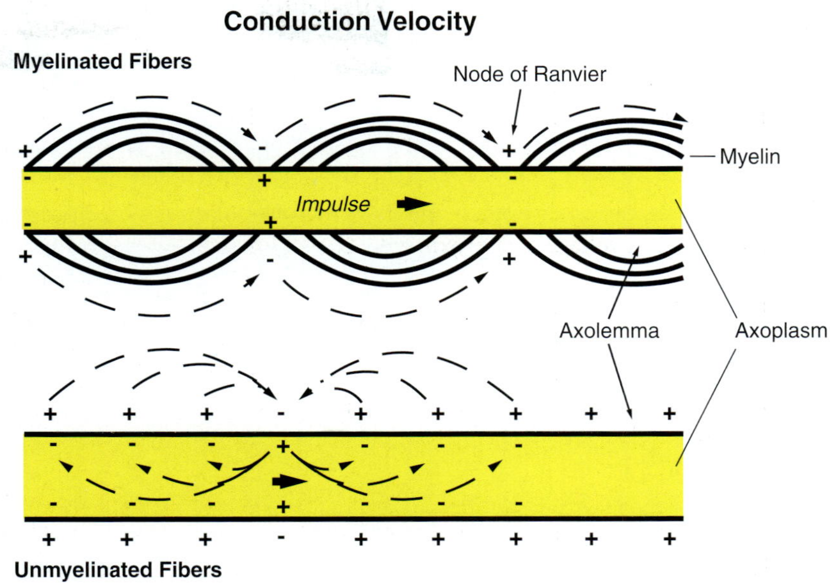

FIG 1-17 The representation of the propagation of the action potential in myelinated and unmyelinated axons.

Synaptic vesicles contain 5000–10,000 molecules of ACh; the number of molecules in a vesicle represents a *quantum*. The vesicles are stored in three areas of the nerve terminal: (1) the area that is closest to the synaptic membrane that contains the vesicles available for immediate release; (2) a mobilization store area that contains 10,000 quanta; and (3) the main storage area, where the packing and resynthesis of the neurotransmitter occur, which contains 300,000 quanta.[20,21]

Vesicle mobilization is triggered by the calcium-dependent phosphorylation of synapsin. These are then transported to the active zone region where they are docked. Interaction of synaptobrevin and syntaxin and NSAP25 start the fusion process with subsequent binding of calcium to synaptotagmin triggered in quanta release.

The arrival of the nerve action potential opens the calcium channel in the *active zone* which induces the vesicles to fuse with the terminal membrane, resulting in ACh release.[22] Approximately 100–200 quanta, each having 5000–10,000 molecules of ACh, are released with the arrival of a nerve action potential (see Fig. 1-12) with the aid of vesicular transporters. The released ACh binds to the receptors in the postsynaptic folds, opening its channels to cations and causing endplate depolarization (the *endplate potential [EPP]*). After the generation of the action potential, ACh is removed by hydrolysis by the enzyme acetylcholinesterase forming acetate and choline, which returns by reuptake to the nerve terminal.

Small spontaneous releases of ACh, which are not triggered by a nerve action potential, produce small electrical changes in the endplate, called the *miniature endplate potentials*.

The EPP has an amplitude of about 70–80 mV, which is more than sufficient to exceed the threshold of −45 mV to generate a *muscle action potential (MAP)*. This causes the activation of voltage sodium channels in the muscle fibers located at the postjunctional folds, allowing more sodium to enter and further depolarizing the membrane. This, in turn, opens the neighboring sodium channels, propagating the action potential along the muscle membrane. The action potential also travels through the tubular system activating calcium channels of the sarcoplasmic reticulum, triggering muscle contractions.[20,21] (Table 1-4).

TABLE 1-4 Events of Neuromuscular Transmission

Invasion of nerve terminal by a nerve action potential
Influx of Ca^{++} to the nerve terminal
Release of ACh through active zones located on the presynaptic nerve terminal
Diffusion of ACh across the synaptic cleft
Binding of ACh to two binding sites of each ACh receptor complex
Generation of an EPP by the depolarization of the endplate
Generation of a muscle AP when the EPP is of sufficient magnitude to exceed AP generation threshold
Removal of ACh from the synaptic cleft from hydrolysis of ACh by acetylcholinesterase to choline and acetate and passive diffusion of neurotransmitter from the area
Transport (active) of choline into the nerve terminal for resynthesis of ACh

ACh, Acetylcholine; *AP*, action potential; *EPP*, endplate potential.

The difference between the threshold to generate an MAP and the EPP amplitude is called the *safety factor (SF)*. The SF can be diminished in presynaptic disorders, affecting the synthesis or packing of ACh, altering the entrance of calcium into the nerve terminal, or blocking the release of the neurotransmitter. The SF can also be decreased in postsynaptic disorders, from a decreased number of available ACh receptors or from abnormalities of channel function.

In normal individuals, repetitive, slow nerve impulses at rates of 2–3 Hz cause a decrease of EPP amplitudes, but this still exceeds the threshold needed to generate MAPs. Fast nerve stimulation with stimulus intervals of less than 200 ms

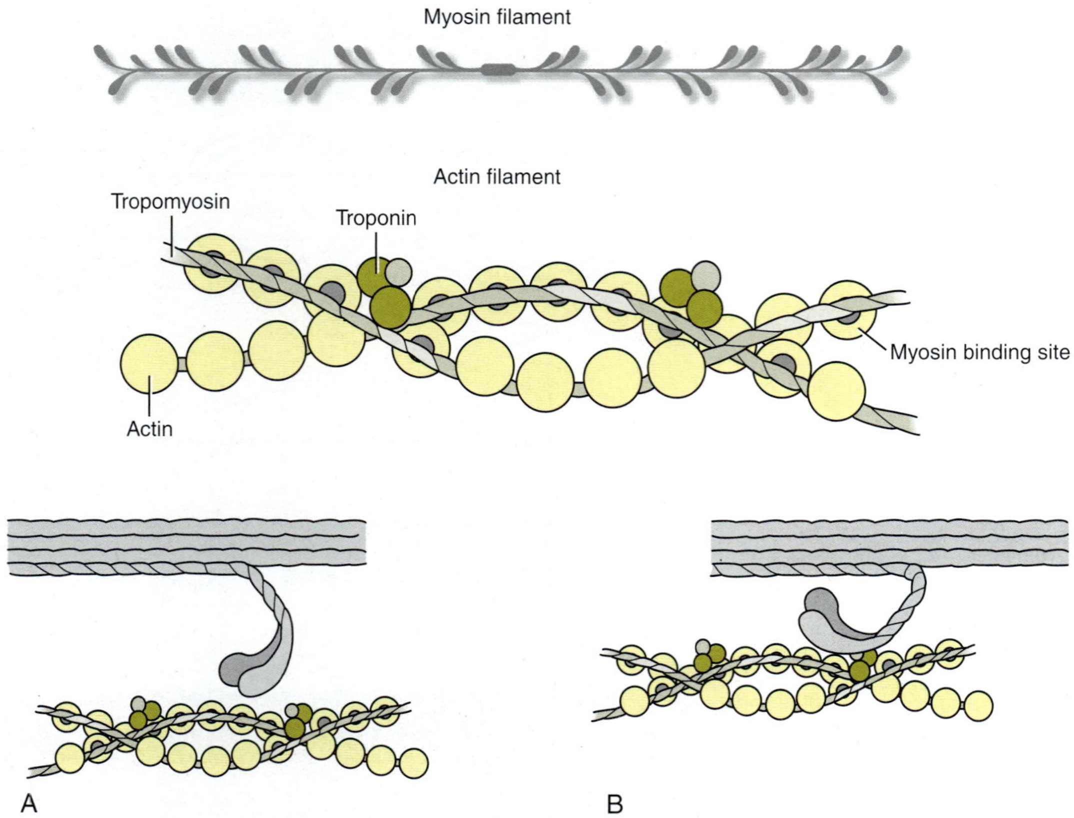

FIG 1-18 The myosin and actin filaments (top and center). Below, notice how the myosin head is not attached to the myosin-binding site during muscle relaxation because it is covered by the troponin and tropomyosin **(A)**. During contraction, the myosin head attaches to its binding site **(B)**.

facilitates the release of the neurotransmitter, increasing the EPP amplitudes but not changing the MAP in normals. In the clinical setting the repetitive stimulation test is done by measuring the CMAP (the summation of individual MAPs generated by a supramaximal electrical stimulation of nerves) using stimulation at different rates.

Muscle Contraction

Contractile proteins of muscle are *actin* and *myosin*, the main components of the *thin* and *thick* filaments, respectively. Each *thick* filament contains about 300 molecules of myosin and is shaped like golf clubs twisted together (Fig. 1-18). The two heads are called the *myosin heads*, or *cross bridges*.[23,24] The tails point toward the center of the sarcomere (toward the M lines), while the head projects toward one of the thin filaments and contains an *actin-binding site*, an *ATP binding site*, and an *ATPase*.

The thin filaments extend from the Z lines; they are formed by the actin molecules twisted in a helix. Each molecule has a *myosin-binding* site for the myosin head.[23]

The *"regulatory"* proteins *troponin* and *tropomyosin* are also part of the thin filament. Troponin has three subunits: TnT, which binds to tropomyosin; TnC, which binds calcium; and TnI, which inhibits the actin–myosin interaction.

At rest, ATP binds ATPase and one myosin molecule; it is hydrolyzed very slowly. During this period, the actin-binding sites of the myosin molecules are blocked by the *troponin–tropomyosin complex*.

TABLE 1-5 Excitation Contraction Coupling

Muscle action potential travels through the muscle membrane, T tubes, and then the SR.
The voltage-gated calcium channel opens causing the release of calcium by the ryanodine calcium-release channel in the SR.
Calcium increases in the cytosol and binds to troponin.
Calcium binding to troponin causes a conformational change of the troponin–tropomyosin complex, exposing the actin-binding site to myosin.
Myosin binds to actin. The power strike is caused by the hydrolysis of ATP. This energizes the movement by releasing ADP and phosphate.
Myosin detaches from actin to bind another molecule of ATP.
Calcium reuptake to the SR by the ATPase pump.
Decreased cytosolic calcium causes the troponin–tropomyosin complex to glide back to cover the myosin-binding site and muscle relaxes.

ATP, Adenosine triphosphate; *SR*, sarcoplasmic reticulum.

Excitation contraction coupling is the process by which an electrical stimulus triggers the release of calcium by the sarcoplasmic reticulum, initiating the mechanism of muscle contraction by sarcomere shortening. These steps are summarized in Table 1-5, which occur in the following.

When the MAP reaches the sarcoplasmic reticulum, it opens the voltage-gated calcium channels, triggering the release of calcium by the ryanodine receptor (Fig. 1-19). Calcium then binds to troponin altering the conformational shape of tropomyosin and exposing the actin-binding sites of myosin and initiates binding of the filaments[23] (see bottom of Fig. 1-18).

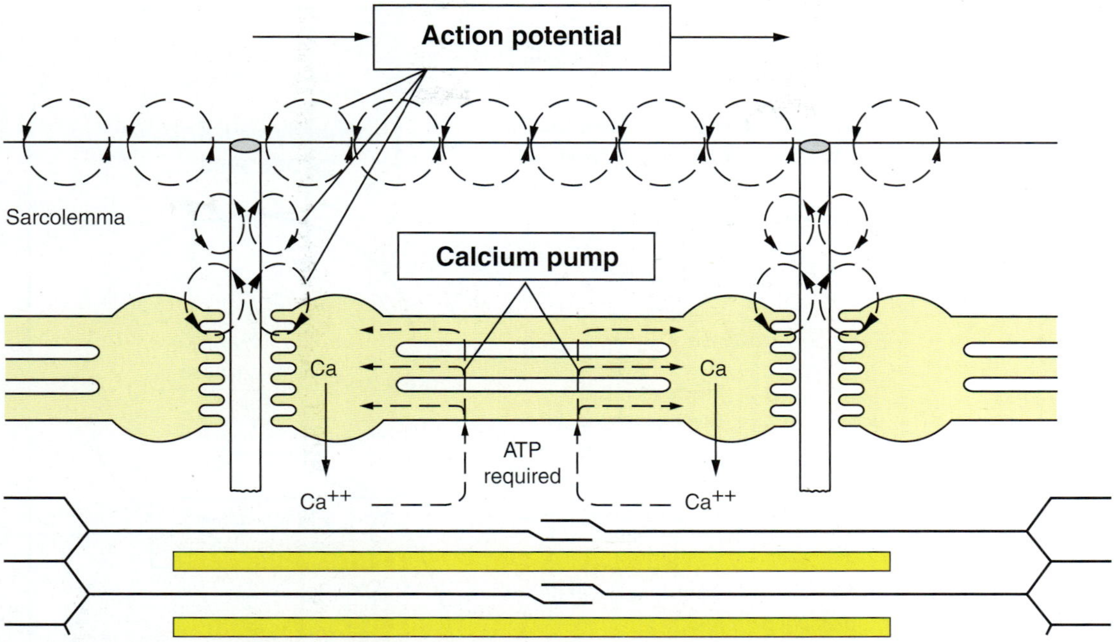

FIG 1-19 Sarcoplasmic calcium release. Action potential is shown propagating into the T tubule system carrying the impulse into the depths of the muscle and producing Ca++ release from the sarcoplasmic reticulum. The cycling of calcium ions is demonstrated following an action potential. (Reprinted with permission from Guyton AC. *Textbook of Medical Physiology*. 9th ed. Philadelphia, PA: WB Saunders; 1996.)

The hydrolysis of ATP releases ADP and phosphate, triggering the "power strike" for the contraction, then actin passes the myosin filament, causing this filament to move toward the M line shortening the sarcomere[24,25] (Fig. 1-20). When new ATP molecules bind to myosin, the head detaches and then hydrolyzes slowly, preparing the head for a new interaction. This process repeats throughout the duration of the action potential.

Muscle relaxation is initiated by the energy-dependent reuptake of calcium by the sarcoplasmic reticulum, which restores muscles to their original configuration. With the drop of calcium in the cytosol, the troponin–tropomyosin complexes glide back to cover the myosin-binding sites, and the muscle fiber relaxes. In the sarcoplasmic reticulum calcium binds to *calsequestrin*, increasing the concentration of calcium, which at rest is 10,000 times higher than in the cytosol.

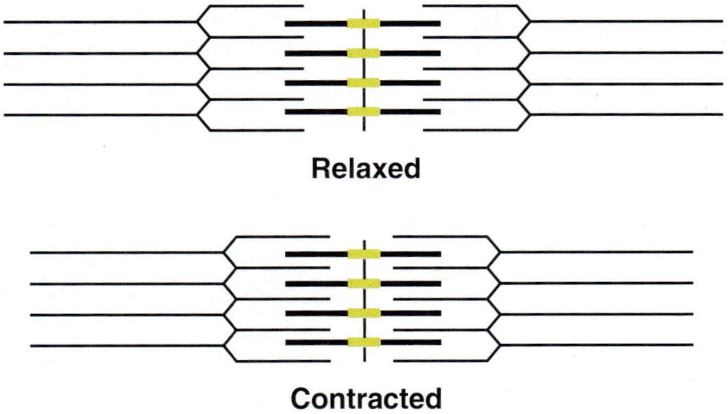

FIG 1-20 Muscle during relaxation and contraction with shortening of the sarcomere.

The Energy Supply for Muscle Contraction. At rest, muscle fibers produce more ATP than the necessary energy from various sources of its metabolism, and some of the excess is used in the synthesis of *creatine phosphate*, which is an energy-rich molecule. This reaction is catalyzed by the enzyme CK, producing the transfer of one high-energy phosphate group from ATP to creatine and forming *creatine phosphate* and ADP.

At the beginning of contractions, particularly during short bursts, CK catalyzes the transfer of energy phosphate groups from creatine phosphate back to ADP forming new ATP molecules. Upon increasing contractions, energy is obtained by two important metabolic pathways: the *anaerobic* (or *glycolytic*) pathway, and the *oxidative, or aerobic* pathway. At maximal exercise, energy for the anaerobic pathway is obtained from glucose (glycolysis) and later from stored glycogen molecules (glycogenolysis), and their end-products pyruvic and lactic acid.[26] Pyruvic acid moves into the mitochondria where it enters the Krebs cycle, forming acetyl CoA for its use in oxidative metabolism. If not enough oxygen is available for mitochondrial oxidation, then more lactic acid is formed. This diffuses to the blood and enters the liver, where some is converted to glucose.[23,24]

Oxygen for aerobic metabolism is obtained from circulating blood, as well as from myoglobin in muscle fibers. The energy necessary for prolonged exercise is then obtained from the metabolism of fat from fatty acids, which are transported into the mitochondria across the membrane as acyl carnitines, with the carrier molecule carnitine. This transport is mediated by the activity of a translocase and the palmitoyl transferase I and II enzymes. The oxidation of fatty acids forms acetyl CoA from beta-oxidation. Acetyl CoA is thus the common metabolite

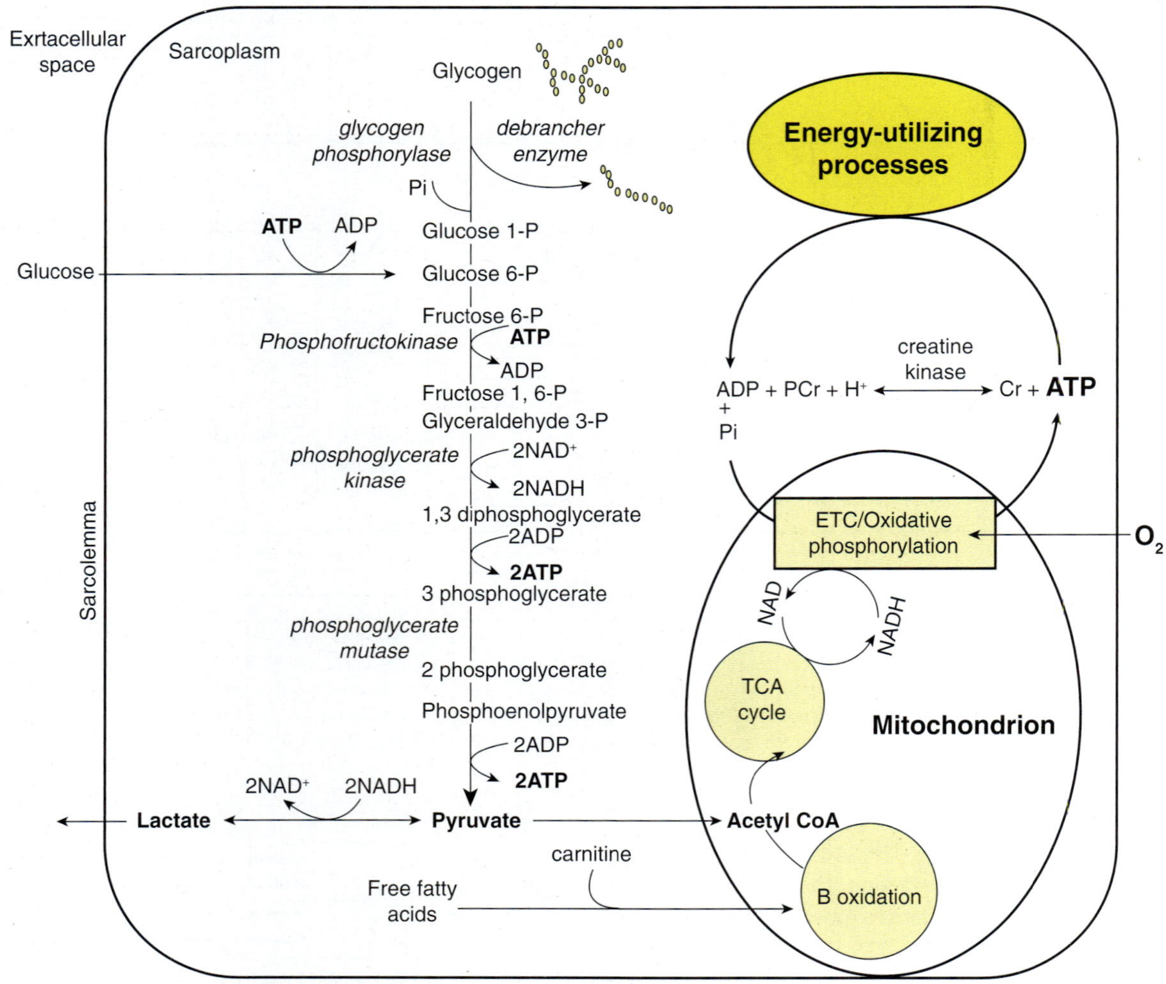

FIG 1-21 Pathways of muscle metabolism. (Reprinted with permission from Lodi R, Taivassalo T. Phosphorus magnetic resonance spectroscopy in the clinical investigation of muscle disorders. In: Bertorini TE, ed. *Clinical Evaluation and Diagnostic Tests for Neuromuscular Disorders.* Boston, MA: Butterworth-Heinemann; 2002.)

between lipid and carbohydrate metabolism.[26] Acetyl CoA is oxidized in the Krebs cycle, providing electrons for mitochondria respiratory chains (Fig. 1-21).

Amino acids, obtained from the metabolism of protein by deamination and in the liver by transamination, provide nitrogen residuals that can be degraded to provide high-energy phosphate bonds.

REFERENCES

1. Kandel ER, Schwartz JH, Jessell TM. The organization of movement. In: *Principles of Neural Science.* 4th ed. New York: McGraw-Hill; 2000:653–673.
2. Kandel ER, Schwartz JH, Jessell TM. The motor unit and muscle action. In: *Principles of Neural Science.* 4th ed. New York: McGraw-Hill; 2000:674–694.
3. Bertorini TE, Stalberg E, Yuson CP, Engel WK. Single-fiber electromyography in neuromuscular disorders: correlation of muscle histochemistry, single-fiber electromyography, and clinical findings. *Muscle Nerve.* 1994;17:345–353.
4. Kandel ER, Schwartz JH, Jessell TM. Ion channels. In: *Principles of Neural Science.* 4th ed. New York: McGraw-Hill; 2000:108–124.
5. Kandel ER, Schwartz JH, Jessell TM. Membrane potential. In: *Principles of Neural Science.* 4th ed. New York: McGraw-Hill; 2000:150–170.
6. Carpenter MB. *Human Neuroanatomy.* Baltimore, MD: Williams & Wilkins; 1976.
7. Haymaker W, Woodhall B. Peripheral nerve injuries. In: Principles of Diagnosis. 2nd ed. Philadelphia, PA: WB Saunders; 1967.
8. Bertorini TE, Horner LH. Histology and histochemistry of muscle and nerve. In: Bertorini TE, ed. *Clinical Evaluation and Diagnostic Tests for Neuromuscular Disorders.* Boston, MA: Butterworth-Heinemann; 2002:595–692.
9. Midroni B, Bilbao JM. The axon: normal structure and pathological alterations. In: Midroni S, Bilbao JM, Cohen SM, eds. *Biopsy: Diagnosis in Peripheral Neuropathy.* Boston, MA: Butterworth-Heinemann; 1995:45–74.
10. Craig R, Padron R. Molecular structure of the sarcomere. In: Engel AG, Franzini-Armstrong C, eds. *Myology.* 3rd ed. New York: McGraw-Hill; 2004:129–166.
11. Krause W. *Uber die Endigung der Muskelnerven. Z Rationelle Med,* 1863:461–464.
12. Engel AG. The neuromuscular junction. In: Engel AG, Franzini-Armstrong C, eds. *Myology.* 3rd ed. New York: McGraw-Hill; 2004:325–372.

13. Gulpill JC, Sanders DV, Evoli A. Anti-MuSK antibody myasthenia gravis: clinical findings and response to treatment in two large cohorts. *Muscle Nerve.* 2011;44:36–40.
14. Pevzner A, Schoser B, Peters K, et al. Anti-LRP antibodies in AchR- and MuSK-antibody- negative myasthenia gravis. *J Neurol.* 2012;259:427–435.
15. Koester J. Resting membrane potential and action potential. In: Kandel ER, Schwartz JH, eds. *Principles of Neural Science.* 2nd ed. New York: Elsevier; 1985:49–57.
16. Koester J. Voltage gated channels and the generation of the action potential. In: Kandel ER, Schwartz JH, eds. *Principles of Neural Science.* 2nd ed. New York: Elsevier; 1985:75–86.
17. Stämpfli R. Overview of studies on the physiology of conduction in myelinated nerve fibers. *Adv Neurol.* 1981;31:11–23.
18. Waxman SG. Action potential propagation and conduction velocity: new perspectives and questions. *Trends Neurosci.* 1983;6: 157–161.
19. Macintosh FC. Formation, storage and release of acetylcholine at nerve endings. *Can J Biochem Physiol.* 1959;37:343–356.
20. Ruffer SW, Yoshikami D. The number of transmitter molecules in a quantum: an estimate from iontophoretic applications of acetylcholine at the neuromuscular junction synapse. *J Physiol.* 1975;251:465–482.
21. Magleby K. Neuromuscular transmission. In: Engel AG, Franzini-Armstrong C, eds. *Myology.* 3rd ed. New York: McGraw-Hill; 2004:373–395.
22. Katz B. *Nerve Muscle and Synapse.* New York: McGraw-Hill; 1968.
23. Guyton AC. *Human Physiology and Mechanism of Disease.* 4th ed. Philadelphia, PA: WB Saunders; 1987.
24. Tortora J, Grabowski SR. *Principles of Anatomy and Physiology.* New York: Wiley; 2000:268–301.
25. Squire JM. Molecular mechanisms of neuromuscular contraction. *Trends Neurosci.* 1983;6:409–413.
26. DiMauro S, Shanske S, Naini A, Krishna S. Biochemical evaluation of metabolic myopathies. In: Bertorini TE, ed. *Clinical Evaluation and Diagnostic Tests for Neuromuscular Disorders.* Boston, MA: Butterworth-Heinemann; 2002:535–564.

2

Neurologic Evaluation and Ancillary Tests

THE HISTORY AND PHYSICAL EXAMINATION

Thorough and detailed medical history and examination are most important in neuromuscular disorders for diagnosis and proper interpretation of ancillary tests, such as electrodiagnostic studies, imaging or nerve and muscle biopsies, and genetic tests. During the evaluation, the clinician needs to determine if the disease is acquired or inherited and needs to localize the affected regions of the neuromuscular system to find out if the process is focal (i.e., mononeuropathy or radiculopathy) or generalized (i.e., polyneuropathies or myopathies).

Weakness is a common manifestation of neuromuscular disorders, and this could be progressive or of rapid onset, as in Guillain–Barré syndrome (GBS) and rhabdomyolysis, or could fluctuate during the day, as in myasthenia gravis (MG). This could also be intermittent and episodic, as in the periodic paralyses. Weakness is proximal in most myopathies (Fig. 2-1) and some motor neuron diseases and is distal in most neuropathies (Fig. 2-2). There are some dystrophies as well as inclusion body myositis that can present with distal weakness. It could be focal or asymmetric in motor neuron diseases, mononeuropathies, plexopathies, or radiculopathies[1] (Table 2-1).

Involvement of the cranial nerves helps in diagnosis. For example, fluctuating ptosis and diplopia could suggest MG, and ptosis, hearing loss, lipomas, and cardiac disease suggest a mitochondrial disorder.

A history of fatigue after physical activity would also suggest a disorder of neuromuscular transmission, whereas exercise intolerance accompanied by pain and contractures suggests a metabolic myopathy as in glycogen storage diseases. Muscle stiffness could suggest myotonia or other disorders of motor unit hyperactivity as in stiff-person syndrome.

Sensory complaints such as pain and numbness are characteristics of diseases affecting the sensory axons in peripheral nerves, roots, or plexus.

A good physical examination will elicit findings that lead to a diagnosis. For example, skeletal abnormalities such as scoliosis or high arches occur in hereditary ataxias and neuropathies, visceromegaly in some polyneuropathies such as the POEMS (polyneuropathy, organomegaly, endocrinopathy, monoclonal gammopathy, and skin changes) syndrome. Mees' lines in fingernails are seen in arsenic poisoning, while a skin rash is seen in dermatomyositis.

The clinical evaluation should also determine if there is autonomic dysfunction as that occurs in Eaton–Lambert syndrome and some neuropathies.

Gait and posture should be observed in order to detect prominent lordosis seen in stiff-person syndrome and some myopathies, the waddling gait seen in myopathies, or the steppage gait seen in polyneuropathies. The examiner should also note if the patient is able to rise up from the floor or a chair, in those with hip extensor weakness, or is unable to step up to or down from a stool from hip flexor or quadriceps muscle weakness.[2]

The presence of selective, or more prominent, weakness in some muscle groups is helpful. For example, ptosis and extraocular weakness are seen in MG, oculopharyngeal dystrophy, and mitochondrial myopathies. Facial weakness is characteristic of facioscapulohumeral dystrophy but can also be seen in sarcoidosis and familial amyloidosis. Tongue weakness with atrophy and fasciculations occurs in motor neuron disease. Tongue weakness without fasciculations can be seen in MG. A large tongue is seen in older children with Duchenne dystrophy as well as in patients with Pompe disease. Proper examination of palatal movement also helps to determine the risk of aspiration in these patients.

Neck flexor weakness is most common in myopathies, but some patients could also present with a head drop because of neck extensor weakness. This can be seen in, among others, myositis, some dystrophies, amyotrophic lateral sclerosis (ALS), mitochondrial myopathies, and MG.[3] Several myopathies may show characteristics of winging of the scapulae, but when this is unilateral, it could be caused by weakness of the rhomboid, trapezius, or serratus muscles in focal nerve disorders.[1,4,5]

Manual muscle testing is always necessary, and the major groups should be quantitated. The grading system used in the cases presented in this book is the standard Medical Research Council scale, which is as follows: 5 = normal strength; 4 = the patient holds the test position against gravity and moderate resistance; 3 = the muscle moves the joint against gravity, but not against resistance to the full extent of mechanical range; 2 = the muscle moves the joint when gravity is eliminated through a partial extent of mechanical range; 1 = there is a flicker of contraction without joint motion; and 0 = no contractions.

The examiner should determine if the weakness is accompanied by focal or generalized atrophy or if there is a lack of significant atrophy as that occurs in disorders of neuromuscular transmission, and frequently in demyelinating neuropathies.

Analysis of muscle strength during repetitive motion helps in diagnosing disorders of neuromuscular transmission, although muscle fatigue can also occur in other diseases.

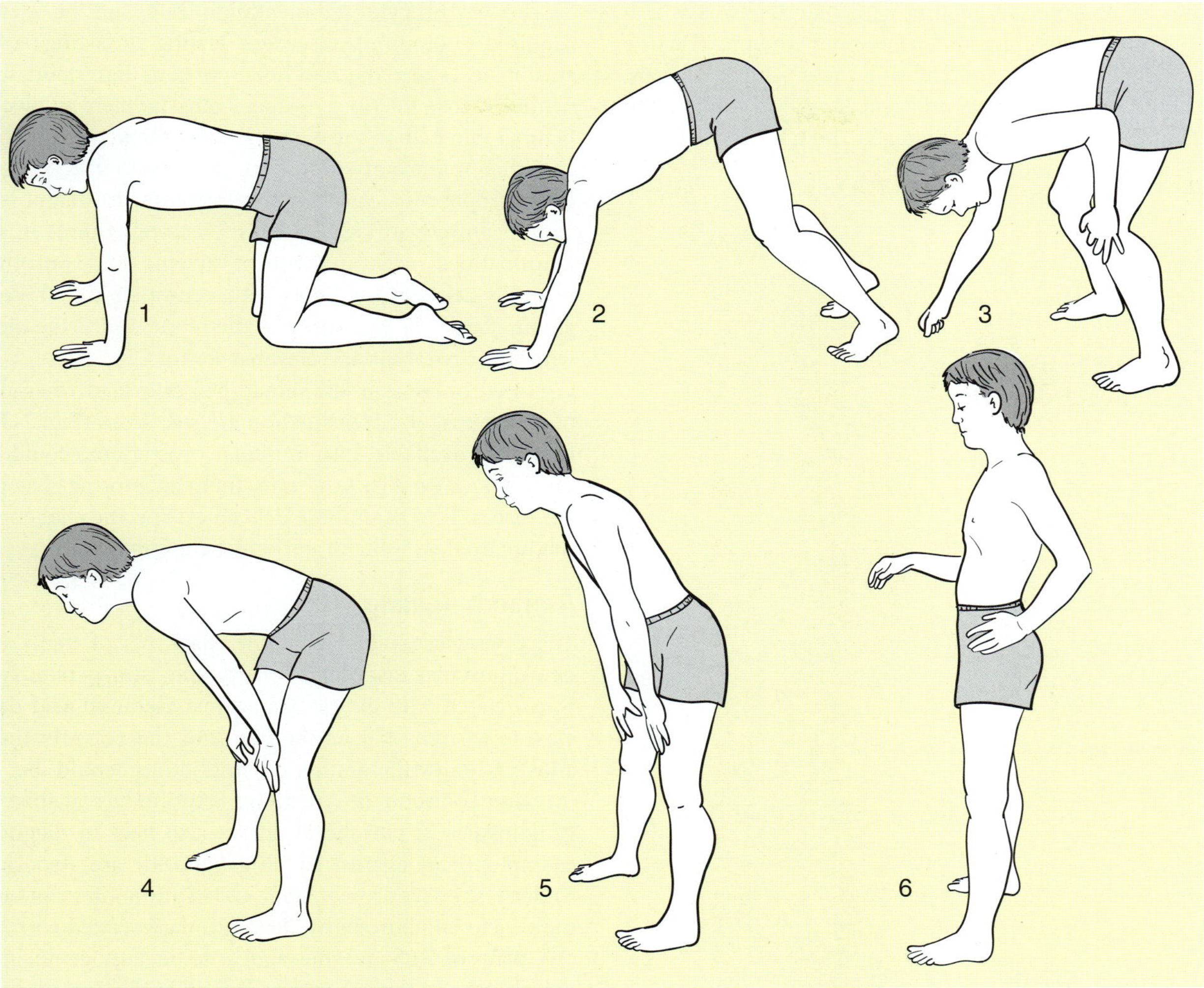

FIG 2-1 Drawing of a patient with muscular dystrophy performing the Gower's maneuver to rise up from the floor.

Muscle stretch reflexes are usually hyperactive in ALS. While distal areflexia is characteristic of axonal neuropathies, generalized areflexia suggests a demyelinating neuropathy. Reflexes are usually normal in myopathies.

Hyporeflexia that improves during repetitive tapping can be observed in Eaton–Lambert syndrome. A focal loss of reflexes, correlating with sensory deficits in territories of nerves, plexuses, or roots, helps in localization.

Reflexes graded in this book are as follows: 0 = absent, 1 = diminished, 2 = normal, 3 = hyperactive normal, and 4 = abnormally increased with clonus. During the examination, the examiner should also determine the presence of Babinski signs in order to diagnose involvement of the corticospinal tracts.[6]

The sensory examination should include the analysis of large myelinated fiber function, such as position and vibratory sense, and the Romberg test and analysis of small fiber function, such as pain and temperature sensations.

Large fiber dysfunction is seen in chronic demyelinating neuropathies, and a preferential impairment of unmyelinated fibers occurs in some neuropathies, like amyloidosis. Touch sensation involves small and large myelinated fibers. The use of the two-point discrimination test and Semmes–Weinstein filaments allows for a better quantitation of touch.

Coordination should be analyzed with the eyes open and closed in order to determine the presence of sensory or cerebellar ataxia.

IMPORTANT ANCILLARY TESTS

Ancillary tests include measurement of pulmonary function, which can be done in the office with portable respirometers, to determine the forced vital capacity and other respiratory parameters[7] that allow for proper quantitation and follow-up.[1,7] Other useful tests include electrocardiography and echocardiography in particular disorders such as muscular dystrophies.

Blood tests should include a complete metabolic panel to determine if there is a treatable electrolyte disturbance or renal and liver disease. Elevated enzymes, such as alanine transaminase (ALT), aspartate transaminase (AST), creatine kinase (CK), and aldolase, are seen in myopathies, whereas ALT and AST are also elevated in liver disease, and gamma-glutamyl transpeptidase is elevated *only* in liver disease. A complete blood count (CBC) should always be done to determine the presence of anemia with macrocytosis which would lead to the diagnosis of pernicious anemia (PA) or folic acid deficiency. Measurement of B_{12} and folic acid levels, homocysteine, and methylmalonic acid is used to confirm the diagnosis of PA and folate deficiencies. The CBC is also used in monitoring immunotherapy.

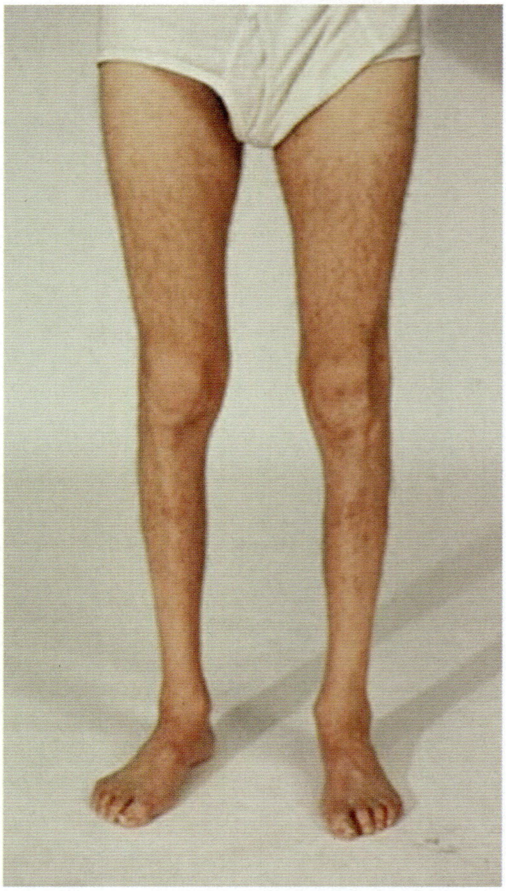

FIG 2-2 A patient with peripheral neuropathy showing distal leg wasting.

The erythrocyte sedimentation rate can be elevated in acquired autoimmune disorders. Testing for fasting blood sugar and, if necessary, the two-hour postprandial blood sugar test or the glucose tolerance test and measurement of glycosylated hemoglobin help in the diagnosis of diabetic neuropathies.

Other important studies include serum and urine immunoelectrophoresis, using immunofixation to diagnose monoclonal gammopathies, and tests for cryoglobulins in acquired neuropathies. Measurement of arsenic and porphyrins in urine[8] is helpful in patients with neuropathies, whereas myoglobin should be measured in the blood and urine of patients with acute paralysis and elevated serum CK.[9]

An edrophonium test should be performed when disorders of neuromuscular transmission are suspected (Fig. 2-3). If this test is not available, intramuscular prostigmine could be used. The forearm exercise test[10] is useful in diagnosing glycogen storage disease and deaminase deficiency. Specific challenge methods are used, as well, for periodic paralysis.[11]

Antibody Testing

These tests are valuable in the diagnosis of many acquired neuromuscular disorders. For example, stiff-person syndrome is associated with antibodies against glutamic acid decarboxylase,[12] whereas Hμ antibodies, and the recently discovered anti-CV2/CRMP5 antineural antibodies, could be elevated in paraneoplastic neuropathies. Antibodies against various gangliosides in peripheral nerves also help in diagnosis. For example, those against *GQ1b* ganglioside are associated with Miller Fisher syndrome, while *GD1a* antibodies can be seen in motor axonal neuropathy. Several are associated with the various forms of GBS and they appear to be pathogenic, including, among others, those against GM1, GM1b, GD1a, glycolipids, and myelin proteins. However, they are not usually measured in the clinical setting.[13–17]

GD1b antibodies can be elevated in some patients with sensory neuropathies, and those against *GM1* ganglioside are frequently high in multifocal motor neuropathy, helping in the

TABLE 2-1 Neuromuscular Disease: Clinical Evaluation

Clinical Parameter	Motor Neuron Disease	Polyneuropathy	Diseases of Neuromuscular Junction	Myopathy
Pattern of weakness	Variable, symmetric in most, often asymmetric in ALS	Distal > proximal	Proximal > distal, fluctuates, often involves extraocular muscles	Proximal > distal
Fasciculations	Yes	Sometimes	No	No
Muscle stretch reflexes	Variable, decreased in most, increased in ALS	Decreased or absent	Normal in postsynaptic disorders (myasthenia gravis), decreased in presynaptic disorders (Eaton–Lambert syndrome and botulism)	Normal initially, may be decreased in later stages (ankle reflexes often preserved until very late)
Sensory loss	No	Usually present	No	No

ALS, Amyotrophic lateral sclerosis.

Reprinted with permission from Bertorini TE, ed. *Clinical Evaluation and Diagnostic Tests for Neuromuscular Disorders.* Boston, MA, Butterworth-Heinemann; 2002:3.

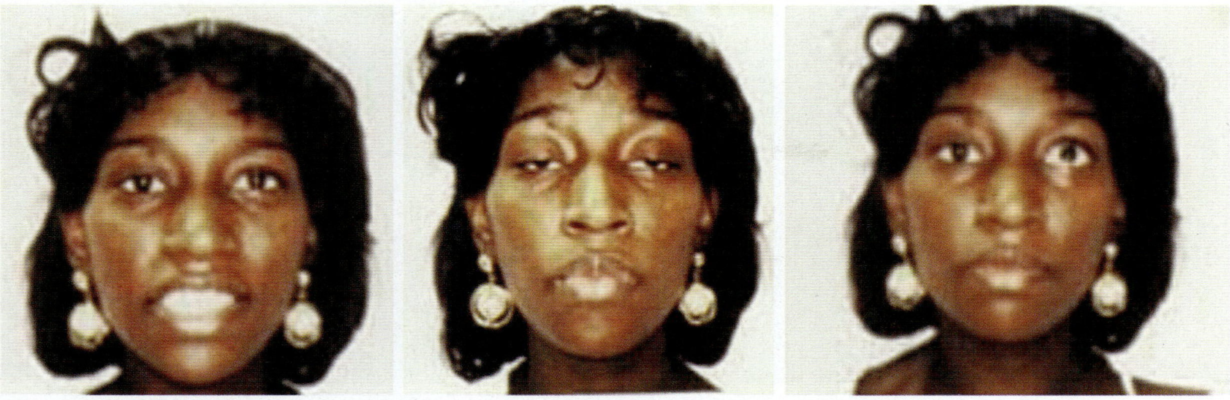

FIG 2-3 A patient with myasthenia gravis (MG) undergoing an edrophonium test: baseline (left); upon sustained upward gaze (center); after receiving 6 mg of intravenous edrophonium (right).

diagnosis. A distal demyelinating neuropathy in older persons is frequently associated with antibodies against myelin-associated glycoprotein (MAG).[18–21] Isaacs syndrome is caused by those that bind the voltage-gated potassium channels in peripheral nerves.[22]

MG is caused by antibodies against the ACh receptors, and patients who are ACh–antibody negative could have them against muscle-specific protein kinase, agrin, or LRP4 antibodies. Eaton–Lambert syndrome is caused by those against the presynaptic voltage-gated Ca channels.[23]

There are several antibodies associated with myositis such as antisynthetase antibodies for which the JO-1 type is particularly important as this can be present in patients with interstitial lung disease.[24] For patients with necrotizing myositis, we should test for signal recognition particle (SRP) antibodies and anti-HMGCR antibodies.

Antinuclear antibodies are seen in lupus erythematosus, and anti-*SS-A/Ro* or anti-*SS-B/La* are elevated in Sjögren's syndrome, a systemic disease which might manifest with a ganglioneuritis or myositis.[25] ANCA titers help in the evaluation of vasculitis. Ganglioneuritis can also occur with neoplasms and anti-Hμ antibodies.[26] Gliadin antibodies help in diagnosing myopathies and neuropathies associated with sprue.[27]

Imaging

Imaging helps to detect structural abnormalities in the spine, plexuses, or even peripheral nerves and to diagnose myeloma associated with neuropathies. Magnetic resonance imaging (MRI) and MR neurography help in the detection of nerve or plexus edema or neoplasm (Figs. 2-4 and 2-5).

MRI of the spine is used to diagnose spinal disease (Fig. 2-6) as shown in several cases in this book and to help rule out a structural disease of the spine that might mimic ALS. MRI can also be used in focal entrapments, for example, to demonstrate structural abnormalities of the carpal tunnel compressing the median nerve. Diagnostic ultrasound is also used with increased frequency in the evaluation of carpal tunnel syndrome (CTS) and other entrapments and muscle atrophy (Fig. 2-7).

Muscle MRI aids in the determination of the presence of inflammation, infarcts, necrosis, or tumors. Inflammation and necrosis are associated with an increased signal in the T2-weighted images (Fig. 2-8), whereas fat replacement is demonstrated in the T1-weighted images (Fig. 2-9). Muscle necrosis also can be shown by radionuclear scanning.[28]

Magnetic spectroscopy is a technique of great value in detecting metabolic myopathies causing muscle fatigue but is now largely used as a research tool.[29]

MRI and ultrasound of muscle help to determine the pattern of muscle involvement in children and to select muscles for biopsies.[30]

Dual-energy x-ray absorptiometry scan is a radiographic method that assesses total-body mineral composition and uses scanners with an x-ray tube with K-edge filtration. Body tissues have varying degrees of absorption ratios, depending on the density, and thus, the technique detects bone mineral content, lean body mass, and fat, and this is used to diagnose osteopenia, measure muscle mass, and determine disease progression in therapeutic trials, having a good correlation with manual muscle testing.[31]

Electrical bioimpedance is a new method that does not provide imaging but analyzes the response of muscles following stimuli of low-intensity electrical currents with a high frequency of 50 kHz. This measures the resistance and reactance of tissue, and the increased capacitance is associated with better muscle mass. The test is done with portable equipment and is simple, safe, rapid, and reproducible.[32,33] Different techniques are used such as measurement of the total body mass, whereas others study selected muscles. We use regional limb impendence using the Quantum V segmental method which provides appendicular (each exam and leg and torso and total body) composition results and has demonstrated lack of variability when normal subjects are tested twice at different dates. We have used the technique to monitor the progression and response to therapy in neuromuscular diseases.[34,35]

CLINICAL ELECTROPHYSIOLOGIC STUDIES

Electrophysiologic tests, such as nerve conduction studies, needle electromyography (EMG), and repetitive stimulation tests, are valuable tools in neuromuscular disease. They are particularly helpful in the localization of focal or segmental disorders, such as radiculopathies and nerve entrapments. These should be used as an expansion of a proper neurologic history and examination for interpretation (Table 2-2).

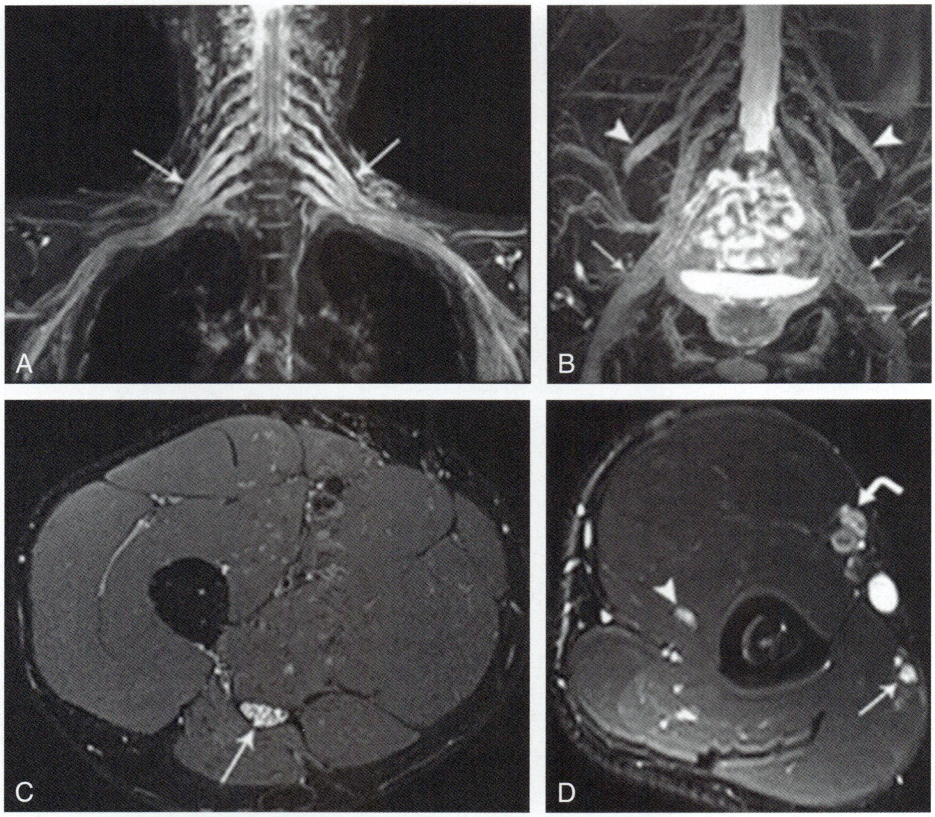

FIG 2-4 In patients with immunoglobulin G4 (IgG4) anti-NF-155 antibodies. Three-dimensional (3D) magnetic resonance (MR) neurography revealed bilateral hypertrophy of brachial and lumbosacral plexi. 3D MR neurography of the brachial **(A)** and lumbosacral plexus **(B)**, coronal views; 2D MR neurography of the right sciatic nerve at mid-thigh **(C)** and of the right arm at mid-humerus **(D)**. **A**, Bilateral, symmetric hypertrophy of the brachial plexus, which is predominant in the nerve roots, with gradual normalization toward the proximal limbs (*arrows*). **B**, Bilateral symmetric hypertrophy of the lumbosacral plexus, involving the terminal branches, intrapelvic femoral nerves (*arrowheads*), and sciatic nerves at the sciatic notch (*arrows*). **C**, Increased signal intensity and size (cross-sectional area [CSA] = 89 mm^2) of the right sciatic nerve, with diffuse fascicular hypertrophy (*arrow*). **D**, Increased signal intensity and size of the right median (CSA = 16 mm^2, *curved arrow*), ulnar (CSA = 10 mm^2, *arrow*), and radial (CSA = 7.6 mm^2, *arrowhead*) nerves. (From El -Abassi R N el al. Chapter 16 In: Bertorini, *Neuromuscular Disorders—Treatment and Management*. 2nd ed. Copyright 2022 by Elsevier.)

Nerve Conduction Tests

Nerve conduction tests are done using conventional EMG equipment which consists of an oscilloscope with differential amplifiers and signal averaging. The equipment has stimulating units connected to the oscilloscope that triggers its sweeps.

Sensory Conduction Studies. These tests provide a direct assessment of the function and population of large myelinated sensory axons. The *sensory nerve action potential* (*SNAP*) represents the summation of the potentials of individual nerve fibers with conduction velocities above 34 m/s that have diameters of about 9 µm. This tests large myelinated sensory axons but not small myelinated or unmyelinated fibers. Near nerve needle recording electrodes allow the study of slow myelinated axons. C fibers can be studied indirectly by measuring the sympathetic skin response that evaluates postganglionic autonomic fibers, and also by using other autonomic tests, and microneurography.

The SNAPs are much smaller than *compound muscle action potentials* (*CMAPs*) and therefore more sensitive to temporal dispersion with increased distances, particularly using proximal stimulation sites. They are used primarily to test distal nerve segments.[36-39]

Stimulations should be just above maximal and are done either distally—for example, in the digits and recording at the wrist (*orthodromic conduction*)—or proximally—for example, at the wrist and recording at the digits (*antidromic conduction*) (Fig. 2-10). The SNAPs obtained with antidromic stimulation are usually larger. The latency is measured at the initial deflection or at the peak of the negative response. In the past, latency to the peak was used, particularly in the orthodromic method, because it was hard to identify the onset of the SNAP. This can now be done easily with signal averaging, allowing measurement of the conduction velocity of faster axons from the SNAP onset.

Because sensory nerve conduction tests do not include the delay of the neuromuscular junction as in the motor conduction test, the *sensory nerve conduction velocity* can be calculated directly by dividing the distal latency by the distance or by dividing it by the difference in latencies when more than one site is stimulated. Some report only the latency measurements at set distances, particularly when using orthodromic methods.

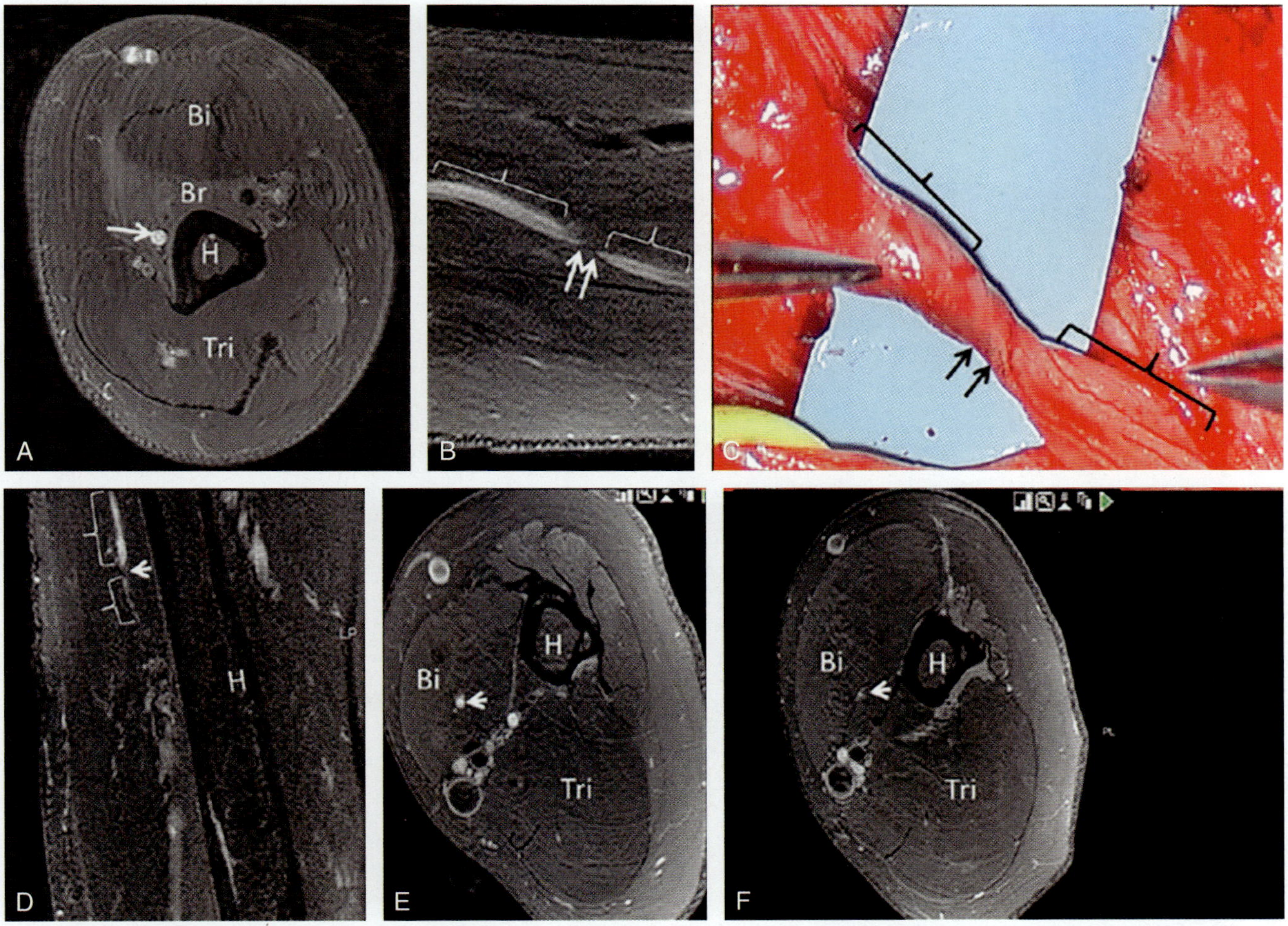

FIG 2-5 Images from a 51-year-old man with left radial nerve and musculocutaneous nerve (MCN) palsy for 1 year. **A** and **B**, Axial two-dimensional (2D) T2-weighted Dixon fat-suppressed image **(A)** reveals enlargement, signal hyperintensity, and a "bullseye" sign of the radial nerve (*arrow*) within the distal arm, just proximal to a severe constriction (*arrows*, **B**) of the nerve demonstrated on the longitudinal 2D Dixon image. There is denervation edema pattern of the brachialis (Br) and sparing of the biceps (Bi) muscles, a classical finding in PTS. **C**, Intraoperative photograph reveals torsed appearance of the radial nerve (*brackets*) with focal constriction (*arrows*) at the same site identified by magnetic resonance imaging **(B)**. **D**, Oblique coronal 2D T2-weighted Dixon fat-suppressed image reveals focal intrinsic constriction (*arrow*) of the MCN (*brackets*), likely distal to the takeoff of the biceps branch within the arm. **E** and **F**, Axial 2D, T2-weighted Dixon fat-suppressed images reveal MCN enlargement immediately proximal (*arrow*, **E**) and collapse immediately distal (*arrow*, **F**), to the site of constriction shown in image (**D**). *H*, Humerus; *Tri*, triceps muscle. (Reproduced with permission from Sneag D, Raney SK, Wolfe SW et al. Brachial plexitis or neuritis? *Muscle Nerve*. 2018;58.)

The *amplitude* of the SNAPs is measured from the baseline to the peak of the negative response or from the peak of the negative wave to the peak of the positive wave (Fig. 2-11). Axonal dropout can cause a decreased SNAP amplitude, whereas prolongation of latencies with diminished conduction velocity is caused by demyelination. Demyelinating neuropathies can cause not only slowing but also low-amplitude SNAPs, and even their disappearance, because of increased temporal dispersion.

The *duration* of the SNAP is measured from the beginning of the negative wave to the end of the negative wave. The *area* is calculated automatically by newer EMG equipment. The area decreases with dropout of axons from axonal degeneration, and its measurement is more accurate than the amplitude to evaluate for axonal dropout, because the latter might be influenced by temporal dispersion.

Decreased SNAP amplitudes and areas can occur in plexopathies and in focal neuropathies, but usually not in radiculopathies, because the sensory axons originate at the posterior ganglia, which are not affected in the latter disorders, thereby helping in the diagnosis (Table 2-3).

Mixed Nerve Conduction. Stimulation over a mixed nerve distally and recording directly in more proximal segments measures mixed nerve conduction, using settings similar to those of sensory conduction tests, and is of value in diagnosing focal entrapments. Palmar stimulation of the ulnar and median nerves and the plantar tibial nerve are mixed nerve conduction techniques. The tests measure the velocity and population of sensory and motor axons directly, but also the 1 alpha afferent axons which are more sensitive to compression.

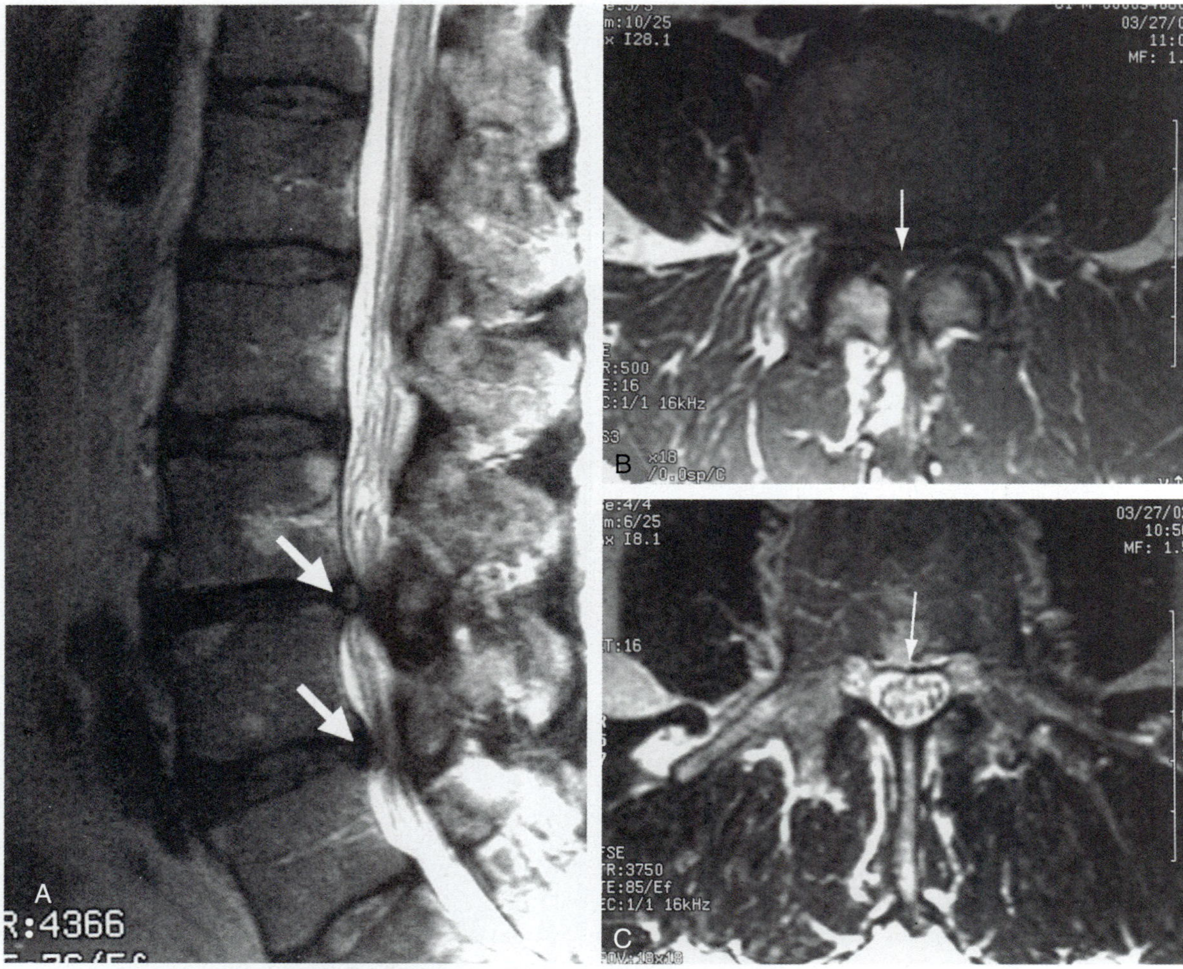

FIG 2-6 **A**, Magnetic resonance imaging (MRI), T2-weighted image (*sagittal view*) prominent disk bulging and canal stenosis at L3–L4, L4–L5 (*arrows*). **B**, Very small canal seen in the axial view on MRI T2-weighted image at the L4–L5 level (*arrow*). **C**, Axial view MRI, T2-weighted image showing minimal stenosis at the L2 level (*arrow*). (From Bertorini TE. *Neuromuscular Case Studies*. Philadelphia, PA: Butterworth-Heinemann; 2008:193.)

Quantitative Sensory Testing. Quantitative sensory tests are psychophysical tests that are used in the determination of sensitivity to pain, temperature, and vibration. These are not electrical tests but help in determining the function of various types of nerve fibers[40] (Fig. 2-12).

Motor Nerve Conduction Tests. Nerve conduction of peripheral motor nerves is studied by stimulating the nerve distally, and at one or more points proximally, while recording the response in a muscle innervated by that nerve (Fig. 2-13A). The stimuli should be supramaximal to allow the stimulation of all motor axons. The motor response is called the *CMAP*, or *M-wave*; this is a biphasic potential with initial negativity.[37,38]

Stimulations and recordings are done with surface disk electrodes, but needle electrodes can also be used. The cathode of the stimulating electrodes should be over the studied nerve and the anode placed at a distance of 2–3 cm. The cathode of the recording electrode is placed over the belly of the tested muscle and the anode over a tendon, usually about 3–4 cm from the cathode.

Motor nerve conduction tests include the measurement of *latency* from the stimulus artifact to the onset of the CMAP, as this represents the conduction of the fastest axons. This latency includes not only axonal conduction but also the delays of neuromuscular transmission and depolarization of muscle fibers. The latency from the distal stimulating point is called *distal latency* or *terminal latency* and those from proximal points are called *proximal latencies*. The distal latency can be prolonged in some entrapments, such as that of the median nerve in CTS or the tibial nerve in tarsal tunnel syndrome. It is also prolonged in demyelinating neuropathies.

The *amplitude* of the negative peak (see Fig. 2-13B), or of the whole wave (peak to peak), is also measured to detect the conduction block from focal demyelination, causing a drop in amplitude obtained from the proximal stimulation compared to the distal response. Changes in amplitude can also occur in cross-innervations, such as in the Martin–Gruber anastomosis. A decreased amplitude of both the proximal and distal responses can be seen in axonal neuropathies.

Measurement of the *duration* of the negative wave is useful in the diagnosis of demyelination which causes a prolonged CMAP. Such a potential might appear dispersed because of different rates of slowing of the axons. The *area* of the CMAP is measured automatically with newer equipment; this represents

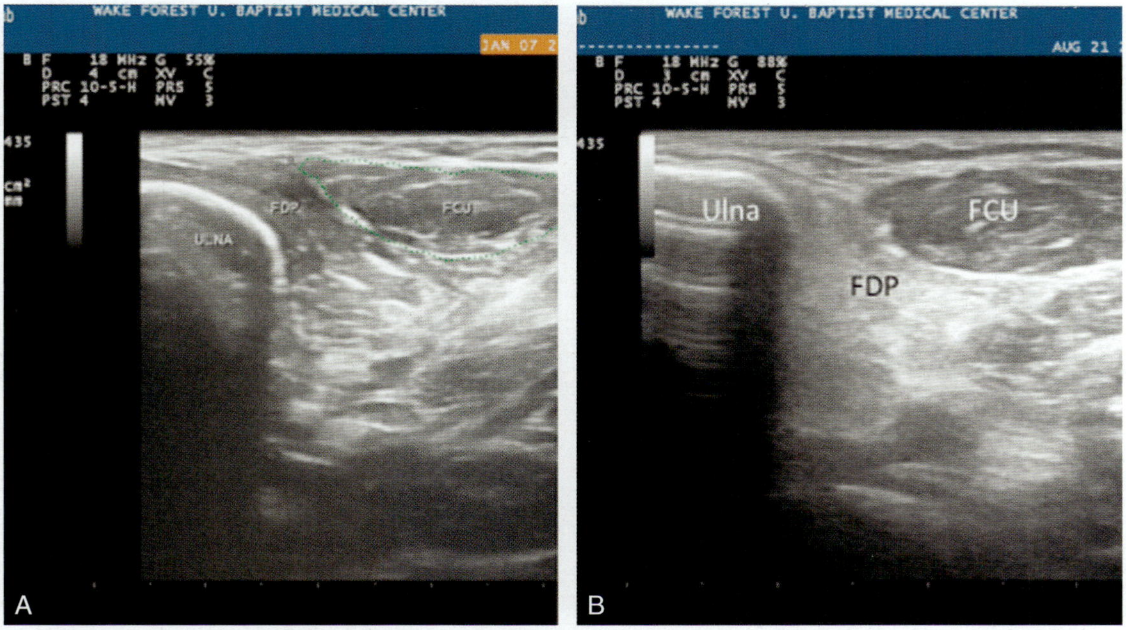

FIG 2-7 Two cross-sectional images using an 18 MHz transducer (Esaote MyLab Gold) taken of the proximal forearm over the flexor carpi ulnaris (FCU) muscle. The left image from a normal control **(A)** shows a "starry night" pattern of muscle architecture with the bulk of the muscle being hypoechoic interspersed with fibrous tissue stroma in both FCU and the flexor digitorum profundus (FDP). The ulna has a bright edge. **B**, From a patient with inclusion body myositis showing the FDP muscle is preferentially involved, showing loss of normal architecture, and is diffusely hyperechoic consistent with chronic muscle diseases. The oval shape FCU is seen with the normal "starry night" pattern with a background of very dark muscle tissue interspersed with bright (hyperechoic) punctate and curvilinear fibrous tissue stroma, but the FDP shows loss of normal architecture and is diffuse hyperechoic. (Courtesy Dr. Michael Cartwright and Dr. Francis Walker.)

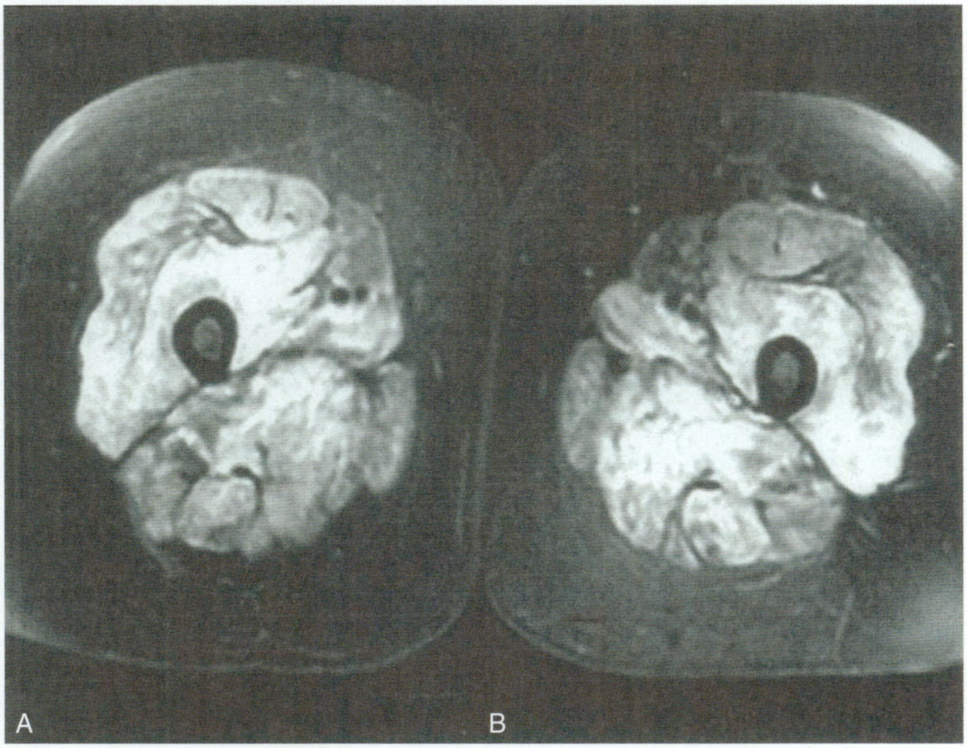

FIG 2-8 Axial **(A)** and coronal **(B)** fast spin echo T2-weighted fat-suppressed magnetic resonance images from a patient with active polymyositis. Fat suppression was performed using a short tau inversion recovery technique (repetition time/echo time =3500/45 ms, inversion time = 160 ms). There is diffuse extensive abnormal signal involving all muscle groups in the thigh. This increased signal is due to muscle edema. (From Bertorini TE, ed. *Clinical Evaluation and Diagnostic Tests for Neuromuscular Disorders*. Woburn, MA, Butterworth-Heinemann; 2002:579.)

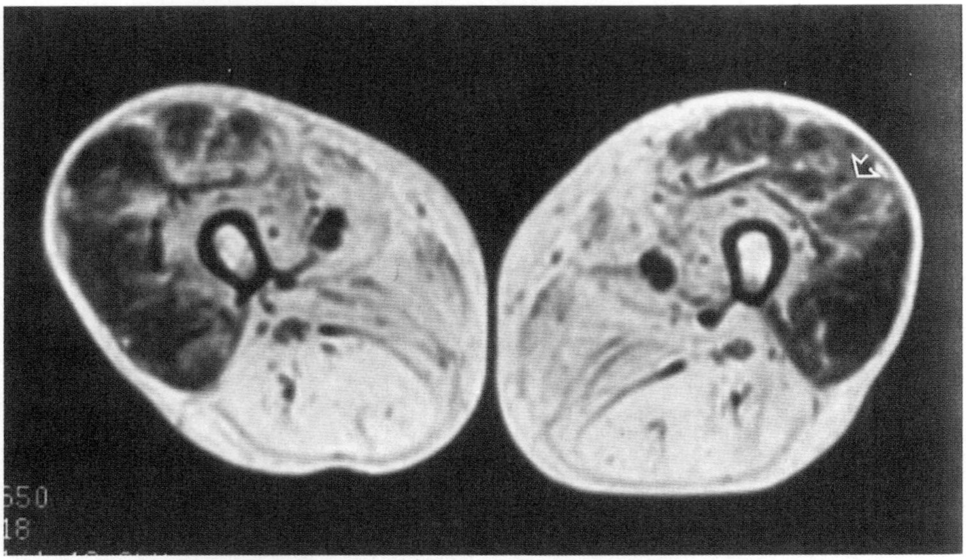

FIG 2-9 Magnetic resonance imaging axial T1-weighted spine echo images of a patient with Becker's muscular dystrophy showing severe involvement and fat replacement in the hamstring muscle, and relatively less involvement of the vastus lateralis (*open arrow*), more involvement of the hamstrings (*arrow*). (From Bertorini TE, ed. *Clinical Evaluation and Diagnostic Tests for Neuromuscular Disorders.* Woburn, MA: Butterworth-Heinemann; 2002:576, Fig. 18 11b.)

TABLE 2-2 Neuromuscular Disease: Laboratory Evaluation

Test	Motor Neuron Disease	Polyneuropathy	Myopathy	Diseases of Neuromuscular Junction
Serum muscle enzymes	Normal or mild elevation	Normal	Increased	Normal
Nerve conduction studies	Normal or low-amplitude CMAPs, normal SNAPs	Usually slow nerve conduction velocities or low-amplitude CMAPs and SNAPs	Normal	Normal
Electromyography	Decreased number of motor units, evidence of denervation and reinnervation (large motor units)	Decreased number of motor units, evidence of denervation and reinnervation (large motor units)	Normal number of motor units with short duration and low amplitude, frequently polyphasic	Normal or small motor units, variability of motor unit size and shape
Repetitive nerve stimulation test	Usually normal, decremental responses can occur	Normal	Normal	Decrement of CMAP at low rate of stimulation, increment at fast rates in presynaptic disorders
Muscle biopsy	Denervation (atrophic angular and target fibers, fiber-type grouping, group atrophy)	Denervation (atrophic angular and target fibers, fiber-type grouping)	"Myopathic" (necrosis, storage material, inflammation)	Normal or some type II muscle fiber atrophy

CMAP, Compound muscle action potential; *SNAP*, sensory nerve action potential.
Reproduced with permission from Bertorini TE, ed *Clinical Evaluation and Diagnostic Tests for Neuromuscular Disorders.* Boston, MA, Butterworth-Heinemann; 2002:5.

the combination of the amplitude and duration and is more accurate in the assessment of conduction block.

Motor nerve conduction velocity is calculated by subtracting the latency from two stimulating points (see Fig. 2-13C). For example, if the CMAP is obtained when the median nerve is stimulated at the wrist (*distal stimulation*) and recorded at the thenar eminence, and is also stimulated at the elbow (*proximal stimulation*) using the same recording site, then the distance between the two stimulating points (elbow to wrist) is measured, and the velocity is calculated by dividing the distance by the latency difference. Stimulation of more proximal segments helps to determine focal slowing, such as in ulnar nerve entrapment at the elbow.

Causes of error in motor and sensory nerve conduction tests include measurements at low body temperature which slows conduction velocity. Inappropriate stimulation sites and improper positioning of electrodes can also cause erroneous results. Age and body size play a role in conduction velocity because very old, very young, and very tall individuals have slower conduction velocities.[38,39]

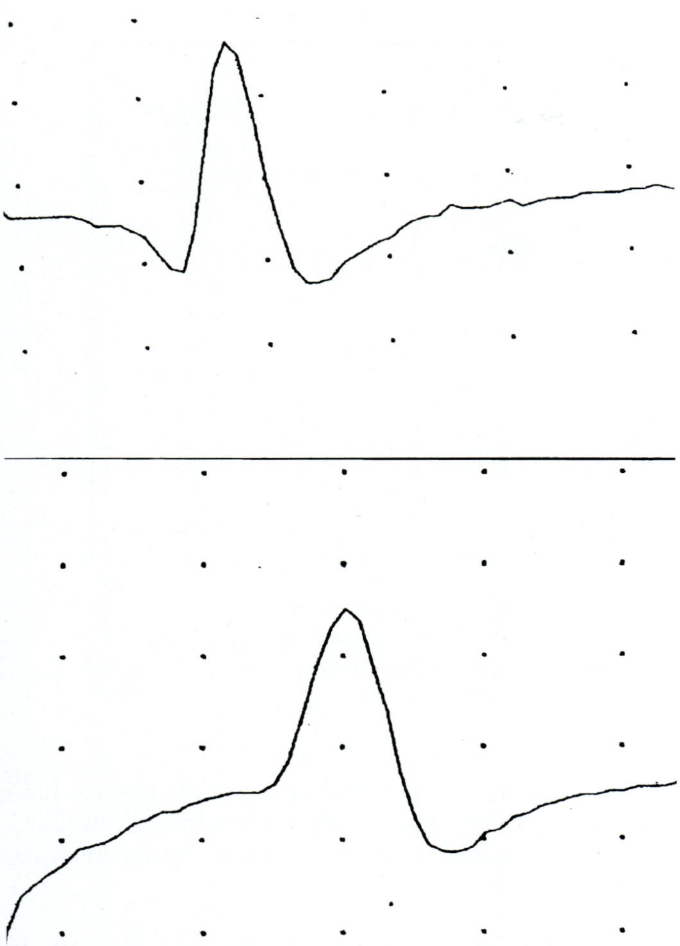

FIG 2-10 Sensory nerve action potentials obtained with orthodromic stimulation (*top*) and antidromic stimulation (*bottom*) (20 mV/2 ms).

Demyelination causes slowing of conduction velocity, usually below 80% of normal or lower. Nonuniform nerve conduction slowing is usually seen in acquired neuropathies, whereas uniform slowing occurs in most hereditary demyelinating neuropathies. Acquired demyelinating neuropathies can also cause conduction block and temporal dispersion, with prolongation of the CMAP from the variability of conduction of the various fibers. Demyelination also causes prolongation of the distal latencies (see Fig. 2-13D), F-wave, and H-reflexes, which could be absent. Several criteria of slowing and conduction block are used in research to diagnose demyelination, as discussed in individual cases of this book.

The *terminal latency index* (*TLI*) is the ratio of the *calculated* over the *measured* latency; it is used to demonstrate prominent demyelination in distal segments, relative to proximal segments,

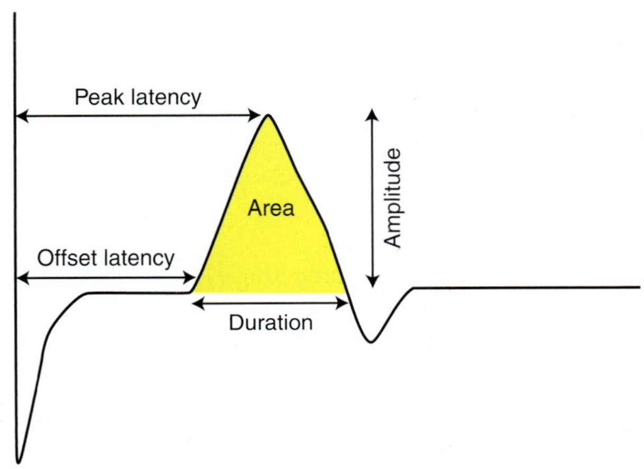

FIG 2-11 The elements of the sensory nerve action potential.

TABLE 2-3 Clinical and Laboratory Descriptions of Segmental Neurologic Disorders

	Mononeuropathy	Plexopathy	Radiculopathy
Muscle weakness and reflexes	Weakness, decreased reflexes in muscles innervated by single nerves	Weakness or reflexes in muscles innervated by roots from affected plexus but by different nerves	Weakness in muscles innervated by the same root but different nerves
Sensory deficit	Follows a single nerve territory	Follows a plexus sensory territory	Follows territory of the involved roots
Limb needle electromyography	Signs of denervation following the territory of one nerve	Signs of denervation in multiple nerves involved in affected plexus area (e.g., lower trunk = hand muscles of ulnar, median nerves)	Signs of denervation in muscles innervated by the same roots or by different nerves
Paraspinal needle electromyography	No paraspinal muscle denervation	No paraspinal muscle denervation	Paraspinal muscle denervation is common
Motor nerve	Slow in affected nerve; CMAP amplitude could be decreased when stimulating the affected nerve; conduction block could be seen	Normal (CMAP amplitude could be decreased when stimulating nerves whose axons travel through the affected plexus), slowing across Erb's point	Normal (CMAP amplitude could be decreased when stimulating nerves whose axons originate in affected roots)
Sensory-evoked responses	Low amplitude and/or prolonged latency SNAP	Low-amplitude SNAP in nerves whose axons travel through the affected plexus area	Normal SNAPs
Proximal responses (F-waves, H-reflexes)	Could be slow or absent in affected nerves	Could be slow or absent in nerves from affected plexus area	Could be slow or absent in nerves from affected root

CMAP, Compound muscle action potential; *SNAP*, sensory nerve action potential.

Reprinted with permission from Bertorini TE, ed. *Clinical Evaluation and Diagnostic Tests for Neuromuscular Disorders.* Boston, MA, Butterworth-Heinemann; 2002:7.

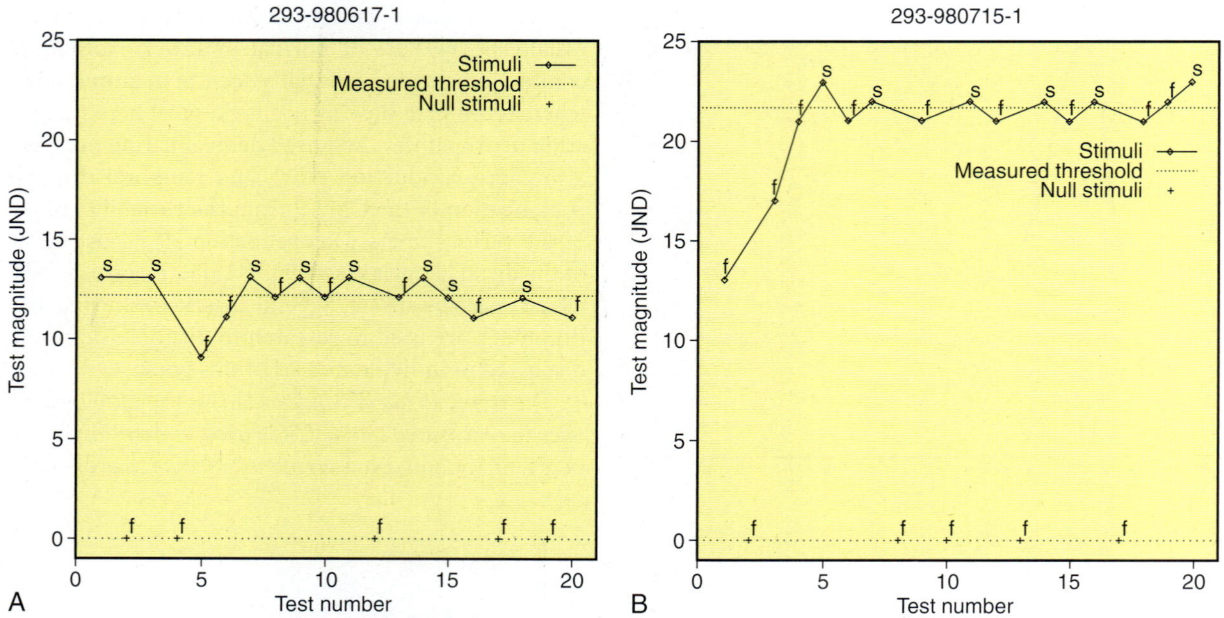

FIG 2-12 **A**, Vibration detection threshold of a normal patient (10th percentile; threshold, 12.4). **B**, Vibration detection threshold on a patient with peripheral neuropathy (98th percentile). Notice the higher detection threshold. (Units represent incremental and decremental steps using the CASE IV system.)

in patients with peripheral neuropathies. A low index indicates disproportionally distal demyelination. This is particularly useful in distinguishing CTS in patients with neuropathies.

The TLI is calculated by determining first the *calculated distal latency*, which is the latency that corresponds to the recorded proximal conduction velocity; this is obtained by dividing the value of the *measured distal distance* by the *proximal conduction velocity*. For example, if the distal distance is 8 cm and the proximal conduction velocity is 50 m/s, *the calculated latency* will be 1.6 ms (8 cm divided by 50 ms). The TLI is then obtained by dividing the value of the *calculated latency* by the *measured latency*. In this example, if the measured latency was 4 ms, the latency index would be 0.4 (1.6/4).[36]

In axonal neuropathies, the CMAP could be of low amplitude, with normal or only mildly decreased velocities, and have normal or mildly decreased latencies. Focal nerve lesions, such as *neurapraxia* (first-degree lesions of Sunderland classification),[36] are caused by edema and focal demyelination, showing conduction block from stimulation above to the lesion. Its recovery time can vary from hours to a few months.

Axonotmesis describes a lesion of the axon causing its degeneration but maintaining the integrity of the connective tissue. This can be subdivided into three types: (1) when the axon is discontinued but the endoneurium is intact (second degree of Sunderland); (2) when the axon and endoneurium are discontinued, but the perineurium and epineurium are preserved (third degree of Sunderland); and (3) when the epineurium remains intact (fourth degree of Sunderland). A lesion affecting the axon and its connective tissue, when the nerve is completely severed, is called *neurotmesis* (fifth degree of Sunderland).[41]

In axonotmesis and neurotmesis the CMAP obtained from stimulation below the lesion remains normal until enough time has elapsed to produce a complete axonal degeneration, but no CMAP is obtained upon proximal stimulation. These findings are accompanied by signs of denervation on EMG, and no elicitable motor units in muscles that are innervated by the affected nerve.

The H-Reflex. This is a late reflex, named after Johann Hoffmann who first described the wave.[42] The H-reflex is obtained by stimulating mixed nerves inframaximally in order to stimulate only sensory axons that have a lower threshold of activation. This stimulus produces a reflex, as the impulse travels orthodromically through the sensory axons, stimulating the posterior root ganglia and then the anterior horns, which depolarizes and produces an electrical impulse. This wave travels orthodromically through its motor axon, producing the late response in muscle (Fig. 2-14). The H-reflex is a monosynaptic reflex, which disappears with the sectioning of the posterior roots in animals.[42]

The stimulus duration used to test the H-reflex should be 0.5–1 ms, as this preferentially stimulates the 1 alpha fibers. During H-reflex tests, either no direct CMAP (or M-wave) is seen or it is very small (as some motor axons might also be stimulated), but the reflex should always be of higher amplitude than the M-wave and have a persistent latency and voltage during sequential stimulation in the same site and in using the same intensity. The H-reflex is usually studied by stimulating the tibial nerve at the knee while recording at the soleus muscle. This has a latency of about 30–35 ms. The reflex can be obtained by stimulating different nerves in young children. In adults this can be studied in the femoral[43] and radial nerves.[44] The tibial H-reflex is useful in diagnosing S1 radiculopathy, in which the reflex could be slow or absent[45] and could also be slow or absent in sciatic, proximal tibial neuropathies, and lumbosacral plexopathies. This is usually, but not always, absent when the

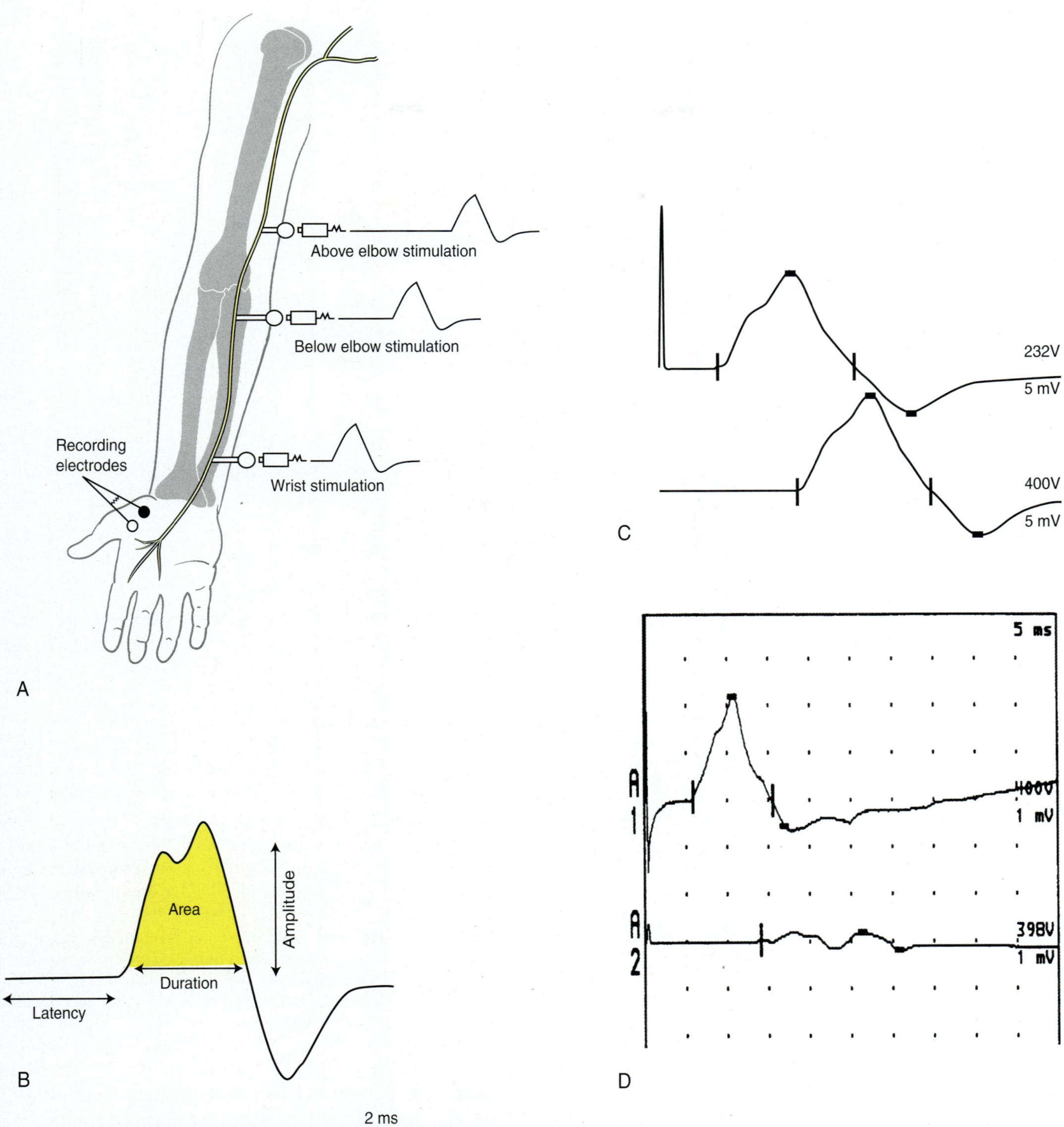

FIG 2-13 **A**, Motor nerve conduction velocity test of the median nerve showing the different compound muscle action potentials (CMAPs) obtained at various stimulation sites. **B**, The elements of the CMAP. **C**, Normal CMAPs of the ulnar nerve stimulating at the wrist (*top*) and at the elbow (*bottom*) (5 mV/2 ms). **D**, Median nerve stimulation at the wrist (*top*) and elbow (*bottom*) on a patient with a demyelinating polyneuropathy. Notice temporal dispersion and partial conduction block (1 mV/5 ms).

ankle reflex disappears. Absent H-reflexes are the earliest findings in GBS.

The F-Response. This is a late response whose name comes from *foot* where it was initially recorded. The wave is obtained by *supramaximal* stimulation of a motor nerve. This stimulus travels orthodromically producing an early CMAP and also travels antidromically toward the spinal cord stimulating motor neurons. Upon depolarization, these neurons send an electrical impulse that travels orthodromically back to the muscle, producing a late motor action potential (Figs. 2-15 and 2-16). Each F-wave represents a stimulated individual motor unit.

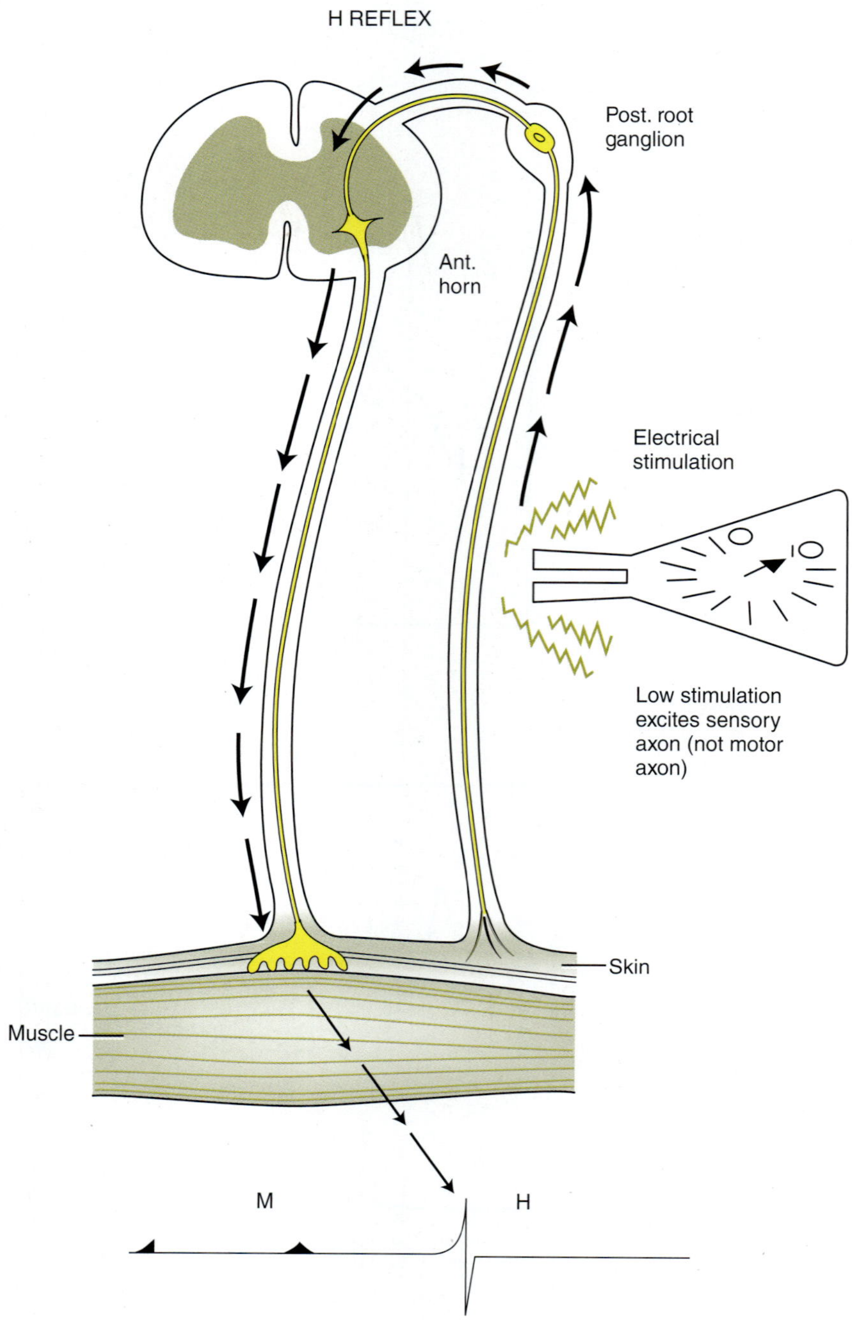

FIG 2-14 Diagram of the H-reflex pathway. Notice that a low-intensity stimulus excites the sensory axon that produces the late H-reflex; notice that there is no M-wave (CMAP) obtained. *CMAP*, Compound muscle action potentials.

They vary in shape and latency, but not all stimulations produce an F-wave (Fig. 2-17).

Supramaximal stimuli also depolarize the sensory axons, but this orthodromic response collides with the motor response.

The F-wave normally has a latency of about 28–30 ms recorded in the hand; in the foot, the latency is 40–55 ms.[46] The individual F-waves are obtained with each stimulation, vary in latency, and are much smaller than the M-wave. Their latency represents the motor conductions of individual motor unit axons.

Conventionally, the shortest latency obtained from several stimulations is measured. Some electromyographers use F-latencies to calculate their conduction velocities.[47,48] The latency could be prolonged in peripheral neuropathies and focally in radiculopathies and plexopathies. They tend to disappear or be prolonged in demyelinating neuropathies.[49] Normally, about 50% of the waves are obtained from various direct motor stimuli, and the number of F-waves (F-wave persistency) is usually diminished in demyelinating neuropathies (Figs. 2-17 and 2-18).

Increased variations of F-wave latencies are seen in demyelinating neuropathies (*chronodispersion*) from variations of conductions of individual axons. The variation in conduction velocities is called *tachydispersion*.[46]

The Axonal Wave. The axonal (A) wave is a response observed sometimes during F-wave studies, and its latency is usually shorter than that of the F-waves (Fig. 2-19), although occasionally they appear late. A-waves persist during most or all sequential

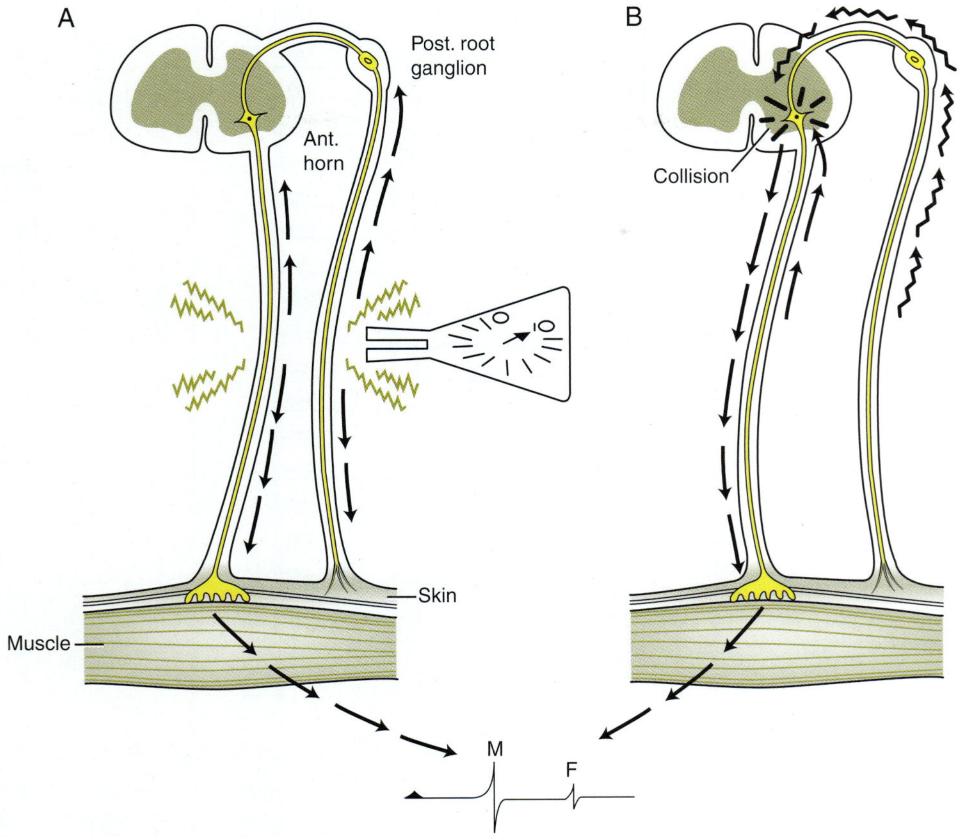

FIG 2-15 Diagram of the F-response. **A**, A supramaximal stimulus produces a direct M-response. **B**, As the stimulus also travels toward the anterior horn cell this is depolarized and its action potential produces a late F-response.

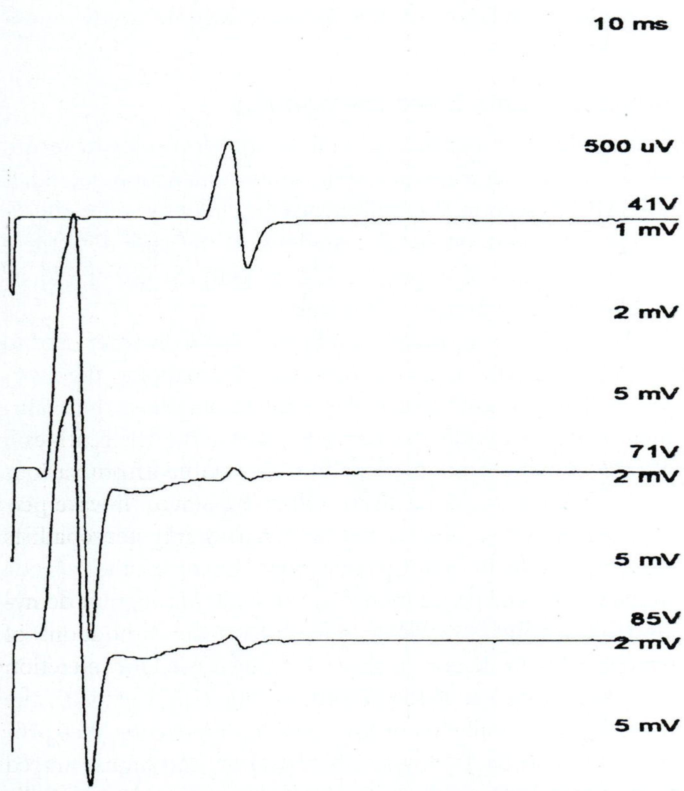

FIG 2-16 A low submaximal stimulation produces a late H-reflex without a direct CMAP (*top*). The bottom two tracings show a normal early CMAP and a late F-wave obtained upon increasing the stimulus strength (*top*, 1 mV/10 ms; *bottom*, 2 mV/10 ms). *CMAP*, Compound muscle action potentials.

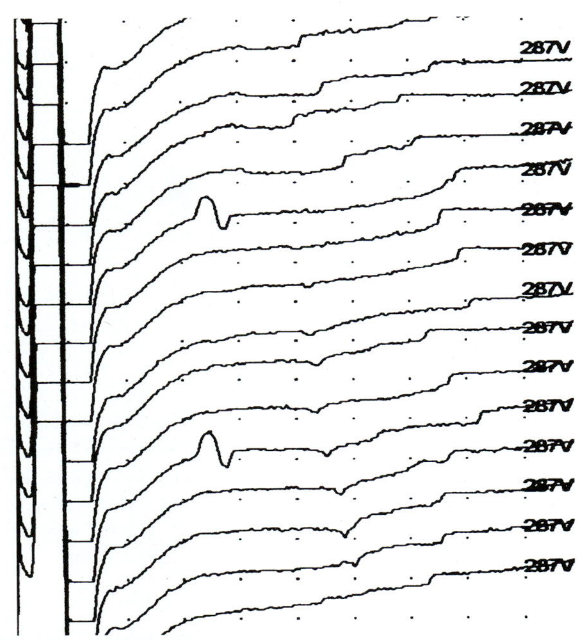

FIG 2-17 A case of demyelinating neuropathy showing a decreased number of F-waves obtained with a series of 20 stimulations of the ulnar nerve and recording in the abductor digiti minimi (ADM) muscle. Only two F-waves were obtained; because they are identical, it is likely that they represent the same motor unit (200 μV/10 ms).

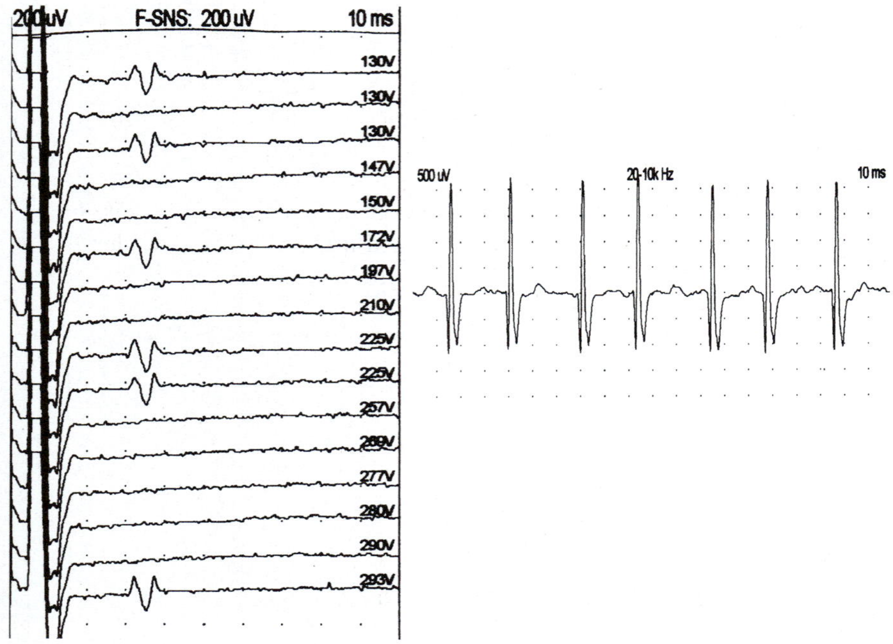

FIG 2-18 Median nerve study of F-waves, stimulating at the wrist and recording at the abductor pollicis brevis muscle in a patient with GBS. Notice several late responses of normal F-latencies; they appear identical and could represent A-waves or repeater F-waves of the same motor unit. No late responses were seen in other tracings (200 μV/10 ms) (*left*). Right, A needle EMG study on the same muscle shows a fast-firing motor unit without recruiting a second motor unit (500 μV/10 ms). *GBS*, Guillain–Barré syndrome.

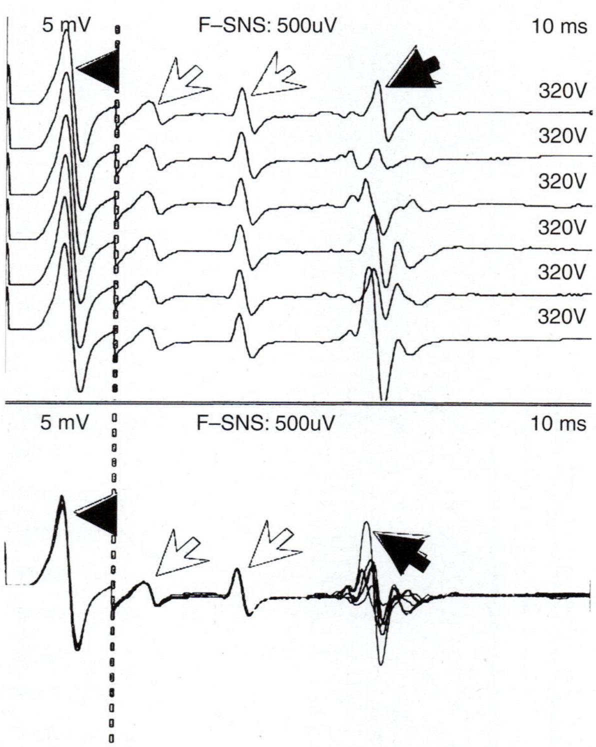

FIG 2-19 Stimulation of the ulnar nerve recording at the abductor digiti minimi (ADM) muscle in a patient with mixed axonal and demyelinating neuropathy. The response is recorded with a roster mode (*top*) and a superimposed mode (*bottom*); notice the direct M-response (*arrowheads*). There are two axonal waves (*white arrows*) and F-waves, some large (*black arrows*) (*left*, 5 mV/10 ms; *right*, 500 μV/10 ms).

stimulations and are of identical shape and latency. The waves are believed to be caused by ephaptic or ectopic discharges of demyelinating axons but may also be caused by axonal sprouting in which the antidromic stimuli activate the regenerating axon.[38,39]

Other Nerve Conduction Tests Used in Neuromuscular Disorders. *Somatosensory-evoked responses* and motor responses obtained during *magnetic stimulation* allow the study of sensory and motor pathways, not only of the brain and spinal cord but also of peripheral nerves; these are used in the diagnosis of proximal nerve, plexus, or root damage. Proximal nerve segments can also be studied by direct root stimulation. Magnetic stimulation of the brain is used to study motor pathways.[50]

Routine Needle Electromyography

Routine EMG is performed with needle electrodes to record the electrical characteristics of the motor unit action potentials (MUAPs) as seen in the oscilloscope and to observe for abnormal spontaneous potentials. Analysis of the sound of these potentials is also of value; this is done with the use of a loudspeaker attached to the oscilloscope.

EMG helps in the diagnosis of generalized disorders and to localize segmental diseases. For example, mapping the myotomal distribution of denervation potentials allows the examiner to localize the affected root and assist in the differentiation of radiculopathy from plexopathies or mononeuropathies.

Recordings are done using either bipolar or monopolar needle electrodes. Bipolar needle electrodes have the anode and the cathode in their tip concentric electrodes, the cathode in the center, and the reference in the shaft. Monopolar needle electrodes, which are Teflon coated, have the cathode in the uncovered tip; a distant surface electrode is used for reference. The characteristics of the recorded potentials vary with the needle. For example, recording with monopolar needles produces more artifacts, a less stable baseline, and higher amplitude motor units with an increased number of polyphasic MUAPs, compared with recordings obtained with concentric electrodes.

During routine EMG, the following are analyzed.

Insertional Activity. The insertion of the needle electrode in the muscle causes a mechanical stimulation that produces discharges that are called *insertional activity* (*IA*). This burst of electrical potentials indicates that the needle is indeed in the muscle. The IA has increased the duration in denervated and necrotic muscles and myotonias. It is decreased if the muscle is replaced by connective tissue or fat. The IA is also decreased during attacks of periodic paralysis or contractures in McArdle's disease, from decreased excitability of the muscle membrane.[51]

After analysis of the IA, the muscle is examined at rest, and, normally, there should be no electrical activity, unless the needle is placed next to the endplate, where there are variations of the baseline or *endplate noise*. Endplate noise is caused by extracellular recordings of miniature endplate potentials (EPPs). *Endplate spike potentials* can also be observed; these are of negative onset biphasic waves which are repetitive and of continuous discharges of individual muscle fibers firing irregularly (5–50 Hz with amplitudes of 100–200 μV) (Fig. 2-20).

Abnormal Spontaneous Potentials. *Fasciculations* are spontaneous depolarizations of *individual motor units* (Fig. 2-21). They usually produce visible movements of the electrode. Fasciculations can occur in healthy people, but when accompanied by muscle atrophy and weakness, they usually indicate a disorder of the motor neuron. Fasciculations, however, can also occur in radiculopathies, in some neuropathies, in some metabolic disorders, and in anticholinesterase overmedication.[52,53]

Differentiation of normal fasciculations from those of neuromuscular disorders is difficult, but in neurogenic disorders, which cause large and polyphasic voluntarily elicited MUAPs, the fasciculations might also show these characteristics. The firing rate is faster in normals than in those with neurogenic disorders, but this is difficult to assess and not reliable in diagnosis.

Myokymic discharges are the spontaneous firing of motor units which usually contain 2–10 spikes discharging at 30–40 Hz in each burst. They occur at regular intervals and have the characteristic sound of "marching soldiers" (Fig. 2-22). Myokymic discharges can be seen in radiculopathies and in plexopathies, particularly those caused by radiation. These are also seen in GBS and in the facial muscles of multiple sclerosis and brainstem gliomas.[54,55]

Fibrillations are spontaneous biphasic potentials of about 1–5 ms duration and of 20–500 μV amplitude (Figs. 2-23 and 2-25). They usually have an initial negative phase, except when the

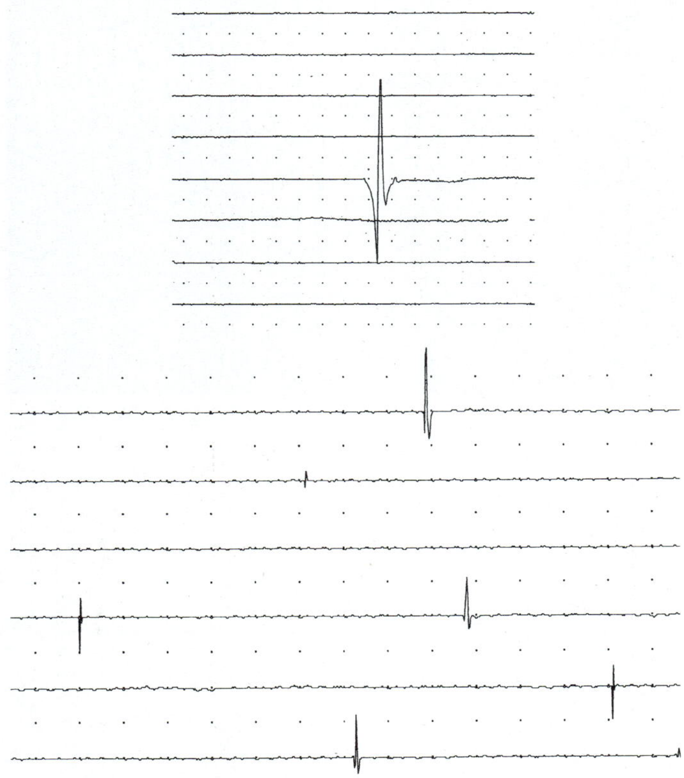

FIG 2-21 A single fasciculation potential recorded (*top*) (200 μV/10 ms); several fasciculations recorded in several tracings using a roster mode (*bottom*) (500 μV/50 ms).

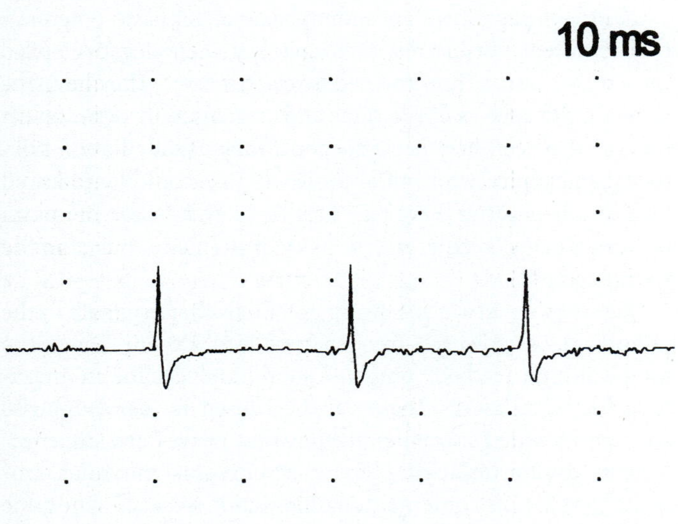

FIG 2-20 Endplate spikes at 100 μV/10 ms.

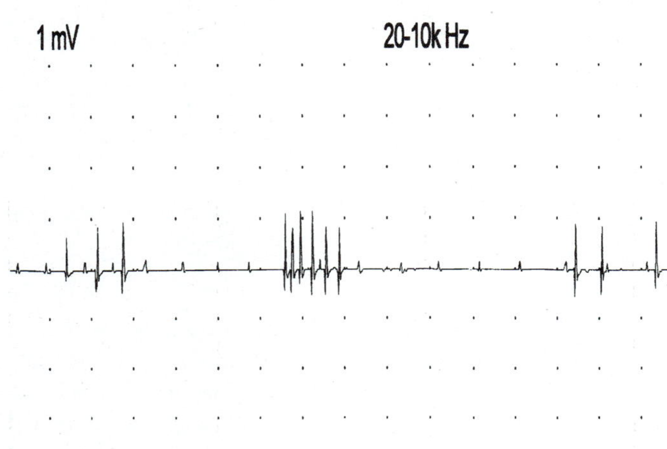

FIG 2-22 Myokymic discharges in the deltoid muscle in a patient with a plexopathy (1 mV/20 ms).

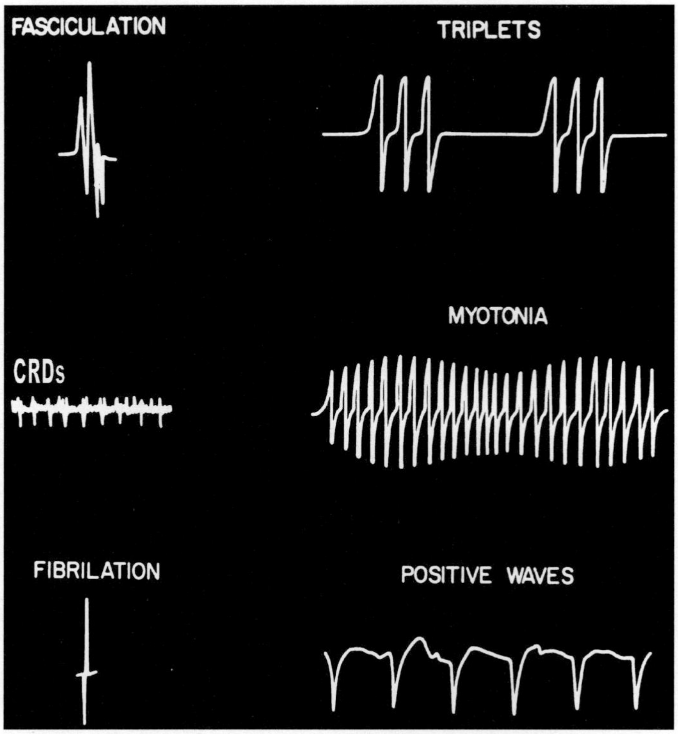

FIG 2-23 Various abnormal spontaneous muscle action potentials.

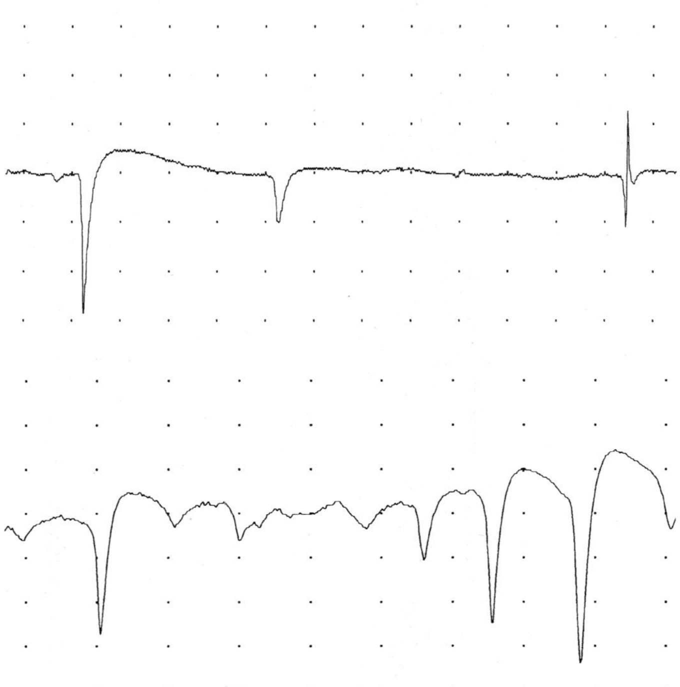

FIG 2-24 Two positive sharp waves and one fibrillation potential (*top*); several positive sharp waves (*bottom*) (200 μV/10 ms).

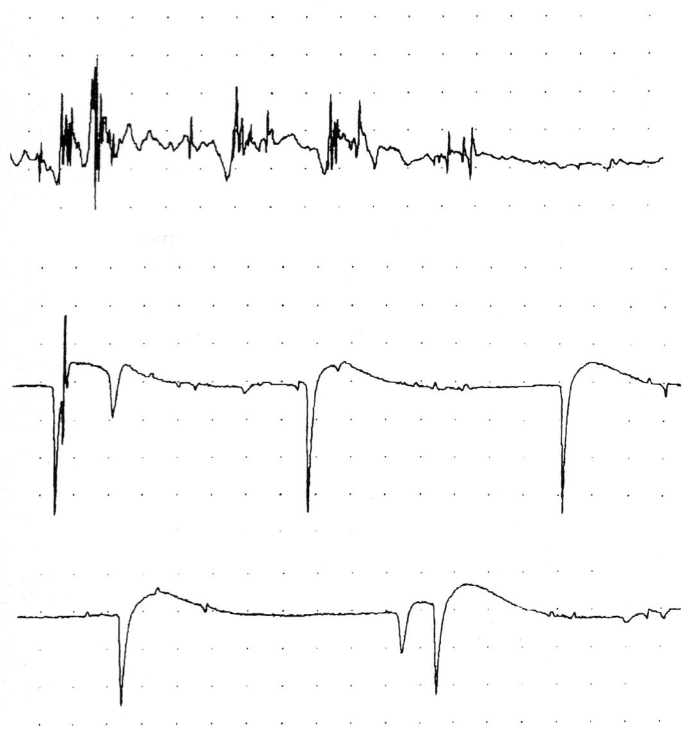

FIG 2-25 Electromyography (EMG) study of the deltoid muscle in a patient with polymyositis. Notice small polyphasic motor units (*top*) and two tracings showing positive sharp waves (100 μV/10 ms).

needle is close to the endplate, in which case they can have a positive onset and may be difficult to differentiate from endplate spikes.[56] Fibrillations are spontaneous depolarizations of individual muscle fiber; these depolarizations are caused by increased sensitivity to acetylcholine (ACh) from diffuse extrajunctional ACh receptors in denervated or necrotic muscle fibers.

Fibrillations usually appear 2 weeks after a nerve injury, but their onset depends on the distance from the site of the injury to the studied muscles. Thus, they appear earlier in more proximal muscles, where they also disappear earlier during recovery. They are smaller in more chronic disorders.

These potentials are characteristically seen in neurogenic disorders but also occur in necrotizing myopathies, particularly polymyositis (Fig. 2-25) and muscular dystrophies. The presence of fibrillations in different muscle groups helps the electromyographer to localize segmental diseases (see Table 2-3).

Positive sharp waves are monophasic or biphasic potentials that represent fibrillations that have lost their negative spike, caused by trauma from the needle electrode.[57,58] They have the same significance as fibrillations and are caused by denervation but are also seen in other disorders. They usually have a saw-tooth appearance with initial positivity that could be followed by a slower negative wave (see Figs. 2-24 and 2-25). These can be seen during needle insertions or movements but also fire spontaneously.

Neuromyotonia are fast-firing potentials that originate in the peripheral nerve with a frequency of 100–300 Hz. They have a typical high-pitched "pinging" sound and decline in amplitude very quickly.[55,56] These can be caused by nerve injuries and are recorded intraoperatively when nerves are stretched. Neuromyotonic discharges can be seen in spinal muscular atrophies (SMAs), in some neuropathies, and in Isaacs syndrome accompanied by other spontaneous discharges.[55]

Complex repetitive discharges (*CRDs*) are discharges that have an abrupt onset and disappearance and do not fluctuate in amplitude, remaining unchanged (Fig. 2-26). These complex and polyphasic waves are formed by several individual fiber potentials. The group fires at 50–100 ms and has amplitudes of 50 μV–1 mV. CRDs are caused by ephaptic transmission of individual muscle fibers that fire nearly synchronously. They are seen in neurogenic diseases but also in myopathies, such as polymyositis, acid maltase deficiency, some muscular dystrophies, and Schwartz–Jampel syndrome.[50,55]

Myotonic discharges are potentials of amplitude from 10 μV to 1 mV and vary in duration and amplitude, waxing, and waning; they do not disappear abruptly (Fig. 2-27). They are characteristically seen in myotonic disorders but also occur in other channelopathies, such as hyperkalemic periodic paralysis, polymyositis, and acid maltase deficiency. Myotonia is caused by abnormalities of the muscle chloride or the sodium channels, which increase membrane excitability.[51]

Cramps are sustained involuntary contractions of nerve origin that are not electrically silent, unlike the muscle contractures seen in metabolic myopathies. The cramp potentials consist of repetitive discharges of normal-appearing motor units, which fire very rapidly at 200–300 Hz.[51,52]

Motor Unit Action Potentials. MUAPs are produced by the summation of electrical potentials of individual muscle fibers innervated by the same motor neuron and are activated by voluntary muscle contractions. The recorded MUAP represents potentials of about 8–10 fibers that are close to the needle electrode[55,58] (Fig. 2-28).

Normally, the motor units discharge at an initial rate of about 4 Hz, and this rate increases as the intensity of contractions increases (Fig. 2-29). Smaller units are recruited first, and, according to experimental studies, they belong to type I motor neurons. With the force of increasing contractions, more motor units are recruited until they fill the oscilloscope. This is called the *interference pattern* (*IP*).

The characteristics of MUAP can be analyzed qualitatively or quantitatively with signal delays, triggers, and averaging, or by the use of automatic methods.

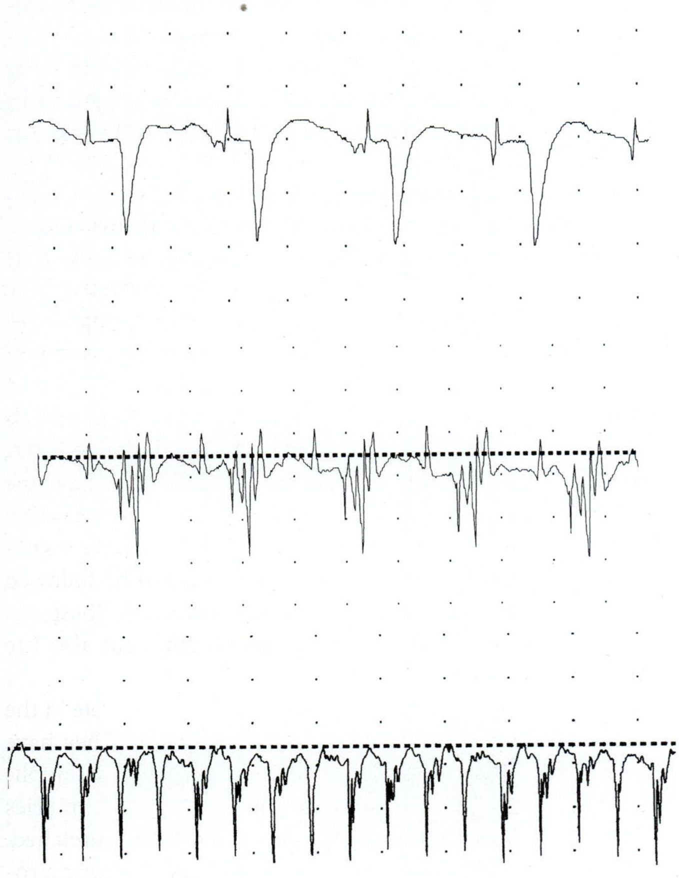

FIG 2-26 Three different complex repetitive discharges (CRDs). Notice the complex but uniform waveforms that do not change in shape: (*top*, 200 μV/10 ms), (*middle*, 100 μV/20 ms), and (*bottom*, 100 μV/50 ms).

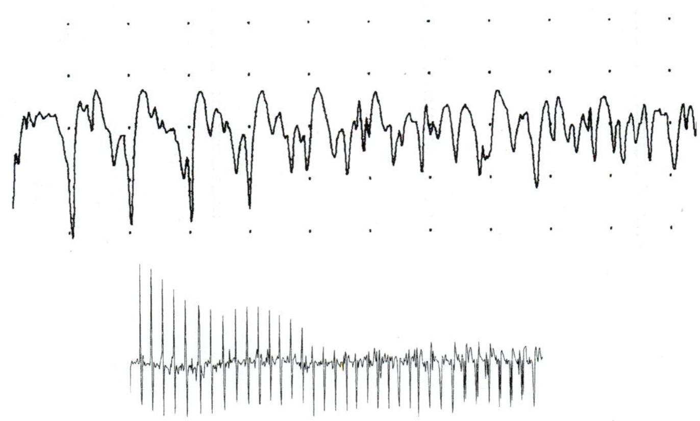

FIG 2-27 Myotonic discharges waxing and waning in amplitude: (*top*, 100 μV/10 ms) and (*bottom*, 200 μV/20 ms).

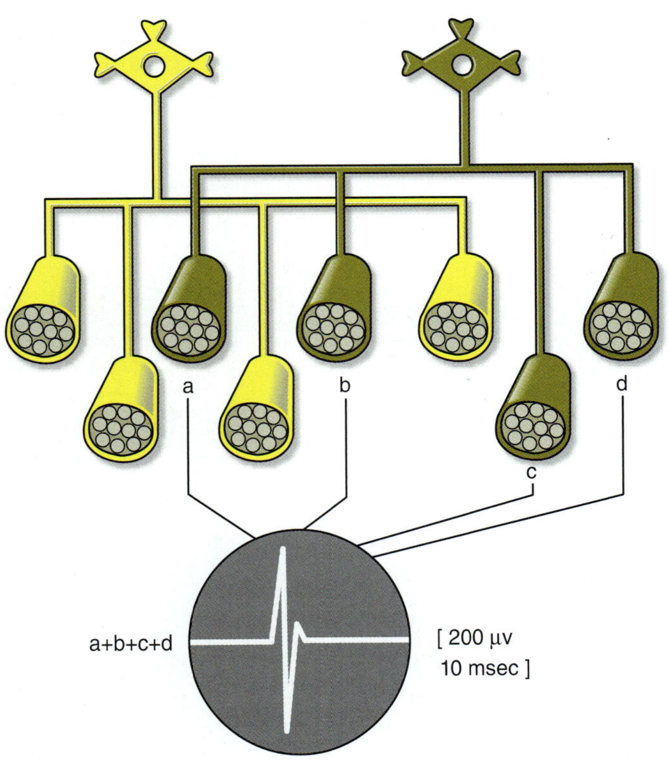

FIG 2-28 The origin of the motor unit action potential. This is formed from summation of individual potentials of muscle fibers (a to d) innervated by the same motor neuron.

Analysis of MUAPs includes the determination of their *duration* from onset to end or from departing to returning to the baseline. The phases represent spikes that cross the baseline. *Turns* are changes in the direction of spikes within the MUAP that have more than 50 µV in amplitude and do not cross the baseline (Fig. 2-30).

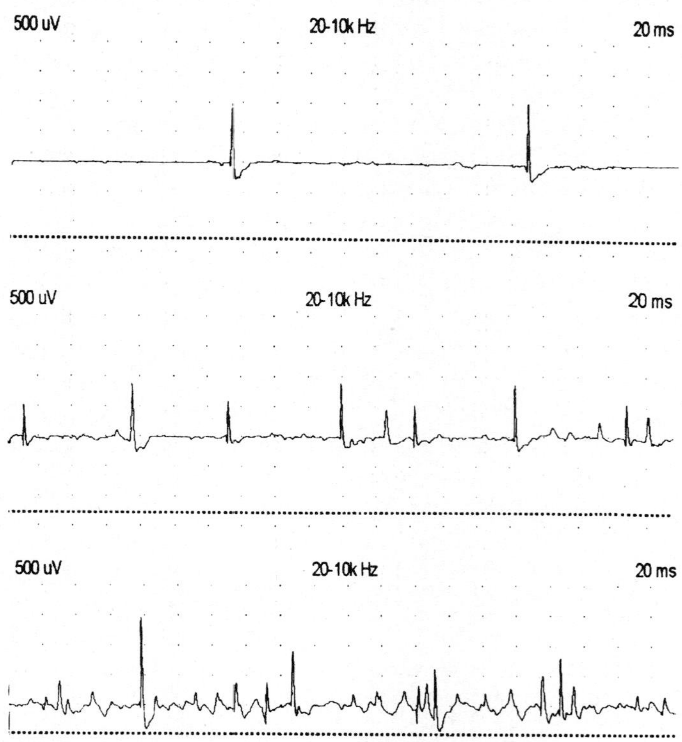

FIG 2-29 Notice an increased recruitment of MUAPs with increasing contractions: motor units firing at a rate of about 5 Hz (*top*); more MUAPs recruited (3) as the firing rate increases to 7–8 Hz (*middle*); several motor units recruited upon increased contraction force (*bottom*) (500 µV/20 ms). *MUAPs,* Motor unit action potentials.

The MUAP *amplitude* is determined by the size and number of muscle fibers within 0.5 mm of the recording electrode, and the *area* is produced by fibers within 2 mm of the recording electrode.[59]

The phases are caused by temporal dispersion of potentials of individual muscle fibers contributing to the MUAP. The number of phases is usually two to three but may sometimes be four; in normal, less than 15% of the recorded motor units should have five or more phases[51,60] (Fig. 2-31).

Individual muscle fiber potentials that appear later and separate from the main MUAP are called *late potentials* or *satellites*[61] (Figs. 2-31 and 2-32). These can be seen in neuropathies, motor diseases, and myopathies, from slow-conducting axons or muscle fibers.

An important characteristic of the MUAPs analyzed during EMG is the ability to recruit other motor units upon increasing the strength of muscle contraction. The recruitment of a second motor unit usually occurs when a MUAP is firing at less than 10 Hz, and more motor units are recruited at faster rates. The *recruitment rate* is the rate of firing of the motor unit when a second motor unit is recruited. The *recruitment ratio* is calculated by dividing the firing rate by the number of motor units seen in the oscilloscope. For example, if 3 motor units are firing at 15 Hz, then the recruitment ratio would be 5. Normally, the recruitment ratio is less than 5.

The IP is also examined during EMG testing and can be analyzed automatically.[62–64] This is usually reduced in neurogenic conditions, causing a dropout of motor neurons or their axons; thus, fewer motor units are recruited that discharge at a faster rate. The IP may be reduced with lack of effort and in upper motor neuron disorders, but in these, the MUAPs fire at slower rates.

MUAP stability represents lack of variability in amplitude and duration. Increased variability is caused by desynchronization of individual fiber potentials in disorders of

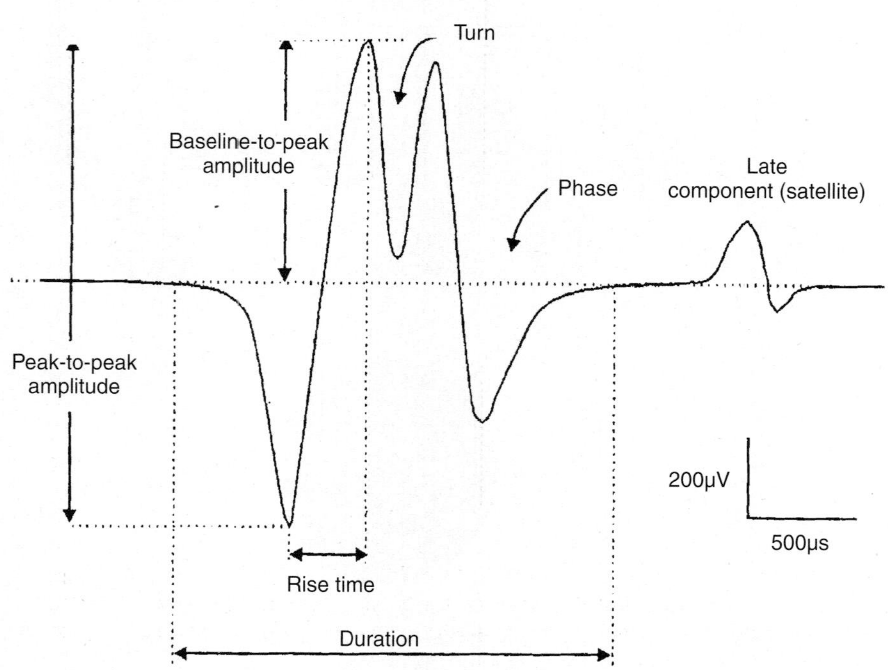

FIG 2-30 The elements of the motor unit action potential. (Reprinted with permission from Kimura J. Routine needle electromyography. In: Bertorini T, ed. *Clinical Evaluation and Diagnostic Tests for Neuromuscular Disorders*. Boston, MA, Butterworth-Heinemann; 2002.)

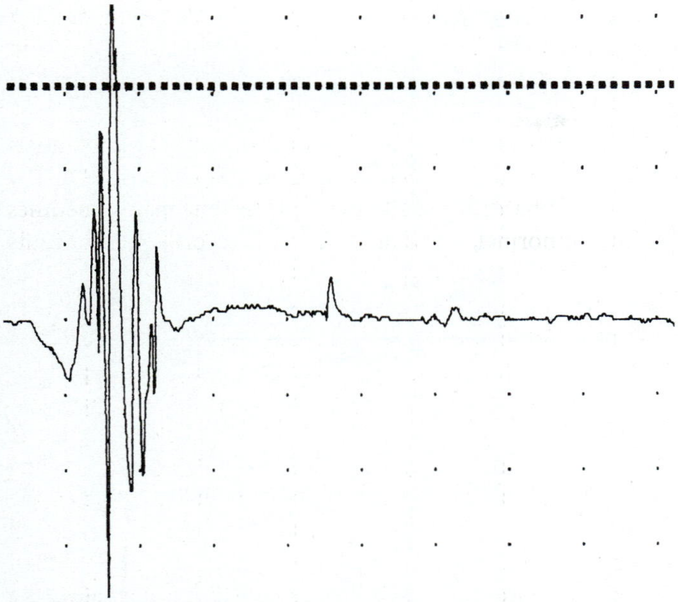

FIG 2-31 A single polyphasic motor unit action potential with a satellite (200 μV/10 ms).

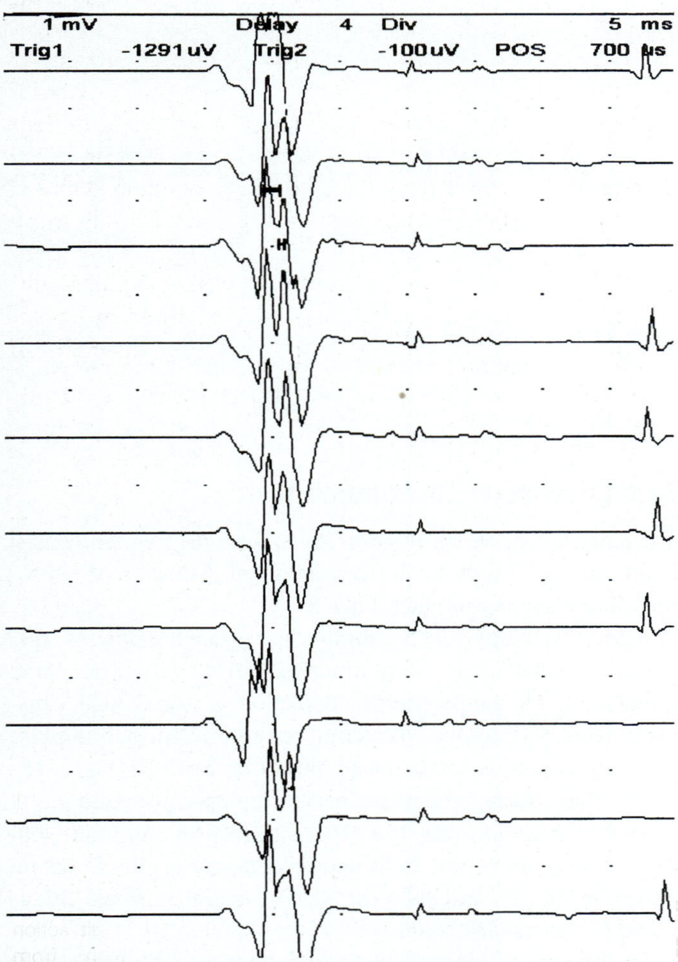

FIG 2-32 A motor unit action potential recorded in the quadriceps muscle from a patient with amyotrophic lateral sclerosis (ALS). Notice two satellite potentials, the second one showing intermittent blocking (1 mV/5 ms).

neuromuscular transmission. This also occurs in neurogenic disorders such as ALS.[55]

Normal MUAPs that discharge spontaneously and not during voluntary contractions are seen in stiff-person syndrome. These disappear with the use of nerve blocks, general anesthesia, and intravenous diazepam.

Characteristics of Motor Unit Action Potentials. In *myopathies*, MUAPs typically have short durations and low amplitudes. These smaller potentials are caused by a decreased number of functional muscle fibers that belong to a motor unit (Fig. 2-33) and that are closer to the electrode.

These MUAPs can be very polyphasic (Fig. 2-34) or serrated (increased number of turns) due to asynchronous firing of the individual potentials. In myopathies, there is rapid recruitment of motor units, and the IPs are usually full and show an increased number of turns with decreased amplitudes during an automatic analysis (Figs. 2-35 and 2-36). The conventional use of the term *myopathic motor units* is not accurate because small polyphasic motor units can also be seen in disorders of neuromuscular transmission and in some neuropathies without complete reinnervation,[65] causing the so-called *nascent* MUAPs that are small and polyphasic but show decreased recruitments (Fig. 2-37).

In *neurogenic disorders*, the MUAPs are larger because reinnervation produces an increased number of muscle fibers that belong to the same motor units close to the needle electrode (Fig. 2-38). The number and recruitment of MUAPs are usually

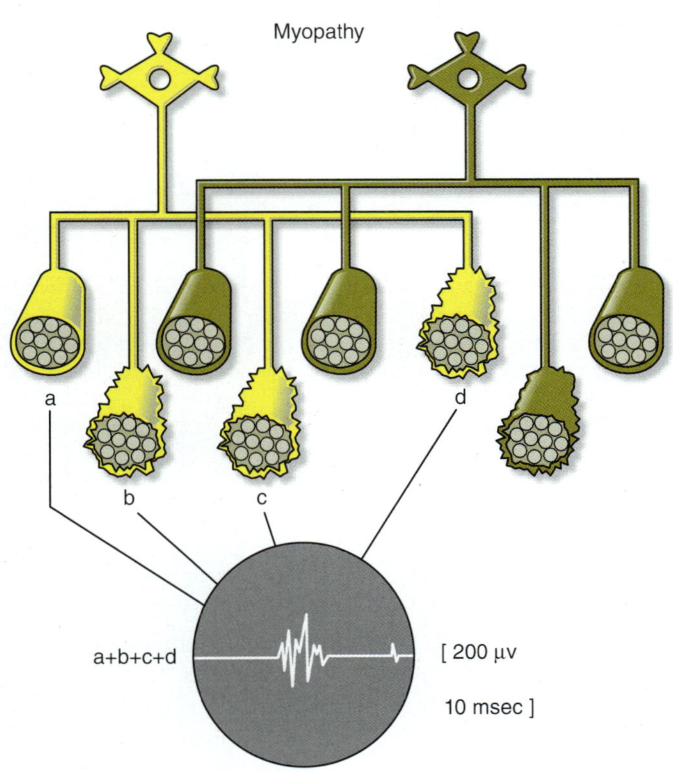

FIG 2-33 The origin of the motor unit action potential in myopathy. Notice that the motor neurons and axons are normal; individual muscle fiber action potentials are formed by damaged muscle fibers that fire asynchronously (a to d).

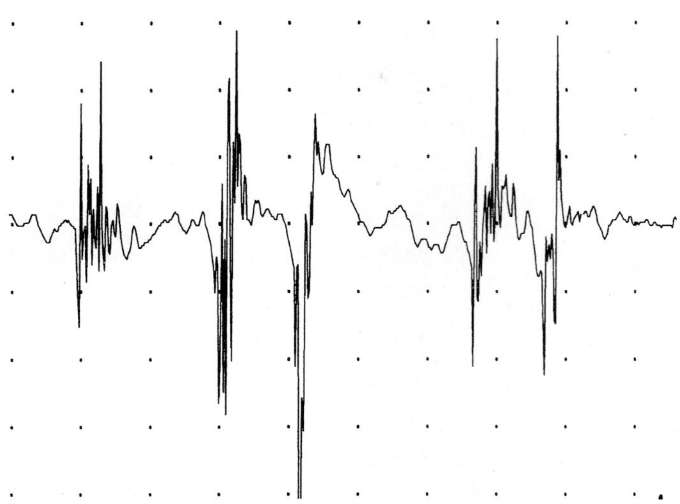

FIG 2-34 Several polyphasic motor units in a patient with inclusion body myositis (100 μV/10 ms).

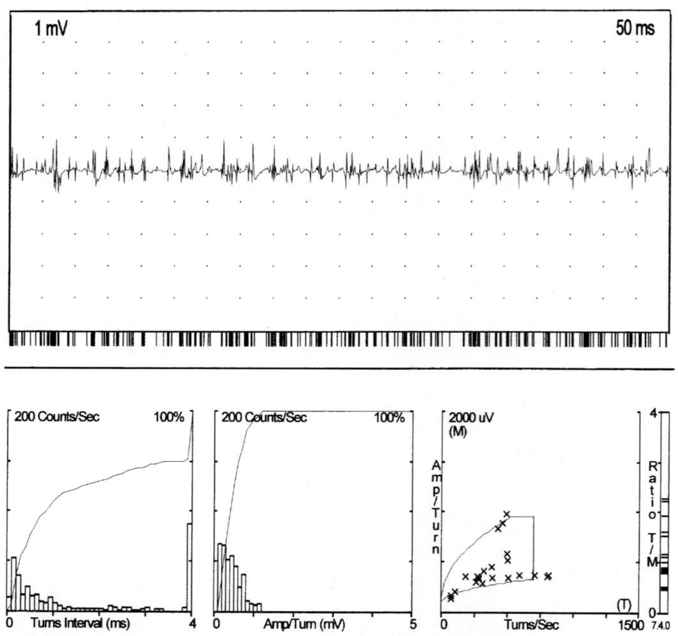

FIG 2-35 Electromyography (EMG) using automatic motor unit "cloud" analysis of the biceps muscle in a patient with polymyositis (the diagram "cloud" represents the normals). Notice amplitudes on the vertical axis and number of turns in the horizontal axis. Notice also that several potentials are smaller than normal (outside the "cloud") (*bottom right*).

decreased because of the reduced number of motor neurons and axons (Figs. 2-39–2-41). The MUAP can also be polyphasic from desynchronization of the individual potentials due to the variation in the conduction of individual axons.[50]

Other abnormal MUAPs are *multiplets*, or paired discharges (Figs. 2-42 and 2-43), which can be seen in some neurogenic conditions and in tetany. These could be *duplets* or *triplets* or *quadruplets*. Multiplets fire two or more times at very short intervals at a rate of about 2–20 Hz, and they maintain the same relationship with one another.[50]

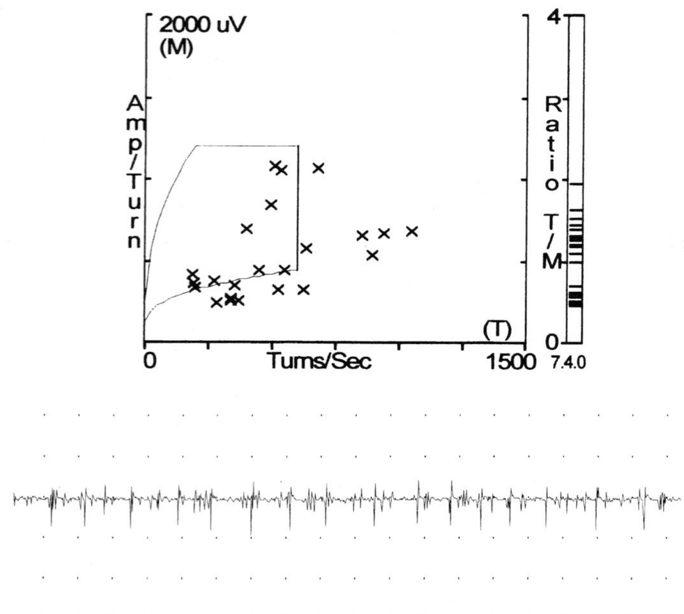

FIG 2-36 Quadriceps muscle "cloud" analysis in another patient with polymyositis. Notice deceased amplitude and also several recordings with increased number of turns (outside the normal "cloud").

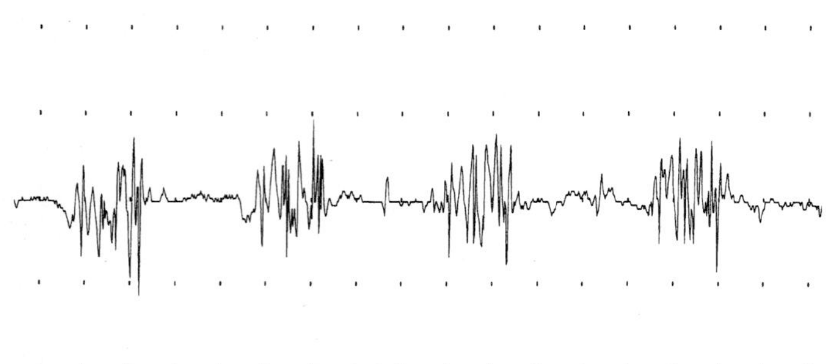

FIG 2-37 Nascent motor unit action potential in the deltoid muscle of a patient with radiculopathy and early reinnervation. These are firing at rates of 20 Hz without recruiting a second motor unit (100 μV/10 ms).

Repetitive Nerve Stimulation Test

The repetitive nerve stimulation test is the most frequently used diagnostic technique in the evaluation of disorders of neuromuscular transmission (see Table 2-2).

The physiology of neuromuscular transmission is discussed in Chapter 1. To summarize, during repetitive nerve impulses, there is a progressive depletion of stored ACh, causing a decreased number of quanta released from each impulse resulting in a reduction in the amplitude of the EPPs (Fig. 2-44). In normals, during repetitive nerve impulses, for example at 2–5 Hz stimulation rate, the EPPs diminish in amplitude, but they remain above the threshold to generate a muscle action potential (MAP), and thus the MAPs remain normal. This is called the *safety factor* (*SF*).[66,67]

In the clinical electrodiagnostic laboratory, the test is performed by stimulating a nerve supramaximally and recording the CMAP (the summation of the stimulated MAP of the studied muscle).

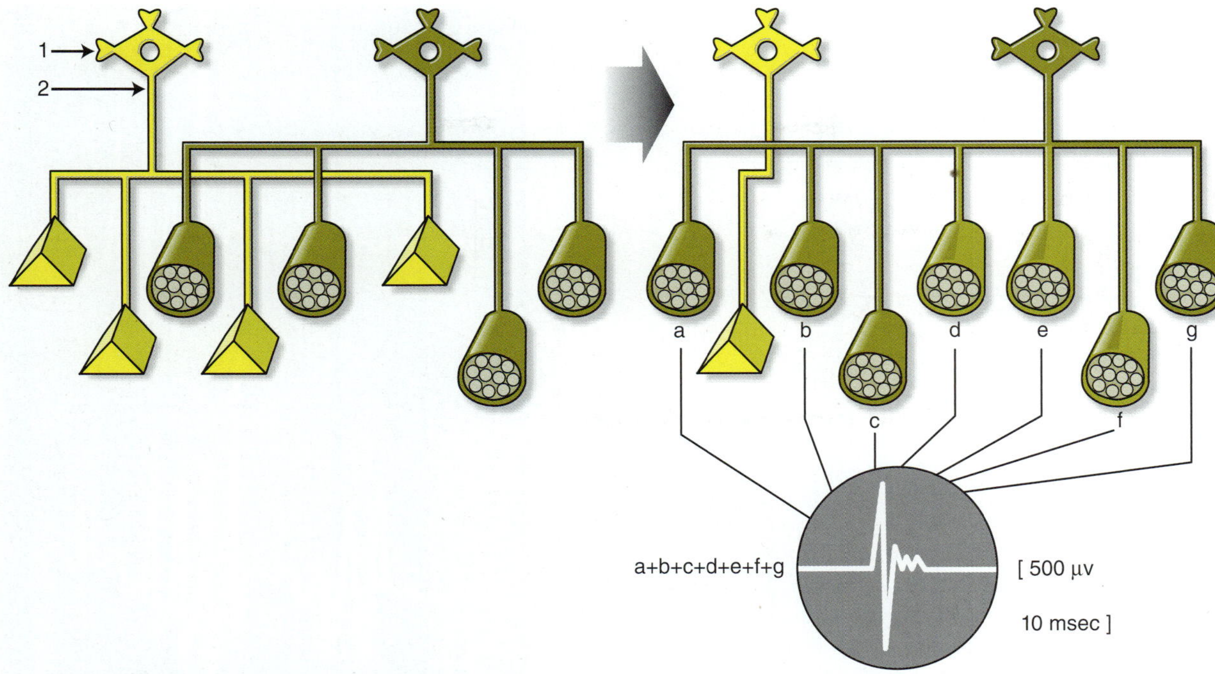

FIG 2-38 The origin of large motor unit action potentials (MUAPs) in neuropathy. Damaged axons on the motor neuron cause angular atrophic fibers (*left*). There is grouping from sprouting, with more muscle fibers belonging to the same motor unit (*right*). The motor unit action potential is produced by the summation of potentials from more muscle fibers (a to g) close to the needle electrode.

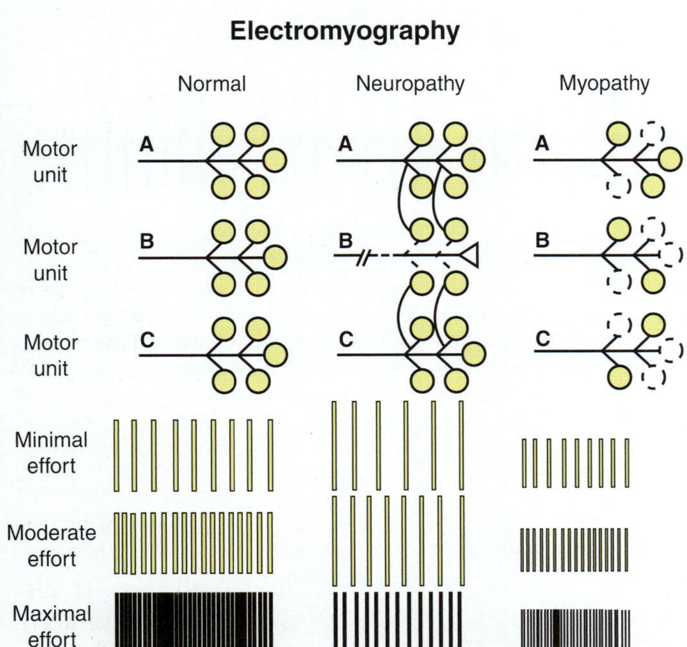

FIG 2-39 A diagram showing recruitment of MUAPs in a normal patient (*left*); a patient with neuropathy (*center*); and a patient with myopathy (*right*). In the normal patient there are few MUAPs recruited initially, these increase in number upon increasing effort. In neuropathy the MUAPs have increased amplitude but there is reduced recruitment. In myopathy the motor units are small, but the recruitment appears to be increased. *MUAPs*, Motor unit action potentials.

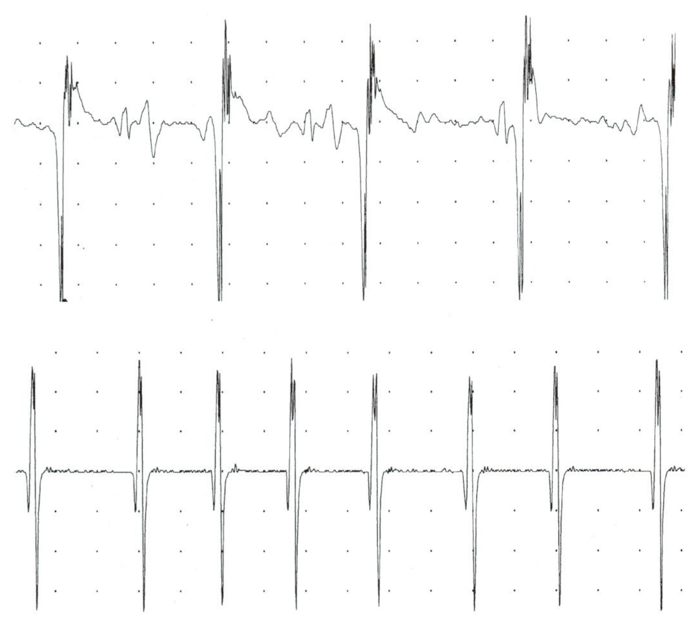

FIG 2-40 EMG in a patient with ALS: notice the MUAPs discharge at 25 Hz without recruiting a second motor unit (top) (500 μV/10 ms). EMG from a patient with previous poliomyelitis (bottom) shows very large MUAPs that fire at an increased rate of 20 Hz without recruiting a second motor unit (1 mV/20 ms). *ALS*, Amyotrophic lateral sclerosis; *EMG*, electromyography; *MUAPs*, motor unit action potentials.

In disorders of neuromuscular transmission, there is a reduction of the SF. At low rates of stimulation, the decrement of the EPP amplitudes makes them become lower than the SF (Fig. 2-45), causing a decreased number of individual MAPs obtained during consecutive stimulations, and in consequence a reduction of the CMAP.[66]

During fast stimulation rates, or after tetanic contractions, there is a significant calcium accumulation of the nerve terminal

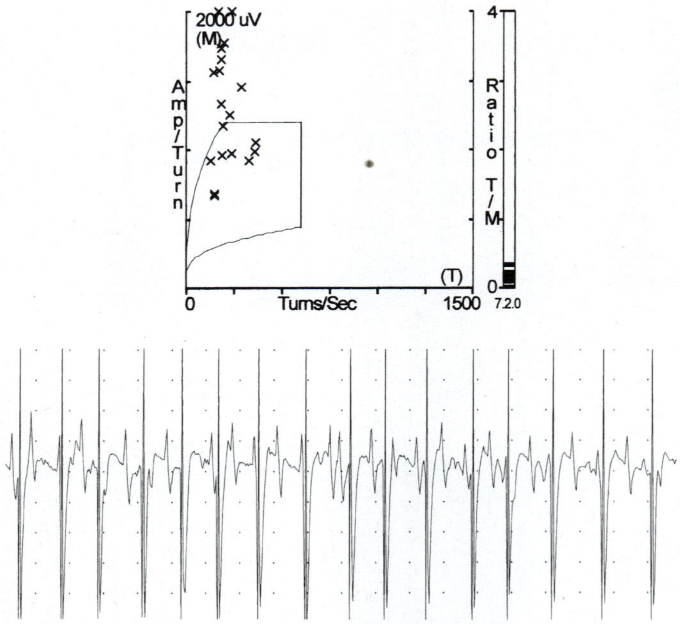

FIG 2-41 Automatic motor unit "cloud" analysis in the quadriceps muscle in a patient with radiculopathy. Notice increased amplitude and decreased number of turns.

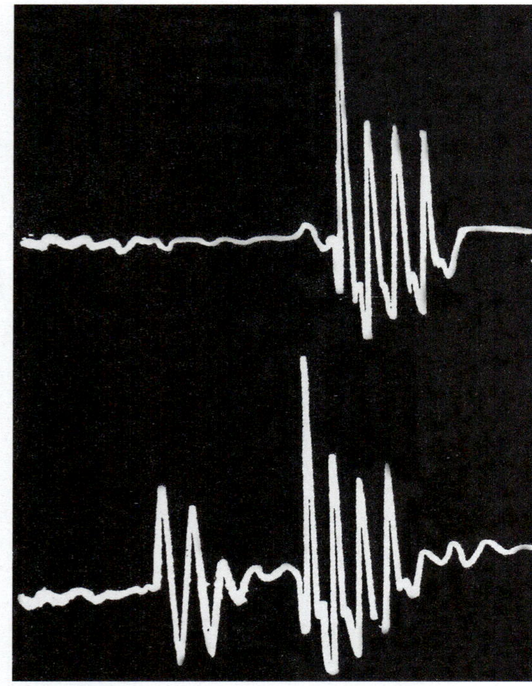

FIG 2-43 Multiplets potential in a patient with tetany (200 μV/10 ms).

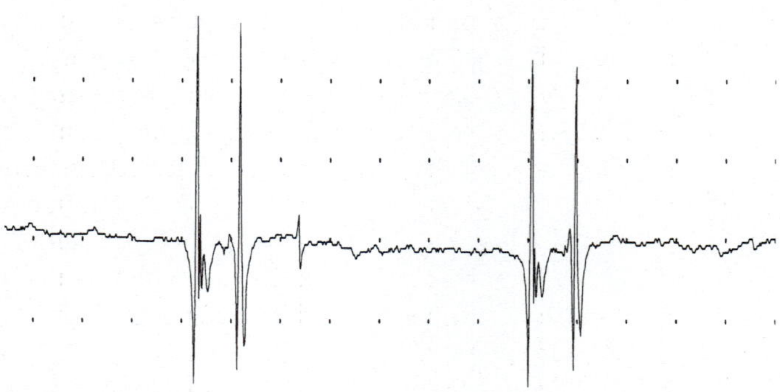

FIG 2-42 Duplets potentials in a patient with a motor neuron disease (200 μV/10 ms).

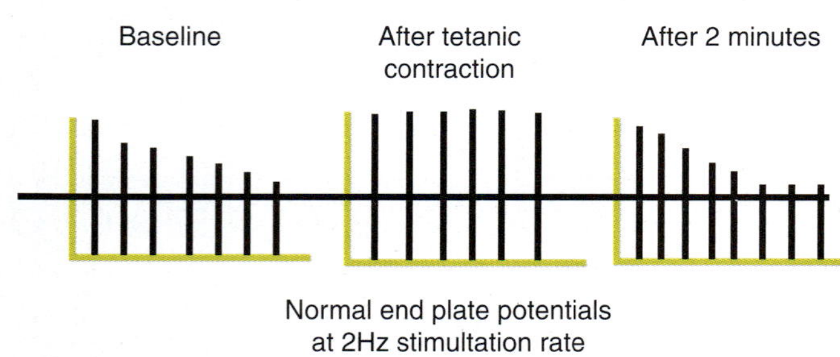

FIG 2-44 Diagram of endplate potentials in normals obtained during stimulation at 2 Hz before, immediately after, and 2 min after a tetanic contraction. The horizontal bar represents the threshold to generate a muscle action potential (safety factor). Notice that the endplate potentials decrease in amplitude during repetitive stimulus, but are all above the safety factor to generate a muscle action potential.

producing increased ACh quantal releases and an incremental response of the EPP (*facilitation*). In normals, as the EPPs remain above the threshold to produce MAPs, the CMAP does not change during consecutive fast stimulations[66] (Figs. 2-46 and 2-47). The amplitude of the CMAP, however, might increase in disorders of neuromuscular transmission, particularly in presynaptic disorders, because the initial EPPs are smaller than normal and below the SF (producing a smaller CMAP). Fast stimulations produce larger EPPs which are above the threshold to generate MAPs, and thus the CMAP becomes larger.

In the clinical setting, the method of the *repetitive stimulation test* consists of stimulating a motor nerve with 4–6 stimuli supramaximally at rates of 2–3 Hz or 5 Hz. This is followed by a 10- to 20-second voluntary tetanic contraction. The nerve is then stimulated again immediately and at 2 and 3 minutes afterward.[67,68] If the test is negative, this could be repeated after 1 minute of tetanic contraction.

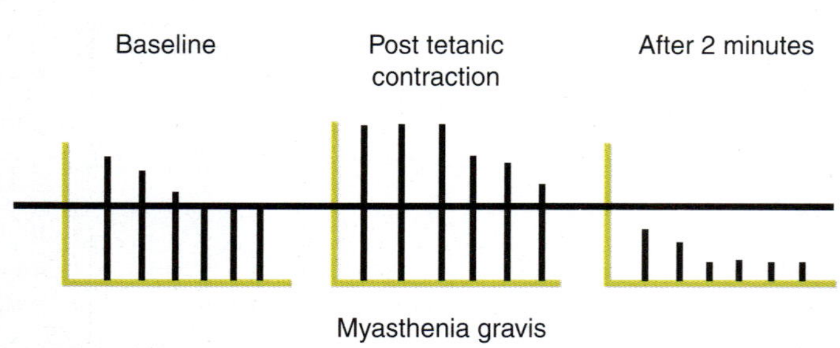

FIG 2-45 Diagram of endplate potentials in MG. The EPPs become smaller and are below the safety factor during repetitive stimulus. Upon tetanic contraction the EPPs increase in amplitude and are above the threshold to generate a muscle action potential (facilitation). Two minutes later they become smaller (postactivation exhaustion). Potentials below the threshold (safety factor) do not produce muscle action potentials. *EPPs*, endplate potentials; *MG*, myasthenia gravis.

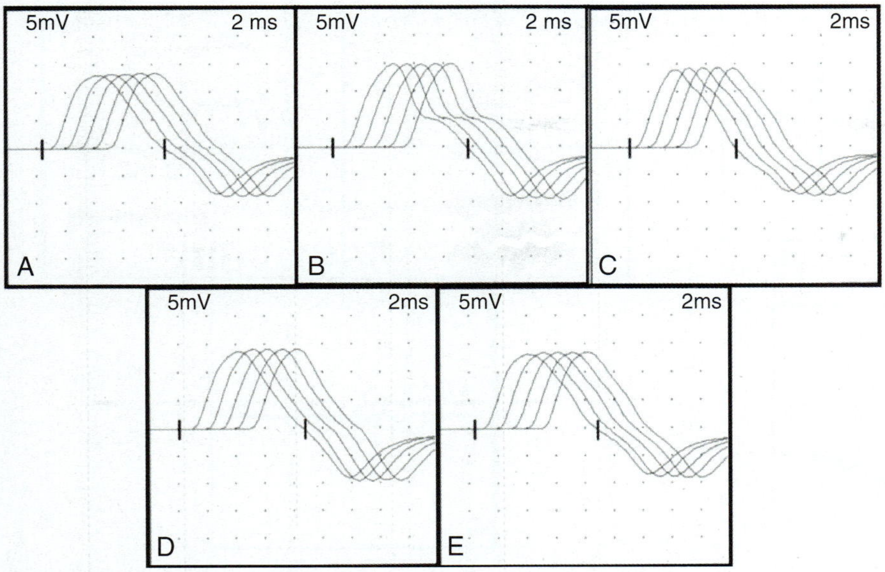

FIG 2-46 Series of repetitive stimulation tests stimulating the ulnar nerve at 3 Hz, recording in the abductor digiti minimi (ADM) muscle of a normal patient. **A**, Baseline; **B**, after tetanic contraction; **C**, 1 min; **D**, 2 min; **E**, 3 min after a tetanic contraction. Notice the lack of change in the compound muscle action potential (CMAP).

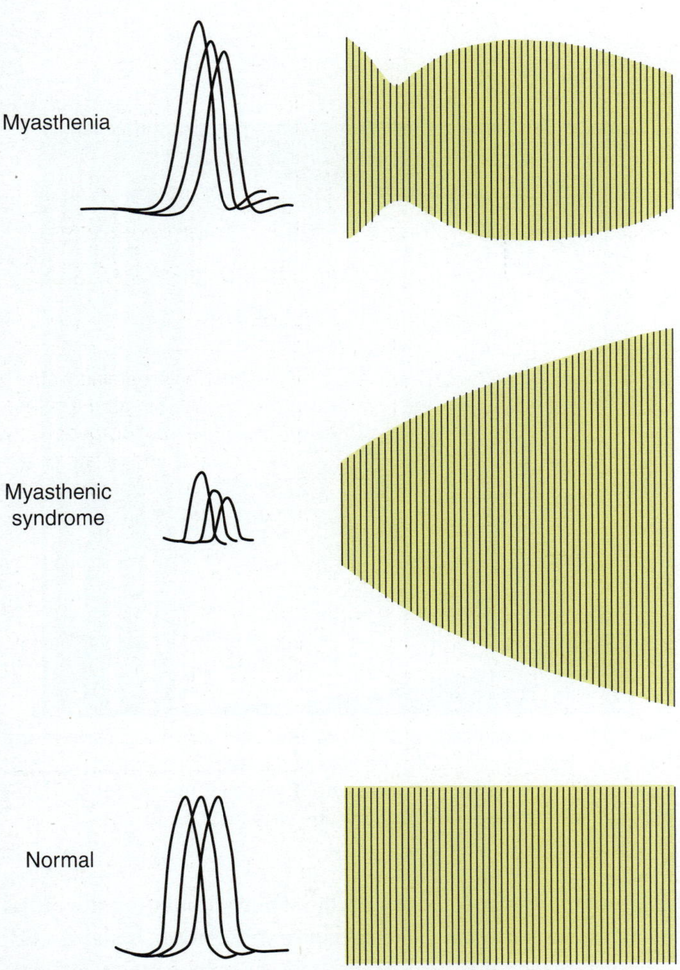

FIG 2-47 Diagram of the repetitive stimulation test showing compound muscle action potentials (CMAPs) obtained with slow stimulation rates (*left*) and with faster stimulation rates (*right*) in myasthenia, normal, and Eaton–Lambert syndrome.

In normal persons the CMAPs do not change during slow repetitive nerve stimulations (2–3 Hz). In postsynaptic disorders, such as MG, the initial CMAP is normal or mildly decreased in amplitude, and there is a *decrement* of the amplitude and area. There is also a *posttetanic facilitation* from the release of previously blocked neuromuscular junctions. The decrement of the CMAP then is larger for about 1–3 minutes after the tetanic contraction (*postactivation exhaustion*)[68,69] (Figs. 2-47–2-49). In some cases the baseline stimulation trend might not produce a decrement, but this becomes evident 1–3 minutes after the tetanic contraction.

In presynaptic disorders such as Eaton–Lambert syndrome, botulism, and some presynaptic congenital myasthenic syndromes, the initial CMAP is of low amplitude. There could also be a decrement at slow stimulation rates, but marked increment of the amplitude and area is evident after a tetanic contraction (*facilitation*) (Fig. 2-50), or during faster stimulation rates of 10 Hz or more (Fig. 2-51). The lower initial CMAP amplitude is caused by an impairment in the release of synaptic vesicles associated with lower amplitude EPPs, and the posttetanic facilitation is caused by increased ACh releases afterward.[66,68]

In congenital myasthenic syndromes caused by *cholinesterase deficiency*, or in the *slow channel syndrome*, the CMAP could have a second or even a third wave or afterdischarge following the main CMAP; there is also decrement at the slow stimulation rates (Fig. 2-52).[67,68] This phenomenon can also occur in cholinergic crisis from overly excessive doses of anticholinesterase drugs and in organophosphate poisoning.[67,68]

The protocol for the repetitive stimulation test consists of first stimulating a distal nerve, such as the ulnar, and recording the CMAP on a muscle innervated by that nerve, such as the adductor digiti minimi, or stimulating the median nerve and recording in the thenar eminence. If this produces normal

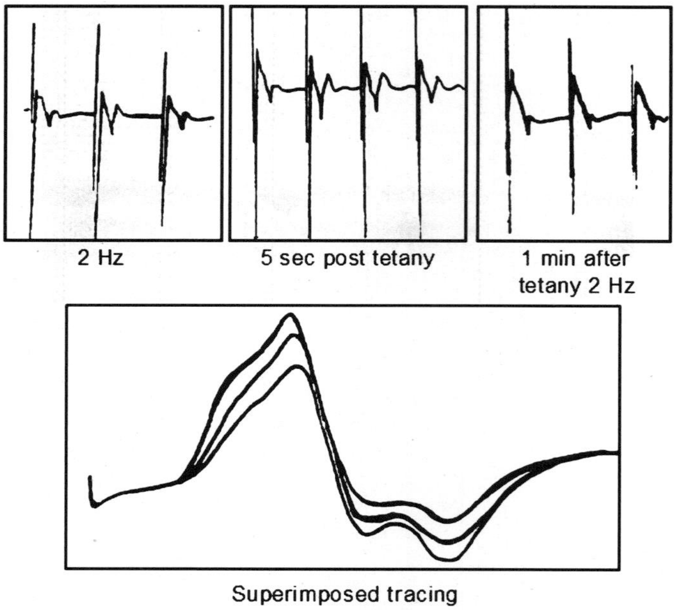

FIG 2-48 Compound muscle action potential recorded in the abductor digiti minimi (ADM) muscle and stimulation of the ulnar nerve at 2 Hz of a patient with myasthenia gravis (MG). Fast sweep recordings (*top*) show a decrement in amplitude, posttetanic facilitation, and postactivation exhaustion. The CMAPs are recorded in superimposed tracings (*bottom*); notice decrease in amplitude in an area of the CMAP (2 mV/2 ms). *CMAPs*, Compound muscle action potential.

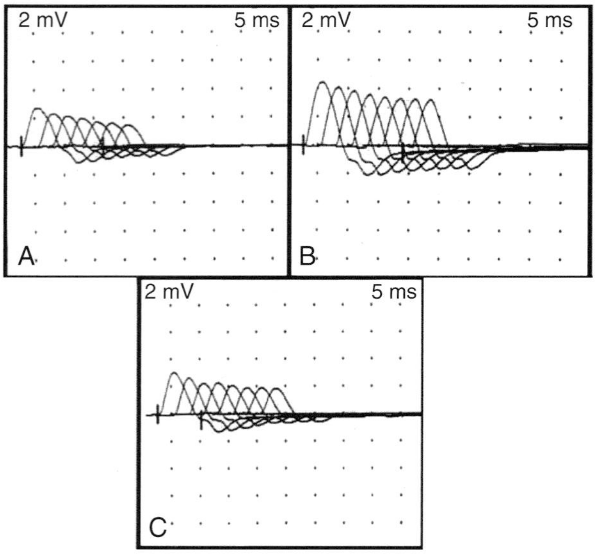

FIG 2-50 CMAP in a patient with Eaton–Lambert syndrome during repetitive stimulation of the ulnar nerve at 2 Hz, recording at the abductor digiti minimi (ADM) muscle. Notice an initial decrement of the CMAP **(A)**, significant posttetanic facilitation **(B)**, and increased decrement 1 min after tetanic contraction **(C)** (2 mV/5 ms). *CMAPs*, Compound muscle action potential.

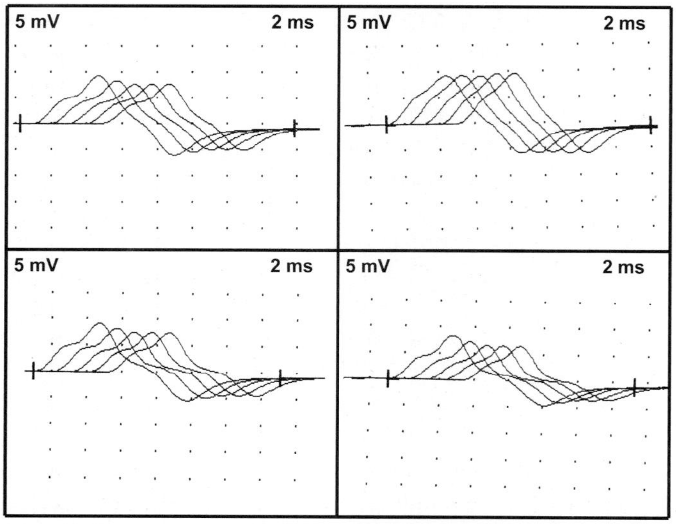

FIG 2-49 Repetitive stimulation test of the ulnar nerve recording the abductor digiti minimi (ADM) muscle on a patient with myasthenia gravis (MG) at 3 Hz stimulation. Notice mild decrement (*top left*), posttetanic facilitation is seen on stimulation immediately after tetanic contraction (*top right*), and increased decrement after 1 min (*bottom left*) and 2 min after tetanic contraction (*bottom right*) (5 mV/2 ms).

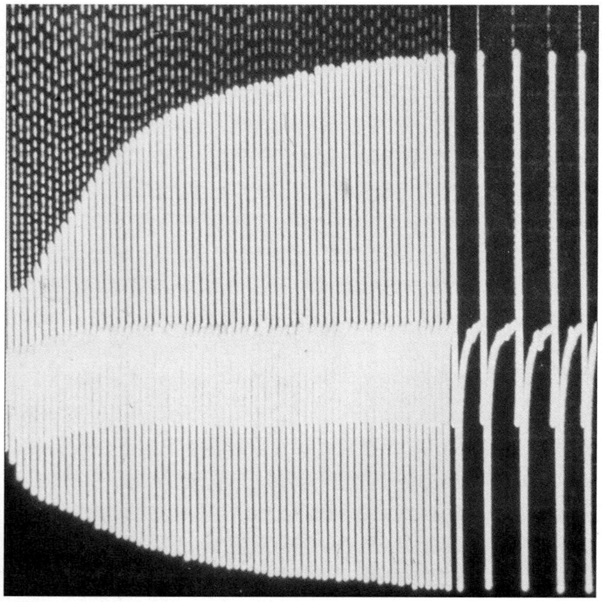

FIG 2-51 Fast stimulation at 20 Hz of the ulnar nerve recording at the abductor digiti minimi (ADM) muscle in a patient with Eaton–Lambert syndrome; notice marked increased amplitude of the CMAP (2 mV/20 ms). *CMAPs*, Compound muscle action potential.

results, a proximal nerve should then be studied. Most recommend recording at the trapezius muscle stimulating the spinal accessory nerve.[69] Others stimulate the musculocutaneous nerve while recording at the biceps muscle, or the axillary nerve while recording at the deltoid muscle, but those are painful and produce movement artifacts.

Studying the anconeus muscle[70] while stimulating the radial nerve above the elbow, or facial nerve stimulation, is also useful; however, the latter is painful and may cause movement artifacts.

As discussed, there is no facilitation during fast stimulation in normals, but there could be a "pseudofacilitation," which consists of an increased CMAP *amplitude* without changing the

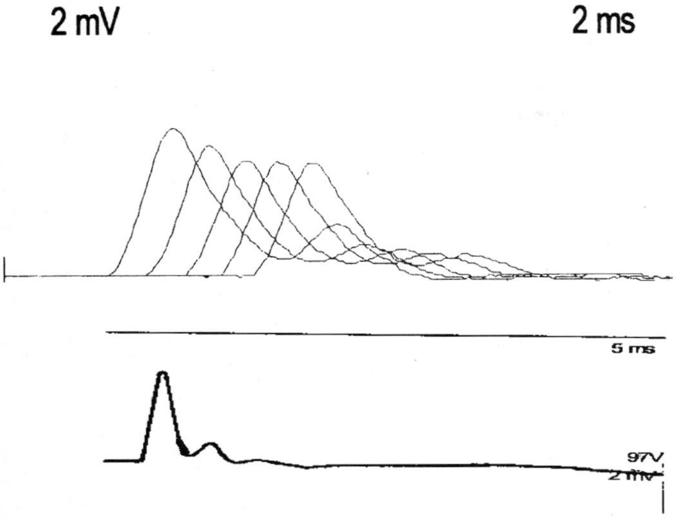

FIG 2-52 CMAP of the abductor digiti minimi (ADM) muscle during repetitive stimulation of the ulnar nerve at 2 Hz in a patient with slow channel myasthenic syndrome (*top*). (Notice a decrement of the CMAP during repetitive stimulation.) The tracing below shows the characteristic after discharge of the CMAP (2 mV/2 ms.) *CMAPs*, Compound muscle action potential.

total area. This is caused by a progressive shortened conduction time in muscle fibers. For this reason the *area* of the CMAP, rather than the amplitude, should be measured.[71]

To enhance the sensitivity, muscles are exercised for 5 minutes prior to the stimulation. The *prolonged stimulation test* also increases sensitivity; this is done by stimulating the nerve supramaximally at 3 Hz for 4–5 minutes and then performing the standard protocol. The *double-step test* consists of prolonged stimulation before and after ischemia of the limb, increasing the diagnostic yield. This is done by recording hand muscles.[72]

At low stimulation rates, CMAP area decrements of over 10% from the initial waveform are considered abnormal and indicative of a defect of neuromuscular transmission. Conventionally, the diagnosis of a disorder of presynaptic transmission is made if there is a posttetanic facilitation of 100% or over or when this occurs during fast stimulation rates. It has recently been suggested that a change of 60% is sufficient to diagnose Eaton–Lambert syndrome.[73]

To perform the test, the examiner should avoid submaximal stimuli or improper positioning of the electrodes. Also, the limb should be properly immobilized. Surface temperature should be at about 34°C, as lower temperatures diminish the decrement.

Abnormal decremental responses could also occur in motor neuron diseases and in some neuropathies due to secondary abnormalities of the motor endplates. This is also observed in myotonia (Fig. 2-53), but in those cases it is caused by a decrease in muscle fiber action potential amplitude and not from a defective neuromuscular transmission. A low amplitude of the initial CMAP is seen in attacks of periodic paralysis, and this amplitude increases after the stimulation of 5–10 Hz. In McArdle's disease a decremental response can be seen during fast stimulation rates.

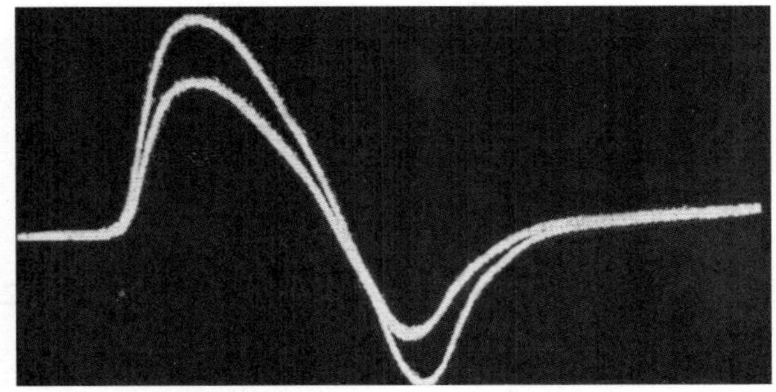

FIG 2-53 Two superimposed CMAPs of the abductor digiti minimi (ADM) muscle while stimulating the ulnar nerve at 2 Hz, in a patient with myotonia congenita. Notice that the action potential becomes smaller (2 mV/2 ms). *CMAPs*, Compound muscle action potential.

Motor Unit Number Estimates

Various techniques use motor unit number estimates (MUNEs) to estimate the number of viable motor units present in a muscle. These methods are usually applied in research, not during routine electrodiagnostic testing.[74–77]

The MUNE techniques include those using nerve stimulation, such as the *incremental stimulation* described initially by McComas et al.,[77] which is based on the stimulation of the nerve, and recording surface individual motor unit potentials (SMUPs), by several incremental submaximal stimulations and then by a supramaximal stimulus (CMAP) to determine how many motor units form the CMAP. This assumes that each potential produced by incremental stimulation corresponds to an individual motor unit. Other techniques include counting the motor units obtained with *multiple-point stimulation* of the nerve using submaximal stimulation, since each stimulation produces an all-or-none response of reproducible motor units. About 10 samples are taken to calculate the mean size of the motor unit. The *F-response method* is performed using supramaximal stimulation and counting the number of F-responses obtained as each F-wave represents an individual motor unit.[76]

The *statistical method* analyzes the variance of a Poisson distribution of the SMUPs obtained with submaximal stimulus at various intensities to determine the mean size of motor units obtained with each stimulus intensity.[78]

The *spike triggering technique*[79] is based on the recording of MUAPs with a needle electrode used as a trigger and recording its corresponding SMUP with a surface electrode; in this way different motor units are counted. All these and several other techniques can be used to estimate the number of viable motor units present in a muscle.[80]

Single Fiber Electromyography

Single fiber electromyography (SFEMG) is a technique used primarily in the study of disorders of neuromuscular transmission, but it is also valuable in analyzing the topography of motor unit territory in a muscle.[81] The test is performed with special electrodes of 25-μm diameter placed in the side of a needle. Recordings can also be made with concentric or monopolar needles.[82] SFEMG tests are done with special settings, increasing

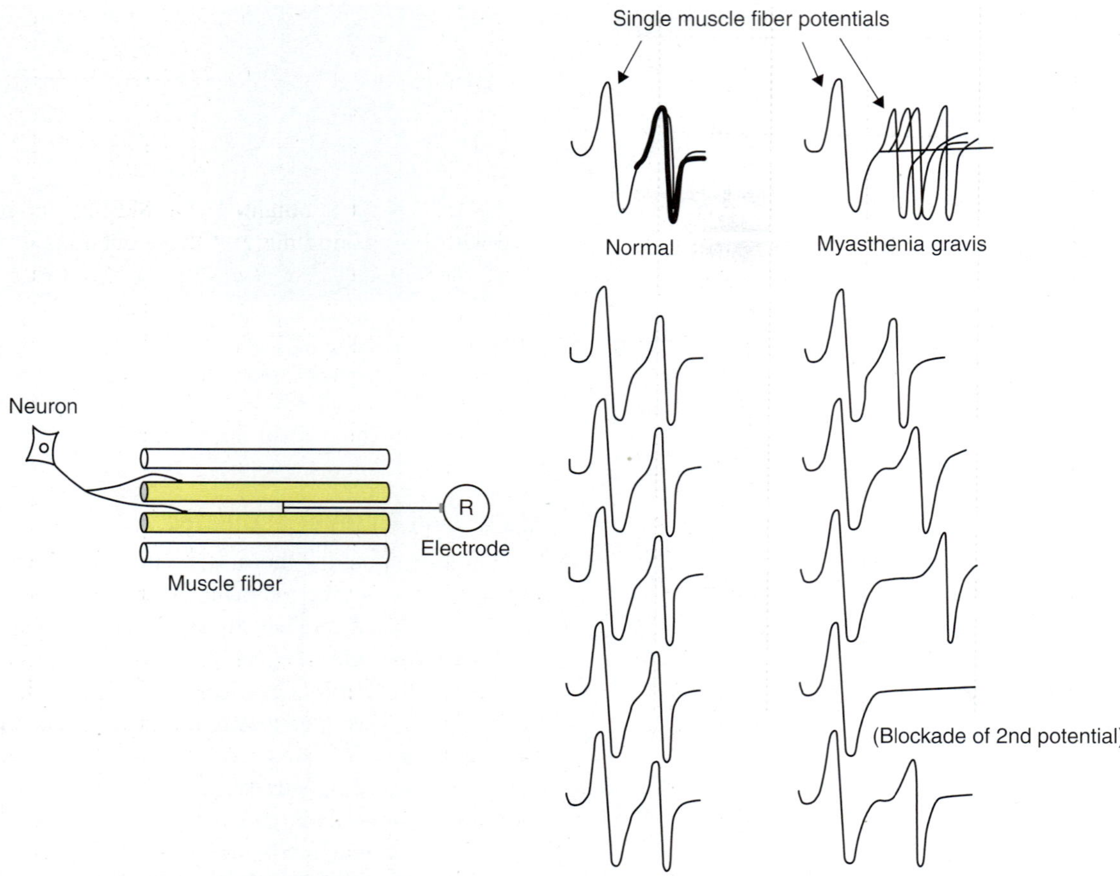

FIG 2-54 Diagram of the single fiber electromyography. Notice the needle electrode between two muscle fibers of the same motor neuron (*left*); single-fiber potentials recordings demonstrated on superimposed mode (*top center*) and roster mode (*bottom center*); and evidence of increased jitter and blocking in myasthenia gravis (MG) on superimposed (*top right*) and roster mode (*bottom right*).

sweep speeds of the oscilloscope, using trigger and delay lines, and raising the low-frequency filters to 500 Hz.[83]

Jitter Analysis. Normally, one or two individual muscle fiber potentials from the same motor units are recorded by the needle electrode during muscle contractions. If one potential is used to trigger the sweep, then the variability of the firing of the second potential, or *jitter*, from the one triggering the sweep is measured. Minimal variabilities that are caused by delays in neuromuscular transmission are recorded in healthy individuals; this is called *normal jitter*. An *increased jitter* is seen in disorders of neuromuscular transmission (Figs. 2-54–2-56), but also in other conditions such as ALS. *Blocking* of one of the potentials is caused by a total failure of transmission (see Figs. 2-55 and 2-56); this is usually accompanied by increased jitter values. Jitter calculation can be performed during voluntary contractions and using axonal stimulation.[83]

The neuromuscular jitter is measured as the mathematical calculation of the mean consecutive differences, which determines the variability of the individual fiber potentials. Usually, 50–100 recordings are done of each pair. Normal values are usually below 55 μs, but values vary in different muscles. The test should determine if the *mean jitter* is above the normal range. The analysis should also determine how many potential pairs have jitter values above the upper limit of the normal range. For

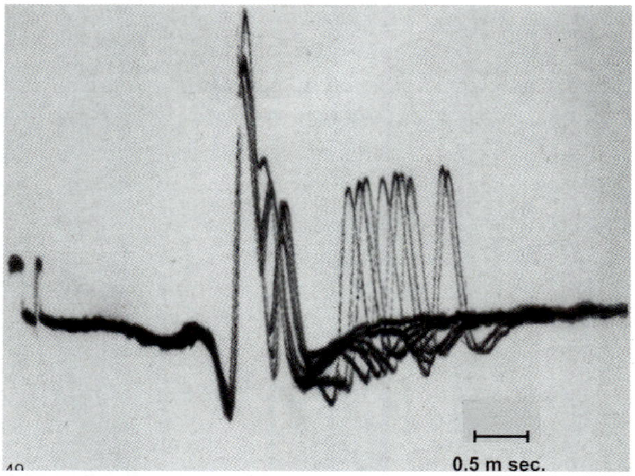

FIG 2-55 Single fiber electromyography of the extensor digitorum communis (EDC) muscle in a patient with myasthenia gravis (MG). Notice variability of the second potential in a superimposed recording mode (500 μV/0.5 ms).

example, the upper limit for the mean jitter of the extensor digitorum communis is 36 μs; if the mean value obtained in a patient is above this, the test is considered abnormal. Also, the maximal individual jitter value for this muscle is 52 ms; if more than one pair exceeds this value, the test is also considered abnormal. The number of potentials with blocks is also determined, and no blocks are seen in normals. The most frequently tested muscle is

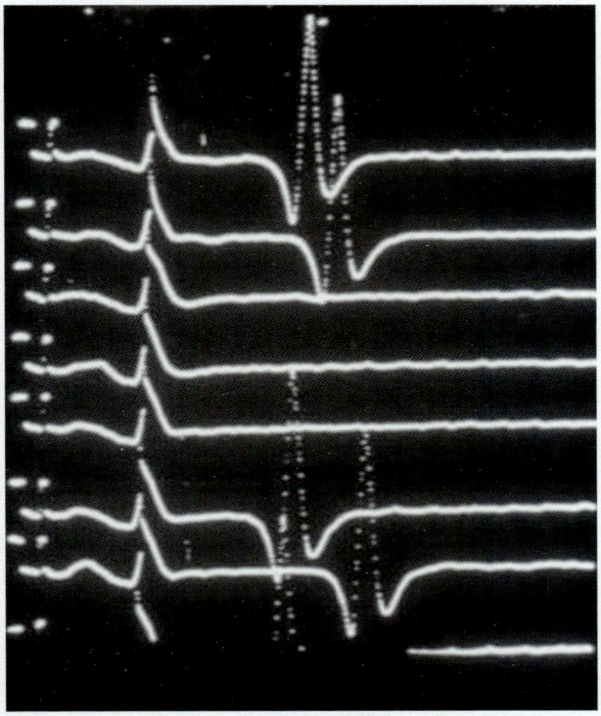

FIG 2-56 A potential pair of the EDC muscle; notice jitter and blocking in a patient with myasthenia gravis (MG) (200 μV/0.5 ms).

the extensor digitorum communis, but the frontalis and orbicularis oculi are more sensitive in diagnosing MG.

Increased jitter and blocking observed during slow contractions and that disappear during fast contractions, or during fast nerve stimulations, are characteristic of Eaton–Lambert syndrome.

The abnormalities obtained with SFEMG should be correlated with clinical findings and those obtained during routine EMG. The test is very sensitive, but not specific, and abnormalities can be seen not only in primary disorders of neuromuscular transmission but also in other diseases.

Fiber Density. During a voluntary contraction, one or two, but rarely three, single muscle fiber potentials that belong to the same motor units are recorded during each needle insertion in normal individuals. The calculated mean number of potentials observed in 30 recordings determines the *fiber density* (*FD*). Increased FD is seen in reinnervation because more muscle fibers of the same motor unit are close to the recording electrode (Figs. 2-57 and 2-58). FD is also increased in atrophy and fiber splitting; thus this test is very sensitive but not specific.[84] FD correlates with clustering of muscle fibers but does not assess the whole territory of the motor unit, which is better studied by *Macro-EMG*.[83]

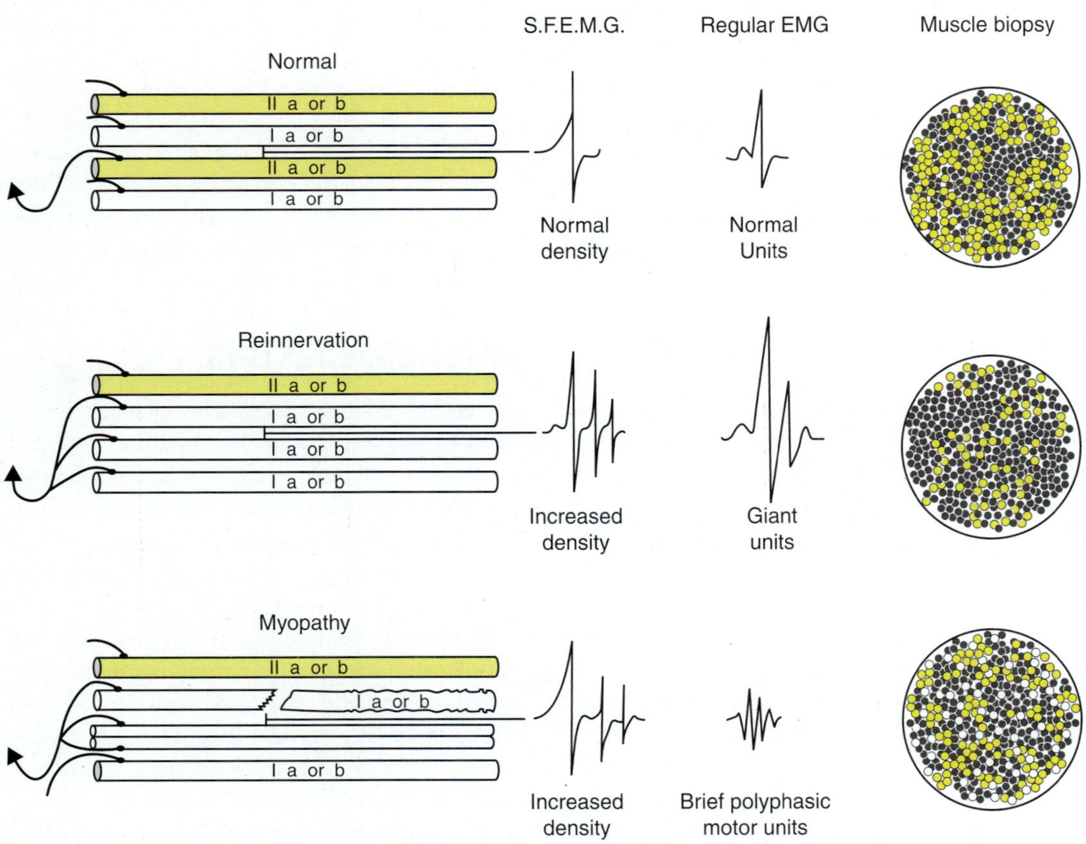

FIG 2-57 Diagram of fiber density recorded with a single fiber electrode and a concentric needle electrode. On the left are diagrams of the normal muscle, on reinnervation, and in myopathy. In the center, tracings demonstrate a fiber density recording with a single fiber needle (*left center*) and with the concentric electrode (*right center*). On the right are the muscle biopsy findings. Notice that with reinnervation there is increased fiber density and large motor units with grouping on the muscle biopsy. In myopathy, there is increased density with small motor units but with fiber atrophy and no grouping.

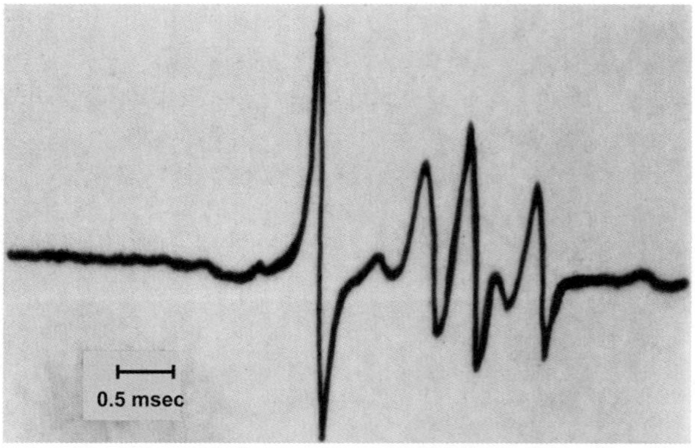

FIG 2-58 Single fiber electromyography (EMG) recording of a patient with amyotrophic lateral sclerosis (ALS). The motor units have increased number of individual potentials (increased density) (200 mV/0.5 ms).

Blink Reflex

The trigeminal nerve can be studied by measurement of the masseter reflex and the blink reflex. The masseter reflex is the electrical equivalent of the myotatic reflex and examines the trigeminal sensory and motor pathways. The blink reflex studies the afferent trigeminal nerve and the efferent response through the seventh nerve to facial muscles.[85]

The electrophysiologic blink reflex studies the electromyographic response of the facial muscles upon electrical or mechanical stimulation of the trigeminal nerve and provides information on the integrity of both the V and VII cranial nerves and their brainstem connections.

The test is usually performed by stimulation of the supraorbital nerve, but other branches of the trigeminal nerve can also be stimulated. This stimulus travels through A-beta myelinated afferent fibers before making connections in the brainstem.

The reflex has two responses. The R1 response with latencies of about 10–13 ms is relayed through an oligosynaptic pathway in the pons. The R2 response is relayed through a polysynaptic pathway via the spinal trigeminal nucleus in the medulla, with connections to the facial nerve motor nucleus in both sides. The R2 has a latency of about 30 ms (Fig. 2-59). There is also a much later, or R3, response, obtained with high stimulus intensity.

The R1 response is recorded only in the stimulated side, whereas R2 response is recorded in both the stimulating and the opposite side. The R2 response has a tendency to disappear or habituate.[86]

Analysis of the blink reflex includes a comparison of side-to-side differences. The test is also valuable in diagnosing demyelinating neuropathies that cause delayed responses.

In trigeminal nerve disorders both the ipsilateral R1 and the ipsilateral and contralateral R2 responses could be absent or delayed when stimulating the affected side. The R1 and both R2 responses are normal when stimulating the normal side.

In seventh nerve lesions, stimulation in the affected side produces abnormal or absent R1 and R2 responses in that side and a normal R2 in the opposite side. Stimulation of the unaffected side produces a normal ipsilateral R1, an R2 response, and an abnormal contralateral R2 (side of the affected seventh nerve).[87]

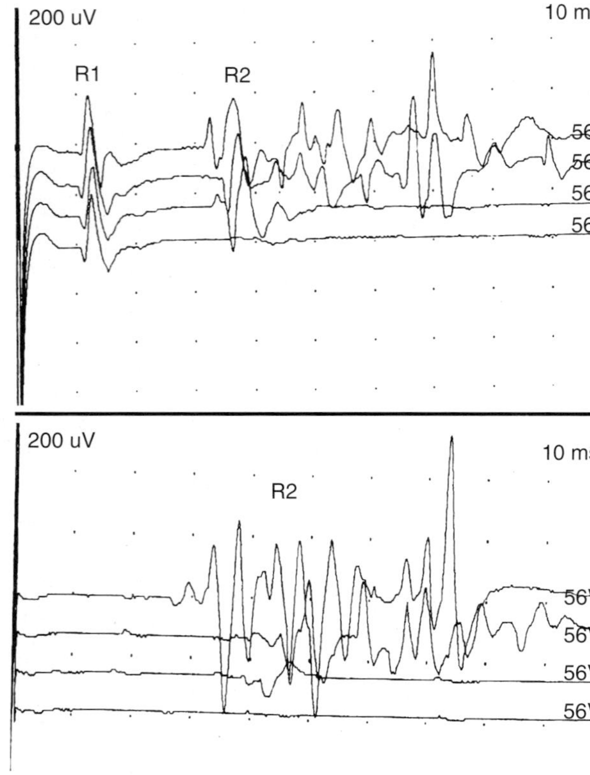

FIG 2-59 Blink reflex in a normal person: ipsilateral R1 and R2 responses (*top*) and normal contralateral R2 responses (*bottom*). Notice that the R2 response in the last tracing disappears after several stimuli (habituation).

The blink reflex has prognostic implications in Bell's palsy. Two weeks after the onset of symptoms, a finding of absent or delayed R1 and R2 responses accompanied by low-amplitude CMAP, obtained during direct facial nerve stimulation, is usually an indication of a poor prognosis.[87]

AUTONOMIC TESTING

The autonomic nervous system can be affected in neuromuscular disorders, particularly neuropathies, such as those from diabetes and amyloidosis, and in some disorders of neuromuscular transmission, such as Eaton–Lambert syndrome.

The autonomic system is a complex network of neurons in the brain and spinal cord with afferent and efferent fibers. It has two divisions, the sympathetic and parasympathetic systems. Both systems have two efferent neurons, the preganglionic ones located centrally and the postganglionic neurons located outside the central nervous system [88] (CNS). The central parasympathetic neurons are located in the brainstem and sacral spinal cord. The postganglionic neurons are located in the ganglia close to the innervated organs. The main neurotransmitter for both is ACh. The sympathetic preganglionic neurons are located in thoracic and lumbar spinal cords. The postganglionic neurons are in the prevertebral ganglia or paravertebral chains. The preganglionic sympathetic neurotransmitter is ACh, while the postganglionic one is neuroepinephrine. (Sweat glands are sympathetic, but their neurotransmitter is ACh.)

The preganglionic axons of both systems emerge from the CNS as small myelinated fibers. (The parasympathetic fibers can also be unmyelinated.) Postganglionic axons are unmyelinated C fibers, and they are usually affected in small fiber neuropathy.[89-91]

Testing of the autonomic system includes evaluations of functions governed mainly by the parasympathetic system, such as changes in heart rate and blood pressure during deep breathing (Fig. 2-60) and heart rate changes during the Valsalva maneuver (the Valsalva ratio), pulse changes during phase IV of the Valsalva maneuver (Fig. 2-61), and heart rate responses upon standing (the 30:15 ratio).

Sympathetic system tests include the determination of blood pressure changes during the forearm isometric exercise test and during the tilt table and sweat tests[90] (Fig. 2-62), as well as the sympathetic skin response (Fig. 2-63) and blood pressure

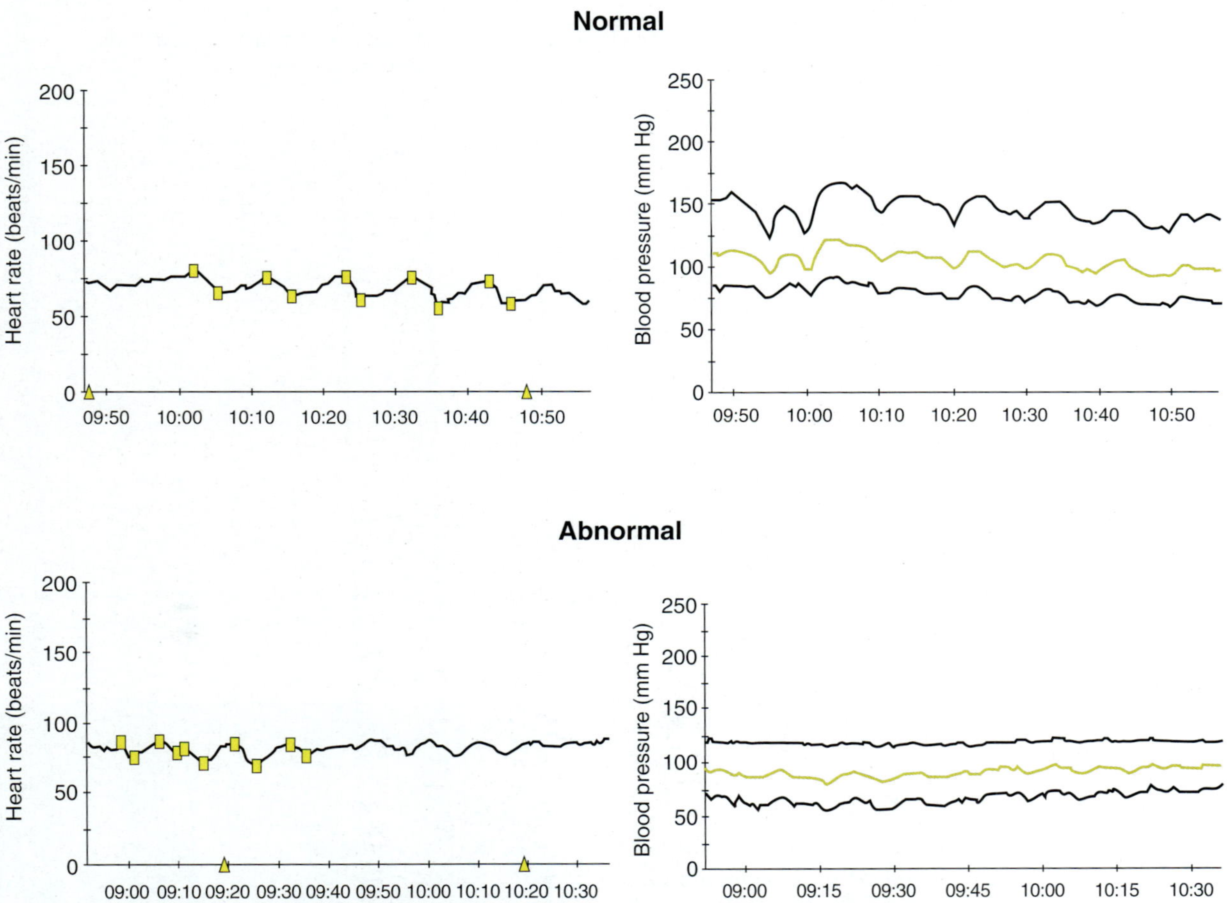

FIG 2-60 Recordings of pulse rates (*left*) and blood pressure (*right*, systolic blood pressure [top line], mean blood pressure [middle line], and diastolic blood pressure [bottom line]) during deep breathing in a healthy subject (*top*) and a patient with diabetic neuropathy (*bottom*). Notice decreased variability of the pulse rate and blood pressure during deep inspiration in the patient with neuropathy.

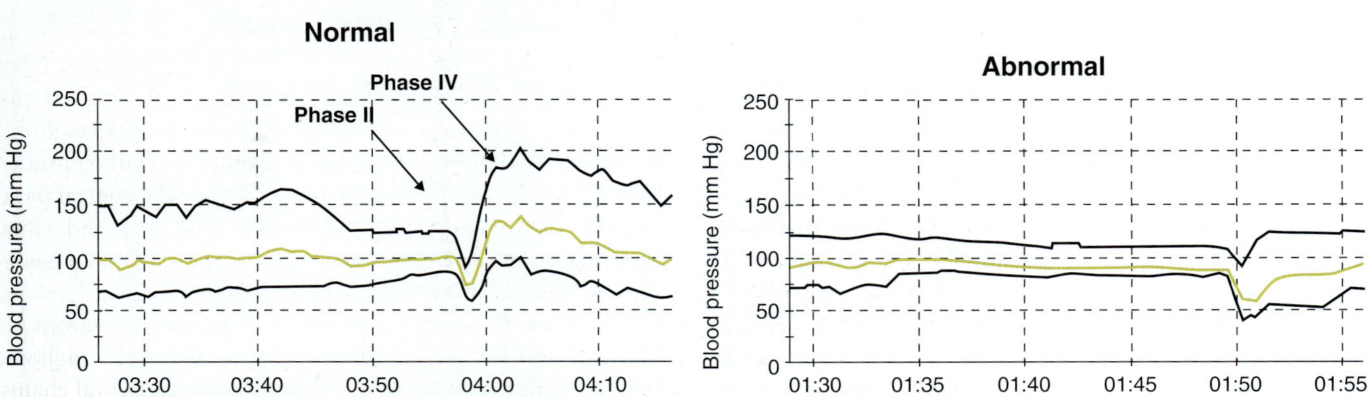

FIG 2-61 Valsalva maneuver of normal subject (*left*) and patient with dysautonomia (*right*). The recordings show systolic blood pressure at the top, mean blood pressure in the middle, and diastolic blood pressure on the bottom. In the normal subject, notice the changes in blood pressure with a drop in phase II of the Valsalva maneuver and increased blood pressure in phase IV. In the patient with dysautonomia there is minimal variation in blood pressure.

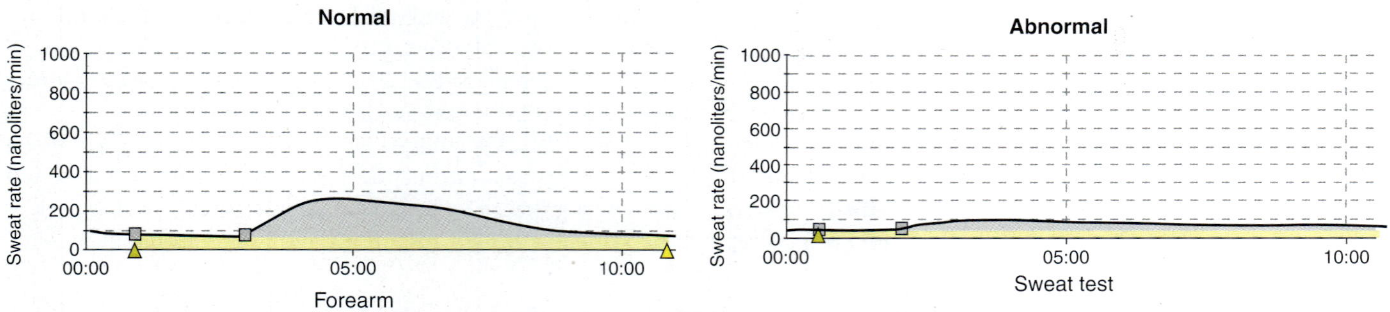

FIG 2-62 Sweat test after acetylcholine given by iontophoresis for 5 min. The figure on the left shows normal sweat; the on the right figure is from a patient with peripheral neuropathy showing decreased sweat.

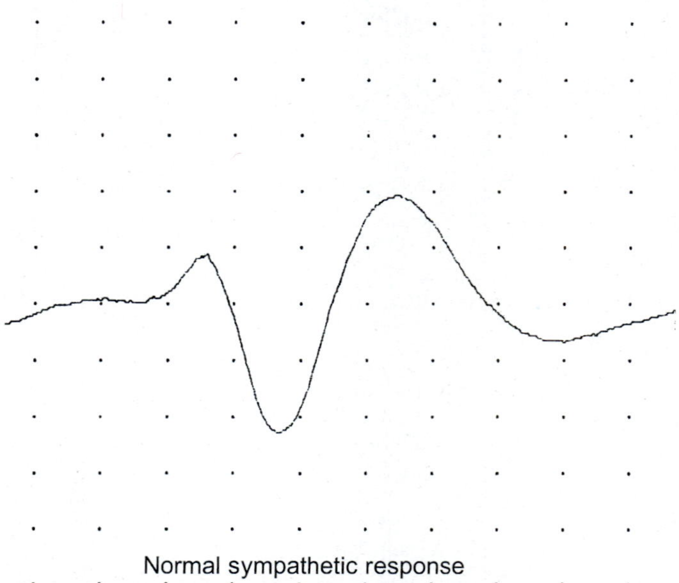

FIG 2-63 Normal sympathetic skin response of the arm after stimulation of the opposite arm (100 μV/20 ms).

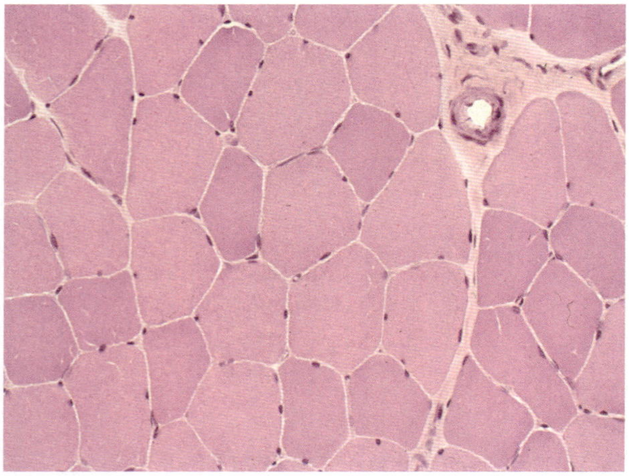

FIG 2-64 Normal muscle histology. Notice that the muscle fibers have a polygonal shape with peripherally located nuclei (H&E stain, ×200).

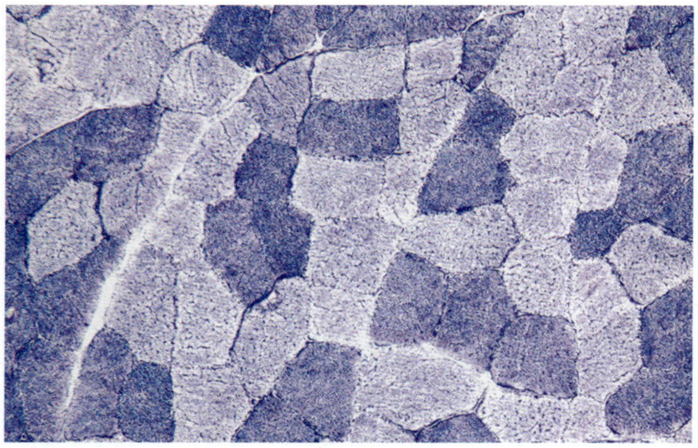

FIG 2-65 Normal muscle biopsy showing an almost checkerboard distribution of muscle fibers (NADH-TR stain, ×200).

changes during phase II of the Valsalva maneuver. Some of these evaluations can be done in standard EMG laboratories, while others, such as the tilt table and sweat test, require a dedicated autonomic laboratory.

MUSCLE/NERVE HISTOPATHOLOGY

Muscle biopsy is very helpful in diagnosing most myopathies and in demonstrating widespread denervation, when the EMG is nondiagnostic in patients suspected to have a motor neuron disease. Muscle biopsies are also useful in the diagnosis of systemic diseases such as sarcoidosis, vasculitis, and amyloidosis. In patients with muscle pain, a fascia biopsy can be used to determine if there is a fascitis causing the symptoms; this should be done in conjunction with a muscle biopsy in patients with myalgias.[92]

The muscle biopsy should be done in a clinically affected muscle, but not in muscles that are severely atrophic, as this could show endstage and nonspecific changes. One usually biopsies muscle that shows EMG abnormalities on the contralateral side. MRI[93] and ultrasound[30] can also help in selecting the proper muscle, based on abnormalities of these tests. The most frequently biopsied muscles are the quadriceps, biceps, and deltoids. Biopsies of the gastrocnemius–soleus should be discouraged because of the frequent nonspecific changes seen in both diseased and normal people. The gastrocnemius–soleus, however, could be used when suspecting vasculitis in conjunction with a sural nerve biopsy.

The specimens are analyzed by the following techniques: (1) histology to detect inflammation, necrosis, dystrophic changes, and structural abnormalities, to diagnose mitochondrial or storage myopathies and enzyme deficiencies (Figs. 2-64–2-66), and to demonstrate changes in muscle histology and histochemistry; (2) biochemistry for the diagnosis of disorders of glycogen

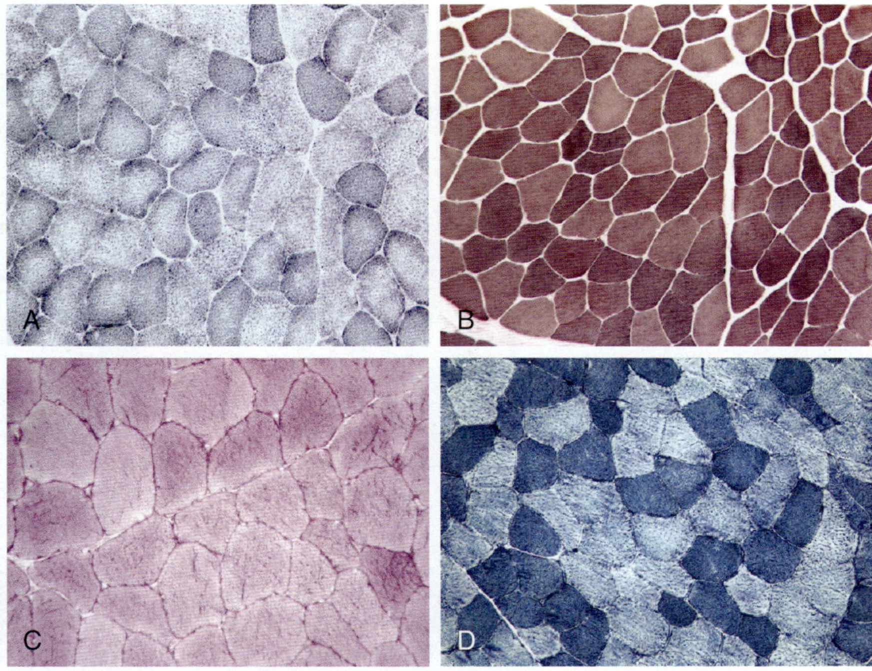

FIG 2-66 Normal histochemical stains using different enzyme staining: succinate dehydrogenase **(A)**; phosphorylase **(B)**; periodic acid Schiff **(C)**; and phosphofructokinase **(D)** (×100).

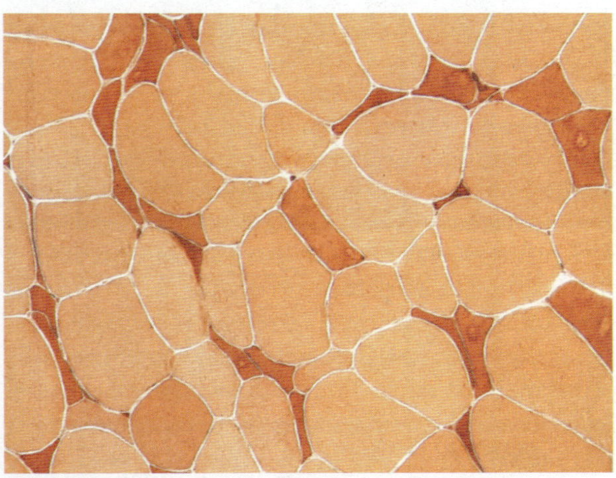

FIG 2-67 Nonspecific esterase stain showing atrophic angular esterase-positive fibers in a neuropathy (×200).

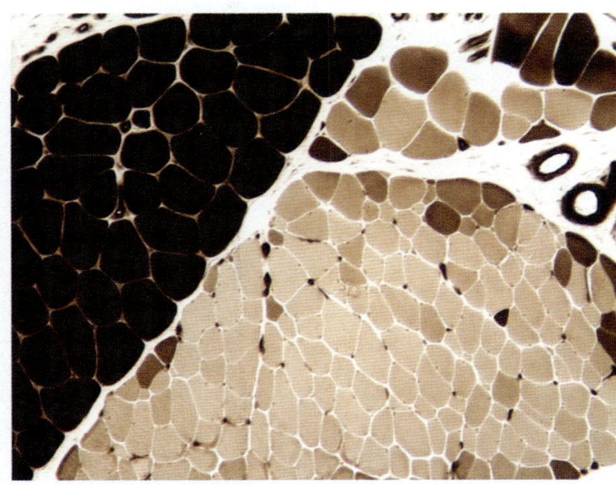

FIG 2-68 Fiber-type grouping in a chronic neuropathy; notice large groups of fibers of both types (ATPase stain at pH 4.6, ×100).

or lipid metabolism,[94,95] myoadenylate deaminase deficiency, and mitochondrial disorders[95]; (3) DNA testing of mitochondrial disorders that affect selected tissues such as muscle; (4) Western blot to determine if there are protein defects, such as of dystrophin or sarcoglycans in muscular dystrophies; (5) electromicroscopy (EM) to analyze structural abnormalities in specific myopathies, such as central core disease and rod myopathy, and to confirm the accumulation of lipid or glycogen or the presence of abnormal mitochondria. EM is also important in observing characteristic inclusions in some myopathies.

Diagnostic findings in neuropathies and motor neuron disorders include atrophic angular fibers that stain positive for nonspecific esterase (Fig. 2-67), pyknotic nuclei, target fibers, and fiber-type grouping in more chronic diseases (Fig. 2-68), and group atrophy (Fig. 2-69 and Table 2-4).

Abnormalities seen in myopathies include necrosis (Fig. 2-70), phagocytosis, regeneration, variation in fiber size with an increased number of internalized nuclei and proliferation of connective tissue and fat (Figs. 2-71 and 2-72), and inflammation in inflammatory myopathies (Fig. 2-73; see also Table 2-5). Staining for C5b9 show its presence in vessels in autoimmune disorders of nerve and muscle. In inflammatory myopathies there is upregulation of the major histocompatibility complex (MHC) in fibers and there could be staining with CD45 mononuclear cells and specific lymphocyte staining.

Specific histologic changes are diagnostic, such as the presence of ragged red fibers in mitochondrial disorders, glycogen lipid accumulation, enzymes, or protein deficiencies, as in dystrophinopathies using immunohistochemistry.[92–95] Examples of these are seen in various cases of this book.

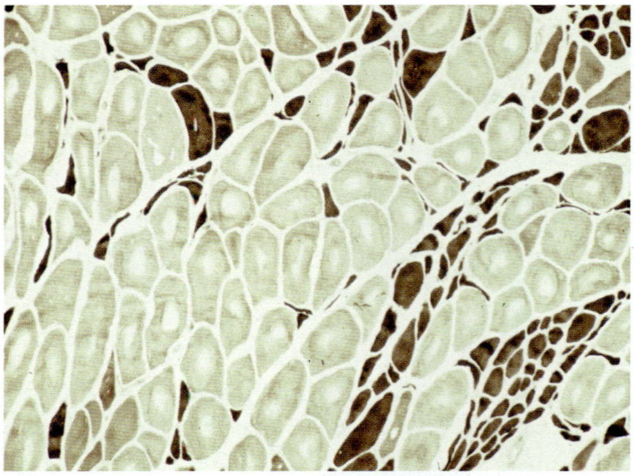

FIG 2-69 Fiber atrophy and targets in type I muscle fibers, there is also fiber-type grouping, and group atrophy, from an ALS patient (ATPase stain at pH 9.4, ×100).

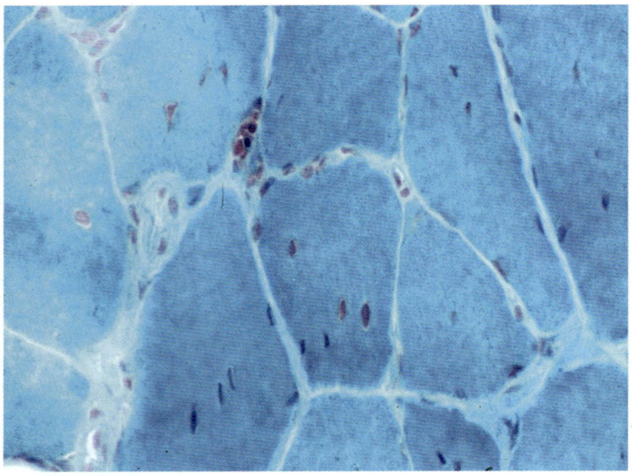

FIG 2-71 A dystrophic muscle with increased internalized nuclei and mildly increased endomysial connective tissue (H&E stain, ×400).

TABLE 2-4 Histologic Changes in Muscle Biopsy Found Predominantly in Neurogenic Disease and Myopathies[a]

Neurogenic Disease	Myopathy
Atrophic, esterase-positive angular fibers	Necrosis, phagocytosis
Targets; targetoids	Regenerating fibers
Large fiber-type grouping	Round atrophic and hypertrophic fibers (variation in fiber size); fiber splitting
Group atrophy	Internalized nuclei and capillaries; lobulated fibers
Pyknotic nuclei[b]	Proliferation of endomysial connective tissue and fat; specific fiber abnormalities (e.g., ragged red fibers, storage, inflammation, vacuoles, protein deficiencies)

[a]Some changes can be seen in both myopathies and neurogenetic disease; the prominence of the findings suggests one or the other in diagnosis.
[b]Can be prominent in some myopathies as well (e.g., myotonic dystrophy).
Reprinted with permission from Bertorini TE. *Clinical Evaluation and Diagnostic Tests for Neuromuscular Disorders*. Boston, MA, Butterworth-Heinemann; 2002:609.

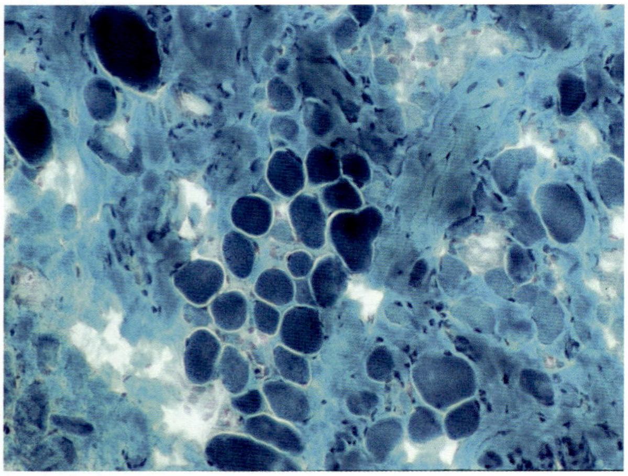

FIG 2-72 A severely dystrophic muscle with prominent proliferation of connective tissue and fiber atrophy (trichrome stain, ×100).

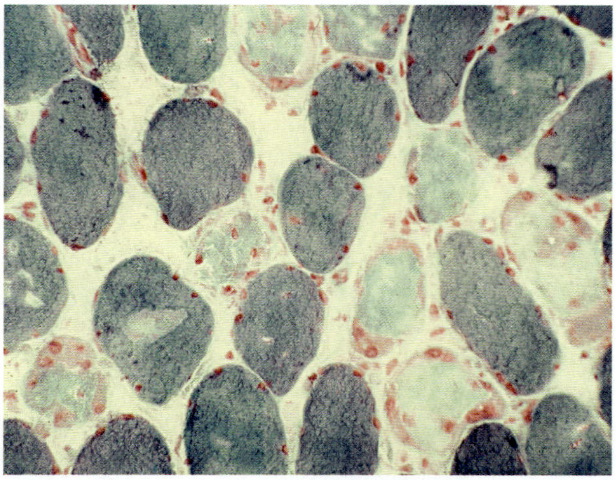

FIG 2-70 Quadriceps muscle biopsy in a patient with polymyositis; notice pale necrotic fibers (modified trichrome stain, ×200).

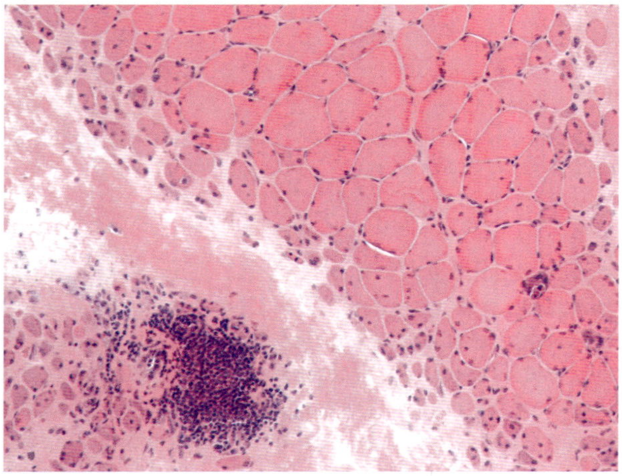

FIG 2-73 Muscle biopsy in a patient with dermatomyositis. Notice perifascicular atrophy and a small perivascular lymphocytic infiltrate (H&E stain, ×100).

Nerve biopsy, particularly of the sural nerve, is done less frequently than muscle biopsies; this helps to determine if there is axonal degeneration versus prominent demyelination, which is well demonstrated using teased nerve preparations, and thick plastic embedded sections (Table 2-5). Figs. 2-74–2-82 show examples of normal nerve and several abnormalities seen in nerve biopsies. EM allows the examiner to study unmyelinated axons. Nerve biopsies help to diagnose vasculitis, storage material, sarcoidosis, and infections such as leprosy and amyloidosis[97]; they also help to observe "onion bulbs" seen in chronic demyelinating neuropathies or tomaculae in hereditary neuropathy with liability to pressure palsy. With inflammatory cells invading the vessel walls and causing vascular necrosis, there could be focal loss of myelinated axons (see Fig. 2-80B), and in chronic cases, deposits of hemosiderin in macrophages of the vessel walls. A widely spaced myelin lamela is seen in some neuropathies, particularly those with antibodies against MAG; characteristic inclusions are seen in some hereditary metabolic neuropathies and those caused by toxins such as amiodarone.[96] Skin biopsies are used to measure the number of epidermal nerve fibers, particularly in small fiber neuropathies.[92] This helps to determine the presence of small fiber neuropathy and helps in research studies to assess response to treatment (Fig. 2-83).

Molecular Genetics

Molecular genetics has become increasingly valuable in understanding and diagnosing inherited neuromuscular disorders; therefore it is important that neuromuscular clinicians know the basic principles of and the diagnostic tests used in molecular diagnosis.[97–102] The following is a brief summary of these.

A *gene*, or *allele*, is the fundamental basis of inheritance that is based on DNA. Genes are located in 46 large molecules of DNA, or *chromosomes*. Humans have two sets of 23 chromosomes; out of which 22 pairs are of autosomes and one pair is of sex chromosomes. The total genetic information in a cell is called the *genome*. (The book *Genome* describes in an entertaining style the interesting history of disorders associated with mutations of different chromosomes.[103])

A gene is a fragment of DNA that encodes a protein or a ribonucleic acid (RNA) with a specific function. The coding regions of the gene are the *exons* which are interspersed with noncoding segments, or *introns*. Exons form mature transcripts of messenger RNA (mRNA) with their removal or splice. *Splicing* refers to the process of the removal of introns to generate an mRNA.[101,102]

Molecules of DNA are formed by nucleotides that consist of a nitrogenous base and deoxyribose with a phosphate group that forms its backbone. These molecules have a double-stranded structure coiled around a common axis (Fig. 2-84). The individual strands run in opposite directions and are held together by hydrogen bonds of the nitrogenous base. The bases are two purines, adenine (A) and guanine (G), and a pyrimidine that is either thymidine (T) or cytosine (C). Their pairing is always predictable: A always pairs with T and G always pairs with C.[102] Amino acids that make a protein are encoded by a sequence of nucleotides called a *codon*.

Transcription is the process that converts the information contained in the DNA sequence into messenger RNA that is then transported out of the nucleus to the cytoplasm. Ribosomes translate this information into an amino acid sequence and the synthesis of proteins. *Translation* refers to the process that decodes mRNA to specify the synthesis of a protein.

Mutations are changes in the nucleotide sequence of a gene that disables or alters the function of a protein. Those that affect protein synthesis or function are called *polymorphisms*.[102]

The chromosomal location of a gene is called a *locus*, and the various loci differentiating individual DNA sequences are called *alleles*. A normal allele is called *wild-type*; a mutation or a change in the nucleotide sequence of a gene that alters the function of the protein is called a *mutant* allele. Inherited diseases are caused by mutant alleles.[104,105]

Subjects affected with *autosomal dominant diseases* have one mutant and one wild-type allele in the affected chromosome pair. Those with autosomal recessive disease have both mutant alleles. When identical alleles occur in both chromosomes, the person is a *homozygote;* when two alleles are different, they are called *heterozygotes*. Individuals with *autosomal recessive disorders* are homozygotes because they have two mutant alleles, and these disorders could be inherited from either autosomes or the sex chromosomes.[97,102]

The *genotype* of a particular disease is the specific mutation of the locus for the disease, whereas a *phenotype* indicates the physical characteristics of the individual with the disease.

When referring to a genetic location, the locus is referred to as the affected chromosome number, for example, 12. In addition, if the gene is located in the short arm, this number is followed by a letter *p*, from the French *petit*, and when it is located in the long arm, the number is followed by a *q*. The letter is followed by a description of the area in the arm of the chromosome where the gene is located.[102] For example, the mutation for Charcot–Marie–Tooth disease 1A is caused by a duplication or a point mutation in chromosome 17p11.2-12.

Unifactorial or *Mendelian inheritance* refers to inheritance caused by mutations of a single gene, and these could be autosomal dominant, autosomal recessive, or X-linked. Most dominant mutations cause a *gain* of function of a protein. Mutations in autosomal recessive disorders usually cause a protein deficiency; for example, a sarcoglycan in some limb-girdle muscular dystrophies, or an enzyme, such as phosphorylase, in McArdle's disease.[102]

Autosomal Dominant and Recessive Disorders

As discussed before, in *autosomal dominant (AD) disorders*, the affected person has a normal and a mutant allele. Therefore, the affected person is a *heterozygote*; however, the mutant allele is dominant, thereby causing the disease. There can be variability in clinical manifestations in AD disorders; this is called *expressivity. Penetrance* indicates the proportion of individuals who carry the mutant gene and manifest the disease. AD diseases affect both sexes and either parent can transmit the condition, thus they appear in consecutive generations. In AD disorders each child has a 50% chance of being affected.

Autosomal recessive (AR) disorders are those in which affected individuals (either male or female) carry both abnormal alleles (homozygotes). The disease is not seen in consecutive generations because both parents of the affected individual are only carriers (heterozygotes) and do not manifest the disease. In AR conditions each offspring has a 25%, or one out of four, chance of being homozygous affected; a 50%, or two

TABLE 2-5 Biopsy Findings That Indicate Axonal Degeneration or Demyelination[a]

Axonal Degeneration	Demyelination
May affect myelinated and unmyelinated fibers	Affects primarily myelinated fibers
Axonal degeneration of myelinated fibers seen on thick plastic sections, teased nerve preparations (large ovoids)	Segmental demyelination Paranodal retraction, variation in internodal length
Axonal atrophy, inclusions	Large axons with thin myelin
Denervated Schwann cell subunits	Onion-bulb formations
Flattened, unmyelinated axons	Some tiny ovoids with variation in internodal length may be seen on teased nerve preparations
Bands of Büngner	–
Regenerating clusters of myelinated fibers	–
Schwann cell processes with increased numbers of small unmyelinated axons	–

[a]These changes are not definitive for diagnosis and, in many neuropathies, could show evidence of both axonal degeneration and demyelination, with the diagnosis based on the predominance of one or the other to determine whether the process is primarily demyelinating or an axonopathy.

Reprinted with permission from Bertorini TE, ed. *Clinical Evaluation and Diagnostic Tests for Neuromuscular Disorders*. Boston, MA, Butterworth-Heinemann; 2002:652.

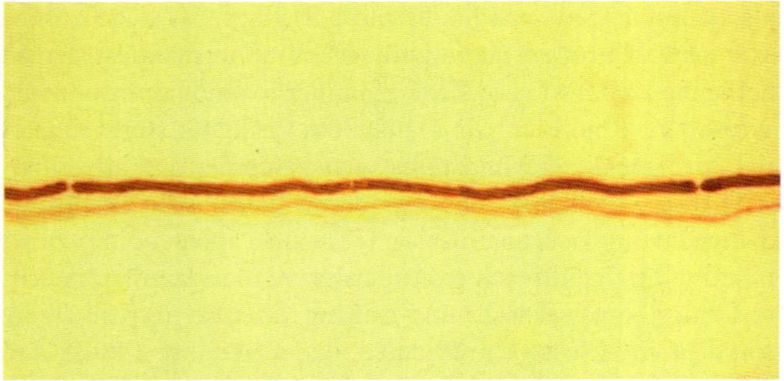

FIG 2-75 Teased nerve preparation; normal internodal length in a myelinated (*top*) and a small myelinated fiber (×400).

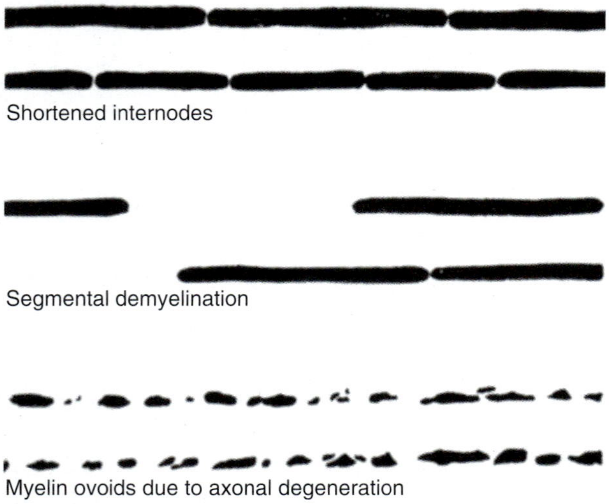

FIG 2-76 Diagram of the different abnormalities detected on teased nerve preparations.

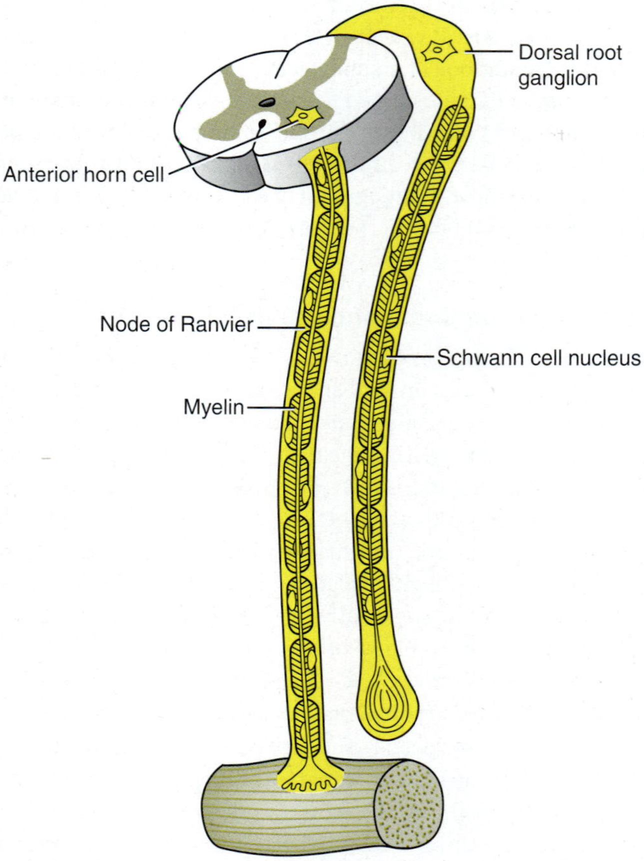

FIG 2-74 Diagram of normal motor and sensory axons and their myelin.

out of four, chance of being heterozygous, or unaffected carriers. Offspring also have a 25%, or one in four, chance of being homozygous unaffected, because they carry both wild-type alleles, and they do not transmit the disease; heterozygotes can sometimes manifest some symptoms of the condition. The occurrence of different mutations on both alleles is known as *compound heterozygosity*.[97]

X-Linked Recessive and Dominant Diseases

X-linked recessive diseases are those caused by mutations of the X chromosome. Only males can inherit the condition, while only females can transmit the disease, but only to their male children; there is no male-to-male transmission.

There are, however, females who are affected in X-linked recessive diseases and these are called *manifest carriers*. The cause may be a chromosomal abnormality, as in Turner syndrome, or a non-random inactivation of the X chromosome. Normally, the inactivation of one of the X chromosomes is random, so that 50% of cells have a maternally inherited chromosome and 50% are paternally derived. In manifest carriers, there is an increased inactivation of the normal X chromosome.

X-linked dominant disorders are rare. In these, both men and women can be affected, but women are usually less affected.

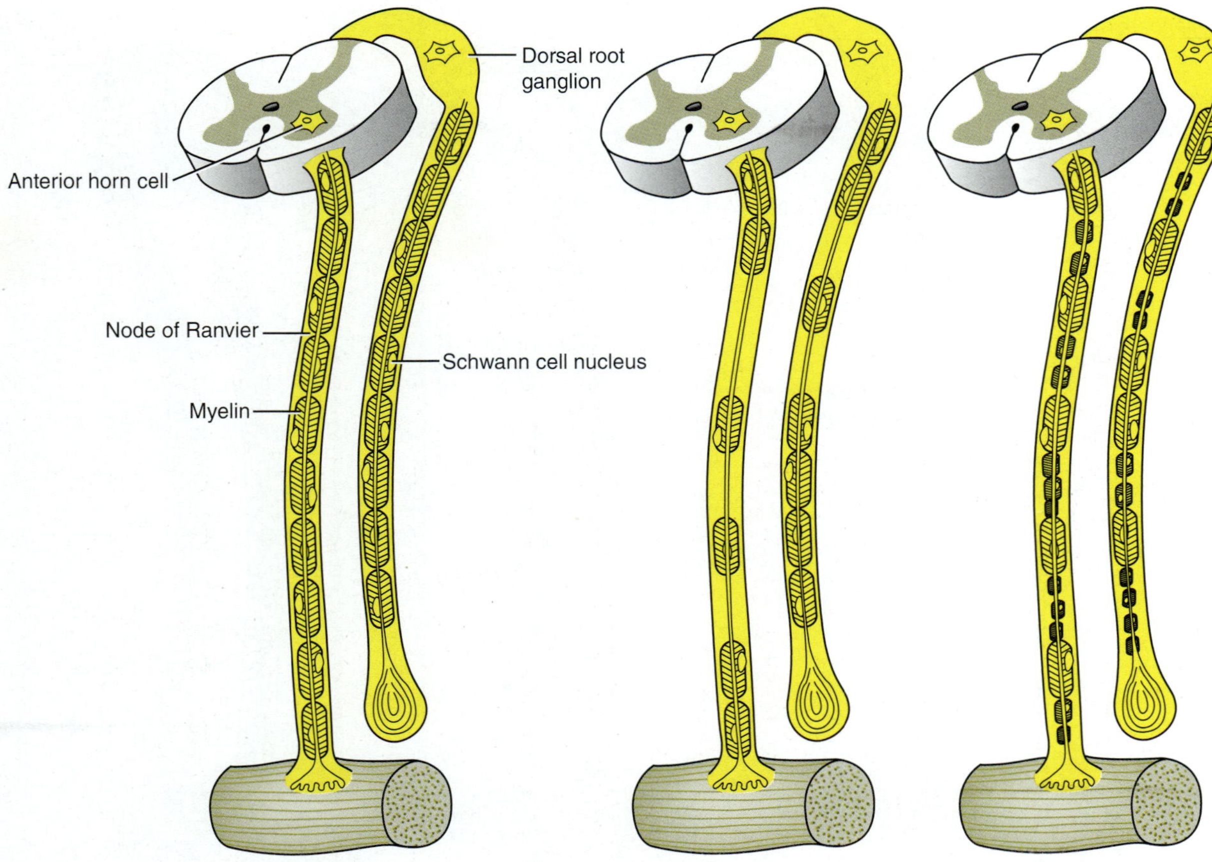

FIG 2-77 Diagram showing segmental demyelination with preservation of axons.

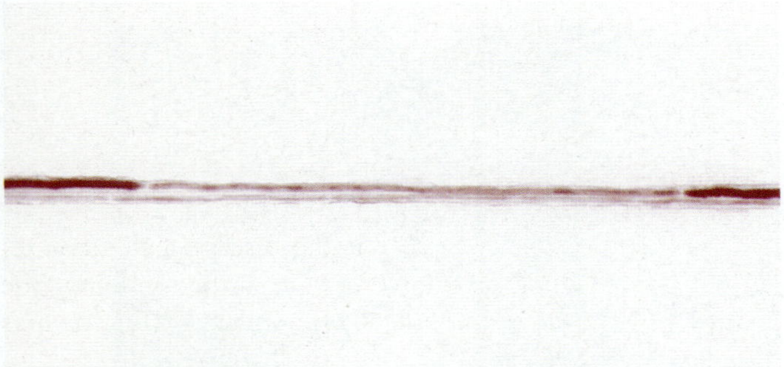

FIG 2-78 Osmicated teased nerve preparation showing segmental demyelination (×200).

Men transmit the disease only to their daughters; usually the cause is dominant alleles in the X chromosome.

Mitochondrial Inheritance

The mitochondria have their own genes, and unlike nuclear DNA, which consists of only two copies per cell (except for the X chromosome in males), mitochondrial DNA varies in each cell. Therefore, mitochondrial DNA mutation results in a mixed population of normal and mutant mitochondria, or *heteroplasmy*. Over time, cell lineages can also have pure mutant or pure normal DNA populations (homoplasmy).[106]

The sperm does not contain mitochondria, so all mitochondrial genes are inherited from the mother; thus, mitochondrial inherited disorders are maternally inherited, and both males and females can be affected. Mitochondrial inheritance can be traced to common female ancestors (for an interesting reading, see Reference 107). The effects of mitochondrial mutations vary among tissues. Clinical manifestations depend on the tissue and organs that are more energy dependent—such as muscle, heart, and brain—are primarily affected. Manifestations depend also on when energy production falls below a minimum (*threshold effect*). The mitochondria have 37 genes, of which 24 are involved in the translation and 13 encode units of the respiratory chain. Importantly, genes for other mitochondrial proteins are encoded by nuclear DNA, so that diseases of mitochondria function might also be caused by mutations of nuclear DNA.

Types of Genetic Mutations

Structural Chromosomal Abnormalities. These include loss or gain of an individual chromosome or extra copies of the entire set of chromosomes; others are ringing, large deletions, and translocations of fragments from different chromosomes.

Single-Gene Mutations. Nucleotide substitutions or deletions, also called *point* mutations, occur during DNA replication.

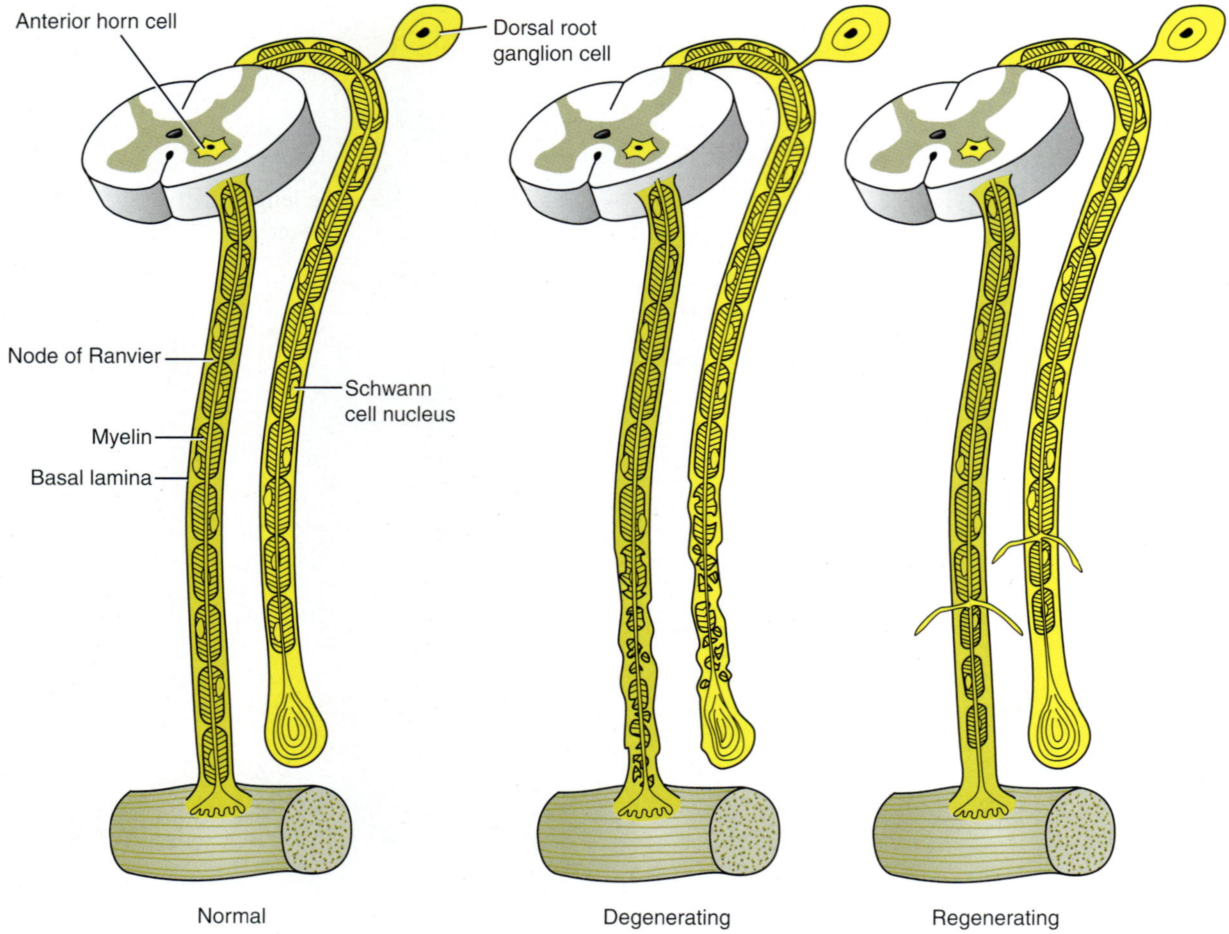

FIG 2-79 Diagram of distal axonal degeneration.

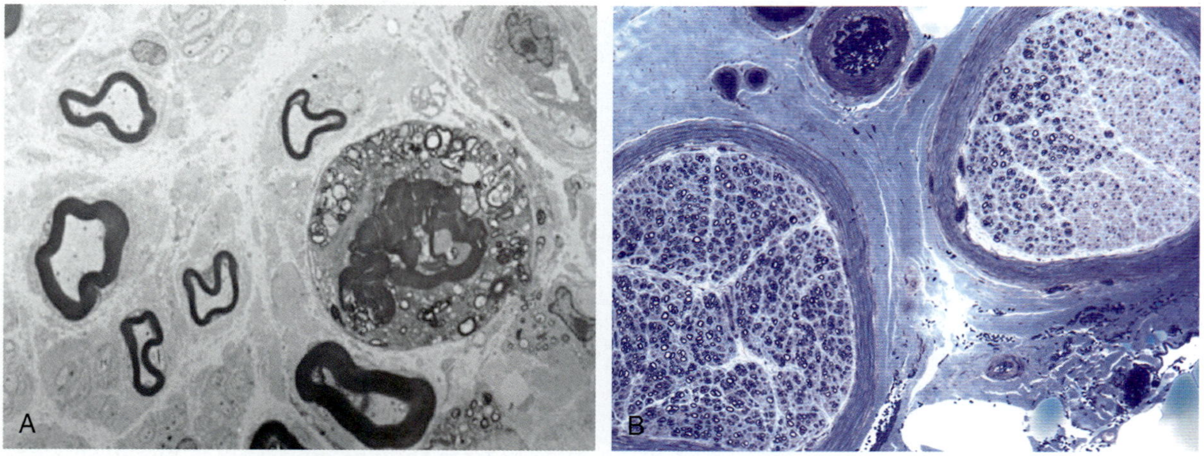

FIG 2-80 **A**, A degenerated axon on electromicroscopy (×4000). **B**, Section of the sural nerve with severe focal loss of myelinated axons in one fascicle (*right*), and a fairly normal population of axons in another (*left*), from a case of vasculitis (toluidine blue stain, ×100).

These result in one amino acid change and are called *missense* mutations. Those producing a change that results in *stop codons* and affects the reading frame for proteins are called *nonsense* mutations (Fig. 2-85).

Other mutations include deletions or insertions of one or a few nucleotides. Those that alter the reading frame are called *frameshift* mutations (Fig. 2-86). Some large mutations that include the whole exon can also occur. Duplications and inversions are other types of mutations. In duplications, mutations are homologous unequal crossovers that may be accompanied by a reciprocal deletion.

Splice mutations are mutations that occur during the processing or removal of the primary transcript. These sometimes consist of deletions of the entire exon, depending on the length of the mutation. These deletions could be *frameshift* mutations or could leave the reading frame intact, that is, *in-frame*.[101,102]

Expansion or Trinucleotide Repeat Sequences. Repeats of trinucleotides are normally found throughout the gene and are stable in various generations. A *trinucleotide sequence expansion* is a phenomenon in which there are expansions of the number of repeats of a nucleotide, and this causes a disease when they exceed certain numbers. For example, CTG repeat expansions within the gene that encodes the dystrophic myotonia protein kinase (*DMPK*) in chromosome 19q13 cause dystrophic myotonia type I; those that have over 100 repeats are more severely affected.

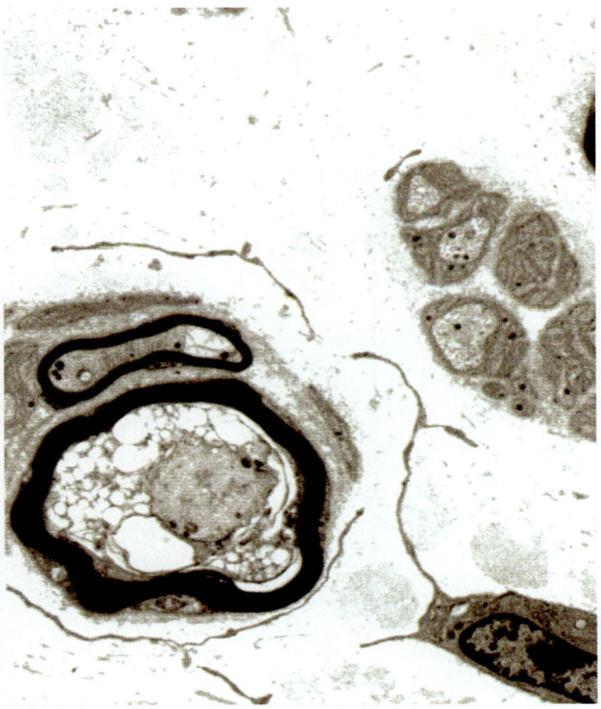

FIG 2-81 An atrophic and degenerating axon; notice normal unmyelinated axons (upper right) (×4000).

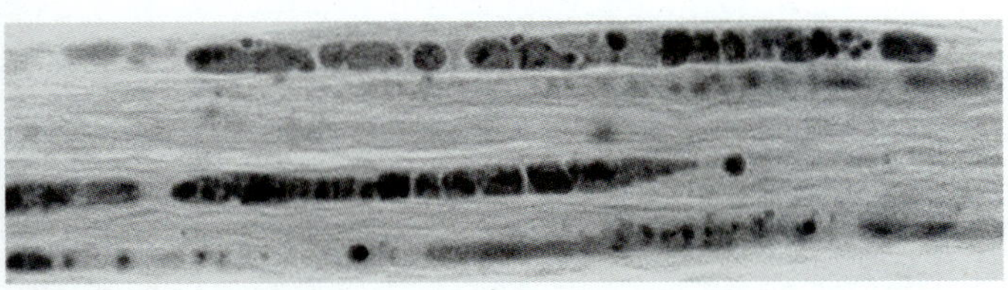

FIG 2-82 Teased nerve preparation showing characteristic myelin ovoids of axonal degeneration (×200).

In these disorders, the length of the repeat correlates with the age of onset and the severity of the disease. Because occurrences tend to increase in each successive generation, there are more-severe phenotypes that start at early ages. This phenomenon is called *anticipation*.

Another genetic mechanism that affects the phenotype is *imprinting* or the dependence of the gene expression on the parent of origin of the mutation. As the gene is transcribed by one allele, the severity of the expression varies according to the sex of the parent who transmitted the disease. By this mechanism, one of the inherited alleles is silenced (maternal or paternal) and only the other causes the disease, that is, the mechanism can be either *maternally imprinted* or *paternally imprinted*. In *uniparental disomy* both members of a chromosome pair are inherited from one parent.[108]

Molecular Genetic Tools

Molecular genetic diagnosis includes a number of tests, from *simple karyotype analysis*, which detects gross chromosomal abnormalities, to more elaborate tests to detect small deletions or mutations (Fig. 2-87). The latter are more important in neuromuscular disorders and are used if the genetic defect or its location has been identified. If the gene has not been identified, but its location is known, linkage analysis can be useful, as discussed later in this chapter.

More sophisticated cytogenetic fluorescence using in situ hybridization (FISH) increases the level of resolution; this method uses pieces of cloned and purified human genomic DNA, which is labeled and hybridized with a cytogenetic spread of the patient's chromosomes. FISH allows the detection of genetic variabilities such as chromosomal deletions and rearrangements.[99,101]

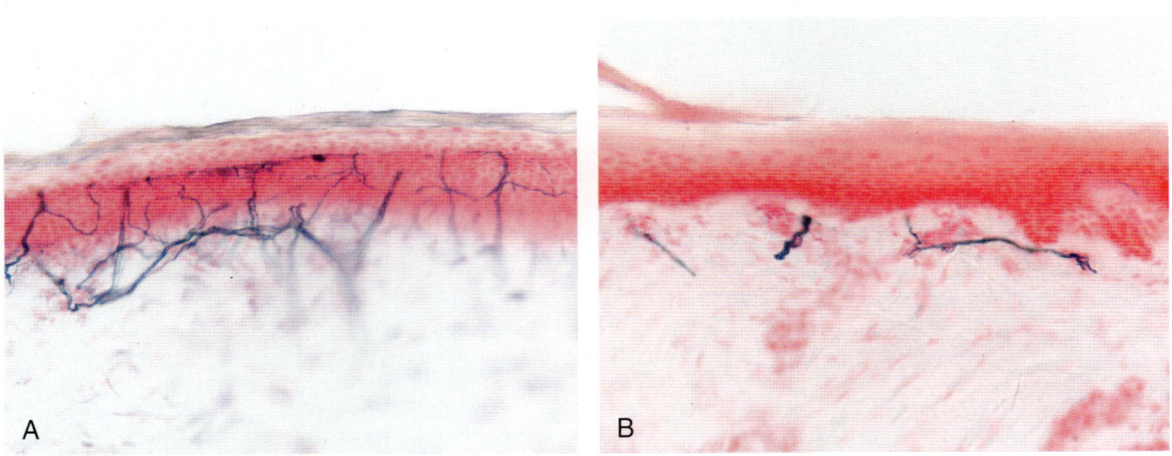

FIG 2-83 **(A)** A punch skin biopsy showing axons staining with protein gene product (PGP) (9.5) antibody contrasted with nuclear fast red, left normal nerve (×200) and **(B)** is diabetic neuropathy, notice the lack of small nerve fibers close to the epidermis (×200).

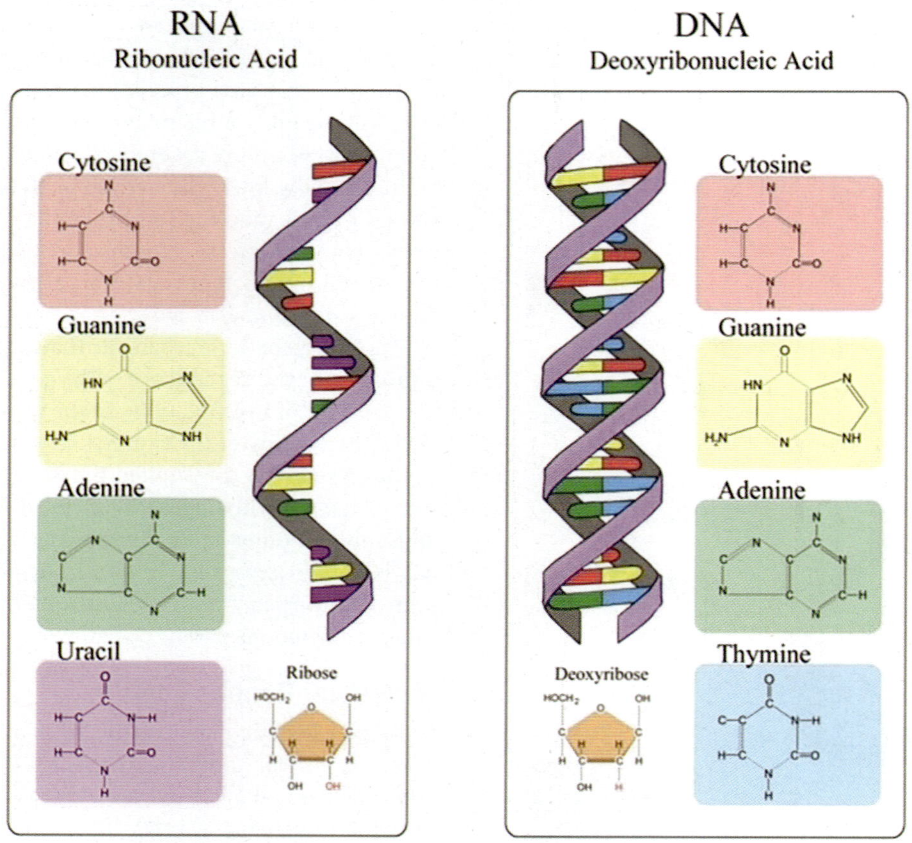

FIG 2-84 Diagram of RNA on the left and DNA on the right. These are made for chains of nucleotides which contain a phosphate base and a sugar which is ribose in RNA and deoxyribose in DNA and an organic base as listed for each. The RNA is opened and DNA is double helix. The RNA is single stranded and the base is uracid that replaces the thymine from DNA which contains thymine guanine and cytosine. (Modified from Narayanaswami, P, Zivkovic S Ch 11 of Bertorini TE ed. Neuromuscular Disorders Treatment and Management, Elsevier 2022.)

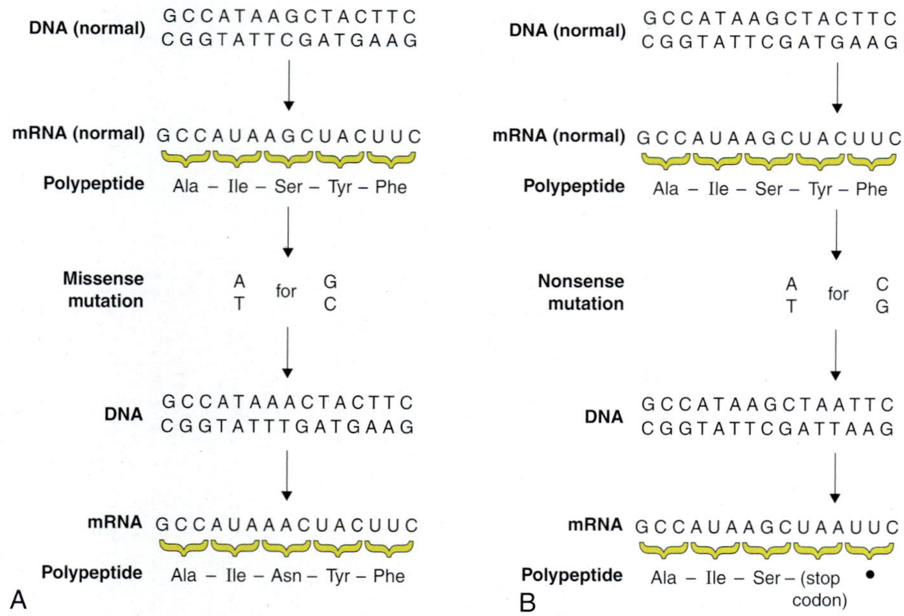

FIG 2-85 Base pair substitution. Missense mutations **(A)** produce a single amino acid change, whereas nonsense mutations **(B)** produce a stop codon in the mRNA. Stop codons terminate translation of the polypeptide. (Reprinted with permission from Jorde LB, Carney JC, Bamshad MJ, White RL, eds. *Medical Genetics*, 3rd ed. Philadelphia, PA, Mosby; 2007.)

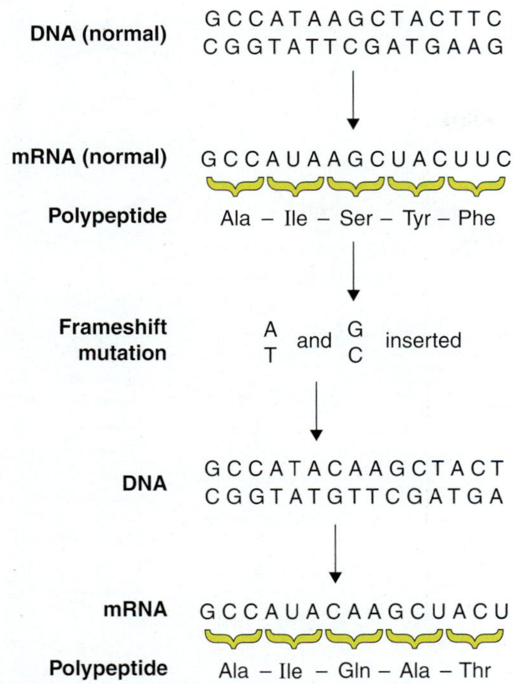

FIG 2-86 Frameshift mutations result from the addition or deletion of a number of bases that is not a multiple of three. This alters all of the codons downstream from the site of insertion or deletion. (Reprinted with permission from Jorde LB, Carney JC, Bamshad MJ, White RL, eds. *Medical Genetics*, 3rd ed. Philadelphia, PA, Mosby; 2007.)

Polymerase Chain Reaction. Polymerase chain reaction (PCR) is used to synthesize larger amounts of DNA for analysis. Many copies of DNA fragments that are generated allow their use in other diagnostic tests. The PCR method consists of the separation of the two strands of DNA into single strands that are then hybridized with *primers* of the sequence to be studied. Primers are synthetic oligonucleotides that serve as templates for the formation of DNA. The method uses *polymerase enzymes* (from bacteria) that synthesize DNA from deoxynucleotide diphosphates that are added to the reaction.[97,102]

Electrophoresis. Electrophoresis is a simple test in which fragments of DNA or RNA can be separated according to their size. This is based on the fact that negatively charged nucleic acid molecules migrate toward the anode in an electric field. A polymer gel matrix is used for the analysis, and the fragments are visualized as bands which are measured using fluorescent- or radioactive-based techniques. For example, in a disease caused by an expansion of CTG repeats, a larger than normal fragment is detected in the gel (Fig. 2-88).

Southern Blotting. The name of this method comes from Dr. Ed Southern who first described the technique that is used to identify DNA with nucleic acid hybridization. In this method, a segment of DNA containing the sequence to be studied is digested using *restriction enzymes*. The DNA is then transferred from a gel to a nitrocellulose filter. The DNA fragments are then hybridized with radioactive-labeled nucleic acid, proven to detect the target sequence (Fig. 2-89). The restriction enzymes are *endonucleases*, bacterial enzymes that recognize DNA sequences and cleave these into fragments of different sizes.[105]

Northern and Western Blotting. Northern blotting is similar to Southern blotting but is used to identify RNA molecules that are separated by gel electrophoresis according to their size. These are recognized using fragments of labeled complementary DNA, or *genomic probes*.

Western blots are used to identify proteins that are separated by polyacrylamide electrophoresis. After transferring to a membrane, the protein is identified by incubation with an antibody that binds to specific recognition sites; this primary antibody is then visualized with a secondary antibody that is labeled with a reagent for colorimetric detection (Fig. 2-90). The terms *Northern* and *Western* blotting do not identify individual scientists but are used to differentiate from *Southern* blotting.

Screening for Known Mutations. *Allele-specific oligonucleotide hybridization*, or dot blotting, is a method for testing known mutations. In this method DNA products generated by PCR are dotted in duplicate membranes: one membrane is dotted, or *hybridized*, with an oligonucleotide corresponding to the wild-type sequence, and the other to a mutant sequence. Normal individuals show hybridization only with the normal probe; homozygous individuals show hybridization only with the mutant probe; and heterozygous individuals hybridize with both probes (normal and wild-type).[97]

Restriction digest is a method that uses several restriction enzymes to detect variations from the expected digestion patterns of sequences.

Microarrays use nucleotide sequences placed in a solid support or chip. Then the test sample undergoes amplification by PCR and is then hybridized and analyzed with computer technology.[101]

Screening for Possible Mutations. *Multiplex PCR* is a technique by which different fragments of DNA are amplified and used for the detection of large mutations depending on their three-dimensional shape. *DNA sequencing* (Fig. 2-91) is used to determine the sequence of nucleotides and to detect mutations and their type.[109] Sequencing is difficult particularly when studying diseases caused by large genes.

Recently, automated simplified methods are used for diagnosing disorders such as muscular dystrophies caused by mutations of a large gene.[110–113] Next-generation sequencing can be done routinely, and this uses massive parallel sequencing to generate a large number of reads at once and is very time efficient and can be less expensive, and is used in genetic diagnostic panels.[114] This identifies mutations providing identification of single nucleotide variations, insertions, and deletions. It is used in screening patients such as those with limb-girdle muscular dystrophy (LGMD) and familial neuropathies. The technique has limitations as it does not detect repeat expansions for which standard PCR and Southern blot analysis are helpful. Examples of this include myotonic dystrophy and some familial forms of ALS. When the tests are not informative, then whole exon sequencing could also be used, but at this time it is very expensive and time consuming. Finally, another alternative

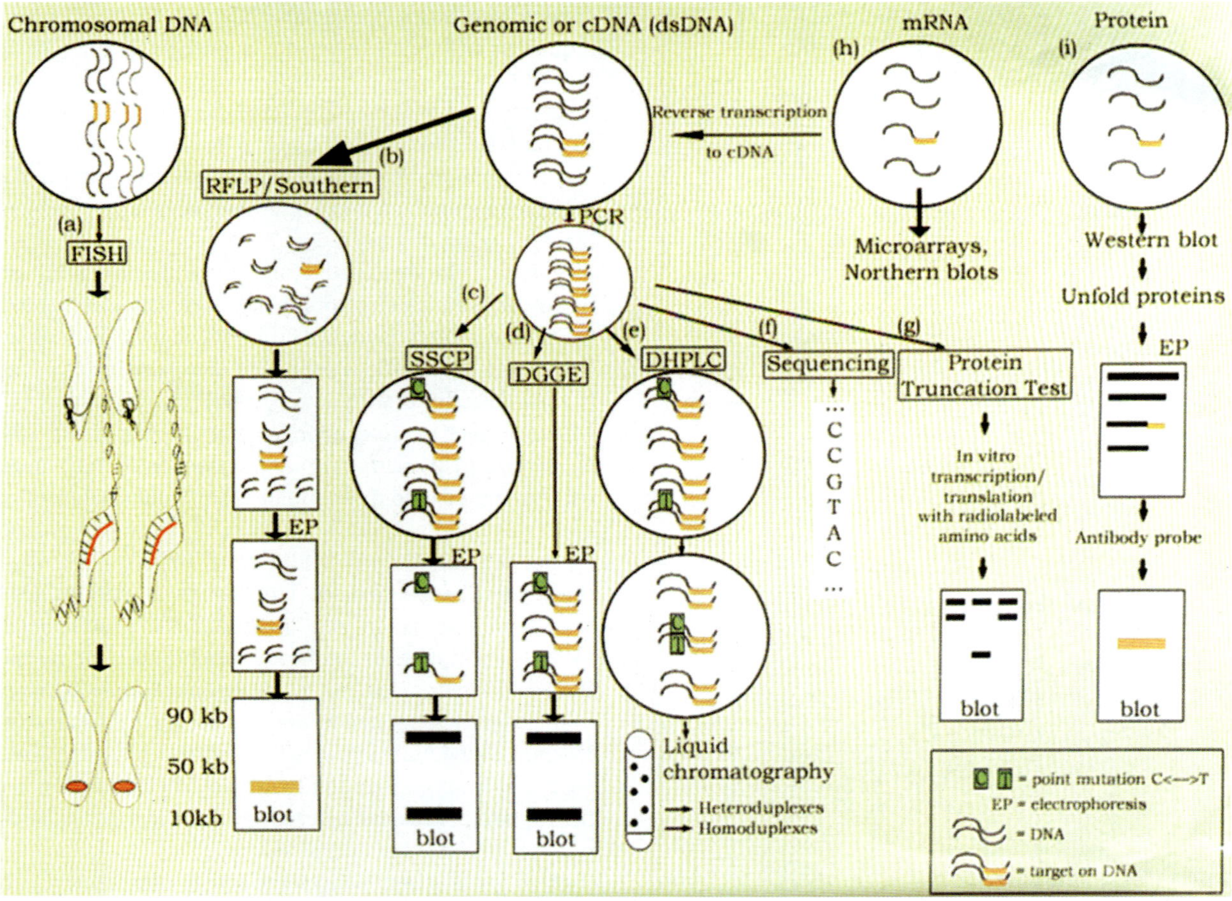

FIG 2-87 Commonly used molecular diagnostic methods. **(a)** Cytogenetic methods, such as fluorescent in situ hybridization (FISH), are done on whole cells or chromosomes; chromosomes are denatured, a probe added, and then renatured. Most other methods start with in vitro genomic DNA, mRNA, or protein. **(b)** Southern analysis: dsDNA is fragmented by restriction enzymes, separated by gel electrophoresis, denatured to single-stranded DNA, and then probed. A number of techniques (c to g) start with PCR amplification to obtain large quantities of the dsDNA sequence of interest. These include the various denaturing techniques, sufficiently sensitive to detect single base mutations, though these will identify both polymorphisms and mutations, requiring subsequent sequencing to define which: **(c)** single-strand conformation polymorphism analysis (SSCP) in which dsDNA is denatured and then separated by electrophoresis (EP); **(d)** denaturing gradient gel electrophoresis (DGGE) in which the denaturing of SSCP is incorporated into a single step with electrophoresis using a denaturing gradient gel; and **(e)** denaturing high-performance liquid chromatography (DHPLC), in which dsDNA is denatured, then annealed, and then separated by liquid chromatography. When a point mutation is present (i.e., c for g in the figure), some dsDNA with a mismatched base pair will form ("heteroduplexes") and have different mobility through the column. **(f)** Sequencing is frequently done with the automated-fluorescent dye-terminator method. **(g)** The protein truncation test, often starting with mRNA that is reverse transcribed to cDNA, involves in vitro synthesis of protein and detects nonsense mutations that result in premature truncation of protein during translation. **(h)** mRNA methods include reverse transcription to cDNA, followed by any of the other dsDNA methods noted, or by microarray analysis, or direct measurements using Northern blots. **(i)** Protein methods include tissue immunohistochemistry (not shown) and, for in vitro isolation of proteins, Western blot, which requires the use of specific antibodies as probes to the protein of interest. (Reprinted with permission from Greenberg S, Walsh RT. Molecular diagnosis of inheritable neuromuscular disorders. Part II: Applications of genetic testing in neuromuscular disease. *Muscle Nerve*. 2005;31:431–451.)

would include whole gene sequencing techniques,[110] but at this time it is also very expensive. Karyotype chromosome microarrays can be used to determine large deletions, duplications, and translocations.

With the use of next-generation sequencing, one frequently encounters variants of unknown significance, which means that they have not been reported in a disease at the time of the test, and may be benign and nonpathogenic variants but is not unlikely that at a later date could be associated with particular diseases.[114] RNA sequencing is a promising tool in genetics, but this is used in tissue samples.

Single confirmation polymorphism: This method is used to detect mutations depending on the three-dimensional shape of single-stranded DNA molecules of the sequence. DNA sequences first undergo amplification by PCR and then are denatured by heating and rapid cooling. The single strands form

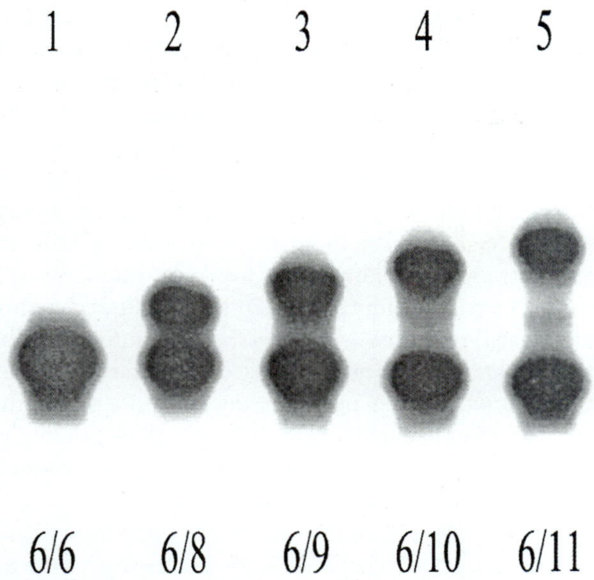

FIG 2-88 Molecular analysis of the poly(A) binding protein 2 (PABP2) gene trinucleotide repeat. Polymerase chain reaction analysis with primers flanking the (GCTGN) repeat in five individuals referred for diagnostic testing for oculopharyngeal muscular dystrophy. Numbers denote GCG sizes. The patient in lane 1 is homozygous normal for two alleles carrying six GCG repeats. Patients in lanes 2–5 carry expanded alleles (GCG8–11) within the *PABP2* gene. Alleles in this size range are associated with the clinical manifestations of oculopharyngeal muscular dystrophy. (Courtesy Dr. Nicholas Potter, Department of Medical Genetics, University of Tennessee Medical Center, Knoxville.)

sequence-specific structures that can be analyzed in standard polyacrylamide gel to observe for variations.

Heteroduplex formation with denaturing gel electrophoresis and high-performance liquid chromatography (DHPLC) are important tests used to detect mutations of DNA after amplification by PCR; these are then denatured, resulting in single strands. Thereafter, these are renatured by cooling, producing combinations of three different products: (1) *homoduplexes* (normal–normal and mutant–mutant); (2) *heteroduplex* (normal–mutant), which does not hybridize at the location of the mutation; (3) change of the motility characteristics of the fragments on electrophoresis. The fragments can also be analyzed by DHPLC instead of electrophoresis.[102]

Linkage Analysis. Methods of linkage analysis are used in pedigrees affecting individuals of various generations and when a gene has not been identified but its location is known. Linkage analysis is based on the principle of *linkage disequilibrium*, determining if two closely linked markers follow each other in one pedigree. The markers used for diagnosis are DNA sequences that are polymorphic and heterozygous in a random population. *Restriction enzymes* are used to detect polymorphisms of different sizes in the restricted fragments, or *restriction fragment length polymorphisms*. These fragments are neutralized and separated, allowing hybridization with primers to detect affected members by tracking the mutations. Tandem repeats are stretches of DNA formed entirely of mono-, di-, tri-, and tetranucleotides. Tetranucleotides are now also used for linkage analysis.[97,98]

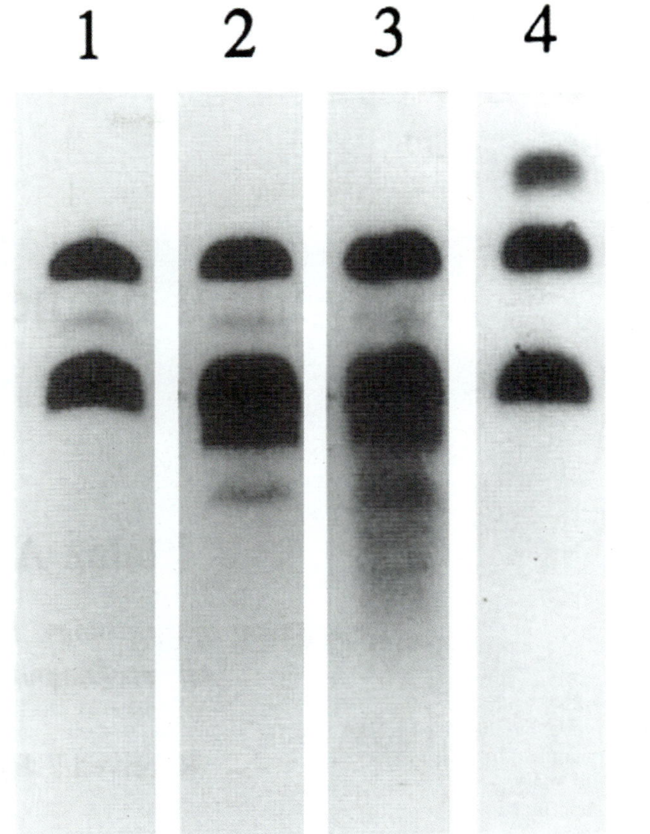

FIG 2-89 Autoradiogram for the direct detection of the type 1A Charcot–Marie–Tooth disease (CMT 1A) mutation and the hereditary neuropathy with liability to pressure palsies (HNPP) mutation by restriction endonuclease digestion and Southern blot analysis of pulse-field gel electrophoresed (FGE) genomic DNA. Lane 1 is a normal control, lanes 2 and 3 are positive CMT 1A, and lane 4 is an HNPP control, respectively. (Reprinted with permission from Almasaddi M, Bertorini TE, Seltzer WK. Demyelinating neuropathy in a patient with multiple sclerosis and genotypical HMSN-1. *Neuromuscul Disord.* 1998;8:87–89.)

When and What Genetic Tests Does One Order?

Genetic tests can be used for direct diagnosis of inherited disorders, sometimes obviating the need for invasive tests such as muscle biopsy, and for identifying the need for genetic counseling.[112] When performing this, proper pedigree should be reported using standard terminology and symbols (Fig. 2-92). Most genetic mutations can be tested in blood, including mitochondrial disorders. However, in mitochondrial disorders the lack of a detectable mutation in leukocytes does not preclude the diagnosis, and analysis of muscle tissue may be necessary.

Genetic tests are done in patients who appear to be affected by a disease that occurs in the family or who have a phenotype that is highly suggestive of a hereditary disease, even if there is no family history, as the subject could represent a new mutation.

Also, tests should be done on individuals who have some features, but not the complete phenotype, of a particular disease. For example, a man with a motor neuron disease with bulbar and limb weakness, fasciculations, and areflexia needs to be tested for the mutation of Kennedy's disease in the

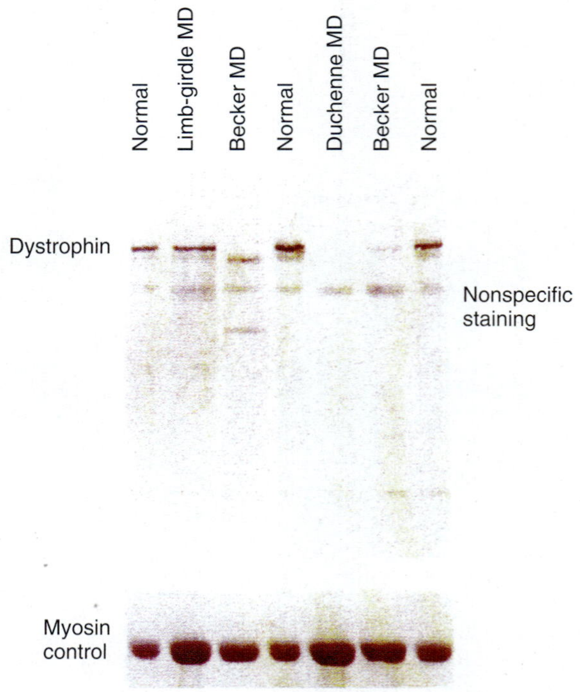

FIG 2-90 An immunoblot analysis showing dystrophin as a large protein present in the muscle biopsy from a normal individual. Duchenne's MD patients do not show any detectable protein, whereas Becker's MD patients may have shorter or less dystrophin (qualitative and quantitative abnormality). (Reprinted with permission from Miller RG, Hoffman EP. Molecular diagnosis and modern management of Duchenne muscular dystrophy. *Neurol Clin.* 1994;12:699–725.)

androgen receptor gene, even if there is no evidence of gynecomastia, testicular atrophy, or other features of the disease. This allows the clinician to diagnose a more benign disorder and to initiate proper genetic counseling. On the other hand, in typical amyotrophic lateral sclerosis (ALS) the diagnosis should be made by clinical observation, electrophysiologic studies, and ancillary tests, such as imaging, because the incidence of inherited ALS is no more than 10%, and, even in those, most genetic tests are not commercially available. Mutations of the Cu/Zn superoxide dismutase (*SOD*) gene,[115] however, should be investigated in those ALS patients with an autosomal dominant inheritance. Other genes to be considered in ALS ere the C9orf72 (chromosome 9 open reading frame) which actually can be detected in sporadic cases. The AR DNA binding protein or TDP43 and the FUS (fuse in sarcoma) genes could also be studied in suspected cases of the disease.

As another example, in the case of a floppy infant with fasciculations suspected to have SMA, proper testing for the SMA mutation in chromosome 5q is diagnostic, avoiding the use of invasive diagnostic methods.

An important consideration when ordering genetic tests is that routine screening tools might not detect the suspected genetic mutation, for example, when there is a point mutation. In those, the diagnosis should be made with immunohistochemistry or Western blot to test for the protein defect, as in dystrophonopathies, or by sequencing.

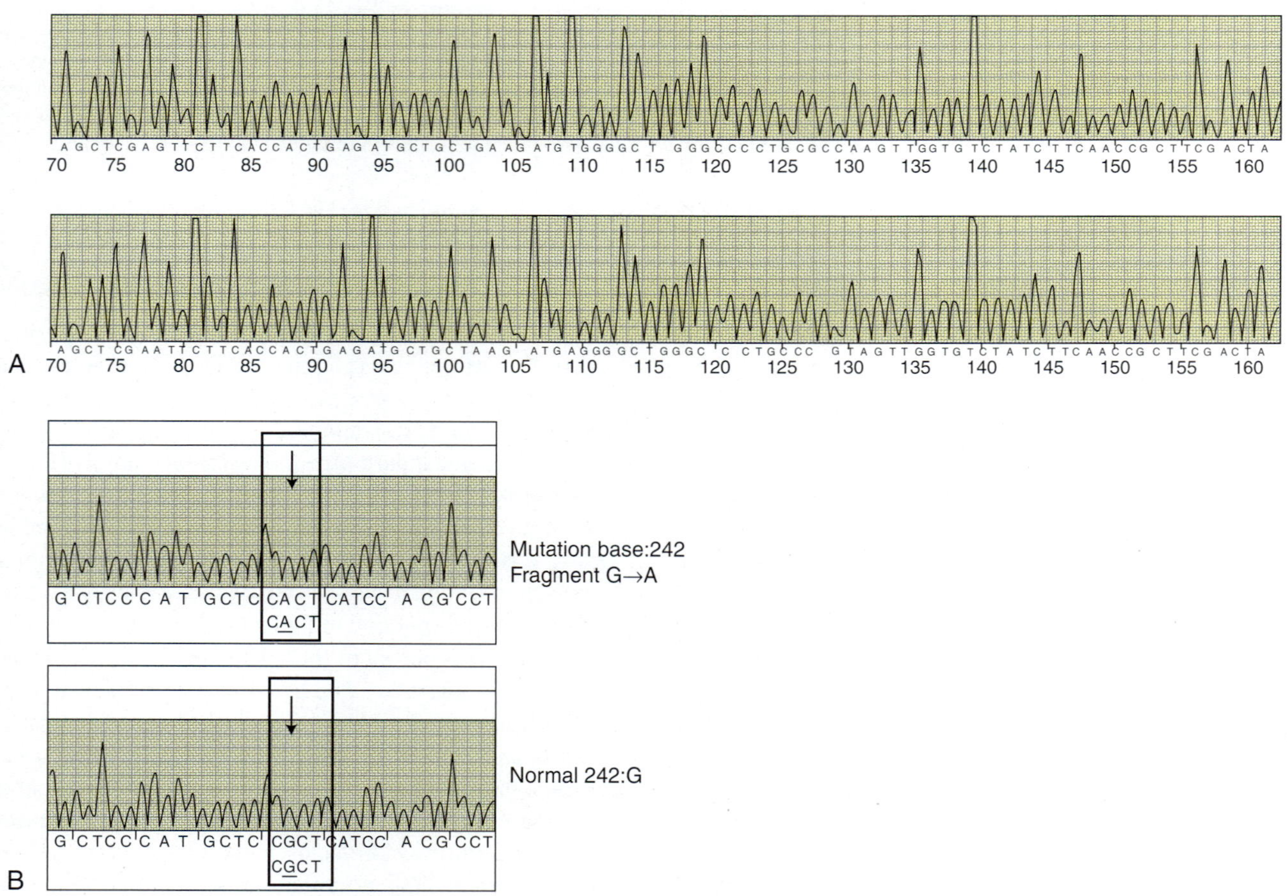

FIG 2-91 **A**, A sequencing analysis of the calcium channel gene (*top*) and normal (*bottom*). This is better demonstrated in the diagram showing a mutation of guanine for adenine in base 242 from a patient with hypokalemic periodic paralysis **(B)**.

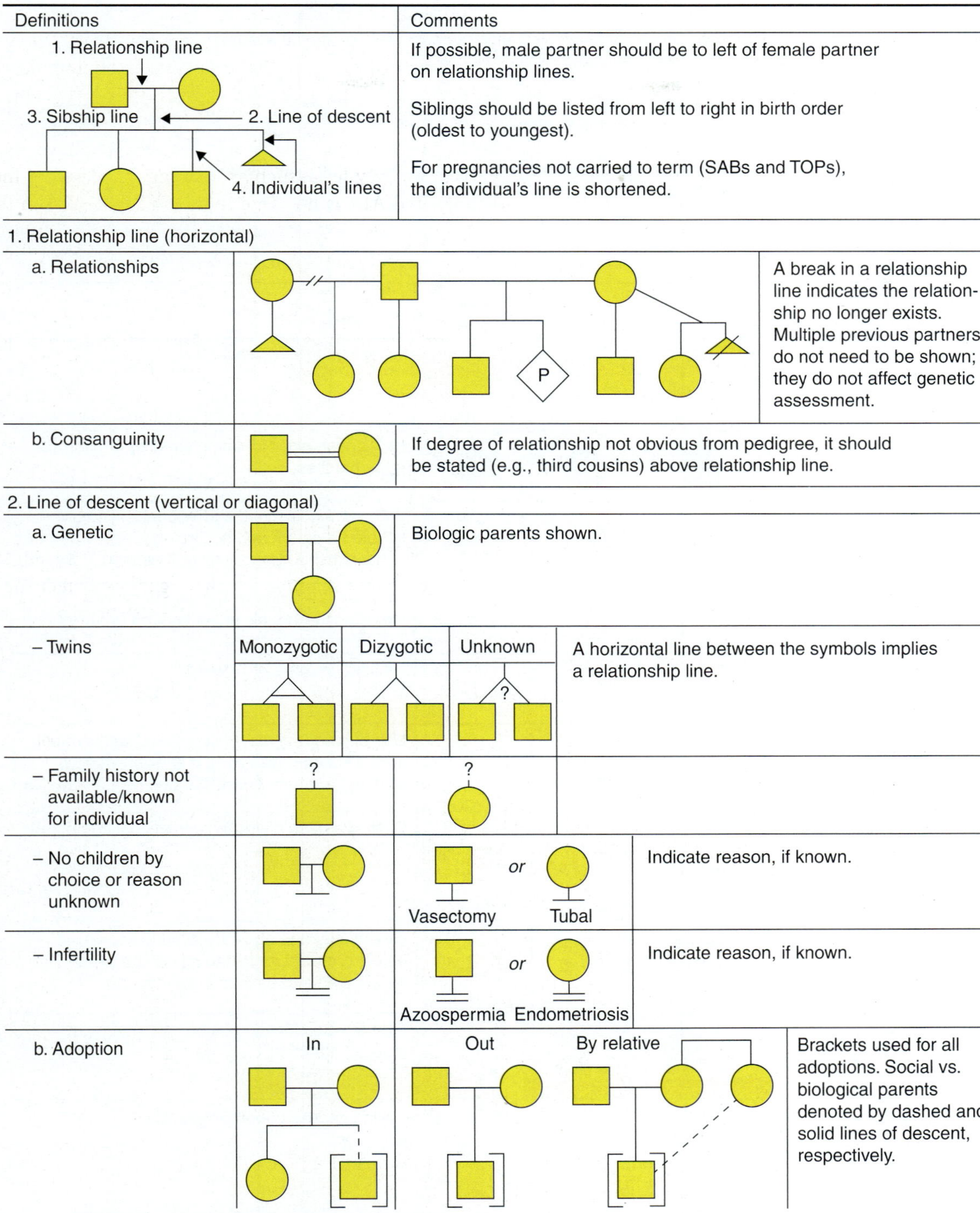

FIG 2-92 Pedigree symbols. (Reprinted with permission from Bennett RL, Steinhaus KA, Uhrich SB, et al. Recommendations for standardized human pedigree nomenclature. Pedigree Standardization Task Force of the National Society of Genetic Counselors. *Am J Hum Genet.* 1995;56:745–752.)

Genetic testing also helps in some disorders when a conclusive diagnosis cannot be made by other methods. For example, in LGMD caused by a sarcoglycan deficiency, the defective sarcoglycan cannot be identified by Western blot or by histology, because the lack of one sarcoglycan causes the absence of the others. Such a case requires genetic tests for individual sarcoglycan mutations. Also, patients with LGMD 2I have mutations of the *FKRP* gene. This is not diagnosed histologically but rather by mutation analysis.

Molecular diagnostic tests may also provide inconclusive data, for example, when the number of CTG repeats in a suspected case of myotonic dystrophy type I is borderline. Another problem arises when the patient has the disease phenotype, but not the genotype. In facioscapulohumeral (FSH) dystrophy, for example, some patients do not have the common genetic defect.

In some inherited diseases, testing for all mutations is not commercially available, or not all genetic defects are known, for example, cerebellar degenerations, Charcot–Marie–Tooth

Instructions:
___ Key should contain all information relevant to interpretation of pedigree (e.g., define shading)
___ For clinical (non-published) pedigrees, include:
a) family names/initials, when appropriate
b) name and title of person recording pedigree
c) historian (person relaying family history information)
d) date of intake/update
___ Recommended order of information placed below symbol (below to lower right, if necessary):
a) age/date of birth or age at death
b) evaluation
c) pedigree number (e.g., 1-1, 1-2, 1-3)

	Male	Female	Sex Unknown	Comments
1. Individual	b. 1925	30 yr	4 mo	Assign gender by phenotype.
2. Affected individual				Key/legend used to define shading or other fill (e.g., hatches, dots).
				With ≥2 conditions, the individual's symbol should be partitioned accordingly, each segment shaded with a different fill and defined in legend.
3. Multiple individuals, number known	5	5	5	Number of siblings written inside symbol. (Affected individuals should not be grouped.)
4. Multiple individuals, number unknown	n	n	n	"n" used in place of "?" mark.
5a. Deceased individual	d. 35 yr	d. 4 mo		Use of cross (†) may be confused with symbol for evaluated positive (+). If known, write "d," with age at death below symbol.
5b. Stillbirth (SB)	SB 28 wk	SB 30 wk	SB 34 wk	Birth of a dead child with gestational age noted.
6. Pregnancy (P)	P LMP: 7/1/94	P 20 wk	P	Gestational age and karyotype (if known) below symbol. Light shading can be used for affected and defined in key/legend.
7a. Proband	P ↗	P ↗	P ↗ P	First affected family member coming to medical attention.
7b. Consultand	↗	↗	Individual(s) seeking genetic counseling/testing.	

FIG 2-92, cont'd. Pedigree symbols.

disease type 2,[110] and limb-girdle dystrophies.[113] In these cases, and when there is a large and informative pedigree, one might consider performing these studies in an academic center.

Information on genetic defects or available tests can be obtained from large university or commercial laboratories or on the Internet using dedicated websites. Examples of these websites are listed below:

www.ataxia.org
www.sem.com
www.veloxmedia.com
www.molgen.ua.ac.be/CMTMutations/
www.dmd.nl/
www.ncbi.nlm.nih.gov
hugo@hugo-international.org
www.genetests.org

REFERENCES

1. Bertorini TE. Clinical evaluation and clinical laboratory tests. In: Bertorini TE, ed. *Clinical Evaluation and Diagnostic Tests for Neuromuscular Disorders*. Boston, MA: Butterworth-Heinemann; 2002.
2. Griggs R, Mendell J, Miller R. Evaluation of the patient with myopathy. In: Griggs R, Mendell J, Miller R, eds. *Evaluation*

and Treatment of Myopathies. Contemporary Neurology Series. Philadelphia, PA: FA Davis; 1995:17–78.
3. Narayanaswami P, Bertorini TE. The dropped head syndrome. *Neuromuscul Disord.* 2000;2(2):106–112.
4. Brooke M. Clinical evaluation of patients with neuromuscular disease. In: Shapria A, Griggs R, eds. *Muscle Diseases.* Boston, MA: Butterworth-Heinemann; 1999:1–30.
5. Brooke M. A clinician's view of neuromuscular disease. In: Brooke M, ed. *The Symptoms and Signs of Neuromuscular Disease.* Baltimore, MD: Williams & Wilkins; 1986:1–33.
6. Haerer AF, DeJong RN. *DeJong's The Neurologic Examination.* Philadelphia, PA: Lippincott-Raven; 1992.
7. Clausen JL. *Pulmonary Function Testing: Guidelines and Controversies.* Orlando, FL: Grune & Stratton; 1983.
8. Moore MR. Biochemistry of porphyria. *Int J Biochem.* 1993;25(10): 1353–1368.
9. Bertorini TE. *Myoglobinuria. Malignant hyperthermia. Neuroleptic malignant syndrome. Serotonin syndrome. Neurology Clinics of North America.* St. Louis, MO: WB Saunders; 1997:649–671.
10. Bertorini TE, Shively V, Taylor B, et al. ATP degradation products after ischemic exercise: hereditary lack of phosphorylase of carnitine palmityl transferase. *Neurology.* 1985;35:1355–1357.
11. McManis PG, Lambert EH, Daube JR. The exercise test in periodic paralysis. *Muscle Nerve.* 1986;9(8):704–710.
12. Solimena M, Folli F, Denis-Donini S, et al. Autoantibodies to glutamic acid decarboxylase in a patient with stiff-man syndrome, epilepsy and type I diabetes mellitus. *N Engl J Med.* 1988;318:1012–1020.
13. Narayanaswami P. Autoantibody testing. In: Bertorini TE, ed. *Clinical Evaluation and Diagnostic Tests for Neuromuscular Disorders.* Boston, MA: Butterworth-Heinemann; 2002:99–130.
14. Ho TW, Willison HJ, Nachamkin I, et al. Anti-GD1a antibody is associated with axonal but not demyelinating forms of Guillain-Barré syndrome. *Ann Neurol.* 1999;45:168–173.
15. Quarles RH, Weiss MD. Autoantibodies associated with peripheral neuropathy. *Muscle Nerve.* 1999;22(7):800–822.
16. Archelos JJ, Hartung HP. Pathogenetic role of autoantibodies in neurological disease. *Trends Neurosci.* 2000;23:317–327.
17. Hartung HP, Willison H, Jung S, et al. Autoimmune responses in peripheral nerve. *Springer Semin Immunopathol.* 1996;18:97–123.
18. Hays AP, Latov N, Takatsu M, Sherman WH. Experimental demyelination of nerve induced by serum of patients with neuropathy and an anti-MAG IgM M-protein. *Neurology.* 1987;37:242–256.
19. Kornberg AJ, Pestronk A. Chronic motor neuropathies: diagnosis, therapy and pathogenesis. *Ann Neurol.* 1995;37(suppl 1):S43–S50.
20. Kissel JT, Mendell JR. Neuropathies associated with monoclonal gammopathies. *Neuromuscul Disord.* 1996;6:3–18.
21. Latov N, Hays P, Sherman WH. Peripheral neuropathy and anti-MAG antibodies. *Crit Rev Neurobiol.* 1988;3:301–332.
22. Hart IK. Acquired neuromyotonia: a new autoantibody mediated neuronal potassium channelopathy. *Am J Med Sci.* 2000;319: 209–916.
23. Lennon VA, Lambert EH, Whittingham S, Fairbanks V. Autoimmunity in the Lambert-Eaton myasthenic syndrome. *Muscle Nerve.* 1982;5(suppl):S21–S25.
24. Sherer Y, Livneh A, Levy Y, et al. Dermatomyositis and polymyositis associated with the antiphospholipid syndrome—a novel overlap syndrome. *Lupus.* 2000;9:42–46.
25. Von Muhlen CA, Tan EM. Autoantibodies in the diagnosis of systemic rheumatic diseases. *Semin Arthritis Rheum.* 1995;24: 323–358.
26. Graus F, Cordon-Cardo C, Posner JB. Neuronal antinuclear antibody in sensory neuronopathy from lung cancer. *Neurology.* 1985;35:538–543.
27. Hadjivassiliou M, Chattopadhyay AK, Grunewald RA, et al. Myopathy associated with gluten sensitivity. *Muscle Nerve.* 2007;35:443–450.
28. Halford H, Graves A. Imaging techniques. In: Bertorini TE, ed. *Clinical Evaluation and Diagnostic Tests for Neuromuscular Disorders.* Boston, MA: Butterworth-Heinemann; 2002: 565–593.
29. Lodi R, Taivassalo T. Phosphorus magnetic resonance spectroscopy in the clinical investigation of muscle disorders. In: Bertorini TE, ed. *Clinical Evaluation and Diagnostic Tests for Neuromuscular Disorders.* Boston, MA: Butterworth-Heinemann; 2002:503–534.
30. Zuberi SM, Matta N, Nawaz S, et al. Muscle ultrasound in the assessment of suspected neuromuscular disease in childhood. *Neuromuscul Disord.* 1999;9(4):203–207.
31. Fuller NJ, Laskey MA, Elia M. Assessment of the composition of major body regions by dual-energy x ray absorptiometry (DEXA) with special reference to limb muscle mass. *Clin Physiol.* 1992;12(3):253–266.
32. Janssen L, Heymsfield SB, Baumgarter RN, Ross R. Estimation of skeletal muscle mass by bioelectrical impedance analysis. *J Appl Physiol.* 2000;89(2):465–471.
33. Rutkove SB. Electrical impedance myography, background current state and future directions. *Muscle Nerve.* 2009;40(6): 936–946.
34. Bertorini T, Knickerbocker J, Meter J. Clinical findings and segmental bioimpedance studies in adults with spinal muscular atrophy receiving intrathecal nusinersen. *Muscle Nerve.* 2019:65–67.
35. Bertorini T., Zhao Y., Meter J., Mays W., Talbot L. Segmental bioimpedance measurements in various neuromuscular diseases. Presented at the American Association of Neuromuscular Diseases and Electrodiagnostic Medicine. *Muscle Nerve.* 2019;60:21.
36. Bertorini TE. Sensory nerve conduction studies. In: Kimura J, editor. *Handbook of Neurophysiology.* Vol. 7. Amsterdam: Elsevier; 2006:155–176.
37. Kimura J. Principles and pitfalls of nerve conduction studies. *Ann Neurol.* 1984;16:415–429.
38. Oh SJ. Nerve conduction velocity tests: their clinical applications. In: Bertorini TE, ed. *Clinical Evaluation and Diagnostic Tests for Neuromuscular Disorders.* Boston, MA: Butterworth-Heinemann; 2002:141–207.
39. Oh SJ. *Clinical Electromyography: Nerve Conduction Studies.* Baltimore, MD: Williams & Wilkins; 1993.
40. Verdugo RJ, Dubrovsky AL. Computerized sensory evaluation. In: Bertorini TE, ed. *Clinical Evaluation and Diagnostic Tests for Neuromuscular Disorders.* Boston, MA: Butterworth-Heinemann; 2002:131–140.
41. Sunderland S. The anatomy and physiology of nerve injury. *Muscle Nerve.* 1990;13:771–784.
42. Hoffman P. Uber die Benziehungen der Schmemreglexe zur Wilkerlichen Bewegung and Tomus Z. *Lietsdar Biol.* 1918;68:307–370.
43. Verhagen WI, Schrooten GJ, Schiphof PR, van Ammers V. The H reflex of the medial vastus muscle: a study in controls and patients with radiculopathy. *Electromyog Clin Neurophysiol.* 1988;28:421–425.
44. Jabre JF. Surface recording of the H reflex of the flexor carpi radialis. *Muscle Nerve.* 1981;4:435–438.

45. Braddom RI, Johnson EW. Standardization of H-reflex and diagnostic use in S1 radiculopathy. *Arch Phys Med Rehabil.* 1974;55:161–166.
46. Panayiotopoulos CP, Chroni E. F-waves in clinical neurophysiology: a review, methodological issues and overall value in peripheral neuropathies. *Electroencephalogr Clin Neurophysiol.* 1996;101:365–374.
47. Fraser JL, Olney RK. The relative diagnostic sensitivity of different F-wave parameters in various polyneuropathies. *Muscle Nerve.* 1992;15:912–918.
48. Fisher MA. AAEM minimonograph #13: H-reflexes and F-waves: physiology and clinical indications. *Muscle Nerve.* 1992;15:1223–1233.
49. Lachman T, Shahani BT, Young RR. Late responses as aids to diagnosis in peripheral neuropathy. *J Neurol Neurosurg Psychiatry.* 1980;43:156–162.
50. Menkes DL. Proximal conduction techniques: somatosensory evoked potentials, magnetic stimulation, root stimulation. In: Bertorini TE, ed. *Clinical Evaluation and Diagnostic Tests for Neuromuscular Disorders.* Boston, MA: Butterworth-Heinemann; 2002:209–238.
51. Kimura J. Routine needle electromyography. In: Bertorini TE, ed. *Clinical Evaluation and Diagnostic Tests for Neuromuscular Disorders.* Boston, MA: Butterworth-Heinemann; 2002:331–364.
52. Layzer RB. The origin of muscle fasciculations and cramps. *Muscle Nerve.* 1994;17:1243–1249.
53. Richardson AT. Muscle fasciculation. *Arch Phys Med Rehabil.* 1954;35:281–286.
54. Albers JW, Allen 2nd AA, Bastron JA, Daube JR. Limb myokymia. *Muscle Nerve.* 1981;4:494–504.
55. Daube JR. AAEE minimonograph #11: needle examination in clinical electromyography. *Muscle Nerve.* 1991;14:685–700.
56. Dumitru D, King JC, Rogers WE, Stegeman DF. Positive sharp wave and fibrillation potential modeling. *Muscle Nerve.* 1999;22:242–251.
57. Kraft GH. Are fibrillation potentials and positive sharp waves the same? No. *Muscle Nerve.* 1996;19:216–220.
58. Stålberg E, Falck B. The role of electromyography in neurology. *Electroencephalogr Clin Neurophysiol.* 1997;103:579–598.
59. Nandedkar SD, Barkhaus PE, Sanders DB, Stålberg EV. Analysis of amplitude and area of concentric needle EMG motor unit actions potentials. *Electroencephalogr Clin Neurophysiol.* 1988;69:561–567.
60. Daube JR. Rubin Di: electrodiagnostics of muscle disorders. In: Engel AG, Franzini-Armstrong C, eds. *Myology.* 3rd ed. New York: McGraw-Hill; 2004:619–654.
61. Finsterer J, Mamoli B. Satellite potentials as a measure of neuromuscular disorders. *Muscle Nerve.* 1997;20:585–592.
62. Liguori R, Dahl K, Fuglsang-Frederiksen A. Turns-amplitude analysis of the electromyographic recruitment pattern disregarding force measurement. I. Method and reference values in healthy subjects. *Muscle Nerve.* 1992;15:1314–1318.
63. Nandedkar SD, Barkhaus PE. Quantitative analysis: objective and interactive assessment in electromyography. In: Bertorini TE, ed. *Clinical Evaluation and Diagnostic Tests for Neuromuscular Disorders.* Boston, MA: Butterworth-Heinemann; 2002:365–416.
64. Stalberg E, Chu J, Bril V, et al. Automatic analysis of the EMG interference pattern. *Electroencephalogr Clin Neurophysiol.* 1983;56:672–681.
65. Engel WK, Warmolts JR. The motor unit. Disease affecting it in toto or in portio. In: Desmedt JE, editor. *New Developments in Electromyography and Clinical Neurophysiology.* Vol. 1. Basel, NY: S Karger; 1973:141–177.
66. Dumitru D. Neuromuscular junction disorders. In: Dumitru D, ed. *Electrodiagnostic Medicine.* Philadelphia, PA: Hanley & Belfus; 1955:929–1029.
67. Ciafaloni E, Massey JM. Repetitive stimulation tests. In: Bertorini TE, ed. *Clinical Evaluation and Diagnostic Tests for Neuromuscular Disorders.* Boston, MA: Butterworth-Heinemann; 2002:81–294.
68. Oh SJ, Eslami N, Nishihira T, et al. Electrophysiological and clinical correlation in myasthenia gravis. *Ann Neurol.* 1982;12:348–354.
69. Schumm F, Stohr M. Accessory nerve stimulation in the assessment of myasthenia gravis. *Muscle Nerve.* 1984;7:147–151.
70. Kennett RP, Fawcett PR. Repetitive nerve stimulation of anconeus in the assessment of neuromuscular transmission disorders. *Electroencephalogr Clin Neurophysiol.* 1993;89:170–176.
71. McComas AJ, Galea V, Einhorn RW. Pseudofacilitation: a misleading term. *Muscle Nerve.* 1994;17:599–607.
72. Gilchrist JM, Sanders DB. Double-step repetitive stimulation in myasthenia gravis. *Muscle Nerve.* 1987;10(3):233–237.
73. Oh SJ, Kurokawa K, Claussen GC, Ryan Jr HF. Electrophysiological diagnostic criteria of Lambert-Eaton myasthenic syndrome. *Muscle Nerve.* 2005;32(4):15–20.
74. Lomen-Hoerth C. Motor unit number estimates. In: Bertorini TE, ed. *Clinical Evaluation and Diagnostic Tests for Neuromuscular Disorders.* Boston, MA: Butterworth-Heinemann; 2002:449–464.
75. Olney RK, Lomen-Hoerth C. Motor unit number estimates: how many it contributes to the diagnosis of ALS? *Amyotroph Lateral Scler Other Motor Neuron Disord.* 2000;23(suppl):S41–S49.
76. Bromberg M. Motor unit number estimations in peripheral neuropathy. In: Kimura J, ed. *Handbook of Clinical Neurophysiology.* Vol. 7. Peripheral Nerve Diseases. Amsterdam: Elsevier; 2006:281–294.
77. McComas AJ, Fawcett PR, Campbell MJ, Sica RE. Electrophysiological estimation of the number of motor units within a human muscle. *J Neurol Neurosurg Psychiatry.* 1971;34:121–131.
78. Olney RK, Yuen EC, Engstrom JW. Statistical motor unit number estimation: reproducibility and sources of error in patients with amyotrophic lateral sclerosis. *Muscle Nerve.* 2000;23:193–197.
79. Bromberg MB. Motor unit estimation: reproducibility of the spike-triggered averaging technique in normal and ALS subjects. *Muscle Nerve.* 1993;16:466–471.
80. Gooch C.L., Henderson R. Motor unit number estimates. Waltham, MA: UpToDate; 2019.
81. Stålberg E, Trontelj JV. *Single fiber electromyography. Studies in Healthy and Diseased Muscle.* 2nd ed. New York: Raven Press; 1994:1–291.
82. Wiechers DO. Single fiber electromyography with a standard monopolar electrode. *Arch Phys Med Rehabil.* 1985;66:47–48.
83. Trontelj JV, Stalberg E. Single-fiber and macro electromyography. In: Bertorini TE, ed. *Clinical Evaluation and Diagnostic Tests for Neuromuscular Disorders.* Boston, MA: Butterworth-Heinemann; 2002:417–449.
84. Bertorini TE, Stalberg E, Yuson CP, Engel WK. Single-fiber electromyography in neuromuscular disorders: correlation of muscle histochemistry, single-fiber electromyography, and clinical findings. *Muscle Nerve.* 1994;17:345–353.
85. Luciano CA. Other useful electrodiagnostic techniques: blink reflex, masseter reflex, and silent periods. In: Bertorini TE, ed.

Clinical Evaluation and Diagnostic Tests for Neuromuscular Disorders. Boston, MA: Butterworth-Heinemann; 2002:239–256.
86. Ongerboer de Visser B. Trigeminal reflex circuits. In: Valls-Sole J, Tolosa E, eds. *Brainstem Reflexes and Function*. Madrid: ENE Publicidad; 1998:67–78. chapter 5.
87. Ghonim M, Gavilan C. Blink reflex: prognostic value in acute peripheral facial palsy. *ORL J Otorhinolaryngol Relat Spec*. 1990;52:75–79.
88. Wang AK, Kaufmann H. Autonomic function testing. In: Bertorini TE, ed. *Clinical Evaluation and Diagnostic Tests for Neuromuscular Disorders*. Boston, MA: Butterworth-Heinemann; 2002:257–280.
89. Stewart JD, Low PA, Fealey RD. Distal small fiber neuropathy: results of tests of sweating and autonomic cardiovascular reflexes. *Muscle Nerve*. 1992;15:661–665.
90. Wang AK, Fealey RD, Gehrking TL, Low PA. Autonomic failure in amyloidosis. *Neurology*. 1999;52:A388.
91. Low PA, Caskey PE, Tuck RR, et al. Quantitative sudomotor axon reflex test in normal and neuropathic subjects. *Ann Neurol*. 1983;14:573–580.
92. Bertorini TE, Horner LH. Histology and histochemistry of muscle and nerve. In: Bertorini TE, ed. *Clinical Evaluation and Diagnostic Tests for Neuromuscular Disorders*. Boston, MA: Butterworth-Heinemann; 2002:595–692.
93. Reimers CD, Schedel H, Fleckenstein JL, et al. Magnetic resonance imaging of skeletal muscles in idiopathic inflammatory myopathies of adults. *J Neurol*. 1994;241(5):306–314.
94. DiMauro S, Shanske S, Naini A, Krishna S. Biochemical evaluation of metabolic myopathies. In: Bertorini TE, ed. *Clinical Evaluation and Diagnostic Tests for Neuromuscular Disorders*. Boston, MA: Butterworth-Heinemann; 2002:535–564.
95. Dubowitz V. Histological and histochemical reactions in muscle biopsy. A practical approach. London, England: Bailliere Tindall; 1993:19–40.
96. Midroni G, Bilbao JM. Peripheral neuropathy and the role of nerve biopsy. In: Midroni G, Bilbao JM, Cohen SM, eds. *Biopsy Diagnosis of Peripheral Neuropathy*. Boston, MA: Butterworth-Heinemann; 1995:1–12.
97. Gorospe JR, Hoffman EP. Basic medical genetics and molecular diagnostics. In: Bertorini TE, ed. *Clinical Evaluation and Diagnostic Tests for Neuromuscular Disorders*. Boston, MA: Butterworth-Heinemann; 2002:693–836.
98. Martin JB, Longo FM. Molecular neurobiology. In: Jameson JL, ed. *Principles of Molecular Medicine*. Totowa, NJ: Humana Press; 1998:871–890.
99. Koop P, Jameson JL. Transmission of human genetic disease. In: Jameson JL, ed. *Principles of Molecular Medicine*. Totowa, NJ: Humana Press; 1998:43–63.
100. Hoffee P, ed. *Medical Molecular Genetics*. Madison, CT: Fence Creek Publishing; 1998.
101. Malcolm S. Molecular methodology. In: Rimoin DL, Conner JM, Pyeritz RE, eds. *Principles and Practice of Medical Genetics*. 3rd ed. New York: Churchill Livingstone; 1996:67–84.
102. Walsh RJ, Greenberg SA. Molecular diagnosis of inheritable neuromuscular disorders. Part 1. *Muscle Nerve*. 2005;31: 418–430.
103. Priddy M. *Genome*. New York: HarperCollins; 2000.
104. Pulst S-M. Introduction to medical genetics. In: Pulst S-M, ed. *Neurogenetics*. New York: Oxford University Press; 2000.
105. Korf B. Molecular diagnosis. Part 2 of 2. *N Engl J Med*. 1995; 332:1499–1502.
106. Schon EA. Mitochondrial genetics and disease. *Trends Biochem Sci*. 2000;25:555–560.
107. Sykes B. *The Seven Daughters of Eve*. New York: WW Norton; 2001.
108. Bartolomei MS, Tilghman SM. Genomic imprinting in mammals. *Annu Rev Genet*. 1997;31:493–525.
109. Rosenthal N. Tools of the trade—recombinant DNA. *N Engl J Med*. 1994;331:315–317.
110. Flanigan KM, von Niederhausern A, Dunn DM, et al. Rapid direct sequence analysis of the dystrophin gene. *Am J Hum Genet*. 2003;72:931–939.
111. Shendure J, Mitra RD, Varma C, Church GM. Advance sequencing technologies: methods and goals. *Nat Rev Gen*. 2004;5:335–344.
112. Blancalana L, Moore SA, Shilling C, et al. Limb girdle muscular dystrophy in United States. *J Neuropath*. 2006;65(10): 995–1003.
113. Richards S, Aziz N, Bale S, Das S, et al. Standards and guidelines for the interpretation of sequence variants: a joint consensus recommendation of the American College of Medical Genetics and Genomics and the Association for Molecular Pathology. *Genet Med*. 2015;17(5):405–424.
114. Lupski JR, Reid JG, Gonzaga-Jauregui C, et al. Whole-genomic sequencing in a patient with Charcot-Marie-Tooth neuropathy. *N Engl J Med*. 2010;362:1181–1191.
115. Pramatarova A, Figlewicz DA, Krizus A, et al. Identification of new mutations in the Cu/Zn superoxide dismutase gene of patients with familial amyotrophic lateral sclerosis. *Am J Hum Genet*. 1995;56:592–596.

3

Therapy in Neuromuscular Diseases

Neuromuscular diseases are treated not only with drugs aiming to reverse the cause, such as the immunosuppressants in autoimmune neuropathies, myopathies, and myasthenia gravis (MG), but also with therapies that ameliorate symptoms such as those of painful neuropathy or dysautonomia. Treatments also consist of using methods that provide comfort, increase mobility, and improve the quality of life.

The therapeutic plan has to be individualized so that it involves a team approach[1] and also aims to manage complications, such as respiratory insufficiency, swallowing problems, and cardiac disease, which occur, for example, in some muscular dystrophies.[2]

An important consideration is the prevention and proper management of perioperative complications, for example, in those with MG who undergo thymectomy or other surgeries, during which weakness may increase and cause respiratory failure.[3,4] Patients with channelopathies and those with metabolic and congenital myopathies are predisposed to develop attacks of malignant hyperthermia syndrome. These patients should be properly monitored and receive both precautionary measurements and treatment for the attacks.[4]

Patients with motor neuron diseases such as amyotrophic lateral sclerosis (ALS) and those with severe myopathies may benefit from noninvasive ventilation as a conservative approach, but some may require tracheostomy for respiratory assistance.[1] This might also be necessary during a myasthenic crisis. Percutaneous endoscopic gastrostomy is also frequently necessary for feeding, particularly in ALS, and should be performed before there is significant respiratory failure.

Patients with muscular dystrophies are treated with tendon stretching and physical therapy which play an important role in management, as do proper exercise programs.[2,5] Tendon releases and scoliosis surgeries are done according to their severity when patients have an acceptable vital capacity. In our center, surgery for scoliosis is performed in curvatures of over 20 degrees with vital capacity over 50% of the predicted values for the body size.[3]

Patients with Duchenne's muscular dystrophy and those with limb-girdle dystrophies that affect the heart can benefit from angiotensin-converting enzyme inhibitors[6], beta-blockers, or mineralocorticoid receptor antagonists. Some might benefit from pacemaker and/or implantable defibrillators. Those with Becker's muscular dystrophy with prominent cardiac disease may sometimes need cardiac transplantation.[2]

There are several important complications in myotonic dystrophy that require symptomatic therapy. These include gastrointestinal dysmotility and cardiac arrhythmia, which may require pacemaker placement.[2] Patients may also develop respiratory insufficiency, show an increased sensitivity to anesthesia, and prove difficult to wean off the ventilator after surgery.[2]

Those with chronic peripheral neuropathies require management to prevent the development of foot ulcers from deformities and decreased pain perception. Proper use of orthosis, such as ankle–foot orthosis, and sometimes osteotomies are important choices in their management. The active participation of physical medicine and rehabilitation specialists is very valuable, and physical therapy and rehabilitation play a very valuable, and physical therapy and rehabilitation play a very important role in the management of patients with neuromuscular diseases.

It must be emphasized the role of stretching exercises and to maintain ambulation to preserve muscle function and also emphasize the need for proper bracing with the contribution of an occupational therapist and orthotists as well as other ambulator assistances and a wheelchair with adjustments.

We must also emphasize the important role of exercise to maintain function in these disorders.

Specific treatments are discussed in individual cases in this book. The remainder of this chapter covers the management of pain and dysautonomia, the treatment of disorders of neuromuscular transmission, and the use of immunosuppressants and newer genetic therapies.

TREATMENT OF PAINFUL NEUROPATHIES

Pain is a common complaint in patients with neuropathies, particularly those that affect small fibers, such as nociceptive C fibers and small myelinated A-delta fibers. Pain is a major problem in diabetics.

The symptoms of painful neuropathies include burning, aching, lancinating pains, and pins/needles paresthesias. Patients may also have allodynia and hyperalgesia.[7]

The pathogenesis of neuropathic pain includes multiple central and peripheral mechanisms. For example, there is increased sensitization of primary nociceptive afferents and increasing axonal excitability with ectopic discharges and ephaptic transmission. There could also be the formation of neuromas and alteration of the expression of ionic channels causing increasing nerve excitability.

Central sensitization occurs in the spinal cord and brain.[8–11] Their mechanisms include the release of cytokines and other inflammatory mediators with increased excitability of spinal sensory neurons and decreased activity of inhibitory neurons. Neuronal damage is caused by an increased activity of the AMPA and glutamate receptors and by the accumulation of calcium through the AMPA receptors. In chronic pain there is an increased expression of micro-opioid receptors and increased activity of substance P through the *N*-methyl-D-aspartic acid (NMDA) receptors, facilitating excitatory responses. There is also evidence of increased connections of nonnociceptive A-beta fibers to nociceptive neurons in the lamina II of the spinal cord.[9,11]

Sympathetic neuronal sprouting occurs in the posterior root ganglia with increased sensitization of C terminals and the release of inflammatory mediators from sympathetic nerve terminals.[12,13]

Finally, connections of sensory pathways with the limbic system might contribute to the emotional effects of chronic pain.

DRUGS USED TO TREAT CHRONIC PAIN

The rational approach for the management of chronic neuropathic pain includes the use of a combination of therapies that act in different areas of pain generation, including central and peripheral sensitization (Fig. 3-1).

First-line drugs are those whose benefit has been demonstrated with well-controlled clinical trials; these include tricyclic antidepressants, gabapentin, duloxetine, and pregabalin (see Fig. 3-1). These drugs can be used alone or in combination, for example, tricyclics in addition to gabapentin. Other therapies can be initiated when there is no response to first-line drugs. (Table 3-1 lists common drugs used in painful neuropathy, their side effects, and mechanisms of action.)

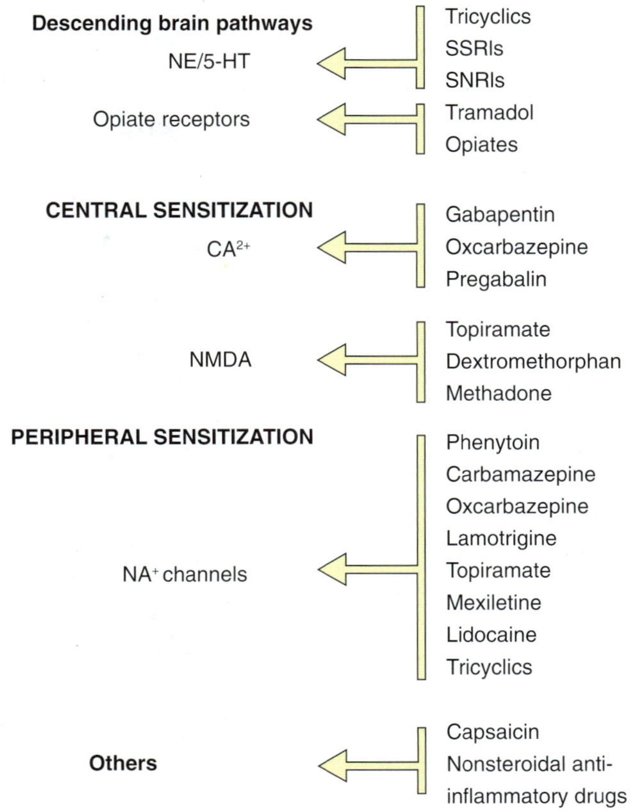

FIG. 3-1 Site of action of the different drugs used to treat neuropathic pain.

TABLE 3-1 Drugs Used in the Treatment of Pain

Drug	Mechanism	Side Effects
Antidepressants		
Tricyclics and tetracyclics	5-HT and NE reuptake inhibitors, Na^+ channel blockage	Sedation, cholinergic effects, glaucoma, dryness, constipation, psychosis, arrhythmias, and seizures; desipramine produces fewer cholinergic effects, nortriptyline fewer cardiac effects
Duloxetine	5-HT and NE reuptake inhibitor	Sedation, cognitive dysfunction, nausea, and minor cholinergic effects
Venlafaxine	5-HT and NE reuptake inhibitor	Sedation, psychosis, lowers seizure threshold, insomnia, nervousness; used in the treatment of tobacco addiction, and weight loss
Anticonvulsants		
Gabapentin	Ca^{2+} channel agonist	Dryness, cognitive dysfunction, and weight gain
Carbamazepine	Modulator of Ca^{2+} channel, blocks Na^+ channel	Sedation, dizziness, hyponatremia, liver toxicity, and leukopenia
Phenytoin	Blocks Na^+ channels	Hirsutism, osteopenia, anemia, rash, liver toxicity, neuropathy, and gingival hyperplasia
Pregabalin	Ca^{2+} channel blocker	Dizziness, weight gain, cognitive dysfunction, and swelling
Topiramate	Na^+ channel blocker	Glaucoma, kidney stones, sedation, and weight loss
Lamotrigine	Na^+ channel stabilization, glutamate release inhibitor, modulate Ca^{2+}, K^+ currents	Rash, Stevens–Johnson syndrome, needs slow titration, and liver toxicity
Mexiletine	Na^+ channel blocker	Leukopenia, arrhythmia
Analgesics		
Opiates (hydroxycodone, oxycodone, codeine)	Opioid agonists, bind opioid receptors, and mainly μ receptors	Sedation, dry mouth, nausea, constipation, respiratory depression, confusion, and addiction
Tramadol	Micro-opioid receptor agonist	Seizures, addictive potential, and nausea
Dextromethorphan	NMDA antagonist	Sedation, addictive potential
Medical marijuana	Acts in GABA and NMDA receptors, but exact mechanism unknown	Delirium, sedation Addiction potentials

5-HT, Serotonin; *GABA*, gamma-aminobutyric acid; *MNDA*, m-methyl-d-aspartic acid; *NE*, norepinephrine; *NMDA*, *N*-methyl-D-aspartic acid.

Tricyclic Antidepressants

These are serotonin (5-HT) and norepinephrine (NE) reuptake inhibitors with some effect on dopa reuptake. The tricyclics have a cyclical structure similar to phenothiazines, but with different mechanisms of action. The first tricyclic used was *imipramine*, which is metabolized to *desipramine*, while another tricyclic, *nortriptyline*, is a metabolite of amitriptyline.

Tricyclics are absorbed in the gut, bind to albumin, and are metabolized in the liver. Their effects in chronic pain include blockade of sodium channels, suppression of ectopic discharges, alterations of central NE and 5-HT reuptake, and central nociceptive modulation.[13,14]

Side effects and benefits of different tricyclics vary. The most common include constipation, orthostatic hypotension (OH), dry mouth, other cholinergic symptoms, and weight gain. They can precipitate attacks of narrow-angle glaucoma or cause urinary retention, particularly in patients with prostatic hypertrophy. These drugs should not be used concomitantly with monoamine oxidase (MAO) inhibitors.

Because of their sedative effects, tricyclics are usually given at nighttime for insomnia and nocturnal symptoms. Nortriptyline has fewer cardiovascular effects, such as arrhythmias, particularly in the elderly, while desipramine is less sedating and has fewer anticholinergic effects (see Table 3-1). The usual dosage of amitriptyline is 10–150 mg, nortriptyline 10–150 mg, desipramine 25–150 mg, and imipramine 50–200 mg.[15,16]

Atypical Antidepressants, Selective Serotonin, and Norepinephrine Reuptake Inhibitors

Venlafaxine is a 5-HT and NE reuptake inhibitor antidepressant also useful in chronic pain syndrome. Side effects include nausea, diarrhea, and sedation. The drug is used in dosages of 75–225 mg a day.[14,17]

Bupropion is a nontricyclic antidepressant that inhibits NE and dopamine reuptake. The drug is used in dosages of 150–300 mg a day for chronic pain. It has also been used for tobacco addiction. Bupropion causes less sexual dysfunction than other antidepressants but might produce hypertension and lower the threshold for seizures. The drug is eliminated primarily by the liver and its metabolism could be affected by other drugs.[18]

Duloxetine hydrochloride is a selective 5-HT and NE reuptake inhibitor introduced recently to treat painful diabetic neuropathy usually in dosages of 60 mg twice a day (higher doses can be used). This drug is eliminated mainly by hepatic metabolism in the P450 system. Side effects include minor cholinergic symptoms, nausea, vomiting, and constipation. Duloxetine may interfere with MAO inhibitors and may produce mild cognitive dysfunction and sedation, similar to tricyclics.[14] Because this drug metabolizes in the liver and kidney, it should be taken with caution in patients with liver or kidney failure.

Selective 5-HT reuptake inhibitors such as *fluoxetine* may help diminish depression but do not have proven effects in pain.[18]

Anticonvulsants

Anticonvulsants have been used extensively in neuropathic pain because of their action of diminishing peripheral and spinal cord pain–mediated mechanisms.[13,14,19,20]

Carbamazepine is closely related to tricyclics and acts by inhibiting sodium channels. The drug is used in doses of 200 mg three times a day, but the dosage should be adjusted slowly by titration, because the drug can cause dizziness and sedation, which is increased according to plasma levels, but tolerability varies. Side effects include not only dizziness but also sedation, hyponatremia, liver toxicity, and particularly aplastic anemia and agranulocytosis. Some patients might develop a rash. Carbamazepine is metabolized in the liver, and its metabolites are eliminated by the kidneys. In chronic users, levels should be monitored and dosage may need to be increased, because the drug is a self-inducer of its metabolism.

Oxcarbazepine is structurally similar to carbamazepine but has different pharmacokinetic and pharmacodynamic properties. It slows the recovery state of voltage-activated sodium channels, inhibits calcium channels, and reduces glutaminergic transmission, thus affecting central and peripheral mechanisms of pain. Oxcarbazepine has fewer bone marrow depressive effects than carbamazepine but can produce significant hyponatremia and sedation.[14]

Phenytoin has some effect in pain reduction by blocking sodium channels[19–21] and, because of its long half-life, can be used in single daily dosages, usually of 300 mg adjusted according to blood levels. Phenytoin is metabolized in the liver by the P450-enzyme system and its levels are affected by other drugs that utilize this system. Side effects of phenytoin are common, for example, hirsutism, gingival hyperplasia, mild peripheral neuropathy, bone marrow suppression, rash, Stevens–Johnson syndrome, macrocytic anemia and vitamin D deficiency, liver disease, and, rarely, cerebellar degeneration.

Valproic acid is a *carboxylic* acid derivative that potentiates gabaminergic neuronal activity. It benefits patients with chronic pain by potentiating inhibitory pathways.[14,19,22] Its starting dose is 15 mg/kg, increased up to 60 mg/kg, adjusting according to blood levels. The usual doses are 250–500 mg three times a day. Side effects include tremor, obesity, hair loss, skin rash, and liver dysfunction. Valproic acid should not be used in patients with liver disease. The drug could also cause bone marrow suppression and can produce teratogenic effects. The metabolism of valproic acid could be influenced by other drugs.

Gabapentin is a gamma-aminobutyric acid (GABA) agonist[23] with very weak antiepileptic activity but has significant effects on chronic pain. It is well tolerated and is eliminated mainly in the kidney, so it is not affected by other drugs that are metabolized in the liver. It competes with L-type amino acids for active transport, has a high affinity binding to the alpha-2-delta subunit of the voltage-activated calcium channels, inhibits sodium channels, and increases 5-HT concentrations. Daily dosages can be raised to 3600 mg a day or even higher, according to clinical response and side effects. Common side effects include dizziness, drowsiness, edema, and weight gain; significant cognitive dysfunction occurs with higher doses.

Lamotrigine is an anticonvulsant that not only stabilizes sodium channels and inhibits glutamate release but also has an effect on calcium and potassium currents. The drug is efficient in chronic pain management and is well tolerated.[24] The usual dosages can vary from 200 to 600 mg daily. The most significant side effect is rash which can be severe, and some patients develop Stevens–Johnson syndrome. The risks can be diminished with slow titration. Lamotrigine metabolizes in the liver and can be affected by other drugs such as valproic acid. Cognitive dysfunction is minimal.

Topiramate works by inhibiting voltage-gated calcium and sodium channels by enhancing GABA receptors and antagonizing glutamate receptors. It is particularly useful in the treatment of diabetic neuropathy[25,26]; side effects include loss of appetite and weight, somnolence, diarrhea, and dizziness. There is a risk of kidney stones, and the drug can precipitate attacks of glaucoma. Dosages vary from 100 to 400 mg a day given in divided doses.

Pregabalin is a new antiepileptic that acts preferentially, binding to the alpha-2-delta subunit of the voltage-gated calcium channels. Its antiepileptic effects are weak but it has a proven beneficial effect in painful neuropathies.[27,28] Pregabalin is eliminated primarily by the kidneys; only 9% is metabolized in the liver. Side effects include dryness, dizziness, weight gain, somnolence, edema, and infections. It can cause decreased cognitive function. The drug should be given with caution in patients with liver and kidney disease. The usual dosages are 75–150 mg two times a day.

Other Treatments

Antiarrhythmic agents such as *tocainide* and *mexiletine* have a peripheral effect, blocking sodium channels and thereby producing significant pain relief.[29] These drugs have also been used in the treatment of myotonia and in patients with muscle spasms of neurogenic origin.[30] Tocainide is no longer used because of its toxic effects. Opioids and other pain medications such as oxycodone and others are useful, but can cause addiction, and should be used with caution. Medical marijuana is now being used increasingly in the treatment of chronic pain. The main metabolites tetrahydroxy cannabinol and cannabidiol and other cannabinoids appear to be very useful in the management of chronic peripheral neuropathy pain.

Methadone is a 5-HT and NE reuptake inhibitor as well as an NMDA receptor antagonist and is very helpful in the management of pain that should be used with caution, because of addiction, and particularly should be given by pain specialists. Levorphanol is a synthetic opioid with NMDA receptor antagonism and is used in painful neuropathies. Tapentadol is a centrally acting drug that has a very strong analgesic effect with opioid and adrenergic features and has been proven to be helpful in diabetic neuropathy.[31]

Opioid analgesics are not only useful mainly in acute pain management but are also prescribed in some chronic pain syndromes, although these drugs cause addiction. Side effects include sedation and cholinergic symptoms, such as constipation and nausea. *Tramadol* is a nonnarcotic, centrally acting synthetic analgesic that has a low addicting potential compared with hydroxycodone or oxycodone. Tramadol is used in doses of 50 mg four times a day starting with slow titration. Higher dosages can be used; it may lower the threshold for seizures, cause constipation, and produce dryness and respiratory problems.[32] Other opiates can also be used in severe pain, but they have higher addictive effects.[33]

NMDA antagonists such as *dextromethorphan* provide mild relief in painful neuropathy and have side effects similar to tramadol.

Skin patches of the local anesthetic *lidocaine* and *capsaicin* are topical therapies for pain.[34–36] Capsaicin depletes substance P in nerve terminals. Magnets[37] and other nonspecific treatments, such as acupuncture, may also be helpful and is free of side effects, because of poor absorption; side effects may include skin irritation.

Topical lidocaine is a therapeutic method used to treat postherpetic neuralgia but can be used to treat chronic pain from neuropathy. High-frequency spinal cord stimulation produces substantial pain relief in diabetic polyneuropathy.[38]

TREATMENT OF AUTONOMIC DYSFUNCTION

Patients with peripheral neuropathy and other neuromuscular disorders might also develop symptoms of dysautonomia which include orthostatic hypotension (OH), constipation, bladder problems, and sexual dysfunction.

OH is treated with a commonsense approach, including proper hydration and by increasing fluid and caffeine intake during the day. Pressurized stockings are also helpful. Drugs that cause OH should be discontinued or used in lower doses.[39]

Midodrine hydrochloride is the drug most frequently used for OH. It is metabolized to desglymidodrine, an alpha-1 agonist that increases vascular tone and blood pressure. Because of this, a potential side effect is supine hypertension that can be severe at night. For this reason, it should be given with caution, avoiding late-night dosages, and patients taking it should sleep with their heads elevated. The usual dosage is 2.5–10 g four times a day.[40] Other similar drugs, such as *phenylpropanolamine and ephedrine*, are sometimes used in patients who cannot take midodrine.

Fludrocortisone is a potent mineralocorticoid that is used in a dosage of 0.1–0.2 mg two times a day. Side effects include hyperglycemia, fluid retention, edema, hypertension, hypokalemia, and, rarely, hypomagnesemia.[39]

Droxidopa in doses of 100–600 mg three times a day has been very useful and is a synthetic precursor of NE that induces peripheral brain and arterial vasoconstriction. The main side effects of concern include hypertension.

Other treatments include *erythropoietin* that might help by increasing blood expansion and is used in those with mild anemia. *Oteoclide*, which can be given in subcutaneous injections, is used in those with severe postprandial hypotension, in dosages of 0.2 mg/kg subcutaneously three times a day with meals. *Desmopressin* is a potent V2 renal vasopressor receptor agonist that produces nocturnal antidiuretic effects. It therefore can be used in patients with severe disease and nocturnal polyuria in a dosage of 10–40 μg transnasal every night.

Pyridostigmine also helps OH by increasing transmission in sympathetic ganglion.[41]

Decreased esophageal and intestinal motility and constipation are treated with proper hydration. Pyridostigmine can be helpful.

Metoclopramide is an anticholinergic and antidopamine agent that acts mainly in GI 5-HT receptors; it is sometimes of benefit in those with decreased esophageal motility. The drug is used in dosages of 5–10 mg three times a day. It can produce dryness, nausea, vomiting, and, particularly, confusion, dystonia, and parkinsonism. It can precipitate malignant neuroleptic syndrome. Proper use of stool softeners, bisacodyl, and senna can be helpful for constipation.

Urinary Symptoms

Urinary retention and particularly urinary incontinence can be caused by detrusor hyperreflexia which is treated with the anticholinergic *oxybutynin* in doses of 2.5–15 mg three times a day, or *tolterodine* in doses of 1–4 mg three times a day. Both drugs have extended-release forms. *Desmopressin* can be used because of its antidiuretic effects, particularly in those with nocturnal enuresis.

Sexual dysfunction in males is treated with a commonsense approach, including avoidance of drugs that can decrease libido and psychotherapeutic measurements.

Sildenafil citrate and similar drugs work by inhibiting cyclic guanosine monophosphate, which is a specific phosphodiesterase inhibitor that produces vasodilation of the corporae smooth muscle. They have several side effects, which include change in color perception, facial flushing, headaches, and, rarely, optic nerve damage. They might decrease platelet aggregability and have the potential to cause intracranial hemorrhage. This drug can also cause severe cardiovascular complications, particularly in patients with heart disease, and can potentiate vasodilation and hypotension caused by nitrates.

Other treatment includes vacuum constriction devices, urethral suppositories, and intracavernous injections of vasoactive drugs.

OTHER SYMPTOMATIC TREATMENTS IN NEUROMUSCULAR DISORDERS

Management of neuromuscular disorders also includes treatment and control of secondary symptoms that are not uncommon in patients with severe weakness, including sialorrhea in ALS and other motor neuron diseases from poor swallowing. This can be treated with anticholinergic drugs such as *glycopyrrolate* in doses of 1–2 mg three times a day and *benztropine* and *trihexyphenidyl* in doses of 2 mg three times a day. Dosages can be increased with caution; side effects include constipation, dryness, and confusion. These drugs can precipitate attacks of glaucoma. *Scopolamine patches* and tricyclics can also be used to decrease sialorrhea.

Antispasticity drugs are frequently used to treat patients with prominent upper motor neuron disorders. These include *baclofen*, a GABA agonist that is used in doses of 10–20 mg four times a day, but this can be increased up to 200 mg per day as tolerated. Baclofen metabolizes in the liver and interacts with other drugs. Side effects include sedation, dizziness, and liver toxicity. Rapid withdrawal can cause hallucinations. A potential problem, as with other muscle relaxants, is the possibility of increasing weakness.

Tizanidine is a centrally acting alpha 2-adrenergic agonist that relieves spasticity by increasing presynaptic inhibition of the motor neurons. The usual starting dosage is 2–4 mg three times a day, increasing to 36 mg a day as tolerated. Tizanidine not only is metabolized in the liver and has interactions with other drugs that utilize the P450 system but is also eliminated in the kidney. Its excretion might be affected in patients with kidney disease. The most significant side effects are sedation and dizziness, but the drug can also cause hypotension, as it has a mechanism of action similar to the antihypertensive clonidine and, rarely, can cause liver failure.

Quinine sulfate, a commonly used muscle relaxant, is also a sodium channel blocker. It is used for peripheral muscle cramps in doses of 260–375 mg a day. It is contraindicated in myasthenia gravis (MG), can produce thrombocytopenia, dizziness, and tinnitus, and could precipitate arrhythmias.

Benzodiazepines are centrally acting GABA agonists. The drug used most commonly is *diazepam*. It has sedating effects and can be addictive. Diazepam can be used in dosages of 5–10 mg three times a day. This and other benzodiazepines are metabolized in the liver, and their metabolism is affected by other drugs. Side effects include sedation and increased muscle weakness.

Dantrolene is a peripherally acting muscle relaxant that works via inhibition of the release of calcium by the sarcoplasmic reticulum in muscle; the usual dosages are 25–50 mg three times a day. This drug is helpful not only in spasticity but also in the prevention and treatment of attacks of malignant hyperthermia in the dosage of 2 mg/kg IV every 5 minutes until the attack is controlled.[4] We have found the drug to be beneficial in the treatment of muscle spasms, particularly in myopathies. Dantrolene is metabolized mainly in the liver and affects the metabolism of other drugs. It can cause severe sedation and, rarely, severe liver disease, particularly in young children.

TREATMENT OF MYASTHENIA GRAVIS AND OTHER DISORDERS OF NEUROMUSCULAR TRANSMISSION

The first-line therapy of MG includes the use of anticholinesterase drugs. Other treatments include immunosuppressants, plasma exchange, and gamma globulin infusions, discussed in the section on immunosuppressants. These are used in patients with generalized myasthenia and those with disabling ocular myasthenia who do not respond to anticholinesterase drugs.

Thymectomy is an effective treatment, particularly in those with generalized myasthenia, even if there is no evidence of thymoma.[42–44] In our center we first stabilize the patient prior to thymectomy, particularly with the use of plasmapheresis 2–3 weeks prior to surgery, depending on the clinical presentation. In patients with significant weakness, corticosteroids are initiated at least 1 month prior to thymectomy. Thymectomy has not been proven beneficial in controlled studies, but the evidence is very suggestive that this is an important therapeutic option. Most recommend a total or a transsternal thymectomy,[45] and this is the approach in our center. Proper management during the pre- and perioperative period is important to prevent complications.[3,45,46]

Pyridostigmine (Mestinon) is the most common anticholinesterase drug used to treat MG. Its pharmacologic effects are produced by inhibition of cholinesterase, the enzyme that metabolizes the neurotransmitter acetylcholine at the neuromuscular junction and the autonomic ganglia. It is given in doses of 60–120 mg every 4 hours; the dosage should be regulated according to the symptoms. A time-released preparation is also available but is not frequently used because of unpredictable absorption, though some give it in dosages of 180 mg three times a day. This preparation is used sometimes only at night to prevent early morning weakness. It should not be broken or split.

Patients who cannot take oral pyridostigmine may be given a parenteral dosage of $^1/_{30}$ of the usual oral dose.[43,44]

Side effects include muscarinic cholinergic symptoms such as increased secretions, bronchial spasms, diarrhea, and cramps. Pyridostigmine can also increase intraocular pressure. Excessive dosages can cause increased weakness and a cholinergic crisis. Allergic reactions to the bromide in the drug can occur. Pyridostigmine is metabolized mainly in the liver.

Neostigmine is another anticholinesterase drug, although used less frequently. It is given in doses of 15–30 mg every 4 hours; the total daily dose should not exceed 150 mg. Neostigmine can be given intravenously or intramuscularly in doses of 0.5–1.5 mg every 4 hours. This drug is also metabolized in the liver.

Ambenonium chloride is a seldom-used anticholinesterase drug that seems to produce fewer cholinergic side effects. The usual dosage is 7.5 mg but could go up to 15 mg every 6 hours as tolerated.

3–4 Aminopyridine is a potassium channel blocker that enhances acetylcholine release and is used in the treatment of Eaton–Lambert syndrome. The dosage is 5–20 mg four times a day. Side effects include tingling paresthesias, spasms, and seizures at a total dosage of 100 mg or more. Immunotherapy could be beneficial in these patients, particularly for those with idiopathic causes.

Ephedrine is helpful in some congenital myasthenic syndromes. *Fluoxetine* and *quinidine* are beneficial in the slow channel myasthenic syndrome.

IMMUNOTHERAPY

Many neuromuscular disorders have an autoimmune etiology whose treatments require the use of either a single or a combination of immunosuppressant drugs and other therapies such as plasma exchange and gamma globulin infusions. The most frequently prescribed immunotherapeutic drugs are described in the following subsections (summarized in Table 3-2).

Corticosteroids

These compounds are used to suppress the immune response and affect inflammation by their action on the glucocorticoid receptors and multiple signaling pathways.

Corticosteroids bind the glucocorticoid receptor complex, moving to the nucleus where they bind to DNA sequences called *glucocorticoid-responsive elements*. The resulting complex recruits coactivator or corepressor proteins that modify the structure of chromatin, facilitating or inhibiting transcription. They also act by signaling membrane-associated receptors and second messengers, using nongenomic pathways.[47]

The antiinflammatory effects are achieved by the inhibition of prostaglandin, by three independent mechanisms: (1) *activation and induction of annexin 1*, (2) *induction of MAPK phosphatase 1*, and (3) the *repression of transcription of cyclooxygenase 2*, as the cortisol–glucocorticoid receptor complex interacts with NF-κB to block its transcriptional activity, thus repressing cyclooxygenase 2. Corticosteroids also increase the activity of nitrous oxide synthetase, resulting in the formation of nitrous oxide.

The consequence of these various effects is decreased T-cell proliferation, macrophage activation, inhibition of the release of cytokine transcription and of proteolytic and lipolytic enzymes, and the transfer of leukocytes to areas of injury. Corticosteroids also increase apoptosis of auto-aggressive T cells.[47] These drugs affect predominantly cell-mediated immunity and have a lesser effect on B cell function.[48,49]

The most frequently used corticosteroid is *prednisone* which is converted in the liver to its active agent prednisolone. Prednisolone is eliminated in the liver, and only 2.5% of a prednisone dose appears in the urine. Enzyme-inducer drugs increase its metabolism. On the other hand, medications such as ketoconazole and some antibiotics and contraceptives delay its elimination. *Deflazacort* is an oral corticosteroid that appears to have lesser side effects than prednisone but is not available in the United States.

The usual dose of prednisone is 0.5–2 mg/kg daily up to 100 mg a day for 1 month and then switching to alternating days, but the dosages are individualized according to the clinical presentation and response to therapy.

Another method of treatment is by intravenous *methylprednisolone*, 1 g daily for 3–5 days. This dosage is repeated monthly tapering toward 1 g monthly. *Dexamethasone* can also be used in equivalent dosages; however, this compound has higher mineralocorticoid effects, causing more complications.

The side effects of corticosteroids are numerous; particularly, they cause Cushing's syndrome. Their chronic use causes adrenal atrophy and insufficiency, an important consideration when withdrawing therapy.

Other side effects include dyslipidemia, thrombosis, changes in behavior, insomnia, psychosis, and depression. Corticosteroids can also affect memory and can cause cortical cerebral atrophy, produce hyperglycemia, possibly increase the incidence of gastrointestinal bleeding from peptic ulcers, and can be associated with pancreatitis.[47,49,50]

TABLE 3-2 **Types of Immunotherapy**

Drug	Dosage	Side Effects	Drug Monitoring	Indications	Evidence Level according to the AAN criteria
Corticosteroids Prednisone	0.5-2 mg/kg po daily then taper	See Box 7-1	Weight, blood pressure, glucose, bone density, eye examination	CIDP Myasthenia gravis Vasculitic neuropathy Dermatomyositis Duchenne MD	C U U U A
Methylprednisolone	1 g IV q day x 3-5 days as initial treatment then 1 g IV weekly for 1 month before tapering or 500 mg po q week	See Box 7-1	As above	Discussed earlier MG PM	A V
IV Immunoglobulin	1-2 g/kg IV over 1-5 days; may be repeated 3-6 weeks	Headaches, chills, myalgias, renal insufficiency, thrombosis, rash, anaphylaxis	Blood pressure Serum creatinine during daily infusions Pseudohyponatremia and falsely elevated sedimentation rate may be seen	AIDP CIDP Myasthenia gravis Dermatomyositis	B B B C B
Subcutaneous IgG	5—mg weekly	Same	Same		
Therapeutic Plasma Exchange	500-5000 mL plasma volume per exchange x 4 exchanges	Pneumo-hemothorax, easy bruising or bleeding, hypotension	Blood pressure Calcium, fibrinogen	AIDP CIDP Myasthenia gravis	B C B
Inhibitors of Purine Synthesis Azathioprine	1-3 mg/kg po q day or divided bid. Initiate with a small dose (e.g. 50 mg) if TPMT assay not available. Reduce dose for those on ACE inhibitors.	Myelotoxicity, Nausea, Idiosyncratic "flu-like" symptoms, Pancreatitis, Infections	Advise assessing TPMT activity before initiating treatment. CBC weekly for 1 month then q 3 months. Liver function studies. Amylase, lipase if pancreatitis is suspected.	Myasthenia gravis CIDP Inflammatory myopathies	C U U
Methotrexate	5 mg/week to 25 mg/week po or IV/IM	Nausea Oral ulcers Hepatotoxicity Pulmonary fibrosis Infections	Screen for hepatits, interstitial lung disease on intitation. CBC and liver functions q 4-12 weeks. Yearly chest X-ray. Folic acid daily.	Inflammatory myopathies Neuromuscular Complications of Rheumatologic Disorders	U U
Mycophenolate mofetil	2-4 or 5 g daily, divided bid	Gastrointestinal upset, paresthesias, bone marrow suppression, liver toxicity (rare)	CBC weekly to monthly initially then tri-monthly	Myasthenia gravis CIDP myositis	B U U
Cyclophosphamide	0.5-1 g/m^2 IV q month	Myelosuppression, myelofibrosis, hemorrhagic cystitis, malignancy (especially bladder)	CBC weekly, liver function tests weekly for a month and then every 1 to 3 months, urinalysis every 1 to 3 months	Vasculitis CIDP Myasthenia gravis Inflammatory myopathies	U U U U
Calcineurin inhibitors Cyclosporin	3-5 mg/kg po q day divided bid	Hypertension, renal insufficiency, CNS toxicity, hirsutism	Trough drug levels weekly at first BMP weekly at first Avoid NSAIDS	Myasthenia gravis dermatomyositis	C U

Drug	Dosage	Side Effects	Drug Monitoring	Indications	Evidence Level according to the AAN criteria
Tacrolimus	3-4 mg up to 1 mg/kg po q day divided bid	Same as discussed earlier but less common, diabetes mellitus	Trough drug levels CMP monthly	Myasthenia gravis dermatomyositis	U U
Rapamycin	2-5 mg po q day	Hyperlipidemia	Periodic CMP	dermatomyositis	U
Monoclononal Antibodies Rituximab	0.375 g/m² IV weekly x 4 or 1 g IV q other week x2	Infusion reactions PML (rare)	CD20 CBC, CMP Brain MRI	MMN Anti-MAG neuropathy CIDP MuSK+ MG Acetylcholine R+ Myasthenia gravis	U U U A B B
Alemtuzumab	Varies	Infusion reaction Idiopathic thrombocytopenic purpura	CBC CMP	CIDP	U
NF-α Blockers Infliximab	3-6 mg/kg IV periodically	Infections Inflammatory neuropathy, vasculitis	CBC, CMP monthly	Dermatomyositis Polymyositis	U
Etanercept	25 mg sq biweekly	As above	As above	Dermatomyositis Polymyositis Myasthenia gravis CIDP	U
Anakinra	100 mg sq q day	Injection site reactions Diarrhea Infections Autoimmune disorders	CBC, CMP monthly	Inflammatory myopathies	U
Interferon-β-1a	30 μg IM q week	Injection site reactions, Flu-like symptoms Mild leucopenia, abnormal LFT's, abnormal thyroid function	CMP, TSH periodically	CIDP	U
Anti-thymocyte globulin	Varies	Serum sickness		Inclusion body myositis	U
Complement inhibitor Eculizumab	900 mg IV weekly x 4 then 1200 mg q 2 weeks	Infections by encapsulated bacteria such as meningococcus, etc	Vaccination for meningococcus, etc.	Acetylchonine R+ Myasthenia gravis MG	A
Ravulizumab	3,300 to 3,600 mg IV every 2 months	Same	CBC, CMP	Myasthenia gravis	A
Ziculoplan	0.3 mg/kg sub q or ER 0.3 mg/kg weekly	Same	CBC, CMP	Myasthenia gravis	A
Neonatal Fc receptor blocker Efgaratigimab Increase IGG and antibody clearance	10 mg/kg Sub q weekly X 4 weeks then repeat after one month if needed.	Low WBC, dehydration	CBC, CMP		A

CBC, Complete blood count; *CIDP*, chronic inflammatory demyelinating polyradiculoneuropathy; *IgG*, immunoglobulin G; *MG*, myasthenia gravis; *MMN*, multifocal motor neuropathy; *MuSK*, muscle-specific kinase; *TNF*, tumor necrosis factor; *WBC*, white blood count. Bold indicates the type of compound.

Additional side effects include skin atrophy, impairment of normal healing, erythema, hypertrichosis, dermatitis, petechiae, acne and striae rubrae distensae, aseptic necrosis of bones, type II muscle fiber atrophy, and osteoporosis and, in children, retardation of longitudinal bone growth. These drugs can also cause cataracts, glaucoma, sodium retention, obesity, hypertension, and hypokalemia and can cause polyhydramnios and fetal growth retardation.[50] Patients are usually given proton pump inhibitors and take calcium, vitamin D, and potassium supplements (if serum potassium is low). Drugs may also be needed to treat osteopenia, if this is significant, with proper monitoring of bone density. The new compound vamorolone has been found to be promising and has been beneficial in Duchenne dystrophy with fewer side effects than conventional corticosteroids. It is a dissociative steroid that has minimal cortical antagonistic effects producing fewer side effects.[51]

These drugs are used in the treatment of vasculitis and neuropathies associated with connective tissue disorders, polymyositis, dermatomyositis,[52,53] MG,[43] and chronic inflammatory demyelinating polyradiculoneuropathy (CIDP).[54,55] They do not help multifocal motor neuropathy (MMN) and in fact might aggravate this disease.[55,56]

Azathioprine

Azathioprine is an immunosuppressant used frequently as a steroid-sparing agent that can also be used as a first-line therapy. But because its effects might be delayed for weeks or even months—as occurs with other immunosuppressants—the drug could be given initially in combination with steroids and then later the steroids can be tapered off.

Azathioprine is absorbed in the gut and then distributed in the body. Thirty percent is bound to protein. The drug is converted by *xanthine oxidase* to form *6-mercaptopurine* which is secreted in the kidneys. Allopurinol, used in the treatment of gout, suppresses xanthine oxidase, and patients taking allopurinol should use reduced doses of azathioprine.[51,55]

The immunotherapeutic effects of azathioprine are mediated by *6-mercaptopurine*, which is a purine analog of hypoxanthine and guanine; this interferes with the synthesis of *purines*, reducing the production of RNA and DNA.[50,57,58]

Azathioprine decreases T- and B-lymphocytes and antibody production from B cell proliferation.[50,55]

The usual dosage is 1–3 mg/kg daily in single or divided doses, which are better tolerated. The doses can be increased up to 5 mg/kg, according to the clinical picture and the total white count. The doses should be lowered if the total white count falls below 3500 mm^3 and withheld if it reaches 2500 mm^3 or if the absolute neutrophil count falls below 1000 mm^3. The therapy should then be reinitiated after 2 weeks using lower dosages.

About 10% of the population is deficient in the enzyme *thiopurine methyltransferase*, which results in the reduction of azathioprine metabolism, increasing its toxicity.[59] This enzyme can now be measured in plasma. If this is not done, the azathioprine dose can be increased by 50 mg every 2 weeks until reaching the standard dose while monitoring the white blood count (WBC) for the first 8–12 weeks and then after 3 months, when the dosages have been stabilized according to the white cell counts and the clinical response. Complete blood count (CBC) and liver function are monitored every 3 months. The drug should be avoided in pregnancy because the active metabolites of azathioprine cross the placenta and can cause chromosomal abnormalities.

An important side effect of azathioprine is bone marrow suppression, which usually occurs in the first month. There is usually a mild leukopenia and macrocytosis, and although there is not a good correlation between the dosages with the erythrocyte mean corpuscular volume (MCV) one usually considers the dose to be therapeutic if this is increased and when it is associated with mild leukopenia of over 4000 mm^3. Nausea and vomiting are not uncommon, and some patients develop elevated liver enzymes. Rarely, they can develop an idiosyncratic reaction with high fever.[60,61] Pancreatitis and infections can occur, and those with long-term use may also develop tumors, particularly lymphomas, and could predispose to skin cancer. Azathioprine is used in the treatment of CIDP and other chronic autoimmune neuropathies,[50,54,55,62,63] stiff-person syndrome, MG,[63,64] and inflammatory myopathies.[65]

Mycophenolate Mofetil

Mycophenolate mofetil, introduced relatively recently, is isolated from penicillium mold cultures. It is used orally, absorbed in the gut, and hydrolyzed in the liver to make *mycophenolic acid* which is a noncompetitive inhibitor of *inositol monophosphate dehydrogenase*, an important enzyme in the synthesis for *guanosine nucleotides* and *purines*. Mycophenolic acid is metabolized to mycophenolic glucoside, which is secreted in the urine. Its immunosuppressant effects are mediated by its action in T- and B-lymphocyte proliferation. It also reduces the adherence of leukocytes to endothelial cells.[66–68] Mycophenolate appears to be more effective than azathioprine in preventing organ transplant rejection.

The usual dosage is 2 g daily in two divided doses; higher doses up to 3500 mg a day can be prescribed if well tolerated.[69] Some use dosages as high as 4–5 g,[56] which should be reduced in the presence of leukopenia.

Side effects include limb swelling with fluid retention, nausea, GI bleeding, vomiting, diarrhea, abdominal pain, pancreatitis, predisposition to infections, leukopenia, thrombocytopenia, and hepatic toxicity. Lymphoma can occur with its chronic use.[70]

The WBC should be monitored weekly for the first month and monthly for 3 months and then every 3 months.

This drug has more rapid therapeutic effects than azathioprine. It is well tolerated and used with increased frequency. Benefit has been reported in MG,[71] polymyositis/dermatomyositis,[52] and CIDP.[49,68,72]

A similar drug, antithymocyte globulin (ATG), a potent antibody against T cells, is promising for inclusion body myositis (IBM).[73]

Methotrexate

Methotrexate inhibits *dihydrofolic acid reductase*, the enzyme that reduces *dihydrofolate* to *tetrahydrofolate*, which is utilized in purine nucleotide synthesis. Thus methotrexate interferes with DNA synthesis, repair, and cellular replication.[74]

The drug interferes particularly with DNA of proliferating lymphocytes and suppresses interleukin 2. It also interferes with the active transport of folate across cell membranes, and folic acid might reduce the activity of methotrexate; on the other hand, folic acid deficiency might increase its toxicity.[75]

The usual dosage is 7.5–25 mg orally weekly, increasing in accordance with the total leukocyte and neutrophil count and red cell MCV. It can be used in doses of 25–50 mg parenterally, also weekly. The dosage should be reduced in renal failure. Acute methotrexate toxicity can be treated with leucovorin and hemodialysis.

Side effects include oral ulcers, skin rash, infections, leukopenia, pancytopenia, pulmonary fibrosis, diarrhea, dermatitis (excessive exposure to sunlight should be avoided), liver disease, and neoplasm.

Methotrexate is used in vasculitis and neuropathies associated with connective tissue disorders,[54,56] polymyositis, and dermatomyositis[52,53,65] and can be used in myasthenia and inflammatory neuropathies when other drugs are contraindicated or produce significant side effects.

Cyclophosphamide

Cyclophosphamide is an alkylating agent, like *chlorambucil* and *melphalan* which act particularly by cross-linking DNA and RNA. It thus inhibits the transcription and translation of proliferating cells, particularly rapidly proliferating T cells. It has a similar effect on resting B and T cells and also reduces antibody production. In low doses, it depletes suppressor and precursor cells and at high dosages reduces T helper cells. It can also reduce cytotoxic T cells and killer cells. In moderate doses, it inhibits mainly B cells.[76–78]

Cyclophosphamide is used orally in dosages of 1–2 mg/kg daily, which can be increased according to the WBC. It can also be given intravenously in doses of 0.5–1 mg/m^2 monthly. The drug is metabolized in the liver to active metabolites which are excreted in the kidney.

During intravenous use the WBC should be monitored carefully for leukopenia after 2 weeks. The total white count should be maintained at above 3500 cells/mm^3.

When using oral therapy, a CBC and a urinalysis should be performed monthly for the first 3 months and then tri-monthly.

Side effects include alopecia, nausea and vomiting, infections, and hemorrhagic cystitis, particularly when used orally; this can be prevented by proper hydration. The use of *2-mercaptoethane sulfate (Mesna)* binds and neutralizes *acrolein*, the toxic metabolite of cyclophosphamide.[50]

Cyclophosphamide can, rarely, cause liver disease. It can cause infertility and predispose to blood and bladder cancers and pulmonary fibrosis.

The risk of permanent bone marrow suppression and cancers increases with total cumulative doses of 80 g or more.

This medication has been used in polymyositis, dermatomyositis,[52,53] MG,[43,79] CIDP,[80] and other autoimmune neuropathies, particularly MMN,[54,56,81] and those associated with monoclonal gammopathy[82] and vasculitides.[73]

Cyclosporine

Cyclosporine is a drug similar to another more potent immunosuppressant, *tacrolimus*. It forms a heterodimeric complex with *cyclophiline* that binds to calcineurin, inhibiting its phosphatase activity, and thus the de novo expression of nuclear regulatory proteins and helper T-cell activation genes that encode interleukin 2. Through this mechanism cyclosporine inhibits the immune response, blocking the production of cytokines.

Oral cyclosporine absorption and metabolism vary in patients, and it is eliminated mainly by the liver.[49] The concentration is influenced by inhibitors of C4D3A4, such as some antibiotics and antifungal agents, or by inducers such as anticonvulsants.

The initial dose is 3–5 mg/kg per day in divided doses with maintenance of 2 mg/kg. Some patients need to receive as much as 7 mg/kg with proper monitoring of blood levels. The common dose of tacrolimus in MG is 3 mg/d.

Side effects include nephrotoxicity, hypertension, hirsutism, nausea, edema, infections, and gingival hyperplasia. The drug should not be given to patients who are breast-feeding because it is eliminated in the milk.[50]

Cyclosporine has been used in myasthenia gravis[43] and, rarely, in inflammatory myopathies. It has also been used in some cases of CIDP[49] and MMN.[83] Tacrolimus has been used particularly in myasthenia; it has similar side effects but can also cause hyperglycemia.

Rituximab

Rituximab is a chimeric monoclonal antibody that eliminates B-lymphocytes by binding the lymphocyte antigen molecule CD20, inducing apoptosis and cytolysis. This antigen is present exclusively in B-lymphocytes, and thus, affects plasma cells. Because of this, rituximab is used in complement and antibody-dependent cytotoxicity.[84,85]

The usual dosage is 375 mg/m^2 weekly for 4 weeks, repeating the cycle every 6 months.

Side effects include hypotension, nausea and vomiting, rash, fever and chills, leukopenia, infections, and thrombocytopenia.[85] WBCs should be measured 1 month after each infusion and in 3 weeks if the WBC is low. There are reports of progressive multifocal leukoencephalopathy developing in patients with lupus and lymphoma that received rituximab.[86]

Rituximab has been used in patients with MG[43] and in myasthenia crisis and stiff-person syndrome and is promising in those that have antibodies against muscle-specific kinase.[87] It is also beneficial in myelin- associated glycoprotein (MAG) associated neuropathy,[54,88] MMN, and refractory CIDP.[54]

Ocrelizumab is another CD20 inhibitor that has been approved to treat multiple sclerosis and potentially can be used in neuromuscular diseases.

Daratumumab is a monoclonal antibody that targets CD38, is used to treat multiple myeloma, and could be potentially helpful in MG, and we have treated one single patient with good response.

Plasma Exchange

Plasma exchange is a method of therapy that consists of removing the patient's plasma which is then replaced with albumin and saline supplement with calcium, acid citrate, dextrose, and heparin. Newer immunoabsorption techniques do not use albumin.

The exchange results in the removal of pathogenic immunoglobulins. One single exchange removes about 3–5 L of plasma, resulting in the reduction of circulatory immunoglobulin G (IgG) by 45%. Three to five exchanges are required to remove 90% of IgG.[49]

Plasmapheresis should be used when patients have large, accessible veins; if not, they may require placement of central catheters.

Side effects include hypotension, anemia, thrombocytopenia, allergic reactions, cardiac arrhythmia, vasovagal reactions, nausea and vomiting, electrolyte imbalance, and coagulopathy. Other complications include pneumothorax and large hematomas.[49]

Plasma exchange has been used in the treatment of Guillain–Barré syndrome, performing 5 plasma exchanges over a seven-day period.[49] In chronic disorders usually 1–2 exchanges are done weekly and afterward every 2 months. The drug is also beneficial in CIDP,[89] Miller–Fisher syndrome, and MG,[43] particularly during exacerbations and prior to thymectomy or other surgeries if necessary.

Gamma Globulin Infusions

Intravenous IgG infusion is a form of immunotherapy used initially in the 1950s for the treatment of patients with immune deficiency. Since then, it has been applied to a variety of autoimmune disorders. Gamma globulin is prepared by cold ethanol fractionation of IgG pooled from about 5000 donors.

The immunotherapeutic benefits of gamma globulin are mediated by its effects in the modulation of complement

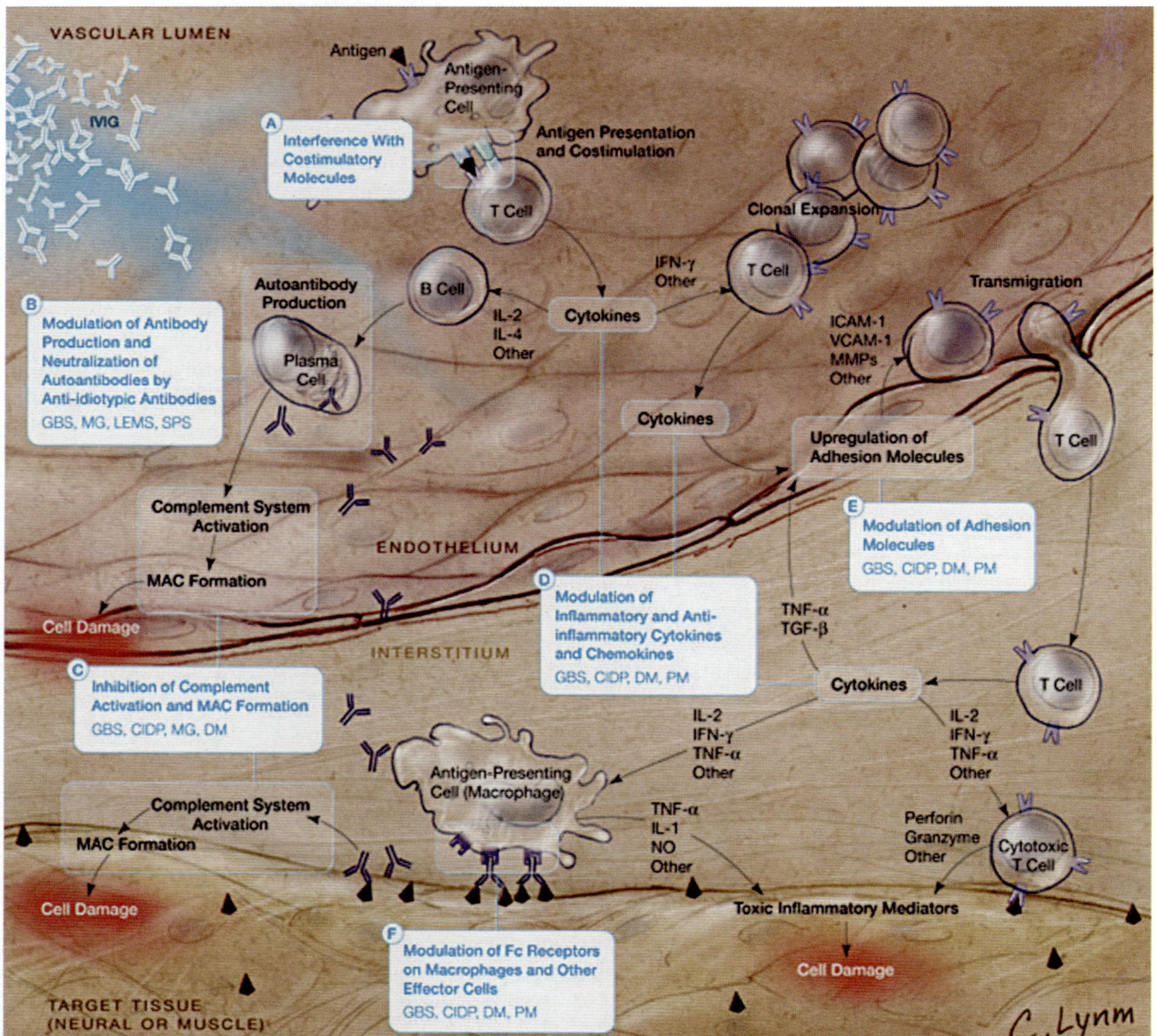

FIG. 3-2 Different mechanisms of the action of immunoglobulin. (Reprinted with permission from Dalakas MC. Intravenous immune globulin therapy for neurologic disease. *Ann Intern Med.* 1997;126:721–730.)

activation pathways with blockade of idiotypic antibodies and saturation of (FC) receptors in macrophages and suppression of various inflammatory mediators, such as cytokines, metalloproteinases, and chemokines[90] (Fig. 3-2).

The usual starting dosage is 2 g/kg which can be given over 2–5 days depending on the patient's size and age. It is usually recommended to begin treatment in the hospital setting, or in a well-equipped and monitored outpatient unit, over 4–5 days with daily measurement of renal function. It is better not to use IgG in patients with impaired renal function, particularly those with diabetes.

Although newer preparations have a lesser IgA content, anaphylactic reactions are still possible, and for this reason, IgA levels should be measured prior to initial infusions.

In chronic disorders IgG infusions are given once a month in doses of 1–2 g/kg over 2 days and, rarely, 500 mg/kg weekly. This form of treatment is expensive, and some preparations may be difficult to obtain.

Side effects include thromboembolic complications, such as pulmonary embolism, myocardial infarction, and strokes. These are rare and are caused by increased viscosity.[91,92] Proper hydration and the use of subcutaneous heparin can help prevent these complications, but this has not been proven. Acute renal failure can occur, particularly with the use of products containing sucrose; this is usually reversible. It is recommended to monitor electrolytes and renal function daily during infusions. Other side effects include headaches, malaise, fever, rash, allergic reactions, and aseptic meningitis.[93] (Table 3-3 lists the commercially available immunoglobulin preparations and their characteristics.)

Gamma globulin infusion has been proven beneficial in Guillain–Barré syndrome (GBS), CIDP, motor and sensory neuropathy, and multifocal neuropathy, and in patients with CIDP associated with monoclonal gammopathy of uncertain significance (MGUS).[53] It also can be used in MG, dermatomyositis, and stiff-person syndrome.[90]

Subcutaneous gamma globulin infusion is a new way of treatment which is very convenient for some patients to avoid recurrent intravenous access as well as the complication of port-a-caths (Table 3-4 lists commonly used subcutaneous preparations).[94,95] It may also provide more steady levels of IgG; this has been approved for the use in CIDP.

Complement Inhibitors. Eculizumab is a humanized monoclonal antibody that binds to the C5 complement protein inhibiting its cleavage to 5A and 5B which results in reduced chemotaxis of pro-inflammatory cells and inhibition of the formation of the membrane attack complex formation, respectively.[96] This is a novel treatment for autoimmune diseases, and it blocks the complement-mediated destruction of acetylcholine receptors in MG and could possibly be beneficial in other autoimmune diseases in which complement has a pathogenic role. Eculizumab was recently approved for the treatment of neuromyelitis optica.[97]

Eculizumab has proven effective in a double-blind controlled study in acetylcholine receptor antibody positive MG,[96] and it has shown long-lasting efficacy.[98] Potential complications include infection by encapsulated bacteria such as meningococcus and gonorrhea, streptococcus, haemophilus, and even fungal agents such as aspergillus. Proper vaccination is recommended and patients should be educated about the risk of such infections. Otherwise, eculizumab appears to be rather safe, and in published trials the most common side effect compared with placebo was musculoskeletal pain.[97] The dosage used is 900 mg IV weekly for 4 weeks and thereafter 1200 mg every 2 weeks. The doses can be adjusted if needed. Supplemental doses can be given in patients receiving plasma exchange. Most myasthenic patients respond well and rapidly, but there are rare nonresponders. The reasons for lack of response are not clear, but in a study of paroxysmal nocturnal hemoglobinuria, it has been reported that some genetic variants of C5 may account for a poor response to eculizumab.[99] This suggests that it may be possible to predict which patients may not respond to this form of treatment.

Zilucoplan is a 15 amino acid synthetic macrocyclic peptide that inhibits C5 and has also been demonstrated to be beneficial in generalized MG.[100] Zilucoplan is self-administered subcutaneously. Possible complications are similar to eculizumab, but because it is not a monoclonal antibody but instead a small synthetic peptide, it may cause less immunogenicity. Zilucoplan has yet to be approved by the FDA. Ravulizumab is another complement inhibitor that is given every 2 months.[101]

Anti–Tumor Necrosis Factor-α Agents

Tumor necrosis factor (TNF)-α is a potent pro-inflammatory cytokine that is likely involved in the pathogenesis of several autoimmune conditions, particularly rheumatoid arthritis and the inflammatory myopathies. Anti-TNF-α agents have been used with varied results in several neuromuscular disorders.

Infliximab is a chimeric monoclonal antibody against TNF-α. The drug has been reported to be of benefit to some patients with refractory inflammatory myopathies,[102,103] but an open-label trial found no improvement in muscle strength.[103] Etanercept is not a monoclonal antibody but rather a TNF-α receptor fusion protein that can bind and inactivate the cytokine. Although anecdotal reports of successful treatment of polymyositis with this agent exist,[103–105] other reports document a uniform worsening of disease status during treatment.[106] A pilot trial of etanercept in IBM found that the drug was well tolerated and a small improvement in hand grip at 1 year was noted.[107] Etanercept has also been used in a small open-label trial for the treatment of steroid-dependent MG. Although 5 of 11 patients improved significantly, 3 patients dropped out of the study, 1 because of a significant exacerbation of disease associated with up-regulation of TNF-α levels.[108] A series of 10 patients with CIDP treated with etanercept showed definite improvement in 3 cases.[109]

Side effects of anti-TNF-α agents are usually mild, but several are of specific concern. Because TNF-α plays an important pro-inflammatory role in the immune system, the incidence of infection, particularly by intracellular organisms such as *Mycobacterium tuberculosis*, is increased. The use of these agents has also been associated with the development or

TABLE 3-3 Types of IgG preparations and their characteristics in bold

Intravenous IgG Preparation	Liquid IVIg									Lyophilized IV IgG
	Flebogamma DIF	Gammagard liquid	Gammaked	Gammaplex	Gamunex-C	Bivicam	Panzyga	Octagam	Privigen	Gammagard S/D with IgA <1 μg/mL
Manufacturer	Grifols	Shire (formerly Baxalta)	Kedrion	Bio Products Laboratory	Grifols	ADMA	Pfizer	Octapharma	CSL Behring	Shire (formerly Baxalta)
Clinical contact	1–888–474–3657	1–866–424–6724	1–855–353–7466	1–800–843–7477	1–800–520–2807	1–800–458–4244	1–888–429–4535	1–888–429–4535	1–800–504–5434	1–866–424–6724
Dosing sizes (g)	• 5%: 0.5, 2.5, 5, 10, and 20 • 10%: 5, 10, and 20	1, 2.5, 5, 10, 20, and 30	1, 2.5, 5, 10, and 20	• 5%: 5, 10, and 20 • 10%: 5, 10, and 20	1, 2.5, 5, 10, and 20	5, 10	2.5, 5, 10, 20, and 30	• 5%: 1, 2.5, 5, 10, and 25 • 10%: 2, 5, 10, and 20	5, 10, 20, and 40	5, 10 (vial sizes)
Concentration (%)	5, 10	10	10	5, 10	10	10	10	10	10	10
Sugar content	5%, 10% D-Sorbitol	Sugar free, stabilized with glycine	Sugar free, stabilized with glycine	• 5%: 5 g D-sorbitol in 100 mL of buffer solution • 10%: sugar free, stabilized with glycine and polysorbate 80	Sugar free, stabilized with glycine	No added sugar	Glycine	100 mg/mL maltose	No sugars, stabilized with L-proline	2% glucose
Sodium content	• 5%: <3.2 mmol/L • 10%: Trace	N/A	Trace	• 5%: 0.2 g sodium acetate and 0.3 g sodium chloride in 100 mL of buffer solution • 10%: <30 mM sodium chloride in 100 mL of buffer solution	Trace amounts	100–140 mmol/L	Trace amounts	<30 mmol/L	<1 mmol/L (10% solution)	0.85% with 5%
Osmolality/Osmolarity (mOsm/kg)	240–370	240–300	258	• 5%: Typically 420–500 (not less than 240) • 10%: Typically 280 (not less than 240)	258	≤510	240–310	310–380	320 (range 240–440)	5%: 636
pH	5–6	4.6–5.1	4–4.6	• 5%: 4.8–5.1 • 10%: 4.9–5.2	4–4.5	4.0–4.6	4.5–5.0	5–6	4.8 (range 4.6–5.0)	6.8 + or − 0.4 (after reconstitution)
IgA content (μg/mL)	• 5%: <50 • 10%: <100	37	46	• 5%: <10 • 10%: <20	46	≤200	Average 100	≤200	<25	<1
% IgG	>97	>98	>98	• 5%: >95 • 10%: >98	>96	>96	>96	>96	>98	>90
Storage requirements	• 2°C–25°C • Protect from light • Do not freeze	• Refrigerate or room temperature • Do not freeze	• Refrigerate or room temperature • Do not freeze	• Refrigerate or room temperature • Do not freeze	• Refrigerate or room temperature • Do not freeze	• 2°C–8°C • Do not freeze	• 2°C–8°C • Do not freeze	Room temperature	Room temperature	Room temperature

TABLE 3-4

Subcutaneous IG

	Cuvitru	Gammagard Liquid	Gammaked	Gamunex-C™	Hizentra	Xembify	Hyquiva
Manufacturer	Shire (formerly Baxalta)	Shire (formerly Baxalta)	Kedrion	Grifols	CSL Behring	Grifols	Shire (formerly Baxalta)
Vial sizes	1 g, 2 g, 4 g, and 8 g	1 g, 2.5 g, 5 g, 10 g, 20 g, and 30 g	1 g, 2.5 g, 5 g, 10 g, and 20 g	1 g, 2.5 g, 5 g, 10 g, and 20 g	1 g (5 mL), 2 g (10 mL), 4 g (20 mL), and 10 g (50 mL)	1 g, 2 g, 4 g, and 10 g	2.5 g/200 U, 5 g/400 U, 10 g/800 U, 20 g/1600 U, and 30 g/2400 U
Concentration (%)	20	10	10	10	20	20	10
Sugar content	Sugar free; stabilized with glycine	Sugar free; stabilized with glycine	Sugar free; stabilized with glycine	Sugar free; stabilized with glycine	Sugar free; stabilized with L-proline	Sugar free; stabilized with glycine	Sugar free; stabilized with glycine
Sodium content	N/A	N/A	Trace amounts	Trace amounts	Trace amounts	Trace amounts	N/A
Osmolality/ Osmolarity (mOsm/kg)	280–292	240–300	258	258	380	280–404	240–300
pH	4.6–5.1	4.6–5.1	4.0–4.5	4.0–4.5	4.6–5.2	4.1–4.8	4.6–5.1
IgA content (μg/mL)	80	37	46	46	<50	<70	37
% IgG	≥98	>98	>98	>98	≥98	>98	>98

IgG, Immunoglobulin G.
Modified from Immunoglobulin Comparison Chart – CVS Speciality and Coram CVS Specialties Infusion Services.

clinical worsening of leukocytoclastic vasculitis, a lupus-like syndrome, and interstitial lung disease.[110] Of particular interest to neuromuscular physicians, these drugs have also been associated with a wide variety of nerve and muscle disorders, including GBS, CIDP, mononeuritis multiplex, axonal sensorimotor polyneuropathy, and inflammatory myopathies.[110,111] Central demyelination during anti-TNF-α treatment has also been observed.[112]

Abatacept is a fusion protein consisting of the Fc region of the immunoglobulin IgG1 fused with the extracellular domain of the cytotoxic T-lymphocyte–associated protein 4. This fusion protein prevents costimulatory signaling required for T-cell activation. It has been approved for rheumatoid arthritis and has also shown some promise in the management of inflammatory myopathies.[113]

Miscellaneous Agents. Anakinra, an IL-1 receptor antagonist, has been reported to be effective in a single patient with the antisynthetase syndrome.[114] Interferon-β-1a has been used successfully and safely for multiple sclerosis for more than a decade. Vallat et al. explored its use for CIDP in a multicenter, open-label trial. They found that the drug was well tolerated, with no serious side effects, and only asthenia and flu-like symptoms. There was a significant improvement in a measure of disability and in conduction velocities, although clinical muscle strength testing was not significantly altered.[115] As such, interferon-β-1a could be considered for patients with CIDP who do not respond to other therapies. ATG is a preparation of polyclonal antihuman T-lymphocyte antibodies that results in apoptosis or complement-mediated cytolysis of T cells.[116] It has been used in a small open-label trial in IBM, and methotrexate was given after induction with ATG to prevent repletion of autoimmune T cells. Patients treated with this combination stabilized muscle strength or had modest gains compared with the patients who were given methotrexate alone, who all showed deterioration. Because ATG is produced in animals (e.g., horses), serum sickness is an expected complication, although it did not occur in the pilot study by Lindberg et al.[117]

IgG **antagonists** can be used in autoimmune diseases by diminishing overall IgG levels as well as inhibiting IgG recycling. They target and block the neonatal Fc receptor, increasing IgG turnover and may help other IgG-related disorders as well. The term *neonatal* is a bit misleading as these receptors were first identified in neonatal rats but are present in adult mice and humans as well. Ravulizumab decreases IgG levels in healthy volunteers and appears to be beneficial in experimental models of MG.[118,119] Another compound, efgartigimod, was reported as beneficial and safe and has been approved by the FDA in generalized myasthenia gravis[120,121]; the dosage is 10 mg/kg weekly for 4 weeks and the series can be repeated after two months of the initial dose. This is being tried in CIDP.[122] Nipocalimat is undergoing therapeutic trials.

Edasalonexent is a small molecule that inhibits NF-κB which plays a role in cell necrosis. Edasalonexent was found to be safe and beneficial in the treatment of Duchenne dystrophy in preliminary studies[123,124] and could become an important addition to other therapies in autoimmune disorders.

Genetic Therapies. Genetic therapies are new revolutionary methods used in the treatment of neuromuscular diseases. These include antisense therapy and small molecular gene therapy, among others. In this section, we will review these treatments. For more details, see Narawasami P and Zukovich, T. Molecular and genetic therapies, Chapter 11 in T. Bertorini, *Neuromuscular Disorders: Treatment and Management*, Elsevier, 2001.

To understand genetic therapies, it is important to remember the steps in protein synthesis. Protein synthesis is regulated by RNA, in which the genetic code is copied from DNA to messenger RNA (mRNA) in the nucleus, and this is controlled by the enzyme RNA polymerase. A nucleotide sequence called pre-mRNA containing both exons and introns is formed, and the pre-mRNA is then edited to remove introns to form mature mRNA by "splicing." Spliceosomes are complexes of proteins that mediate splicing. Splice enhancers and silencers play a role in this process. mRNA travels from nucleus to cytoplasm where protein "translation" occurs in the ribosomes, and this requires ribosomal RNA and transfer RNA.

RNA-Based Therapies

These therapies target RNA for treatment, and these include antisense oligonucleotides (ASOs), RNA interference with small-interfering RNA (siRNA) as well as micro-RNAs (miRNAs).

Antisense Oligonucleotide Therapy. ASOs are sequences that can bind to selected sequences of RNA and regulate the expression of genes. They are complementary to the "sense strand" that encodes protein synthesis.[125,126] Thus, for this reason, they are called "antisense." ASOs are modified chemicals that are modified to improve stability and prevent enzymatic degradation and increase protein production. The ASOs can restore protein expression or can be used to reduce expression of a toxic protein or to modify the effect of proteins to reduce their toxicity.[127] Genetic diseases are frequently caused by mutations that modify splicing, and for this, they are amendable to ASO treatment (see Fig. 3-3).

Duchenne Muscular Dystrophy

ASO therapies are used to skip the mutated exons to convert the "out of frame" transcript into an "in frame" transcript producing a shorter but functional protein, as it occurs in Becker's dystrophy.[128] Because of this, several mutations in Duchenne muscular dystrophy (DMD) can be amenable for this therapy.[129] Eteplirsen was first approved to skip exon 51 during splicing, and is beneficial to about 14% of DMD cases.[130–133] Viltolarsen is another ASO that also skips exon 53 and is also approved by the FDA.[133]

Casimersen skips exon 45 and has been recently approved for patients who are amendable for this ASO treatment.[134] Another ASO, golodirsen, is used for skipping exon 53.[130]

ASO therapies are given intravenously once a week; they are well tolerated. These, unfortunately, can be applied only for a small number of patients. They, however, appear very promising and have been demonstrated to produce benefits, and for this reason, other ASOs have been tested.

Spinal Muscular Atrophy

Most cases of spinal muscular atrophy (SMA) are produced by loss of function from a deletion of the survival motor neuron gene SMN1, on chromosome 5q13 affecting the production of motor neuron proteins.[135] There is a closely related gene (SMN2) that expresses low levels of the protein in normals but is rapidly degradable.[136] The number of functional SMN proteins produced depends on the number of copies of the SMN2, thus milder cases (SMA3) have higher quantities of the protein.

A nucleotide substitution in exon 7 affects the splicing in SMN2 with exclusion of exon 7 producing a truncated protein. The ASO treatment aims to increase the inclusion of exon 7 in the mRNA of SMN2 increasing the functional protein. An intronic splicing–silencer N1 (ISS-N1) inhibits inclusion of exon 7 into the pre-SMN2-blockage of the ISS-N1 producing greater inclusion of SMN2 mRNA transcript. The ASO, nusinersen, which blocks ISS-N1 is given intrathecally every 4 months in children and adults and has produced significant benefits with few detrimental effects.[137]

Transthyretin Amyloidosis (ATTR)

Transthyretin amyloidosis (ATTR) is caused by mutations that affect TTR encoding with aggregation of monomers into insoluble amyloid deposits. In hereditary transthyretin amyloidosis, there are deposits of amyloids in nerves and heart affecting function, and for this, treatment with the ASO, inotersen, that knocks down the hepatic production of transthyretin,[138] has been approved and is used in the treatment for this condition.

Intrathecal administration of the ASO tofersen reduced SOD levels in spinal fluid and neurofilament light chain in plasma in familial ALS caused by SOD mutations, and produced a clinical benefit (140) which was confirmed by the open label extension of the trial, leading to an approval by the FDA. There are also trials for the C9orf72 ALS and in myotonic dystrophy.

Small Molecules. Small molecules are also used in therapeutic trials in disorders from nonsense mutations of stop codons by substitution of single-based pairs affecting the sequence of protein formation resulting in truncated proteins.[136] For this treatment to bypass stop codons, PTC (ataluren) has been used in patients with Duchenne muscular dystrophy.[139–142] This type of mutation affects about 10%–15% of these patients.

Risdiplam (EVRYSDI) is an orally administered small molecule of SMN2 mRNA–splicing modifier that produces increased

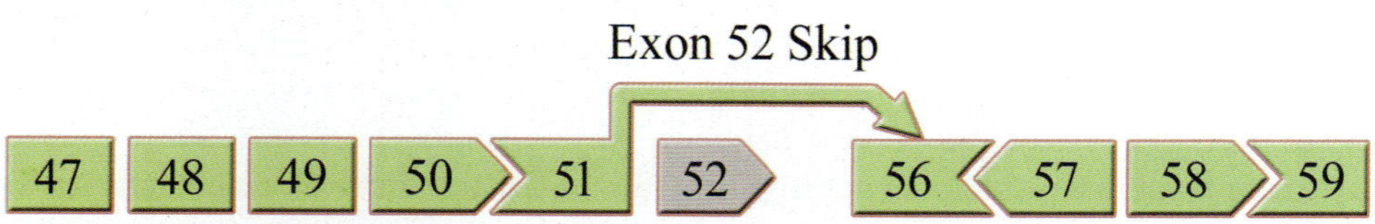

FIG. 3-3 Exon-skipping treatment in a patient with Duchenne dystrophy who had a deletion in exon 53–55. Skipping exon 52 restores the reading frame.

protein, has been beneficial in SMA, and has been approved for this use.[143]

A single small molecule, tafamidis meglumine stabilizes the TTR tetramer preventing its dissociation into amyloidogenic monomers in amyloidosis, and this ASO has been approved in patients with TTR amyloidosis.[144]

Small-Interfering RNA (SiRNA). This another therapeutic approach that involves the introduction of a synthetic siRNA into the target cells to produce RNA inhibition of expression of mRNA to silence the corresponding gene.[145] Patisiran is a lipid nanoparticle produced for delivery to hepatocytes to reduce the expression of mutant and wild-type TTR and for this reason has been used intravenously for familial amyloidosis.[146] Vutisiran is a subcutaneous preparation that was just approved by the FDA for ATTR amyloidosis. In acute intermittent porphyria, liver-directed siRNA targeting the enzyme 5-aminolaevulinic acid synthesis, givosiran, has been approved for the treatment of patients with hepatic porphyria.[147]

Micro-RNA (miRNA)

This inhibits posttranscriptional gene expression on multiple miRNAs. There are three types of miRNAs that inhibit multiple pathogenic genes.[148] These can be used in disorders caused by toxic gain-of-function and appear promising in neuromuscular diseases, particularly in gain of function disorders.

DNA-Based Therapies

Gene-based replacement therapies include the use of gene replacement with viral vectors or use a gene editing technology that has CRISPR-CAS9 editing activity.

Gene Replacement. Gene therapy has been used to correct a mutant gene by introducing and expressing its corrected copy by exogenous nucleic acids within living cells aiming to reverse the genetic defects. This can be delivered by viral and nonviral delivery systems termed "vectors." The expression of the transgene is then regulated by "promoters" that are applied for this treatment, and for this reason, they are very useful in gene therapy.

AA viral therapy also requires helper genes provided by coinfection such as adenovirus or herpes virus. AAVs are small viruses with nonenveloped capsid and linear strands. In SMA, AAV-9 vector–associated gene delivery has been demonstrated to replace the mutated gene and rescue the phenotype. In this disorder, the onasemnogene abeparvovec-xioi has been approved for use in children, and this is given in a single one-time dose.[149] Gene therapy is now being tried in Duchenne dystrophy and other myopathies.[150–152]

Gene Editing. ***Gene editing*** uses the clusters of regulatory interspace short palindromic repeats associated with caspase 9 (CRISPR-CAS9) with an endonuclease guided by single-guided RNA that binds targeted locus producing modifications requiring an exogenous template using AVV vector.[153,154] This method has been used in preclinical trials of SMA, Charcot–Marie–Tooth disease, and some familial cases of ALS.[155]

REFERENCES

1. Anderson PM, Borasio GD, Deregler R, et al. EFNS task force on management of amyotrophic lateral sclerosis: guidelines for diagnosing and clinical care of patients and relatives. *Eur J Neurol.* 2005;12:921–938.
2. Bertorini TE. Muscular dystrophies. In: Pourmand R, ed. *Neuromuscular Disease: Expert Clinicians Views.* Boston: Butterworth-Heinemann; 2001:227–294.
3. Bertorini TE. Perisurgical management of patients with neuromuscular disorders. *Neurol Clin.* 2004;22(2):293–313.
4. Bertorini TE. Malignant hyperthermia in neuromuscular disorders. In: Kaminski HJ, ed. *Clinical Practice.* Boston: Butterworth-Heinemann; 2002:1021–1027.
5. Lovering RM, Porter NC, Bloch RJ. The muscular dystrophies from genes to therapies. *Phys Ther.* 2005;85:1372–1388.
6. Duboc D, Meune C, Lerebours G, et al. Effect of perindopril on the onset and progression of left ventricular dysfunction in Duchenne muscular dystrophy. *J Am Coll Cardiol.* 2005;45(6):855–857.
7. Smith TE, Chong MS. Neuropathic pain. *Hosp Med.* 2000;61(11):760–766.
8. Galer BS. Painful polyneuropathy. *Neurol Clin.* 1998;16:791–812.
9. Woolf CJ, Mannion RJ. Neuropathic pain: Etiology, symptoms, mechanisms and management. *Lancet.* 1999;353:1959–1964.
10. Merskey H, Bogduk N. *Classification of Chronic Pain: Descriptions of Chronic Pain Syndromes and Definitions of Pain Terms.* 2nd ed. Seattle: IASP Press; 1994.
11. Gracely RH, Lynch SA, Bennett GJ. Painful neuropathy: Altered central processing maintained dynamically by peripheral input. *Pain.* 1992;51:175–194.
12. Galer BS. Neuropathic pain of peripheral origin: Advances in pharmacologic treatment. *Neurology.* 1995;45(suppl 9): S17–S25.
13. Nodera H, Herrmann DN. A diagnostic and treatment approach of painful neuropathy. In: Bromberg MB, Smith AG, eds. *Handbook of Peripheral Neuropathy.* Boca Raton, FL: Taylor and Francis; 2005:599–620.
14. Wolfe S. Medical management of painful peripheral neuropathy. *American Academy of Neurology Educational Program.* 2006:104–123.
15. Kieburtz K, Simpson D, Yiannoutsos C, et al. A randomized trial of amitriptyline and mexiletine for painful neuropathy in HIV infection: AIDS Clinical Trial Group 242 Protocol Team. *Neurology.* 1998;51:1682–1688.
16. Max MB, Culnane M, Schafer SC, et al. Amitriptyline relieves diabetic neuropathy pain in patients with normal or depressed mood. *Neurology.* 1987;37:589–596.
17. Brunton L, Lazo J, Parker K, eds. *Goodman and Gilman's The Pharmacological Basis of Therapeutics.* 2nd ed. New York, NY: McGraw-Hill; 2005.
18. Max MB, Lynch SA, Muir J, et al. Effects of desipramine, amitriptyline and fluoxetine on pain in diabetic neuropathy. *N Engl J Med.* 1992;326:1250–1256.
19. Jensen TS. Anticonvulsants in neuropathic pain: Rationale and clinical evidence. *Eur J Pain.* 2002;6:61–68.
20. Backonja M. Use of anticonvulsants for treatment of neuropathic pain. *Neurology.* 2002;59(Suppl):S14–S17.
21. Saudek CD, Werns S, Reidenberg MM. Phenytoin in the treatment of diabetic symmetrical polyneuropathy. *Clin Pharmacol Ther.* 1977;22:196–199.
22. Kochar DK, Jain N, Agarwal RP, et al. Sodium valproate in the management of painful neuropathy in type 2 diabetes—A

randomized placebo-controlled study. *Acta Neurol Scand.* 2002;106:248–252.
23. Gorson KC, Schott C, Herman R, et al. Gabapentin in the treatment of painful diabetic neuropathy: A placebo-controlled, double blind, crossover trial. *J Neurol Neurosurg Psychiatry.* 1999;66:251–252.
24. Simpson DM, Olney R, McArthur JC, et al. A placebo-controlled trial of lamotrigine for painful HIV-associated neuropathy. *Neurology.* 2000;54:2115–2119.
25. Raskin P, Donofrio PD, Rosenthal NR, et al. Topiramate vs. placebo in painful diabetic neuropathy: Analgesic and metabolic effects. *Neurology.* 2004;63:865–873.
26. Thienel U, Neto W, Schwabe SK, et al. Topiramate in painful diabetic polyneuropathy: Findings from three double blind, placebo-controlled trials. *Acta Neurol Scan.* 2004;110:221–231.
27. Lesser H, Sharma U, LaMoreaux L, Poole RM. Pregabalin relieves symptoms of painful diabetic neuropathy: A randomized controlled trial. *Neurology.* 2004;63:2104–2110.
28. Richter RW, Portenoy R, Sharma U, et al. Relief of diabetic peripheral neuropathy with pregabalin: A randomized, placebo-controlled trial. *J Pain Symptom Manage.* 2005;6:253–260.
29. Oskarsson P, Ljunggren J-G, Lins P-E. Efficacy and safety of mexiletine on the treatment of painful diabetic neuropathy Mexiletine study group. *Diabetes Care.* 1997;20:1594–1597.
30. Puniani TS, Bertorini TE. Tocainide therapy in muscle cramps and spasms due to neuromuscular disease. *Muscle Nerve.* 1991;14:280–285.
31. Dworkin RH, Backonja M, Rowbotham MC, et al. Advances in neuropathic pain: Diagnosis, mechanisms, and treatment recommendations. *Arch Neurol.* 2003;60:1524–1534.
32. Semenchuk MR, Sherman S, Davis B. Double-blind, randomized trial of bupropion SR for treatment of neuropathic pain. *Neurology.* 2001;57:1583–1588.
33. Nelson KA, Park KM, Robinovitz E, et al. High-dose dextromethorphan versus placebo in painful diabetic neuropathy and postherpetic neuralgia. *Neurology.* 1997;48:1212–1218.
34. Galer BS, Rowbotham MC, Perander J, Friedman E. Topical lidocaine patch relieves postherpetic neuralgia more effectively than a vehicle topical patch: Results of an enriched enrollment study. *Pain.* 1999;80:533–538.
35. Low PA, Opfer-Gehrking TL, Dyck PJ, et al. Double-blind, placebo-controlled study of the application of capsaicin cream in chronic distal painful polyneuropathy. *Pain.* 1995;62:163–168.
36. The Capsaicin Study Group Treatment of painful diabetic neuropathy with topical capsaicin: A multicenter, double-blind, vehicle-controlled study. *Arch Intern Med.* 1991;151(11):2225–2229.
37. Weintraub MI, Wolfe GI, Barohn RA, et al. Static magnetic field therapy for symptomatic diabetic neuropathy: A randomized, double-blind, placebo-control trial. *Arch Phys Med Rehabil.* 2003;84:736–746.
38. Petersen EA, Stauss TG, Scowcroft JA. Effect of High-Frequency (10-kHz) Spinal Cord Stimulation in Patients With Painful Diabetic Neuropathy: A Randomized Clinical Trial. *JAMA Neurol.* 2021;78(6):687–699.
39. Fealey RD. Neurogenic orthostatic hypotension. In: Johnson RT, Griffin JW, McArthur JC, eds. *Current Therapy in Neurologic Diseases.* Philadelphia: Elsevier; 2006:8–13.
40. Low PA. Neurogenic orthostatic hypotension. In: Noseworthy JH, ed. *Neurologic Therapeutics: Principles and Practice.* New York, NY: Martin Dunitz; 2003:2267–2274.
41. Sandroni P, Opfer-Gehrking TL, Singer W, Low PA. Pyridostigmine for treatment of neurogenic orthostatic hypotension [correction of hypertension]—A follow-up survey study. *Clin Auton Res.* 2005;15(1):51–53.
42. Wolfe GI, Kaminksi HJ, Aban IB, Minisman MA, et al. Randomized Trial of Thymectomy in Myasthenia Gravis. *N Engl J Med.* 2016;375:511–522.
43. Sieb JP. Myasthenia gravis: Emerging new therapy, options. *Curr Opin Pharmacol.* 2005;5:303–307.
44. Saperstein DS, Barohn RJ. Management of myasthenia gravis in myasthenia gravis. *Semin Neurol.* 2004;24(1):41–48.
45. Jaretzki A, Steinglass KM, Sonett JR. Thymectomy in the management of myasthenia gravis. *Semin Neurol.* 2004;24(2):49–62.
46. Juel VC. Management of myasthenia crisis and perioperative care. *Semin Neurol.* 2004;24(1):75–81.
47. Rhen T, Cidlowski JA. Anti-inflammatory action of glucocorticoids—New mechanisms for old drugs. *N Engl J Med.* 2005;353(16):1711–1723.
48. Bromberg MB, Carter O. Corticosteroid use in the treatment of neuromuscular disorders: Empirical and evidence-based data. *Muscle Nerve.* 2004;30(1):20–37.
49. Vardesy O, Smith SA. Treatment of immune mediated peripheral neuropathy. In: Bromberg MB, Smith AG, eds. *Handbook of Peripheral Neuropathy.* Boca Raton FL: Taylor and Francis; 2005:639–656.
50. Min DI, Monaco AP. Complications associated with immunosuppressive therapy and their management. *Pharmacotherapy.* 1991;11(Suppl 5):119S–125S.
51. Mah JK, Clemens PR, Guglieri M, et al. Efficacy and Safety of Vamorolone in Duchenne Muscular Dystrophy. A 30-Month Nonradomized Controlled Open-Label Extension. *JAMA Netw Open.* 2022;5(2):E2144178. https://doi.org/10.1001/jamanetworkopen.2021.44178.
52. Dalakas MC. Therapeutic targets in patients with inflammatory myopathies: Present approaches and a look to the future. *Neuromuscul Disord.* 2000;16:223–236.
53. Bertorini TE. Inflammatory myopathies (polymyositis, dermatomyositis, inclusion body myositis). *Compr Ther.* 1998;24:494–502.
54. Finsterer J. Treatment of immune-mediated, dysimmune neuropathies. *Acta Neurol Scand.* 2005;112(2):115–125.
55. Dalakas MC, Engel WK. Chronic relapsing (dysimmune) polyneuropathy: Pathogenesis and treatment. *Ann Neurol.* 1981(Suppl 9):S134–S145.
56. Pollard JD, Hartung H-P, Hughes RA. Principles of immunotherapy. In: Dyck PJ, Thomas PK, eds. *Peripheral Neuropathy.* 4th ed. Philadelphia: WB Saunders/Elsevier; 2005:635–648.
57. Suthanthiran M, Morris RE, Strom TB. Immunosuppressants: Cellular and molecular mechanisms of action. *Am J Kidney Dis.* 1996;28(2):159–172.
58. Anstey A, Lear JT. Azathioprine: Clinical pharmacology and current indications in autoimmune disorders. *BioDrugs.* 1998;9(15):33–47.
59. Holme SA, Duley JA, Sanderson J, et al. Erythrocyte thiopurine methyl transferase assessment prior to azathioprine use in the UK. *QJM.* 2002;95(7):439–444.
60. Kissel JT, Levy RJ, Mendell JR, Griggs RC. Azathioprine toxicity in neuromuscular disease. *Neurology.* 1986;36:35–39.
61. Hohlfeld R, Michels M, Heininger K, et al. Azathioprine toxicity during long-term immunosuppression of generalized myasthenia gravis. *Neurology.* 1988;38(2):258–261.
62. Yuill GB, Swinburn WR, Liversedge LA. Treatment of polyneuropathy with azathioprine. *Lancet.* 1970;2:854–856.

63. Bertorini TE, Narayanaswami P. Autoimmune neuropathies. *Compr Ther*. 2003;29:134–209.
64. Mantegazza R, Antozzi C, Peluchette D, et al. Azathioprine as a single drug or in combination with steroids in the treatment of myasthenia gravis. *J Neurol*. 1988;235(8):449–453.
65. Bromberg MB. Advances in diagnosis and management of inflammatory myopathies. *Neuromuscul Disord*. 2005;6:167–179.
66. Lipsky JJ. Mycophenolate mofetil. *Lancet*. 1996;348:1357–1359.
67. Chang CC, Aversa G, Punnonen J, et al. Brequinar sodium, mycophenolic acid, and cyclosporin A inhibit different stages of IL-4 or IL-13 induced human IgG4 and IgE production in vitro. *Ann NY Acad Sci*. 1993;696:108–122.
68. Chaudry V, Cornblath DR, Griffin JW, et al. Mycophenolate mofetil: A safe and promising immunosuppressant in neuromuscular disease. *Neurology*. 2001;56:94–96.
69. Solinger MW. Mycophenolate mofetil. *Kidney Int*. 1995;52(Suppl):S14–S17.
70. Vernino S, Salomao DR, Habermann TM, O'Neill BP. Primary CNS lymphoma complicating treatment of myasthenia gravis with mycophenolate mofetil. *Neurology*. 2005;65:639–641.
71. Meriggioli MN, Rowin J, Richman JG, Leurgans S. Mycophenolate mofetil for myasthenia gravis: A double-blind, placebo-controlled pilot study. *Ann NY Acad Sci*. 2003;998: 494–499.
72. Gorson KC, Ropper AH. Chronic inflammatory demyelinating polyradiculoneuropathy (CIDP): A review of syndromes and treatment approaches in clinical practice. *Neuromuscul Disord*. 2003;4:174–189.
73. O'Dell JR. Drug therapy: Therapeutic strategies for rheumatoid arthritis. *N Engl J Med*. 2004;350:2591–2602.
74. Marder W, McCune WJ. Advances in immunosuppressive drug therapy for use in autoimmune disease and systemic vasculitis. *Semin Respir Crit Care Med*. 2004;25(5):581–594.
75. Zhu LP, Cupps TR, Whalen G, Fauci AS. Selective effects of cyclophosphamide therapy on activation, proliferation, and differentiation of human B cells. *J Clin Invest*. 1987;79(4):1082–1090.
76. Hengst JC, Kempf RA. Immunomodulation by cyclophosphamide. *Clin Immunol Allergy*. 1984;14:199.
77. Cupps TR, Edgar LC, Fauci AS. Suppression of human B lymphocyte function by cyclophosphamide. *J Immunol*. 1982;128:2453–2457.
78. Drachman DB, Jones RJ, Brodsky RA. Treatment of refractory myasthenia: "Rebooting" with high-dose cyclophosphamide. *Ann Neurol*. 2003;53:29–34.
79. Good JL, Chehrenama M, Mayer RF, Koski CL. Pulse cyclophosphamide therapy in chronic inflammatory demyelinating polyradiculoneuropathy. *Neurology*. 1998;51(6):1735–1738.
80. Brannagan III TH, Alaedini A, Gladstone DE. High-dose cyclophosphamide without stem cell rescue for refractory multifocal motor neuropathy. *Muscle Nerve*. 2006;34(2):246–250.
81. Notermans NC, Lokhorst HM, Franssen H, et al. Intermittent cyclophosphamide and prednisone treatment of polyneuropathy associated with monoclonal gammopathy of undetermined significance. *Neurology*. 1996;47:1227–1233.
82. Brodsky RA, Petri M, Smith BD, et al. Immunoablative high-dose cyclophosphamide without stem-cell rescue for refractory, severe autoimmune disease. *Ann Intern Med*. 1998;129:1031–1035.
83. Nemni R, Santuccio G, Calabrese E, et al. Efficacy of cyclosporine treatment in multifocal motor neuropathy. *J Neurol*. 2003;250:1118–1120.
84. Grillo-Lopez AJ, Hedrick E, Rashford M, Benyunes M. Rituximab: Ongoing and future clinical development. *Semin Oncol*. 2002;29(Suppl):S105–S112.
85. Maloney DG, Smith B, Rose A. Rituximab: Mechanism of action and resistance. *Semin Oncol*. 2002;29(Suppl):S2–S9.
86. U.S. Food and Drug Administration (FDA): FDA warns of safety concern regarding Rituxan in new patient preparations. FDA News. Accessed at www.fda.gov/medwatch/.
87. Hain B, Jordan K, Deschauer M, Zierz S. Successful treatment of MuSK antibody positive myasthenia gravis with rituximab. *Muscle Nerve*. 2006;33:575–580.
88. Renaud S, Fuhr P, Gregor M, et al. High dose rituximab and anti-MAG-associated polyneuropathy. *Neurology*. 2006;66(5):742–744.
89. Dyck PJ, Litchy WJ, Kratz KM, et al. A plasma exchange versus immune globulin infusion trial in chronic inflammatory demyelinating polyradiculoneuropathy. *Ann Neurol*. 1994;36:838–845.
90. Dalakas MC. Intravenous immune globulin therapy for neurologic disease. *Ann Intern Med*. 1997;126:721–730.
91. Dalakas MC. High-dose intravenous immunoglobulin and serum viscosity: Risk of precipitating thromboembolic events. *Neurology*. 1994;44:223–226.
92. Koffman B, Dalakas MC. Effect of high-dose intravenous immunoglobulin (IVIG) on hematologic and serum chemistry profiles in the treatment of patients with neuromuscular disease. *Neurology*. 1996;45:A235.
93. Bertorini TE, Nance AM, Horner LH, et al. Complications of intravenous gamma globulin in neuromuscular and other disease. *Muscle Nerve*. 1996;19:388–391.
94. Alonso A, Vandebert P, Lang J, Yuzuik J, et al. Immune globulin subcutaneous, human 20%solution (Xembify), a new high concentration immunoglobulin product for subcutaneous administration. *Biologicals*. 2020;64:34–40.
95. Lamb YN, Syed YY, Dhillon S. Immune Globulin Subcutaneous (Human) 20% (Hizentra): A Review in Chronic Inflammatory Demyelinating Polyneuropathy. *CNS Drugs*. 2019;33(8):831–838.
96. Howard JF JR, Utsugisawa K, Benatar M, Murai H, Barohn RJ, Illa L, et al. Safety and efficacy of eculizumab in anti-acetylcholine receptor antibody-positive refractory generalised myasthenia gravis (REGAIN): a phase 3, randomised, double-blind, placebo-controlled, multicentre study. *Lancet Neurol*. 2017;16(12):976–986.
97. Pittock SJ, Berthele A, Fujihara K, Kim HJ, Levy M, Palace J, et al. Eculizumab in Aquaporin-4-positive Neuromyelitis Optica Spectrum Disorder. N Eng. *J Med*. 2019;381(7):614–625.
98. Muppidi S, Utsugisawa K, Benatar M, Murai H, Barohn RJ, Illa L, et al. Long-term safety and efficacy of eculizumab in generalized myasthenia gravis. *Muscle Nerve*. 2019;60(1): 14–24.
99. Nishimura J, Yamamoto M, Hayashi S, Ohyashiki K, et al. Genetic variants in C5 and poor response to eculizumab. *N Engl J Med*. 2014;370(7):632–639. /NEJMoa13110084.
100. Howard JF JR, Nowak RJ, Wolfe GI, et al. Clinical effects of the self-administered subcutaneous complement inhibitor zilucoplan in patients with moderate to severe generalized myasthenia gravis: results of a phase 2 randomized, double-blind, placebo-controlled, multicenter clinical trial. *JAMA Neurol*. 2020;77(5):582–592.
101. Vu T, Meisel A, Mantegazza R, et al. Terminal Complement Inhibitor Ravulizumab in Generalized Myasthenia Gravis. *NEJM Evid*. 2022;1(5):April 26, 2022.

102. Hengstman GJD, van den Hoogen FHJ, Barrera P, Netea MG, Pieterse A, van de Putte LBA, et al. Successful treatment of dermatomyositis and polymyositis with anti-tumor-necrosis-factor-alpha: preliminary observations. *Eur Neurol.* 2003;50(1):10–15.
103. Riley P, McCann LJ, Maillard SM, Woo P, Murray KJ, Pilkington CA. Effectiveness of infliximab in the treatment of refractory juvenile dermatomyositis with calcinosis. *Rheumatology (Oxford).* 2008;47(6):877–880.
104. Iannone E, Scioscia C, Falappone PC, Covelli M, Lapadula G. Use of etanercept in the treatment of dermatomyositis: A case series. *J Rheumatol.* 2006;339(9):1802–1804.
105. Sprott H, Glatzel M, Michel BA. Treatment of myositis with etanercept (Enbrel), a recombinant human soluble fusion protein of TNF-alpha type II receptor and IgG1. *Rheumatology.* 2004;43(4):524–526.
106. Dastmalchi M, Grundtman C, Alexanderson H, Mavragani CP, Einarsdottir H, Helmers SB, et al. A high incidence of disease flares in an open pilot study of infliximab in patients with refractory inflammatory myopathies. *Ann Rheum Dis.* 2008;12:1670–1677.
107. Barohn RJ, Herbelin L, Kissel JT, King W, McVey AL, Saperstein DS, et al. Pilot trial of etanercept in the treatment of inclusion-body myositis. *Neurology.* 2006;66(2 suppl 1):S123–S124.
108. Rowin J, Meriggioli MN, Tuzun E, Leurgans S, Christadoss P. Etanercept treatment in corticosteroid-dependent myasthenia gravis. *Neurology.*. 2004;63(12):2390–2392.
109. Chin RL, Sherman WH, Sander HW, Hays AP, Latov N. Etanercept (Enbrel) therapy for chronic inflammatory demyelinating polyneuropathy. *J Neurol Sci.* 2003;210(1-2): 19–21.
110. Remos-Casals M, Brito-Zeron P, Munoz S, Soria N, Galiana D, Bertolaccini L, et al. Autoimmune diseases induced by TNF-targeted therapies: Analysis of 233 cases. *Medicine.* 2007;86(4):242–251.
111. Stubgen JP. Tumor necrosis factor-alpha antagonists and neuropathy. *Muscle Nerve.* 2008;37(3):281–292.
112. Robinson WH, Genovese MC, Moreland LW. Demyelinating and neurologic events reported in association with tumor necrosis factor alpha antagonism: By what mechanism could tumor necrosis factor alpha antagonists improve rheumatoid arthritis but exacerbate multiple sclerosis? *Arthritis Rheum.* 2001;44(9):1977–1983.
113. Tjarnlund A., Tang Q., Wick C., Dastmalchi M., Mann H., Tomasova Studynkova J. et al. Abatacept in the treatment of adult dermatomyositis and polymyositis: A randomized phase IIb treatment delayed-start trial. Ann Rheum Dis. 77(1), 55-62.
114. Furlan A, Botsios C, Ruffatti A, Todesco S, Punzi L. Antisynthetase syndrome with refractory polyarthritis and fever successfully treated with the IL-1 receptor antagonist, anakinra: A case report. *Joint Bone Spine.* 2008;75(5):366–367.
115. Vallat JM, Hahn AF, Leger JM, Cros DP, Magy L, Tabaraud F, et al. Interferon beta-la as an investigational treatment for CIDP. *Neurology.* 2003;60(8 suppl 3):S23–S28.
116. Dalakas MC. Therapeutic targets in patients with inflammatory myopathies: Present approaches and a look to the future. *Neuromuscul Disord.* 2006;16(4):223–236.
117. Lindberg C, Trysberg E, Tarkowski A, Oldfors A. Anti-T-lymphocytic globulin treatment in inclusion body myositis: A randomized pilot study. *Neurology.* 2003;61(2):260–262.
118. Kiessling P, Liedo-Garcia R, Watanabe S, Langdon G, Tran D, Bari M, et al. The FcRn inhibitor rozanolixizumab reduces human serum IgG concentration: A randomized phase 1 study. *Sci Transl Med.* 2017((414) aan 1208.
119. Liu L, Garcia AM, Santoro H, Zhang Y, McDonnell K, Dumont J, et al. Amelioration of experimental myasthenia gravis in rats by neonatal RcR blockade. *Journal of Immunology.* 2007;178(8):5390–5398.
120. Howard JF, Bril V, Burns TM, Mantegazza R, Bilinska M, Szczudlik A, et al. Randomized phase 2 study of FcRn antagonist efgartigimod in generalized myasthenia gravis. *Neurology. 92(23).* 2019:e2661–e2673.
121. Howard Jr J.F., Tuan V., Bril V., DeMantegazza J.L., Meiisel M., Peric S., et al ADAPT: a phase 3 sdtudy of the FcRn antagonist efgartigimod in generalized Myasthenia Gravis. Presented at the AANEM Congress. 2020.
122. Donofrio P, Gorson K, Hofman E, Karan CH, et al. Diagnostic adjudication of chronic inflammatory demyelinating polyneuropathy in the ADHERE Trial: Review of the first 100 cases. *Muscle Nerve.* 2021;560
123. Finanger E, Vandenbourne K, Finkel RS, Sweeney HL, Tennekoon G, Yum S, et al. Phase I study of Edasalonexent (CAT-1004) an Oral NF kB inhibitor in Pediatric Patients with Duchenne Muscular Dystrophy. *J Neuromuscul Dis.* 2019;6(1):43–54.
124. Monici MC, Aguennouz M, Mazzeo A, Messina C, Vita G. Activation of nuclear factor-kappa B in inflammatory myopathies and Duchenne muscular dystrophy. *Neurology.*. 2003;60(6):993–997.
125. Goyal N, Narayanaswami P. Making sense of antisense oligonucleotides: A narrative review. *Muscle and Nerve.* 2018;57(3):356–370.
126. Cherry J. RNA therapeutics: RNAi and antisense mechanisms and clinical applications. *Postdoc J.* 2016;4(7):35–50.
127. Evers MM, Tran HD, Zalachoras I, Pepers BA, Meijer OC, den Dunnen JT, et al. Ataxin-3 protein modification as a treatment strategy for spinocerebellar ataxia type 3: removal of the CAG containing exon. *Neurobiol Dis.* 2013;58:49–56.
128. Bladen CL, Salgado D, Monges S, Foncuberta ME, et al. The TREAT-NMD DMD Global Database: analysis of more than 7,000 Duchenne muscular dystrophy mutations. *Hum Mutat.* 2015;36(4):395–402.
129. Cirak S. Arechavala-Gomeza V, Guglieri M, Feng L, Torelli S, Anthony K, et al. Exon skipping and dystrophin restoration in patients with Duchenne muscular dystrophy after systemic phosphorodiamidate morpholino oligomer treatment: an open-label, phase 2, dose-escalation study. *Lancet.* 2011;378(9791):595–605.
130. Mendell JR, Rodino-Klapac LR, Sahenk Z, Roush K, Bird L, Lowes LP, et al. Eteplirsen for the treatment of Duchenne muscular dystrophy. *Ann Neurol.* 2013;74(5):637–647.
131. Mendell JR, Goemans N, Lowes LP, Alfano LN, Berry K, Shao J, et al. Longitudinal effect of eteplirsen versus historical control on ambulation in Duchenne muscular dystrophy. *Ann Neurol.* 2016;79(2):257–271.
132. Dowling J, Gonorazky H, Cohn R. Campbell. Treating pediatric neuromuscular disorders: The future is now. *Am J Med Genet A.*. 2018;176(4):804–841.
133. Wood MJ, Gait MJ, Yin H. RNA-targeted splice-correction therapy for neuromuscular disease. *Brain.*. 2010;133(Pt 4): 957–972.
134. Roshmi RR, Yokota T. Viltolarsen for the treatment of Duchenne muscular dystrophy. *Drugs of Today (Barc).* 2019;55(10): 627–639.

135. Shirley M. Casimersen: First Approval. *Drugs. May.* 2021;81(7):875–887.
136. Lefebvre S, Burglen L, Reboullet S, Clermont O, Burlet P, Viollet L, et al. Identification and characterization of a spinal muscular atrophy-determining gene. *Cell.* 1995;80(1):155–165.
137. Burnett BG, Munoz E, Tandon A, Kwon DY, Sumner CJ, Fischbeck KH. Regulation of SMN protein stability. *Mol Cell Biol.* 2009;29(5):1107–1115.
138. Chiriboga GA, Swoboda KJ, Darras BT, Iannaccone ST, Montes J, DeVivo DC, et al. Results from a phase 1 study of nusinersen (ISIS-SMN (Rx)) in children with spinal muscular atrophy. *Neurology.* 2016;86(10):890–897.
139. Benson MD, Waddington-Cruz M, Berk JL, Polydefkis M, Dyck PJ, Wang AK, et al. Inotersen Treatment for Patients with Hereditary Transthyretin Amyloidosis. *N Engl J Med..* 2018;379(1):22–31.
140. Miller TM, Cudkowicz ME, Genge A, et al. Trial of Antisense Oligonucleotide Tofersen for SODI ALS. *N Engl J Med.* 2022;387:1099–1110.
141. Siddiqui N, Sonenberg N. Proposing a mechanism of action for ataluren. *Proc Natl Acad Sci U.S.A.* 2016;113(44):12353–12355.
142. Celik A, Kervestin S, Jacobson A. NMD: At the crossroads between translation termination and ribosome recycling. *Biochimie..* 2015;114:2–9.
143. Finkel RS, Flanigan KM, Wong B, Bönnemann C, Sampson J, Sweeney HL, et al. Phase 2a study of ataluren-mediated dystrophin production in patients with nonsense mutation Duchenne muscular dystrophy. *PLoS One.* 2013;8(12):e81302.
144. McDonald CM, Campbell C, Torricelli RE, Finkel RS, Flanigan KM, Goemans N, et al. Ataluren in patients with nonsense mutation Duchenne muscular dystrophy (ACT DMD): A multicentre, randomized, double-blind, placebo-controlled, phase 3 trial. *Lancet.* 2017;390(10101):1489–1498.
145. Dhillon S. Risdiplam: First Approval. *Drugs.* 2020;80(17):1853–1858.
146. Maurer MS, Schwartz JH, Gundapaneni B, Elliott PM, Merlini G, Waddington-Cruz M, et al. Tafamidis Treatment for Patients with Transthyretin Amyloid Cardiomyopathy. *N Engl J Med.* 2018;379(11):1007–1016.
147. Behlke MA. Progress towards in vivo use of siRNAs. *Mol Ther.* 2006;13(4):644–670.
148. Adams D, Gonzalez-Duarte A, O'Riordan WD, Yang CC, Ueda M, et al. Patisiran, an RNAi Therapeutic, for Hereditary Transthyretin Amyloidosis. *N Engl J Med.* 2018;379(1):11–21.
149. Scott LJ. Givosiran: First Approval. *Drugs..* 2020;80(3):335–339.
150. Lam J.K., Chow M.Y., Zhang Y. & Leung S.W. siRNA Versus miRNA as Therapeutics for Gene Silencing. Mol Ther Nucleic Acids, Sept 15 (4), e252, doi. 1038/mtna. 23. 2015.
151. Aguiti S, Marlerba A, Zhaou H. The progress of AAV-mediated gene therapy in neuromuscular disorders. *Expert Opin Biol Ther.* 2018;18(6):681–693.
152. Hoy SM. Onasemnogene Abeparvoc: First Global Approval. *Drugs..* 2019;79(11):1255–1262.
153. Daya S, Berns K. Gene therapy using adeno-associated virus vectors. *Clin Microbiol Rev.* 2008;21(4):583–593.
154. Chamberlain JR, et al. Progress towards gene therapies for Duchenne muscular dystrophy. *Mol Ther.* 2017;25(5):1125–1131.
155. Long C, Amoasii L, Bassel-Duby R, Olson EN. Genome editing of monogenic neuromuscular diseases: a systematic review. *JAMA Neurol.* 2016;73(11):1349–1355.

Case Studies

1 CASE

An Elderly Woman With Numbness in the Hands

An 82-year-old woman with a long-standing history of rheumatoid arthritis (RA) recently suffered a hip fracture that caused difficulty walking, forcing her to use a walker. She presented with numbness and tingling of the hands that had persisted for the previous 6 weeks.

Examination revealed mild limitation of neck movements. Strength and reflexes were normal. She had mild atrophy of the right thenar muscles. There were joint deformities at the hands and wrists. Pain sensation was decreased in the median nerve distribution of the hands; the patient also had a bilateral positive Phalen test.

Neurologic examination was otherwise negative.

WHAT IS THE DIFFERENTIAL DIAGNOSIS?

This patient's symptoms are characteristic of a median neuropathy at the wrist. There are other possibilities to be considered, including C6–C7 radiculopathy, other median neuropathies, and brachial plexopathy, but these are less likely.

AN ELECTROMYOGRAPHY (EMG) TEST WAS PERFORMED

Motor Nerve Studies

Nerve and Site	Latency(ms)	Amplitude (mV)	Conduction Velocity (m/s)
Median Nerve R.	**Normal ≤ 4.2**	**Normal ≥ 6**	**Normal ≥ 50**
Wrist	**7.8**	**1.7**	–
Elbow	12.2	**1.7**	55
Ulnar Nerve R.	**Normal ≤ 3.6**	**Normal ≥ 8**	**Normal ≥ 50**
Wrist	3.0	11	–
Elbow	6.4	10	56

WHAT WERE THE EMG FINDINGS?

This test was done following the practice parameters recommended by the American Association of Neuromuscular and Electrodiagnostic Medicine.[1] It showed prolonged median nerve distal motor latency on the right with a low-amplitude compound muscle action potential (CMAP). The elbow-to-wrist conduction velocity was normal. The right ulnar conduction velocity, CMAP amplitude, and distal latency were normal. The right median sensory nerve action potential (SNAP) had a prolonged latency and slow conduction velocity. The left median CMAP distal latency was mildly prolonged and of normal amplitude; the conduction velocity was normal. The left median SNAP was prolonged and had slow conduction velocity. The ulnar SNAP was normal.

The F-response on the right median nerve was prolonged, likely secondary to the prolonged distal motor latency.

Motor Nerve Studies—cont'd

Nerve and Site	Latency (ms)	Amplitude (mV)	Conduction Velocity (m/s)
Median Nerve L.	**Normal ≤ 4.2**	**Normal ≥ 6**	**Normal ≥ 50**
Wrist	**4.3**	6	–
Elbow	8.4	6	55

F-Wave Studies

Nerve	Latency (ms)	Normal Latency ≤ (ms)
Median nerve R.	**39.4**	30
Ulnar nerve R.	27.2	30
Median nerve L.	28.1	30

Sensory Nerve Studies

Nerve	Onset Latency (ms)	Normal Onset Latency ≤ (ms)	Peak Latency (ms)	Normal Peak Latency ≤ (ms)	Amp (μV)	Normal Amp ≥ (μV)	Conduction Velocity (m/s)	Normal Conduction Velocity ≥ (m/s)
Median nerve R.	**6.5**	2.6	**7.0**	3.1	**5**	20	**20**	50
Ulnar nerve R.	2.4	2.6	2.9	3.1	25	13	50	50
Median nerve L.	**3.4**	2.6	**3.9**	3.1	26	20	**38**	50

EMG Data

Muscle	Insrt Activity	Fibs	Pos Waves	Fasc	Amp	Dur	Poly	Pattern
Brachioradialis R.	Norm	None	None	None	Norm	Norm	None	Full
Flexor carpi ulnaris R.	Norm	None	None	None	Norm	Norm	None	Full
Extensor dig. communis R.	Norm	None	None	None	Norm	Norm	None	Full
Abductor pollicis brevis R.	Norm	None	None	None	**Lg**	**Inc**	None	**Red**
First dorsal interosseous R.	Norm	None	None	None	Norm	Norm	None	Full

Amp, Amplitude; *ms*, milliseconds; *mV*, millivolts; *μV*, microvolts; *m/s*, meters per second; *Dur*, duration; *Fasc*, fasciculations; *Fibs*, fibrillation potentials; *Inc*, increased; *Insrt*, insertional; *Lg*, large; *Poly*, polyphasic; *Pos Waves*, positive sharp waves. These abbreviations apply to all EMG reports in this book. Values in bold are abnormal.

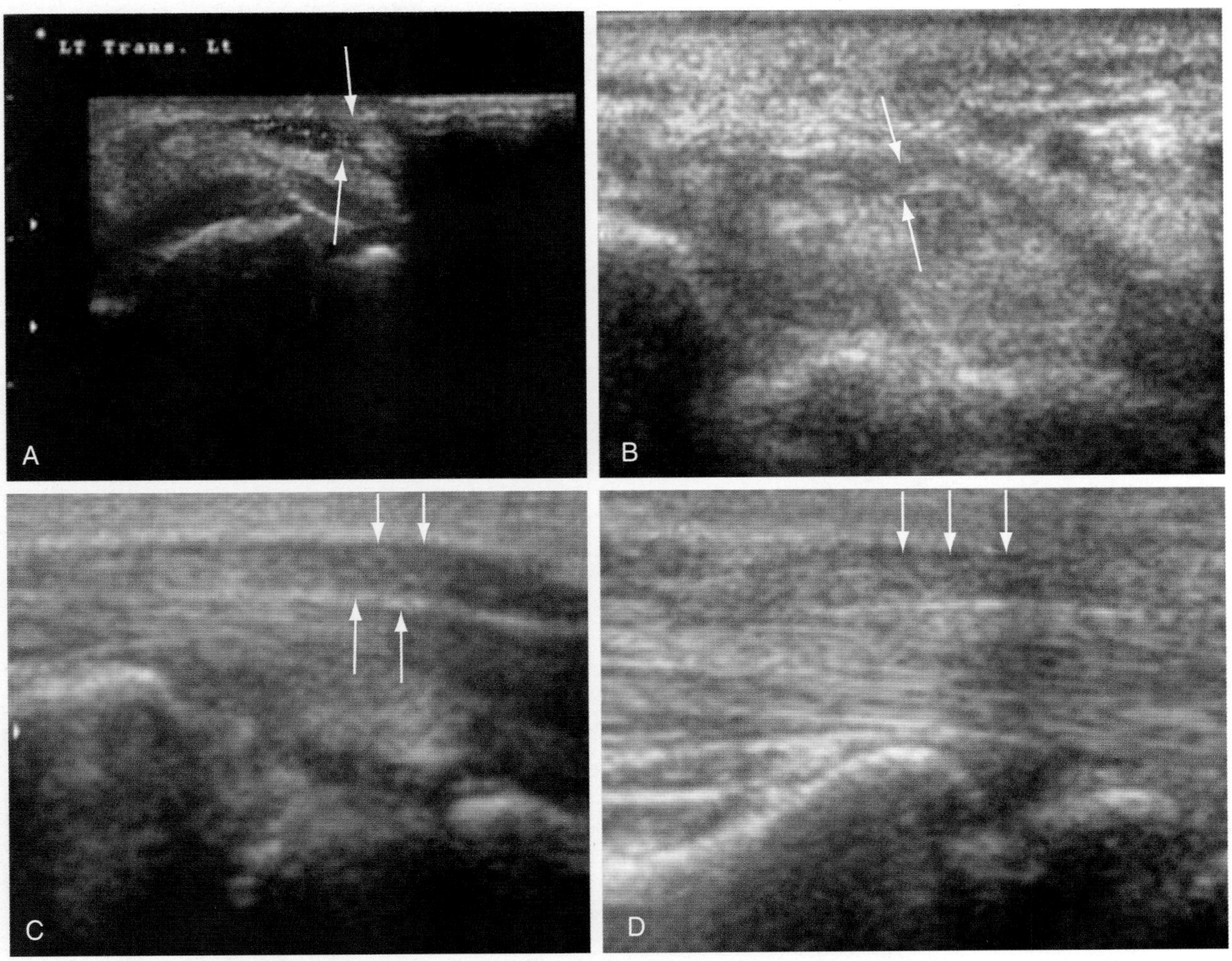

FIG. 1-1 A and B, Ultrasound of the left wrist showing narrowing of the median nerve diameter marked with arrows. **C and D**, Normal ultrasound of the median nerve in a control subject.

The needle test showed large motor unit potentials only in the abductor pollicis brevis muscle.

There was thus distal median nerve demyelination and chronic axonal degeneration in the right, causing a low-amplitude CMAP and large motor unit potentials with reduced recruitment.

It was concluded that this patient had carpal tunnel syndrome from RA and likely also from a compression from the use of a walker.

An ultrasound of the wrist showed evidence of compression deformity at the median nerve at the wrist (Fig. 1-1).

For further discussion, important points, and references, see Case 2.

SUMMARY

This elderly woman, who has RA and uses a walker to ambulate, developed symptoms of median neuropathy at the wrist, documented electrophysiologically. Nerve conduction tests were diagnostic of carpal tunnel syndrome. She was treated conservatively with wrist splints.

For further discussion, important points, and references, see Case 2.

A Diabetic Man With Arm Swelling, Pain, and Numbness

A 65-year-old insulin-dependent diabetic developed end-stage renal disease. He had undergone hemodialysis therapy through a catheter in the left arm for the past 3 years. He presented with pain and swelling of the arm and had evidence of infection in the hemodialysis fistula by *Neisseria*.

Neurologic examination revealed the swelling of the left arm with hand weakness and sensory deficits in the median and ulnar distributions. The examination was difficult because of the patient's severe pain. He also had decreased sensation in the median nerve distribution of the right hand, where he had a positive Phalen test. There was also distal leg weakness and areflexia in the legs with absent vibration sense in the feet and ankles and with decreased pinprick sensation up to the midcalf. The neurologic examination was otherwise normal.

AN ELECTROMYOGRAPHY TEST WAS PERFORMED

Motor Nerve Studies

Nerve and Site	Latency(ms)	Amplitude (mV)	Conduction Velocity (m/s)
Peroneal Nerve L.	**Normal ≤ 5.7**	**Normal ≥ 3**	**Normal ≥ 40**
Ankle	**NR**	**NR**	–
Fibular head	**NR**	**NR**	**NR**

All bolded values are abnormal.

Peroneal Nerve L. (Tibialis Anterior, Recording With a Needle Electrode)

Fibular head	4.2	**3**	–
Knee	6.8	**3**	**39**
Tibial Nerve L.	**Normal ≤ 5.3**	**Normal ≥ 4**	**Normal ≥ 40**
Ankle	5.2	**3**	–
Pop. fossa	16.5	**2**	**38**

Median Nerve L.	**Normal ≤ 4.2**	**Normal ≥ 6**	**Normal ≥ 50**
Wrist	**5.9**	**1.0**	–
Elbow	10.8	**1.0**	**48**
Nerve and Site	**Latency (ms)**	**Amplitude (mV)**	**Conduction Velocity (m/s)**
Ulnar Nerve L.	**Normal ≤ 3.6**	**Normal ≥ 8**	**Normal ≥ 50**
Wrist	**4.2**	**0.4**	–
Below elbow	9.7	**0.3**	**43**
Above elbow	22.8	**0.3**	9
Median Nerve R.	**Normal ≤ 4.2**	**Normal ≥ 6**	**Normal ≥ 50**
Wrist	4.0	6	–
Elbow	8.3	6	52
Ulnar Nerve R.	**Normal ≤ 3.6**	**Normal ≥ 8**	**Normal ≥ 50**
Wrist	2.7	8	–
Below elbow	6.0	8	63
Above elbow	8.0	8	60

F-Wave and Tibial H-Reflex Studies

Nerve	Latency (ms)	Normal Latency ≤ (ms)
Peroneal nerve L.	**NR**	54
Tibial nerve L.	**NR**	54
Median nerve L.	**NR**	30
Ulnar nerve L.	**NR**	30
Median nerve R.	**32.6**	30
Ulnar nerve R.	**31.2**	30
H-reflex L.	**NR**	34
H-reflex R.	**NR**	34

Sensory Nerve Studies

Nerve	Onset Latency (ms)	Normal Onset Latency ≤ (ms)	Peak Latency (ms)	Normal Peak Latency ≤ (ms)	Amp (μV)	Normal Amp ≥ (μV)	Conduction Velocity (m/s)	Normal Conduction Velocity ≥ (m/s)
Median nerve L.	**NR**	2.6	**NR**	3.1	**NR**	20	**NR**	50
Ulnar nerve L.	**NR**	2.6	**NR**	3.1	**NR**	13	**NR**	50

Sensory Nerve Studies—cont'd

Nerve	Onset Latency (ms)	Normal Onset Latency ≤ (ms)	Peak Latency (ms)	Normal Peak Latency ≤ (ms)	Amp (μV)	Normal Amp ≥ (μV)	Conduction Velocity (m/s)	Normal Conduction Velocity ≥ (m/s)
Median nerve R.	2.4	2.6	2.9	3.1	21	20	54	50
Ulnar nerve R.	2.3	2.6	2.8	3.1	13	13	52	50
Sural nerve L.	**NR**	3.5	**NR**	4.0	**NR**	11	**NR**	40

Electromyography Data

Muscle	Insrt Activity	Fibs	Pos Waves	Fasc	Amp	Dur	Poly	Pattern
Extensor dig. communis L.	Norm	None	None	None	Norm	Norm	None	Full
Flexor carpi ulnaris L.	Norm	None	None	None	Norm	Norm	None	Full
Abductor pollicis brevis L.	**Inc**	None	**2+**	None	Norm	Norm	None	**Red**
First dorsal interosseous L.	**Inc**	None	**2+**	None	**Lg**	**Inc**	None	**Red**
Pronator quadratus L.	Norm	None	None	None	Norm	Norm	None	Full
Abductor pollicis brevis R.	Norm	None	None	None	Norm	Norm	None	Full
First dorsal interosseous R.	Norm	None	None	None	Norm	Norm	None	Full
Tibialis anterior L.	Norm	None	None	None	**Lg**	**Inc**	None	**Red**

WHAT WERE THE ELECTROMYOGRAPHY FINDINGS?

Motor nerve conduction tests showed nonrecordable compound muscle action potentials (CMAP) when stimulating the left peroneal nerve and recording on the extensor digitorum brevis muscle and borderline conduction velocity when recording at the tibialis anterior muscle with a needle electrode. The tibial nerve motor conduction velocity was mildly slow with a borderline CMAP amplitude. The left median nerve conduction velocity was slow, and the CMAP was of low amplitude and of prolonged latency; ulnar nerve conduction velocity was slow, particularly across the elbow, and the CMAP was of very low amplitude. Tests of both median and ulnar nerves were normal on the right.

The left median and ulnar sensory nerve action potentials (SNAPs) were absent, and they were both normal on the right. There were absent H-reflexes and sural SNAPs. F-responses were absent on the left arm and leg and were mildly prolonged on the right arm.

Needle electromyography (EMG) revealed denervation potentials with large motor unit potentials in the median-and ulnar-innervated muscles of the hand, indicating axonal degeneration. Large motor unit potentials with a reduced recruitment pattern were also seen in the tibialis anterior muscle secondary to the patient's polyneuropathy.

WHAT IS THE MOST LIKELY DIAGNOSIS?

It was concluded that this patient had diffuse polyneuropathy from uremia and diabetes. The hand symptoms and EMG findings were diagnostic of a shunt-related ischemic monomelic neuropathy (IMN). The shunt was replaced by one placed in the inguinal area. The patient received aggressive antibiotic therapy.

IMN, a condition reported initially by Wilbourn in 1983,[1] is caused by complete occlusion of the shunt after placement or infection and manifests by burning paresthesias and weakness in the median- and ulnar-innervated muscle; there could also be swelling. IMN occurs most frequently in diabetics,[2] particularly those with peripheral neuropathy and atherosclerotic disease.[3,4] As in this case, treatment consists of surgical removal of the affected shunt.[5,6]

Other shunt-related neuropathies include a vascular steal neuropathy[7] that occurs several months after shunt placement and is caused by reverse arterial flow away from the digits. There are also shunt-related compression neuropathies of the median and ulnar nerves.[8] Other mononeuropathies in uremics include carpal tunnel syndrome (CTS) and other entrapments. Uremic patients can also have damage to nerves during kidney transplants.[9]

FOLLOW-UP

The patient got progressively better and did well until 1 year later, when he presented with paresthesias and mild swelling in both hands.

Neurologic examination then was essentially normal except for a motor sensory neuropathy with a bilateral positive Phalen test and mild decreased sensation in both median nerve distribution and mild swelling of the digits.

A SECOND ELECTROMYOGRAPHY TEST WAS PERFORMED

Motor Nerve Studies

Nerve and Site	Latency (ms)	Amplitude (mV)	Conduction Velocity (m/s)
Median Nerve R.[a]	Normal ≤ 4.2	Normal ≥ 6	Normal ≥ 50
Wrist	**8.7**	**0.8**	–
Elbow	15.6	**0.8**	**39**

Motor Nerve Studies—cont'd

Ulnar Nerve R.[b]	Normal ≤ 3.6	Normal ≥ 8	Normal ≥ 50
Wrist	2.6	8	–
Below elbow	5.9	8	63
Above elbow	7.9	8	60
Median Nerve L.[c]	**Normal ≤ 4.2**	**Normal ≥ 6**	**Normal ≥ 50**
Wrist	**4.9**	**4**	–
Elbow	11.3	**3**	**44**
Ulnar Nerve L.[d]	**Normal ≤ 3.6**	**Normal ≥ 8**	**Normal ≥ 50**
Wrist	3.2	**0.6**	–
Below elbow	14.7	**0.5**	**49**

[a]Terminal latency index 0.020; normal 0.343–0.353.
[b]Terminal latency index 0.042; normal 0.396–0.414.
[c]Terminal latency index 0.032; normal 0.343–0.353.
[d]Terminal latency index 0.044; normal 0.396–0.414.

Motor Nerve Studies—cont'd

Nerve and Site	Latency (ms)	Amplitude (mV)	Conduction Velocity (m/s)
Peroneal Nerve R.	**Normal ≤ 5.7**	**Normal ≥ 3**	**Normal ≥ 40**
Ankle	**NR**	**NR**	–
Fibular head	**NR**	**NR**	**NR**
Knee	**NR**	**NR**	**NR**

Motor Nerve Studies—cont'd

Tibial Nerve R.	Normal ≤ 5.3	Normal ≥ 4	Normal ≥ 40
Ankle	5.2	**1**	–
Pop. fossa	21.8	**0.7**	**32**

F-Wave and Tibial H-Reflex Studies

Nerve	Latency (ms)	Normal Latency ≤ (ms)
Median nerve R.	**NR**	30
Ulnar nerve R.	**30.5**	30
Median nerve L.	**37**	30
Ulnar nerve L.	**32.6**	30
Peroneal nerve R.	**NR**	54
Tibial nerve R.	**NR**	54
H-reflex R.	**NR**	34
H-reflex L.	**NR**	34

Sensory Nerve Studies

Nerve	Peak Latency (ms)	Normal Peak Latency ≤ (ms)	Amp (μV)	Normal Amp ≥ (μV)
Median nerve R.	**NR**	3.1	**NR**	20
Ulnar nerve R.	2.8	3.1	**11**	13
Median nerve L.	**NR**	3.1	**NR**	20
Ulnar nerve L.	**3.2**	3.1	**12**	13
Sural nerve R.	**NR**	4.0	**NR**	11

Electromyography Data

Muscle	Insrt Activity	Fibs	Pos Waves	Fasc	Amp	Dur	Poly	Pattern
Flexor carpi ulnaris R.	Norm	None	None	None	**Lg**	**Inc**	**Few**	Full
Abductor pollicis brevis R.	**Inc**	**2+**	**2+**	None	**Lg**	**Inc**	**Few**	**Red**
First dorsal interosseous R.	Norm	None	None	None	**Lg**	**Inc**	None	Full
Pronator quadratus L.	Norm	None	None	None	Norm	Norm	None	Full
Extensor digitorum communis L.	Norm	None	None	None	Norm	Norm	None	Full
First dorsal interosseous L.	Norm	None	None	None	Norm	Norm	None	Full
Abductor pollicis brevis L.	Norm	None	None	None	Norm	Norm	None	Full

WHAT DID THE SECOND ELECTROMYOGRAPHY SHOW?

This test showed absent peroneal CMAP and low-amplitude tibial CMAP with slow conduction velocity. The H-reflex and sural SNAPs were absent. F-responses were absent in the right leg and right median nerve and were prolonged in the left median and ulnar nerves.

There was markedly prolonged right median distal motor latency with a low-amplitude CMAP. The left median distal latency was prolonged, the velocity was slow, and the CMAP had low amplitude. The conduction velocity latency and CMAP were normal in the right ulnar nerve. The left ulnar nerve showed borderline low conduction velocity and low CMAP amplitude. The median nerves' terminal latency indexes were low, indicating distal demyelination in those.

The needle test showed denervation of the right abductor pollicis brevis muscle with decreased motor unit recruitment.

It was concluded that this patient had bilateral median neuropathy at the wrist—likely from CTS—more severe on the right with axonal degeneration, in addition to polyneuropathy.

WHAT OTHER TESTS SHOULD BE DONE?

Erythrocyte sedimentation rate was normal; ANCA titers, immunoelectrophoresis, and FANA were normal. Creatinine was 8 mg/dL (normal, <1.5 mg/dL) and blood urea nitrogen was 48 mg/dL (normal, <20 mg/dL); fasting blood sugar was 148 mg/dL (normal, <120 mg/dL) and glycosylated hemoglobin was 5% (normal, 5.3%–7.5%).

WHAT IS THE MOST LIKELY DIAGNOSIS?

This patient with diabetic and uremic polyneuropathy developed CTS in both hands with swelling. β_2-Microglobulin levels were 26,574 µg/L (normal, <3000 µg/L). He was treated with wrist splints and hemodialysis with microfiltration. Three months later, he underwent kidney and pancreas transplantation, and his symptoms improved slowly. He has now been completely asymptomatic for 2 years.

SUMMARY

This patient with diabetic and uremic polyneuropathy developed an ischemic shunt-related neuropathy and later had bilateral CTS thought to be caused by β_2-microglobulin deposits. He improved with pancreas/kidney transplant. He is no longer a diabetic, his renal function is normal, and he is asymptomatic.

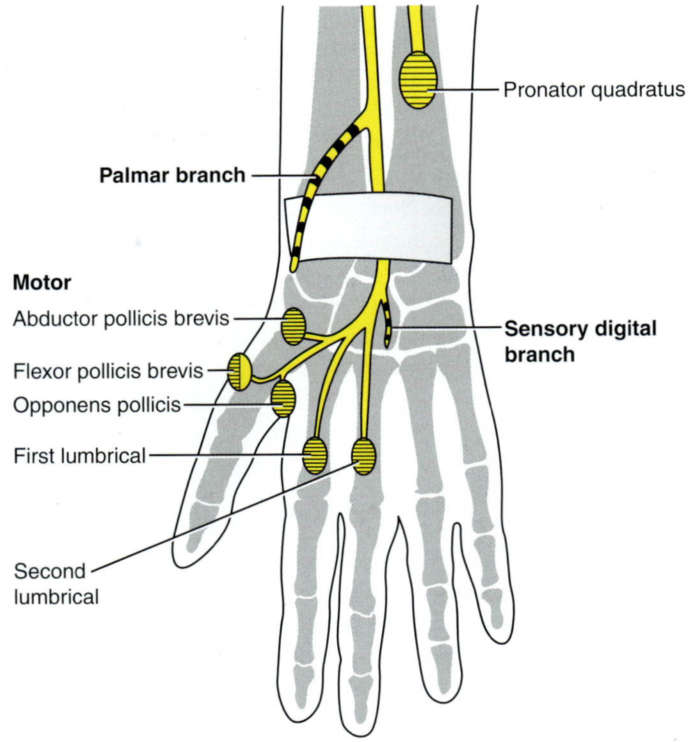

FIG. 2-1 Anatomy of the median nerve and its branches at the wrist and hand.

DISCUSSION (CASES 1 AND 2)

Case 1 had CTS, likely related to her rheumatoid arthritis (RA) and compression of the median nerve from the use of a walker was also contributory.

To understand CTS, it is important to remember the anatomy of the median nerve at the wrist. After giving off the cutaneous branch that covers the skin of the thenar eminence, the median nerve passes through the carpal tunnel. Here the carpal bones form a concavity which is covered by the transverse carpal ligament (Fig. 2-1). Through this tunnel also pass the tendons of the finger flexors and the flexor pollicis longus. This is a relatively narrow canal where the nerve is predisposed to compression.

After passing through the tunnel, the median nerve gives off the motor recurrent branch that innervates the muscles of the thenar eminence and then divides into median and lateral branches. These subdivide to provide innervation of the other median hand muscles, as well as the skin of the palmar surface of the hand, the palmar surface of the first three digits and part of the fourth, and the dorsal surface of the distal phalanx of the first three digits and part of the fourth.

Compressions of the median nerve in the carpal tunnel cause CTS, which is the most common entrapment neuropathy. This condition has a prevalence in the general population of about 0.6 in men and 6.8 in women[10] and has an estimated incidence in the United States of about 55–125 cases in 100,000 people.[11,12] CTS is commonly associated with neuropathies as in uremic diabetes and thyroid disorders.

Compression of the median nerve was first described in 1913 by Marie and Foix.[12] It was recognized later as a clinical entity[13,14] and as one of the most frequently seen neurologic disorders.[15–17]

CTS has many causes, particularly frequent flexion and extension movements and typing.[15–18] It is associated with endocrine disorders,[19,20] pregnancy,[21] compression by tumors, congenital narrowing of the canal,[22] and particularly RA caused by thickening of the tendons or osteophytes.[23,24] Amyloidosis,[25] and particularly β_2-microglobulin accumulation in uremia, can also cause CTS.[26] Cyclists and persons in wheelchairs may develop CTS from wrist compression[27] similar to what was likely the mechanism caused by the use of a walker in Case 1.

The symptoms of CTS are tingling and numbness in the hands with pain frequently occurring at night. Patients report temporary improvement when they shake their hands.[22] Later, with progression, there could be persistent numbness in the digits as well as weakness and atrophy of the thenar eminence.

The clinical diagnosis is based on the history and the sensory deficit in the median digits, as well as a positive Phalen test. This consists of flexing the hand for 30–60 seconds, which produces numbness and tingling.[28,29] The reverse Phalen test, done by extending the wrist, produces the symptoms in a similar manner.[30] Tinel's sign is also used in the diagnosis; this consists of percussing the median nerve at the wrist, thereby producing a shooting pain. Compression of the median nerve at the wrist by the examiner's thumb is another useful test which when positive causes tingling and numbness in the hand.[28]

The differential diagnosis of CTS includes radiculopathies and brachial plexopathy, as well as other median neuropathies caused by trauma, vasculitis, and entrapments at the axilla, arm, or forearm.[31,32] Patients with CTS might have an associated radiculopathy, the diagnosis of which should be established with needle EMG.

There are several electrophysiologic tests used in the diagnosis of CTS.[33–36] These include the commonly used technique of measurement of the CMAP latency of the median nerve while recording at the abductor pollicis brevis muscle. The test can also be done by stimulating the palm to compare with the CMAP amplitude obtained during wrist stimulation. In this way the examiner can determine whether or not there is a conduction block, as palmar stimulation is distal to the site of compression.[33–36] Inching techniques can also be used to detect the site of conduction block.[36]

Sensory tests, particularly those measuring the SNAP latencies and conduction velocity of the median nerve to the digits and then comparing them with those of the ulnar and radial nerves, are very useful and sensitive.[37] Measurement of the medial palmar cutaneous mixed nerve latency is also a valuable test and is the most sensitive test for CTS.

The terminal latency index is used to diagnose CTS in patients who also have a neuropathy, to determine if there is more distal demyelination in the median nerve, particularly when compared with the ulnar.[35] Other tests include comparisons of the median and ulnar nerve latencies while recording at the thenar eminence.[36] Comparison of the motor latencies with the second lumbrical/interosseous when stimulating the median and ulnar nerves is another useful diagnostic method.[38,39]

Needle EMG is not absolutely necessary in the diagnosis of CTS, but it is often done to determine the presence of axonal degeneration in patients who have significant prolongation of the distal latency. It is also helpful in diagnosing other associated conditions such as radiculopathy.

Imaging studies such as MRI[39–41] and ultrasonography[42] are useful in detecting structural abnormalities. One study demonstrated a high sensitivity of ultrasonography when compared with electrodiagnostic tests and documented changes in the carpal tunnel morphology in 35% of cases. It suggested that this could lead to a different therapeutic approach.[43]

The treatment of CTS includes removal of the causes, as in the case of tumors or the treatment of hypothyroidism. Weight loss can help. Wrist splinting can relieve the symptoms,[44] and if that yields no response, local steroid injections are helpful.[22] Surgical release can be curative.[45] This can now be done with endoscopic techniques.[46]

Case 2 is interesting because the patient had two forms of focal neuropathies that occur in uremics. He presented initially with a shunt-related ischemic neuropathy and later developed bilateral CTS with some swelling in the hands. He had an elevation of β_2-microglobulin plasma levels, and it was thought that his CTS was caused by β_2-microglobulin accumulation,[47–49] although this was not confirmed. This cause of CTS occurs frequently in patients with chronic hemodialysis and has been reported to have an incidence of 100% of patients who undergo dialysis for over 25 years.[49] In these cases, during surgery, the carpal tunnel is found to be full of soft gold-brown material, which is demonstrated to be amyloid.[49] This form of dialysis-induced amyloid deposits results from the accumulation of the abnormal protein that is not filtered by cellulose dialysis membranes. Dialysis with ultrafiltration may be helpful, but the best treatment is kidney transplantation. Surgical release may be beneficial.

IMPORTANT POINTS

- CTS has many causes, including frequent repetitive movements, swelling, tumors, hypothyroidism, diabetes and amyloid deposits, and RA, among others, and can be aggravated by compression such as that caused by the use of walkers.
- CTS is diagnosed by the history of tingling paresthesias and pain associated with numbness in the hand in the median nerve distribution; if severe, there could also be thenar muscle atrophy. Patients might show positive Phalen test and Tinel signs.
- Electrophysiologic tests in CTS should include testing median CMAP latency and conduction velocity, and SNAP and mixed nerve latencies and velocities; this should be done in both sides. Ulnar sensory and motor conduction tests should also be done in the affected side.
- The SNAP latency and mixed nerve conduction tests are most sensitive for documenting CTS. If peripheral neuropathy is suspected, other nerves should be studied. The terminal latency index is helpful in diagnosing CTS in patients with peripheral neuropathy.
- Needle EMG can be used to document or rule out an associated disease, such as radiculopathy. This includes testing of median-innervated muscles in the hand and forearm and of muscles that are not innervated by the median nerve but share the same roots, cords, or trunks of the brachial plexus.
- The treatment of CTS is conservative with splinting and steroid injections; surgery is used in cases that do not respond to conservative management.
- Uremics usually have a peripheral neuropathy and can also be predisposed to entrapments and compression from shunts and shunt-related ischemic neuropathy.
- CTS in uremics can be caused by deposits of β_2-microglobulin in the carpal tunnel. Its incidence increases with the duration of renal failure.
- The best treatment for β_2-microglobulin accumulation is kidney transplantation. Surgical release is also helpful.

REFERENCES

1. Jablecki CK, Andary MT, Floeter MK, et al. Practice parameter: electrodiagnostic studies in carpal tunnel syndrome. Report of the American Association of Electrodiagnostic Medicine, the American Academy of Neurology, and the American Academy of Physical Medicine and Rehabilitation. *Neurology*. 2002;58:1589–1592.
2. Wilbourn AJ, Furlan AJ, Hulley W, Ruschhaupt W. Ischemic monomelic neuropathy. *Neurology*. 1983;33(4):447–451.
3. Riggs JE, Moss AH, Labosky DA, et al. Upper extremity ischemic monomelic neuropathy: a complication of vascular

access procedures in uremic diabetic patients. *Neurology.* 1989;39(7):997–998.
4. Bolton CF, Driedger AA, Lindsay RM. Ischaemic neuropathy in uremic patients caused by bovine arteriovenous shunt. *J Neurol Neurosurg Psychiatry.* 1979;42(9):810–814.
5. Hebl JR, Horlocker TT. Brachial neuropathy after haemodialysis shunt placement under axillary blockade. *Anesth Analg.* 1999; 89(4):1025–1026.
6. Hye RJ, Wolf YG. Ischemic monomelic neuropathy: an under-recognized complication of hemodialyses access. *Ann Vasc Surg.* 1994;8(6):578–582.
7. Wytrzes L, Markley HG, Fisher M, Alfred HJ. Brachial neuropathy after brachial artery antecubital vein shunts for chronic hemodialysis. *Neurology.* 1987;37(8):1398–1400.
8. Miles AM. Vascular steal syndrome and ischemic monomelic neuropathy: two variants of upper limb ischemia after haemodialysis vascular access surgery. *Nephrol Dial Transplant.* 1999;14(2):297–300.
9. Delmez JA, Holtmann B, Sicard GA, et al. Peripheral nerve entrapment syndromes in chronic hemodialysis patients. *Nephron.* 1982;30(2):118–123.
10. Al-Hayk K, Bertorini TE. Neuromuscular complications in uremics: a review. *Neurologist.* 2007;13:188–196.
11. Dumitru D, Zwarts MJ. Focal peripheral neuropathies. In: Dumitru D, Amato AA, Zwarts MJ, eds. *Electrodiagnostic Medicine.* 2nd ed. Philadelphia, PA: Hanley & Belfus; 2002:1044–1045.
12. de Krom MC, Knipschild PG, Kester AD, et al. Carpal tunnel syndrome: prevalence in the general population. *J Clin Epidemiol.* 1992;45:373–376.
13. Marie P, Foix C. Atrophic isolee de l'eminence thenar d'origine nevritque: role du ligament annulaire anterieur dans la localization de la lesion. *Rev Neurol (Paris).* 1913;26:647–649.
14. Cannon BW, Save JG. Tardy median palsy, median neuritis, median thenar neuritis, amenable to surgery. *Surgery.* 1946;20:210–216.
15. Brain WR, Wright AD, Wilkerson M. Spontaneous compression of both median nerves in the carpal tunnel. *Lancet.* 1947;1:277–288.
16. Silverstein BA, Fine LJ, Armstrong TJ. Occupational factors and carpal tunnel syndrome. *Am J Ind Med.* 1987;11:343–358.
17. Werner RA, Armstrong TJ. Carpal tunnel syndrome: ergonomic risk factors and intra carpal canal pressure, carpal tunnel syndrome. *Phys Med Rehabil Clin N Am.* 1997;8:555–569.
18. Roquelaure Y, Mechali S, Dano C, et al. Occupational and personal risk factors for carpal tunnel syndrome in industrial workers. *Scand J Work Environ Health.* 1997;23:364–369.
19. Koskimies K, Farkkila M, Pyykko I, et al. Carpal tunnel syndrome in vibration disease. *Br J Ind Med.* 1990;47:411–416.
20. Murray IP, Simpson JA. Acroparaesthesia in myxoedema: a clinical and electromyographic study. *Lancet.* 1958;1:1360–1363.
21. Melvin JL, Burnett CN, Johnson EW. Median nerve conduction in pregnancy. *Arch Phys Med Rehabil.* 1969;50:75–80.
22. Stewart JD. *Peripheral Neuropathies.* 3rd ed. Philadelphia, PA: Lippincott, Williams & Wilkins; 2000:183–239.
23. Phalen GS. The carpal tunnel syndrome: 17 years experience in diagnosis and treatment of 654 hands. *J Bone Joint Surg Am.* 1966;48:211–228.
24. Vemireddi NK, Redford JB, PombeJara CN. Serial nerve conduction studies in carpal tunnel syndrome secondary to rheumatoid arthritis: preliminary study. *Arch Phys Med Rehabil.* 1979;60:393–396.
25. Gertz MA, Kyle RA. Primary systemic amyloidosis: a diagnostic primer. *Mayo Clin Proc.* 1989;64:1505–1519.
26. Shirahama T, Skinner M, Cohen AS, et al. Histochemical and immunohistochemical characterization of amyloid associated with chronic hemodialysis as beta-2 microglobulin. *Lab Invest.* 1985;53:705–709.
27. Boninger ML, Robertson RN, Wolff M, Cooper RA. Upper limb nerve entrapments in elite wheelchair racers. *Am J Phys Med Rehabil.* 1996;75:170–176.
28. de Krom MC, Knipschild PG, Kester AD, Spaans F. Efficacy of provocative tests for diagnosis of carpal tunnel syndrome. *Lancet.* 1990;335:393–395.
29. Seror P. Phalen's test in the diagnosis of carpal tunnel syndrome. *J Hand Surg [Br].* 1988;13:383–385.
30. Werner RA, Bir C, Armstrong TJ. Reverse Phalen's maneuver as an aid in diagnosing carpal tunnel syndrome. *Arch Phys Med Rehabil.* 1994;75:783–786.
31. Gessini L, Jandolo B, Pietrangeli A. Entrapment neuropathies of the median nerve at and above the elbow. *Surg Neurol.* 1983;19:112–116.
32. Bilge T, Yalaman O, Bilge S, et al. Entrapment neuropathy of the median nerve at the level of the ligament of Struthers. *Neurosurgery.* 1990;27:787–789.
33. Kimura J. *Assessment of individual nerves.* In: *Electrodiagnosis in Diseases of Nerve and Muscle: Principles and Practice.* 3rd ed. Oxford: Oxford University Press; 2001:130–177.
34. Sander HW, Quinto C, Saadeh PB, Chokroverty S. Sensitive median-ulnar motor comparative techniques in carpal tunnel syndrome. *Muscle Nerve.* 1999;22:88–98.
35. Simovic D, Weinberg DH. Terminal latency index in the carpal tunnel syndrome. *Muscle Nerve.* 1997;20:1178–1180.
36. Kimura J. The carpal tunnel syndrome: localization of conduction abnormalities within the distal segment of the median nerve. *Brain.* 1979;102:619–635.
37. Pease WS, Cannell CD, Johnson EW. Median to radial latency difference test in mild carpal tunnel syndrome. *Muscle Nerve.* 1989;12:905–909.
38. Preston DC, Logigian EL. Lumbrical and interossei recording a carpal tunnel syndrome. Muscle Nerve. 1992;15:1253–1257.
39. Britz GW, Haynor DR, Kuntz C, et al. Carpal tunnel syndrome: correlation of magnetic resonance imaging, clinical, electrodiagnostic, and intraoperative findings. *Neurosurgery.* 1995;37:1097–1103.
40. Allmann KH, Horch R, Uhl M, et al. MR imaging of the carpal tunnel. *Eur J Radiol.* 1997;25:141–145.
41. Horch RE, Allmann KH, Laubenberger J, et al. Median nerve compression can be detected by magnetic resonance imaging of the carpal tunnel. *Neurosurgery.* 1997;41:76–82.
42. Chen P, Maklad N, Redwine M, Zelitt D. Dynamic high-resolution sonography of the carpal tunnel. *Am J Roentgenol.* 1997;168(2):533–537.
43. Kele H, Verheggen R, Bittermann HJ, Reimers CD. The potential value of ultrasonography in the evaluation of carpal tunnel syndrome. *Neurology.* 2003;61(3):389–391.
44. Burke DT, Burke MM, Stewart GW, Cambre A. Splinting for carpal tunnel syndrome: in search of the optimal angle. *Arch Phys Med Rehabil.* 1994;75:1241–1244.
45. Armstrong MB, Villalobos RE. Surgical treatment of carpal tunnel syndrome. *Phys Med Rehabil Clin N Am.* 1997;8:529–539.
46. Jimenez DF, Gibbs SR, Clapper AT. Endoscopic treatment of carpal tunnel syndrome: a critical review. *J Neurosurg.* 1998;88:817–826.
47. Kessler M, Hestin D, Aymard B, et al. Carpal tunnel syndrome with beta 2-microglobulin amyloid deposits and erosive

arthropathy of the wrist and spine in an uremic patient before chronic hemodialysis. *Nephrol Dial Transplant*. 1995;10(2): 298–299.
48. Charra B, Calemard E, Laurent G. Chronic renal failure treatment duration and mode: their relevance to the late dialysis periarticular syndrome. *Blood Purif*. 1988;6(2):117–124.
49. Naito M, Ogata K, Goya T. Carpal tunnel syndrome in chronic renal dialysis patients: clinical evaluation of 62 hands and results of operative treatment. *J Hand Surg [Br]*. 1987;12(3):366–374.

A Diabetic Man With Hand Numbness and Fainting Spells

A 66-year-old insulin-dependent diabetic man was seen because of mild hand tremors and numbness in the first three fingers of his right hand, which made it difficult for him to play the clarinet.

Past medical history included hyperthyroidism 20 years previously for which he received radiation. He was on thyroid replacement.

He used to smoke but did not drink. Several family members had diabetes mellitus (DM). He was taking tamsulosin for prostatic hypertrophy.

General physical examination, mentation, cranial nerves, and muscle strength were normal; he had no rigidity, bradykinesia, or muscle atrophy. Reflexes were absent at the ankles, trace at the knees, and normal in the upper extremities. He had decreased vibration sense in the toes and ankles and decreased pain sensation up to the ankles. He also had marked decreased pain sensation in the right median nerve distribution. A Phalen test was positive in both upper extremities. Neck motility was normal. The rest of the neurologic examination was normal.

AN EMG TEST WAS PERFORMED

Motor Nerve Studies

Nerve and Site	Latency (ms)	Amplitude (mV)	Conduction Velocity (m/s)
Median Nerve R.[a]	**Normal ≤ 4.2**	**Normal ≥ 6**	**Normal ≥ 50**
Wrist	**8.5**	6	–
Elbow	13.3	6	**42**
Ulnar Nerve R.[b]	**Normal ≤ 3.6**	**Normal ≥ 8**	**Normal ≥ 50**
Wrist	3.4	**7**	–
Below elbow	7.3	**5**	**47**
Above elbow	10.4	**5**	**39**
Median Nerve L.[c]	**Normal ≤ 4.2**	**Normal ≥ 6**	**Normal ≥ 50**
Wrist	**6.2**	**5**	–
Elbow	10.8	**4**	**45**

[a]Terminal latency index 0.188; normal 0.343–0.353.
[b]Terminal latency index 0.411; normal 0.396–0.414.
[c]Terminal latency index 0.241; normal 0.343–0.353.

Motor Nerve Studies—cont'd

Nerve and Site	Latency (ms)	Amplitude (mV)	Conduction Velocity (m/s)
Ulnar Nerve L.[d]	**Normal ≤3.6**	**Normal ≥ 8**	**Normal ≥ 50**
Wrist	2.9	16	–
Below elbow	6.5	15	**48**
Above elbow	8.7	15	54
Peroneal Nerve L.[e]	**Normal ≤ 5.3**	**Normal ≥ 4**	**Normal ≥ 40**
Ankle	**6.1**	**0.6**	–
Fibular head	13.2	**0.6**	40
Knee	15.5	**0.6**	**39**

[d]Terminal latency index 0.482; normal 0.396–0.414.
[e]Terminal latency index 0.327; normal 0.386–0.406.

F-Wave Studies

Nerve	Latency (ms)	Normal Latency ≤ (ms)
Median nerve R.	**38.3**	30
Ulnar nerve R.	**32.2**	30
Median nerve L.	**36.3**	30
Ulnar nerve L.	28.6	30
Peroneal nerve L.	**63.3**	54

Sensory Nerve Studies

Nerve	Peak Latency (ms)	Normal Peak Latency ≤ (ms)	Amp (μV)	Normal Amp ≥ (μV)
Median nerve R.	**NR**	3.1	**NR**	20
Ulnar nerve R.	**NR**	3.1	**NR**	13
Median nerve L.	**NR**	3.1	**NR**	20
Ulnar nerve L.	**NR**	3.1	**NR**	13
Sural nerve L.	**NR**	4.0	**NR**	11

EMG Data

Muscle	Insrt Activity	Fibs	Pos Waves	Fasc	Amp	Dur	Poly	Pattern
Deltoid R.	Norm	None	None	None	Norm	Norm	None	Full
Biceps brachii R.	Norm	None	None	None	Norm	Norm	None	Full
Flexor carpi radialis R.	Norm	None	None	None	Norm	Norm	None	Full
Flexor carpi ulnaris R.	Norm	None	None	None	**Lg**	**Inc**	None	**Red**
Abductor poll. brevis	Norm	None	None	None	**Lg**	**Inc**	None	**Red**
Abductor dig. minimi	Norm	None	None	None	**Lg**	**Inc**	None	**Red**
First dorsal interosseous R.	Norm	None	None	None	**Lg**	**Inc**	None	**Red**
Tibialis anterior R.	Norm	None	None	None	**Lg**	**Inc**	None	**Red**

WHAT WERE THE EMG FINDINGS?

This electrophysiologic study demonstrated slow motor conduction velocities of the ulnar and median nerves and low-amplitude CMAPs with borderline conduction velocity of the peroneal nerve also with low-amplitude CMAP. The median, ulnar, and sural SNAPs were absent. Median nerve distal motor latencies were markedly prolonged in both sides; the ulnar latencies were normal, and the difference between median and ulnar CMAP latencies was 4.1 ms on the right and 3.5 ms on the left (normal, 1.6 ms). Both median and ulnar motor conduction velocities were slow, with more prominent slowing of the ulnar nerve across the elbow. There were prolonged median nerve F-responses corresponding to prolonged distal latencies.

Comparison of CMAP latencies while recording at the thenar eminence and stimulating the median and ulnar nerves showed that the ulnar latency was 4.2 ms whereas the median latency was 8.5 ms on the right, with a difference of 4.3 ms (normal upper limit of latency difference is 0.8 ms).[1] The latency difference on the left was 2.1 ms. Also, the difference of CMAP latency while recording in the second interossei-lumbrical muscles when stimulating the right median and ulnar nerves was 4.1 ms (normal, <0.4 ms)[2] (Not shown in the table).

The terminal latency index was low in the median nerves but not in the ulnar nerves, indicating more distal demyelination of the median nerve, likely from carpal tunnel syndrome (CTS).[3] There were large motor unit potentials with decreased recruitment in the distal muscles, but no active denervation.

In conclusion, the findings indicated a chronic sensory motor polyneuropathy and a superimposed median neuropathy at both wrists, likely from CTS.

The patient declined surgery and was treated with splinting resulting in some improvement.

His tremor improved with low doses of trihexyphenidyl. He did not tolerate primidone, and beta-blockers were avoided because of his diabetes.

He returned 4 years later, complaining of fainting spells after standing up. His neurologic examination was essentially unchanged. There was a drop in blood pressure from 120/70 mm Hg to 105/60 mm Hg during tilt.

WHAT SHOULD BE DONE NEXT?

Autonomic nervous system testing revealed absent sympathetic skin responses in the foot and hand (Table 3-1). He developed presyncopal symptoms during the tilt table test, and his blood pressure dropped from 130/66 mm Hg supine to 79/60 mm Hg after 14 minutes of tilt (normal, <20 mm Hg) with stable pulse rates of 72 and 75 per minute.

His heart rate during deep inspiration changed 10 beats per minute (normal, >15), while his Valsalva ratio was 1.1 (normal, >1.21). After 5 minutes of isometric exercise, his diastolic blood pressure increased only 5 mm Hg (normal, >16 mm Hg). The patient also had decreased sweat response in the legs and absent in the foot during the quantitative sudomotor axon reflex test.[4]

The abnormal tilt table test, absent sympathetic skin response, and lack of significant increase in blood pressure during sustained handgrip indicate impairment of the sympathetic nervous system. Similarly, the abnormal Valsalva ratio

TABLE 3-1 Autonomic Testing

	Normal Range	Patient's Values
Change in HR with deep respirations	>15 bpm	**10 bpm**
Valsalva ratio	>1.21	**1.1**
Sympathetic Isometric Exercise Test: Diastolic BP		
Baseline	–	68 mm Hg
After 5 min	–	73 mm Hg
Difference after 5 min	>16 mm Hg	**5 mm Hg**
Sympathetic Skin Responses		
Upper limb	Present	**Absent**
Lower limb	Present	**Absent**
QSART (sweat test)		
Forearm	2.67–5.06 mL/cm	**0.8** mL/cm
Leg	1.83–3.82 mL/cm	**0.5** mL/cm
Foot	1.75–3.65 mL/cm	**0.0** mL/cm

bpm, Beats per minute; *HR*, heart rate; *QSART*, quantitative sudomotor axon reflex test.

and the abnormal heart rate changes during deep inspiration indicate impairment of the parasympathetic nervous system, all likely from his diabetic neuropathy and from the effects of medications.

WHAT SHOULD BE THE MANAGEMENT?

The trihexyphenidyl and tamsulosin were discontinued with some improvement of his orthostatic hypotension. The addition of midodrine 5 mg three times daily and elastic stockings provided further improvement.

SUMMARY

This diabetic patient with a polyneuropathy had bilateral CTS, demonstrated by significant distal motor median nerve slowing compared with that of the ulnar nerve. He later developed dysautonomia, likely due to his diabetic neuropathy. He was treated with midodrine and elastic stockings.

DISCUSSION

This patient had a diabetic polyneuropathy and bilateral CTS, an entrapment neuropathy commonly seen in diabetics and also in musicians. Electrophysiologic testing demonstrated a more distal median nerve slowing at the wrist from the demyelination caused by CTS.

He later developed orthostatic hypotension caused from autonomic dysfunction, which is also not unusual in diabetes.[5] Other symptoms of dysautonomia in diabetics include constipation, incontinence, gastroparesis, and impotence. It was thought that his autonomic symptoms were exacerbated by trihexyphenidyl and tamsulosin. He responded to discontinuation of medications and the addition of midodrine.

Peripheral neuropathy is a common complication of DM. This usually manifests with burning, pins-and-needles paresthesias, numbness, autonomic symptoms, and, later, weakness.

In one study peripheral polyneuropathy was seen in 54% of patients with insulin-dependent DM, of which only 50% had symptoms. CTS was seen in 33% and autonomic neuropathy in 7%.[6] In patients with noninsulin-dependent DM, peripheral neuropathy was demonstrated in 45%, CTS in 35%, and autonomic dysfunction in 5%. Thus all of the most common peripheral nerve manifestations in diabetics occurred in this patient.

Patients with DM can also develop other entrapments and mononeuropathies, such as diabetic ophthalmoplegia, diabetic femoral neuropathy, facial palsy, and diabetic truncal neuropathy. A mononeuritis multiplex can also occur, affecting different individual nerves at the same time,[7,8] and diabetic proximal neuropathy or diabetic amyotrophy.[8,9] Diabetics may also develop autoimmune neuropathies.

Those with DM are most predisposed to nerve entrapments, but mononeuropathies, mononeuritis multiplex, and diabetic amyotrophy all can develop, likely caused by vasculopathy and in some cases vasculitis.[9,10]

The diabetic polyneuropathy has several possible pathogenic mechanisms. These include intracellular accumulation of glycosylated proteins that deposit in several tissues, particularly the vasa nervorum, causing vascular insufficiency that can result in nerve infarcts.[10–12] There is also evidence that the accumulation of glycosylated agents causes oxidative damage.

Pathologically, diabetic vessels show endothelial swelling and thickening of the basal lamina.[11] This and arteriosclerosis predispose diabetics to vascular insufficiency.

An abnormal accumulation of the sugar–alcohol sorbitol and fructose causes nitrous oxide deficiency and oxidative injury. These occur because the excessive intracellular glucose is processed through the polyol pathway, producing sorbitol and fructose in a series of reactions catalyzed by the enzyme aldose-reductase.[13,14] Excessive fructose and sorbitol also cause a defect of sodium myoinositol cotransporter and decreased myoinositol in cells. Myoinositol is a precursor of phosphoinositide, and its deficit lowers the production of this element, impairing the pathway necessary for sodium–potassium ATPase pump activity, and regulation of the membrane potential.[15,16] Abnormalities of the Na–K ATPase pump affect diabetic nerve membrane potential, and calcium channel dysfunction also plays a role in cellular injury from excessive voltage-dependent calcium activity.[17]

Increased consumption of aldose-reductase depletes its cofactor the reduced form of nicotinamide adenine dinucleotide phosphate (NADPH), nitrous oxide (NO) synthetase, and glutathione which requires NADPH as a cofactor. A deficiency of this cofactor limits the production of NO, which is a potent vasodilator, whereas reduced glutathione predisposes to oxidative stress.[16]

Other contributing factors in diabetic neuropathy include deficiency of nerve growth factors, such as the insulin-derived growth factor that correlates with the severity of nerve injury. These proteins are essential in maintaining neuronal function and repair.[18,19]

Also in DM, there is impairment in the conversion of linoleic acid to δ-linoleic acid, a precursor of arachidonic acid, which is essential for the production of prostacyclin, a potent vasodilator and platelet inhibitor.[20]

The most important treatment of DM polyneuropathy is tight control of glycemia.[21] Administration of nerve growth factors has not been proven beneficial.[15] Therapy with aldose-reductase inhibitors has been disappointing, and has produced significant side effects. A beneficial effect has been demonstrated in only one study.[22] γ-Linoleic acid and alpha-lipoic acid appear to be helpful.[22–26]

Immunotherapy has been found effective in some patients with diabetic mononeuropathy or diabetic mononeuritis multiplex, particularly those who show evidence of vasculitis.[9]

The treatment of pain and dysautonomia in diabetic neuropathy is discussed in the section on treatment in Chapter 3.

IMPORTANT POINTS

- Diabetics frequently develop several types of neuropathies. In particular, patients with polyneuropathy can also manifest with a CTS and dysautonomia.

- To diagnose CTS in patients with a polyneuropathy it is necessary to demonstrate a more severe distal demyelination in the median nerve compared with the ulnar nerve.
- Diabetic polyneuropathy has several possible etiologies linked to hyperglycemia. These include, particularly, the accumulation of glycosylated end-products, accumulation of sorbitol, and reduced myoinositol, causing oxidative stress. The deposits of glycosylated end-products appear to cause vascular damage, and in diabetes there is endothelial swelling and a thick basal lamina of vessels. There are also deficiencies of nerve growth factors, abnormalities of the calcium channels, and defects in the production of δ-linoleic acid.
- The best treatment of diabetic polyneuropathy is tight glycemic control. The use of linolenic and lipoic acids appears to be beneficial.
- Some focal neuropathies in diabetics may be caused by a vasculitis which may respond to immunotherapy.

REFERENCES

1. Sander HW, Quinto C, Saadeh PB, Chokroverty S. Sensitive median-ulnar motor comparative techniques in carpal tunnel syndrome. *Muscle Nerve.* 1999;22:88–98.
2. Preston DC, Logigian EL. Lumbrical and interossei recording in carpal tunnel syndrome. *Muscle Nerve.* 1992;15:1253–1257.
3. Simovic D, Weinberg DH. Terminal latency index in the carpal tunnel syndrome. *Muscle Nerve.* 1997;20:1178–1180.
4. Low PA. Testing the autonomic nervous system. *Semin Neurol.* 2003;23:407–421.
5. Vinik AI, Freeman R, Erbas T. Diabetic autonomic neuropathy. *Semin Neurol.* 2003;23:365–372.
6. Dyck PG, Kratz KM, Karnes JL, et al. The prevalence by staged severity of various types of diabetic neuropathy, retinopathy and nephropathy in a population-based cohort: the Rochester Diabetic Neuropathy Study. *Neurology.* 1993;43:817–824.
7. Said G, Lacroix C, Lozeron P, et al. Inflammatory vasculopathy in multifocal diabetic neuropathy. *Brain.* 2003;126:376–385.
8. Kelkar P, Parry GJ. Mononeuritis multiplex in diabetes mellitus: evidence for underlying immune pathogenesis. *J Neurol Neurosurg Psychiatry.* 2003;74:803–806.
9. Dyck PJ, Windebank AJ. Diabetic and nondiabetic lumbosacral radiculoplexus neuropathies: new insights into pathophysiology and treatment. *Muscle Nerve.* 2002;25:477–491.
10. Krendal DA. Diabetic neuropathies. In: Brown WF, Bolton CF, Aminoff MG, eds. *Neuromuscular Function and Disease: Basic Clinical and Electrodiagnostic Aspects.* Philadelphia, PA: WB Saunders; 2002:1061–1080.
11. Malik RA, Tesfaye S, Thompson SD, et al. Endoneurial localization of microvascular damage in human diabetic neuropathy. *Diabetologia.* 1993;36:454–459.
12. Bassam B, Bertorini TE. Chapter 21: Neuromuscular manifestations of acquired metabolic, endocrine, and nutritional disorders. In: Bertorini, TE, ed. *Neuromuscular Disorders: Treatment and Management.* 2nd ed. Amsterdam, Netherlands: Elsevier; 2022:528–553.
13. Oates PJ. Polyol pathway and diabetic peripheral neuropathy. *Int Rev Neurobiol.* 2002;50:325–392.
14. Yagihashi S, Yamagishi SI, Wada RI, et al. Neuropathy in diabetic mice overexpressing human aldose reductase and effects of aldose reductase inhibitor. *Brain.* 2001;124:2448–2458.
15. Gooch C, Podwall D. The diabetic neuropathies. *Neurologist.* 2004;10:311–321.
16. Martinez P, Bertorini TE. La neuropatia diabetica. *Rev Neurol Argent.* 29200472–84.
17. Hall KE, Liu J, Sima AA, et al. Impaired inhibitory G-protein function contributes to increased calcium currents in rats with diabetic neuropathy. *J Neurophysiol.* 2001;86:760–770.
18. Verrotti A, Giuva T, Morgese G, et al. New trends in the etiopathogenesis of diabetic peripheral neuropathy. *J Child Neurol.* 2001;6:389–394.
19. Faradji V, Sotelo J. Low serum levels of nerve growth factor in diabetic neuropathy. *Acta Neurol Scand.* 1990;81:402–406.
20. Horrobin D. Essential fatty acids in the management of impaired nerve function in diabetes. *Diabetes.* 1997;46(Suppl):S90–S93.
21. The Diabetes Control and Complications Trial Research Group. The effect of intensive diabetes therapy on the development and progression of neuropathy. *Ann Intern Med.* 1995;122:561–568.
22. Hotta N, Toyota T, Matsuoka K, et al. Clinical efficacy of fidarestat, a novel aldose reduction inhibitor, for diabetic peripheral neuropathy: a 52-week multicenter placebo-controlled double-blind parallel group study. *Diabetes Care.* 2001;24:1776–1782.
23. Keen H, Payan J, Allawi J, et al. Treatment of diabetic neuropathy with gamma-linolenic acid. *Diabetes Care.* 1993;16:8–15.
24. Cameron NE, Cotter MA, Horrobin DH, et al. Effects of alpha lipoic acid on neurovascular function in diabetic rats: interaction with essential fatty acids. *Diabetologia.* 1998;41:390–399.
25. Ametov AS, Barinov A, Dyck PJ, et al. The sensory symptoms of diabetic polyneuropathy are improved with alpha-lipoic acid: the SYDNEY trial. *Diabetes Care.* 2003;26(3):770–776.
26. Ziegler D, Ametov A, et al. Oral treatment with alpha-lipoic acid improves symptomatic diabetic polyneuropathy: the SYDNEY 2 trial. *Diabetes Care.* 2006;29(11):2365–2370.

A Man With Hand Pain

A 48-year-old man had a 6-month history of pain in the right hand, occasionally radiating to the shoulder. He also had numbness with tingling in the first two digits and was referred for an EMG.

The neurologic examination was normal, except for mild weakness of the thenar muscle on the right and a positive Phalen test. There was a sensory deficit in the median nerve distribution on the right and left hands. Strength, reflexes, and sensory examinations in the legs were essentially normal.

AN EMG TEST WAS PERFORMED

Motor Nerve Studies

Nerve and Site	Latency(ms)	Amplitude (mV)	Conduction Velocity (m/s)
Median Nerve R.	**Normal ≤4.2**	**Normal ≥ 6**	**Normal ≥ 50**
Wrist	**6.4**	6.9	–
Elbow	8.4	**10.9**	**120**
Ulnar Nerve R.	**Normal ≤ 3.6**	**Normal ≥ 8**	**Normal ≥ 50**
Wrist	2.8	18.0	–
Below elbow	6.4	**14.4**	63

Motor Nerve Studies—cont'd

Median Nerve L.	Normal ≤ 4.2	Normal ≥ 6	Normal ≥ 50
Wrist	**5.2**	13	–
Elbow	9.2	12	55
Nerve and Site	**Latency (ms)**	**Amplitude (mV)**	**Conduction Velocity (m/s)**
Ulnar Nerve L.	**Normal ≤ 3.6**	**Normal ≥ 8**	**Normal ≥ 50**
Wrist	2.8	18	–
Below elbow	6.6	18	62
Median Nerve R. Recording at Adductor Digiti Minimi Muscle			
Wrist	NR	NR	–
Elbow	8	3	–

F-Wave Studies

Nerve	Latency (ms)	Normal Latency ≤ (ms)
Median nerve R.	**31.2**	30
Ulnar nerve R.	26.2	30
Median nerve L.	30.0	30
Ulnar nerve L.	27.2	30

Sensory Nerve Studies

Nerve	Onset Latency (ms)	Normal Onset Latency ≤ (ms)	Peak Latency (ms)	Normal Peak Latency ≤ (ms)	Amp (μV)	Normal Amp ≥ (μV)	Conduction Velocity (m/s)	Normal Conduction Velocity ≥ (m/s)
Median nerve R.	**4.2**	2.6	**4.7**	3.1	4	20	**31**	50
Ulnar nerve R.	1.9	2.6	2.4	3.1	16	13	63	50
Median nerve L.	**4.2**	2.6	**4.7**	3.1	**12**	20	**31**	50
Ulnar nerve L.	1.8	2.6	2.3	3.1	14	13	67	50

EMG Data

Muscle	Insrt Activity	Fibs	Pos Waves	Fasc	Amp	Dur	Poly	Pattern
Deltoid R.	Norm	None	None	None	Norm	Norm	None	Full
Biceps brachii R.	Norm	None	None	None	Norm	Norm	None	Full
Flexor carpi radialis R.	Norm	None	None	None	Norm	Norm	None	Full
Flexor carpi ulnaris R.	Norm	None	None	None	Norm	Norm	None	Full
Extensor dig. communis R.	Norm	None	None	None	Norm	Norm	None	Full
Abductor pollicis brevis R.	Norm	None	None	None	Norm	Norm	None	Full
1st dorsal interosseous R.	Norm	None	None	None	Norm	Norm	None	Full

WHAT WERE THE EMG FINDINGS?

This test revealed prolonged SNAP latencies and slow velocities of both median nerves but not the ulnar nerve, indicating the patient had bilateral median neuropathy at the wrist. The motor studies were unusual: although there was prolongation of the distal latencies of both median CMAPs, supporting the diagnosis of median entrapment, the conduction velocity of the right median nerve from elbow to wrist was *faster than normal.* There was also a higher amplitude of the median CMAP when stimulated at the elbow compared with the response obtained with stimulation at the wrist. There was a positive "dip" at the beginning of the right median CMAP when stimulating at the elbow but not at the wrist (Fig. 4-1). The right ulnar CMAP was larger from wrist stimulation than from elbow stimulation (Fig. 4-2). The needle test was normal.

These electrophysiologic findings are highly suggestive that the patient not only had bilateral carpal tunnel syndrome (CTS) but also a right Martin–Gruber anastomosis (MGA). The larger amplitude CMAP from median elbow stimulation is caused by the contribution to the CMAP of ulnar-innervated muscles that receive innervation from the anomaly above the wrist. The initial positive deflection of the median CMAP obtained from elbow stimulation is caused by volume-conducted responses of the ulnar muscles innervated by the anomaly. The abnormally fast median motor conduction velocity is explained by the contribution of axons traveling within the ulnar nerve that crosses above the wrist and does not pass through the carpal tunnel.

The higher amplitude of the ulnar nerve CMAP from wrist stimulation compared with that obtained from the elbow stimulation is caused by the stimulation of axons that incorporate in the ulnar nerve from the crossover *below* the elbow but *above* the wrist. This finding should always be considered with caution as it can be confused with a conduction block. The stimulation should always be supramaximal, as less-than-supramaximal stimulation can also cause low-amplitude CMAPs.

HOW DOES ONE PROVE THE DIAGNOSIS OF A MARTIN–GRUBER ANASTOMOSIS?

In this case the anastomosis was proved by stimulating the median nerve at the elbow and recording a response in the abductor digiti minimi (ADM) muscle (Fig. 4-3) not obtained by stimulating the wrist. This indicates that the fibers from the median nerve travel through the anastomosis to the ADM muscle.

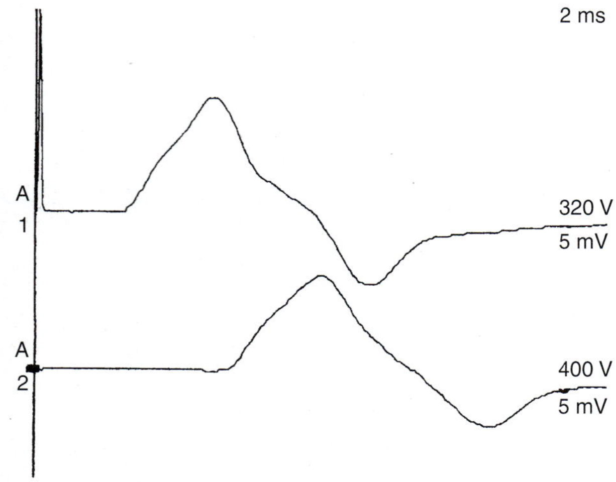

FIG. 4-2 Normal CMAP configuration of the ADM muscle with a lower amplitude on ulnar elbow stimulation compared with wrist stimulation. *ADM*, Adductor digiti minimi.

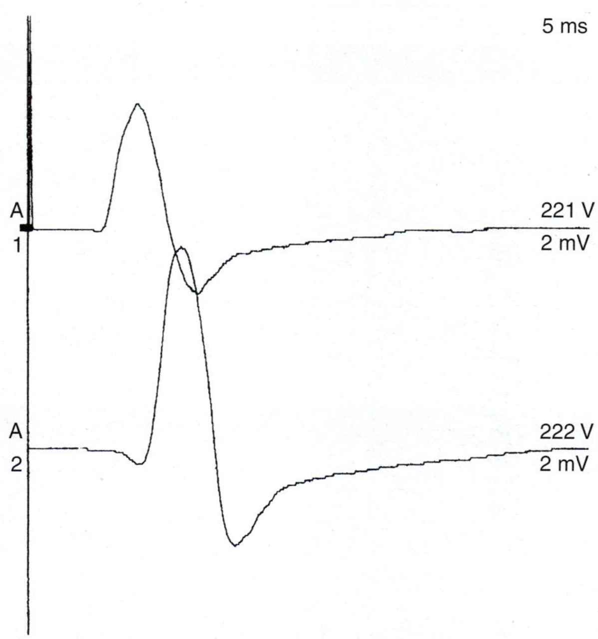

FIG. 4-1 Right median nerve motor conduction studies. Notice large amplitude median CMAP on elbow stimulation with an initial positive deflection.

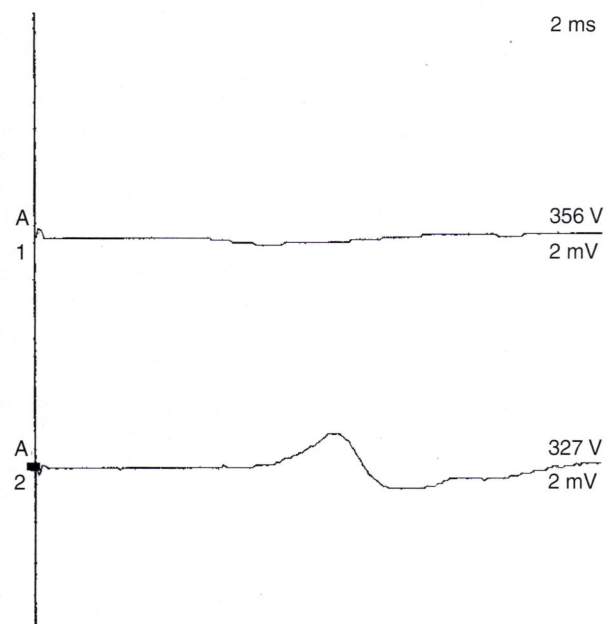

FIG. 4-3 CMAP obtained from median nerve stimulation at the elbow (A2) but not at the wrist when recording at the ADM muscle (A1).

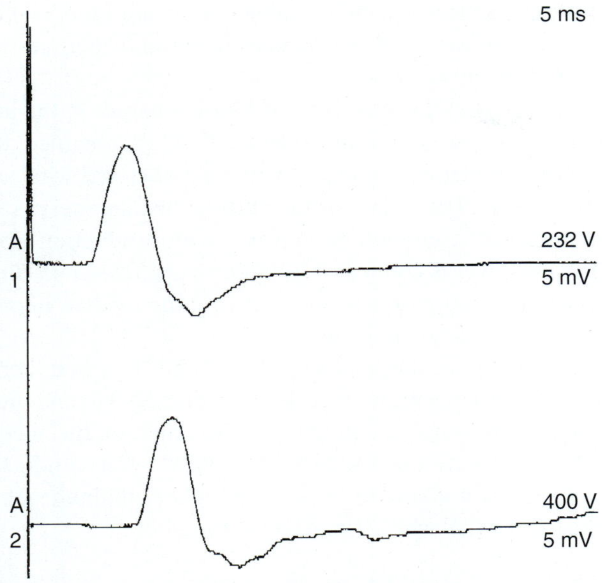

FIG. 4-4 Normal configuration of both median nerve CMAP responses on the left side.

In suspected cases, ulnar stimulation while recording at the first dorsal interosseous muscle could demonstrate the abnormality not seen using the standard recording at the ADM muscle.

There was no cross-innervation in the left median nerve, which had equal CMAPs from proximal and distal stimulation (Fig. 4-4).

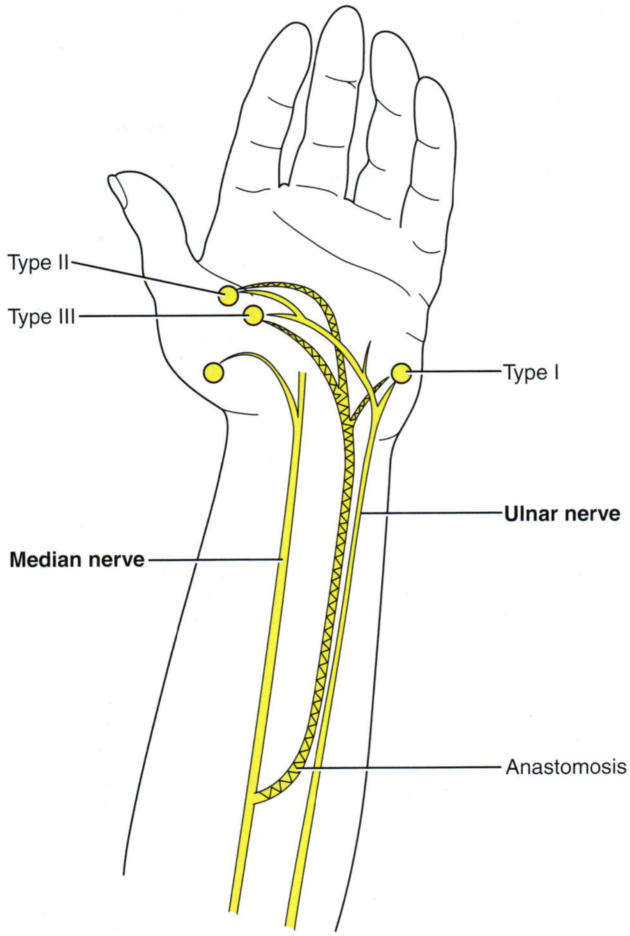

FIG. 4-5 Diagram of the different median-ulnar anatomies of the forearm (MGA types I, II, III). *MGA*, Martin–Gruber anastomosis.

WHAT IS THE MARTIN–GRUBER ANASTOMOSIS?

This anomalous cross-innervation from median to ulnar nerves was initially described by Martin in 1763[1] and later by Gruber in 1870.[2] The MGA consists of a crossover of fibers going from the median to the ulnar nerve in the forearm (Fig. 4-5). It has been reported that more frequently the anomalous axons go through the anterior interosseous nerve.[3] In a recent cadaveric study, however, it was found that the most common anastomosis was between the branches to the flexor digitorum profundus muscle.[4] This study also demonstrated that some cases of anomalous innervation cannot be demonstrated by EMG.

In MGA, there is cross-innervation of motor axons, but the crossover of sensory axons can also occur.[5] MGA has been found in about 31% of subjects.[6] In one study, it was present in 62% of family members, suggesting an autosomal dominant inheritance.[7] The crossover is bilateral in 68% of cases,[8] and its presence is demonstrated by the methods described earlier and by the use of collision techniques.[9]

In a group of 22 subjects, Wilbourn and Lambert[6] found that the anomaly innervated the ADM in 9 cases (this is considered MGA type I), the first dorsal interosseous in 21 cases (MGA type II), and the thenar muscles normally innervated by the ulnar nerve in 3 cases (MGA type III) (Fig. 4-6). There are variations of these, and they can also occur in combination. In addition, there are variations in the site of the anomalous connection in the forearm. In an anatomical

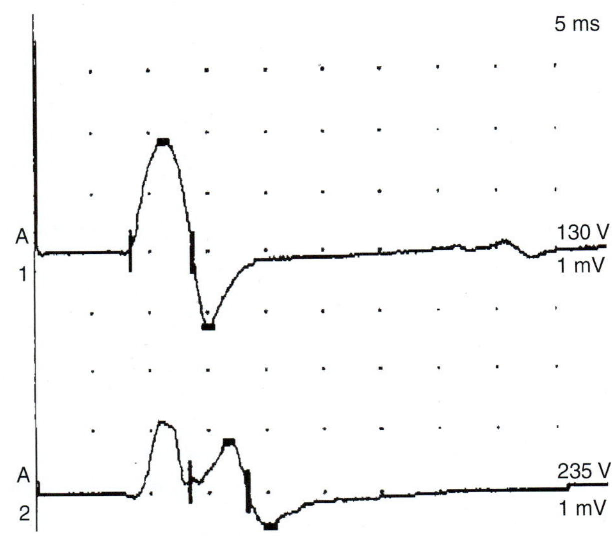

FIG. 4-6 Another patient with CTS. Notice the normal CMAP median nerve with prolonged latency on wrist stimulation and a double wave CMAP with stimulation at the elbow. *CTS*, Carpal tunnel syndrome.

study in 100 forearms, MGA was found in 27 and the most common communication originated from the anterior interossei nerve.[10]

MGA is only one of the various anomalous nerve connections; some persons have an anastomosis from the ulnar to the median nerve, and in some, all muscles of the hand are innervated by the median nerve. Variations of innervation occurring in the hand were described by Riche and by Cannieu.[11,12] These cross-innervations have not been studied in detail but should be taken under consideration when unusual electrophysiologic findings are being interpreted. For example, Dumitru et al.[13] documented denervation of the abductor pollicis brevis muscle (normally innervated by the median nerve) in a patient with ulnar neuropathy at the elbow.

To summarize, type I MGA is demonstrated by the presence of a response in the ADM upon stimulating the median nerve at the elbow. Type II is demonstrated by the presence of a response in the first dorsal interosseous upon stimulation at the median nerve at the elbow. Type III is difficult to document but sometimes is recognized by a double hump of the median response upon stimulation at the elbow (see Fig. 4-6).

SUMMARY

This patient with bilateral CTS had unusual electrophysiologic findings caused by an MGA. He responded to surgery.

MGA should be suspected when there is a higher amplitude CMAP of the median nerve from elbow stimulation, compared with the one obtained with stimulation at the wrist, and a lower amplitude of the ulnar nerve CMAP when stimulated at the elbow compared with the wrist.

MGA in a patient with CTS is suggested by the following:

1. Prolonged distal median motor and SNAP latencies
2. A higher proximal than distal median CMAP amplitude
3. A positive deflection of the median CMAP during elbow stimulation[14,15]
4. A larger ulnar CMAP with wrist stimulation compared with elbow stimulation (this and numbers 2 and 3 are seen in MGA without CTS)
5. A falsely fast elbow-to-wrist median motor conduction velocity[16]
6. A double response of the median nerve CMAP, when stimulated at the elbow, caused by a much slower conduction of the median nerve than the ulnar nerve[17]

The treatment of CTS in patients with MGA is the same as in those without the anomaly.

This patient was treated unsuccessfully with wrist splints and later underwent carpal tunnel release surgery with excellent response.

IMPORTANT POINTS

- MGA occurs in about 31% of all people. This anomalous innervation consists of a crossover of axons from the median nerve to the ulnar nerve in the forearm, so that muscles normally innervated by the ulnar nerve are innervated by axons traveling with the median nerve and then crossing over to the ulnar nerve.
- Electrophysiologic diagnosis of MGA is based on the presence of larger amplitude median CMAPs obtained with elbow stimulation compared with that obtained with wrist stimulation. The reverse occurs during the ulnar nerve stimulation and should not be confused with conduction block.
- The crossover is confirmed by observing a CMAP in ulnar-innervated muscles, when stimulating the median nerve at the elbow and not at the wrist.
- MGA should be suspected in cases with CTS when there is not only prolongation of the distal median SNAPs and motor latencies but also an initial positive "dip" of the median CMAP with elbow stimulation, a falsely fast conduction velocity from elbow to wrist, and higher amplitude of the median CMAP when stimulated at the elbow.

REFERENCES

1. Martin R. *Tal om Nervus allmam na Egenskaperi Manniskans Kropp*. Stockholm: L Salviu; 1763.
2. Gruber W. Uber die Verbindung des Nervus medianus mit dem Nervus Ulnaris am Unteerarme des Menschen und der Saugetiere. *Arch Anat Physiol Med Leipzig*. 1870;37:501–522.
3. Srinivasan R, Rhodes J. The median-ulnar anastomosis (Martin-Gruber) in normal and congenitally abnormal fetuses. *Arch Neurol*. 1981;38:418–419.
4. Lee KS, Oh CS, Chung IH, Sunwoo IN. An anatomic study of the Martin-Gruber anastomosis: electrodiagnostic implications. *Muscle Nerve*. 2005;31:95–97.
5. Santoro L, Rosato R, Caruso G. Median-ulnar nerve communications: electrophysiological demonstration of motor and sensory fibre cross-over. *J Neurol*. 1983;229:227–235.
6. Wilbourn J, Lambert EH. The forearm median to ulnar nerve communication: electrodiagnostic aspects. *Neurology*. 1976;26:368.
7. Crutchfield CA, Gutmann L. Hereditary aspects of median-ulnar nerve communications. *J Neurol Neurosurg Psychiatry*. 1980;43:53–55.
8. Kimura J, Murphy MJ, Varda DJ. Electrophysiological study of anomalous innervation of intrinsic hand muscles. *Arch Neurol*. 1976;33(12):842–844.
9. Kimura J. Collision technique: physiologic block of nerve impulses in studies of motor nerve conduction velocity. *Neurology*. 1976;26:680–682.
10. Cavalheiro CS, Filho MR, Pedro G, Caetano MF, et al. Clinical repercussions of Martin-Gruber anastomosis: anatomical study. *Rev Bras Ortop*. 2016;51(2):214–223. https://doi.org/10.1016/j.rboe.2016.01.003.
11. Riche P. Le nerf cubital et less muscles de l'eminece thenar. *Bull Mem Soc Anat Paris*. 1897;5:251–252.
12. Cannieu JMA. Note sur une anastomose entre la branch profonde du cubital et le median. *Bull Soc d'Anat Physiol Bordeaux*. 1897;18:339–349.
13. Dumitru D, Walsh NE, Weber CF. Electrophysiologic study of the Riche-Cannieu anomaly. *Electromyogr Clin Neurophysiol*. 1988;28:27–31.

14. Gutmann L, Gutierrez A, Riggs JE. The contribution of median to ulnar communication in diagnosis of mild carpal tunnel syndrome. *Muscle Nerve*. 1986;9:319–321.
15. Gutmann L. Median-ulnar communications and carpal tunnel syndrome. *J Neurol Neurosurg Psychiatry*. 1977;40:982–986.
16. Iyer V, Fenichel GM. Normal median nerve proximal latency in carpal tunnel syndrome: a clue to coexisting Martin-Gruber anastomosis. *J Neurol Neurosurg Psychiatry*. 1976;39:449–452.
17. Lambert EH. Diagnostic value of electrical stimulation of motor nerves. *Electroencephalogr Clin Neurophysiol*. 1962;22(Suppl):9–16.

5 CASE

A Woman With Hand Weakness, Numbness, and Pain After Cardiac Catheterization

A 65-year-old diabetic woman underwent coronary arteriogram through left elbow catheterization. Shortly afterward, she developed severe pain in the left hand and numbness in the first three digits of the left hand and was referred for evaluation 1 month later. The patient was hypertensive and had thyroid disease; she was taking medicines for these conditions.

Neurologic examination revealed normal mentation and cranial nerves. Strength was normal except for diminished flexion of the left thumb; she could not completely flex digits 2 and 3 when asked to make a fist, and she could not oppose the thumb to the index finger to perform the O sign (Fig. 5-1). She also had weakness of the toe dorsiflexors bilaterally. Reflexes were normal, except in the ankles where they were absent. Sensory examination revealed decreased pain sensation in the median nerve distribution of the left hand, decreased vibration sense in the toes, and decreased pain sensation up to the ankles. The neurologic examination was otherwise normal.

WHAT IS THE DIFFERENTIAL DIAGNOSIS?

This patient appeared to have a diabetic neuropathy and a median neuropathy at the elbow. The motor findings localized the lesion, or affected, mainly at the anterior interosseous nerve, but the sensory findings suggested that the main trunk of the median nerve was affected.

AN EMG TEST WAS PERFORMED

Motor Nerve Studies

Nerve and Site	Latency (ms)	Amplitude (mV)	Conduction Velocity (m/s)
Peroneal Nerve L.	**Normal ≤ 5.7**	**Normal ≥ 3**	**Normal ≥ 40**
Ankle	4.8	**2**	–
Fibular head	12.7	**2**	**35**
Knee	14.5	**2**	40
Tibial Nerve L.	**Normal ≤ 5.3**	**Normal ≥ 4**	**Normal ≥ 40**
Ankle	4.2	**3**	–
Pop. fossa	14.5	**2**	**37**
Median Nerve L.	**Normal ≤ 4.2**	**Normal ≥ 6**	**Normal ≥ 50**
Wrist	4.1	14	–
Elbow	8.5	7	**45**
Nerve and Site	**Latency (ms)**	**Amplitude (mV)**	**Conduction Velocity (m/s)**
Ulnar Nerve L.	**Normal ≤ 3.6**	**Normal ≥ 8**	**Normal ≥ 50**
Wrist	3.5	8	–
Below elbow	8.0	8	**48.8**

F-Wave Studies

Nerve	Latency (ms)	Normal Latency ≤ (ms)
Peroneal nerve L.	**54.8**	54
Tibial nerve L.	**55.6**	54
Median nerve L.	**30.5**	30
Ulnar nerve L.	**30.2**	30

Sensory Nerve Studies

Nerve	Onset Latency (ms)	Normal Onset Latency ≤ (ms)	Peak Latency (ms)	Normal Peak Latency ≤ (ms)	Amp (μV)	Normal Amp ≥ (μV)	Conduction Velocity (m/s)	Normal Conduction Velocity ≥ (m/s)
Sural nerve L.	3.4	3.5	3.9	4.0	**4**	11	41	40
Median nerve L.	**NR**	2.6	**NR**	3.1	**NR**	20	**NR**	50
Ulnar nerve L.	2.6	2.6	3.1	3.1	24	13	50	50

EMG Data

Muscle	Insrt Activity	Fibs	Pos Waves	Fasc	Amp	Dur	Poly	Pattern
L. cervical paraspinals L.	Norm	None	None	None	Norm	Norm	None	Full
Biceps brachii L.	Norm	None	None	None	Norm	Norm	None	Full
Pronator teres L.	Norm	None	None	None	Norm	Norm	None	Full
Flexor carpi radialis L.	**Inc**	**1+**	**1+**	None	Norm	Norm	None	**Red**
Flexor dig. profundus L.	**Inc**	**2+**	**2+**	None	Norm	Norm	None	**Red**
Flexor dig. superficialis L.	**Inc**	**1+**	**1+**	None	Norm	Norm	None	Full
Pronator quadratus L.	**Inc**	**2+**	**2+**	None	Norm	Norm	None	**Red**
Palmaris longus L.	**Inc**	**2+**	**2+**	None	Norm	Norm	None	Full
Flexor carpi ulnaris L.	Norm	None	None	None	Norm	Norm	None	Full
Extensor dig. com. L.	Norm	None	None	None	Norm	Norm	None	Full
1st dorsal interosseous L.	Norm	None	None	None	Norm	Norm	None	Full
Abductor pollicis brevis L.	**Inc**	**1+**	**1+**	None	Norm	Norm	None	Full
Flexor pollicis brevis L.	**Inc**	**2+**	**2+**	None	Norm	Norm	None	**Red**
Tibialis anterior L.	Norm	None	None	None	**Lg**	**Inc**	None	Full
Gastrocnemius L.	Norm	None	None	None	**Lg**	**Inc**	None	Full

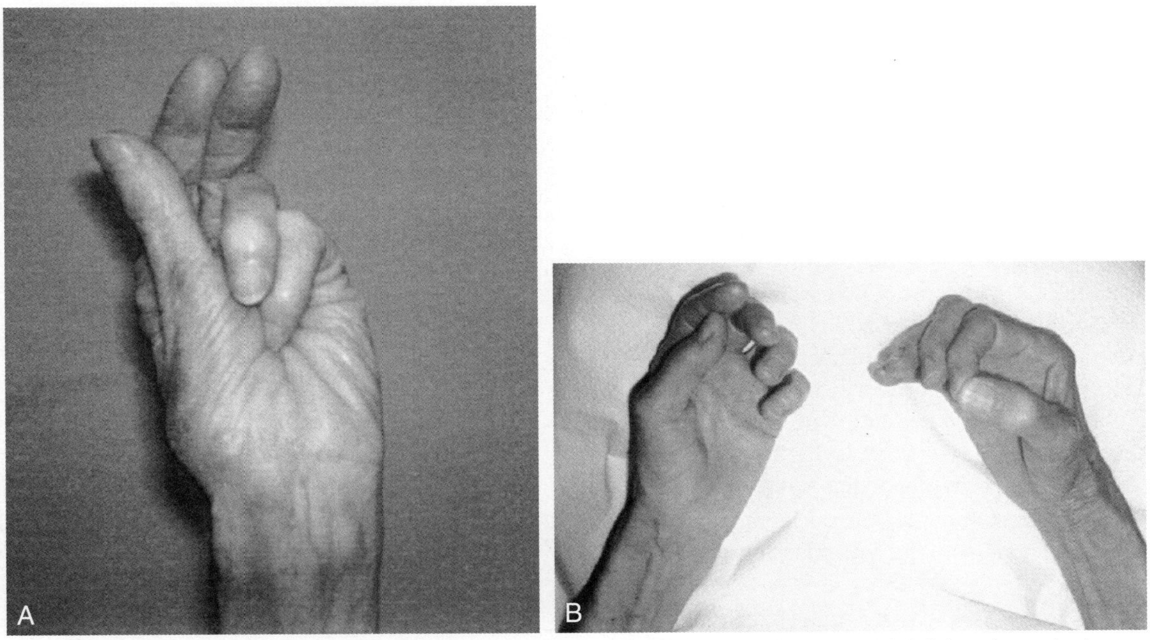

FIG. 5-1 **A**, The patient cannot flex the distal phalanx of the thumb or the second and third digits when asked to make a fist. **B**, The patient cannot make the O sign in the left hand.

WHAT WERE THE EMG FINDINGS?

This test showed a peripheral neuropathy with low-amplitude CMAPs and slowing nerve conduction velocity of the peroneal nerve. The sural SNAP was of low amplitude. The test also showed no left median digital SNAP with a normal ulnar SNAP. There was a low-amplitude median CMAP with conduction block at the elbow, with slowing of the median nerve motor nerve conduction velocity from elbow to wrist. There was evidence of active denervation in the median-innervated muscles of the forearm, the flexor carpi radialis, flexor digitorum superficialis, and palmaris longus. This was more severe in the pronator quadratus, flexor pollicis longus, and flexor digitorum profundus (I and II). A median neuropathy at the elbow was diagnosed; this affected mainly the anterior interosseous nerve fibers and caused axonal degeneration. She also had a mild sensorimotor peripheral neuropathy, likely from diabetes.

WHAT SHOULD BE DONE NEXT?

An MRI could have been done to document any edema or mass. It was decided that the lesion was likely traumatic, and the patient was treated conservatively. After 6 months she had only mild weakness with numbness in the median nerve distribution.

For further discussion, important points, and references, see Case 6.

SUMMARY

This patient had a traumatic median neuropathy just at the elbow caused by catheterization. She had weakness in the forearm and hand muscles. The neuropathy was documented by EMG. She responded to conservative treatment.

6 CASE

A Man Who Practices Karate and Has Forearm Pain

A 33-year-old man came in with left arm pain and numbness in the hand for 5 weeks. He practiced karate. His past medical history was negative.

There was weakness without atrophy of the thumb flexion at the distal phalanx and mild weakness of the first two finger flexors. Pain sensation was decreased in the first three digits and median palmar area of the hand and thumb. There was mild tenderness of the forearm. A Phalen test was negative. No Tinel's sign was elicited at the elbow, arm, or wrist. The rest of the neurologic examination was normal.

WHAT IS THE DIFFERENTIAL DIAGNOSIS?

This patient developed symptoms suggestive of a median neuropathy. The differential diagnosis was a plexopathy or radiculopathy, but because of the focal pain in the forearm, a proximal median neuropathy in this area was a strong consideration. A carpal tunnel syndrome (CTS) seemed less likely.

The sensory abnormality in the hands also included the palmar area of the thumb which should not be affected in CTS, as the sensory branch to this area comes from above the flexor retinaculum.

This patient practiced karate and had frequent pronation movement of the forearm while playing the sport. It was thought that he had damage to the median nerve as it passes to the pronator teres muscle. Other possible causes include masses, fibrous bands, or hypertrophy of the teres muscle.

AN EMG TEST WAS PERFORMED

Motor Nerve Studies

Nerve and Site	Latency (ms)	Amplitude (mV)	Conduction Velocity (m/s)
Median Nerve L.	**Normal ≤ 4.2**	**Normal ≥ 6**	**Normal ≥ 50**
Wrist	3.9	12	–
Elbow	8.5	8	58
Above elbow	10.5	8	51

Motor Nerve Studies—cont'd

Nerve and Site	Latency (ms)	Amplitude (mV)	Conduction Velocity (m/s)
Ulnar Nerve L.	**Normal ≤ 3.6**	**Normal ≥ 8**	**Normal ≥50**
Wrist	2.9	19	–
Below elbow	6.4	18	58
Above elbow	8.3	18	63
Axilla	11.2	18	53
Erb's point	14.5	16	63
Median Nerve R.	**Normal ≤ 4.2**	**Normal ≥ 6**	**Normal ≥ 50**
Wrist	3.6	11	–
Elbow	8.0	11	55
Above elbow	10.2	11	55
Ulnar Nerve R.	**Normal ≤ 3.6**	**Normal ≥ 8**	**Normal ≥ 50**
Wrist	2.9	18	–
Below elbow	6.7	18	57

F-Wave Studies

Nerve	Latency (ms)	Normal Latency ≤ (ms)
Median nerve L.	29.7	30
Ulnar nerve L.	29.0	30
Median nerve R.	29.3	30
Ulnar nerve R.	28.6	30

Sensory Nerve Studies

Nerve	Onset Latency (ms)	Normal Onset Latency ≤ (ms)	Peak Latency (ms)	Normal Peak Latency ≤ (ms)	Amp (μV)	Normal Amp ≥ (μV)	Conduction Velocity (m/s)	Normal Conduction Velocity ≥ (m/s)
Median nerve L.	2.3	2.6	2.8	3.1	**16**	20	57	50
Ulnar nerve L.	2.3	2.6	3.0	3.1	28	13	52	50
Median nerve R.	2.3	2.6	2.8	3.1	36	20	57	50
Ulnar nerve R.	2.3	2.6	2.8	3.1	37	13	52	50

EMG Data

Nerve	Insrt Activity	Fibs	Pos Waves	Fasc	Amp	Dur	Poly	Pattern
Biceps brachii L.	Norm	None	None	None	Norm	Norm	None	Full
Pronator teres L.	Norm	None	None	None	Norm	Norm	None	Full
Extensor dig. communis L.	Norm	None	None	None	Norm	Norm	None	Full
Flexor carpi radialis L.	**Inc**	**1+**	**1+**	None	Norm	Norm	None	Full
Pronator quadratus L.	**Inc**	**2+**	**2+**	None	Norm	Norm	None	Full
Flexor carpi ulnaris L.	Norm	None	None	None	Norm	Norm	None	Full
Abductor pollicis brevis L.	**Inc**	None	None	None	Norm	Norm	None	Full
First dorsal int. L.	Norm	None	None	None	Norm	Norm	None	Full
Flexor dig. profundus 2 and 3 L.	**Inc**	**2+**	**2+**	None	Norm	Norm	None	Full
Flexor pollicis longus L.	**Inc**	**2+**	**2+**	None	Norm	Norm	None	Full

WHAT WERE THE EMG FINDINGS?

The nerve conduction test showed a drop in the CMAP amplitude of the left median nerve obtained from elbow stimulation without slowing the conduction velocity or prolonged motor or sensory latencies at the wrist. The digital SNAP of the median nerve was decreased in amplitude. Both ulnar nerves and right median nerve studies were normal.

The needle test showed denervation potentials not only in muscles innervated by the anterior interosseous nerve but also in the flexor carpi radialis (FCR) muscle. There was also increased insertional activity in the abductor pollicis brevis (APB) muscle. Both the FCR and APB muscles are innervated by the main trunk of the median nerve.

It was concluded that this patient had a median neuropathy from repetitive pronation and supination movements, affecting the main trunk of the median nerve at the level of the pronator teres muscle. The patient improved with clinical management including immobilization.

SUMMARY

This patient was a karate athlete and developed pain and dysfunction of the hand and forearm. He was diagnosed as having pronator teres syndrome. His condition improved after discontinuing the practice of karate and receiving steroid injections in the area of the pronator teres muscle.

DISCUSSION, CASES 5 AND 6

Case 5 presented with hand numbness from a traumatic injury to the left median nerve just above the elbow (Fig. 6-1) affecting predominantly fibers going to the anterior interosseous motor branch. The differential diagnosis is rather limited.[1–6] This patient's clinical examination also indicated a peripheral neuropathy. She had weakness and numbness in the median nerve territory of the hand; the thenar eminence weakness was mild and there was weakness of the distal phalanx of the first three digits, particularly the thumb. It appeared that her neuropathy affected the anterior interosseous nerve more, and she could not perform the O ("OK" or circle) sign due to lack of flexion of the distal phalanges of the thumb and index fingers. Also, she could not oppose the thumb to the fifth digit due to weakness. This is characteristic of an anterior interossei lesion, but it may also be seen in median neuropathy at the elbow.

When the patient was asked to make a fist, she could not completely flex digits 2 and 3. Her hand resembled the "benediction sign," "preacher hand," or "orator hand," similar to what occurs in ulnar nerve lesions, but in ulnar neuropathy the sign is seen when the fingers are *extended* with a lack of flexion of the last two fingers. Actually, the initial description of the sign referred to combined median and ulnar nerve lesions.[7]

The needle test showed denervation in muscles innervated by the anterior interosseous nerve, a purely motor branch of the median nerve. The FCR, palmaris longus, and APB were also affected, indicating that the lesion affected the main trunk. Muscles innervated by other nerves in the forearm were normal.

Median neuropathy at the elbow is much less common than CTS and may be caused by trauma such as fractures, dislocations, masses, entrapment at the ligament of Struthers,[1,6] and angiography-related injuries,[8] as in patient #5. Preferential damage of fascicles to the anterior interosseous nerve could mimic an anterior interosseous syndrome.[9]

The median nerve may also be compressed by thickened bicipital aponeurosis and hypertrophy of the pronator teres, abnormal vessels, masses or fibrous bands in this area, or repetitive elbow motions causing the pronator teres syndrome, as in *Case 6*.[10–13] Distal to the proximal edge of the bicipital aponeurosis, the median nerve passes between the two heads of the pronator muscles, where it could be compressed,[12] then immediately passes the sublimis bridge, which is a fibrous arch of the flexor digitorum superficialis muscle, then continues distally under this muscle where the nerve may be compressed.[1,13]

Patients with pronator teres syndrome, as did *Case 6*, usually have a diffuse dull, aching pain in the forearm, and occasionally some may have an acute onset of a sharp pain during pronation and supination. (12) On palpation there is tenderness in the pronator teres area. Electrophysiologic studies show abnormal SNAPs of the median nerve. The median nerve motor conduction velocity may be abnormal, but this is not consistent.[13–15] Measurement of the motor latency to the FCR compared with

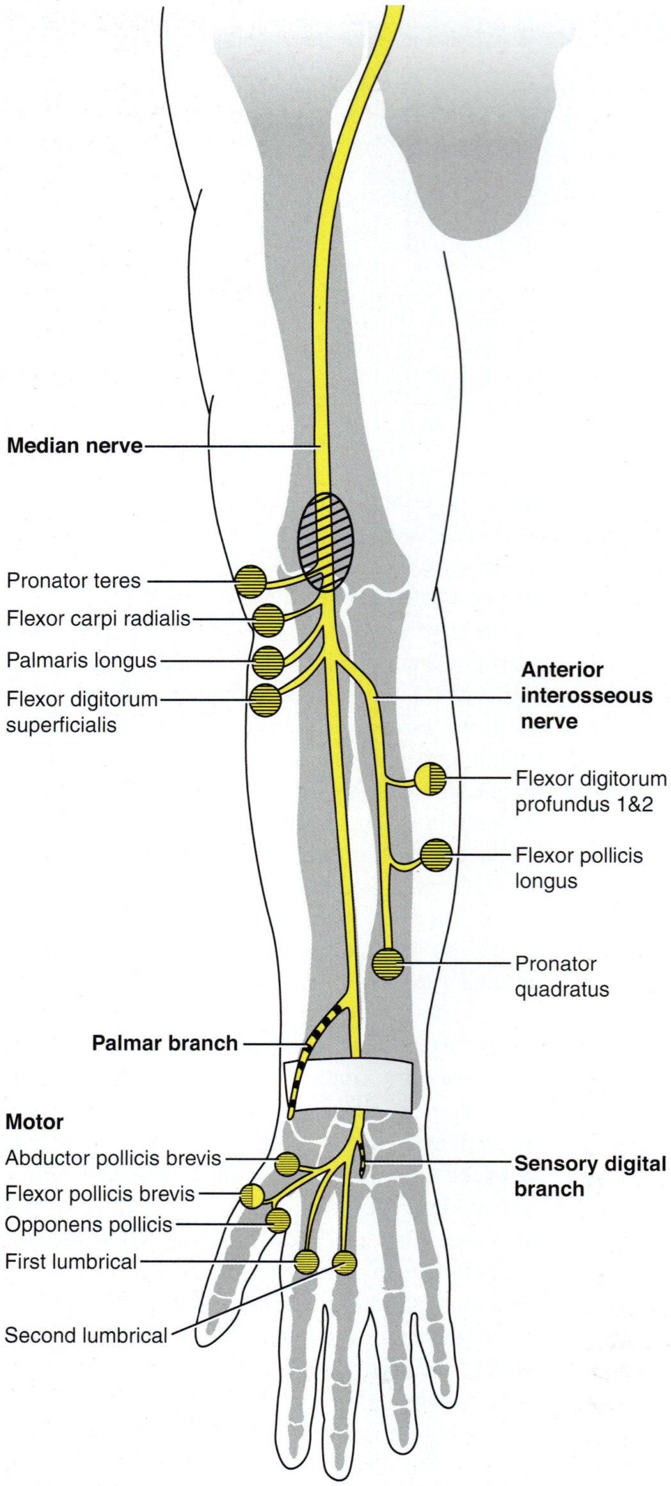

FIG. 6-1 Anatomy of the median nerve. The circle shows the level of the lesion (see Case 5).

the opposite side is often of value. There could be denervation present in nerves in muscles innervated by the main trunk distal to the pronator teres muscle, which is usually spared because it is innervated by axonal branches prior to entering the muscle.[13,14]

The treatment consists of conservative management, avoiding repetitive trauma, and corticosteroids. Surgical release sometimes is useful.[12,14,16]

IMPORTANT POINTS FOR CASES 5 AND 6

- Median neuropathy at or just above the elbow can be caused by trauma, masses, hypertrophy of the pronator teres, and entrapment of the ligament of Struthers.
- Patients with median neuropathy at the elbow usually have sensory deficits in the median nerve distribution, as well as weakness of the wrist flexors and thenar muscles, and of muscles innervated by the anterior interosseous nerve.
- Patients with predominantly anterior interosseous nerve lesions are usually unable to perform the O ("OK" or circle) sign from lack of strength of the distal thumb and the index finger and are not able to oppose the thumb to the fifth digit. Patients also make a benediction sign when they attempt to make a fist because the distal phalanx of the second and third fingers does not flex. This is different from the sign seen in ulnar neuropathy when the patient is asked to extend the fingers and the last two digits do not extend.
- The EMG in suspected median neuropathy of the arm and forearm should include measurement of motor conductions of both median nerves below and above the elbow, compared with the opposite side, and measurement of SNAPs of the median and ulnar nerves. Measurement of the motor latencies of the CMAP amplitude of the median nerve to the FCR, with stimulation at and above the elbow and compared with the opposite side, can also be helpful. If a polyneuropathy is suspected, one nerve of the lower extremity should be studied. The needle test should include median-, ulnar-, and radial-innervated muscles to rule out radiculopathy and plexopathy.
- Lesions at the pronator teres area characteristically spare the pronator teres muscle but affect muscles of the median nerve at the hand and forearm.
- Pronator teres syndrome may be caused by fibrous bands, hypertrophy of the muscle, and frequent pronation and supination movements.
- Treatment of a median neuropathy at the forearm including the pronator teres syndrome consists of rest, removal of precipitating cause, and steroid injections. Surgery is beneficial in severe cases.

REFERENCES FOR CASES 5 AND 6

1. Stewart JD. Median nerve. In: Stewart JD, ed. *Focal Peripheral Neuropathies*. 3rd ed. Philadelphia, PA: Lippincott Williams & Wilkins; 2000:183–239.
2. Suranyi L. Median nerve compression by Struthers ligament. *J Neurol Neurosurg Psychiatry*. 1983;46:1047–1049.
3. Gessini L, Jandolo B, Pietrangeli A. Entrapment neuropathies of the median nerve at and above the elbow. *Surg Neurol*. 1983;19:112–116.
4. Bilge T, Yalaman O, Bilge S, et al. Entrapment neuropathy of the median nerve at the level of the ligament of Struthers. *Neurosurgery*. 1990;27:787–789.
5. Laha RK, Dujovny M, DeCastro SC. Entrapment of median nerve by supracondylar process of the humerus: case report. *J Neurosurg*. 1977;46:252–255.

6. Martinelli P, Gabellini AS, Poppi M. Pronator syndrome due to thickened bicipital aponeurosis. *J Neurol Neurosurg Psychiatry*. 1982;45:181–182.
7. La Mesa M, Marks MM, Segal E. The two histories of the "sign of benediction": neurological literature vs art history. *Neurology*. 2007;68(Suppl 1):A7.
8. Kennedy AM, Grocott M, Schwartz MS, et al. Median nerve injury: an underrecognised complication of brachial artery cardiac catheterisation? *J Neurol Neurosurg Psychiatry*. 1997; 63:542–546.
9. Wertsch JJ, Sanger JR, Matloub HS. Pseudo-anterior inter-osseus nerve syndrome. *Muscle Nerve*. 1985;8:68–70.
10. Ul Haq MA, Rashid M, Kwok CS, Wong CW, et al. Hand dysfunction after transradial artery catheterization for coronary procedures. *World J Cardiol*. 2017;9(7):609–619. https://doi.org/10.4330/wjc.v9.i7.609.
11. Morris HH, Peters BH. Pronator syndrome: clinical and electrophysiological features in seven cases. *J Neurol Neurosurg Psychiatry*. 1976;39:461–464.
12. Hartz CR, Linscheid RL, Gramse RR, Daube JR. The pronator teres syndrome: compressive neuropathy of the median nerve. *J Bone Joint Surg Am*. 1981;63:885–890.
13. Dididze M, Tafti D, Sherman AI. *Pronator teres syndrome. StatPearls [Internet]*. Treasure Island, FL: StatPearls Publishing; 2022.
14. Beaton LE, Anson BJ. The relation of the median nerve to the pronator teres muscle. *Anat Rec*. 1939;75:23–26.
15. Gessini L, Jandolo B, Pietrangeli A. Entrapment neuropathies of the median nerve at and above the elbow. *Surg Neurol*. 1983;19:112–116.
16. Cho DS, MacLean IC. Pronator syndrome: establishment of electrophysiological parameters. *Arch Phys Med Rehabil*. 1981;62:531–535.

7 CASE

A Man With a History of Polio Who Developed Hand Weakness and Numbness

A 61-year-old hypertensive man presented with a 2-month history of progressive weakness and wasting in the left hand and mild numbness in the fifth digit.

His past medical history was positive for poliomyelitis as a child, which left residual weakness in both legs. He had an almost complete recovery except for a mild deformity of the left foot. He did have occasional fasciculations in the leg. Family history was noncontributory. He denied alcohol or tobacco use.

On examination the left-hand interossei muscles were wasted but without fasciculations. He had a positive Froment sign (Fig. 7-1A) and a Tinel's sign right below the left elbow. When extending his fingers, the last two digits had a tendency to remain flexed (Fig. 7-1B). He could not "cup" the left hand. Adson's maneuver was negative. On sensory examination, there was decreased pain sensation in the left fifth digit and the ulnar half of the fourth with questionably decreased pain sensation in the ulnar aspect of the dorsum of the hand. Sensation in the lower extremities was normal. The left foot had an equinovarus deformity. All reflexes were mildly depressed.

WHAT IS THE CLINICAL DIAGNOSIS?

Patients with polio may develop progressive weakness and atrophy or post-polio amyotrophy, but it is unlikely in this patient who had symptoms and clinical findings suggestive of an ulnar neuropathy at the elbow.[1,2] This is consistent with the numbness in the last two digits, atrophy of the first dorsal interosseous muscle and the Froment sign, and the inability to cup the hand from palmaris brevis muscle weakness.

Another finding in ulnar neuropathy is the *benediction sign*, characterized by the tendency of the last two digits to flex when the patient is asked to extend the wrist and the fingers (see Fig. 7-1B). This sign is produced by hyperextension of the metacarpophalangeal joints of the last two fingers from weakened lumbrical muscles and unopposed extension of the extensor digitorum communis. The flexion of the distal phalanges is caused by flexion of the stretched tendons of the flexor digitorum. The name "benediction," "orator sign," or "papal benediction sign" originates from catholic priests who extend the thumb and first two fingers and flex the last two fingers during benediction. A similar position occurs in median neuropathy (see Case 5); in this, the patient is asked to *flex* the fingers, or make a fist but cannot do so because of an inability to flex the first three digits due to weakness of the median-innervated finger flexors. Patients with ulnar neuropathy could also show wasting of the ulnar-innervated hand muscles and have a characteristic "claw hand."

AN EMG TEST WAS PERFORMED

Motor Nerve Studies

Nerve and Site	Latency (ms)	Amplitude (mV)	Conduction Velocity (m/s)
Median Nerve L.	**Normal ≤ 4.2**	**Normal ≥ 6**	**Normal ≥ 50**
Wrist	**4.7**	11	–
Elbow	9.8	10	53
Ulnar Nerve L.	**Normal ≤ 3.6**	**Normal ≥ 8**	**Normal ≥ 50**
Wrist	3.5	**3**	–
Below elbow	8.3	**3**	57
Above elbow	11.4	**1**	**39**
Axilla	13.2	**1**	67
Peroneal Nerve L.	**Normal ≤ 5.7**	**Normal ≥ 3**	**Normal ≥ 40**
Ankle	5.2	4	–
Fibular head	12.3	4	44
Knee	14.3	4	50
Median Nerve R.	**Normal ≤ 4.2**	**Normal ≥ 6**	**Normal ≥ 50**
Wrist	**4.3**	15	–
Elbow	9.3	14	54
Ulnar Nerve R.	**Normal ≤ 3.6**	**Normal ≥ 8**	**Normal ≥ 50**
Wrist	2.7	10	–
Below elbow	7.2	10	58
Above elbow	9.6	10	50

F-Wave Studies

Nerve	Latency (ms)	Normal Latency ≤ (ms)
Median nerve L.	**30.7**	30
Ulnar nerve L.	**33.0**	30
Peroneal nerve L.	**54.9**	54
Median nerve R.	**30.8**	30
Ulnar nerve R.	**32.1**	30

Inching Technique: Ulnar Nerve L.

Stimulation Site	Latency (ms)	Amplitude (mV)
4 cm below elbow	8.1	3.3
3 cm below elbow	8.3	3.1
2 cm below elbow	**9.0**[a]	**1.4**
1 cm below elbow	**9.7**[a]	**1.3**
Ulnar groove	9.8	**1.3**
1 cm above elbow	9.9	**1.3**
2 cm above elbow	10.0	**1.1**
3 cm above elbow	10.1	**1.1**

[a]0.2 ms difference allowed between stimulation sites.

Sensory Nerve Studies

Nerve	Onset Latency (ms)	Normal Onset Latency ≤ (ms)	Peak Latency (ms)	Normal Peak Latency ≤ (ms)	Amp (μV)	Normal Amp ≥ (μV)	Conduction Velocity (m/s)	Normal Conduction Velocity ≥ (m/s)
Median nerve L.	**3.2**	2.6	**3.7**	3.1	**11**	20	**41**	50
Ulnar nerve L.	**NR**	2.6	**NR**	3.1	**NR**	13	**NR**	50
Dorsal ulnar cut. L.	**NR**	[b]	**NR**	2.3	**NR**	12	**NR**	[b]
Sural nerve L.	2.9	3.5	3.4	4.0	14	11	48	40
Median nerve R.	2.6	2.6	3.1	3.1	**9**	20	50	50
Ulnar nerve R.	2.1	2.6	2.6	3.1	**5**	13	57	50
Dorsal ulnar cut. R.	1.5	[b]	2.0	2.3	12	12	53	[b]

[b]Normal data not available.

EMG Data

Muscle	Insrt Activity	Fibs	Pos Waves	Fasc	Amp	Dur	Poly	Pattern
Biceps brachii L.	Norm	None	None	None	Norm	Norm	**Few**	Full
Triceps L.	Norm	None	None	None	**Lg**	**Inc**	None	Full
Flexor carpi radialis L.	Norm	None	None	None	Norm	Norm	None	Full
Flexor carpi ulnaris L.	Norm	None	None	None	Norm	Norm	None	Full
1st dorsal interosseous L.	**Inc**	**2+**	**2+**	None	**Lg**	**Inc**	None	**Red**
Abductor pollicis brevis L.	Norm	None	None	None	Norm	Norm	None	Full
Flexor digitorum profundus L.	**Inc**	**2+**	**2+**	None	**Lg**	**Inc**	None	**Red**
Vastus lateralis L.	**Inc**	None	**2+**	None	**Lg**	**Inc**	None	**Red**
Tibialis anterior L.	Norm	None	None	None	**Lg**	**Inc**	None	**Red**
Gastrocnemius L.	**Inc**	None	**1+**	None	**Lg**	**Inc**	None	Full

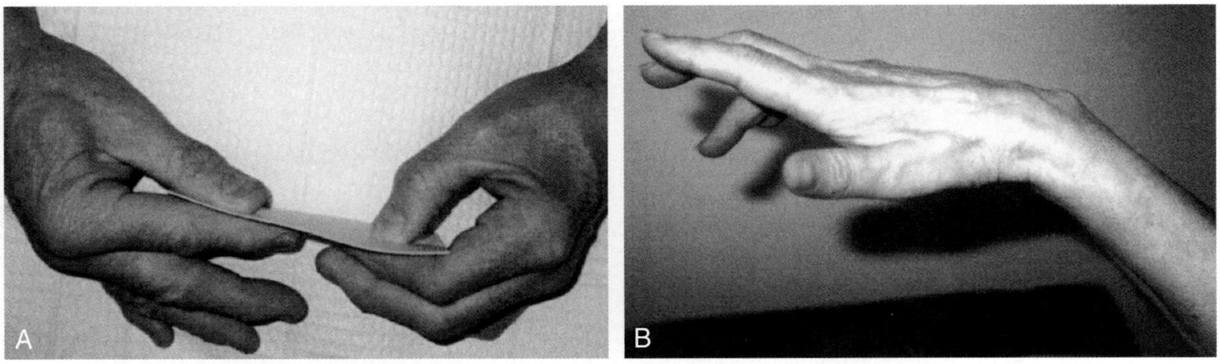

FIG. 7-1 **A**, Patient showing the Froment sign in the left hand. He has to flex the distal phalanx to hold the paper, secondary to adductor weakness and a normal median-innervated flexor pollicis longus. There is also atrophy of the first dorsal interosseous muscle. **B**, The benediction sign, showing partial flexion of the last two digits when the patient extends his fingers and hand.

WHAT WERE THE EMG FINDINGS?

This electrophysiologic study was done following the standards recommended by the American Association of Neuromuscular and Electrodiagnostic Medicine to examine the ulnar nerve for entrapment at the elbow.[3] Absent were the left digital ulnar and dorsal cutaneous SNAPs. The SNAP of the medial antebrachial cutaneous nerve, which helps to differentiate ulnar nerve lesions from plexopathy, was not tested. The motor ulnar nerve conduction velocity from elbow to wrist was normal but was slow at 39 m/s across the elbow. Conduction velocity of less than 50 m/s, 10 m/s slower than the elbow–wrist segment, or 10 m/s slower than the velocity across the elbow in the opposite side is considered abnormal. A recent study indicated that an absolute velocity of below 48 m/s across the elbow is suggestive of an ulnar entrapment in this area.[4]

The "inching," or short (1 cm) segment increment study,[5] revealed a significant prolongation of 0.7 ms (normal, ≤0.5 ms) at 2 cm distal to the medial epicondyle where there was also a drop in amplitude over 50%. The needle test showed denervation potentials in the left ulnar-innervated intrinsic hand muscles, but not in the median-innervated muscles. There were also denervation potentials in the flexor digitorum profundus although not in the flexor carpi ulnaris. The lack of denervation of the flexor carpi ulnaris does not necessarily localize the exact site of an ulnar nerve lesion at the elbow, as this depends more on the severity than on the site.[6]

The test also showed electrophysiologic evidence of bilateral median neuropathy at the wrist. In addition, there were electrophysiologic findings consistent with the previous history of polio, characterized by large motor unit potentials in the lower extremities with mild active denervation in the gastrocnemius muscle.[7]

WHAT IS THE DIFFERENTIAL DIAGNOSIS?

This patient had entrapments in both median nerves and one ulnar nerve; thus the possibility of familial neuropathy with liability to pressure palsy was considered, but DNA testing was not done. Other considerations included diabetes and hypothyroidism, but chemistry profile, glycosylated hemoglobin, erythrocyte sedimentation rate, fluorescent antinuclear antibody, and thyroid studies were normal. It was concluded that there was no predisposing disease.

WHAT WAS THE MANAGEMENT?

Because of the severity of symptoms, the patient underwent surgical decompression. During surgery, the ulnar nerve was found to be compressed at the cubital tunnel and also at a higher level by a fibrous band adjacent to the medial head of the triceps, the arcade of Struthers. This arcade is an unusual site of compression, found mainly in patients who have had a previous surgical transposition of the nerve.

DISCUSSION

This patient had an ulnar neuropathy at the elbow. Electrophysiologic findings suggested a compression at the ulnar tunnel; surgical exploration revealed an additional compression above the elbow.

Damage of the ulnar nerve can have various etiologies. The term *tardive ulnar palsy* was used in the past to describe ulnar

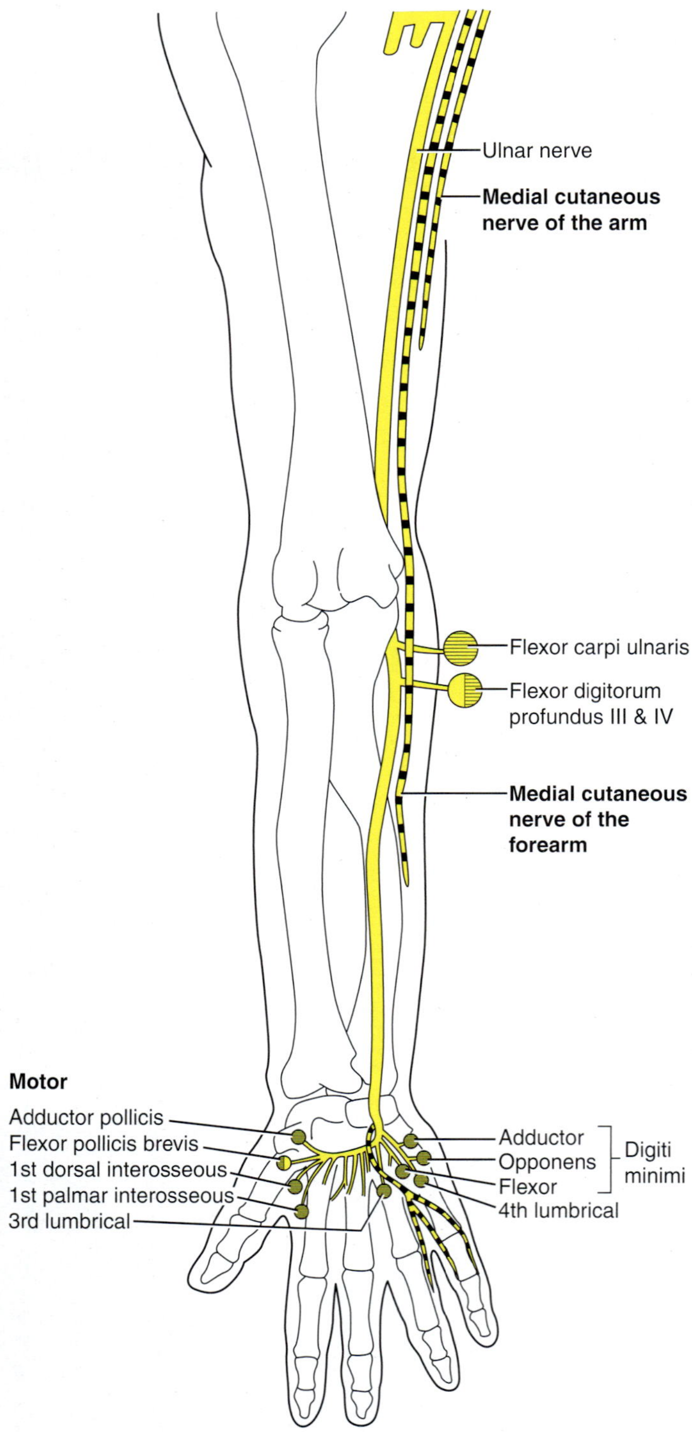

FIG. 7-2 Diagram of the ulnar nerve and its sensory and motor branches.

neuropathies at the elbow, following the initial description by Panas in 1878 of a patient who developed an ulnar neuropathy years after a fracture.[8] The generalized use of this term is not recommended, as trauma is not a common cause of ulnar neuropathy. Later, Buzzard described a compression of the ulnar nerve as it passes the aponeurotic humeroulnar arcade formed by the median and ulnar heads of the flexor carpi ulnaris muscle.[9] The term *cubital tunnel syndrome* was later coined by Feindel and Stratford to describe lesions at this level.[10] The term, however, is also sometimes used erroneously to describe all ulnar neuropathies at the elbow.

The ulnar nerve can be compressed at the axilla (e.g., from crutches). Below the axilla it can be compressed at different levels in the upper extremity. The *first location* is at the intramuscular septum dividing the anterior and posterior compartments of the upper arm, or as the nerve passes beneath the arcade of Struthers.[11] This arcade is formed by fibrous tissue between the intramuscular septum and the medial head of the triceps[12] and should not be confused with the ligament of Struthers, which is another anatomic structure. This uncommon compression is usually a secondary entrapment syndrome after a surgical transposition of the nerve at the elbow.

The *second location* of compression occurs as the nerve passes the condylar groove, where it is susceptible to trauma, subluxation, or bony abnormalities.[13] The *third location* occurs when the nerve enters the ulnar tunnel, where it can be compressed by the humeral ulnar arcade,[14] or cubital tunnel. This results from hypertrophy of the fibrous band or from frequent flexion movements which decreases the tunnel diameter. The nerve can also be compressed by an anomalous muscle, the anconeus epitrochlearis, which occasionally replaces the flexor retinaculum.[15]

Finally, the *fourth location* occurs as the nerve passes between the flexor carpi ulnaris and the flexor digitorum profundus in the forearm.[16] (The anatomy of the ulnar nerve and its different branches can be seen in Fig. 7-2, and the various sites of compression can be seen in Fig. 7-3.)

Causes of ulnar nerve entrapment include hypertrophic fibrous bands, anomalous muscles, bony deformities, fractures, rheumatoid arthritis, chronic subluxation, trauma, prolonged or repetitive elbow flexion, and external compressions.

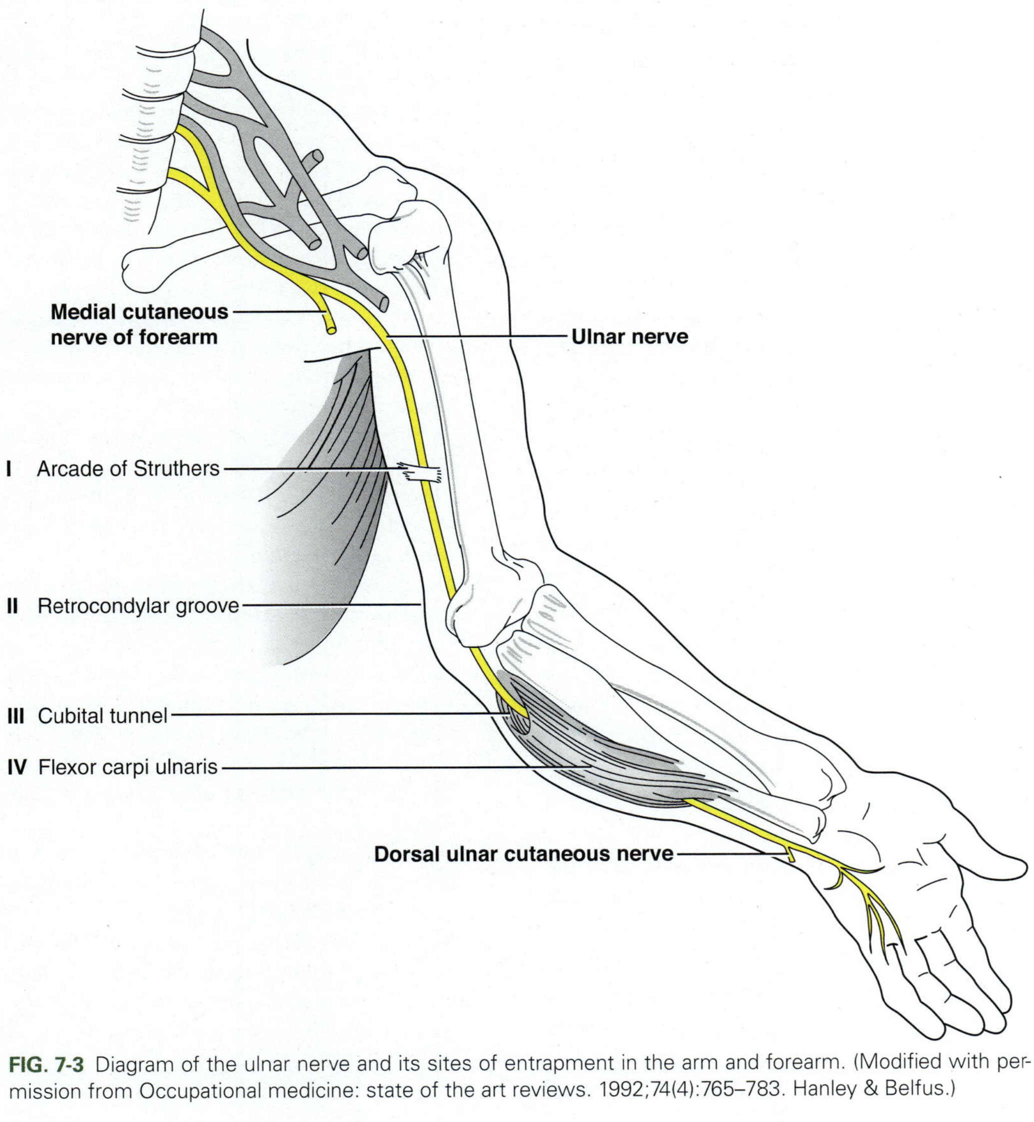

FIG. 7-3 Diagram of the ulnar nerve and its sites of entrapment in the arm and forearm. (Modified with permission from Occupational medicine: state of the art reviews. 1992;74(4):765–783. Hanley & Belfus.)

WHAT SHOULD BE THE TREATMENT?

The treatment of mild ulnar compression is usually conservative and consists of bracing and avoiding prolonged flexion.[17] Surgical release is performed if there is significant dysfunction.

There are several approaches for ulnar nerve surgery at the elbow. These include simple decompression,[18] medial epicondylectomy,[19,20] subcutaneous transposition,[20] and sub/intramuscular or anterior transmuscular positioning of the nerve.[16] Simple decompression provides results similar to transposition but with fewer complications.[21]

Preoperative MRI[22] and inching measurements during surgery[23] can be used to localize the lesion.[23] This case illustrates that during surgery there should be a generous incision that allows for good observation of the nerve.

IMPORTANT POINTS

- Ulnar entrapment at the elbow can manifest sensory deficits in the ulnar nerve territory in the hand as well as the dorsal cutaneous branch, and by weakness of the ulnar-innervated hand and forearm muscles. Patients may have the Froment's sign, characterized by flexion of the thumb to hold paper, due to weakness of the thumb adductor muscles, and also have the "benediction" sign. The patient may also be unable to cup the palm due to weakness of the palmaris brevis and may have a Tinel's sign at the elbow.
- Electrophysiologic studies for suspected ulnar neuropathy should include measurement of the SNAPs of the fifth digit, as well as of the dorsal cutaneous branch, and measurement of the motor ulnar nerve conduction across the elbow, with proper arm positioning. Testing with the use of the short segment intervals is very useful. When a plexopathy is a consideration in the diagnosis, the medial antebrachial cutaneous nerve of the forearm is evidence against a lesion of the lower trunk of the brachial plexus but does not rule it out. Needle electromyography studies should be done not only in ulnar-innervated muscles but also in various C8, lower trunk, medial cord muscles innervated by other nerves, and in the cervical paraspinal muscles to rule out lesions in the root or plexus.
- The ulnar nerve can be compressed at various levels in the upper extremity above the wrist, including the transmuscular septum of the arm (the arcade of Struthers), the condylar groove, and the cubital tunnel, and as it passes between the flexor carpi ulnaris and the flexor digitorum profundus.
- Common causes of entrapment include arthritis, trauma, hypertrophic bands, chronic subluxation, and anomalous muscles.
- The treatment of ulnar compression is usually conservative, but in severe cases where surgical decompression is indicated, inching studies during surgery help to better localize the lesion. MRI and ultrasound are also useful.

REFERENCES

1. Kincaid JC. AAEE minimonograph 31: the electrodiagnosis of ulnar neuropathy at the elbow. *Muscle Nerve*. 1988;11: 1005–1015.
2. Bradshaw DY, Shefner JM. Ulnar neuropathy at the elbow. *Neurol Clin*. 1999;17:447–461. v–vi.
3. [No authors listed] Practice parameter for electrodiagnostic studies in ulnar neuropathy at the elbow: summary statement. American Association of Electrodiagnostic Medicine, American Academy of Neurology, American Academy of Physical Medicine and Rehabilitation. *Muscle Nerve*. 1999;22:408–411.
4. Shakir A, Micklesen PJ, Robinson LR. Which motor nerve conduction study is best in ulnar neuropathy at the elbow? *Muscle Nerve*. 2004;29(4):585–590.
5. Campbell WW, Pridgeon RM, Sahni KS. Short segment incremental studies in the evaluation of ulnar neuropathy at the elbow. *Muscle Nerve*. 1992;15:1050–1054.
6. Campbell WW, Pridgeon RM, Riaz G, et al. Sparing of the flexor carpi ulnaris in ulnar neuropathy at the elbow. *Muscle Nerve*. 1989;12:965–967.
7. Wiechers DO, Hubbell SL. Late changes in the motor unit after acute poliomyelitis. *Muscle Nerve*. 1981;4(6):524–528.
8. Panas J. Sur une cause peu connue de paralysie du nerf cubital. *Arch Gen Med*. 1878;1:5–15.
9. Buzzard EF. Some varieties of toxic and traumatic ulnar neuritis. *Lancet*. 1922;1:317–319.
10. Feindel W, Stratford J. Cubital tunnel compression in tardy ulnar nerve palsy. *Can Med Assoc J*. 1958;78:351–353.
11. Ochiai N, Hayashi T, Ninomiya S. High ulnar nerve palsy caused by the arcade of Struthers. *J Hand Surg*. 1992;17:629–631.
12. Spinner M, Kaplan EB. The relationship of the ulnar nerve to the medial intermuscular septum in the arm and its clinical significance. *Hand*. 1976;8:239–242.
13. Campbell WN, Landaw M. Treatment and management of segmental neuromuscular disorders (Chapter 17). In: Bertorini T, ed. *Neuromuscular Disorders: Treatment and Management*. Amsterdam: Elsevier; 2021. 2nd ed.
14. Sutherland S. *Nerves and Nerve Injuries*. 2nd ed. Philadelphia, PA: WB Saunders; 1978.
15. Masear VR, Hill Jr JJ, Cohen SM. Ulnar compression neuropathy secondary to the anconeus epitrochlearis muscle. *J Hand Surg [Am]*. 1988;13(5):720–724.
16. Campbell WW. AAEE case report no. 18: ulnar neuropathy in the distal forearm. *Muscle Nerve*. 1989;12:347–352.
17. Lowe JB, Novak CB, Mackinnon SE. Current approach to cubital tunnel syndrome. *Neurosurg Clin N Am*. 2001;12:267–284.
18. Gellman H, Campion DS. Modified in situ decompression of the ulnar nerve at the elbow. *Hand Clin*. 1996;12:405–410.
19. King T, Morgan FP. Late results of removing the medial humeral epicondyle for traumatic ulnar neuritis. *J Bone Joint Surg Br*. 1959; 41B:51–55.
20. Dinh PT, Gupta R. Subtotal medial epicondylectomy as a surgical option for treatment of cubital tunnel syndrome. *Tech Hand Up Extrem Surg*. 2005;9(1):52–59.
21. Bartels RH, Verhagen WI, van der Wilt GJ, et al. Prospective randomized controlled study comparing simple decompression versus anterior subcutaneous transposition for idiopathic neuropathy of the ulnar nerve at the elbow: Part 1. *Neurosurgery*. 2005; 56(3):522–530.

22. Britz GW, Haynor DR, Kuntz C, et al. Ulnar nerve entrapment at the elbow: correlation of magnetic resonance imaging, clinical, electrodiagnostic and intraoperative findings. *Neurosurgery*. 1996;38:458–465.
23. Campbell WW, Sahni SK, Pridgeon RM, et al. Intraoperative electroneurography: management of ulnar neuropathy at the elbow. *Muscle Nerve*. 1988;11:75–81.

8 CASE

A Young Woman With Multiple Sclerosis and Hand Numbness

A 30-year-old woman was diagnosed with multiple sclerosis 8 years earlier when she presented with tingling, paresthesias, and weakness in her arms and legs. MRI showed patchy demyelinating plaques of the brain and spinal cord. Upper and lower extremity somatosensory-evoked responses were abnormal, but visual and brain stem–evoked responses were normal. Her spinal fluid showed evidence of oligoclonal bands and IgG elevation. Treatment with intravenous methylprednisolone produced marked improvement. Six months later, she developed an acute episode of optic neuritis. Repeat MRI showed new enhancing plaques in the brain, whereas the spinal cord lesions had disappeared. There was a complete resolution of symptoms with steroid treatment. Since then, she has had several episodes of exacerbations and remissions characterized mainly by leg numbness, weakness, and vertigo. She is currently on β-interferon therapy.

The patient presented this time with a 3-week history of numbness and paresthesias in the ulnar nerve distribution of the right hand. She denied neck pain or trauma.

Her medical history was unremarkable except for chickenpox infection during childhood. She worked as a secretary and did not smoke or drink alcohol.

Examination revealed normal mentation and cranial nerves except for mild pallor of the right optic disk. Strength was intact except for weakness of the interossei muscles on the right hand with first dorsal interosseous (FDI) muscle wasting. On finger extension, the right fifth digit is adducted and separated from the other fingers (Fig. 8-1A) or Wartenberg sign. This is caused by weak third lumbrical and strong hypothenar muscles. This is also seen in more proximal ulnar lesions. Even though the hypothenar muscles are not weak, patients may still have the Wartenberg sign for which the patient did complain of the little finger getting "stuck" when she put her hands in her pocket. She could perform normal "cupping" of the hand indicating a normal palmaris brevis muscle function (Fig. 8-1B). The adductor digiti minimi (ADM), thumb, finger, and wrist flexor strength were normal as were all other right upper extremity muscles. There was no focal tenderness in the wrist or elbow. She had decreased sensation in the ulnar nerve distribution involving the palmar surfaces of the fifth digit and ulnar half of the fourth digit; the dorsum of the hand was normal. Adson's maneuver was negative. There was mild tenderness at the ulnar area of the wrist, but no swelling or masses were detected. No Tinel's sign was elicited at the elbow or the wrist. Muscle stretch reflexes were normal; there were no Babinski signs. Coordination was normal.

WHAT ARE THE MOST LIKELY POSSIBILITIES?

This patient had multiple sclerosis, and her recent symptoms could suggest a spinal cord lesion causing numbness and weakness. However, they corresponded to the distribution of the left ulnar nerve, making a spinal cord lesion unlikely. Other possibilities include a C8 radiculopathy or a lesion of the lower trunk or medial cord of the brachial plexus. Ulnar entrapment at the elbow is a consideration as this is the most common site of entrapment of this nerve, but the lack of involvement of the dorsal cutaneous nerve territory and normal palmaris brevis function suggest that the lesion was distal to the elbow.

AN EMG TEST WAS PERFORMED

Motor Nerve Studies

Nerve and Site	Latency (ms)	Amplitude (mV)	Conduction Velocity (m/s)
Median Nerve R.	**Normal ≤ 4.2**	**Normal ≥ 6**	**Normal ≥ 50**
Wrist	3.2	18	–
Elbow	7.0	18	59
Ulnar Nerve R. (ADM)	**Normal ≤ 3.6**	**Normal ≥ 8**	**Normal ≥ 50**
Wrist	2.8	14	–
Below elbow	6.0	14	66
Above elbow	7.9	13	63
Axilla	10.5	12	63
Erb's point	13.5	12	67
Ulnar Nerve R.[a]	**Normal ≤ 3.6**	**Normal ≥ 8**	**Normal ≥ 50**
Wrist	3.4	**6**	–
Below elbow	7.2	**4**	61

[a]Recording at the first dorsal interosseous.

Motor Nerve Studies—cont'd

Nerve and Site	Latency (ms)	Amplitude (mV)
Ulnar Nerve L.[b]	**Normal ≤ 3.6**	**Normal ≥ 8**
Wrist	3.0	24

[b]Recording at the first dorsal interosseous.

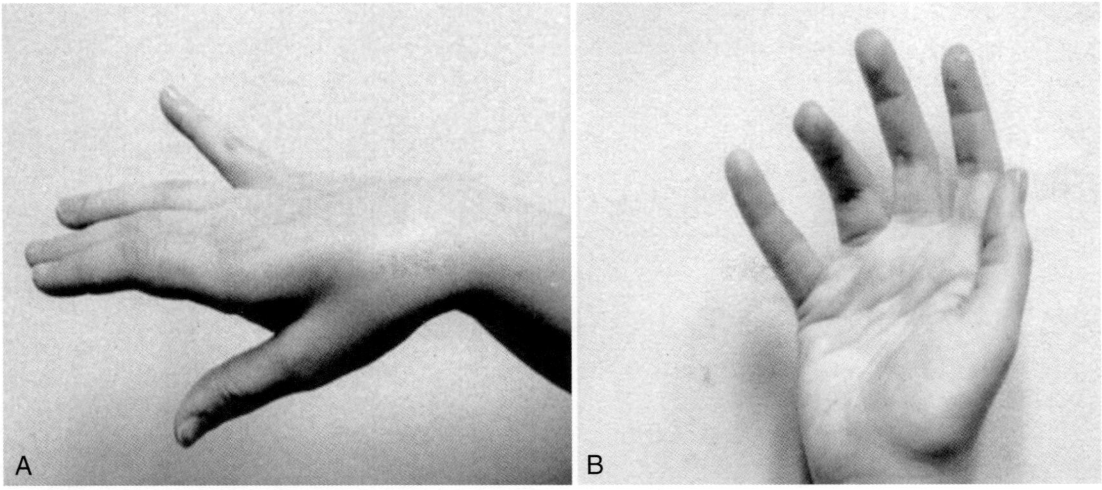

FIG. 8-1 **A**, Mild atrophy of the first dorsal interosseous and a tendency to adduct the fifth digit when extending the fingers from relatively preserved hypothenar muscles. **B**, Normal "cupping" of the hand indicating normal function of the palmaris brevis.

F-Wave Studies

Nerve	Latency (ms)	Normal Latency ≤ (ms)
Median nerve R.	24.4	30
Ulnar nerve R.	24.6	30

Sensory Nerve Studies

Nerve	Onset Latency (ms)	Normal Onset Latency ≤ (ms)	Peak Latency (ms)	Normal Peak Latency ≤ (ms)	Amp (μV)	Normal Amp ≥ (μV)	Conduction Velocity (m/s)	Normal Conduction Velocity ≥ (m/s)
Median nerve R.	2.5	2.6	3.0	3.1	81	20	52	50
Ulnar nerve R.	2.2	2.6	2.7	3.1	21	13	55	50
Ulnar dorsal cut. R.	1.3	–	1.8	2.3	42	12	61	50
Ulnar palmar R.	**1.5**	**1.0**	**2.0**	1.5	20	13	**46**	50
Medial antebrachial R.	1.5	–	2.0	2.2	10	10	50	50

EMG Data

Muscle	Insrt Activity	Fibs	Pos Waves	Fasc	Amp	Dur	Poly	Pattern
Cervical paraspinals R.	Norm	None	None	None	Norm	Norm	None	Full
Biceps brachii R.	Norm	None	None	None	Norm	Norm	None	Full
Flexor carpi radialis R.	Norm	None	None	None	Norm	Norm	None	Full
Flexor carpi ulnaris R.	Norm	None	None	None	Norm	Norm	None	Full
Triceps R.	Norm	None	None	None	Norm	Norm	None	Full
Pronator quadratus R.	Norm	None	None	None	Norm	Norm	None	Full
Flexor dig. pro. R.	Norm	None	None	None	Norm	Norm	None	Full
Abductor dig. min. R.	**Inc**	None	**1+**	None	Norm	Norm	None	Full
First dorsal interosseous R.	**Inc**	**3+**	**3+**	None	Norm	Norm	None	**Red**
Third dorsal interosseous R.	**Inc**	**3+**	**3+**	None	Norm	Norm	None	**Red**

WHAT WERE THE EMG FINDINGS?

The ulnar and median motor conduction velocities, CMAP amplitude, and latency to the ADM and F-wave latencies were normal. However, the CMAP of the ulnar nerve to the FDI was of much lower amplitude on the right compared with the left. There were denervation potentials in the ulnar hand muscles, most severe in the FDI.

These electrophysiologic findings indicated a lesion of distal branches of the motor ulnar nerve in the hand with axonal degeneration more severe in the FDI. Inching studies were not done, but the lower CMAP amplitude of the right FDI, and mild latency difference compared with the other side, suggested a lesion at the wrist.[1] In spite of her sensory complaints and findings, the ulnar SNAP was normal, indicating only partial involvement of the sensory branch of the nerve, without significant axonal degeneration in this. The dorsal cutaneous branch was normal, and the medial antebrachial cutaneous nerve SNAP was present. The opposite side was not tested for amplitude comparison.

WHAT WOULD BE THE NEXT TEST?

An MRI of the wrist showed a ganglion cyst at the base of the right fourth metacarpal bone adjacent to the hamate (Fig. 8-2).

WHAT WOULD BE THE MANAGEMENT?

After surgical removal of the ganglion, her symptoms were resolved.

DISCUSSION

This patient had a distal ulnar neuropathy. For a better understanding of this case, we will summarize anatomy of the distal ulnar nerve. In the forearm, the ulnar nerve gives off the dorsal cutaneous branch about 8 cm above the wrist. Then at the wrist the nerve enters the canal of Guyon which is formed proximally by the pisiform bone and distally by the hook of the hamate, with a thick ligament between the two bones or at the outlet of pisohamate hiatus.

In the canal the nerve divides into two branches: the superficial and the deep motor branches. The superficial branch leaves the canal and innervates the palmaris brevis muscle and then continues superficially to provide sensory innervation to the palmar area of the fifth digit and the medial half of the fourth. The deep branch, which is purely motor, loops around the hook of the hamate and innervates the ADM, flexor digiti minimi, and opponens digiti quinti. This branch then travels through the palm, innervating the lumbricals and interossei, terminating at the FDI, adductor, and flexor pollicis brevis, which is also innervated by the median nerve.

Ulnar nerve lesions at the wrist and hand are difficult to diagnose and localize clinically, although compressions at different sites present with different symptoms that can aid in localization.[1,2] These have numerous etiologies including compression from bicycle riding[3] or driving, trauma, ganglion cysts,[4] tumors, anomalous muscles, fibrotic material, and abnormal vessels.[2]

In a review of 56 cases of ulnar neuropathy at the wrist,[5] the most common etiology was a ganglion cyst (41%), followed by anomalous muscles (10.7%). In another review of 20 cases, however, trauma was the most common cause.[4–6]

Distal ulnar nerve lesions are categorized by lesion location[5] into five different types (Fig. 8-3):

Type I lesion is proximal to the bifurcation of the ulnar nerve into the Guyon's canal and affects both the superficial sensory and the deep motor branches, but spares the dorsal cutaneous branch. The lesion is located just outside or at the proximal level of the canal of Guyon.

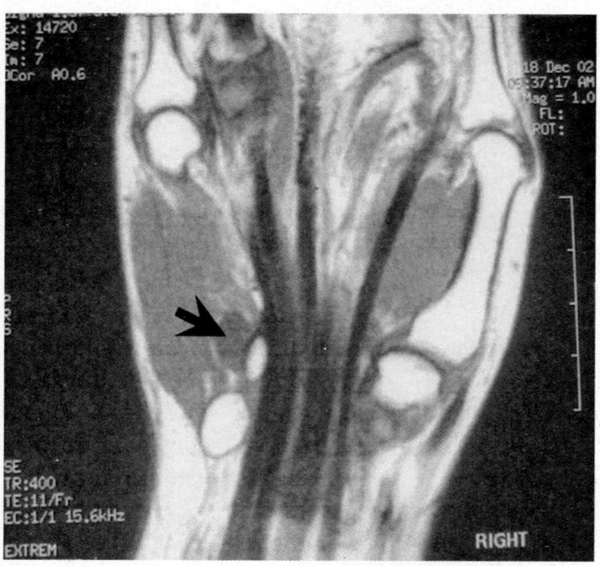

FIG. 8-2 MRI of the wrist. T1-weighted image showing the ganglion cyst (*arrow*).

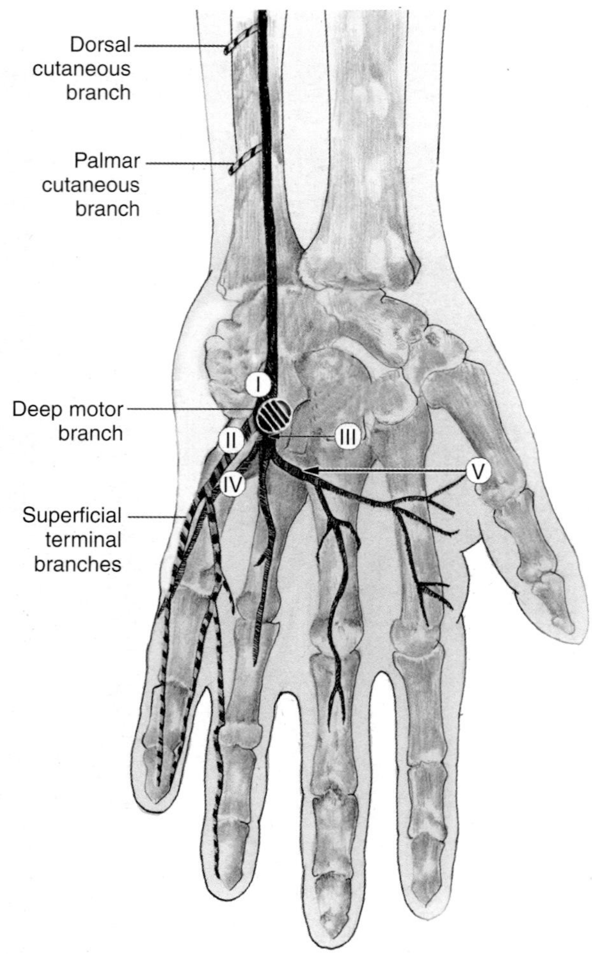

FIG. 8-3 The ulnar nerve in the hand demonstrating the location of different distal lesions. Notice the anatomic distribution of the ulnar nerve and its branches at the wrist and hand and the site of compression indicated by a circle.

Type II lesion involves only the superficial branch distal to the palmaris brevis muscle and thus causes a purely sensory neuropathy.
Type III lesion is distal to the superficial sensory branch and is a purely motor neuropathy involving all motor fibers, including those fibers going to the hypothenar eminence.
Type IV lesion involves the deep motor nerve branch to the hypothenar eminence, affecting these muscles only.
Type V lesion is more distal and involves only fibers going to the FDI and the adductor pollicis brevis muscles.

When performing electrophysiologic tests in a patient with suspected ulnar neuropathy at the wrist, it is important to record the SNAPs to the palm and fifth digit, which could be affected in plexus and ulnar lesions at the elbow or wrist, and the ulnar dorsal cutaneous branch (which is not affected by lesions at the wrist). Motor studies to the ADM and the FDI should be studied in both hands to compare latencies and amplitudes.[7] The medial antebrachial cutaneous SNAP should be studied if a plexus lesion is a consideration.

Inching techniques at the wrist may be used to determine the lesion site.[4,6,8,9] Needle electromyography is used to document denervation in the muscles innervated by different branches of the ulnar nerve, as well as other C8, lower trunk, and medial cord innervated muscles.

This patient appeared to have an atypical or incomplete type I distal ulnar lesion. She had clinical involvement of the superficial sensory branch, in spite of a normal SNAP of the ulnar nerve to the fifth digit. Further, the hypothenar muscles were not weak and showed only mild denervation. The ganglion cyst was located adjacent to the hamate bone and above the division of motor and sensory branches.

Ganglion cysts are accumulations of synovial fluid that occur spontaneously, from trauma or from defects in the joint capsular sheath, usually at the base of the hand[10] or the anterior wrist. They may manifest as masses[10,11] which might not be obvious clinically. The treatment includes the old-fashioned "bible therapy" (smashing of the cyst) and, more properly, needle aspiration or surgery.[9,12]

SUMMARY

This case presented with a distal ulnar neuropathy caused by a ganglion cyst between the fourth and fifth metacarpal bones, compressing the motor fibers to the FDI and/or with relative sparing of the hypothenar eminence and distally with mild damage of the sensory branch.

If there is no obvious trauma or compression, an MRI of the hand may help to evaluate for mass lesions.

IMPORTANT POINTS

- The differential diagnosis of patients presenting with numbness in the last two digits and/or weakness of the dorsal interossei muscles include C8 radiculopathy, lower trunk or medial cord plexopathy, and ulnar entrapment at the elbow, wrist, or palm.
- The neurologic examination should determine if there is weakness in other C8, lower trunk, or medial cord innervated muscles. Sensory examination should assess if there is sensory splitting of the fourth finger, involvement of the dorsal cutaneous branch, or involvement of the medial antebrachial cutaneous nerve in the forearm, which can confirm the site of the lesion.
- An ulnar lesion at the wrist can cause purely motor ulnar deficits of the hand without sensory findings. The differential diagnosis should also include other conditions such as a motor neuron disorder, a radiculopathy, and plexopathy. A distal ulnar neuropathy should be considered in those patients with ulnar sensory deficit in the hand sparing the dorsal cutaneous branch area.
- Electrophysiologic studies of ulnar neuropathy at the wrist demonstrate normal ulnar conduction across the elbow and from elbow to wrist. The dorsal cutaneous branch and medial antebrachial cutaneous nerve SNAPs are normal. There is lack of denervation in ulnar-innervated forearm muscles and other nonulnar-innervated C8, lower trunk, and medial cord muscles. The test could show denervation in hypothenar eminence muscles and on the FDI. In wrist or hand lesions depending on the level, the ulnar digital SNAP could be affected. Similarly, the CMAP of the ADM and/or FDI could be of lower amplitude compared with the opposite side, depending on the level of the lesion.
- Causes of ulnar lesions at the wrist or hand include ganglion cysts, tumors, trauma, or mass lesions, including abnormal muscles.
- Ganglion cysts can be aspirated or removed surgically.

REFERENCES

1. Ebeling P, Gilliatt RW, Thomas PK. A clinical and electrical study of ulnar nerve lesions in the hand. *J Neurol Neurosurg Psychiatry.* 1960;23:1–9.
2. Shea JD, McClain EJ. Ulnar-nerve compression syndromes at and below the wrist. *J Bone Joint Surg.* 1969;51(6):1095–1103.
3. Eckman PB, Perlstein S, Altrocchi P. Ulnar neuropathy in bicycle riders. *Arch Neurol.* 1975;32:130–132.
4. Wu S, Morris JD, Hogan GR. Ulnar neuropathy at the wrist: case report and review of literature. *Arch Phys Med Rehabil.* 1985;66:785–788.
5. Lo YL, Ratnagopal P, Leoh TH, et al. Clinical and electrophysiological aspects of distal ulnar neuropathy. *Acta Neurol Scand.* 2002;105:390–394.
6. Preston DC, Shapiro BE, Schecht HIM. Ganglion cyst at Guyon's canal: electrophysiology and pathology. *J Clin Neuromuscul Dis.* 2001;3:89–91.
7. Olney RK, Wilbourn AJ. Ulnar nerve conduction study of the first dorsal interosseous muscle. *Arch Phys Med Rehabil.* 1985;66:16–18.
8. McIntosh KA, Preston DC, Logigian EL. Short segment incremental studies to localize ulnar nerve entrapments at the wrist. *Neurology.* 1998;50:303–306.
9. Padua L, Insola A, LoMonaco M, et al. A case of Guyon syndrome with neuroapraxic block resolved after surgical decompression. *Electroencephalogr Clin Neurophysiol.* 1998;109:191–193.
10. Angelides AC, Wallace PF. The dorsal ganglion of the wrist: its pathogenesis, gross and microscopic anatomy, and surgical treatment. *J Hand Surg [Am].* 1976;1(3):228–235.
11. Wright TW, Cooney WP, Ilstrup DM. Anterior wrist ganglion. *J Hand Surg [Am].* 1994;19(6):954–958.
12. Richmond DA. Carpal ganglion with ulnar nerve compression. *J Bone Joint Surg Am.* 1963;45B:513–515.

9 CASE

A Woman With a Wrist Drop and a Mass in the Arm

A 56-year-old woman had a 4-month history of left shoulder and arm pain, and a 3-week history of numbness in the dorsum of the hand with some arm weakness. She awakened one morning with a wrist drop and was evaluated the next day by an orthopedic surgeon, who found a mass in the left arm. The patient had no systemic symptoms or history of trauma and no family history of neurologic disorders. She did have a history of hypertension and had undergone a decompressive laminectomy for a lumbar radiculopathy in the past.

Examination showed normal mental status and cranial nerves. She had severe weakness of the brachioradialis muscle, wrist, and finger extensors on the left. Strength of the triceps muscle was difficult to evaluate because of severe pain. The left brachioradialis reflex was absent, and ankle reflexes were diminished bilaterally; other reflexes were normal. There was decreased sensation in the left radial nerve distribution in the hand. The remainder of her neurologic examination was normal. There was a tender, indurated mass in the lower aspect of the left arm.

WHAT IS THE DIFFERENTIAL DIAGNOSIS?

Wrist drop is usually caused by a lesion of the radial nerve. Wrist extensor weakness could also be caused by a C7 radiculopathy or a lesion of the middle trunk of the brachial plexus, but these conditions can also sometimes affect wrist flexion (through median and ulnar innervation). A posterior cord lesion can also cause a wrist drop. It also causes shoulder weakness from involvement of the axillary nerve.

Clinically, this patient appeared to have a radial neuropathy caused by compression from a mass in the arm. Other causes of a radial neuropathy in the arm include external compression, fractures of the humerus, inflammations, and infections. In this case the motor and sensory branches of the radial nerve were affected, but it was not clear if the triceps muscle was involved, because it was difficult to examine. The involvement of the radial sensory branch and weakness of the brachioradialis and extensor carpi radialis indicate a lesion of the main trunk of the radial nerve from the mass likely compressing the nerve, rather than a posterior interosseous neuropathy, which occurs at the elbow and is usually caused by fracture of the radius, entrapment at the supinator or extensor carpi radialis muscle, or post-traumatic injury.

AN EMG TEST WAS PERFORMED

Motor Nerve Studies

Nerve and Site	Latency (ms)	Amplitude (mV)	Conduction Velocity (m/s)
Median Nerve L.	**Normal ≤ 4.2**	**Normal ≥ 6**	**Normal ≥ 50**
Wrist	3.5	17	–
Elbow	6.8	16	61

This case was reported by Alzagatiti BI, Bertorini TE, Horner LH, Maccarino VS, O'Brien T. Focal myositis presenting with radial nerve palsy. *Muscle Nerve.* 1999;22:956–959.

Motor Nerve Studies—cont'd

Nerve and Site	Latency (ms)	Amplitude (mV)	Conduction Velocity (m/s)
Ulnar Nerve L.	**Normal ≤ 3.6**	**Normal ≥ 8**	**Normal ≥ 50**
Wrist	3.0	14	–
Below elbow	6.4	14	57

F-Wave Studies

Nerve	Latency (ms)	Normal Latency ≤ (ms)
Median nerve L.	26.8	30
Ulnar nerve L.	25.6	30

Sensory Nerve Studies

Nerve	Onset Latency (ms)	Normal Onset Latency ≤ (ms)	Peak Latency (ms)	Normal Peak Latency ≤ (ms)	Amp (μV)	Normal Amp ≥ (μV)	Conduction Velocity (m/s)	Normal Conduction Velocity ≥ (m/s)
Median nerve L.	2.1	2.6	2.6	3.1	40	20	62	50
Ulnar nerve L.	2.1	2.6	2.6	3.1	26	13	57	50
Radial nerve L.	**NR**	2.6	**NR**	3.1	**NR**	30	**NR**	50
Radial nerve R.	2.3	2.6	2.8	3.1	36	30	60	50

EMG Data

Muscle	Insrt Activity	Fibs	Pos Waves	Fasc	Amp	Dur	Poly	Pattern
Cervical paraspinals L.	Norm	None	None	None	Norm	Norm	None	Full
Deltoid L.	Norm	None	None	None	Norm	Norm	None	Full
Biceps brachii L.	Norm	None	None	None	Norm	Norm	None	Full
Flexor carpi radialis L.	Norm	None	None	None	Norm	Norm	None	Full
Brachioradialis L.	**Inc**	**1+**	**1+**	None	Norm	Norm	**Few**	**Red**
Extensor digitorum com. L.	**Inc**	**3+**	**3+**	None	[a]	[a]	[a]	[a]
Extensor carpi radialis L.	**Inc**	**3+**	**3+**	None	[a]	[a]	[a]	[a]
First dorsal interosseous L.	Norm	None	None	None	Norm	Norm	None	Full

[a]No motor units recruited.

WHAT WERE THE EMG FINDINGS?

The left median and ulnar nerve SNAPs, conduction velocities and amplitudes were normal, whereas the superficial radial SNAP was absent. Radial nerve motor conduction could not be studied because of discomfort.

The needle test showed denervation potentials in radial-innervated muscles, including wrist extensor and the brachioradialis, indicating that the lesion occurred above the elbow. The normal median- and ulnar-innervated muscles negate a C7 radiculopathy or a lesion of the middle trunk of the brachial plexus. The normal EMG of her deltoid is evidence against a posterior cord lesion.

Denervation in the brachioradialis and extensor carpi radialis and the absent radial SNAP indicate that the main trunk of the radial nerve was affected with axonal degeneration.

WHAT OTHER TESTS SHOULD BE DONE?

A magnetic resonance imaging (MRI) scan of the left arm showed a mass within the left triceps muscle, located about 6 cm below the glenohumeral joint and measuring about 4 cm (Fig. 9-1). There was cortical destruction of the humerus along the mass margin, which favored the diagnosis of soft tissue sarcoma. Biopsy of this mass showed skeletal muscle with a diffuse mononuclear inflammatory cell infiltrate, fibrosis, and rare necrotic muscle fibers (Fig. 9-2).

Laboratory test results were normal, including erythrocyte sedimentation rate, serum creatine kinase level, blood chemistry profile, tests for antinuclear antibodies, and rheumatoid factor.

WHAT ARE THE DIAGNOSES AND TREATMENT?

The patient was found to have a focal myositis (FM) and was treated with corticosteroids at a dose of 60 mg a day for 1 week, with tapering over an additional 1 month until discontinued. The mass disappeared after 2.5 months, and the patient slowly recovered strength. By 6 months the radial nerve palsy resolved completely. After 9 months a repeat MRI revealed normal triceps muscle and no mass (Fig. 9-3). (Fig. 9-4 shows the radial nerve and its branches.) An EMG at that time showed no abnormalities except for large motor unit potentials in the brachioradialis, the extensor digitorum communis, and the extensor carpi radialis muscles from reinnervation. There was no recurrence of the radial nerve palsy or the mass after 2 years.

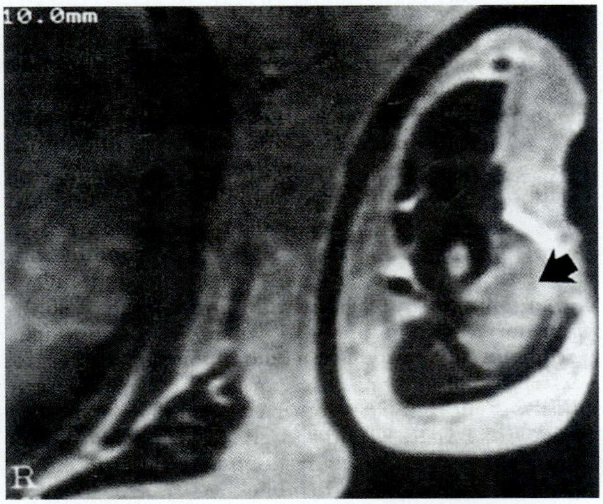

FIG. 9-1 T2-weighted MRI showing the mass with increased signal intensity within the triceps muscle (*arrow*).

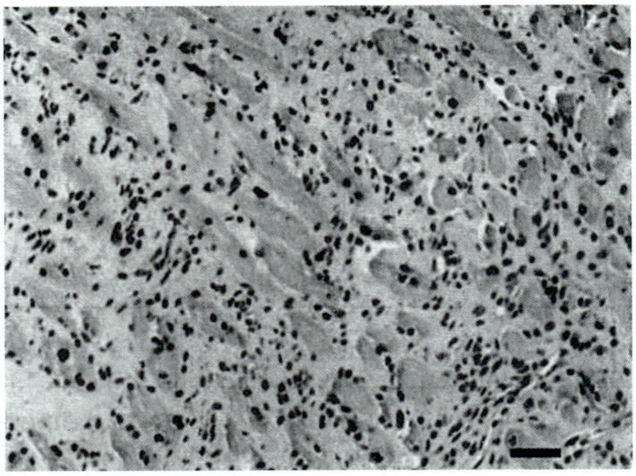

FIG. 9-2 Biopsy of the mass showing inflammatory cell infiltrate, fibrosis, and rare necrotic fibers (H&E stain, ×200).

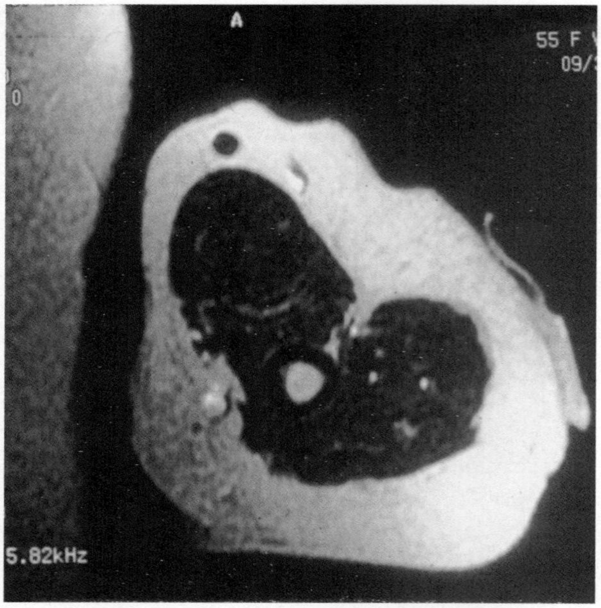

FIG. 9-3 T2-weighted MRI showing normal signal intensity and no mass in the triceps muscle after 9 months.

DISCUSSION

This patient had an FM that manifested as a mass compressing the radial nerve and producing severe paralysis of the muscles innervated by this nerve. The symptoms improved and the mass disappeared with corticosteroid treatment; the paralysis resolved without recurrence.

Since the initial report by Heffner et al. in 1977,[1] FM is recognized as a benign inflammatory disorder of muscle that presents as an isolated soft tissue mass and resembles a sarcoma,[2,3] but unlike sarcomas, it frequently regresses spontaneously. FM may be a manifestation of vasculitis[4] or may later show evidence of diffuse spread (polymyositis)[5,6] but usually does not have peripheral nerve symptomatology.[7–15]

There is one reported case of FM that had calf enlargement secondary to S1 radiculopathy, but which also had focal inflammation, necrotic muscle fibers, and fiber-type grouping on muscle biopsy.[14] The hypertrophy, therefore, could have been secondary to chronic and partial denervation, and the authors suggest that denervated calf muscles may be predisposed to damage during walking, causing a secondary inflammatory process. Edema and fibrosis may also have contributed to the enlargement. Denervation and reinnervation changes have been reported in other cases,[12] and it is possible that these findings are secondary to the inflammation affecting or compressing intramuscular nerves.

The etiology of most cases of FM is not apparent, but it has been suggested that it is secondary to trauma[13] or infection.[16,17] Rheumatoid arthritis, sarcoidosis, and connective tissue disease may also manifest as an FM.[16,18] In a recent study, matrix metalloproteinase (MMP)-A was consistently increased in all inflammatory myopathies, including FM, whereas MMP-Z and MMP-7 were not increased in FM.[19]

Imaging studies, such as computed tomography and MRI, are used in the evaluation of focal soft tissue masses and FM.[20,21] MRI usually reveals an increased signal intensity on T2-weighted images in myositis and is useful for directing a muscle biopsy or identifying the location and extent of the disease process, providing a noninvasive method for follow-up. A muscle biopsy, however, is necessary for a definitive diagnosis.

FM usually disappears spontaneously, but some cases persist or are recurrent.[11,22] Surgical excision is useful for removal of the mass.[13] Immunosuppressive therapy and radiation may be beneficial in progressive cases.[14] This patient was treated aggressively with corticosteroids because of her neurologic impairment, caused by the compression of the radial nerve.

SUMMARY

This case presented with a radial neuropathy of the arm caused by a mass, which proved to be an FM.

FM is an idiopathic inflammation that can be posttraumatic or caused by rheumatoid arthritis and sarcoidosis. The condition usually disappears spontaneously or responds to steroids. In some cases, surgical treatment may be necessary.

IMPORTANT POINTS

- Radial neuropathies at the arm affect the finger extensors, supinator, brachioradialis, and wrist extensor muscles, sparing other nonradial-innervated C6–C7 roots, middle trunk, and posterior cord muscles. These neuropathies usually also affect the sensory branch at the radial nerve.
- Radial neuropathy could be caused by external compression, masses, fracture of the humerus, blunt injuries, or injections.
- FM is a relatively benign inflammatory disease but presents as a soft tissue mass that either could be caused by inflammation or could be idiopathic secondary to trauma, denervation, sarcoidosis, or rheumatoid arthritis.
- FM may disappear spontaneously or respond to steroids. Occasionally, surgical removal may be necessary.

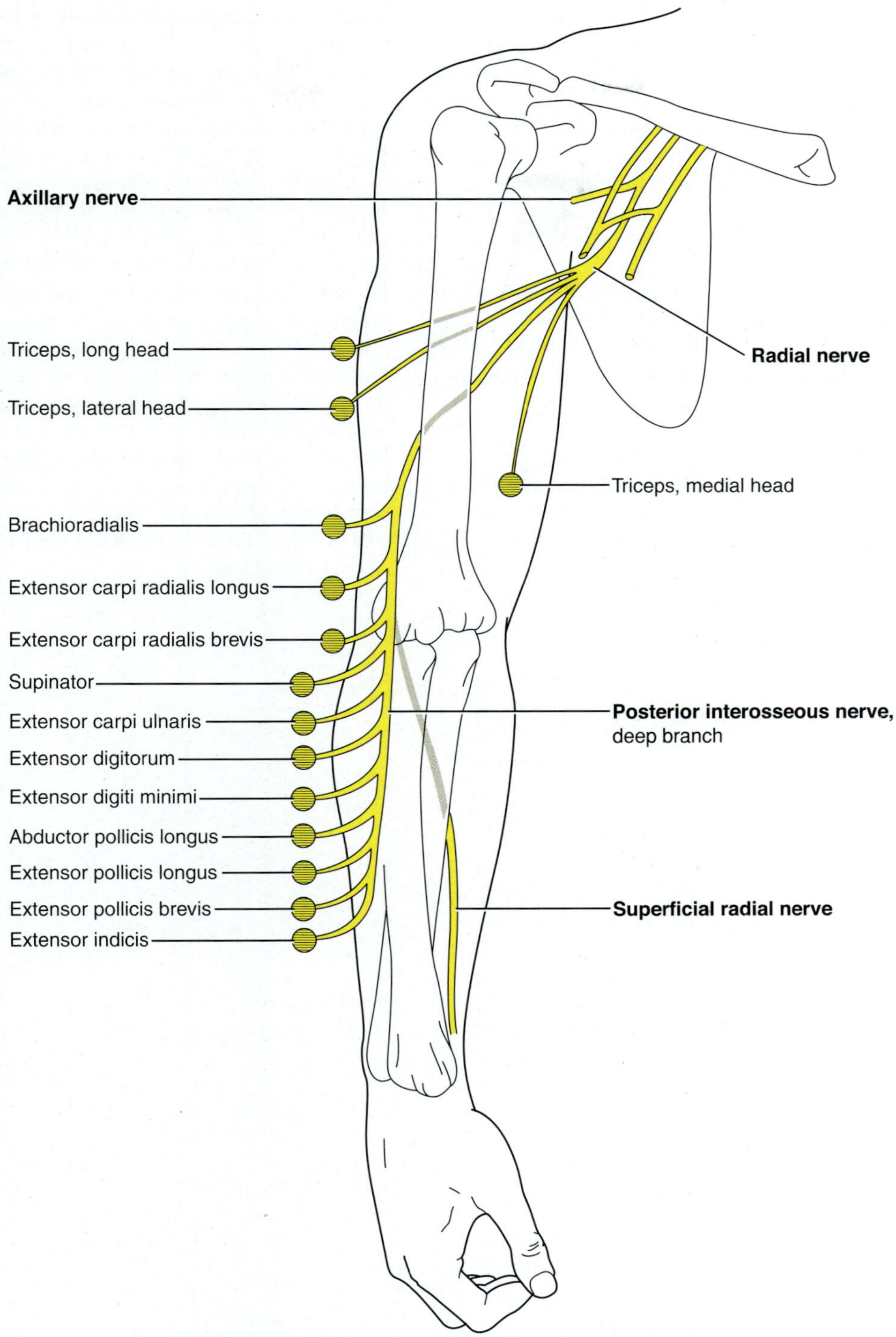

FIG. 9-4 The radial nerve, its branches, and innervated muscles.

REFERENCES

1. Heffner RR Jr, Armbrustmacher VW, Earle KM. Focal myositis. *Cancer*. 1977;40:301–306.
2. Caldwell CJ, Swash M, Van der Walt JD, Geddes JF. Focal myositis: a clinicopathological study. *Neuromuscul Disord*. 1995;5:317–321.
3. Liefeld PA, Ferguson AB Jr, Fu FH. Focal myositis: a benign lesion that mimics malignant disease: a case report. *J Bone Joint Surg Am*. 1982;64(9):1371–1374.
4. Allen I, Mullally B, Mawhinney H, et al. The nodular form of polymyositis—a possible manifestation of vasculitis. *J Pathol*. 1980;131:183–191.
5. Cumming WJ, Weiser R, Teoh R, et al. Localised nodular myositis: a clinical and pathological variant of polymyositis. *QJM*. 1977;46:531–546.
6. Heffner RR Jr, Barron SA. Polymyositis beginning as a focal process. *Arch Neurol*. 1981;38:439–442.
7. Azuma T, Komori A, Nagayama M. Focal myositis of the tongue. *J Oral Maxillofac Surg*. 1987;45:953–955.

8. Flaisler F, Blin D, Asencio G, et al. Focal myositis: a localized form of polymyositis? A case report. *J Rheumatol.* 1993;20:1414–1416.
9. Hansen LB, Baekgaard N, Reske-Nielsen E. Focal myositis of the rectus abdominal muscles. *Acta Chir Scand.* 1985;151:77–80.
10. Gomez Rodriguez N, Formigo Rodriguez E, Ibañez Ruan J, et al. Pseudotumor in the forearm caused by focal myositis: a rare form of idiopathic inflammatory myopathy. *An Med Interna.* 1996;13:398–400.
11. Hassell AB, Plant MJ, Dawes PT. Focal myositis: another cause of pseudothrombophlebitis. *Br J Rheumatol.* 1994;33:687.
12. Heffner RR Jr, Barron SA. Denervating changes in focal myositis, a benign inflammatory pseudotumor. *Arch Pathol Lab Med.* 1980;104:261–264.
13. Isaacson G, Chan KH, Heffner RR Jr. Focal myositis: a new cause for the pediatric neck mass. *Arch Otolaryngol Head Neck Surg.* 1991;117:103–105.
14. Krendel DA, Hedaya EV, Gottleib AJ. Calf enlargement, S1 radiculopathy, and focal myositis. *Muscle Nerve.* 1992;15:517–518.
15. Vercelli-Retta J, Ardao G, DeCabrera M. Focal myositis and its differential diagnosis: a case report and review of the literature. *Ann Pathol.* 1988;8:54–56.
16. Walton J. The inflammatory myopathies. *J R Soc Med.* 1983;76:998–1010.
17. Auerbach A, Fanburg-Smith JC, Wang G, Rushing EJ. Focal myositis: a clinicopathologic study of 115 cases of an intramuscular mass-like reactive process. *Am J Surg Pathol.* 2009;33(7):1016–1024. https://doi.org/10.1097/PAS.0b013e31819e63fe.
18. Mastaglia FL, Walton JN. Inflammatory myopathies. In: Mastaglia FL, Walton JN, eds. *Skeletal Muscle Pathology*. Edinburgh: Churchill Livingstone; 1992:453–491.
19. Rodolico C, Mazzeo A, Toscano A, et al. Specific matrix metalloproteinase expression in focal myositis: an immunopathological study. *Acta Neurol Scand.* 2005;112(3):173–177.
20. Fraser DD, Frank JA, Dalakas M, et al. Magnetic resonance imaging in the idiopathic inflammatory myopathies. *J Rheumatol.* 1991;18:1693–1700.
21. Moskovic E, Fisher C, Westbury G, Parsons C. Focal myositis, a benign inflammatory pseudotumor: CT appearances. *Br J Radiol.* 1991;64:489–493.
22. Sieb JP, Ries F, Träber F, et al. Recurrent focal myositis. *Muscle Nerve.* 1997;20:1205–1206.

CASE 10

A Man With Bilateral Arm Weakness After Lumbar Surgery

A 42-year-old man was referred with a 3-week history of weakness in both arms after he underwent a complicated lumbar laminectomy for severe chronic, posttraumatic low back pain and a disk rupture. The surgery lasted longer than normal. When he woke up from surgery he could not flex his arms but had no other neurologic problems. Past medical history was unremarkable except for hypertension. There was a strong family history of diabetes. The patient did not smoke or drink.

Examination revealed normal mentation and cranial nerves. Strength was normal and symmetric except for significant weakness and atrophy (Fig. 10-1) in both biceps with normal brachioradialis muscles, and he used his brachioradialis to flex the arms. Other upper extremity muscles appeared grossly normal. Reflexes were 2+ in the triceps, knees, and ankles and left brachioradialis; both biceps and right brachioradialis reflexes were absent. There was decreased pain sensation in the lateral aspect of the forearm. The rest of the examination was normal except for the lumbar laminectomy scar.

MRI of the neck and the brachial plexus with and without gadolinium done prior to referral was normal.

AN EMG TEST WAS PERFORMED

Motor Nerve Studies

Nerve and Site	Latency (ms)	Amplitude (mV)	Conduction Velocity (m/s)
Median Nerve R.	**Normal ≤ 4.2**	**Normal ≥ 6**	**Normal ≥ 50**
Wrist	4.0	13	–
Elbow	9.4	13	51
Ulnar Nerve R.	**Normal ≤ 3.6**	**Normal ≥ 8**	**Normal ≥ 50**
Wrist	3.0	11	–
Below elbow	8.5	11	**48**
Above elbow	10.8	11	52
Axilla	13.7	11	62
Erb's point	**NR**	**NR**	**NR**

Motor Nerve Studies—cont'd

Nerve and Site	Latency (ms)	Amplitude (mV)	Conduction Velocity (m/s)
Median Nerve L.	**Normal ≤ 4.2**	**Normal ≥ 6**	**Normal ≥ 50**
Wrist	**4.4**	10	–
Elbow	10.4	9	**48**
Ulnar Nerve L.	**Normal ≤ 3.6**	**Normal ≥ 8**	**Normal ≥ 50**
Wrist	2.6	12	–
Below elbow	7.9	12	50
Above elbow	9.5	12	68
Axilla	12.3	12	54
Erb's point	**NR**	**NR**	**NR**
Peroneal Nerve R.	**Normal ≤ 5.7**	**Normal ≥ 3**	**Normal ≥ 40**
Ankle	3.5	6	–
Fibular head	12.7	5	**36**
Knee	15.6	5	**31**
Musculocutaneous nerve R.		**Normal ≥ 8**	
	8.6[a]	2	–
Musculocutaneous nerve L.		**Normal ≥ 8**	
	4.5[a]	3	–

[a]Side-by-side comparison: more than 2 ms difference is significant.

F-Wave Studies

Nerve	Latency (ms)	Normal Latency ≤ (ms)
Median nerve R.	**33.1**	30
Ulnar nerve R.	**34.2**	30
Median nerve L.	**33.4**	30
Ulnar nerve L.	**34.0**	30
Peroneal nerve R.	**58.2**	54

Sensory Nerve Studies

Nerve	Onset Latency (ms)	Normal Onset Latency ≤ (ms)	Peak Latency (ms)	Normal Peak Latency ≤ (ms)	Amp (μV)	Normal Amp ≥ (μV)	Conduction Velocity (m/s)	Normal Conduction Velocity ≥ (m/s)
Median nerve R. (thumb)	2.6	2.6	3.1	3.1	21	20	50	50
Ulnar nerve R.	1.9	2.6	2.4	3.1	11	13	63	50

(Continued)

Sensory Nerve Studies—cont'd

Nerve	Onset Latency (ms)	Normal Onset Latency ≤ (ms)	Peak Latency (ms)	Normal Peak Latency ≤ (ms)	Amp (μV)	Normal Amp ≥ (μV)	Conduction Velocity (m/s)	Normal Conduction Velocity ≥ (m/s)
Median nerve L.	**2.9**	2.6	**3.4**	3.1	28	20	45	50
Ulnar nerve L.	2.1	2.6	2.6	3.1	11	13	57	50
Sural nerve R.	3.1	3.5	3.5	4.0	17	11	45	40
Superficial peroneal R.	**3.7**	3.5	**4.2**	4.0	11	8–10	41	40
Lateral ante. cut. R.	1.5	[b]	2.0	2.3	11	11	[b]	[b]
Lateral ante. cut. L.	1.8	[b]	2.3	2.3	**4**	10	[b]	[b]

[b]Normal data not available.

EMG Data

Muscle	Insrt Activity	Fibs	Pos Waves	Fasc	Amp	Dur	Poly	Pattern
L. cervical paraspinals R.	Norm	None	None	None	Norm	Norm	None	Full
Serratus anterior R.	Norm	None	None	None	Norm	Norm	None	Full
Supraspinatus R.	**Inc**	None	None	None	Norm	Norm	None	Full
Infraspinatus R.	**Inc**	None	None	None	Norm	Norm	**Few**	Full
Deltoid R.	**Inc**	**1+**	**2+**	None	Norm	Norm	None	Full
Biceps brachii R.	**Inc**	**3+**	**3+**	None	[c]	[c]	[c]	**Absent**
Triceps R.	**Inc**	None	None	None	Norm	Norm	None	Full
Brachioradialis R.	**Inc**	**4+**	**4+**	None	Norm	Norm	**Few**	Full
Brachialis R.	**Inc**	**4+**	**4+**	None	Norm	Norm	None	**Red**
Flexor carpi radialis R.	**Inc**	None	None	None	Norm	Norm	**Few**	Full
Abductor pollicis brevis R.	**Inc**	None	None	None	Norm	Norm	None	Full
First dorsal interosseous R.	**Inc**	**1+**	**1+**	None	Norm	Norm	None	Full
Supraspinatus L.	Norm	None	None	None	Norm	Norm	None	Full
Deltoid L.	**Inc**	None	None	None	Norm	Norm	**Few**	Full
Biceps brachii L.	**Inc**	**3+**	**3+**	None	[c]	[c]	[c]	**Absent**
Brachialis L.	**Inc**	**4+**	**4+**	None	Norm	Norm	None	**Red**
Triceps L.	**Inc**	None	None	None	Norm	Norm	None	Full
Flexor carpi radialis L.	Norm	None	None	None	Norm	Norm	None	Full
Flexor carpi ulnaris L.	Norm	None	None	None	Norm	Norm	None	Full
First dorsal interosseous L.	Norm	None	None	None	Norm	Norm	**Few**	Full
Vastus lateralis R.	Norm	None	None	None	Norm	Norm	None	Full
Tibialis anterior R.	**Inc**	None	**1+**	None	**Lg**	**Inc**	None	Full
Gastrocnemius R.	**Inc**	None	**1+**	None	Norm	Norm	None	Full

[c]No motor unit potentials detected.

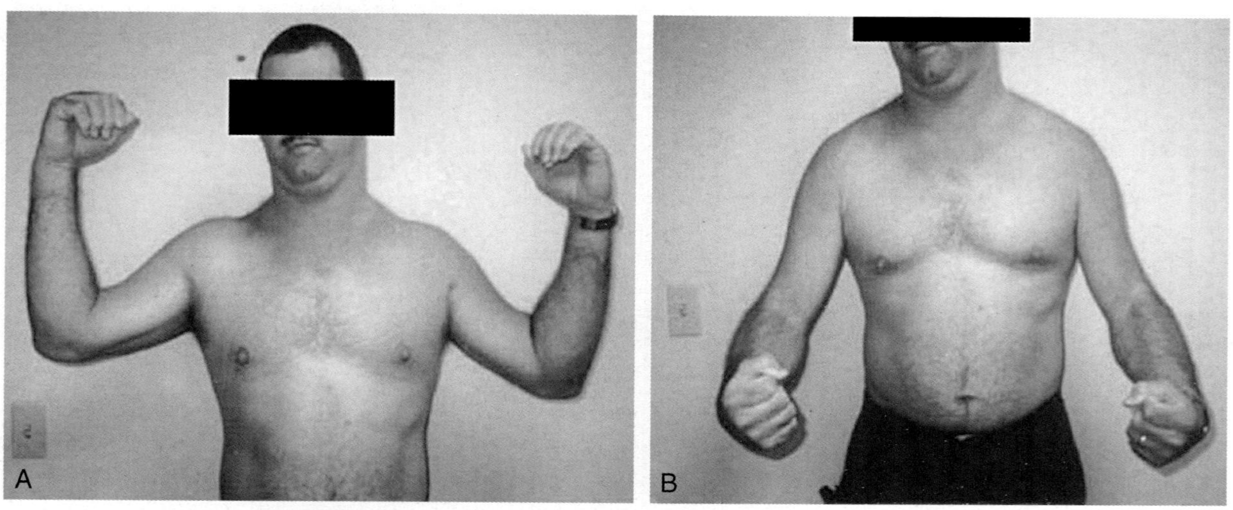

FIG. 10-1 **A**, Patient showing atrophy of the biceps muscle. **B**, Patient flexes his arms by using the brachioradialis muscle; also notice the atrophic biceps.

WHAT WERE THE EMG FINDINGS?

This test showed mild slowing of the left median, right ulnar, and right peroneal nerve motor conduction velocities with normal CMAP amplitudes; this indicated a mild neuropathy. The ulnar CMAP response from the Erb's point was absent on both sides, but this was technically difficult due to the patient's size and pain. Median and ulnar F-responses were prolonged. SNAPs had mildly prolonged latencies in the median nerve and the superficial peroneal nerves but had normal amplitudes. There was prolonged distal latency of the right musculocutaneous nerve and both sides had low-amplitude CMAPs; the amplitude of the right lateral cutaneous nerve of the forearm was decreased compared with that of the left; both latencies were normal. This could be seen in musculocutaneous neuropathy and in lesions of the upper trunk of the brachial plexus; the normal median nerve SNAP in the thumb was somewhat against the latter.

Needle electromyography detected significant denervation in the brachialis and biceps brachii bilaterally with no motor unit potentials recorded in the biceps muscles. There was increased insertional activity and mild denervation in the gastrocnemius. There was 1+ denervation in the deltoid and cervical paraspinal muscles.

This nerve conduction test showed bilateral musculocutaneous neuropathy with axonal degeneration, likely from compression. The lesion, thus, appeared more severe than only a neuropraxia. The findings in other areas indicated that the damage was more diffuse and could have been caused by prolonged traction of the plexus or could be from the polyneuropathy. There were findings that favored an upper trunk plexopathy such as the involvement of the brachioradialis. Absent lateral cutaneous SNAP can occur in both upper trunk lesions and musculocutaneous neuropathy. It could be concluded that there was a partial upper trunk plexopathy in addition to the musculocutaneous nerve lesion.

WHAT SHOULD BE DONE NEXT?

A fluorescent antinuclear antibody test was normal. Immunoelectrophoresis, B_{12}, and antineutrophil cytoplasmic antibodies were normal. The only abnormality on the blood tests was an elevation of fasting blood sugar. Serum glucose was 200 mg/dL (normal, 70–115 mg/dL), and glycosylate hemoglobin was 8% (normal, 4.3%–6.1%).

DNA test for hereditary neuropathy with liability to pressure palsies (HNPP) deletion analysis was negative.

It was concluded that the patient had a polyneuropathy and severe compression of the musculocutaneous nerves during surgery.

DISCUSSION

This patient not only developed severe weakness of the elbow flexion indicating a preferential involvement of the musculocutaneous nerve but also had signs of an upper trunk plexopathy. The possibility that he had a bilateral C5–C6 radiculopathy was unlikely, as this usually occurs unilaterally with pain, which was not present. Also, there was no paraspinal or serratus denervation. It appears that his problems were caused by compression or traction during surgery as it was noted immediately afterward.

The possibility of a neuropathy that predisposed him to compression, such as HNPP or diabetes, was a consideration, and he had elevated blood sugar and glycosylated hemoglobin.

The musculocutaneous nerve arises from the lateral cord and upper trunk of the brachial plexus from fibers originating mainly from C5 to C6. The nerve travels in the fascia between the biceps and the brachialis muscles; after this, it passes anterior to the coracobrachialis innervating these muscles, then gives off the cutaneous sensory branch that originates proximal to the elbow, and runs deep into the fascia over the brachialis muscle and innervates the skin of the lateral half of the forearm (Fig. 10-2).

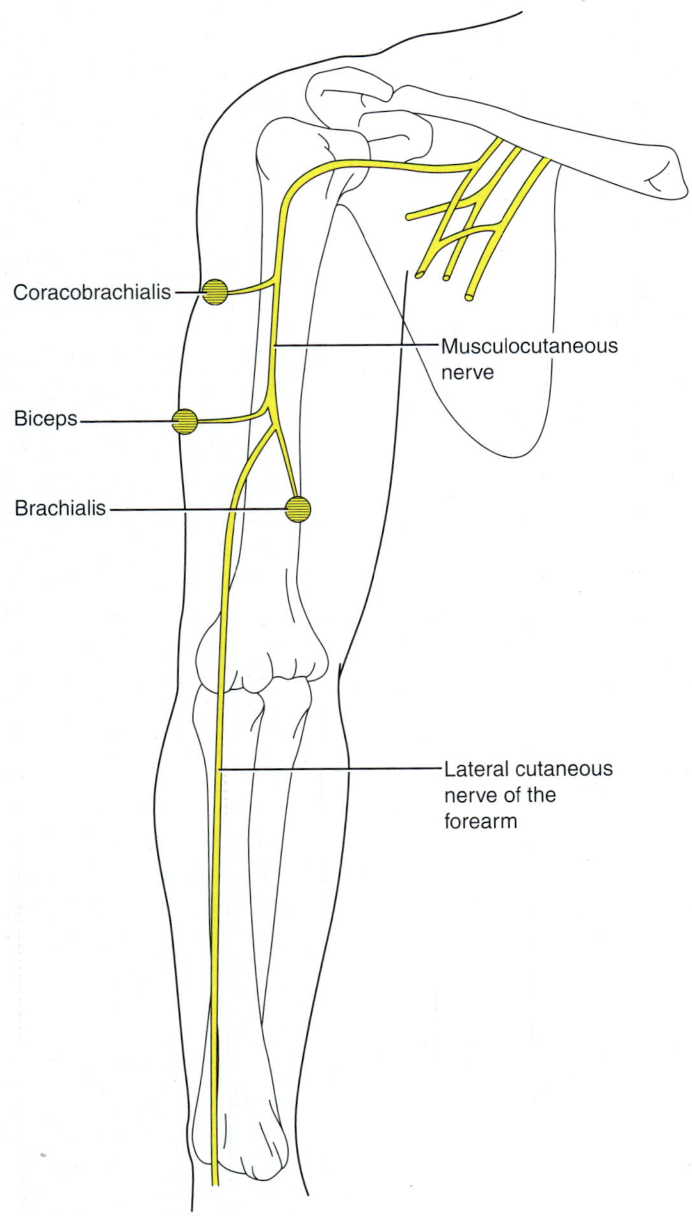

FIG. 10-2 Diagram of the musculocutaneous nerve and its branches.

Musculocutaneous neuropathies are rare and could be caused by trauma, shoulder dislocation, and fractures of the upper arm. The nerve could be affected in brachial neuritis[1] and has been reported to be compressed during general anesthesia similar to this case.[2] Sports, weight lifting and lifting heavy objects, traumatic arm extension, or pitching a baseball,[3–6] can also cause a musculocutaneous nerve injury. Other causes include tumors, anomalous muscles, or bony formations and shoulder dislocations[7–9] when it could be damaged together with the axillary nerve.[10]

Clinical findings of musculocutaneous neuropathy include weakness of elbow flexion and paresthesias from numbness in the lateral aspect of the forearm and absent biceps reflex.

The differential diagnoses include traumatic upper trunk lesions, mononeuritis multiplex, upper cervical radiculopathy, and brachial neuritis.

Electromyography might detect prolonged and low-amplitude CMAP of the biceps muscle compared with the opposite side, absent or low-amplitude SNAP of the lateral antebrachial cutaneous nerve, and denervation of the musculocutaneous-innervated muscles. The findings depend on the severity of the nerve damage and if there is only neuropraxia or axonotmesis. This helps to determine the prognosis.

As in this patient, positioning during anesthesia,[11,12] particularly for prolonged surgery,[13,14] can affect any area of the brachial plexus but more commonly the lower trunk.[14,15] Traction and pressure appear to be the major reasons for dysfunction, caused by neuropraxia and a conduction block that improves after several weeks.

Several nerves can be affected during surgery, including those of the lower extremities. Five percent of patients undergoing median sternotomy for cardiac surgery develop some form of brachial plexus injury, and most lesions affect the lower trunk.[16–18] In those, there could be denervation in muscles innervated by the lower trunk and low-amplitude SNAPs, particularly of the ulnar nerve which seems to be preferentially affected. During electrophysiologic evaluation, one should carefully assess the ulnar nerve, particularly at the elbow region, to rule out an entrapment. Paraspinal examination is also important to rule out a radiculopathy, and other predisposing causes should be considered.[19]

SUMMARY

This patient had back surgery with prolonged positioning during a lengthy procedure and developed compressive neuropathy affecting mainly the musculocutaneous nerve bilaterally. He also had a polyneuropathy, likely from diabetes. The patient responded to conservative treatment and slowly improved.

IMPORTANT POINTS

- The musculocutaneous nerve originates from the C5 to C6 root fibers that travel through the upper trunk and lateral cord of the brachial plexus. It innervates the biceps, coracobrachialis, and brachialis, and has a sensory branch, the lateral antebrachial cutaneous nerve of the forearm.
- Neuropathies during surgery are usually caused by compression from positioning.
- Neuropathies of the musculocutaneous nerve affect elbow flexion and cause numbness in the lateral aspect of the forearm.
- Other perioperative lesions include nerve damage during orthopedic surgery or medial sternotomy which usually affects the lower trunk of the plexus.
- In compressive neuropathies, one should also look for a possible predisposing cause.
- Most, but not all, musculocutaneous nerve compressions are neuropraxic and usually have a favorable prognosis. The treatment is conservative.

REFERENCES

1. Fisher M. Other mononeuropathies of the upper extremity. In: Brown WF, Bolton CF, eds. *Clinical Electromyography*. 2nd ed. Stoneham, MA: Butterworth-Heinemann; 1993:271–304.
2. Dundore DE, DeLisa JA. Musculocutaneous nerve palsy: an isolated complication of surgery. *Arch Phys Med Rehabil.* 1979;60(3):130–133.
3. Sander HW, Quinto CM, Elinzano H, Chokroverty S. Carpet carrier's palsy: musculocutaneous neuropathy. *Neurology.* 1997; 48(6):1731–1732.
4. Braddom RL, Wolfe C. Musculocutaneous nerve injury after heavy exercise. *Arch Phys Med Rehabil.* 1978;59(6):290–293.
5. Mastaglia FL. Musculocutaneous neuropathy after strenuous physical activity. *Med J Aust.* 1986;145(3–4):153–154.
6. Simonetti S. Musculocutaneous nerve lesion after strenuous physical activity. *Muscle Nerve.* 1999;22(5):647–649.
7. Juel VC, Kiely JM, Leone KV, et al. Isolated musculocutaneous neuropathy caused by a proximal humeral exostosis. *Neurology.* 2000;54(2):494–496.
8. Bassett III FH, Nunley JA. Compression of the musculocutaneous nerve at the elbow. *J Bone Joint Surg Am.* 1982;64(7): 1050–1052.
9. Kim SM, Goodrich JA. Isolated proximal musculocutaneous nerve palsy: case report. *Arch Phys Med Rehabil.* 1984;65(11): 735–736.
10. Stewart J. Nerves arising from the brachial plexus. In: Stewart J, ed. *Focal Peripheral Neuropathies*. 3rd ed. Philadelphia, PA: Lippincott Williams & Wilkins; 2000.
11. Kuhlman KA, Batley RJ. Bilateral musculocutaneous nerve palsy: a case report. *Am J Phys Med Rehabil.* 1996;75(3):227–231.
12. Lincoln JR, Sawyer HP Jr. Complications related to body positions during surgical procedures. *Anesthesiology.* 1961;22:800–809.
13. Cheney FW, Domino KB, Caplan RA, Posner KL. Nerve injury associated with anesthesia: a closed claims analysis. *Anesthesiology.* 1999;90(4):1062–1069.
14. Clausen EG. Postoperative anesthetic paralysis of the brachial plexus: a review of the literature and report on nine cases. *Surgery.* 1942;12:933–942.
15. Cooper DE, Jenkins RS, Bready L, Rockwood CA Jr. The prevention of injuries of the brachial plexus secondary to malposition of the patient during surgery. *Clin Orthop.* 1988; 228:33–41.
16. Graham JG, Pye IF, McQueen IN. Brachial plexus injury after median sternotomy. *J Neurol Neurosurg Psychiatry.* 1981;44(7): 621–625.

17. Hanson MR, Breuer AC, Furlan AJ, et al. Mechanism and frequency of brachial plexus injury in open-heart surgery: a prospective analysis. *Ann Thorac Surg*. 1983;36(6):675–679.
18. Jackson L, Keats AS. Mechanism of brachial plexus palsy following anesthesia. *Anesthesiology*. 1965;26:190–194.
19. Pareyson D, Solari A, Taroni F, et al. Detection of hereditary neuropathy with liability to pressure palsies among patients with acute painless mononeuropathy or plexopathy. *Muscle Nerve*. 1998;21:1686–1691.

11 CASE

A Woman With Acute Onset of Shoulder Pain and Weakness

A 35-year-old woman presented with a 3-week history of right shoulder pain with numbness in the forearm and difficulty raising her arm. She had an upper respiratory infection 2 weeks before presentation.

Past medical history was unremarkable. She drank alcohol occasionally but did not smoke. She denied using illegal drugs.

Examination revealed winging of the right scapula toward the middle when the arm was extended forward, indicating weakness of the serratus (Fig. 11-1) rather than the trapezius muscle. (Fig. 11-2 demonstrates another patient who had spinal accessory neuropathy and trapezius weakness.) There was mild weakness of the right deltoid and only flexion of the distal phalanx of the first two fingers of the right hand. Also, the patient had difficulty opposing the thumb to the fifth digit. She had patchy decreased pain sensation in the shoulder. Reflexes were 2+ throughout, except for the right biceps and brachioradialis reflexes which were 1+. The rest of the examination was normal.

WHAT IS THE CLINICAL DIAGNOSIS?

The arm pain with weakness in muscles innervated by the upper trunk of the brachial plexus and C5–C6 roots suggested a radiculopathy or an upper trunk brachial plexopathy. She, however, also had weakness in muscles not innervated by the C5–C6 roots and the upper trunk of the brachial plexus. The lack of neck pain is somewhat against the diagnosis of radiculopathy.

The acute presentation with pain and weakness of muscles involved by several nerves, preceded by a recent viral infection, is in favor of this being an acute brachial neuritis (BN).

Other possibilities to consider include a hematoma or a tumor in the upper plexus or roots, but as discussed earlier, she also had weakness of the flexors of the fingers, particularly the thumb and index finger, which are not innervated by the C5–C6 roots or the upper trunk. These muscles, the flexor digitorum profundus and flexor pollicis longus, are innervated by the median nerve, particularly through its anterior interosseous branch, from axons coming off the C7 and C8 roots and middle and lower trunks of the plexus.

AN EMG TEST WAS PERFORMED

Motor Nerve Studies

Nerve and Site	Latency (ms)	Amplitude (mV)	Conduction Velocity (m/s)
Median Nerve R.	**Normal ≤ 4.2**	**Normal ≥ 6**	**Normal ≥ 50**
Wrist	3.8	16	–
Elbow	7.8	16	56
Ulnar Nerve R.	**Normal ≤ 3.6**	**Normal ≥ 8**	**Normal ≥ 50**
Wrist	3.3	12	–
Below elbow	6.8	12	60
Above elbow	8.9	12	60

Side-to-Side Comparison[a]

Nerve and Site	Latency (ms)	Amplitude (mV)	Conduction Velocity (m/s)
Axillary nerve R.	6.2	1	–
Axillary nerve L.	2.9	5	–

[a]2 ms difference in latencies is significant.

F-Wave Studies

Nerve	Latency (ms)	Normal Latency ≤ (ms)
Median nerve R.	26.8	30
Ulnar nerve R.	26.4	30

Sensory Nerve Studies

Nerve	Onset Latency (ms)	Normal Onset Latency ≤ (ms)	Peak Latency (ms)	Normal Peak Latency ≤ (ms)	Amp (μV)	Normal Amp ≥ (μV)	Conduction Velocity (m/s)	Normal Conduction Velocity ≥ (m/s)
Median nerve R.	2.1	2.6	2.6	3.1	25	20	62	50
Ulnar nerve R.	1.9	2.6	2.4	3.1	20	13	63	50
Lat. cut. nerve R.	1.8	b	2.3	2.6	**11**	12	b	b
Lat. cut. nerve L.	1.6	b	2.2	2.6	19	12	b	b

[b]Normal data not available.

EMG Data

Muscle	Insrt Activity	Fibs	Pos Waves	Fasc	Amp	Dur	Poly	Pattern
Cervical paraspinals R.	**Inc**	**1+**	**1+**	None	Norm	Norm	None	Full
Supraspinatus R.	**Inc**	**1+**	**1+**	None	Norm	Norm	None	Full
Infraspinatus R.	**Inc**	None	None	None	Norm	Norm	None	Full
Serratus anterior R.	**Inc**	**1+**	**1+**	None	Norm	Norm	None	Full
Deltoid R.	**Inc**	**2+**	**2+**	None	**Lg**	**Inc**	**Few**	**Red**
Biceps brachii R.	Norm	None	None	None	Norm	Norm	None	Full
Triceps R.	Norm	None	None	None	Norm	Norm	None	Full
Flexor carpi radialis R.	Norm	None	None	None	Norm	Norm	None	Full
Flexor dig. profundus R.	**Inc**	**1+**	**1+**	None	Norm	Norm	None	Full
Flexor carpi ulnaris R.	Norm	None	None	None	Norm	Norm	None	Full
Pronator quadratus R.	**Inc**	**2+**	**2+**	None	**Lg**	**Inc**	**Few**	**Red**
Flexor pollicis longus R.	**Inc**	**2+**	**2+**	None	**Lg**	**Inc**	**Few**	**Red**
First dorsal interosseous R.	Norm	None	None	None	Norm	Norm	None	Full

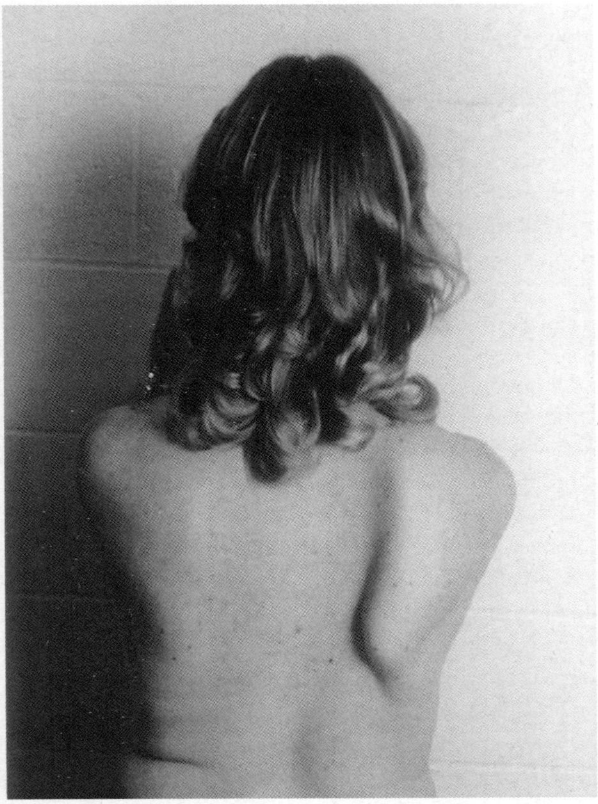

FIG. 11-1 Patient shows medial and posterior deviation of the angle of the scapula characteristic of serratus weakness.

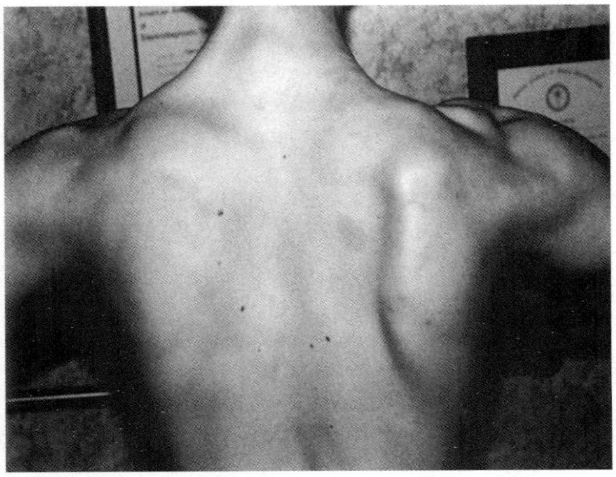

FIG. 11-2 Another patient with scapular winging secondary to spinal accessory neuropathy, showing lateral deviation of the right scapula when raising the arm from trapezius weakness. Notice atrophy of the trapezius.

WHAT WERE THE EMG FINDINGS?

The test showed normal median and ulnar motor nerve conduction velocities, CMAP amplitudes, and distal latencies. The axillary nerve CMAP latency was prolonged on the left side and had low amplitude, indicating damage to that nerve with demyelination and axonal degeneration. The F-responses of the median and ulnar nerves were normal. Sensory-evoked responses in the hand were normal, but the SNAP of the lateral antebrachial cutaneous nerve on the left had a low amplitude compared with the right. These findings are more supportive of a peripheral nerve or plexus lesion. The normal median and ulnar SNAPs indicate that the sensory fibers of these nerves were not affected.

The needle test showed denervation potentials in some, but not all, muscles innervated by the upper trunk of the brachial plexus; rather, the pattern of denervation seemed to follow the territories of individual nerves such as the long thoracic, the suprascapular, axillary, and, in particular, the anterior interosseous. There was denervation in some muscles innervated by the same nerve roots or plexus territories, but not in others. For example, there was denervation in the deltoid and supraspinatus, from the upper trunk (C5–C6 roots) but not in the musculocutaneous; there was also denervation from the upper trunk (C5–C6), the pronator quadratus (C8, T1) but not the first dorsal interosseous (C8, T1). There was denervation in the flexor digitorum profundus and particularly the flexor pollicis longus innervated by the anterior interosseous nerve from the middle trunk and C7 root, but not other C7, middle trunk, and median nerve-innervated muscles. The paraspinal muscles also showed mild denervation, and there were denervation potentials in the serratus that comes directly from the C6 to C7 roots to the long thoracic nerve and not from the plexus, indicating a patchy individual nerve and root involvement, with axonal degeneration.

The lower amplitude of the right lateral antebrachial cutaneous nerve SNAP when compared with the other side, as well as the prolonged axillary nerve motor latency, also suggested a more peripheral lesion. Because a radiculopathy rarely affects the posterior root ganglia, thereby causing abnormal SNAPs, a cervical spine lesion could not be completely ruled out, particularly as there was cervical paraspinal denervation. Thus the process most likely involved roots and individual nerves.

WHAT OTHER TESTS SHOULD BE DONE?

An MRI of the neck was normal. An MRI or magnetic resonance neurography, useful in studying the brachial plexus,[1] was not done.

It was concluded that the acute onset of shoulder pain and weakness, as well as the EMG abnormalities, indicated an acute BN.

TREATMENT

The patient was treated with 30 mg of prednisone; her pain disappeared after 1 month, and she improved clinically. At the 6-month follow-up, she had marked improvement with only mild winging of the scapulae.

DISCUSSION

This patient presented with an acute onset of pain and weakness in the right shoulder. She was diagnosed as having acute BN, or Parsonage–Turner syndrome.[2] Other names of this condition include brachial plexitis, neuralgic amyotrophy, and paralytic BN.[3,4]

BN is believed to be an autoimmune disorder usually preceded by a generalized viral infection or an upper respiratory infection,[2] and in 45% of the cases, BN has a preceding event such as an infection, vaccination, or a surgical procedure. It also occurs after botulinum toxin injections for dystonia and in HIV-infected patients.[4] BN, usually unilateral, is bilateral in 34% of the cases.[5,6]

The characteristic clinical presentation consists of the acute onset of sharp pain in the shoulder, which is followed after weeks by a duller pain.[4] There is weakness and sometimes atrophy of the shoulder muscles, and also in muscles innervated by the anterior interosseous, axillary, suprascapular, and thoracic nerves, and, rarely, the phrenic nerve.[7] A prominent involvement of the anterior interosseous nerve, in some cases, could suggest an entrapment of this nerve, but the shoulder pain and weakness are usually indicative of BN.[8] Rarely, patients also develop vocal cord paralysis[9] or weakness of muscles of other cranial nerves.[3,10]

Routine motor nerve conduction studies may be normal, but proximal nerve stimulation could reveal low-amplitude responses in muscles innervated by an affected nerve with conduction block indicating a demyelination. There is also axonal degeneration, indicated by the presence of denervation potentials. The EMG findings demonstrate a pattern of mononeuropathy or plexopathy, or a combination of both, but more characteristically, there is a single or multiple mononeuropathy.[3,4,11–13] These could be caused by inflammation or nerve constrictions. Typically, there is no paraspinal denervation,[14] but this can occur,[15] as in this patient.

In BN the median nerve SNAPs of the thumb could be abnormal, whereas the SNAP recorded in the middle finger is usually normal in suspected BN. The lateral antebrachial cutaneous nerve should be tested, as it is frequently affected.[16]

MR neurography can be useful in the diagnosis.[1,17]

The prognosis of BN is usually benign and most patients improve within 1 month. Thirty-six percent improve during the first year, whereas 89% show improvement after the third year.[5]

Most cases of BN are believed to be autoimmune, but there is also recurrent familial brachial plexopathy in individuals with dysmorphic features associated with a genetic defect in chromosome 17q24–25.[18] Patients with hereditary neuropathy with liability to pressure palsy, caused by defects in chromosome 17p112–12, could also develop a brachial neuropathy similar to BN[19] without dysmorphic features and without pain.

Although there is no demonstrated therapy for BN, corticosteroids appear to be helpful, and improvement has been reported even in later cases[20] and some patients respond to immunoglobulin infusions.[4]

SUMMARY

This young woman presented with an acute onset of shoulder pain and weakness.

The EMG studies showed normal conduction velocities, but low-amplitude axillary nerve CMAP and low-amplitude lateral antebrachial cutaneous nerve SNAP. This indicated that the pathology was distal to the root, but the presence of paraspinal denervation suggested that widespread involvement was included in the roots and various nerves. The patient was diagnosed as having acute BN, or neuralgic amyotrophy. She was treated with steroids and recovered satisfactorily.

IMPORTANT POINTS

- Neuralgic amyotrophy, or acute BN, is a focal autoimmune disorder affecting predominantly the upper trunk of the brachial plexus or individual nerves such as the axillary, long thoracic, suprascapular, and anterior interossei. A familial recurrent brachial neuropathy is associated with a defect in chromosome 17q24–25, and neuralgic amyotrophy can also occur in patients with the familial neuropathy having liability to pressure palsy.
- Patients with BN present with acute pain and weakness in the shoulder with winging of the scapulae.
- The anterior interosseous-innervated muscles are frequently involved in BN; the median-innervated muscles of the hand and forearm are usually spared.
- Abnormalities of SNAPs of the lateral antebrachial cutaneous nerve or of the median SNAP of the thumb, but not of other

fingers, help localize the lesion to the plexus rather than the roots, although evidence of mild root involvement may be seen.

- BN usually has a benign prognosis; immunotherapy may be helpful.

REFERENCES

1. Zhou L, Yousem DM, Chaudhry V. Role of magnetic resonance neurography in brachial plexus lesions. *Muscle Nerve*. 2004;30(3): 305–309.
2. Parsonage MJ, Turner AJW. Neuralgic amyotrophy: the shoulder-girdle syndrome. *Lancet*. 1948;1:973–978.
3. Wilbourn AJ. Brachial plexus disorders. In: Dyck PJ, Thomas PK, eds. *Peripheral Neuropathy*. 3rd ed. Philadelphia, PA: WB Saunders; 1993:911–950.
4. Dumitru D, Zwarts MJ. Brachial plexopathies and proximal mononeuropathies. In: Dumitru D, Amato AA, Zwarts MJ, eds. *Electrodiagnostic Medicine*. 2nd ed. Philadelphia, PA: Hanley & Belfus; 2002:777–836.
5. Tsairis P, Dyck PJ, Mulder DW. Natural history of brachial plexus neuropathy: report on 99 cases. *Arch Neurol*. 1972;27:109–117.
6. Tsairis P. Brachial plexus neuropathies. In: Dyck PJ, Thomas PK, Lambert EH, eds. *Peripheral Neuropathy*. Philadelphia, PA: WB Saunders; 1975:659–681.
7. Mulvey DA, Aquilina RJ, Elliott MW, et al. Diaphragmatic dysfunction in neuralgic amyotrophy: an electrophysiologic evaluation of 16 patients presenting with dyspnea. *Am Rev Respir Dis*. 1993;147:66–71.
8. Rennels GD, Ochoa J. Neuralgic amyotrophy manifesting as anterior interosseous nerve palsy. *Muscle Nerve*. 1980;3:160–164.
9. Sanders EA, Van den Neste VM, Hoogenraad TU. Brachial plexus neuritis and recurrent laryngeal nerve palsy. *J Neurol*. 1988;235:323.
10. England JD. The variations of neuralgic amyotrophy. *Muscle Nerve*. 1999;22:435–436.
11. Ferrante MA, Wilbourn AJ. Electrodiagnostic approach to the patient with suspected brachial plexopathy. *Neurol Clin*. 2002;20: 423–450.
12. James JL, Miles DW. Neuralgic amyotrophy: a clinical and electromyographic study. *Br Med J*. 1966;2:1042–1043.
13. Ferrante MA. Brachial plexopathies: classification, causes, and consequences. *Muscle Nerve*. 2004;30:547–568.
14. Sumner A. Parsonage-Turner revisited. *J Clin Neuro Musc Dis*. 2007;8(4):237–239.
15. Marra TR. The clinical and electrodiagnostic features of idiopathic lumbosacral and brachial plexus neuropathy: a review of 20 cases. *Electromyogr Clin Neurophysiol*. 1987;27(5):305–315.
16. Watson BV, Nicolle MW, Brown JD. Conduction block in neuralgic amyotrophy. *Muscle Nerve*. 2001;24:559–563.
17. Sarikaya S, Sumer M, Ozdolap S, Erdem CZ. Magnetic resonance neurography diagnosed brachial plexitis: a case report. *Arch Phys Med Rehabil*. 2005;86(5):1058–1059.
18. Van Alfen N, Van Engelen BG, Reinders JW, et al. The natural history of hereditary neuralgic amyotrophy in the Dutch population: two distinct types? *Brain*. 2000;123:718–723.
19. Pareyson D, Solari A, Taroni F, et al. Detection of hereditary neuropathy with liability to pressure palsies among patients with acute painless mononeuropathy or plexopathy. *Muscle Nerve*. 1998;21:1686–1691.
20. Butt MA. Successful management of Parsonage-Turner syndrome with steroids in the post-acute weakness phase: a case report. *EMJ Neurol*. 2021;9(1):81–87. https://doi.org/10.33590/emjneurol/21-00068.

12 CASE

A Man With Lymphoma and Numbness in the Fingers of One Hand

A 52-year-old man with a history of non-Hodgkin's lymphoma presented with pain of 1-month duration in the left chest that radiated to the arm with intermittent numbness in the left two fingers.

He drank approximately six beers per week and smoked one pack of cigarettes per day. Past medical history was unremarkable.

Neurologic examination revealed normal mentation and cranial nerves, except for slight droopiness of the left eyelid, and the left pupil was smaller than the right (Fig. 12-1). Both pupils were reactive to light and accommodation. There was decreased sweat in the left hemiface. Extraocular movements and other cranial nerves were normal. He had weakness of the interossei muscles in the left hand and mild weakness of the thenar and finger extensor muscles of the left. There was also left interossei atrophy. No fasciculations were detected. Reflexes were equal in the arms and legs at about 1 to 2+. There were no Babinski signs. There was mildly decreased vibration sense in the toes, decreased pain sensation and two-point discrimination in the last two fingers and dorsum of the left hand, and some questionable decreased pain sensation in the inner forearm. Adson's maneuver was negative. Coordination was normal.

WHAT IS THE DIFFERENTIAL DIAGNOSIS?

This patient's symptoms and clinical findings indicate a mild polyneuropathy and a focal disorder involving muscles innervated by C8 and T1 roots through the ulnar, median, and also apparently the radial nerves on the left.

The sensory findings are also suggestive of a C8 and T1 radiculopathy or a lesion in the medial cord or lower trunk of the brachial plexus. The eye findings indicate Horner syndrome, characterized by ptosis, myosis, and anhidrosis[1–3] from the involvement of the sympathetic ganglia or the T1 root. The sympathetic fibers that dilate the pupils originate in the hypothalamus, extend to the spinal cord, and then exit to the sympathetic ganglia. Thereafter, they run in the wall of the carotid artery and go through the cavernous sinus and the superior orbital fissure (Fig. 12-2). The parasympathetic fibers that direct the constriction of the pupil travel via the third cranial nerve.

AN EMG TEST WAS PERFORMED

Motor Nerve Studies

Nerve and Site	Latency(ms)	Amplitude (mV)	Conduction Velocity (m/s)
Median Nerve L.	**Normal ≤ 4.2**	**Normal ≥ 6**	**Normal ≥ 50**
Wrist	3.7	10	–
Elbow	8.3	10	53
Ulnar Nerve L.	**Normal ≤ 3.6**	**Normal ≥ 8**	**Normal ≥ 50**
Wrist	2.9	9	–
Below elbow	7.7	8	51
Above elbow	9.7	8	60
Axilla	13.2	8	52
Erb's point	17.6	**7**	**42**

Nerve and Site	Latency (ms)	Amplitude (mV)	Conduction Velocity (m/s)
Ulnar Nerve R.	**Normal ≤ 3.6**	**Normal ≥ 8**	**Normal ≥ 50**
Wrist	2.8	10	52
Below elbow	7.6	10	52
Above elbow	9.6	10	59
Axilla	13.0	10	53
Erb's point	15.0	9	60

F-Wave Studies

Nerve	Latency (ms)	Normal Latency ≤ (ms)
Median nerve L.	29.8	30
Ulnar nerve L.	**32.0**	30
Ulnar nerve R.	28.8	30

Sensory Nerve Studies

Nerve	Onset Latency (ms)	Normal Onset Latency ≤ (ms)	Peak Latency (ms)	Normal Peak Latency ≤ (ms)	Amp (μV)	Normal Amp ≥ (μm)	Conduction Velocity (m/s)	Normal Conduction Velocity ≥ (m/s)
Median nerve L.	2.5	2.6	3.0	3.1	40	20	52	50
Ulnar nerve fifth digit L.	2.3	2.6	2.8	3.1	**8**	13	52	50
Dorsal ulnar cutaneous L.	1.7	1.8	2.2	2.3	**4**	12	59	50
Medial ante. cutaneous L.	[a]	[a]	**2.8**	2.6	**6**	12	[a]	[a]

Sensory Nerve Studies—cont'd

Nerve	Onset Latency (ms)	Normal Onset Latency ≤ (ms)	Peak Latency (ms)	Normal Peak Latency ≤ (ms)	Amp (μV)	Normal Amp ≥ (μm)	Conduction Velocity (m/s)	Normal Conduction Velocity ≥ (m/s)
Ulnar nerve fifth digit R.	2.4	2.6	2.9	3.1	18	13	50	50
Dorsal ulnar cutaneous R.	1.7	1.8	2.2	2.3	15	12	59	50
Medial ante. cutaneous R.	[a]	[a]	2.2	2.6	14	12	[a]	[a]

[a]Normal data not available.

EMG Data

Muscle	Insrt Activity	Fibs	Pos waves	Fasc	Amp	Dur	Poly	Pattern
Cervical paraspinals L.	Norm	None	None	None	Norm	Norm	None	Full
Supraspinatus L.	Norm	None	None	None	Norm	Norm	None	Full
Deltoid L.	Norm	None	None	None	Norm	Norm	None	Full
Biceps brachii L.	Norm	None	None	None	Norm	Norm	None	Full
Brachioradialis L.	Norm	None	None	None	Norm	Norm	None	Full
Triceps L.	Norm	None	None	None	Norm	Norm	None	Full
Extensor digitorum communis L.	**Inc**	**2+**	**2+**	None	Norm	Norm	None	**Red**
Extensor indicis proprius L.	**Inc**	**2+**	**2+**	None	Norm	Norm	None	**Red**
Flexor carpi radialis L.	Norm	None	None	None	Norm	Norm	None	Full
Pronator teres	Norm	None	None	None	Norm	Norm	None	Full
Flexor carpi ulnaris L.	**Inc**	**2+**	**2+**	None	Norm	Norm	None	Full
First dorsal interosseous L.	**Inc**	**2+**	**2+**	None	Norm	Norm	None	**Red**
Abductor pollicis brevis L.	**Inc**	**2+**	**2+**	None	**Inc**	**Inc**	None	**Red**

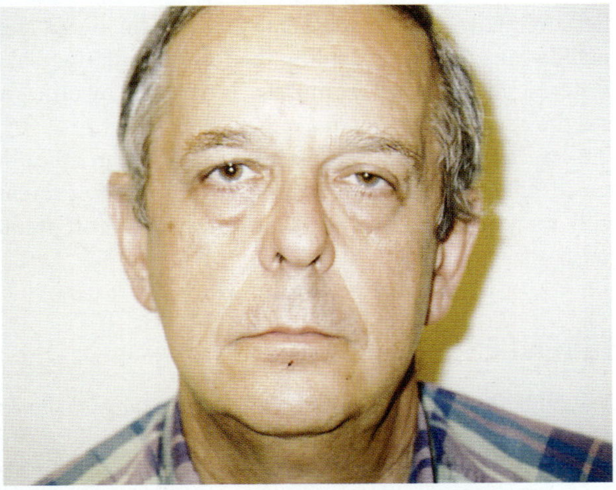

FIG. 12-1 Notice the patient's ptosis on the left with smaller pupil.

WHAT WERE THE EMG FINDINGS?

The nerve conduction tests showed that the SNAPs were normal on the right and left median nerves. The ulnar nerve, the dorsal cutaneous, and the medial anterior cutaneous nerve of the forearm had low-amplitude SNAPs; the ulnar nerve had a mild drop in CMAP amplitude and slower conduction velocity across the Erb's point.

There were denervation potentials in the median-, ulnar-, and some radial-innervated muscles, indicating a lesion of the

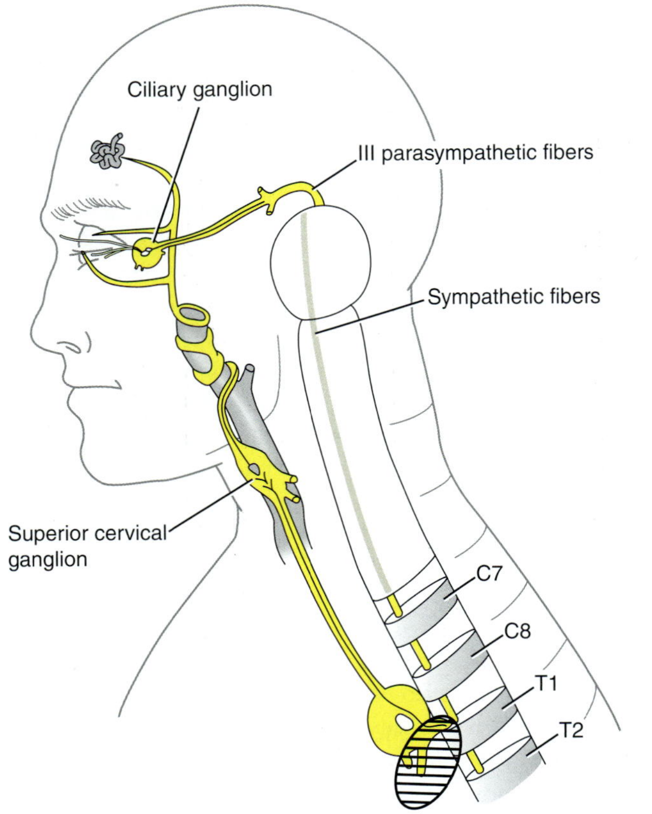

FIG. 12-2 Diagram of sympathetic innervation of the eye and the site of the lesion in Case 12.

lower trunk and/or C8 root. Some muscles innervated by the posterior cord but not the lower trunk were normal.

The denervation of the C8 and T1 lower trunk muscles suggests a lesion in these structures. This was unlikely at the cord level, because the test showed denervation in muscles innervated by the posterior cord and lower trunk (extensor digitorum communis and extensor indicis proprius), but not in the medial cord; and there was no denervation in other muscles from the posterior cord, innervated by other roots, trunks, or nerves (brachioradialis: radial, upper trunk, C5–C6; deltoid: axillary, C5–C6; also upper trunk). Similarly, the flexor carpi radialis and pronator teres, which come primarily from the middle trunk, and the medial and lateral cords were not denervated. The lack of paraspinal denervation is against, but does not rule out, a radiculopathy, particularly because the sympathetic involvement suggested that the T1 root or sympathetic ganglion was affected.

The abnormal ulnar, dorsal cutaneous, and medial cutaneous nerve SNAPs and the drop in ulnar CMAP amplitude across Erb's point indicate that the lesion involved the lower trunk of the brachial plexus.

An MRI of the chest and supraclavicular area demonstrated a mass, which was biopsied and found to be a recurrent lymphoma. The patient received radiation and chemotherapy with the improvement of neurologic symptoms after 6 months.

In conclusion, this patient had a malignant lymphoma that invaded the lower trunk of the brachial plexus but also the T1 root fibers affecting sympathetic axons, causing Horner syndrome.

DISCUSSION

This case presented with hand muscle weakness and Horner syndrome. This syndrome is caused by lesions of the sympathetic fibers going through the T1 root or the sympathetic ganglia, causing myosis, ptosis, and anhidrosis.

The differential diagnosis of this presentation includes a tumor in the apex of the lung, presenting as Pancoast syndrome.[3,4] This could also be caused by other tumors like lymphomas or neurofibromas.[3,5,6] The Pancoast syndrome characteristically produces a Horner syndrome and sensory deficits with weakness of muscles innervated by the lower trunk of the brachial plexus. The tumor can also expand to the epidural space producing a myelopathy. The abnormalities in this patient were caused by a mass from his lymphoma.

Lower trunk lesions also manifest as the so-called thoracic-outlet syndrome, affecting axons and/or vascular structures. When this presents with neurologic deficits, it is called a *neurologic thoracic-outlet syndrome*.[6–9] The *vascular thoracic-outlet syndrome* manifests with brachial arterial insufficiency[10–12] or affects the subclavian vein, producing swelling of the arm.[3,6] This syndrome can also be mixed.

There are also patients who have what is called "disputed thoracic-outlet syndrome" or "nonspecific thoracic-outlet syndrome."[13,14] These do not have clear vascular or neurologic symptoms, but only chronic aches and hypoesthesia in the shoulder and arms, and have nondiagnostic electrophysiologic findings.

Common causes of thoracic-outlet syndrome include fibroid bands, cervical ribs, a hypertrophic transverse process of the C7 vertebrae, tumors, and hypertrophied subclavius muscle.[6,7]

SUMMARY

This patient had a lymphoma and developed symptoms and findings that localize to the lower trunk of the brachial plexus and sympathetic fibers, likely affecting the sympathetic ganglia or the T1 root. These were caused by a recurrent tumor.

IMPORTANT POINTS

- Tumor invasions of the lower trunk and T1 roots produce hand wasting and Horner syndrome.
- The thoracic-outlet syndrome is characterized by neurogenic symptoms causing numbness and weakness, or arterial insufficiency or swelling in the arm from venous obstruction. The syndrome can also be mixed.
- The term *nonspecific thoracic-outlet syndrome* refers to patients who have nonspecific pain and nondiagnostic electrophysiological tests.
- The diagnostic workup for patients with suspected lower trunk or C8–T1 radiculopathy includes measuring SNAPs of ulnar nerves and the medial cutaneous nerve of the forearm, comparing the results with those of the opposite side. The median nerve SNAP to the thumb and index finger should be normal. Motor conduction studies should include ulnar nerve recording with stimulation at the Erb's point and measurement of its F-wave latency. Needle EMG should include muscles innervated by the lower trunk, medial and posterior cords, as well as muscles innervated by other roots and the cervical paraspinals.
- The Pancoast syndrome is usually caused by an apical lung tumor affecting the lower trunk and T1 roots, presenting with weakness and Horner syndrome. The most frequent cause is a carcinoma.

REFERENCES

1. Walsh FB, Hoyt WT, Miller NR, eds. *Clinical Neurophthalmology*. 4th ed. Baltimore, MD: Williams & Wilkins; 1982.
2. Wilkins RH, Brody IA. Horner's syndrome. *Arch Neurol*. 1968; 19(5):540–542.
3. Wilbourn A. Brachial plexopathies. In: Brown WF, Bolton F, Aminoff MJ, eds. *Neuromuscular Function and Disease*. Philadelphia, PA: WB Saunders; 2002:831–851.
4. Lederman RJ, Wilbourn AJ. Brachial plexopathy: recurrent cancer or radiation. *Neurology*. 1984;34:1331–1335.
5. Hepper NG, Herskovic T, Witten DM, et al. Thoracic inlet tumors. *Ann Intern Med*. 1966;64:979–989.
6. Stewart JD. Brachial plexus. In: Stewart JD, ed. *Focal Peripheral Neuropathies*. 3rd ed. Philadelphia, PA: Lippincott Williams & Wilkins; 2000:117–154.
7. Gilliatt RW, LeQuesne PM, Logue V, Sumner AJ. Wasting of the hand associated with a cervical rib or band. *J Neurol Neurosurg Psychiatry*. 1970;33:615–624.

8. Ranney D. Thoracic outlet: an anatomical redefinition that makes clinical sense. *Clin Anat*. 1996;9:50–52.
9. Gilliatt RW, Willison RG, Dietz V, Williams IR. Peripheral nerve conduction in patients with a cervical rib and band. *Ann Neurol*. 1978;4:124–129.
10. Cormier JM, Amrane M, Ward A, et al. Arterial complications of the thoracic outlet syndrome: fifty-five operative cases. *J Vasc Surg*. 1989;9:778–787.
11. Hood DB, Kuehne J, Yellin AE, Weaver FA. Vascular complications of thoracic outlet syndrome. *Am Surg*. 1997;63:913–917.
12. Sanders RJ, Haug C. Review of arterial thoracic outlet syndrome with a report of five new instances. *Surg Gynecol Obstet*. 1991;173: 415–425.
13. Wilbourn AJ. Thoracic outlet syndrome is overdiagnosed. *Muscle Nerve*. 1999;22:130–136.
14. Dawson DH, Hallett M, Wilbourn AJ, et al. *Entrapment Neuropathies*. 3rd ed. Philadelphia, PA: Lippincott-Raven; 1999. 3rd ed.

13 CASE

A Woman With Arm Weakness After Treatment for Breast Cancer

A 68-year-old woman with left breast cancer presented with some discomfort in the left shoulder and weakness with difficulty raising the arm for 6 months after she had been treated with chemotherapy and radiation.

Examination revealed weakness in the left deltoid 3/5, spinati 4/5, biceps 4+/5, and brachioradialis 4/5; other muscles of the arms and legs were normal. Sensory examination showed a patchy sensory deficit in the lateral forearm. Reflexes were 2+, except for the left biceps and brachioradialis where they were absent. The rest of the neurologic examination was normal.

WHAT IS THE DIFFERENTIAL DIAGNOSIS?

This patient with a history of left breast cancer developed weakness in the left upper extremity, particularly in muscles innervated by the C5–C6 roots and the upper trunk of the brachial plexus. The differential diagnosis includes a radiculopathy, a plexopathy caused, for example, by a brachial neuritis, but the progressive course and previous history of cancer and radiation suggest that the etiology would be either neoplastic invasion or a postradiation plexopathy.

Neoplastic invasion of the plexus affects mainly the lower trunk, whereas radiation affects mainly the upper trunk. Although the patient had some discomfort, she had no severe pain, also favoring a diagnosis of radiation plexopathy because, in carcinomatous plexopathy, pain can be significant.

AN EMG TEST WAS PERFORMED

Motor Nerve Studies

Nerve and Site	Latency(ms)	Amplitude (mV)	Conduction Velocity (m/s)
Median Nerve L.	**Normal ≤ 4.2**	**Normal ≥ 6**	**Normal ≥ 50**
Wrist	3.9	8	–
Elbow	7.9	8	51

Motor Nerve Studies—cont'd

Nerve and Site	Latency (ms)	Amplitude (mV)	Conduction Velocity (m/s)
Ulnar Nerve L.	**Normal ≤ 3.6**	**Normal ≥ 8**	**Normal ≥ 50**
Wrist	3.2	9	–
Below elbow	6.8	8	53
Above elbow	9.5	8	50
Axilla	12.3	8	50
Erb's point	15.4	8	47
Ulnar Nerve R.	**Normal ≤ 3.6**	**Normal ≥ 8**	**Normal ≥ 50**
Wrist	2.8	16	–
Below elbow	5.9	16	58
Above elbow	7.8	16	63
Axilla	11.2	13	60
Erb's point	13.5	12	61
Musculocutaneous Nerve L.			
Erb's point	4.2	0.5[a]	–
Musculocutaneous Nerve R.			
Erb's point	3.8	8[a]	–

[a]Normal limit amplitude is 8 mV.

F-Wave Studies

Nerve	Latency (ms)	Normal Latency ≤ (ms)
Median nerve L.	29.2	30
Ulnar nerve L.	29.9	30
Ulnar nerve R.	28.6	30

Sensory Nerve Studies

Nerve	Onset Latency (ms)	Normal Onset Latency ≤ (ms)	Peak Latency (ms)	Normal Peak Latency ≤ (ms)	Amp (μV)	Normal Amp ≥ (μV)	Conduction Velocity (m/s)	Normal Conduction Velocity ≥ (m/s)
Median nerve L.	2.2	2.6	2.7	3.1	21	20	59	50
Ulnar nerve L.	2.4	2.6	2.9	3.1	18	13	50	50
Lat. ante. cut. L.	**NR**	–	**NR**	2.6	**NR**	12	**NR**	–
Ulnar nerve R.	2.2	2.6	2.6	3.1	17	13	55	50

EMG Data

Muscle	Insrt Activity	Fibs	Pos Waves	Fasc	Amp	Dur	Poly	Pattern
Paraspinal L.	Norm	None	None	None	Norm	Norm	None	Full
Infraspinatus L.	**Myokymia**	None	**1+**	None	Norm	Norm	**Few**	**Red**
Deltoid L.	**Myokymia**	None	None	None	Norm	Norm	**Few**	**Red**
Biceps brachii L.	**Inc**	None	**1+**	None	Norm	Norm	None	Full
Brachioradialis L.	**Inc**	**1+**	**1+**	None	Norm	Norm	None	Full
Extensor carpi radialis L.	Norm	None	None	None	Norm	Norm	None	Full
Flexor carpi radialis L.	Norm	None	None	None	Norm	Norm	None	Full
Flexor carpi ulnaris L.	Norm	None	None	None	Norm	Norm	None	Full
Pronator quadratus L.	Norm	None	None	None	Norm	Norm	None	Full
Triceps L.	Norm	None	None	None	Norm	Norm	None	Full
Abductor pollicis brevis L.	Norm	None	None	None	Norm	Norm	None	Full
First dorsal interosseous L.	Norm	None	None	None	Norm	Norm	None	Full

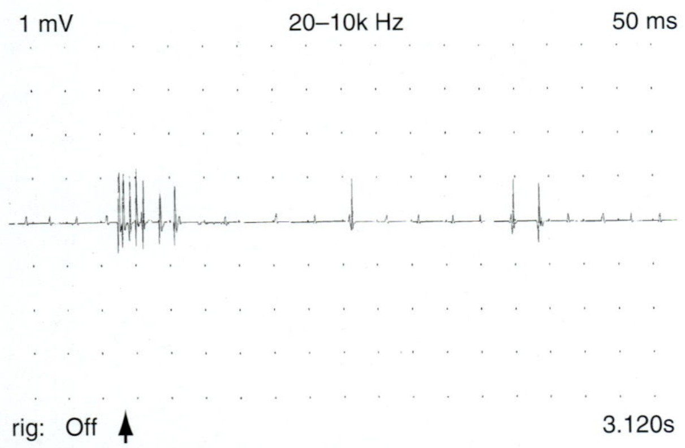

FIG. 13-1 Myokymic discharges in the left deltoid muscle (1 mV/50 ms).

WHAT DID THE EMG SHOW?

This test showed normal nerve conduction velocities, CMAP amplitudes and latencies, except for absent left lateral cutaneous SNAP and the left musculocutaneous nerve that had low-amplitude CMAP; F-responses were normal. The needle test showed evidence of denervation and myokymic discharges (Fig. 13-1) in muscles innervated by C5–C6 roots and the upper trunk of the brachial plexus, but not in muscles innervated by other roots or areas of the plexus, and not in the paraspinal muscles.

An MRI of the plexus area with and without contrast did not reveal a tumor invasion of the plexus. MRI of the neck was normal.

DISCUSSION

This patient with cancer treated by radiation presented with a brachial plexopathy of the upper trunk. The most likely diagnosis is radiation plexopathy.[1,2]

The time of onset, in this case, is characteristic, as her symptoms manifested months after treatment.[3] In this condition, the risk of developing a plexopathy is higher as radiation dosage increases.[4–6] The pathology includes fibrosis with secondary constriction of the vessel walls and ischemia to axons and Schwann cells.[5,6]

In a large study, 80% of the patients with recurrent tumors presented with pain, whereas only 19% of those with radiation plexopathy had pain. The lower trunk was involved in 72% of cases of tumors; those secondary to radiation involved the upper trunk in 78%.[1]

The best diagnostic tests to differentiate these conditions are electromyography and imaging with an MRI or CT.[7]

A clue in the diagnosis of radiation plexopathy is the presence of conduction block and myokymic discharges in the upper trunk muscles.[8–10] The SNAPs in the affected area of the hands could be decreased in amplitude without changes in latency or velocity.[11,12] These changes are characteristic but are not always present, and when in doubt, exploration might be necessary. The prognosis of radiation plexopathy is relatively benign, and the treatment is usually conservative, as in this case.[13] Omentoplasty could be helpful in refractory cases.[14]

SUMMARY

This patient with breast cancer treated with radiation developed a brachial plexopathy later, affecting the upper trunk. No tumor was found on MRI, and electrophysiologic findings were consistent with radiation plexopathy.

IMPORTANT POINTS

- Radiation plexopathy usually affects the upper trunk, whereas tumor invasion involves the lower trunk of the brachial plexus.
- Patients with tumor invasion usually have significant pain, whereas pain is not as frequent or severe in radiation plexopathy.
- Conduction block, myokymia, and fasciculations are seen more frequently in plexopathies caused by radiation therapy, whereas denervation potentials are seen more frequently in cases of tumor invasion.
- The prognosis of radiation plexopathy is relatively benign, but a tumor invasion should also be considered and ruled out.

REFERENCES

1. Stoll BA, Andrews JT. Radiation-induced peripheral neuropathy. *Br Med J*. 1966;1:834–837.
2. Ampil FL. Radiotherapy for carcinomatous brachial plexopathy: a clinical study of 23 cases. *Cancer*. 1985;56:2185–2188.
3. Dumitru D, Zwarts MJ. Brachial plexopathies and proximal mononeuropathies. In: Dumitru D, Amato AA, Zwarts MJ, eds. *Electrodiagnostic Medicine*. 2nd ed. Philadelphia, PA: Hanley & Belfus; 2002:777–836.
4. Match RM. Radiation-induced brachial plexus paralysis. *Arch Surg*. 1975;110:384–386.
5. Bagley FH, Walsh JW, Cady B, et al. Carcinomatous vs radiation-induced brachial plexus neuropathy in breast cancer. *Cancer*. 1978;41:2154–2157.
6. Greenfield MM, Stark FM. Post-irradiation neuropathy. *Am J Roentgenol*. 1948;60:617–622.
7. Kori SH, Foley KM, Posner JB. Brachial plexus lesions in patients with cancer: 100 cases. *Neurology*. 1981;31:45–50.
8. Allbers JW, Allen 2nd AA, Bastron JA, Daube JR. Limb myokymia. *Muscle Nerve*. 1981;4:494–504.
9. Harper CM Jr, Thomas JE, Cascino TL, Litchy WJ. Distinction between neoplastic and radiation-induced brachial plexopathy with emphasis on the role of EMG. *Neurology*. 1989;39:502–506.
10. Lederman RJ, Wilbourn AJ. Brachial plexopathy: recurrent cancer or radiation? *Neurology*. 1984;34:1331–1335.
11. Wilbourn AJ. Electrodiagnosis of plexopathies. *Neurol Clin*. 1985;3:511–529.
12. Levin KH, Lederman RJ, Wilbourn AJ. Spectrum of EMG changes in radiation brachial plexopathy. *Muscle Nerve*. 1987;10:656.
13. Schierle C, Winograd JM. Radiation-induced brachial plexopathy review: complication without a cure. *J Reconstr Microsurg*. 2004;20:149–152.
14. De Oliveira AJM, Castro JPS, Foroni LH, Siqueira MG, et al. Treatment of radiation-induced brachial plexopathy with omentoplasty. *Autops Case Rep*. 2020;10(3):e2020202. https://doi.org/10.4322/acr.2020.202. [Internet].

A Diabetic Man With Shoulder Pain and Weakness

A 42-year-old, type 2 diabetic man on oral antidiabetics developed a sudden onset of pain and weakness in the left shoulder. The pain worsened with movement. The patient states that he woke up with these symptoms and went to the ER where he had X-rays of the neck that were normal. He was treated with common analgesics and was referred to us by his internist after 3 weeks.

He stated that before the onset of symptoms he was carrying some boxes but he did not carry excessive weight.

Physical examination revealed normal mentation and cranial nerves. There was mild tenderness to palpation of the left shoulder over the scapular area. The shoulder joint was not tender. The patient also had weakness of external rotation and abduction, particularly in the initial 15 degrees of movement of the arm. The deltoid muscle and other arm muscles were normal. There was mild flattening of the infraspinatus muscle. Reflexes were equal and symmetric, except for trace at the ankles. There were no Babinski signs. There was decreased vibration sense at the toes and pinprick was normal. Upper extremity sensory examination was normal.

WHAT IS THE DIFFERENTIAL DIAGNOSIS?

The shoulder pain could suggest an orthopedic process, such as rotator cuff syndrome, but the pain on examination was not in the rotator area but in the scapulae. The weakness was out of proportion to the pain, making this diagnosis unlikely. The possibility of brachial neuritis needed to be considered, but the process seemed to involve only the spinati muscles. The sparing of deltoids, serratus, and other muscles in the arm argues against a diagnosis of radiculopathy or a plexopathy.

F-Wave and Tibial H-Reflex Studies

Nerve	Latency (ms)	Normal Latency ≤ (ms)
Median nerve L.	**31.5**	30
Ulnar nerve L.	**30.3**	30
Peroneal nerve L.	**54.8**	54
H-reflex L.	**NR**	34
H-reflex R.	**NR**	34

AN EMG TEST WAS PERFORMED

Motor Nerve Studies

Nerve and Site	Latency(ms)	Amplitude (mV)	Conduction Velocity (m/s)
Median Nerve L.	**Normal ≤ 4.2**	**Normal ≥ 6**	**Normal ≥ 50**
Wrist	3.8	11	–
Elbow	8.7	11	50
Ulnar Nerve L.	**Normal ≤ 3.6**	**Normal ≥ 8**	**Normal ≥ 50**
Wrist	3.0	17	–
Below elbow	7.5	15	51
Above elbow	9.5	15	52

Nerve and Site	Latency (ms)	Amplitude (mV)	Conduction Velocity (m/s)
Peroneal Nerve L.	**Normal ≤ 5.7**	**Normal ≥ 3**	**Normal ≥ 40**
Ankle	4.6	**2**	–
Fibular head	13.1	**1**	**38**
Knee	14.6	**1**	45
Suprascapular Nerve L.[a]			
Supraspinatus L.	**4.9**	**1**	–
Infraspinatus L.	**4.0**	**2**	–
Suprascapular Nerve R.[a]			
Supraspinatus R.	3.1	5	–
Infraspinatus R.	3.0	4	–

[a]Side-to-side comparison.

Sensory Nerve Studies

Nerve	Onset Latency (ms)	Normal Onset Latency ≤ (ms)	Peak Latency (ms)	Normal Peak Latency ≤ (ms)	Amp (μV)	Normal Amp ≥ (μV)	Conduction Velocity (m/s)	Normal Conduction Velocity ≥ (m/s)
Median nerve L.	2.5	2.6	3.0	3.1	20	20	52	50
Ulnar nerve L.	2.4	2.6	2.9	3.1	13	13	50	50
Sural nerve L.	**3.7**	3.5	**4.2**	4.0	**8**	11	**38**	40

EMG Data

Muscle	Insrt Activity	Fibs	Pos Waves	Fasc	Amp	Dur	Poly	Pattern
L. cervical paraspinals L.	Norm	None	None	None	Norm	Norm	None	Full
Supraspinatus L.	**Inc**	**3+**	**3+**	None	**Lg**	**Inc**	None	**Red**
Infraspinatus L.	**Inc**	**3+**	**3+**	None	**Lg**	**Inc**	None	**Red**
Deltoid L.	Norm	None	None	None	Norm	Norm	None	Full
Biceps brachii L.	Norm	None	None	None	Norm	Norm	None	Full
Flexor carpi radialis L.	Norm	None	None	None	Norm	Norm	None	Full
Flexor carpi ulnaris L.	Norm	None	None	None	Norm	Norm	None	Full
Extensor digitorum communis L.	Norm	None	None	None	Norm	Norm	None	Full
Tibialis anterior L.	**Inc**	**1+**	**1+**	None	**Lg**	**Inc**	None	**Red**
Gastrocnemius L.	**Inc**	**1+**	**1+**	None	**Lg**	**Inc**	None	**Red**

WHAT WERE THE EMG FINDINGS?

The nerve conduction velocities were normal, except for mildly low amplitude and slowing of sural nerve SNAP. H-reflexes were absent; there was slow conduction velocity and low-amplitude peroneal nerve CMAP; F-responses were mildly prolonged. All these are likely related to a diabetic neuropathy. Also, the CMAPs of the spinati muscles were of lower amplitude and prolonged latency when compared to the right.

Needle EMG showed mild denervation in the distal muscles of the legs compatible with a peripheral neuropathy. In the left arm, denervation was noted in the supra- and infraspinatus muscles but not in other C5–C6 muscles or the paraspinals; this localized the lesion to the suprascapular nerve.

WHAT OTHER TESTS SHOULD BE ORDERED?

An MRI of the shoulder was normal. The chemistry profile was normal, except for a blood sugar of 250 mg/dL (normal, <110 mg/dL) and glycosylated hemoglobin of 7% (normal, <6%). The sedimentation rate and the fluorescent antinuclear antibody test were normal.

WHAT IS THE TREATMENT?

The pain subsided after 3 weeks of conservative treatment.

WHAT IS THE MOST LIKELY DIAGNOSIS?

This patient had a suprascapular neuropathy with involvement of the supra- and infraspinatus muscles; this suggests a lesion at the suprascapular notch.[1,2] Another site of entrapment of this nerve is at the spinoglenoid notch involving only the infraspinatus muscle. It is possible that pulling boxes might have produced the lesion with stretching of the nerve. Since the patient improved with rest, we could not rule out a mononeuropathy caused by diabetes, or that diabetes made the nerve more sensitive to injury.

DISCUSSION

This patient had a lesion of the suprascapular nerve, which receives fibers from the C5 and C6 roots passing through the upper trunk of the brachial plexus. After crossing the posterior triangle of the neck, the nerve passes under the trapezius muscle and goes to the supraspinatus muscle through the suprascapular notch. After innervation to the supraspinatus, the inferior branch nerve curves around the spinoglenoid notch and then supplies the infraspinatus muscle (Fig. 14-1).[2]

Weakness of the supraspinatus and infraspinatus muscles impairs external rotation of the arm and its abduction, although this function could appear normal because the unaffected deltoid muscle also contributes to this movement.

The suprascapular nerve may be damaged by trauma to the shoulder with fractures of the scapulae, and from shoulder dislocation when it can be damaged alone or in combination with the axillary nerve.[3,4] The suprascapular nerve can also be affected in brachial neuropathy which is usually accompanied by dysfunction of other nerves.

Other causes include ganglion cysts, neuromas, a tight ligament at both the suprascapular and the spinoglenoid notches, bony spurs, masses, and calcifications.[5–11] A suprascapular neuropathy is also caused by a variety of activities such as baseball pitching.[12] This also occurs in wrestlers and weight lifters.[13,14]

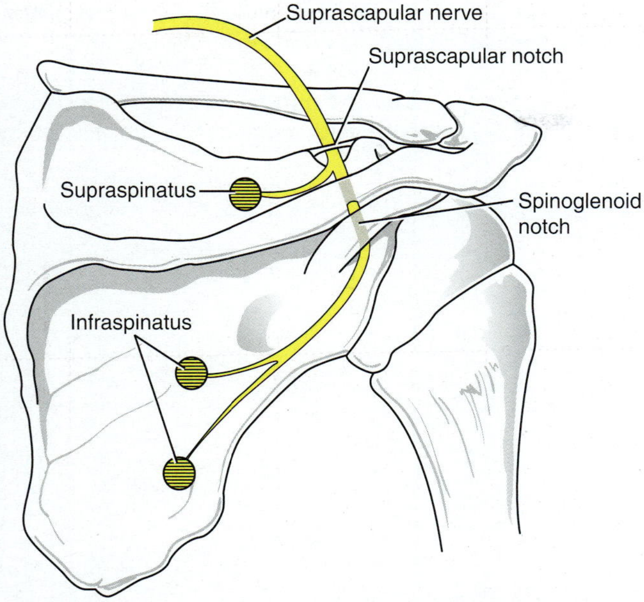

FIG. 14-1 Diagram of the suprascapular nerve and its branches.

Lesions affecting only the infraspinatus muscle are more frequently seen in volleyball players,[15–17] and 12.5% might have asymptomatic wasting and weakness on the dominant side.[18]

The clinical presentation of suprascapular neuropathy includes pain in the shoulder and atrophy with weakness of the supra- and infraspinatus. The weakness is evident on external rotation of the shoulder.

Electrophysiologic testing is a simple way to confirm the diagnosis, documenting low-amplitude and prolonged latencies of the CMAP of the supra- and infraspinatus muscles while stimulating at the Erb's point, and demonstrating denervation in these muscles but not in other shoulder girdle and paraspinal muscles. MRI might be helpful to determine whether there are abnormalities at the notches, as well as to demonstrate muscle wasting.[19–21]

Management includes resting, physical therapy, and injections of corticosteroids which might relieve the pain. Surgical decompression may be helpful in those with thick ligaments or if there is a tumor, which should be removed with careful dissection.[22]

SUMMARY

This diabetic man who presented with a history of pain in the shoulder had evidence of suprascapular nerve damage. The neuropathy was likely related to stretching from lifting boxes; however, the possibility that it was caused by diabetes should also be considered. He responded well to rest. He also had a diabetic polyneuropathy.

IMPORTANT POINTS

- Suprascapular neuropathy causes pain and weakness of the supraspinatus and/or the infraspinatus muscles. Depending on the level of the lesion, this could be at the suprascapular or spinoglenoid notch.
- The differential diagnosis includes C5–C6 radiculopathy, brachial plexopathy, and rotator cuff syndrome.
- The causes of suprascapular neuropathy may include compression, trauma, stretching, neuromas, ganglion cysts, and tumors.
- The treatment depends on the cause; entrapments may improve with rest, steroid injections, or decompression, depending on their severity.

REFERENCES

1. Lichtenberg S, Magosch P, Habermeyer P. Compression of the suprascapular nerve by a ganglion cyst of the spinoglenoid notch: the arthroscopic solution. *Knee Surg Sports Traumatol Arthrosc.* 2004;12:72–79.
2. Kim DH, Murovic JA, Tiel RL, et al. Management and outcomes of 42 surgical suprascapular nerve injuries and entrapments. *Neurosurgery.* 2005;57:120–127.
3. Stewart JD. Nerves arising from the brachial plexus. In: *Focal Peripheral Neuropathies.* Philadelphia, PA: Lippincott Williams & Wilkins; 2000:157–181. 3rd ed.
4. Solheim LF, Roaas A. Compression of the suprascapular nerve after fracture of the scapular notch. *Acta Orthop Scand.* 1978;49: 338–340.
5. Gelmers HJ, Buys DA. Suprascapular entrapment neuropathy. *Acta Neurochir (Vienna).* 1977;38:121–124.
6. Post M, Mayer J. Suprascapular nerve entrapment diagnosis and treatment. *Clin Orthop Relat Res.* 1987;225:126–136.
7. Kiss G, Komar J. Suprascapular nerve compression at the spinoglenoid notch. *Muscle Nerve.* 1990;13:556–557.
8. Callahan JD, Scully TB, Shapiro SA, Worth RM. Suprascapular nerve entrapment: a series of 27 cases. *J Neurosurg.* 1991;74: 893–896.
9. Antoniadis G, Richter HP, Rath S, et al. Suprascapular nerve entrapment: experience with 28 cases. *J Neurosurg.* 1996;85: 1020–1025.
10. Cohen SB, Dines DM, Moorman CT III. Familial calcification of the superior transverse scapular ligament causing neuropathy. *Clin Orthop Relat Res.* 1997;334:131–135.
11. Thompson RC, Schneider W, Kennedy T. Entrapment neuropathy of the inferior branch of the suprascapular nerve by ganglia. *Clin Orthop Relat Res.* 1983;166:185–187.
12. Ringel SP, Treihaft M, Carry M, et al. Suprascapular neuropathy in pitchers. *Am J Sports Med.* 1990;18:80–86.
13. Zeiss J, Woldenberg LS, Saddemi SR, Ebraheim NA. MRI of suprascapular neuropathy in a weight lifter. *J Comput Assist Tomogr.* 1993;17:303–308.
14. Bird SJ, Brown MJ. Acute focal neuropathy in male weight lifters. *Muscle Nerve.* 1996;19:897–899.
15. Ferretti A, Cerullo G, Russo G. Suprascapular neuropathy in volleyball players. *J Bone Joint Surg [Am].* 1987;69:260–263.
16. Montagna P, Colonna S. Suprascapular neuropathy restricted to the infraspinatus muscle in volleyball players. *Acta Neurol Scand.* 1993;87:248–250.
17. Tengan CH, Oliveira AS, Kiymoto BH, et al. Isolated and painless infraspinatus atrophy in top-level volleyball players: report of two cases and review of the literature. *Arq Neuropsiquiatr.* 1993;51:125–129.
18. Dramis A, Pimpalaevillar A. Suprascapular neuropathy in volleyball players. *Acta Orthop Belg.* 2005;71:269–272.

19. Inokuchi W, Ogawa K, Horiuchi Y. Magnetic resonance imaging of suprascapular nerve palsy. *J Shoulder Elbow Surg*. 1998;7: 223–227.
20. Bousquet JC, Denjean S, Faure C, et al. Synovial cyst involving isolated paralysis of the infraspinatus muscle: ultrasonographic diagnosis and MRI. *J Radiol*. 1996;77:275–277.
21. Yu JS, Fischer RA. Denervation atrophy caused by suprascapular nerve injury: MR findings. *J Comput Assist Tomogr*. 1997;21: 302–303.
22. Rask MR. Suprascapular nerve entrapment: a report of two cases treated with suprascapular notch resection. *Clin Orthop Relat Res*. 1977;123:73–75.

A Woman With Arm Weakness and a Skin Rash

A 70-year-old woman developed pain in the right arm and shoulder with some neck discomfort. Four days later, she presented with a rash on the arm and could no longer raise the arm. Past medical and social histories were unremarkable.

Examination revealed an erythematous vesicular rash in the outer aspect of the right arm, and she had weakness of the right deltoid of 2/5 (Fig. 15-1). Supraspinatus was 5/5 and brachioradialis was 3/5. Biceps strength was 3/5; triceps, forearm, and hand muscles were normal. The left arm and leg strength were normal. The right biceps and brachioradialis reflexes were absent; the triceps was normal. Reflexes in the legs and left arm were normal. Sensory examination showed diffuse hypoalgesia in the right lower arm; the affected dermatome was hard to localize. The rest of the neurologic examination was normal.

WHAT IS THE DIFFERENTIAL DIAGNOSIS?

This woman had weakness in muscles innervated by C5–C6 roots and upper trunk of the brachial plexus with decreased brachioradialis and biceps reflexes. These can be caused by a focal lesion, such as a tumor in the plexus, brachial neuritis, a herniated disk, or other lesion in the cervical spine. However, the acute onset accompanied by a rash is very suggestive of a herpes zoster (HZ) infection.

AN EMG TEST WAS PERFORMED

Motor Nerve Studies

Nerve and Site	Latency(ms)	Amplitude (mV)	Conduction Velocity (m/s)
Median Nerve R.	**Normal ≤ 4.2**	**Normal ≥ 6**	**Normal ≥ 50**
Wrist	4.1	10	–
Elbow	7.0	10	62
Ulnar Nerve R.	**Normal ≤ 3.7**	**Normal ≥ 8**	**Normal ≥ 50**
Wrist	3.7	9	–
Below elbow	6.9	9	53
Above elbow	9.2	9	52

F-Wave Studies

Nerve	Latency (ms)	Normal Latency ≤ (ms)
Median nerve R.	26.4	30
Ulnar nerve R.	27.6	30

Sensory Nerve Studies

Nerve	Onset Latency (ms)	Normal Onset Latency ≤ (ms)	Peak Latency (ms)	Normal Peak Latency ≤ (ms)	Amp (μV)	Normal Amp ≥ (μV)	Conduction Velocity (m/s)	Normal Conduction Velocity ≥ (m/s)
Median nerve R.	2.4	2.6	2.9	3.1	25	20	54	50
Ulnar nerve R.	2.3	2.6	2.8	3.1	18	13	52	50

EMG Data

Muscle	Insrt Activity	Fibs	Pos Waves	Fasc	Amp	Dur	Poly	Pattern
Cervical paraspinals R.	**Inc**	**2+**	**2+**	None	Norm	Norm	**Few**	Full
Infraspinatus R.	Norm	None	None	None	Norm	Norm	None	Full
Rhomboids R.	Norm	None	None	None	Norm	Norm	None	Full
Deltoid R.	**Inc**	**2+**	**2+**	None	**Lg**	**Inc**	**Few**	**Red**
Biceps brachii R.	**Inc**	**2+**	**2+**	None	**Lg**	**Inc**	**Few**	**Red**
Brachioradialis R.	**Inc**	**2+**	**2+**	None	**Lg**	**Inc**	**Few**	**Red**
Extensor digitorum comm. R.	Norm	None	None	None	Norm	Norm	None	Full
Flexor carpi radialis R.	Norm	None	None	None	Norm	Norm	None	Full
Flexor carpi ulnaris R.	Norm	None	None	None	Norm	Norm	None	Full
First dorsal interosseous R.	Norm	None	None	None	Norm	Norm	None	Full

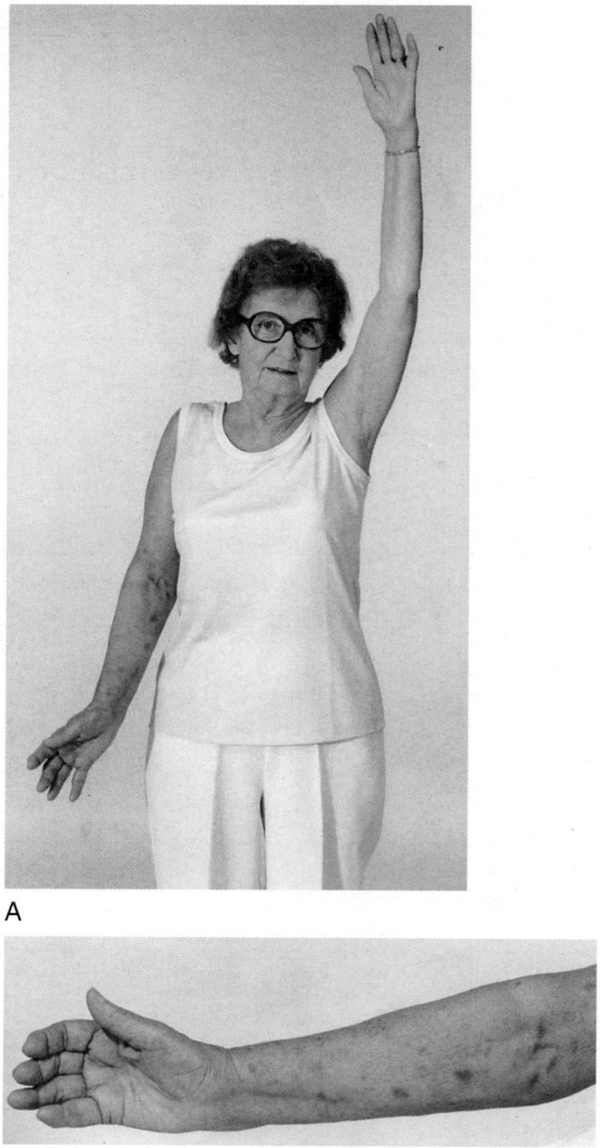

FIG. 15-1 Notice the patient's inability to raise the right arm (**A**) and the characteristic rash, which is better seen in (**B**).

WHAT WERE THE EMG FINDINGS?

The sensory and motor nerve conduction studies were normal. The needle test showed denervation potentials with reduced recruitment of motor units in the deltoid, biceps, brachioradialis, and cervical paraspinal muscles, indicating axonal degeneration of the C6 roots sparing the infraspinatus and rhomboids, as well as forearm and intrinsic hand muscles.

WHAT SHOULD BE DONE NEXT?

The patient was treated with acyclovir 10 mg/kg IV q 8 hours and oral prednisone 50 mg daily for 8 days. She improved slowly; the rash disappeared, and after 3 months, she regained strength.

DISCUSSION

This elderly woman had weakness raising her right arm accompanied by a rash caused by HZ infection involving the motor and sensory C6 roots.

The herpes virus typically manifests with a herpetic rash which usually affects one or two dermatomes. The lesions become vesicular with pustules crusting after 5–10 days. Acute zoster is almost always associated with pain, paresthesias, and hyperesthesias. If the ophthalmic division of cranial nerve V is involved and not treated, this could cause blindness from keratitis or central retinal arteritis and ischemia.[1,2] Other complications of HZ infections include Bell's palsy, encephalitis, and myelitis.[3,4] When Bell's palsy manifests with a rash in the external auditory canal, it is called zoster oticus or Ramsay Hunt syndrome.[1,5–7]

Cervical root zoster infections can be associated with weakness[8,9] and with diaphragmatic paralysis.[10] Lumbosacral HZ can also produce leg weakness.

Pathologically, there is intense lymphocytic inflammation with vasculitis and axonal degeneration of motor and sensory roots which may involve the adjacent spinal cord.[11]

HZ is exclusively a human DNA virus that also causes varicella or chickenpox. The virus resides in ganglionic cells,[12–14] where it remains latent. It is found primarily in the dorsal root ganglion neurons[15] but could be found throughout the neuraxis and, more frequently, in the thoracic, cervical, and trigeminal ganglia. MRI could reveal increased signal at the anterior horns, roots, or plexus.[16]

HZ occurs 10 times more frequently in people over age 60 and particularly in those who are immunosuppressed. The infection can occur after chickenpox or after immunization with a live virus, especially in immunocompromised hosts. The typical rash might precede, accompany, or follow the symptoms and may not occur in some patients (zoster sine herpete).

The treatment consists of acyclovir orally or intravenously according to the severity. Famciclovir can also be used orally. The addition of prednisone is helpful.

Postherpetic neuralgia is described as a pain that persists for 6 weeks after the rash and is usually a severe, burning sensation in the affected area. Therapy includes drugs such as antidepressants, topical lidocaine, carbamazepine,[15] gabapentin,[16] and pregabalin.[17] New HZ vaccines are now being used to prevent the condition in individuals at risk.[18]

SUMMARY

This 70-year-old woman developed weakness and an inability to raise her arm. She had evidence of a C6 radiculopathy clinically and by EMG and a characteristic herpetic rash. She improved with acyclovir and prednisone therapy.

IMPORTANT POINTS

- HZ can both manifest by pain and rash and produce radicular muscle weakness.

- Other manifestations include ophthalmic zoster, Ramsay Hunt syndrome, arteritis with stroke, encephalitis, myelitis, and meningitis.
- Acute zoster is treated with acyclovir or famciclovir; the addition of steroids can diminish the chance of developing postherpetic neuralgia.
- Postherpetic neuralgia is a later complication, treated with drugs such as gabapentin, pregabalin, or amitriptyline and analgesics.

REFERENCES

1. Gilden DH, Kleinschmidt-DeMasters BK, LaGuardia JJ, et al. Neurological complications of the reactivation of varicella-zoster virus. *N Engl J Med.* 2000;342(9):635–645.
2. Tenser RB. Herpes simplex and herpes zoster: nervous system involvement. *Neurol Clin.* 1984;2(2):215–240.
3. de Silva SM, Mark AS, Gilden DH, et al. Zoster myelitis: improvement with antiviral therapy in two cases. *Neurology.* 1996;47:929–931.
4. Gilden DH, Beinlich BR, Rubinstein EM, et al. Varicella-zoster virus myelitis: an expanding spectrum. *Neurology.* 1994;44: 1818–1823.
5. Crabtree JA. Herpes zoster oticus. *Laryngoscope.* 1968;78: 1853–1878.
6. Steffen R, Selby G. "Atypical" Ramsay Hunt syndrome. *Med J Aust.* 1972;1:227–230.
7. Nogueira RG, Seeley WW. Ramsay Hunt syndrome associated with spinal trigeminal nucleus and tract involvement on MRI. *Neurology.* 2003;61(9):1306–1307.
8. Tilki HE, Mutluer N, Selcuki D, Stalberg E. Zoster paresis. *Electromyogr Clin Neurophysiol.* 2003;43(4):231–234.
9. Thomas JE, Howard FM. Segmental zoster paresis—a disease profile. *Neurology.* 1972;22:459–466.
10. Stowasser M, Cameron J, Oliver WA. Diaphragmatic paralysis following cervical herpes zoster. *Med J Aust.* 1990;153(9):555–556.
11. Denny-Brown D, Adams RD, Fitzgerald PJ. Pathologic features of herpes zoster: a note on "geniculate herpes". *Arch Neurol Psychiatry.* 1944;51:216–231.
12. Gilden DH, Rozenman Y, Murray R, et al. Detection of varicella-zoster virus nucleic acid in neurons of normal human thoracic ganglia. *Ann Neurol.* 1987;22:377–380.
13. Mahalingam R, Wellish M, Wolfe W, et al. Latent varicella-zoster viral DNA in human trigeminal and thoracic ganglia. *N Engl J Med.* 1990;323:627–631.
14. Lungu O, Annunziato PW, Gershon A, et al. Reactivated and latent varicella-zoster virus in human dorsal root ganglia. *Proc Natl Acad Sci USA.* 1995;92:10980–10984.
15. Kost RG, Straus SE. Postherpetic neuralgia—pathogenesis, treatment, and prevention. *N Engl J Med.* 1996;335(1):32–42.
16. Liu Y, Wu BY, Ma ZS, Xu JJ, et al. A retrospective case series of segmental zoster paresis of limbs: clinical, electrophysiological and imaging characteristics. *BMC Neurology.* 2018;18(1):121. https://doi.org/10.1186/s12883-018-1130-4.
17. Rowbotham M, Harden N, Stacey B, et al. Gabapentin for the treatment of postherpetic neuralgia: a randomized controlled trial. *JAMA.* 1998;280:1837–1842.
18. Sabatowski R, Galvez R, Cherry DA, et al; 1008-045 Study Group. Pregabalin reduces pain and improves sleep and mood disturbances in patients with post-herpetic neuralgia: results of a randomized, placebo-controlled clinical trial. *Pain.* 2004;109(1–2):26–35.

A Woman With Neck and Arm Pain

A 41-year-old woman came with a 10-month history of neck pain radiating to the right arm.

Neurologic examination showed normal mentation and cranial nerves. There was no weakness, but there was diminished brachioradialis reflex on the right compared with the left. Sensory examination was normal. The rest of the examination was also normal. She was referred for an EMG.

AN EMG TEST WAS PERFORMED

Motor Nerve Studies

Nerve and Site	Latency (ms)	Amplitude (mV)	Conduction Velocity (m/s)
Median Nerve R.	**Normal ≤ 4.2**	**Normal ≥ 6**	**Normal ≥ 50**
Wrist	3.6	13	–
Elbow	7.3	12	59

Motor Nerve Studies—cont'd

Ulnar Nerve R.	Normal ≤ 3.6	Normal ≥ 8	Normal ≥ 50
Wrist	2.8	18	–
Below elbow	6.0	16	61

F-Wave Studies

Nerve	Latency (ms)	Normal Latency ≤ (ms)
Median nerve R.	23.4	30
Ulnar nerve R.	25.2	30

Sensory Nerve Studies

Nerve	Onset Latency (ms)	Normal Onset Latency ≤ (ms)	Peak Latency (ms)	Normal Peak Latency ≤ (ms)	Amp (μV)	Normal Amp ≥ (μV)	Conduction Velocity (m/s)	Normal Conduction Velocity ≥ (m/s)
Median nerve R.	2.5	2.6	3.0	3.1	34	20	52	50
Ulnar nerve R.	2.1	2.6	2.6	3.1	33	13	57	50

EMG Data

Muscle	Insrt Activity	Fibs	Pos Waves	Fasc	Amp	Dur	Poly	Pattern
Cervical paraspinals R.	Norm	None	None	None	Norm	Norm	None	Full
Rhomboids R.	**Inc**	None	**2+**	None	Norm	Norm	None	Full
Supraspinatus R.	**CRDs**	None	None	None	Norm	Norm	None	Full
Infraspinatus R.	**Inc**	None	None	None	Norm	Norm	None	Full
Deltoid R.	**Inc**	None	**1+**	None	Norm	Norm	None	Full
Biceps brachii R.	**Inc**	None	**2+**	None	Norm	Norm	None	**Red**
Flexor carpi radialis R.	Norm	None	None	None	Norm	Norm	None	Full
Flexor carpi ulnaris R.	Norm	None	None	None	Norm	Norm	None	Full
Extensor dig. communis R.	Norm	None	None	None	Norm	Norm	None	Full
First dorsal interosseous R.	Norm	None	None	None	Norm	Norm	None	Full

CRD=complex repetiotive discharges.

WHAT WERE THE EMG FINDINGS?

The median and ulnar motor conduction velocities, distal latencies, compound muscle action potential amplitudes, F-responses, and sensory nerve action potentials were normal. Needle EMG showed denervation potentials in the right biceps, deltoid, and rhomboids and complex repetitive discharges in the supraspinatus muscle. The motor units appeared normal in these muscles. Paraspinal muscles were normal.

This EMG was suggestive of a C5 radiculopathy in spite of there being no paraspinal denervation. This was concluded because there was involvement of muscles innervated only by C5; in particular, the rhomboid that is innervated by the dorsal scapular nerve that originates *directly* from the C5 root and not the brachial plexus.

A cervical MRI was done and showed a right lateral C5–C6 disk herniation. The patient received oral steroids without benefit, and because of severe intermittent pain, she had a diskectomy and spinal fusion with marked relief of symptoms.

For further discussion, important points, and references, see Case 17.

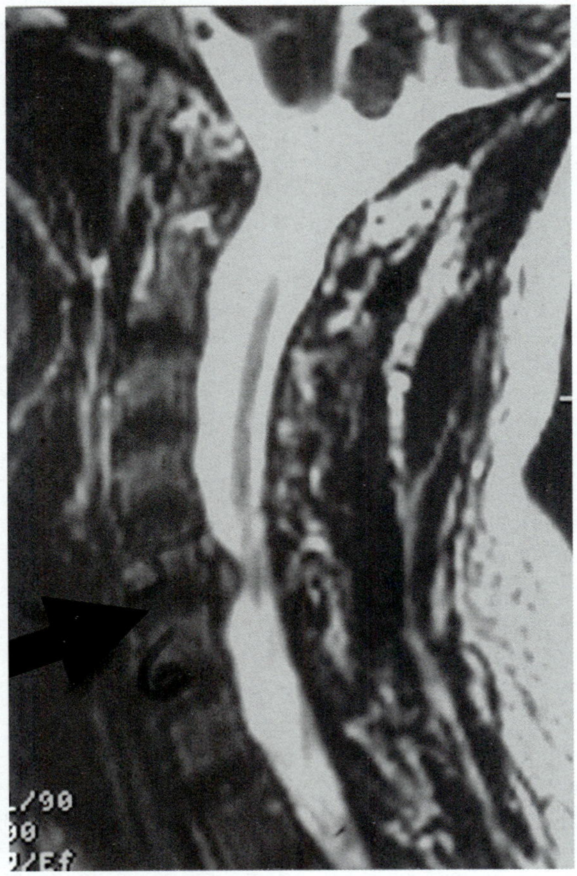

FIG. 16-1 MRI, T2-weighted image (sagittal view) showing the C5–C6 disk herniation (*arrow*).

SUMMARY

This woman presented with neck and arm pain with a diminished brachioradialis reflex. The EMG demonstrated a C5 radiculopathy, and the MRI showed a C5–C6 disk herniation (Fig. 16-1). She did not respond to conservative management but improved with surgery.

For further discussion, important points, and references, see Case 17.

17 CASE

A Woman With Neck Pain and a Weak Arm

A 24-year-old woman presented to her family doctor complaining of difficulty rotating the neck and pain in the left shoulder; she received corticosteroid injections into the neck with some relief. Five months later, she developed left upper extremity pain radiating from the shoulders to the forearm, and she presented to the emergency room because of the increased pain.

Past medical and social histories were unremarkable.

Neurologic examination showed decreased strength of 4/5 in the left triceps and wrist extensors and mild 5−/5 finger extensor weakness. All other upper extremity and lower extremity muscles, including biceps and brachioradialis, were normal. Reflexes were symmetric and normal, except for absent left triceps reflex. Plantar reflexes were flexor. The sensation was intact to pain, vibration, and light touch. Her pain was reproduced when the neck was tilted laterally and slightly rotated and the crown of the head pushed down (Spurling test). The rest of the examination was normal.

WHAT IS THE DIFFERENTIAL DIAGNOSIS?

This woman presented with neck pain and weakness in the triceps and wrist extensor muscles and absent triceps reflex, suggesting a C7 radiculopathy.[1] This was most likely caused by a ruptured disk.[2] Other lesions that can cause radiculopathy are neurofibromas, tumors, vascular malformations, hematomas, spondylosis with bony spurs, and infections, including herpes zoster.[2] The combination of neck pain and muscle weakness makes the diagnosis of a middle trunk, posterior cord, or radial nerve lesion unlikely, particularly as radial nerve-innervated muscles that originate from other roots, such as the brachioradialis (C5–C6), were clinically intact. The foraminal compression on the Spurling test reproduced the pain as it alters the size of the neuroforaminal opening, aggravating nerve irritation.[1–3] On the other hand, tilting the head in the opposite direction and abducting the symptomatic arm relieve the pain due to opening the foramina.

AN EMG TEST WAS PERFORMED

Motor Nerve Studies

Nerve and Site	Latency (ms)	Amplitude (mV)	Conduction Velocity (m/s)
Median Nerve L.	**Normal ≤ 4.2**	**Normal ≥ 6**	**Normal ≥ 50**
Wrist	3.7	12	–
Elbow	8.5	12	53
Ulnar Nerve L.	**Normal ≤ 3.6**	**Normal ≥ 8**	**Normal ≥ 50**
Wrist	2.8	10	–
Below elbow	6.7	10	54
Above elbow	8.7	10	60
Nerve and Site	**Latency (ms)**	**Amplitude (mV)**	**Conduction Velocity (m/s)**
Radial Nerve L.	**Normal ≤ 3.5**	**Normal ≥ 4.4**	**Normal ≥ 51**
Forearm	3.3	6	–
Axilla	6.8	6	63

F-Wave Studies

Nerve	Latency (ms)	Normal Latency ≤ (ms)
Median nerve L.	29.2	30
Ulnar nerve L.	28.8	30

Sensory Nerve Studies

Nerve	Onset Latency (ms)	Normal Onset Latency ≤ (ms)	Peak Latency (ms)	Normal Peak Latency ≤ (ms)	Amp (μV)	Normal Amp ≥ (μV)	Conduction Velocity (m/s)	Normal Conduction Velocity ≥ (m/s)
Median nerve L. (index)	2.4	2.6	2.9	3.1	28	20	54	50
Median nerve L. (middle)	2.2	2.6	2.7	3.1	32	20	59	50
Ulnar nerve L.	2.3	2.6	2.8	3.1	16	13	52	50
Radial nerve L.	1.8	2.6	2.3	3.1	45	30	56	50

EMG Data

Muscle	Insrt Activity	Fibs	Pos Waves	Fasc	Amp	Dur	Poly	Pattern
Cervical paraspinals L.	**Inc**	**2+**	**2+**	None	Norm	Norm	None	Full
Supraspinatus L.	Norm	None	None	None	Norm	Norm	None	Full
Infraspinatus L.	Norm	None	None	None	Norm	Norm	None	Full
Serratus anterior L.	**Inc**	**1+**	**1+**	None	Norm	Norm	None	Full
Deltoid L.	Norm	None	None	None	Norm	Norm	None	Full
Biceps brachii L.	Norm	None	None	None	Norm	Norm	None	Full
Triceps L.	**Inc**	**3+**	**3+**	None	Norm	Norm	None	**Red**
Flexor carpi radialis L.	**Inc**	**2+**	**2+**	None	Norm	Norm	None	**Red**
Flexor carpi ulnaris L.	Norm	None	None	None	Norm	Norm	None	Full
Extensor digitorum communis L.	**Inc**	**2+**	**2+**	None	Norm	Norm	None	**Red**
Extensor indicis proprius L.	**Inc**	**2+**	**2+**	None	Norm	Norm	None	**Red**
Pronator teres L.	**Inc**	**2+**	**2+**	None	Norm	Norm	None	Full
Pronator quadratus L.	Norm	None	None	None	Norm	Norm	None	Full
First dorsal interosseous L.	Norm	None	None	None	Norm	Norm	None	Full

WHAT NERVE CONDUCTION TESTS SHOULD BE DONE AND WHAT MUSCLES ARE STUDIED ON EMG?

Motor and sensory nerve conduction velocities were studied in the radial, ulnar, and median nerves. The tests were normal, particularly the median SNAP of the middle finger.

The needle test showed active denervation in the left triceps, the median-innervated flexor carpi radialis, the extensor digitorum communis and extensor indicis proprius, and cervical paraspinals. All affected muscles are supplied by the C7 root. Because the paraspinal muscles come directly from the dorsal rami of C7 ventral roots, the denervation localized a lesion to the root. In patients like this, but in which there is no paraspinal denervation, the presence of denervation in the serratus anterior, which comes directly from the roots, helps in the diagnosis of a radiculopathy.

An MRI showed intervertebral disk bulge, a large herniated nucleus pulposus at the left C6–C7 in the left posterior paracentral region (Fig. 17-1).

SUMMARY

This woman with neck pain and weakness of the triceps and wrist extensor muscles having decreased triceps reflexes had denervation at C7-innervated limb and paraspinal muscles. She had a large C6–C7 disk and responded well to decompressive surgical intervention.

DISCUSSION (CASES 16 AND 17)

Case 16 had C5 radiculopathy caused by a lateral disk herniation between C5 and C6. The C5 root innervates mainly the spinati, the clavicular part of the pectoralis major, the teres minor, brachialis, and rhomboid. The biceps and brachioradialis have not only C5 but also C6 innervation.[4]

A ruptured medial or lateral disk between C4 and C5 of the cervical spine usually affects the C5 root, and if between C5 and C6, usually damages the C6 root. A far lateral disk fragment, however, could affect the upper root. The most frequent cervical radiculopathy is C7, which occurs in 60% of the cases, whereas the C6 root is affected in 17.6%; other roots are affected in about 10% of cases.[5,6]

Case 17 had a C7 radiculopathy caused by a disk rupture at C6–C7. The triceps muscle is usually involved in a C7 radiculopathy,[7] and the triceps reflex is abnormal in about 70% of patients.[2] (Table 17-1 lists neurologic findings in cervical radiculopathies; Table 17-2 lists the muscles involved in cervical radiculopathy.)

Electromyography is the best electrodiagnostic test in the evaluation of radiculopathy.[7,8] Myotomal distribution of denervation is the most important clue to the diagnosis. Paraspinal muscle denervation is seen in 50% of patients and should always be examined when it is suspected.[9] The presence of paraspinal denervation alone without other findings, should, however, be interpreted with caution, because this can rarely occur in normal people.[10] Sensory and motor nerve conduction studies are almost always normal; however, if the lesion affects the posterior root ganglia, the SNAP can be of low amplitude.[9–11] Measurement of F-wave latency can be useful for lower cervical (C8–T1) radiculopathy. Root stimulation[12] and magnetic stimulation[13] can be useful, but the results have not been validated and these tests are not routinely done.

MRI of the spine is the best imaging test and predicts 88% of surgically proven lesions, compared with 81% with post-myelogram CT.[14]

The combination of EMG and MRI is very important in localizing the lesion and determining the degree of damage.

The initial treatment of radiculopathy is conservative,[15,16] as even patients with motor deficits can improve after the disk desiccates. Surgery may provide more prompt symptom relief, but the long-term benefits of surgery and conservative

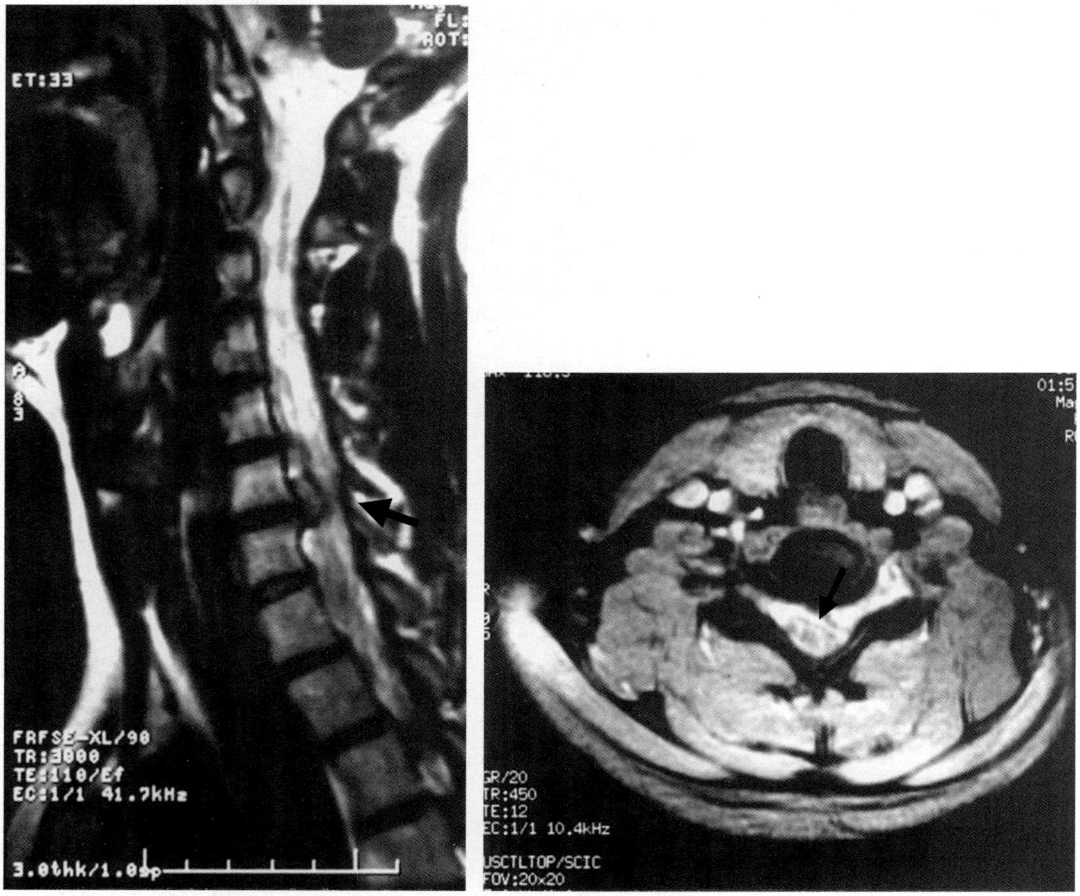

A B

FIG. 17-1 **A**, Sagittal view MRI, T2-weighted image showing a large C6–C7 herniated disk (*arrow*). **B**, Cervical MRI, T2-weighted image (axial view) showing the large protruded disk in the left (*arrow*).

TABLE 17-1 Motor Weakness and Reflex Changes Produced by Acute and Subacute Cervical Radiculopathies[a]

Disk Level	Root	Weakness	Reflex Depressed
C3–C4	C4	None	–
C4–C5	C5	Rhomboid, supraspinatus, infraspinatus, deltoid, biceps, brachioradialis	Biceps, brachioradialis
C5–C6	C6	As for C5 plus extensor carpi radialis longus, supinator, pronator	Biceps, brachioradialis
C6–C7	C7	Triceps, wrist and finger extensors, pronator	Triceps
C7–T1	C8	As for C7 plus wrist and finger flexors, intrinsic hand muscles	Triceps, finger reflex
T1–T2	T1[b]	Intrinsic hand muscles	Finger reflex

[a]Variations are to be expected from one patient to another.
[b]May also have Horner syndrome.
Modified with permission from Stewart JD. Lower cervical nerve roots and spinal nerves. In: Stewart JD, ed. *Focal Peripheral Neuropathies*. 3rd ed. Philadelphia, PA: Lippincott Williams & Wilkins; 2000:100.
Frequency figures from Refs. 5–8.

management are similar.[17] Surgery is indicated in cases with severe persistent pain and neurologic deficits.

IMPORTANT POINTS

- A ruptured cervical disk typically damages the root exiting at its level (e.g., a C5–C6 disk damages the C6 root), but a lateral disk rupture could affect the upper root.
- The rhomboids are innervated directly from the C5 root, so denervation at this muscle suggests a C5 radiculopathy.
- Triceps muscle weakness can be caused by a C7 radiculopathy, a lesion of the middle trunk or posterior cord of the brachial plexus, or the radial nerve.
- EMG of suspected cervical radiculopathy should always include paraspinal muscles and those innervated by different nerves and the same root. Denervation in the triceps, extensor digitorum communis (radial), flexor carpi radialis (median), and paraspinals with lack of denervation in limb muscles innervated by C6 and C8 localized the lesion to the C7 root.
- Paraspinal denervation may be absent in 50% of patients with cervical radiculopathy. The presence of denervation, however, should be correlated with the clinical presentation and other EMG findings, as this could be present in normal people.

TABLE 17-2 Myotomal Chart of Muscles Useful to Test in Patients With Suspected Cervical Radiculopathy

Roots/Spinal Nerves	Muscles
C5	Rhomboid
C5, C6*	**Supraspinatus**
	Infraspinatus
	Deltoid
	Pectoralis major (clavicular head)
	Biceps
	Brachioradialis*
C5, C6, and C7	Serratus anterior
	Teres major
C6, C7	Triceps
	Supinator
	Pronator teres
	Extensor carpi radialis
	Flexor carpi radialis
C6, C7, and C8*	**Latissimus dorsi**
	Pectoralis major (sternal head)
	Extensor digitorum communis*
C7, C8*	**Extensor carpi ulnaris and radialis**
	Extensor indicis proprius*
	Extensor pollicis longus, brevis*
C7, C8, and T1	**Flexor carpi ulnaris**
C8, T1*	**Flexor pollicis longus**
	Flexor digitorum superficialis and profundus
	Abductor pollicis brevis*
	First dorsal interosseous
	Abductor digiti minimi

Muscles in bold type derive their major innervation from the corresponding spinal nerve in bold type. Muscles identified by an asterisk derive their major innervation from the spinal nerves that are similarly identified. Muscles that are not identified are innervated equally by the two or three spinal nerves listed.
Reprinted with permission from Stewart JD. Lower cervical nerve roots and spinal nerves. In: Stewart JD, ed. *Focal Peripheral Neuropathies*. 3rd ed. Philadelphia, PA: Lippincott Williams & Wilkins; 2000:102.

- Cervical MRI is the best imaging modality for the cervical spine.
- The treatment of cervical radiculopathy is conservative, although in patients with severe, persistent pain or neurologic deficits, surgical treatment is indicated.

REFERENCES

1. Yoss RE, Corbin KB, MacCarty CS, Love JG. Significance of symptoms and signs in localization of involved root in cervical disk protrusion. *Neurology*. 1957;7:673–683.
2. Stewart JD. Lower cervical nerve roots and spinal nerves. In: Stewart JD, ed. *Focal Peripheral Neuropathies*. 3rd ed. Philadelphia, PA: Lippincott Williams & Wilkins; 2000.
3. Viikari-Juntura E, Porras M, Laasonen EM. Validity of clinical tests in the diagnosis of root compression in cervical disc disease. *Spine*. 1989;14:253–257.
4. Bertorini TE. Clinical evaluation and clinical diagnostic tests. In: Bertorini TE, ed. *Clinical Evaluation and Diagnostic Tests for Neuromuscular Disorders*. Boston, MA: Butterworth-Heinemann; 2004:15–97.
5. Rahdakrishnan K, Litchy WJ, O'Fallon WM, Kurland LT. Epidemiology of cervical radiculopathy: a population-based study from Rochester, Minnesota, 1976–1990. *Brain*. 1994;117: 325–335.
6. Kelsy JL, Githens PB, Walter SD, et al. An epidemiological study of acute prolapsed cervical intervertebral disk. *J Bone Joint Surg [AM]*. 1984;66A:907–914.
7. Gough J, Koepke G. Electromyographic determination of motor root levels in erector spinae muscles. *Arch Phys Med Rehabil*. 1966;47:9–11.
8. Wilbourn AJ, Aminoff MJ. AAEM minimonograph 32: the electrodiagnostic examination in patients with radiculopathies. *Muscle Nerve*. 1998;21:1612–1631.
9. Levin KH, Maggiano HJ, Wilbourn AJ. Cervical radiculopathies: comparison of surgical and EMG localization of single-root lesions. *Neurology*. 1996;46:1022–1025.
10. Levin KH. Cervical radiculopathies in neuromuscular disorders in clinical practice. In: Katirji B, Kaminski HJ, Preston DC, eds. *Neuromuscular Disorders in Clinical Practice*. Boston, MA: Butterworth-Heinemann; 2004:838–858.
11. Date ES, Kim BJ, Yoon J, Park BK. Cervical paraspinal spontaneous activity in asymptomatic subjects. *Muscle Nerve*. 2006;34:361–364.
12. Berger AR, Busis NA, Logigian EL, et al. Cervical root stimulation in the diagnosis of radiculopathy. *Neurology*. 1987;37:329–332.
13. Cros D, Chiappa KH, Gominak S, et al. Cervical magnetic stimulation. *Neurology*. 1990;40:1751–1756.
14. Modic MT, Masaryk TJ, Mulopulos GP, et al. Cervical radiculopathy: prospective evaluation with surface coil MR imaging, CT with metrizamide, and metrizamide myelopathy. *Radiology*. 1986;161:753–759.
15. Saal JS, Saal JA, Yurth EF. Nonoperative management of herniated cervical intervertebral disc with radiculopathy. *Spine*. 1996;21:1877–1883.
16. Maigne JY, Deligne L. Computed tomographic follow-up study of 21 cases of nonoperatively treated cervical intervertebral soft disc herniation. *Spine*. 1994;19:189–191.
17. Persson LC, Moritz U, Brandt L, Carlsson CA. Cervical radiculopathy: pain, muscle weakness and sensory loss in patients with cervical radiculopathy treated with surgery, physiotherapy or cervical collar: a prospective, controlled study. *Eur Spine J*. 1997;6:256–266.

18 CASE

A Woman With Back Pain and Leg Weakness

A 45-year-old woman without significant past medical history developed numbness in the inner aspect of the left leg and nonradiating back pain. She also had left leg weakness and locking with instability resulting in a fall, causing a fracture of the left second toe 3 weeks prior to her evaluation.

Neurologic examination revealed normal mentation and cranial nerves. Motor and sensory examinations were normal in both upper extremities and right leg. In the left lower extremity the left quadriceps muscle was weak at 4+/5 and the adductors were 5−/5. All reflexes were 2+ (normal), except in the left patellar and left adductor reflexes that were 1+. There was a patchy area of decreased sensation in the anterior left thigh. Straight leg raising and femoral stretch[1] tests were normal. The rest of the neurologic examination was unremarkable.

WHAT IS THE DIFFERENTIAL DIAGNOSIS?

This healthy woman had back pain and weakness limited to muscles innervated by L3–L4.[2] She appeared to have a lumbosacral radiculopathy most likely caused by a disk herniation. A lumbosacral radiculoplexopathy from diabetes is unlikely as she is not diabetic; there are, however, instances of nondiabetic idiopathic or autoimmune lumbosacral plexopathy.[3] Lumbosacral radiculoplexopathy could also be caused by herpes zoster and CMV infection in HIV-positive individuals.[4–6] Other possibilities include tumors, abscesses, and hematomas of the retroperitoneal space and pelvis causing a plexopathy. The weak adductors and decreased adductor reflex argue against a femoral neuropathy. (Table 18-1 outlines the neurologic findings in the various lumbosacral radiculopathies; Table 18-2 outlines their differential diagnosis.)

WHAT SHOULD BE THE DIAGNOSTIC WORKUP?

The patient had a normal comprehensive metabolic panel and glycosylated hemoglobin and erythrocyte sedimentation rate.

AN EMG TEST WAS PERFORMED

Motor Nerve Studies

Nerve and Site	Latency(ms)	Amplitude (mV)	Conduction Velocity (m/s)
Peroneal Nerve L.	**Normal ≤ 5.3**	**Normal ≥ 3**	**Normal ≥ 40**
Ankle	3.7	3	–
Fibular head	11.9	**2**	45
Knee	13.4	**2**	66
Tibial Nerve L.	**Normal ≤ 5.3**	**Normal ≥ 4**	**Normal ≥ 40**
Ankle	3.5	19	–
Pop. fossa	13.4	12	43

Nerve and Site	Latency (ms)	Amplitude (mV)	Conduction Velocity (m/s)
Peroneal Nerve R.	**Normal ≤ 5.7**	**Normal ≥ 3**	**Normal ≥ 40**
Ankle	4.9	5	–
Fibular head	11.2	4	46
Knee	12.8	4	56

F-Wave Studies

Nerve	Latency (ms)	Normal Latency ≤ (ms)
Peroneal nerve L.	50.4	54
Tibial nerve L.	50.2	54
Peroneal nerve R.	49.0	54
H-reflex L.	33.9	34
H-reflex R.	33.8	34

Sensory Nerve Studies

Nerve	Onset Latency (ms)	Normal Onset Latency ≤ (ms)	Peak Latency (ms)	Normal Peak Latency ≤ (ms)	Amp (μV)	Normal Amp ≥ (mV)	Conduction Velocity (m/s)	Normal Conduction Velocity ≥ (m/s)
Sural nerve L.	3.0	3.5	3.5	4.0	**7**	11	47	40
Superficial peroneal L.	**NR**	3.5	**NR**	4.0	**NR**	10	**NR**	40
Sural nerve R.	3.2	3.5	3.7	4.0	12	11	44	40
Superficial peroneal R.	3.4	3.5	3.9	4.0	9	8–10	41	40

EMG Data

Muscle	Insrt Activity	Fibs	Pos Waves	Fasc	Amp	Dur	Poly	Pattern
Lumbar paraspinal L.	**Inc**	None	**1+**	None	Norm	Norm	None	Full
Iliopsoas L.	Norm	None	None	None	Norm	Norm	None	Full
Tensor fasciae latae L.	Norm	None	None	None	Norm	Norm	None	Full
Adductor magnus L.	**Inc**	**1+**	**1+**	None	Norm	Norm	None	Full
Adductor longus L.	**Inc**	None	**1+**	None	Norm	Norm	None	Full
Vastus medialis L.	**Inc**	None	**1+**	None	Norm	Norm	None	**Red**
Vastus lateralis L.	**Inc**	None	**2+**	None	Norm	Norm	None	**Red**
Biceps femoris short-head L.	Norm	None	None	None	Norm	Norm	None	Full
Tibialis posterior L.	Norm	None	None	None	Norm	Norm	None	Full
Tibialis anterior L.	**Inc**	None	None	None	Norm	Norm	None	Full
Peroneus longus L.	Norm	None	None	None	Norm	Norm	None	Full
Gastrocnemius L.	Norm	None	None	None	Norm	Norm	None	Full
Lumbar paraspinal R.	Norm	None	None	None	Norm	Norm	None	Full
Vastus lateralis R.	Norm	None	None	None	Norm	Norm	None	Full
Tibialis anterior R.	Norm	None	None	None	Norm	Norm	None	Full

TABLE 18-1 Neurologic Findings in Lumbosacral Monoradiculopathies

Root Level	Pain	Sensory Loss (Paresthesias)	Motor Abnormalities/ Weakness	Deep Tendon Reflex Abnormalities
L1	Inguinal region	Inguinal region	None	None
L2	Groin, anterior thigh	Anterolateral thigh	Iliopsoas	None
L3	Anterior thigh to knee	Medial thigh and knee	Quadriceps, iliopsoas, and hip adductors	Knee jerk
L4	Anterior thigh to medial foreleg	Medial leg	Tibialis anterior, quadriceps, and hip adductors	Knee jerk
L5	Lateral thigh and leg to dorsum foot	Lateral leg, dorsum foot, and great toe	Toe extensors, ankle dorsiflexors, evertor and invertors, and hip abductors	None (unless S1 involved)
S1	Posterior thigh, calf, and heel	Sole, lateral foot and ankle, and lateral two toes	Toe flexors, gastrocnemii, hamstrings, and gluteus maximus	Ankle jerk
S2–S4	Medial buttocks	Medial buttocks, perineal and perianal region	None unless S1 through S2 involved	Bulbocavernosus and anal wink (ankle jerk if S1 involved)

From Raynor EM, Kleiner-Fisman G, Nardin R. Lumbosacral and thoracic radiculopathies. In: Katirji B, Kaminski HJ, Preston DC, et al., eds. *Neuromuscular Disorders in Clinical Practice*. Boston, MA: Butterworth-Heinemann; 2002:864.

TABLE 18-2 Differential Diagnosis of Lumbosacral Monoradiculopathies

Root Level	Nerve Lesion	Plexus Lesion	Differential Features
L1	Ilioinguinal neuropathy; genitofemoral neuropathy	Unlikely	Sensory loss outside single nerve territory
L2	Lateral femoral cutaneous neuropathy (meralgia paresthetica)	High lumbar plexopathy	Strength normal in meralgia paresthetica; quadriceps more involved with femoral neuropathy
L3	Femoral neuropathy	High lumbar plexopathy; diabetic amyotrophy	Adductor weakness not seen with femoral neuropathy
L4	Femoral neuropathy	Mid lumbar plexopathy	Tibialis anterior, hip adductors not involved in femoral neuropathy; quadriceps not involved in peroneal neuropathy
L5	Common peroneal neuropathy	Mid lumbar plexopathy	Ankle inversion not involved in peroneal neuropathy; hip abduction also normal with peroneal neuropathy
S1	Sciatic neuropathy	Lower lumbosacral plexopathy	Hamstrings not involved in tibial neuropathy; glutei not involved in sciatic neuropathy

From Raynor EM, Kleiner-Fisman G, Nardin R. Lumbosacral and thoracic radiculopathies. In: Katirji B, Kaminski HJ, Preston DC, et al., eds. *Neuromuscular Disorders in Clinical Practice*. Boston, MA: Butterworth-Heinemann; 2002:865.

WHAT WERE THE EMG FINDINGS?

The only abnormalities on nerve conduction tests were borderline amplitude peroneal CMAP from ankle stimulation, and this was lower at the knee. Her superficial peroneal SNAP was absent. The low-amplitude peroneal CMAP in conjunction with an absent left superficial peroneal SNAP could indicate a common peroneal nerve lesion.

Needle electromyography demonstrated denervation potentials in muscles that share innervation by the left L4 root (quadriceps, adductors, and tibialis anterior) and not those that are innervated by L5 or S1 (tensor fasciae latae, peroneus longus, and gastrocnemius) or mainly by L3 but not L4 (iliopsoas). The spontaneous activity of the lumbosacral paraspinal muscles was consistent with a radiculopathy. In addition, the patient had entrapment of the peroneal nerve at the fibular head (Fig. 18-1).

An MRI of the lumbosacral spine showed a paracentral L3–L4 disk herniation (Fig. 18-2).

Physical therapy and oral corticosteroids improved her symptoms after 1 month without surgery being required.

For further discussion and the references, see Case 20.

SUMMARY

This woman with back pain had muscle weakness in the left quadriceps and adductor muscles, which was consistent with an L4 radiculopathy. A paracentral herniated L3–L4 disk impinged the L4 root. A mild peroneal nerve entrapment was found incidentally. The patient responded to conservative management.

IMPORTANT POINTS

- Weakness of the quadriceps and adductors may be caused by a lumbosacral radiculopathy or a plexopathy.
- L4 radiculopathy is usually caused by a centrally herniated L3–L4 disk, but it can also be caused by a laterally herniated L4–L5 disk.

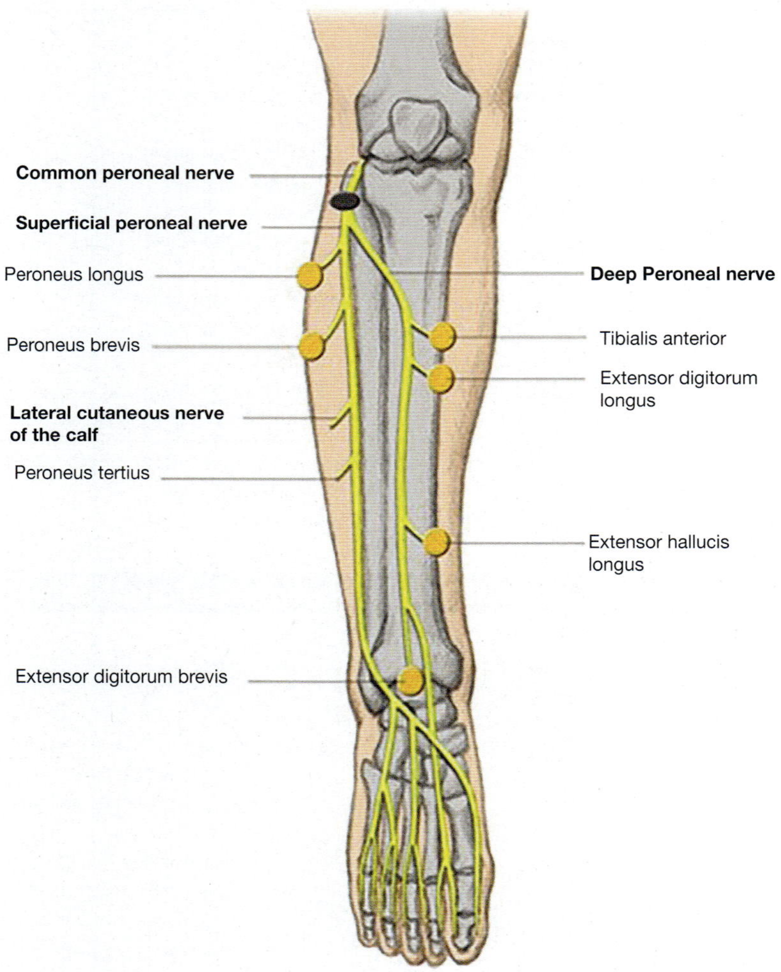

FIG. 18-1 Diagram of the peroneus nerve at site of the lesion.

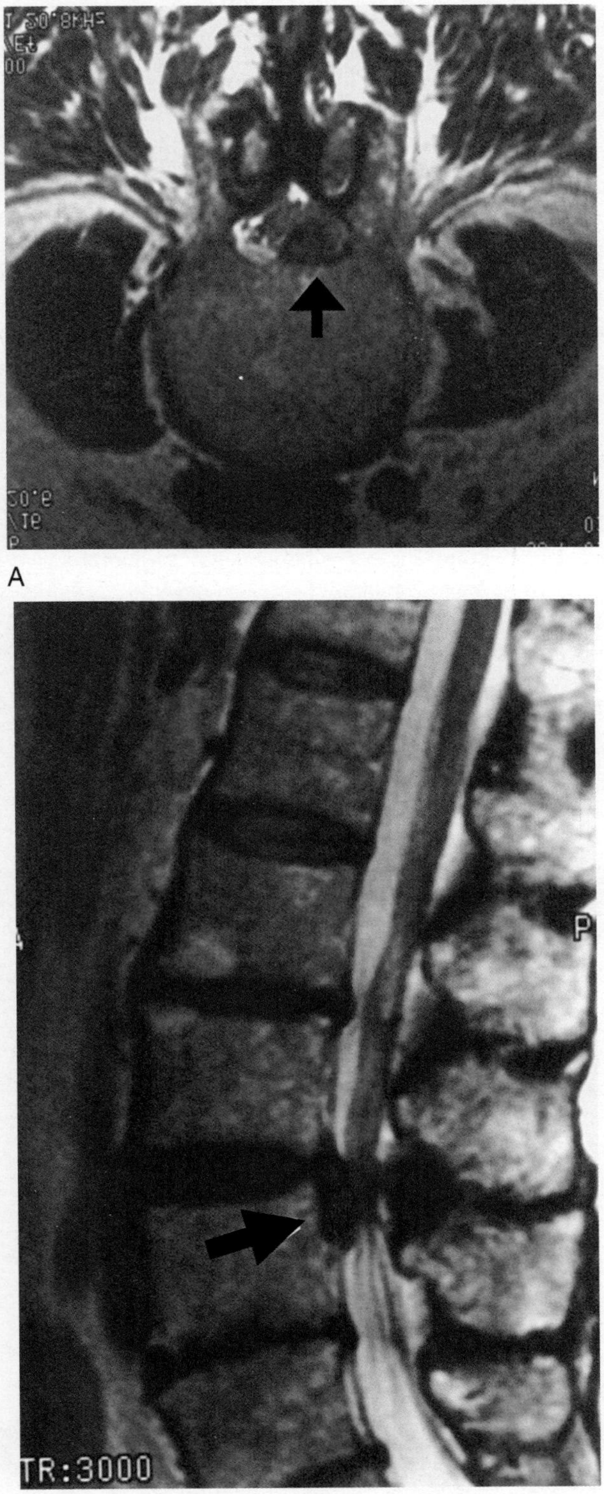

FIG. 18-2 A, MRI (axial view) T1-weighted image showing a paracentral disk herniation (*arrow*). **B**, MRI (sagittal view) T2-weighted image showing the large L3–L4 disk (*arrow*).

- In an L4 radiculopathy, there could be denervation in the paraspinal muscles and muscles sharing innervation by the L4 root, such as quadriceps and adductors (L2–L4), while sparing the iliopsoas (L3) and muscles innervated by L5 and S1 roots, such as the tensor fasciae latae, gluteus maximus, posterior tibial, gastrocnemius, and peronei.
- Conservative therapy can be beneficial in radiculopathy.

19 CASE

A Woman With Back Pain and Weakness

A 52-year-old woman presented with a 1-year history of weakness and pain of the left lower back radiating to the hip and thigh. She occasionally had pain in the other leg. Past medical history was significant for gallbladder surgery and a C-section.

Examination revealed no demonstrable muscle weakness despite her complaints. The straight leg raising test was positive on the left. Reflexes were 2+, symmetrical except for a decreased (trace) left ankle jerk.

She had decreased sensation in the posterior and outer aspect of the leg. The rest of the neurologic examination was normal.

WHAT IS THE DIFFERENTIAL DIAGNOSIS?

The low back pain, positive straight leg raising test, and absent left ankle reflex indicate an S1 radiculopathy, most likely caused by a ruptured disk. Other causes include masses, infections, or canal stenosis from osteoarthritis. The back pain argues against a diagnosis of sciatic neuropathy.

WHAT TESTS SHOULD BE DONE?

An imaging study such as an MRI or CAT scan of the lumbar spine and an EMG should be done.

AN EMG TEST WAS PERFORMED

Motor Nerve Studies

Nerve and Site	Latency (ms)	Amplitude (mV)	Conduction Velocity (m/s)
Peroneal Nerve R.	**Normal ≤ 5.7**	**Normal ≥ 3**	**Normal ≥ 40**
Ankle	3.7	8	–
Fibular head	9.5	7	42
Tibial Nerve R.	**Normal ≤ 5.3**	**Normal ≥ 4**	**Normal ≥ 40**
Ankle	3.2	6	–
Pop. fossa	11.6	5	45

F-Wave and Tibial H-Reflex Studies

Nerve	Latency (ms)	Normal Latency ≤ (ms)
Peroneal nerve R.	43.1	54
Tibial nerve R.	45.9	54
H-reflex R.	32.6	34
H-reflex L.	**34.3**	34

Sensory Nerve Studies

Nerve	Latency (ms)	Normal Latency ≤ (ms)	Amplitude (µV)	Normal Amplitude ≥ (µV)
Sural nerve R.	3.8	4.0	20	11

EMG Data

Muscle	Insrt Activity	Fibs	Pos Waves	Fasc	Amp	Dur	Poly	Pattern
Lumbar paraspinals R.	**Inc**	**2+**	**2+**	None	Norm	Norm	None	Full
Gluteus medius R.	Norm	None	None	None	Norm	Norm	None	Full
Tensor fasciae latae R.	Norm	None	None	None	Norm	Norm	None	Full
Vastus lateralis R.	Norm	None	None	None	Norm	Norm	None	Full
Biceps femoris–short head R.	Norm	None	None	None	Norm	Norm	None	Full
Tibialis anterior R.	Norm	None	None	None	Norm	Norm	None	Full
Tibialis posterior R.	Norm	None	None	None	Norm	None	None	Full
Gastrocnemius R.	**Inc**	None	None	None	Norm	Norm	None	Full

WHAT WERE THE EMG FINDINGS?

These studies revealed normal motor nerve conduction velocities, compound muscle action potential latencies and amplitudes, normal F-responses, and sural nerve sensory nerve action potential. The H-reflex test showed a prolonged latency on the left of 1.7 ms compared with the right. This difference is above the upper limits used in our laboratory (1.5 ms).

A prolonged or absent H-reflex is seen in S1 radiculopathy, plexopathy, and tibial or sciatic neuropathy. The patient also had denervation in the lower paraspinal muscles and mildly increased insertional activity in the gastrocnemius muscle indicating an S1 radiculopathy.[7,8]

An MRI showed an L5–S1 disk protrusion (Fig. 19-1). The patient was treated unsuccessfully to relieve her symptoms with steroids and physical therapy and subsequently required laminectomy and disk removal.

For further discussion and the references, see Case 20.

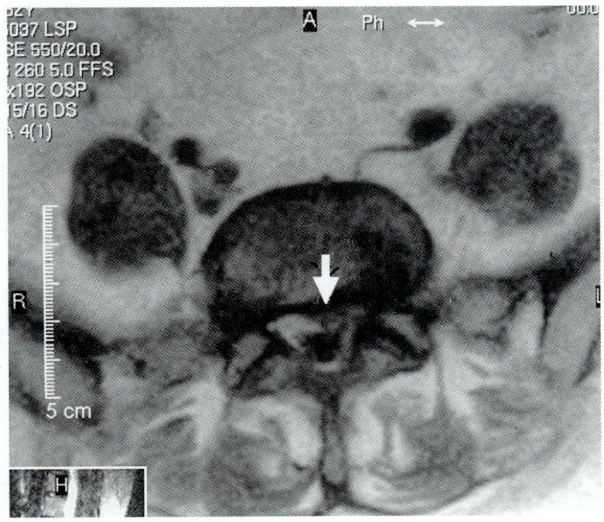

FIG. 19-1 T2-weighted MRI image (axial view) showing an L5–S1 disk herniation (*arrow*).

SUMMARY

This patient had back pain and decreased sensation in the posterior and outer aspect of the legs. She also had a decreased left ankle jerk and positive straight leg raising test. The electrophysiologic study revealed a mildly prolonged H-reflex on the left and denervation in the lumbar paraspinal and gastrocnemius muscles. She was diagnosed as having an S1 radiculopathy. Her lumbosacral spine MRI showed a disk protrusion, likely causing the radiculopathy. She did not respond to physical therapy and required surgery.

IMPORTANT POINTS

- S1 radiculopathy may produce sensory deficits in the posterior aspect of the leg and lateral aspect of the foot.
- Patients can have a positive straight leg raising test and absent or decreased ankle jerks and weakness of the gastrocnemius and hamstring muscles.
- The H-reflex is useful in the diagnosis of S1 radiculopathy, in which case it could be absent or have a prolonged latency.
- Surgery is beneficial in patients who do not respond to physical therapy.

20 CASE

A Woman With Back Pain and Unusual Nerve Conduction Tests

A 36-year-old woman had a 2-month history of pain in her left hip and back radiating to her left leg, particularly during straining.

Past medical history was unremarkable.

Her general and neurologic examinations were normal except for mild weakness of the toe dorsiflexion of the left. Reflexes and sensory examination and straight leg raising test were normal.

WHAT IS THE DIFFERENTIAL DIAGNOSIS IN THIS CASE?

The presentation with pain when straining suggests a lumbosacral radiculopathy likely caused by a ruptured disk, but other causes need to be ruled out. A plexopathy and a focal neuropathy are somewhat unlikely because of back pain and lack of sensory deficits. Other possibilities include spinal canal stenosis and facet hypertrophy, but the lack of classical symptoms of stiffness and back pain in the early morning and the patient's young age are against these diagnoses. The lack of more diffuse findings and sphincter disturbances is somewhat against a lumbosacral tumor.[9]

WHAT WOULD BE THE MOST APPROPRIATE DIAGNOSTIC TEST?

The most important diagnostic tests include imaging of the spine, particularly by MRI. Electrodiagnostic tests are helpful in delineating the affected structures. For example, motor nerve conduction velocities are usually abnormal in focal neuropathies and normal in radiculopathies and plexopathies, but both may show low-amplitude CMAPs, and the SNAPs may be abnormal in plexopathies. Testing of H-reflex and F-responses is also helpful in the evaluation of patients with radiculopathy and plexopathy, although these studies provide variable results. Somatosensory responses with stimulation of nerve trunks or dermatomal stimulation can be of help, but these are not done routinely, and the results are variable.[10,11] Needle electromyography studies are most useful in differentiating radiculopathy from plexopathy or peripheral nerve disease, particularly based on the myotomal distribution of denervation, which is usually present in the paraspinal muscles in radiculopathy.

A NERVE CONDUCTION STUDY WAS PERFORMED

Motor Nerve Studies

Nerve and Site	Latency (ms)	Amplitude (mV)	Conduction Velocity (m/s)
Peroneal Nerve L.	**Normal ≤ 5.7**	**Normal ≥ 3**	**Normal ≥ 40**
Ankle	3.5	11	–
Fibular head	9.9	15	52
Lateral malleolus	3.7	7	–
Nerve and Site	**Latency (ms)**	**Amplitude (mV)**	**Conduction Velocity (m/s)**
Tibial Nerve L.	**Normal ≤ 5.3**	**Normal ≥ 4**	**Normal ≥ 40**
Ankle	2.9	18	–
Pop. fossa	11.2	18	49
Peroneal Nerve R.	**Normal ≤ 5.7**	**Normal ≥ 3**	**Normal ≥ 40**
Ankle	3.7	9	–
Fibular head	10.1	9	52

F-Wave and Tibial H-Reflex Studies

Nerve	Latency (ms)	Normal Latency ≤ (ms)
Peroneal nerve L.	54.0	54
Tibial nerve L.	47.6	54
H-reflex L.	30.3	34
H-reflex R.	30.1	34

Sensory Nerve Studies

Nerve	Onset Latency (ms)	Normal Onset Latency ≤ (ms)	Peak Latency (ms)	Normal Peak Latency ≤ (ms)	Amp (μV)	Normal Amp ≥ (μV)	Conduction Velocity (m/s)	Normal Conduction Velocity ≥ (m/s)
Sural nerve L.	2.8	3.5	3.3	4.0	17	11	50	40

WHAT WERE THE NERVE CONDUCTION TEST FINDINGS?

The left peroneal nerve had normal motor conduction velocity and distal and F-wave latencies, but the CMAP response on knee stimulation was larger than on ankle stimulation (Fig. 20-1A). The left tibial motor nerve had normal conduction velocity, CMAP amplitude, distal latency, and F-wave latency. The right peroneal conduction test, left sural SNAP, and both H-reflexes were normal.

WHAT IS THE SIGNIFICANCE OF THE FINDINGS OF THIS TEST AND WHAT SHOULD BE DONE NEXT?

The tests were normal except for low-amplitude distal peroneal CMAP response compared with the CMAP obtained with proximal stimulation. This could be technical from poor stimulating techniques, as the distal CMAP normally should be close to 100%, compared with results obtained during proximal stimulation; this could also be caused by an accessory peroneal nerve.

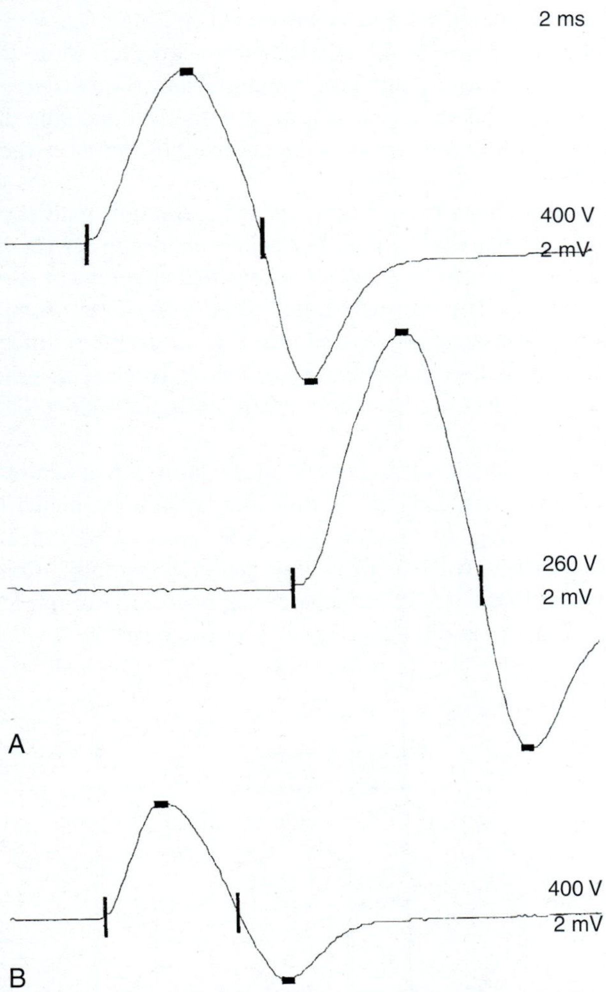

FIG. 20-1 **A**, CMAP of the peroneal nerve, stimulating at the ankle (top) and fibula head (bottom). Note the larger response from the proximal stimulation. **B**, Notice a CMAP of the peroneal nerve stimulating partially across the external malleolus.

The stimuli strength of the peroneal nerve was increased by 25% without an increased CMAP amplitude. The stimulating electrode was then moved to the lateral aspect of the ankle and then behind the lateral malleolus when a small CMAP appeared in the extensor digitorum brevis (EDB) muscle (see Fig. 20-1B).

These findings indicate an accessory deep peroneal nerve, a normal variant that occurs in up to 28% of normal people.[12] In this, one or both EDB muscles are partially innervated by an accessory deep peroneal nerve, a branch of the superficial peroneal nerve (Fig. 20-2). This is the most common cross-innervation of the lower extremity.

A NEEDLE EMG TEST WAS PERFORMED

What Were The EMG Findings?

Electromyography showed denervation potentials in the left tibialis anterior, tensor fasciae latae, and tibialis posterior muscles;

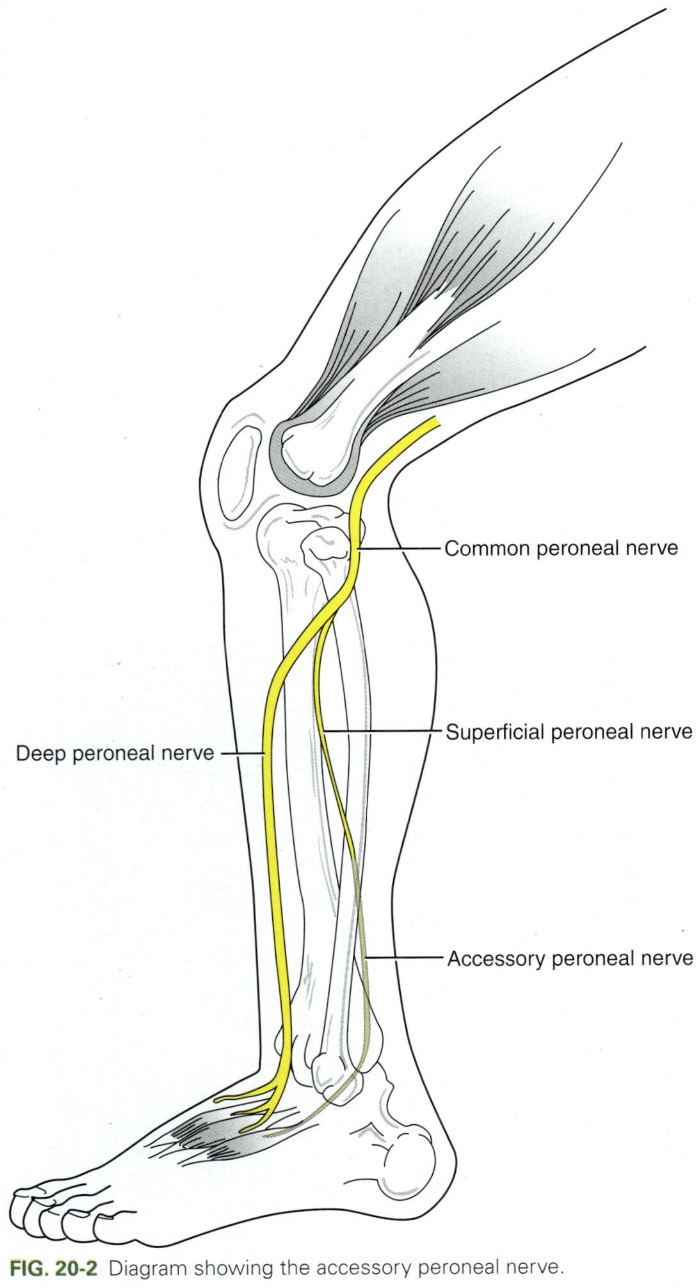

FIG. 20-2 Diagram showing the accessory peroneal nerve.

some large motor unit potentials were seen in the extensor hallucis longus. These muscles are innervated mainly by L4 and L5 roots. The lack of denervation in the vastus lateralis suggests that the L4 was not affected, and the negative findings in the gastrocnemius ruled out an S1 root involvement. Thus all denervated muscles originate from the L5 root, particularly the tensor fasciae lata which is innervated primarily by this root. Although the paraspinal muscles were normal, the electrophysiologic diagnoses were a left L5 radiculopathy and an accessory deep peroneal nerve.

WHAT SHOULD BE THE NEXT TEST FOR THIS PATIENT?

MRI has become the most important imaging study of the lumbosacral spine; CT, lumbar myelography, and post-myelogram CT are also useful. Because spinal abnormalities can be found in normal persons, the findings of these tests should be correlated with the clinical presentation and the results of electrophysiologic tests.

An MRI of the lumbosacral spine showed a herniated lateral L5–S1 disk compressing the L5 root (Fig. 20-3).

The patient was treated with conservative management with physiotherapy without improvement. She was referred to neurosurgery and underwent removal of the disk using laser surgery.

SUMMARY

A 34-year-old female with leg pain was found to have an L5 radiculopathy caused by a herniated disk seen on MRI. She also had an accessory deep peroneal nerve.

IMPORTANT POINTS

- An accessory deep peroneal nerve is a normal anatomic variant that occurs in up to 28% of individuals. The diagnosis is suspected because of lower-amplitude CMAP obtained with distal peroneal nerve stimulation compared with the CMAP obtained with proximal stimulation. To confirm this variation, the examiner should stimulate the nerve laterally, behind the lateral malleolus.
- The most important electrodiagnostic finding in radiculopathy is the presence of myotomal denervation, particularly if there is sparing of the paraspinal muscles. Paraspinal denervation helps in the diagnosis, but its absence does not rule out radiculopathy.
- MRI of the spine is valuable in the evaluation of patients with a lumbosacral radiculopathy, but as abnormalities can be seen in normal people, the interpretation of the findings should be correlated with the clinical presentation and the results of the electrophysiologic tests.
- Radiculopathies caused by herniated lumbar disks can be treated conservatively. Surgery should be considered if there is persistent pain or progressive and prolonged deficits.

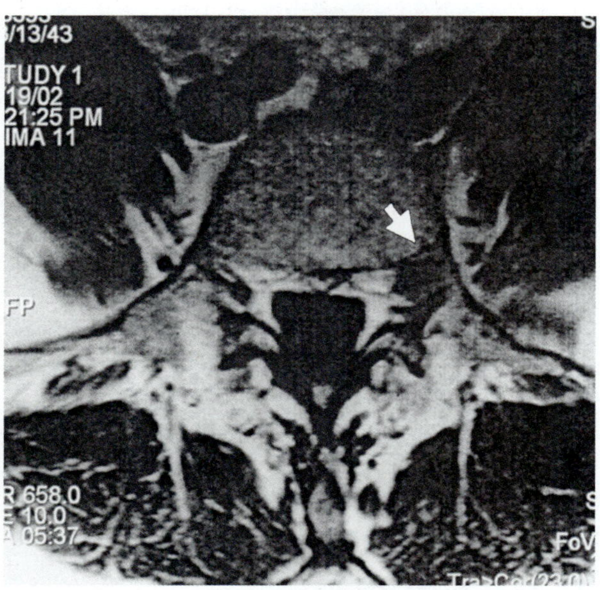

FIG. 20-3 Axial T2-weighted MRI image of the spine showing a lateral L5, S1 disk herniation (*arrow*).

DISCUSSION (CASES 18–20)

In *Case 18*, a woman presented with a history of back pain and leg weakness and numbness in the territory of the L4 root, and muscles supplied by L4 were denervated on EMG. Thus she was diagnosed to have an L4 radiculopathy; however, while these findings are most useful in the diagnosis, they should always be interpreted with some caution for a definitive anatomic diagnosis because of the variable innervation of the lower extremity muscles.[13,14]

In radiculopathies, motor nerve conduction studies and SNAPs are usually normal, but occasionally the SNAPs may be abnormal from large lateral lesions that affect the posterior root ganglia. The routinely tested SNAPs do not evaluate the upper lumbosacral plexus and thus are not useful in differentiating upper lumbosacral plexus lesions from root lesions. Needle EMG is the most important study for lesions of the upper roots.

An L4 radiculopathy is most likely caused by a central or paracentral herniated L3–L4 disk or a laterally herniated L4–L5 disk[14,15] (Fig. 20-4). Other causes of radiculopathy include, among others, osteoarthritis with facet hypertrophy, tumors, and infections.[14,15] MRI is the best imaging technique in lumbar radiculopathy, and CT myelogram can also be useful.[9]

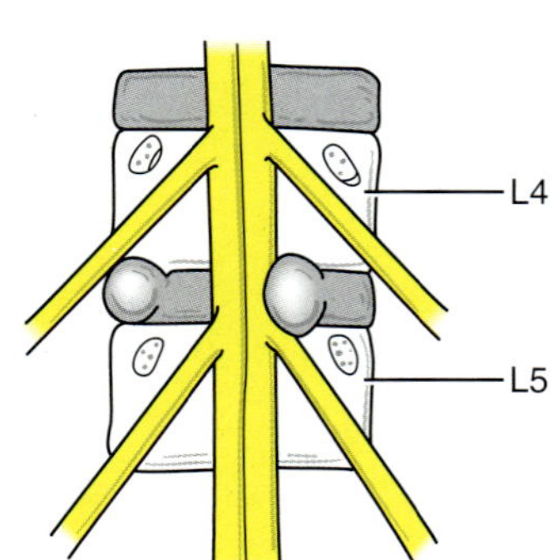

FIG. 20-4 Diagram showing a lateral disk compressing the upper root.

Case 19 had symptoms involving the left S1 dermatome and decreased/absent left ankle jerk and positive straight leg raising. Her H-reflex was prolonged in the left. This case underscored the utility of the H-reflex in diagnosis, with its absence or prolonged latency only in the affected limb compared with the unaffected leg in S1 radiculopathy.[7,8] Abnormal H-reflexes, however, may also occur in tibial and sciatic neuropathies and plexopathies.

Case 20 had an accessory left peroneal nerve, which was proved by stimulating the deep peroneal nerve at the lateral ankle. The anomaly is important to recognize as the changes in amplitude of the peroneal CMAP between distal and proximal stimulation sites can cause difficulties in the diagnosis of peroneal neuropathies.

Other anomalous innervations of the legs include a tibial-to-peroneal nerve communication in which stimulation of the tibial nerve produces a CMAP in the peroneus longus muscles.[16] There are also reports of an "all tibial foot," a variant in which the tibial motor axons travel within the sural nerve.[16]

The accessory deep peroneal nerve arises from the superficial peroneal nerve midway of the lateral aspect of the leg and passes deep and posterior to the peroneus brevis tendon behind the lateral malleolus[17–19] (see Fig. 20-2). This anomaly appears to have an autosomal dominant inheritance, and Crutchfield and Gutmann[18] found that 78% of relatives had this anomaly compared with 22% of unrelated individuals.[18]

This case was also diagnosed as having an L5 radiculopathy despite the lack of paraspinal muscle denervation, as this does not rule out a radiculopathy, because the lesion could spare the posterior rami.[20–22] On the other hand, denervation in the paraspinal muscles could also occur in other conditions such as peripheral neuropathies, myopathies, and motor neuron disorders[23–25] and even in normal people.[26] Thus their presence alone does not provide a definitive diagnosis of a radiculopathy.

The initial treatment of radiculopathies is conservative. Surgery is indicated in those with severe deficits or cauda equina syndrome, intractable pain, or progressive symptoms. Otherwise, the long-term outcome is similar with either conservative or surgical treatment.[15,27–30]

REFERENCES

1. Dyck P. The femoral nerve traction test with lumbar disc protrusions. *Surg Neurol*. 1976;6:163–166.
2. Thage O. The myotomes L2-S2 in man. *Acta Neurol Scand*. 1965;41(suppl 13):241–243.
3. Hinchey JA, Preston DC, Logigian EL. Idiopathic lumbosacral neuropathy: a cause of persistent leg pain. *Muscle Nerve*. 1996;19:1484–1486.
4. Eidelberg D, Sotrel A, Vogel H, et al. Progressive polyradiculopathy in acquired immune deficiency syndrome. *Neurology*. 1986;36:912–916.
5. Behar R, Wiley C, McCutchan JA. Cytomegalovirus polyradiculoneuropathy in acquired immune deficiency syndrome. *Neurology*. 1987;37:557–561.
6. Said G, Lacroix C, Chemouilli P, et al. Cytomegalovirus neuropathy in acquired immunodeficiency syndrome: a clinical and pathological study. *Ann Neurol*. 1991;29:139–146.
7. Kuruoglu R, Oh SJ, Thompson B. Clinical and electromyographic correlations of lumbosacral radiculopathy. *Muscle Nerve*. 1994; 17(2):250–251.
8. Oh SJ. Nerve conduction velocity tests: their clinical applications. In: Bertorini TE, ed. *Clinical Evaluation and Diagnostic Tests for Neuromuscular Disorders*. Boston, MA: Butterworth-Heinemann; 2002:141–208.
9. Wilbourn AJ, Aminoff MJ. Radiculopathies. In: Brown WF, Bolton CF, eds. *Clinical Electromyography*. 2nd ed. Boston, MA: Butterworth-Heinemann; 1993:177–209.
10. Wilbourn AJ. The value and limitation of electromyographic examination in the diagnosis of lumbosacral radiculopathy. In: Hardy RW, ed. *Lumbar Disc Disease*. New York, NY: Raven Press; 1982:65–109.
11. Deschuytere J, Rosselle N. Electromyographic and neurophysiological investigation in root compression syndromes in man. *Electromyography*. 1970;10(4):339–340.
12. Gutmann L. Atypical deep peroneal neuropathy in presence of accessory deep peroneal nerve. *J Neurol Neurosurg Psychiatry*. 1970;33:453–456.
13. Phillips LH, Park TS. Electrophysiological mapping of the segmental anatomy of the muscles of the lower extremity. *Muscle Nerve*. 1991;14:1213–1218.
14. Andersson GB, Deyo RA. History and physical examination in patients with herniated lumbar discs. *Spine*. 1996;21: 10S–18S.
15. Stewart JD. Cauda equina, lumbar and sacral nerve roots, and spinal nerves. In: Stewart JD, ed. *Focal Peripheral Neuropathies*. 3rd ed. Philadelphia, PA: Lippincott Williams & Wilkins; 2000: 315–353.
16. Oh SJ. *Clinical Electromyography: Nerve Conduction Studies*. 3rd ed. Philadelphia, PA: Lippincott Williams & Wilkins; 2003: 345–364.
17. Crutchfield C. *Variation in Innervation of the Extensor Digitorum Brevis Muscle* [Ph.D. thesis]. West Virginia University; 1970.
18. Crutchfield C, Gutmann L. Hereditary aspects of accessory deep peroneal nerve. *J Neurol Neurosurg Psychiatry*. 1973;36: 989–990.
19. Lambert EH. The accessory deep peroneal nerve: a common variation in innervation of extensor digitorum brevis. *Neurology*. 1969;19:1169–1176.
20. Czyrny JJ, Lawrence J. Importance of paraspinal muscle electromyography in cervical and lumbosacral myopathies. *Am J Phys Med Rehabil*. 1995;74:458–459.
21. Kuruoglu R, Oh SJ, Thompson B. Clinical and electromyographic correlations of lumbosacral radiculopathy. *Muscle Nerve*. 1994;17:250–251.
22. Levin K. L5 radiculopathy with reduced superficial peroneal sensory response: intraspinal and extraspinal causes. *Muscle Nerve*. 1998;21(1):3–7.
23. Wilbourn AJ, Aminoff MF. AAEM minimonograph 32: the electrodiagnostic examination in patients with radiculopathies. *Muscle Nerve*. 1998;21:1612–1631.
24. Dumitru D. *Electrodiagnostic Medicine*. Philadelphia, PA: Hanley & Belfus; 1995.
25. Wilbourn AJ. The diabetic neuropathies. In: Brown WF, Bolton CF, eds. *Clinical Electromyography*. 2nd ed. Boston, MA: Butterworth-Heinemann; 1993:477–515.
26. Nardin RA, Raynor EM, Rutkove SB. Fibrillations in lumbosacral paraspinal muscles of normal subjects. *Muscle Nerve*. 1998;21(10):1347–1349.

27. Epstein NE. Evaluation of varied surgical approaches used in the management of 170 far-lateral lumbar disc herniations: indications and results. *J Neurosurg*. 1995;83:648–656.
28. Andersson GB, Brown MD, Dvorak J, et al. Consensus summary of the diagnosis and treatment of lumbar disc herniation. *Spine*. 1996;21:75S–78S.
29. Weber H. Lumbar disc herniation: a controlled, prospective study with ten years of observation. *Spine*. 1983;8:131–140.
30. Hakelius A. Prognosis in sciatica: a clinical follow-up of surgical and non-surgical treatment. *Acta Orthop Scand Suppl*. 1970;41(suppl 129):1–76.

A Man With Pheochromocytoma and Back Pain

A 46-year-old male was referred for evaluation because of intense low back pain and tingling in the anterior aspect of the right thigh for about 3 weeks' duration.

He was diagnosed to have pheochromocytoma 3½ years earlier. At that time he presented with an abdominal mass which was resected, but he did not have systemic manifestations of pheochromocytoma, as the tumor was nonfunctional. He received chemotherapy for 2 years. Past medical history was otherwise unremarkable.

Family history was noncontributory except for a sister who had Hodgkin disease.

General physical examination was unremarkable except for mild tenderness on palpation of the back. Cranial nerves were normal. Strength and reflexes were normal, except for the right knee and adductor reflexes which were trace. There was decreased sensation to light touch and pinprick over the anterior aspect of the right thigh.

WHAT IS THE DIFFERENTIAL DIAGNOSIS?

The distribution of symptoms and findings suggests a disorder affecting nerve roots L2–L4, particularly because of the decreased knee and adductor reflexes on the right and decreased sensation in the anterior aspect of the thigh.

The possibility that this is produced by tumor invasion to the spine is an important consideration. The differential diagnosis includes a disk herniation.

AN EMG TEST WAS PERFORMED

Motor Nerve Studies

Nerve and Site	Latency (ms)	Amplitude (mV)	Conduction Velocity (m/s)
Peroneal Nerve R.	**Normal ≤ 5.7**	**Normal ≥ 3**	**Normal ≥ 40**
Ankle	5.5	3	–
Fibular head	13.0	3	43
Tibial Nerve R.	**Normal ≤ 5.3**	**Normal ≥ 4**	**Normal ≥ 40**
Ankle	4.5	20	–
Pop. fossa	14.7	16	42

F-Wave and Tibial H-Reflex Studies

Nerve	Latency (ms)	Normal Latency ≤ (ms)
Peroneal nerve R.	54.0	54
Tibial nerve R.	52.5	54
H-reflex R.	29.1	34
H-reflex L.	29.0	34

Sensory Nerve Studies

Nerve	Onset Latency (ms)	Normal Onset Latency ≤ (ms)	Peak Latency (ms)	Normal Peak Latency ≤ (ms)	Amp (μV)	Normal Amp ≥ (μV)	Conduction Velocity (m/s)	Normal Conduction Velocity ≥ (m/s)
Sural nerve R.	3.4	3.5	3.9	4.0	22	13	41	40

EMG Data

Muscle	Insrt Activity	Fibs	Pos Waves	Fasc	Amp	Dur	Poly	Pattern
Lumbar paraspinals R.	**Inc**	None	**2+**	None	Norm	Norm	None	Full
Iliopsoas R.	**CRDs**	None	None	None	None	Norm	None	Full
Vastus lateralis R.	Norm	None	None	None	Norm	Norm	None	Full
Adductor longus R.	**Inc**	**1+**	**1+**	None	Norm	Norm	None	Full
Adductor magnus R.	**Inc**	None	None	None	Norm	Norm	None	Full
Gracilis R.	**Inc**	**1+**	**1+**	None	Norm	Norm	None	Full
Tibialis anterior R.	Norm	None	None	None	Norm	Norm	None	Full
Peroneus longus R.	Norm	None	None	None	Norm	Norm	None	Full
Gastrocnemius R.	Norm	None	None	None	Norm	Norm	None	Full

WHAT WERE THE EMG FINDINGS?

The nerve conduction tests were normal, and EMG was normal in muscles innervated by L4–S1, but there were denervation potentials in the adductor longus (mainly L2–L3 root) and the gracilis that is innervated mainly by L2; there was only mild increased insertional activity in the adductor magnus (L3–L4).

There was no denervation in the quadriceps muscle (L2–L4, but mainly L3–L4). There was mild denervation in the iliopsoas (L1–L3). Denervation was also seen in the paraspinal muscles.

This electrophysiologic study localized a lesion at the L2 and L3 roots, but mainly L2.

MRI of the spine showed pathologic fracture from tumor invasion (Fig. 21-1).

The patient underwent back surgery with resection of the lesion and reconstruction of the spine, as well as an anterior fixation.

It was concluded that this L2 radiculopathy was caused by tumor invasion.

DISCUSSION

This patient with a pheochromocytoma had a radiculopathy, and his EMG showed denervation in limb muscles innervated by L2, and the lower paraspinal muscles. This case underscores the fact that focal radiculopathies are not always caused by disk disease, and that other causes, such as tumors, should be considered in the diagnosis.

The most common symptoms of pheochromocytomas are related to hypertension and cardiac arrhythmias.[1] Other symptoms include palpitations, headache, anxiety and panic disorders, and diaphoresis, and physicians usually suspect this disorder in patients with severe hypertension. However, some are normotensive, as was this patient.[2]

Extraadrenal tumors have an increased risk of being malignant. Nonfunctional tumors are found sometimes incidentally on autopsy.[3] Twenty-five percent of pheochromocytomas result from genetic mutations.[4] The tumor is seen more frequently in males, and 10% of these are malignant, 10% are bilateral, and 10% are extraadrenal.

The best diagnostic laboratory markers for functional pheochromocytomas include measurement of plasma metanephrine, which is 99% sensitive and 89% specific. Other laboratory tests include measurement of catecholamines in plasma and urine, and urinary vanillylmandelic acid.[5]

MRI and CT scanning of the abdomen are useful in diagnosis. Radionuclear scanning with metaiodobenzylguanidine is 100% specific for this type of tumor.

The prognosis of malignant pheochromocytomas is not determined by the histology, but primarily by the location of the tumor and evidence of invasion.

The treatment requires proper management of blood pressure, using alpha 1-adrenergic antagonist therapy, and tumor removal.

The 10-year survival rate is 45%.[2,6] Metastatic lesions tend to grow slowly and respond poorly to chemotherapy.[7] They may respond to radiation therapy but can recur even 15 years after resection.[2,6]

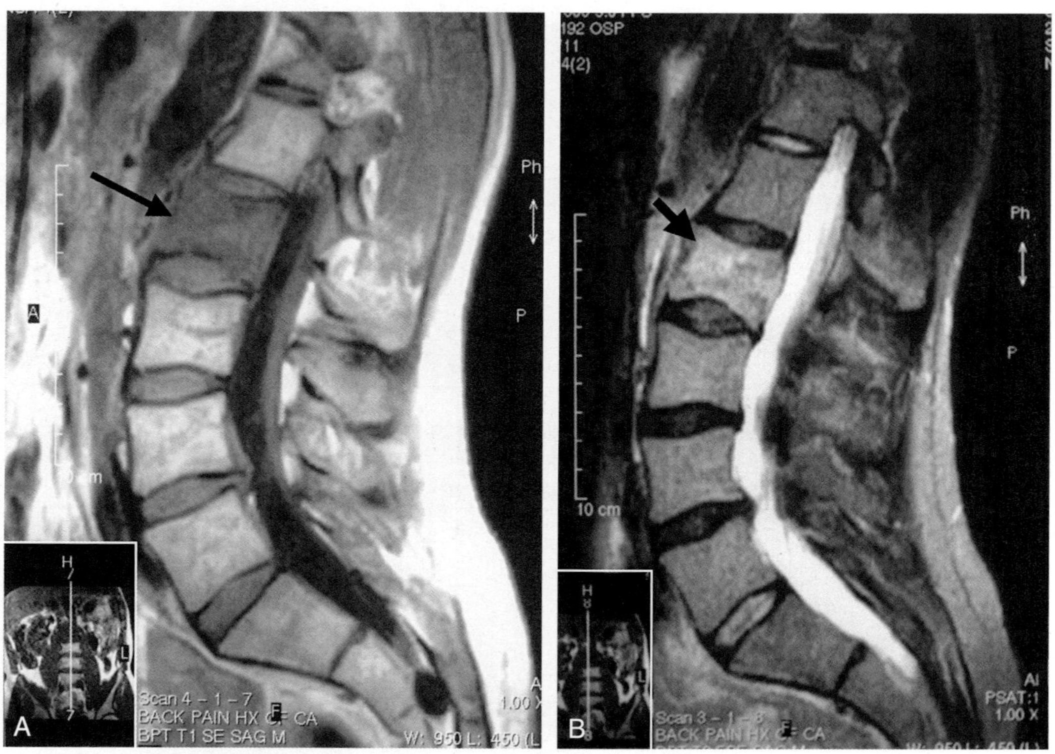

FIG. 21-1 **A**, T1-weighted MRI (sagittal view) showing the L2 vertebral body replaced by tumor (*arrow*). **B**, T2-weighted MRI (sagittal view) showing the hyperintense tumor in the vertebral body (*arrow*).

SUMMARY

This man presented with an L2 radiculopathy caused by recurrent pheochromocytoma invading the L2 vertebra. He was treated with reconstruction surgery and later with radiation.

IMPORTANT POINTS

- The diagnosis of L2 radiculopathy was based on the presence of denervation in the iliopsoas, gracilis, adductor longus, and lumbar paraspinal muscles, but not in the quadriceps or L5- and S1-innervated muscles.
- L2 radiculopathies are rarely caused by disks but can be caused by tumors.
- Pheochromocytoma is a neuroendocrine tumor of the adrenal gland associated with hypertension, but some patients may have normal blood pressure.
- Some pheochromocytomas can be located outside the adrenal glands.
- The best way to diagnose functional pheochromocytoma is by measurement of plasma metanephrine levels and imaging.
- The treatment of pheochromocytoma consists of removal of the tumor and radiation, as it does not respond well to chemotherapy.
- Pheochromocytomas might recur and be metastatic even after many years.

REFERENCES

1. O'Riordain DS, Young WF, Grant CS, et al. Clinical spectrum and outcome of functional extraadrenal paraganglioma. *World J Surg.* 1996;20:916–921.
2. Goldstein RE, O'Neill JA, Holcomb GW III, et al. Clinical experience over 48 years with pheochromocytoma. *Ann Surg.* 1999;229:755–764.
3. Mannelli M, Ianni L, Cilotti A, et al. Pheochromocytoma in Italy: a multicentric retrospective study. *Eur J Endocrinol.* 1999; 141:619–624.
4. Neumann HPH, Bausch B, McWhinney SR, et al. for the Freiburg-Warsaw-Columbus Pheochromocytoma Study Group. Germ-line mutations in nonsyndromic pheochromocytoma. *N Engl J Med.* 2002;346:1459–1466.
5. Lenders JW, Pacak K, Walther MM, et al. Biochemical diagnosis of pheochromocytoma: what test is best? *JAMA.* 2002;287: 1427–1434.
6. Bertorini TE, Perez A. Neurologic complications of disorders of the adrenal glands. *Handb Clin Neurol.* 2014;120:749–771.
7. Lam KY, Lo CY, Wat NM, et al. The clinicopathological features and importance of p53, Rb, and mdm2 expression in pheochromocytomas and paragangliomas. *J Clin Pathol.* 2001;54:443–448.

22 CASE

A Diabetic Man With Back and Leg Pain

A 60-year-old, type 2 diabetic man woke up 2 months prior to admission with back pain that radiated to the left leg below the knee, particularly in the inner side of the leg. It was a nonspecific ache, not a shooting pain. This worsened when having bowel movements. He was more uncomfortable when he sat or stretched out his legs to sleep at night. He took nonsteroidal antiinflammatories without relief.

Past medical history was unremarkable. His diabetes was controlled with oral agents. Family history was noncontributory. He did not smoke, drink, or use recreational drugs.

General physical examination was essentially unremarkable. Neurologic examination showed normal mentation, cranial nerves, and muscle strength; reflexes were 2+ in the upper extremities and the right knee, the left knee reflex was absent, and they were trace at both ankles. There were no pathologic reflexes. Sensory examination showed diminished vibration and touch sensations in the toes and normal pinprick sensation throughout, except for the left anterior thigh. Straight leg raising and femoral stretch were negative. Coordination was normal.

WHAT IS THE DIFFERENTIAL DIAGNOSIS?

This diabetic patient presented with pain in the back and leg, decreased sensation in the anterior left thigh, and an absent knee jerk, which are highly suggestive of an L3–L4 root disease. A mild femoral neuropathy or lumbosacral plexopathy could not be ruled out clinically.

The increased pain with effort might suggest a root compression, and clinically the patient also had signs of a peripheral neuropathy.

Various etiologies should be considered for his presentation, including a ruptured disk, facet hypertrophy, spinal or plexus tumor, and diabetic lumbosacral radiculoplexopathy.[1–4] However, the back pain and lack of significant weakness are against this diagnosis.

WHAT DIAGNOSTIC TESTS SHOULD BE DONE?

His fasting blood sugar was 180 mg/dL (normal, 65–120 mg/dL) and his glycosylated hemoglobin was 6.2% (normal, 5%–9%). Erythrocyte sedimentation rate, chemistry profile, and thyroid-stimulating hormone levels were normal.

AN EMG TEST WAS PERFORMED

Motor Nerve Studies

Nerve and Site	Latency(ms)	Amplitude (mV)	Conduction Velocity (m/s)
Peroneal Nerve L.	**Normal ≤ 5.7**	**Normal ≥ 3**	**Normal ≥ 40**
Ankle	5.0	5	–
Fibular head	15.4	3	**32**
Knee	17.3	3	47

Nerve and Site	Latency (ms)	Amplitude (mV)	Conduction Velocity (m/s)
Tibial Nerve R.	**Normal ≤ 5.3**	**Normal ≥ 4**	**Normal ≥ 40**
Ankle	4.9	8	–
Pop. fossa	18.2	7	**32**

Nerve and Site	Latency (ms)	Amplitude (mV)	Conduction Velocity (m/s)
Ulnar Nerve L.	**Normal ≤ 3.6**	**Normal ≥ 8**	**Normal ≥ 50**
Wrist	3.0	15	–
Below elbow	7.3	13	51

F-Wave and Tibial H-Reflex Studies

Nerve	Latency (ms)	Normal Latency ≤ (ms)
Peroneal nerve L.	53.2	54
Tibial nerve R.	52.8	54
Ulnar nerve L.	28.7	30
H-reflex L.	33.6	34
H-reflex R.	33.2	34

Sensory Nerve Studies

Nerve	Onset Latency (ms)	Normal Onset Latency ≤ (ms)	Peak Latency (ms)	Normal Peak Latency ≤ (ms)	Amp (µV)	Normal Amp ≥ (µV)	Conduction Velocity (m/s)	Normal Conduction Velocity ≥ (m/s)
Sural nerve L.	3.5	3.5	4.0	4.0	16	11	40	40
Ulnar nerve L.	2.4	2.6	2.9	3.1	13	13	50	50

EMG Data

Muscle	Insrt Activity	Fibs	Pos Waves	Fasc	Amp	Dur	Poly	Pattern
Lumbar paraspinals L.	**Inc**	**None**	2+	None	Norm	Norm	None	Full
Iliopsoas L.	**Inc**	2+	2+	None	Norm	Norm	None	Full
Tensor fasciae latae L.	**Inc**	2+	2+	None	Norm	Norm	None	**Red**
Vastus lateralis L.	**Inc**	**None**	2+	None	Norm	Norm	None	**Red**
Adductor longus L.	**Inc**	1+	1+	None	Norm	Norm	None	Full
Tibialis anterior L.	**Inc**	None	1+	None	Norm	Norm	None	**Red**
Peroneus longus L.	**Inc**	None	1+	None	Norm	Norm	None	Full
Gastrocnemius L.	Norm	None	None	None	Norm	Norm	None	Full
Lumbar paraspinals R.	Norm	None	None	None	Norm	Norm	None	Full
Tensor fasciae latae R.	Norm	None	None	None	Norm	Norm	None	Full
Vastus lateralis R.	Norm	None	None	None	Norm	Norm	None	Full
Tibialis anterior R.	Norm	None	None	None	Norm	Norm	None	Full
Gastrocnemius R.	Norm	None	None	None	Norm	Norm	None	Full

WHAT WERE THE EMG FINDINGS?

The nerve conduction test showed mild slowing of tibial and peroneal nerve motor conduction velocities with normal distal latencies and CMAP amplitudes. Latencies of the F-responses and H-reflexes were prolonged, and the sural nerve SNAP was normal. The ulnar SNAP was of low amplitude, but the motor test of this nerve was normal. The needle test showed denervation of the muscles innervated by L4 (tibialis anterior, adductors, and vastus lateralis) and L5 (tensor fasciae latae, tibialis anterior, and peroneus longus); reduced motor unit recruitment was also seen in the muscles, and there was denervation in the iliopsoas, which is usually innervated by L3, but could cause partial innervation by L4. Muscles innervated by the S1 root were spared.[5]

These findings are suggestive of a lumbosacral radiculopathy affecting mainly L3–L4, but also L5, innervated muscles. He also had paraspinal muscle denervation. A lumbosacral radiculopathy was diagnosed. Diabetic lumbosacral radiculoplexopathy or diabetic amyotrophy, however, can also show denervation in the paraspinal muscles.[2,6] There were also findings of a mild polyneuropathy with some mild demyelinating features.

WHAT WOULD BE THE NEXT TEST?

The next test was an MRI of the lumbosacral spine which showed an L4–L5 disk herniation that obliterated the foramina, extended laterally (Fig. 22-1), and was compressing the L4 root; and there was a disk fragment that migrated upward. The denervation in the iliopsoas could not completely be explained. It is likely that in this case this muscle received innervation from the L4 root.

WHAT WOULD ONE DO NEXT?

The patient was given conservative management with physical therapy and improved significantly. After 6 months he was back to normal, except for evidence of a mild neuropathy on examination.

DISCUSSION

This diabetic man presented with back pain and sensory deficit in the left thigh without weakness, and his knee jerk was absent. This suggests an L3–L4 radiculopathy, and indeed, he had denervation in L4, but also L5, innervated muscles. A diabetic lumbosacral plexopathy was a consideration, but patients with this disease usually do not have back pain and have thigh muscle weakness.[6] The MRI showed a lateral disk herniation at L4–L5, compressing the L5 nerve root and extending laterally and upward, also affecting the L4 root, likely causing his symptoms. He was treated conservatively with muscle relaxants, antiinflammatory drugs, and physical therapy. He has done very well for the past 3 years. This case emphasizes that diabetics with focal neurologic problems should always be worked up for other causes and that discogenic disease responds to conservative treatment. (See also discussions of *Cases 18–20*.)

SUMMARY

This diabetic patient had a radiculopathy and had denervation in L4 and L5 innervated muscles, but also in the iliopsoas (L3). MRI showed a lateral disk from L4 to L5 compressing the L4 and L5 roots, which was likely the cause of his symptoms.

IMPORTANT POINTS

- In a diabetic patient with limb and back pain the differential diagnoses include a ruptured disk, spinal stenosis, a spinal tumor or other masses, and diabetic amyotrophy, but this condition usually manifests with weakness.
- L4–L5 disk herniation usually affects the L5 root, but if it is located laterally, it could affect the L4 root.
- Conservative management is frequently beneficial in disk herniation; surgery is performed if there is no improvement or if there is persistent pain or deterioration.

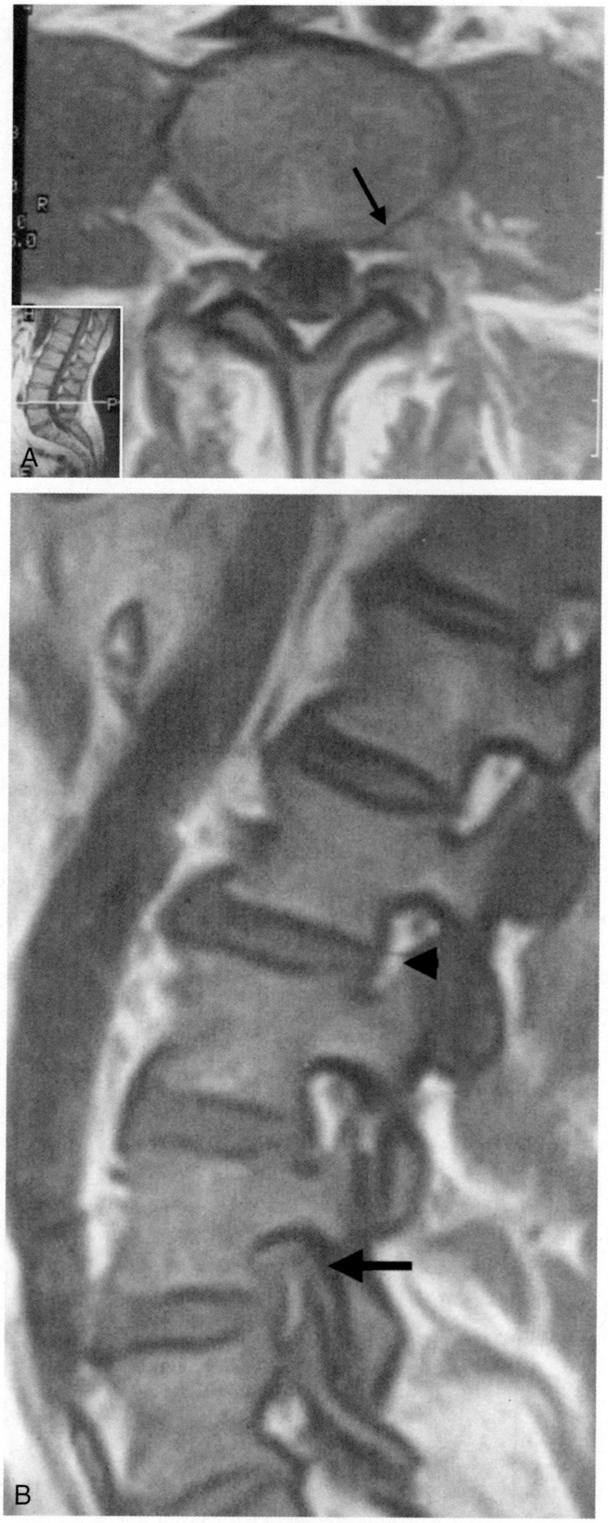

FIG. 22-1 **A**, MRI of lumbosacral spine, axial view; notice large lateral disk herniation (*arrow*). **B**, Sagittal view, T2-weighted image; notice the herniated disk between L4 and L5 with an upward migrated fragment and the disappearance of the root canal fat (*arrow*). Compare this with the normal fat in an unaffected area (*arrowhead*).

REFERENCES

1. Bertorini TE. Clinical evaluation and clinical laboratory tests. In: Bertorini TE, ed. *Clinical Evaluation and Diagnostic Tests for Neuromuscular Disorders*. Boston, MA: Butterworth-Heinemann; 2002:15–98.
2. Chokroverty S, Reyes MG, Rubino FA, Tonata H. The syndrome of diabetic amyotrophy. *Ann Neurol*. 1977;2:181–194.
3. Hardy RW, Plank NM. Clinical diagnosis of the lumbosacral herniated lumbar disc. In: Hardy RW, ed. *Lumbar Disc Disease*. New York, NY: Raven Press; 1982:17–28.
4. Stewart JD, Caude TU. The cauda equina, lumbar and sacral nerve root and spinal nerves. In: Stewart JD, ed. *Focal Peripheral Neuropathies*. New York, NY: Elsevier; 1987:718–719.
5. Raynor EM, Kleiner-Fisman G, Nardin R. Lumbosacral thoracic radiculopathies. In: Katirji B, Kaminski HJ, Preston DC, eds. *Neuromuscular Disorders in Clinical Practice*. Boston, MA: Butterworth-Heinemann; 2002:859–883.
6. Dyck PJ, Windebank AJ. Diabetic and nondiabetic lumbosacral radiculoplexus neuropathies: new insights into pathophysiology and treatment. *Muscle Nerve*. 2002;25:477–491.

A Man With Leg Pain While Walking

A 52-year-old man was referred for evaluation of intermittent pain in the legs and back for 12 years which was associated with leg numbness. The pain radiated to the right hip and leg. Initially, he was found to have an L3–L4 disk herniation, and this was treated conservatively with improvement.

During the last 5 years, he again developed pain in the legs that worsened when he walked and improved with rest, particularly when seated. He also had numbness in the right first and second toes, which had become persistent for a 6-month period, and complained of paresthesias in the soles of his feet. In addition, he gave a 3-week history of numbness in the perianal area and penis.

His past medical history was remarkable for mild glucose intolerance which improved with diet. He was involved in a motor vehicle accident and sustained a fractured clavicle in the remote past and had a history of migraine headaches. Family history was pertinent for a grandmother with diabetes.

Neurologic examination revealed normal mentation and cranial nerves. Strength was normal except for weakness of both toe dorsiflexors, worse on the right with atrophy of the extensor digitorum brevis (EDB) muscles. He was able to walk on his tiptoes and heels. Reflexes were trace at the left ankle, absent on the right, and 1+ in both knees. There were no Babinski signs. Straight leg raising was negative. He had absent vibration sense in the toes and decreased at the ankle on the right but not on the left. There were decreased vibration and pinprick sensations up to the ankles bilaterally. Penile and perianal sensation were normal, but he had no bulbocavernosus reflex. The anal sphincter tone was mildly decreased. Arterial pulses were normal. The rest of the neurologic examination was normal.

WHAT IS THE DIFFERENTIAL DIAGNOSIS?

This patient had a history of chronic back pain with leg pain that increased while walking. This is suggestive of neurogenic claudication which could be caused by spinal stenosis but could have other causes, such as intraspinal masses.[1] There was also a clinical suggestion of a neuropathy likely from diabetes, although other causes should also be considered. The back and leg pain were not from a neuropathy, as this usually is a distal burning pain with tingling paresthesias that occurs mainly at night and does not worsen with activity. His presentation with the asymmetric findings in the neurologic examination is suggestive of a lumbosacral disease which could have several causes, such as diabetic radiculoplexopathy, or a diabetic neuropathy with superimposed radiculopathy. A spinal canal disease is the more likely diagnosis due to the chronic nature of his condition, the back pain, lack of muscle weakness, and the history of claudication.

The pain increased over 3 weeks and was accompanied by numbness in the perianal area and penis. This could be from a mid-low cauda equina syndrome caused by spinal stenosis, or a large L4–L5 disk, or by other lesions affecting the sacral nerve roots.

WHAT SHOULD BE DONE?

The fasting blood sugar and glycosylated hemoglobin were normal. Erythrocyte sedimentation rate, factor antinuclear antibodies (FANA), protein electrophoresis, and thyroid-stimulating hormone (TSH) and B_{12} levels were normal.

AN EMG TEST WAS PERFORMED

What Were the EMG Findings?

Motor Nerve Studies

Nerve and Site	Latency (ms)	Amplitude (mV)	Conduction Velocity (m/s)
Peroneal Nerve R.	**Normal ≤ 5.7**	**Normal ≥ 3**	**Normal ≥ 40**
Ankle	4.2	**1**	–
Fibular head	12.4	**1**	**39**
Knee	14.4	**1**	48

Nerve and Site	Latency (ms)	Amplitude (mV)	Conduction Velocity (m/s)
Tibial Nerve L.	**Normal ≤ 5.3**	**Normal ≥ 4**	**Normal ≥ 40**
Ankle	4.8	10	–
Pop. fossa	16.1	8	**39**

Nerve and Site	Latency (ms)	Amplitude (mV)	Conduction Velocity (m/s)
Ulnar Nerve R.	**Normal ≤ 3.6**	**Normal ≥ 8**	**Normal ≥ 50**
Wrist	3.2	13	–
Below elbow	6.9	13	57
Above elbow	9.2	13	52
Peroneal Nerve L.	**Normal ≤ 5.7**	**Normal ≥ 3**	**Normal ≥ 40**
Ankle	5.7	**2**	–
Fibular head	12.1	**2**	48

F-Wave and Tibial H-Reflex Studies

Nerve	Latency (ms)	Normal Latency ≤ (ms)
Peroneal nerve R.	**59.9**	54
Tibial nerve L.	**60.7**	54
Ulnar nerve R.	30.0	30
H-reflex R.	**39.2**	34
H-reflex L.	**39.0**	34

Sensory Nerve Studies

Nerve	Onset Latency (ms)	Normal Onset Latency ≤ (ms)	Peak Latency (ms)	Normal Peak Latency ≤ (ms)	Amp (μV)	Normal Amp ≥ (μV)	Conduction Velocity (m/s)	Normal Conduction Velocity ≥ (m/s)
Sural nerve R.	3.5	3.5	4.0	4.0	14	11	40	40
Superficial peroneal R.	**3.7**	3.5	**4.2**	4.0	9	8–10	40	40
Ulnar nerve R.	2.3	2.6	2.8	3.1	17	13	52	50

EMG Data

Muscle	Insrt Activity	Fibs	Pos Waves	Fasc	Amp	Dur	Poly	Pattern
Lumbar paraspinals R.	**Inc**	None	**1+**	None	Norm	Norm	**Few**	Full
Gluteus medius R.	Norm	None	None	None	**Lg**	**Inc**	None	Full
Tensor fasciae latae R.	Norm	None	None	None	**Lg**	**Inc**	None	Full
Vastus lateralis R.	Norm	None	None	None	Norm	Norm	None	Full
Tibialis anterior R.	Norm	None	None	None	**Lg**	**Inc**	None	Full
Peroneus longus R.	Norm	None	None	None	Norm	Norm	None	Full
Gastrocnemius R.	Norm	None	None	None	Norm	Norm	None	Full
Tensor fasciae latae L.	Norm	None	None	None	**Lg**	**Inc**	None	**Red**
Tibialis anterior L.	Norm	None	None	None	**Lg**	**Inc**	None	**Red**
Gastrocnemius L.	Norm	None	None	None	**Lg**	**Inc**	None	Full
Deltoid R.	Norm	None	None	None	Norm	Norm	None	Full
1st dorsal interosseus R.	Norm	None	None	None	**Lg**	**Inc**	None	**Red**

The EMG findings suggested a mild neuropathy with slow motor conduction velocities of the peroneal and tibial nerves and slightly prolonged superficial peroneal SNAP latency on the right. There was a low-amplitude peroneal CMAP which could have been caused by a neuropathy or could be secondary to an L5 radiculopathy. The prolonged F-responses and H-reflexes in the legs could be secondary to his neuropathy, but the F-latencies were normal in both arms, and although the legs are usually more affected in neuropathies, the prolongation seemed out of proportion to the conduction velocities. It is likely that the prolonged latencies were related to a lumbosacral disorder.

There were large motor units with reduced recruitment in the legs indicating a chronic neurogenic process, such as a neuropathy, as this was also present in the first dorsal interosseous muscle in the right. Large motor units were also present in the proximal leg muscles. In a patient with such a mild neuropathy, this is also more compatible with a spinal problem. This was reinforced by the presence of paraspinal denervation,[2–4] which was not present in the legs. Because of the overlap of the innervation of paraspinal muscles, electromyography cannot exactly localize the level of the lesion based on this alone.[5] Furthermore, as denervation in these muscles might also be seen in other conditions, and even in normal persons,[5] this is not necessarily diagnostic of a lumbosacral spinal problem. This should be correlated with clinical and other EMG findings.

Because of the clinical presentation, the prolonged late responses only in the legs and out of proportion with his nerve conduction studies, and the large motor unit potentials in proximal and distal muscles of the legs, it was concluded that he had a spinal canal disease in addition to a mild diabetic neuropathy.

WHAT SHOULD BE DONE NEXT?

An MRI of the lumbosacral spine showed severe spinal stenosis with prominent disk bulging, facet hypertrophy with canal compromise with stenosis at L3–L4 and L4–L5 (Fig. 23-1A and B), with only mild narrowing in the S1 area (Fig. 23-1C).

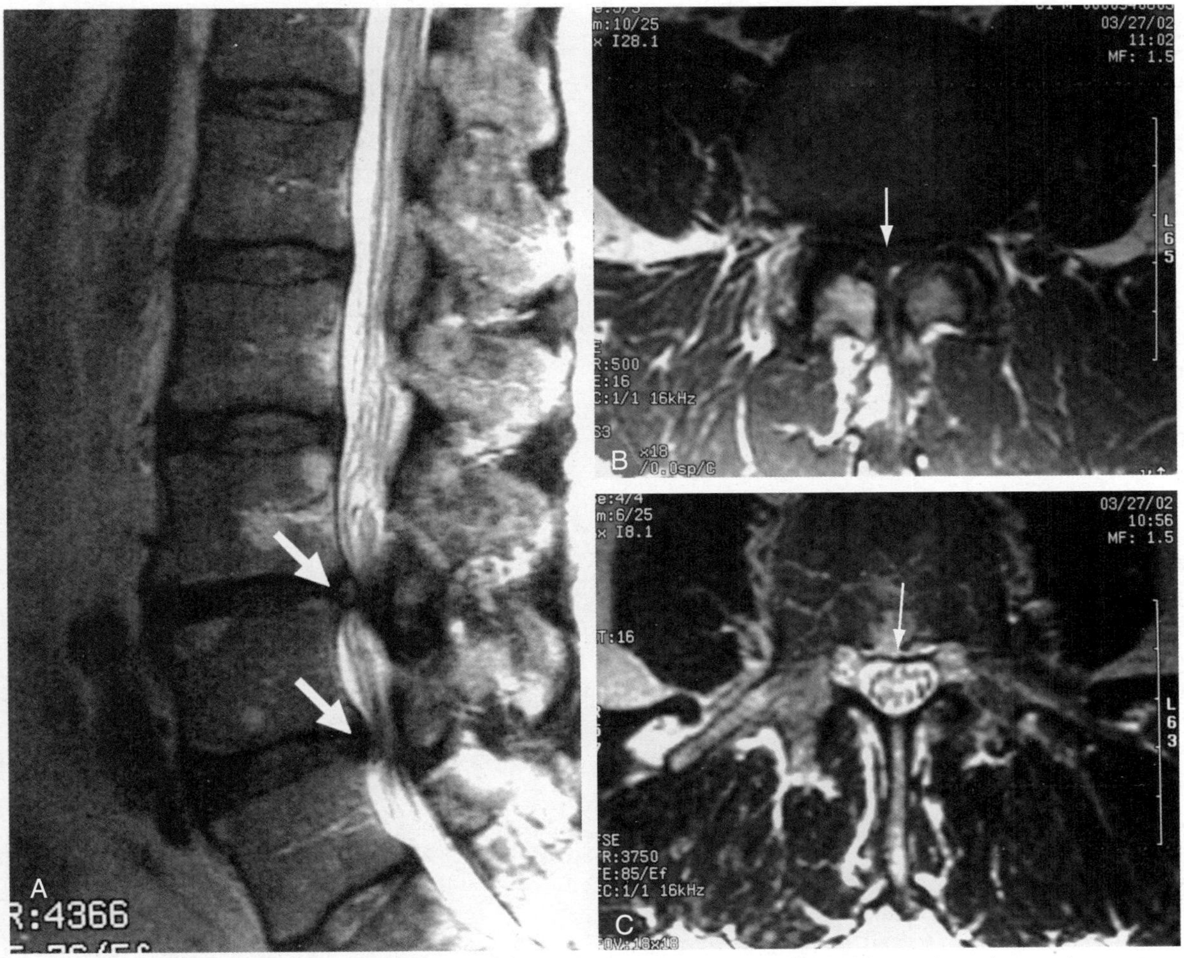

FIG. 23-1 A, MRI, T2-weighted image (sagittal view) showing prominent disk bulging and canal stenosis at L3–L4, L4–L5 (*arrows*). **B**, Very small canal seen in the axial view on MRI T2-weighted image at the L4–L5 level (*arrow*). **C**, Axial view MRI, T2-weighted image showing minimal stenosis at the L2 level (*arrow*).

WHAT SHOULD BE THE TREATMENT?

The patient underwent a lumbar decompression with bilateral hemilaminectomy at L2–L3, L3–L4, and L4–L5 with medial fasciotomies and foraminotomies using microdissection. This produced marked improvement of his symptoms. He is functioning normally now, 3 years after surgery.

DISCUSSION

This patient had a mild neuropathy likely from glucose intolerance and a cauda equina claudication caused by spinal canal stenosis.

This syndrome manifests by back and leg pain which increases or develops during physical activity and might be accompanied by weakness, numbness, paresthesias, and sphincter disturbances.[6,7] Sometimes, there could also be persistent weakness that resembles a neuropathy; the pain usually improves with rest. The pain increases with extension and the pain may decrease with flexion. The patient may have to walk with thoracic flexion or "Simian stance."

Acquired canal stenosis and cauda equina syndrome are often caused by severe degenerative osteoarthritis and disk herniation, which could be accompanied by a congenitally narrowed canal.[8] Large L4–L5 disks could also compress the sacral spinal roots of the central canal causing cauda equina syndrome. Other causes include rheumatoid arthritis, ankylosing spondylitis, arachnoiditis, infections, and interspinal tumors.[9–12]

The symptoms of neurogenic claudication can be insidious, but sometimes present abruptly. Patients may develop paralysis of the legs, which requires emergency neurosurgery. When the lesion includes the conus medullaris, patients have similar manifestations, with sphincter disturbance but also Babinski signs, which were not evident in this patient.

In most cases of symptomatic spinal stenosis, the best treatment is surgical decompression,[12–15] which should be done as a neurologic emergency in patients with acute cauda equina syndrome.

SUMMARY

A 52-year-old diabetic man with a mild neuropathy presented with back and leg pain aggravated by exercise. He was diagnosed as having neurogenic claudication caused by lumbar canal stenosis. He improved after surgical decompression.

IMPORTANT POINTS

- Neurogenic claudication or cauda equina syndrome manifests with pain in the back and legs during physical activity. The findings of the neurologic examination might be nonspecific or show weakness and decreased reflexes.
- The cauda equina syndrome results from a narrow spinal canal with compression of roots at the central canal, such as at the large L4–L5 disk, or from other conditions such as tumors affecting lumbosacral roots and spinal stenosis. Higher lesions might include the conus medullaris, which has a similar presentation, but also Babinski signs.
- Spinal stenosis simply refers to a narrowed spinal canal and may be asymptomatic. Stenosis is often caused by degenerative arthritis but also by other conditions such as rheumatoid arthritis or ankylosing spondylitis.
- Patients with cauda equina syndrome typically present with pain, bowel/bladder problems, and saddle anesthesia.
- Paraspinal muscles have overlap innervation, and thus it is hard to localize the level of the lesion based on denervation in these muscles in electromyography.
- Early recognition and treatment of cauda equina claudication is important to avoid progression and disability; an acute cauda equina syndrome is a neurosurgical emergency.

REFERENCES

1. Hardy RW, Plank NM. Clinical diagnosis of lumbosacral herniated lumbar disc. In: Hardy RW, ed. *Lumbar Disc Disease*. New York, NY: Raven Press; 1982:17–28.
2. Kirkaldy-Willis WH, Wedge JH, Young-Hing K, Reilly J. Pathology and pathogenesis of lumbar spondylosis and stenosis. *Spine*. 1978;3:319–328.
3. Johnson EW, Melvin JL. Value of electromyography in lumbar radiculopathy. *Arch Phys Med Rehabil*. 1971;52(6):239–243.
4. Leyshon A, Kirwan EO, Parry CB. Electrical studies in the diagnosis of compression of the lumbar root. *J Bone Joint Surg Br*. 1981;63(1):71–75.
5. Wilbourn AJ, Aminoff MJ. The electrodiagnostic examination in patients with radiculopathies. AAEM minimonograph 32. *Muscle Nerve*. 1998;21(12):1612–1631.
6. Blau JN, Logue V. The natural history of intermittent claudication of the cauda equina: a long-term follow-up study. *Brain*. 1978;101: 211–222.
7. Jellinger K, Neumayer E. Claudication of the spinal cord and cauda equina. In: Vinken PJ, Bruyn GW, eds. *Handbook of Clinical Neurology*. Amsterdam, North Holland; 1972:504–547.
8. Yates DA. Spinal stenosis. *J R Soc Med*. 1981;74:334–342.
9. Verbiest H. Further experiences of the pathological influence of a developmental narrowness of the bony lumbar vertebral canal. *J Bone Joint Surg Br*. 1955;37:576–583.
10. Bartleson JD. Cauda equina syndrome secondary to long-standing ankylosing spondylitis. *Ann Neurol*. 1983;14:662–669.
11. Fearnside MR, Adams CB. Tumors of the cauda equina. *J Neurol Neurosurg Psychiatry*. 1978;41:24–31.
12. Binder DK, Schmidt MH, Weinstein PR. Lumbar spinal stenosis. *Semin Neurol*. 2002;22(2):157–166.
13. Epstein NE. Surgical management of lumbar stenosis: decompression and indications for fusion. *Neurosurg Focus*. 1997;3(2):e1, discussion.
14. Hutchinson JL. Spinal stenosis. *J Natl Med Assoc*. 2004;96:384.
15. Munakomi S, Foris LA, Varacallo M. Spinal Stenosis and Neurogenic Claudication. In: *StatPearls (Internet)*. Last updated 04.07.22.

A Man With Foot Pain

A 60-year-old man came with a 12-month history of shooting pains in the sole of the left foot along with numbness in the sole and occasional pain which radiated from the hip down. This was worse when he remained seated for a long time.

Previous workup included a normal MRI of the lumbosacral spine and an EMG, upon which he was diagnosed as having a tarsal tunnel syndrome (TTS). He was treated with steroid injections and then later received a nonsteroidal antiinflammatory drug and amitriptyline.

Past medical history was positive for coronary stent placement 5 years previously. Family history was positive for diabetes.

Examination revealed an obese man who had normal mental function and cranial nerves. Muscle strength was normal. Reflexes were equal and symmetrical. Sensory examination was normal. There was no Tinel's sign in the retromalleolar area, but he had mild tenderness in the left hip. No mass was palpable, but this was hard to assess because of the patient's size. Straight leg raising was negative. Back examination was normal.

WHAT IS THE DIFFERENTIAL DIAGNOSIS?

This patient's pain was indeed suggestive of TTS; however, the radiation to his hip might suggest an S1 radiculopathy or sciatic nerve lesion, particularly due to the tenderness in the hip. The diagnosis of TTS was made by EMG previously. His lumbosacral MRI done prior to referral was reviewed, and it was negative.

WHAT IS A TARSAL TUNNEL SYNDROME?

TTS is produced by compression of the tibial nerve at the ankle, causing shooting pains in the ankle and foot; later, patients might develop numbness in the sole of the foot and atrophy in the tibial-innervated foot muscles.

The diagnosis could be suggested by a positive Tinel's sign in the retromalleolar area, but this is not always present. The differential diagnosis includes S1 radiculopathy, sciatic nerve lesions, other tibial nerve lesions, and a plantar neuropathy in the foot. Common causes of TTS are compression, neuromas, fibromas, fractures or other trauma, varicose veins, hypertrophy of the abductor hallucis muscle, lipoma, rheumatoid arthritis, and cysts.[1]

The most useful diagnostic test for this patient was an EMG.

AN EMG TEST WAS PERFORMED

Motor Nerve Studies

Nerve and Site	Latency (ms)	Amplitude (mV)	Conduction Velocity (m/s)
Peroneal Nerve L.	**Normal ≤ 5.7**	**Normal ≥ 3**	**Normal ≥ 40**
Ankle	5.1	5	–
Fibular head	12.8	4	42
Tibial Nerve L.	**Normal ≤ 5.3**	**Normal ≥ 4**	**Normal ≥ 40**
Ankle	4.2	15	–
Pop. fossa	14.8	8	43

Nerve and Site	Latency (ms)	Amplitude (mV)	Conduction Velocity (m/s)
Tibial Nerve L. (ADQP)	**Normal ≤ 5.3**	**Normal ≥ 4**	**Normal ≥ 40**
Ankle	**5.9**	7	–
Pop. fossa	16.4	3	41

F-Wave and Tibial H-Reflex Studies

Nerve	Latency (ms)	Normal Latency ≤ (ms)
Peroneal nerve L.	51.7	54
Tibial nerve L.	48.0	54
H-reflex L.	**34.2**	34
H-reflex R.	33.8	34

Sensory Nerve Studies

Nerve	Onset Latency (ms)	Normal Onset Latency ≤ (ms)	Peak Latency (ms)	Normal Peak Latency ≤ (ms)	Amp (μV)	Normal Amp ≥ (μV)	Conduction Velocity (m/s)	Normal Conduction Velocity ≥ (m/s)
Sural nerve L.	3.5	3.5	4.0	4.0	15	11	40	40
Medial plantar L.	**5.0**	3.2	5.5	3.7	12	10	**28**	40
Lateral plantar L.	**NR**	3.2	**NR**	3.7	**NR**	8	**NR**	40
Medial plantar R.	3.1	3.2	3.6	3.7	13	10	45	40
Lateral plantar R.	3.2	3.2	3.7	3.7	8	8	44	40

EMG Data

Muscle	Insrt Activity	Fibs	Pos Waves	Fasc	Amp	Dur	Poly	Pattern
Lumbar paraspinals L.	Norm	None	None	None	Norm	Norm	None	Full
Tibialis anterior L.	**Inc**	None	None	None	Norm	Norm	None	Full
Peroneus longus L.	**Inc**	None	None	None	Norm	Norm	None	Full
Gastrocnemius L.	Norm	None	None	None	**Lg**	**Inc**	None	Full
Extensor hallucis longus L.	Norm	None	None	None	**Lg**	**Inc**	None	Full
Abductor digiti quinti pedis L.	Norm	None	None	None	Norm	Norm	None	Full
Abductor hallucis L.	**Inc**	None	None	None	Norm	Norm	None	Full

WHAT WERE THE EMG FINDINGS?

The test showed normal tibial CMAP amplitude motor latencies to the foot, but the CMAP latency to the abductor digiti quinti pedis (ADQP) muscle was prolonged; the mixed median plantar nerve action potential (NAP) was prolonged, and the lateral plantar nerve NAP was absent on the left and normal on the right. There was increased insertional activity in the peroneal nerve innervated muscles, and large amplitude motor unit potentials were seen in the tibial-innervated muscles; paraspinal muscles were normal. These findings suggest a more proximal, chronic, likely, sciatic nerve dysfunction, but the prolonged median plantar latency of normal amplitude suggested that this patient did have TTS. The low-amplitude CMAP latency to the ADQP could be caused by a TTS or a sciatic neuropathy. He had a normal sural SNAP, but left H-reflex was mildly prolonged.

WHAT ARE THE EMG FINDINGS OF TARSAL TUNNEL SYNDROME?

A prolongation of the tibial motor distal latencies compared with the contralateral asymptomatic side is diagnostic.[2] This test, however, is not sensitive and is abnormal in only half of the patients with TTS.[3] Measurements of the medial and lateral plantar nerve motor latencies are the most widely used tests to determine the diagnosis; mixed nerve latencies and conduction velocities are also useful. Abnormalities consist of asymmetric slowing or an absent response in the symptomatic side.[4] Some clinicians use digital sensory nerve studies, which are very sensitive, but these lack specificity as low-amplitude responses can be seen in normal persons. The mixed plantar response is more specific, but less sensitive; this would be normal in 85% of patients with TTS. Like in this patient, the lateral plantar response is more frequently abnormal.[3] The medial response could also be abnormal in medial plantar neuropathy.

As discussed, CMAP and SNAP amplitudes can be used for diagnosis, and the most reliable diagnostic finding is a drop in amplitude in the symptomatic side by 50% or more.[5]

The near nerve needle recording technique is also useful.[6] An MRI of the tarsal tunnel area aids in diagnosis.[7] Ultrasound can also be helpful.[8]

The treatment of the TTS consists of conservative management, such as immobilization, local steroid injections, and, if necessary, surgical decompression.[9,10]

WHAT SHOULD BE THE NEXT DIAGNOSTIC TEST IN THIS PATIENT?

This patient is not known to be diabetic and has pain in the hip area. He had a normal MRI of the spine previously and an EMG that suggested a sciatic neuropathy. He underwent an MRI of the sciatic nerve area that revealed a cystic mass measuring 5–7 cm (Fig. 24-1A and B).

Exploratory surgery was performed and a nerve sheath tumor involving the sciatic nerve was excised successfully. The tumor was a neurofibroma with marked myxoid changes (Fig. 24-1C).

DISCUSSION

This patient presented with a previous diagnosis of TTS because of his foot symptoms and abnormal initial electrophysiologic findings.

The abnormalities in the leg seen in the repeated EMG suggested a higher located lesion, such as in the sciatic nerve. He had a mass in the hip area which was found to be a neurofibroma. Sciatic nerve lesions are not only caused by tumors; other causes include injections, prolonged periods of standing, surgery, fractures, contusions, gunshot wounds, aneurysms, muscle fibrosis, abscess, hematomas, and diabetes.[11–15] (Fig. 24-2 demonstrates the anatomy of the sciatic nerve and the circle indicates the site of the lesion in this patient.)

The so-called *piriformis syndrome* is also a consideration in a patient with these presentations, although this is a somewhat vague entity believed to be caused by compression of the sciatic nerve by a hypertrophic piriformis muscle.[16]

This patient had a benign neurofibroma. Neurofibromas are nerve sheath tumors that are well encapsulated. These tumors are formed by Schwann cells, fibroblasts, or perineural cells. They can be completely removed without damaging the nerve.[17,18] In the great majority of cases the tumors are isolated, but in a minority they occur in neurofibromatosis and might be multiple.

This case emphasizes the need for a good history and careful examination when performing electrophysiologic testing, particularly as abnormalities on nerve conduction studies could provide false localization or there could be more than one medical problem.

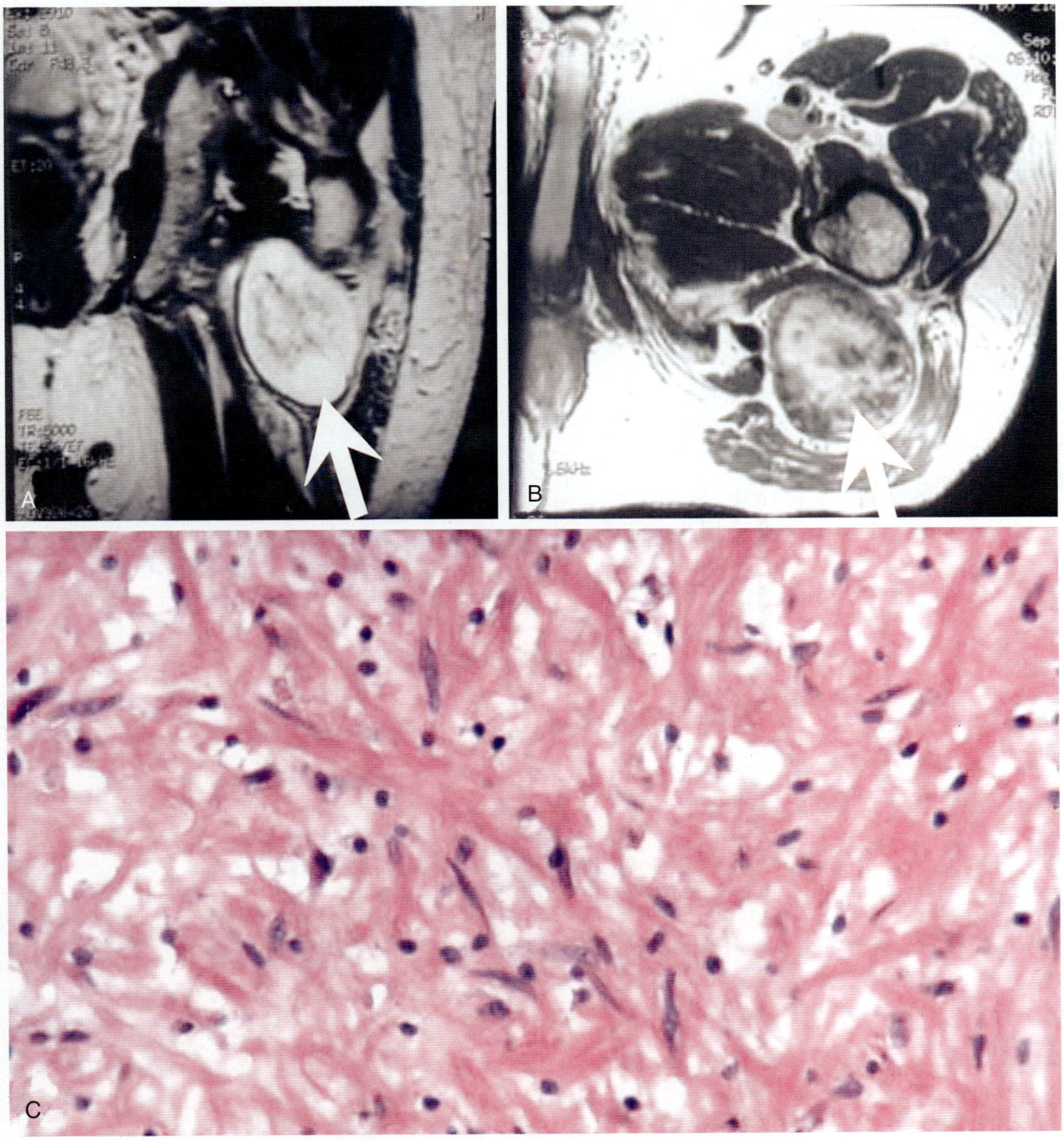

FIG. 24-1 **A**, T1-weighted MRI image of the hip (coronal view) showing the mass in the hip. **B**, Axial view of the hip, T1-weighted image showing the mass (*arrow*). **C**, Histology of the tumor showing the characteristic neurofibromas with their spindle appearance (H&E stain, ×100).

SUMMARY

This patient had a benign neurofibroma in the leg with symptoms affecting the foot, giving false localization and diagnosis of TTS. Examination and electrophysiologic studies were suggestive of a lesion above the tarsal tunnel. The neurofibroma was demonstrated by MRI; the patient improved with surgical removal of the tumor.

IMPORTANT POINTS

- The EMG examination should always be done together with a good history and clinical examination.
- The most sensitive test for TTS is measuring of SNAP and mixed nerve latencies and amplitudes. This is improved with the use of near nerve conduction techniques.

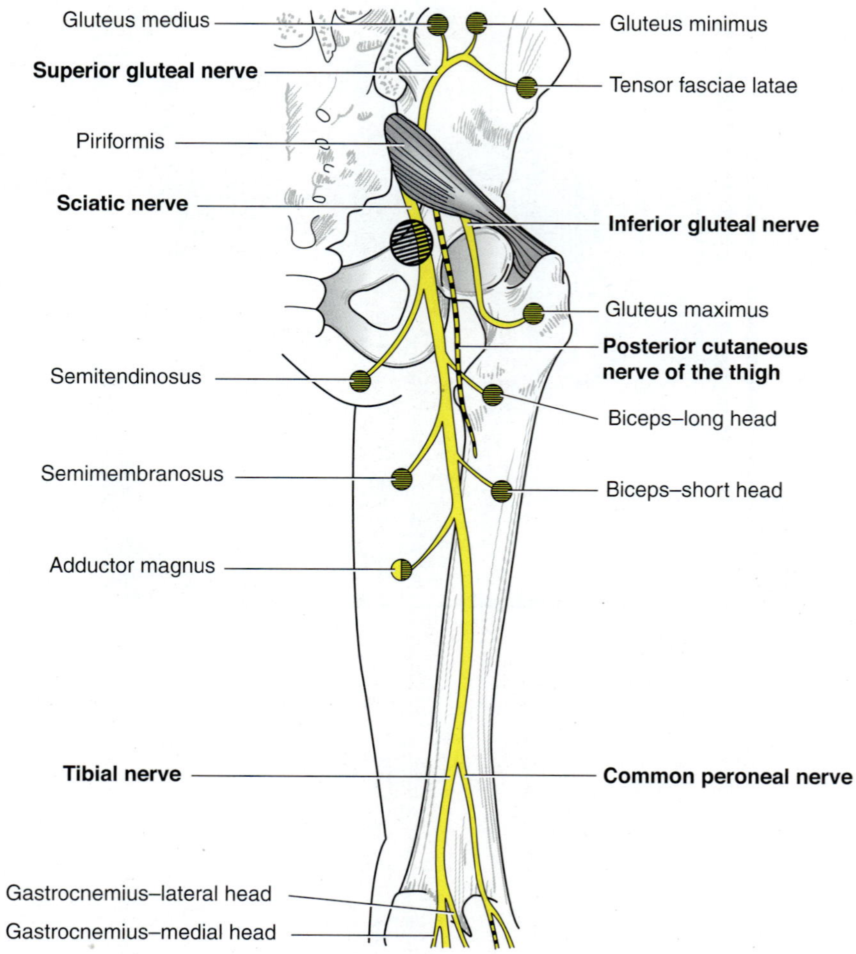

FIG. 24-2 A diagram of the sciatic nerve showing the site of the lesion (*circled mark*).

- Detailed analysis of the patient and EMG findings should be done prior to making the diagnosis that abnormal SNAPs in the feet are caused by TTS.
- Schwannomas or neurofibromas are nerve sheath tumors that can be completely removed.

REFERENCES

1. Katirji B. Compressive and entrapment neuropathies of the lower extremity. In: Katirji B, Kaminski HJ, Preston DC, et al., eds. *Neuromuscular Disorders in Clinical Practice*. Boston, MA: Butterworth-Heinemann; 2002:774–819.
2. Goodgold J, Kopell HP, Spielholz NI. The tarsal tunnel syndrome: objective diagnostic criteria. *N Engl J Med*. 1965;273(14):742–745.
3. Galardi G, Amadio S, Maderna L, et al. Electrophysiologic studies in tarsal tunnel syndrome: diagnostic reliability of motor distal latency, mixed nerve and sensory nerve conduction studies. *Am J Phys Med Rehabil*. 1994;73:193–198.
4. Saeed MA, Gatens PF. Compound nerve action potentials of the medial and lateral plantar nerves through the tarsal tunnel. *Arch Phys Med Rehabil*. 1982;63:304–307.
5. Bromberg MB, Jaros L. Symmetry of normal motor and sensory nerve conduction measurements. *Muscle Nerve*. 1998;21:498–503.
6. Oh SJ, Kim HS, Ahmad BK. The near-nerve sensory nerve conduction in tarsal tunnel syndrome. *J Neurol Neurosurg Psychiatry*. 1985;48(10):999–1003.
7. Erickson SJ, Quinn SF, Kneeland JB, et al. MR imaging of the tarsal tunnel syndrome and related spaces: normal and abnormal findings with anatomic correlation. *Am J Roentgenol*. 1990;155:323–328.
8. Nagaoka M, Matsuzaki H. Ultrasonography in tarsal tunnel syndrome. *J Ultrasound Med*. 2005;24(8):1035–1040.
9. Bailie DS, Kelikian AS. Tarsal tunnel syndrome: diagnosis, surgical technique and functional outcome. *Foot Ankle Int*. 1998;19(2):65–72.
10. Sammarco GJ, Chang L. Outcome of surgical treatment of tarsal tunnel syndrome. *Foot Ankle Int*. 2003;24(2):125–131.
11. Goh KJ, Tan CB, Tjia HT. Sciatic neuropathies: a retrospective review of electrodiagnostic features in 29 patients. *Ann Acad Med Singapore*. 1996;25:566–569.
12. Thomas JE, Piepgras DG, Scheithauer B, et al. Neurogenic tumors of the sciatic nerve: a clinicopathological study of 35 cases. *Mayo Clin Proc*. 1983;58:640–647.
13. McManis PG. Sciatic nerve lesions during cardiac surgery. *Neurology*. 1994;44:684–687.
14. Schmalzried TP, Amstutz HC, Dorey FJ. Nerve palsy associated with total hip replacement: risk factors and prognosis. *J Bone Joint Surg*. 1991;73(7):1074–1080.
15. Edwards MS, Barbaro NM, Asher SW, Murray WR. Delayed sciatic palsy after total hip replacement: case report. *Neurosurgery*. 1981;9:61–63.
16. Silver JK, Leadbetter WB. Piriformis syndrome: assessment of current practice and literature review. *Orthopedics*. 1998;21:1133–1135.
17. Russell DS, Rubenstein LJ, eds. Tumors of cranial and spinal and peripheral nerve. *Pathologies of Tumors of the Nervous System*. 5th ed. Baltimore, MD: Williams & Wilkins; 1988:533–585.
18. Donner TR, Voorhies RM, Kline DG. Neural sheath tumors of major nerves. *J Neurosurg*. 1994;81:362–373.

A Man With Unilateral Proximal Leg Weakness After Heart Catheterization

A 79-year-old diabetic man developed acute pain in the right hip and knee immediately after a heart catheterization. Past medical history included kidney stones, atrial fibrillation, and hypertension. He did not smoke, drink alcohol, or use illicit drugs.

Mental function and cranial nerve examination were normal. He had normal strength and sensation in the upper extremities; there was a profound weakness of the right iliopsoas and quadriceps muscles which did not overcome gravity. Adductors, hamstrings, and gluteal muscles were normal. There was a mild bilateral weakness of toe dorsiflexors. Reflexes were 2+ in the upper extremities, 1+ in the left knee, and 0 at the right knee. Adductor reflexes were 1+ bilaterally. Both ankle jerks were absent. There was absent vibration sense in the toes and decreased pinprick in a stocking distribution to the mid-leg in both sides. There was also a patchy decreased pain sensation in the anterior right thigh. Femoral stretch produced mild pain, and a straight leg raising test was negative. No masses were present in the inguinal area or pelvis. The rest of the examination was unremarkable.

WHAT IS THE MOST LIKELY DIAGNOSIS?

This patient had unilateral weakness in the femoral-innervated muscles, with sparing of the adductors innervated by the obturator nerve. This finding is suggestive of a femoral neuropathy, rather than a lumbosacral plexopathy or an L2–L4 radiculopathy. The most likely cause of this neuropathy is trauma to the femoral nerve during catheterization. Another possibility is a hematoma compressing this nerve. The patient also had evidence of a polyneuropathy, likely from diabetes. It was not clear if the right saphenous nerve was affected by this because the sensory loss in the legs was equal in both sides.

WHAT TESTS SHOULD BE DONE?

A CT scan or an MRI of the pelvis and retroperitoneal area should be done, as should routine blood tests, including a complete metabolic panel (CMP), particularly glucose, a complete blood count (CBC), prothrombin time (PT), partial thromboplastin time, glycosylated hemoglobin, blood urea nitrogen, and creatinine, and an EMG.

CBC, CMP, and PT were normal, except for his blood sugar that was 242 mg/dL (normal, 70–115 mg/dL) and his glycosylated hemoglobin that was 7% (normal, <6.0%).

AN EMG TEST WAS PERFORMED

Motor Nerve Studies

Nerve and Site	Latency(ms)	Amplitude (mV)	Conduction Velocity (m/s)
Peroneal Nerve R.	**Normal ≤ 5.7**	**Normal ≥ 3**	**Normal ≥ 40**
Ankle	5.7	**1**	–
Fibular head	14.8	**1**	**33**
Knee	17.9	**1**	**32**

Nerve and Site	Latency (ms)	Amplitude (mV)	Conduction Velocity (m/s)
Tibial Nerve R.	**Normal ≤ 5.3**	**Normal ≥ 4**	**Normal ≥ 50**
Ankle	4.7	4	–
Pop. fossa	17.5	**3**	**30**

Nerve and Site	Latency (ms)	Amplitude (mV)	Conduction Velocity (m/s)
Ulnar Nerve R.	**Normal ≤ 3.6**	**Normal ≥ 8**	**Normal ≥ 50**
Wrist	**4.4**	8	–
Below elbow	9.8	**7**	**42**
Above elbow	14.9	**6**	**38**
Median Nerve R.	**Normal ≤ 4.2**	**Normal ≥ 6**	**Normal ≥ 50**
Wrist	**5.2**	6	–
Elbow	10.8	**5**	**45**

Femoral Nerve (Side-to-Side Comparison)

Nerve	Latency (ms)	Amplitude (mV)	Distance (cm)
Femoral nerve R.	**6.4**	**0.1**	22
Femoral nerve L.	4.0	4	22

F-Wave and Tibial H-Reflex Studies

Nerve	Latency (ms)	Normal Latency ≤ (ms)
Peroneal nerve R.	**NR**	54
Tibial nerve R.	**61.5**	54
Ulnar nerve R.	**34.6**	30
Median nerve R.	**33.4**	30
H-reflex R.	**NR**	34
H-reflex L.	**NR**	34

Sensory Nerve Studies

Nerve	Latency (ms)	Normal Latency ≤ (ms)	Amp (μV)	Normal Amp ≥ (μV)
Sural nerve R.	**NR**	4.0	**NR**	11
Superficial peroneal nerve R.	**NR**	4.0	**NR**	8–10
Saphenous nerve R.	**NR**	3.7	**NR**	4–6
Saphenous nerve L.	**NR**	3.7	**NR**	4–6
Median nerve R.	**NR**	3.1	**NR**	20
Ulnar nerve R.	**NR**	3.1	**NR**	13

EMG Data

Muscle	Insrt Activity	Fibs	Pos Waves	Fasc	Amp	Dur	Poly	Pattern
Lumbar paraspinals R.	Norm	None	None	None	Norm	Norm	None	Full
Iliopsoas R.	**Inc**	**3+**	**3+**	None	Norm	Norm	None	**Red**
Vastus lateralis R.	**Inc**	**3+**	**3+**	None	Norm	Norm	**Few**	**Red**
Adductor longus R.	Norm	None	None	None	Norm	Norm	None	Full
Tensor fasciae latae R.	Norm	None	None	None	Norm	Norm	None	Full
Tibialis anterior R.	**Inc**	None	None	None	Norm	Norm	None	**Red**
Peroneus longus R.	Norm	None	None	None	Norm	Norm	None	**Red**
Gastrocnemius R.	**Inc**	None	None	None	Norm	Norm	None	**Red**
First dorsal interosseous R.	Norm	None	None	None	**Lg**	**Inc**	None	**Red**

WHAT WERE THE EMG FINDINGS?

This EMG showed slowing of conduction velocities of the ulnar, median, and tibial nerves with low-amplitude CMAPs. The distal latencies were prolonged in the ulnar and median nerves. The peroneal nerve conduction velocity was mildly slow and the CMAP had a low amplitude. A good response was obtained in the left femoral nerve, but a very low-amplitude CMAP was seen in the right femoral nerve. Superficial peroneal, sural, saphenous, median, and ulnar sensory–evoked responses were absent. Needle EMG showed evidence of denervation only on the right femoral-innervated muscles but sparing the thigh adductors and paraspinals. There was reduced motor unit recruitment in the distal legs and first dorsal interossei and markedly reduced motor unit recruitment in the right quadriceps and iliopsoas muscles. These findings indicate a sensory motor neuropathy in addition to a femoral neuropathy.

A CT scan of the pelvis showed a hematoma over the psoas muscle compressing the femoral nerve (Fig. 25-1). He was managed conservatively with physical therapy and improved slowly.

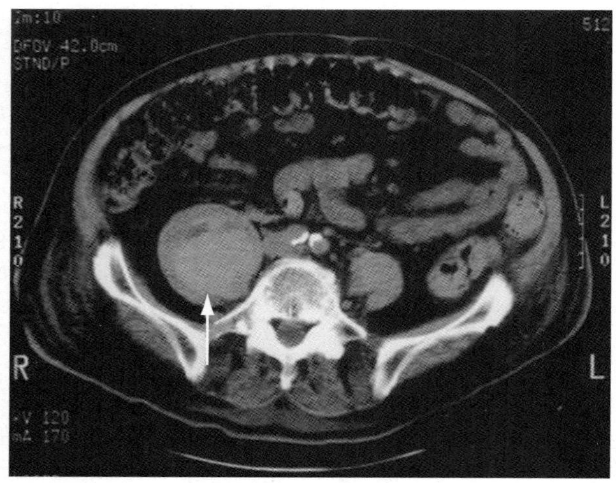

FIG. 25-1 CT scan of the pelvis demonstrates a large hematoma over the psoas muscle (*arrow*).

DISCUSSION

Unilateral quadriceps muscle weakness could be caused by L3–L4 radiculopathy, lumbar plexopathy, or femoral neuropathy.

The femoral nerve arises at the lumbosacral plexus from the posterior divisions of the ventral rami of L2–L3 and L4 roots. The nerve then passes between the border of the psoas and iliacus muscles and is covered by the iliacus fascia; it innervates these muscles and then passes under the inguinal ligament lateral to the femoral artery and vein to the thigh. Then the nerve gives motor branches to the quadriceps muscles and sensory branches to the anterior thigh. The saphenous nerve is a sensory nerve that originates from the femoral nerve and innervates the skin of the anterior and medial leg[1] (Fig. 25-2).

This patient had a femoral neuropathy secondary to a hematoma from catheterization. Femoral neuropathies from catheterization are caused by local trauma, and most are transient.[2] When severe, they are usually caused by a hematoma.[3] Hematomas can also be caused by bleeding from anticoagulation, resulting in a plexopathy or an isolated femoral neuropathy.[4,5] The diagnosis is made clinically and electrophysiologically on the basis of the presentation with involvement of only the femoral-innervated muscles. Additional involvement of the adductor muscles is seen in a plexopathy. In either case imaging studies are mandatory.[6,7]

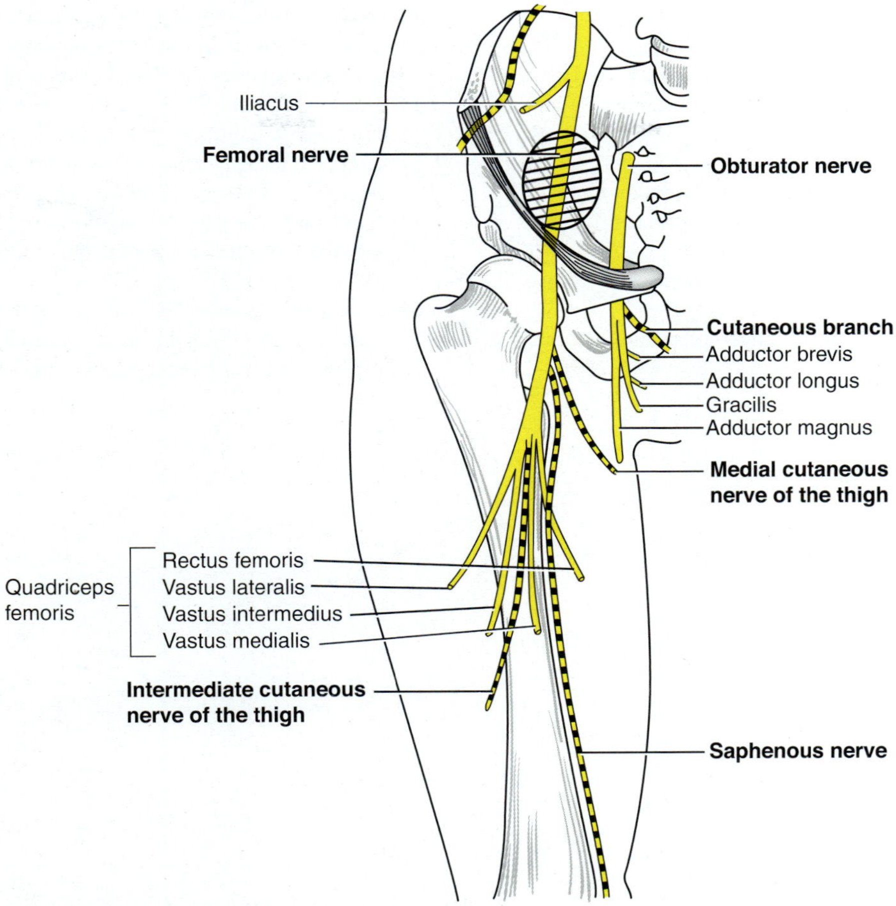

FIG. 25-2 Diagram of the femoral nerve, its innervated muscles, and sensory branches. The circle indicates the site of the lesion in this patient.

The femoral nerve can also be damaged by inguinal, pelvic, and hip surgery,[8,9] hysterectomy[10] or tuboplasty,[11] and renal transplantation and other surgeries of the abdomen,[12] such as herniorrhaphies[13] and hip surgery.[14] Other causes include hip fractures, gunshot wounds, stretch injuries, tumors, abscess, injury or spontaneous hematoma,[2] diabetes, vasculitis, and trauma.

The treatment of femoral neuropathy depends on the cause. Evacuation of hematomas is mandatory when symptoms worsen or the mass enlarges and there is a drop in the hematocrit.

SUMMARY

This patient had a sensorimotor polyneuropathy, likely from diabetes, and has a superimposed femoral neuropathy secondary to a hematoma from catheterization. He was treated conservatively.

IMPORTANT POINTS

- Weakness of the quadriceps muscle while sparing of the thigh adductors localizes a lesion in the femoral nerve rather than in the lumbosacral plexus or lumbar roots.
- The workup in a patient who presents with femoral neuropathy after catheterization should include a CT scan or MRI of the pelvis and retroperitoneal area and coagulation studies, as well as an EMG.
- Causes of femoral neuropathy include, among others, diabetes, vasculitis, trauma, surgery, hernia, masses, and hematomas.
- The treatment of a psoas hematoma is usually conservative, unless there is progression, enlargement of the hematoma, or a significant drop in the hematocrit, in which case evacuation is necessary.

REFERENCES

1. Stewart JD, ed. *Focal Peripheral Neuropathies*. 3rd ed. Philadelphia, PA: Lippincott Williams & Wilkins; 2000:457–473.
2. Jarosz JM, McKeown B, Reidy JF. Short-term femoral nerve complications following percutaneous transfemoral procedures. *J Vasc Intervent Radiol*. 1995;6:351–353.
3. Kent KC, Moscucci M, Gallagher SG, et al. Neuropathy after cardiac catheterization: incidence, clinical patterns, and long-term outcome. *J Vasc Surg*. 1994;19:1008–1013.
4. Gertzbein SD, Evans DC. Femoral nerve neuropathy complicating iliopsoas hemorrhage in patients without hemophilia. *J Bone Joint Surg Br*. 1972;54:149–151.

5. Mastroianni PP, Roberts MP. Femoral neuropathy and retroperitoneal hemorrhage. *Neurosurgery*. 1983;13:44–47.
6. Reinstein L, Alevizatos AC, Twardzik FG, DeMarco SJ III. Femoral nerve dysfunction after retroperitoneal hemorrhage: pathophysiology revealed by computed tomography. *Arch Phys Med Rehabil*. 1984;65:37–40.
7. Eutace S, McCarthy C, O'Byrne J, et al. Computed tomography of the retroperitoneum in patients with femoral neuropathy. *Can Assoc Radio J*. 1994;45:277–282.
8. Walsh C, Walsh A. Postoperative femoral neuropathy. *Surg Gynecol Obstet*. 1992;174:255–263.
9. Kuntzer T, van Melle G, Regli F. Clinical and prognostic features in unilateral femoral neuropathies. *Muscle Nerve*. 1997;20:205–211.
10. Kvist-Poulsen H, Borel J. Iatrogenic femoral neuropathy subsequent to abdominal hysterectomy: incidence and prevention. *Obstet Gynecol*. 1982;60:516–520.
11. Hassan AA, Reiff RH, Fayez JA. Femoral neuropathy following microsurgical tuboplasty. *Fertil Steril*. 1986;45:889–891.
12. Kim DH, Kline DG. Surgical outcome for intra- and extrapelvic femoral nerve lesions. *J Neurosurg*. 1995;83:783–790.
13. Van Hoff J, Shaywitz BA, Seashore JH, Collins WF. Femoral nerve injury following inguinal hernia repair. *Pediatr Neurol*. 1985;1:195–196.
14. Simmons C Jr, Izant TH, Rothman RH, et al. Femoral neuropathy following total hip arthroplasty: anatomic study, case reports, and literature review. *J Arthroplasty*. 1991;6(Suppl):S57–S66.

A Woman With Uterine Cancer and Unilateral Leg Weakness

A 42-year-old woman with invasive carcinoma of the cervix presented with progressive pain and weakness in her left lower extremity of 2 months' duration; she was referred for an EMG.

She had a history of heart disease and had had a coronary artery bypass graft 6 years previously. She had been on warfarin therapy for 1 month because of a recent deep venous thrombosis in the left leg.

Social history revealed no tobacco, alcohol, or illicit drug use. The family history was unremarkable for neurologic complaints. On review of systems she reported some weight loss and intermittent fever.

On physical examination, she was alert and oriented. There were no cranial nerve abnormalities. Severe pain in her left lower extremity interfered with her motor examination. She was felt to have 2/5 left hip flexor strength, 4−/5 knee flexor, 5/5 knee extensor, 5/5 plantar flexion, and 3+/5 dorsiflexion. Strength was normal in the right leg and the upper extremities. There was a sensory loss in the L5 dermatome distribution in her left lower extremity. She had no left patellar and ankle reflexes; these were normal on the right lower extremity. The rest of the neurologic examination was unremarkable. There was evidence of a well-healed old midline abdominal incision.

WHAT IS THE DIFFERENTIAL DIAGNOSIS?

This patient had uterine cancer and a history of deep venous thrombosis for which she received anticoagulation. She presented with unilateral left leg pain and weakness which followed the territories of several myotomes, with absent knee and ankle reflexes representing roots at L2–L4 and S1 and a sensory deficit that seemed to correspond to the L5 dermatome. The possibility of tumor invasion of the lumbosacral plexus was very likely, but a retroperitoneal hematoma might also have a similar presentation, particularly in patients on anticoagulation. The lack of acute abdominal pain, however, is against this diagnosis. The lack of back pain is also against the possibility of tumor invasion of the lumbosacral spine, and she did not have involvement of the other leg to suggest meningeal carcinomatosis. The distribution findings could also suggest a mononeuritis multiplex, but the involvement is only of one limb.

A complete metabolic panel and FANA were normal. Hematocrit was 32% (normal, 36%–48%), and INR was 1.4 (normal, 1.4 or less).

AN EMG TEST WAS PERFORMED

Motor Nerve Studies

Nerve and Site	Latency(ms)	Amplitude (mV)	Conduction Velocity (m/s)
Peroneal Nerve L.	**Normal ≤ 5.7**	**Normal ≥ 3**	**Normal ≥ 40**
Ankle	4.1	**1**	–
Fibular head	11.8	**1**	**39**
Knee	14.1	**1**	43
Tibial Nerve L.	**Normal ≤ 5.3**	**Normal ≥ 4**	**Normal ≥ 40**
Ankle	4.4	13	–
Pop. fossa	13.5	8	43

Nerve and Site	Latency (ms)	Amplitude (mV)	Conduction Velocity (m/s)
Peroneal Nerve R.	**Normal ≤ 5.7**	**Normal ≥ 3**	**Normal ≥ 40**
Ankle	4.1	8	–
Fibular head	10.5	7	46
Knee	12.7	7	50

Peroneal Nerve L.

Ankle, before exercise	1	–	–
Ankle, posttetanic	1	–	–

F-Wave and Tibial H-Reflex Studies

Nerve	Latency (ms)	Normal Latency ≤ (ms)
Peroneal nerve L.	**NR**	54
Tibial nerve L.	51.6	54
Peroneal nerve R.	46.5	54
H-reflex L.	**NR**	34
H-reflex R.	29.6	34

Sensory Nerve Studies

Nerve	Onset Latency (ms)	Normal Onset Latency ≤ (ms)	Peak Latency (ms)	Normal Peak Latency ≤ (ms)	Amp (μV)	Normal Amp ≥ (μV)	Conduction Velocity (m/s)	Normal Conduction Velocity ≥ (m/s)
Sural nerve L.	3.1	3.5	3.6	4.0	16	13	45	40
Superficial peroneal L.	3.4	3.5	3.9	4.0	**6**	11	41	40
Sural nerve R.	3.5	3.5	4.0	4.0	16	13	40	40
Superficial peroneal R.	2.7	3.5	3.2	4.0	23	11	52	40

EMG Data

Muscle	Insrt Activity	Fibs	Pos Waves	Fasc	Amp	Dur	Poly	Pattern
Lumbar paraspinals L.	Norm	None	None	None	Norm	Norm	None	Full
Gluteus maximus L.	**Inc**	**+1**	**1+**	None	Norm	Norm	None	**Red**
Gluteus medius L.	**Inc**	**+1**	**1+**	None	Norm	Norm	None	**Red**
Tensor fasciae latae L.	**Inc**	**+1**	**1+**	None	Norm	Norm	None	**Red**
Adductor magnus L.	**Inc**	**+1**	**1+**	None	Norm	Norm	None	**Red**
Adductor longus L.	**Inc**	**+1**	**1+**	None	Norm	Norm	None	Full
Rectus femoris L.	**Inc**	**+1**	**1+**	None	Norm	Norm	None	**Red**
Vastus lateralis L.	**Inc**	None	**1+**	None	Norm	Norm	None	**Red**
Gastrocnemius L.	**Inc**	None	**1+**	None	Norm	Norm	None	**Red**
Tibialis anterior L.	**Inc**	**+1**	**1+**	None	Norm	Norm	None	**Red**
Tibialis anterior R.	Norm	None	None	None	Norm	Norm	None	Full
Gastrocnemius R.	Norm	None	None	None	Norm	Norm	None	Full

WHAT WERE THE EMG FINDINGS?

The test showed normal motor conduction results, except for low-amplitude left peroneal CMAP with borderline motor conduction velocity, which could be secondary to a dropout of the fast-conducting motor axons. The sensory tests were all normal, except for a low-amplitude left superficial peroneal SNAP. These findings are against a polyneuropathy or a mononeuritis multiplex, and the normal SNAPs mitigate against but do not rule out a lumbosacral plexopathy. An absent left H-reflex with normal tibial motor nerve conduction velocity, however, suggested a more proximal lesion, such as in the sciatic nerve, the sacral plexus, or S1 root.[1] Measurement of femoral nerve conduction velocity and the H-reflex of this nerve could also have been helpful in this case, but these were not done.

The left peroneal nerve F-response was absent, which could be secondary to a proximal lesion. This also could be explained by axonal dropout, which also caused the low-amplitude CMAP.

Needle studies demonstrated active denervation in muscles innervated by several nerves and roots on the left, but sparing the paraspinal muscles. This suggested a lesion in the plexus.[1] Although the paraspinal muscles could sometimes be spared, in lumbosacral radiculopathy the presence of widespread denervation in one limb, sparing the paraspinals, was rather suggestive of a plexopathy. The sensory action potentials are usually affected in plexopathies, but in this case only the superficial peroneal SNAP was of low amplitude, and the sural SNAP was normal. This indicates that the axons to that nerve were spared or that the significant axonal degeneration was not yet developed.

WHAT SHOULD ONE DO NEXT?

In a suspected neoplasm an MRI or CT scan of the lumbosacral plexus area is important in diagnosing a tumor.[2] In this case a CT scan of the abdomen and pelvis showed evidence of invasion by tumor in several areas involving the plexus (Fig. 26-1). (Fig. 26-2 is a diagram of the lumbosacral plexus and the tumor invasion.)

The patient was treated with chemotherapy and radiation.

DISCUSSION

This woman had lumbosacral plexopathy with relative sparing of the sensory-evoked responses that are usually affected in this, but the diffuse denervation in one limb, sparing the lumbosacral paraspinal muscles, was rather suggestive of a plexus involvement. In this case the plexopathy was secondary to tumor invasion, but it can also be caused by hemorrhages and traumatic postoperative aneurysms,[3,4] as well as noncompressive disorders such as diabetic amyotrophy,[5] radiation,[6] idiopathic lumbosacral plexitis,[7,8] vasculitis, infections, toxins (heroin),[9–11] and pregnancy.[12] Various tumors have been

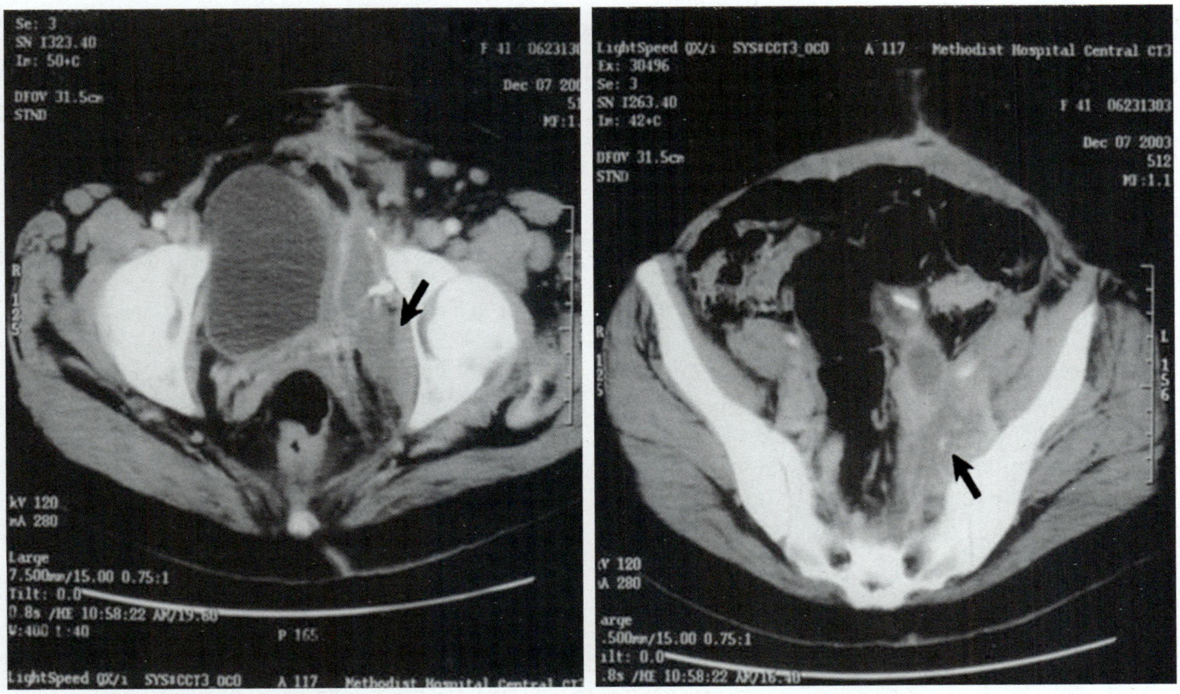

FIG. 26-1 CT scan of the pelvis showing the tumor invasion more prominent on the left with involvement of the psoas muscle (*arrows*).

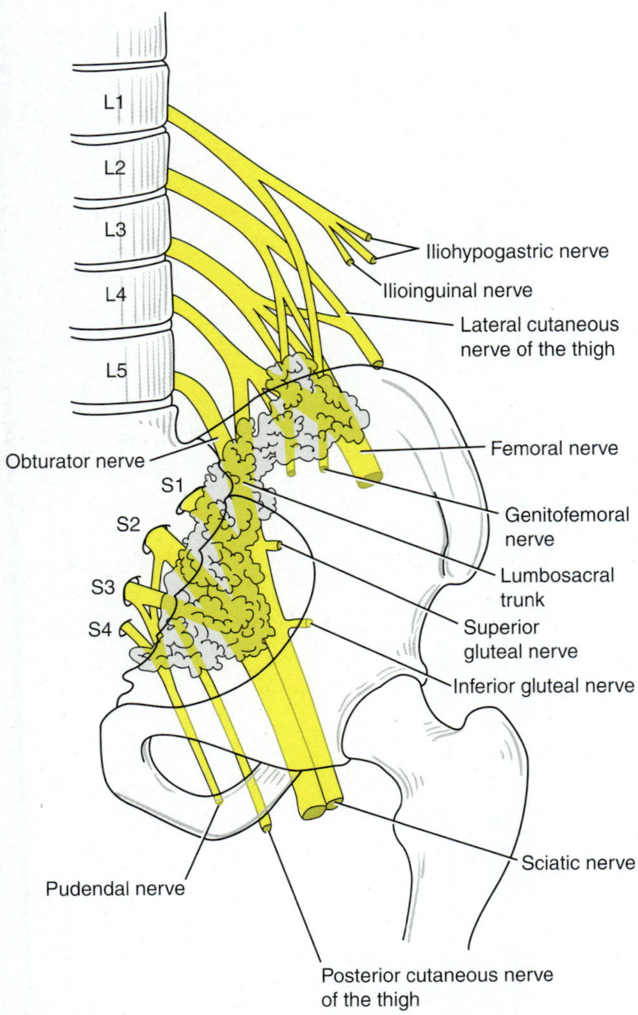

FIG. 26-2 Diagram of the lumbosacral plexus and the tumor invasion, as in this patient.

reported to invade the plexus, as in this case.[13,14] Also, cancer-related plexopathy was the most common cause in a recently reported large series.[15]

Clinical characteristics of lumbosacral plexopathies include pain in the hip and leg with weakness following the involved territory of the lumbosacral plexus.

In lumbosacral plexopathies the nerve conduction tests could be normal or the velocities mildly slow, accompanied by low-amplitude CMAPs from axonal degeneration; the sensory-evoked responses are usually abnormal, but not always. The SNAPs are almost always normal in radiculopathies.

For proper diagnosis an EMG should include detailed nerve conduction tests. In particular, one should compare the SNAP amplitudes with the opposite side and measure proximal responses, as well as perform detailed limb and paraspinal muscle needle tests. In a retrospective study, Tavee and colleagues outlined the difficulties of obtaining a definitive diagnosis of sacral plexopathies.[15] These researchers found that the SNAPs could be absent from other causes, such as the presence of a neuropathy or even from the radiculopathies affecting the posterior root ganglia. Furthermore, some cases of radiculopathy showed no paraspinal denervation.

Treatment of plexopathies usually includes analgesia, decompression, and/or chemotherapy and radiotherapy, according to the cause.

SUMMARY

This patient had carcinomatous involvement of the lumbosacral plexus. She had denervation in muscles innervated by different nerves of the plexus and sparing the paraspinal muscles. The CT of the pelvis demonstrated a mass. She was treated with chemotherapy and radiation.

IMPORTANT POINTS

- The clinical characteristics of lumbosacral plexopathies include pain in the hip and leg with weakness, according to the involved territory; there could be areflexia and sensory deficits in different nerve and root territories.
- Electrodiagnostic studies in lumbosacral plexopathy should include detailed nerve conduction tests, measurement of SNAPs, and comparison with the opposite side. The test should include H-reflexes and F-responses as well as detailed limb and paraspinal muscle needle EMG.
- In lumbosacral plexopathies the motor nerve conduction tests could be normal or mildly slow with low-amplitude CMAPs, but the SNAPs are frequently abnormal. The SNAPs are usually normal in root lesions. Paraspinal denervation is usually seen in radiculopathy and not in plexopathy.
- The differential diagnosis of a lumbosacral plexopathy includes hemorrhages, neoplasms, pregnancy, traumatic postoperative aneurysms, radiation, diabetic amyotrophy, and autoimmune plexopathy.

REFERENCES

1. Eisen AA. The electrodiagnosis of plexopathies. In: Brown WF, Bolton CF, eds. *Clinical Electromyography*. 2nd ed. Boston, MA: Butterworth-Heinemann; 1993:211–225.
2. Taylor BV, Kimmel DW, Krecke KN, Cascino TL. Magnetic resonance imaging in cancer-related lumbosacral plexopathy. *Mayo Clin Proc*. 1997;72:823–829.
3. Crosby ET, Reid DR, DiPrimio G, Grahovac S. Lumbosacral plexopathy from iliopsoas haematoma after combined general-epidural anesthesia for abdominal aneurysmectomy. *Can J Anaesth*. 1998;45:46–51.
4. Jaeckle KA. Nerve plexus metastases. *Neurol Clin*. 1991;9:857–866.
5. Chokroverty S, Reyes MG, Rubino FA, Tonaki H. The syndrome of diabetic amyotrophy. *Ann Neurol*. 1977;2:181–194.
6. Glantz MJ, Burger PC, Friedman AH, et al. Treatment of radiation-induced nervous system injury with heparin and warfarin. *Neurology*. 1994;44:2020–2027.
7. Sander JE, Sharp FR. Lumbosacral plexus neuritis. *Neurology*. 1981;31:470–473.
8. Bradley WG, Chad D, Verghese JP, et al. Painful lumbosacral plexopathy with elevated erythrocyte sedimentation rate: a treatable inflammatory syndrome. *Ann Neurol*. 1984;15:457–464.
9. Challenor YB, Richter RW, Bruun B, Pearson J. Nontraumatic plexitis and heroin addiction. *JAMA*. 1973;225:958–961.
10. Rutkove SB, Sax TW. Lumbosacral plexopathies. In: Katirji B, Kaminski HJ, Preston DC, Ruff RL, Shapiro BE, eds. *Neuromuscular Disorders in Clinical Practice*. Boston, MA: Butterworth-Heinemann; 2002:907–915.
11. Chad DA, Bradley WG. Lumbosacral plexopathy. *Semin Neurol*. 1987;7:97–107.
12. Delarue MW, Vles JS, Hasaart THE. Lumbosacral plexopathy in the third trimester of pregnancy: a report of three cases. *Eur J Obstet Gynecol Reprod Biol*. 1994;53:67–68.
13. Pettigrew LC, Glass JP, Maor M, Zornoza J. Diagnosis and treatment of lumbosacral plexopathies in patients with cancer. *Arch Neurol*. 1984;41:1282–1285.
14. Gilchrist JM, Moore M. Lumbosacral plexopathy in cancer patients. *Neurology*. 1985;35:1392–1393.
15. Tavee J, Mays M, Wilbourn AJ. Pitfalls in the electrodiagnostic studies of sacral plexopathies. *Muscle Nerve*. 2007;35:725–727.

A Man With Burning Sensations in the Thigh

A 48-year-old, mildly obese man developed burning paresthesias in the outer aspect of the right thigh of an insidious onset. This increased when he was working. He denied weakness or other neurologic problems.

Past medical history was unremarkable. Family history was noncontributory; the patient drank moderately.

Examination revealed normal mentation and cranial nerves. Motor examination was normal. Reflexes were normal and equal. There was a patchy area in the right lateral thigh where he had an unusual sensation when touched and felt somewhat numb when compared with the rest of the leg or the other side. The examination was otherwise unremarkable.

WHAT IS THE DIFFERENTIAL DIAGNOSIS?

A lumbar radiculopathy, plexopathy, or femoral neuropathy should be included in the differential diagnosis, but the lack of back pain, weakness, and normal reflexes make these unlikely. The symptoms suggest a lateral femoral cutaneous neuropathy.

WHAT TESTS SHOULD BE ORDERED?

A complete metabolic panel, a 2-hour postprandial blood sugar test, and the sedimentation rate were normal.

AN EMG TEST WAS PERFORMED

Motor Nerve Studies

Nerve and Site	Latency (ms)	Amplitude (mV)	Conduction Velocity (m/s)
Peroneal Nerve R.	**Normal ≤ 5.7**	**Normal ≥ 3**	**Normal ≥ 40**
Ankle	3.7	8	–
Fibular head	10.9	8	45

Motor Nerve Studies—cont'd

Tibial Nerve R.	Normal ≤ 5.3	Normal ≥ 4	Normal ≥ 40
Ankle	4.7	6	–
Pop. fossa	14.3	6	42

F-Wave and Tibial H-Reflex Studies

Nerve	Latency (ms)	Normal Latency ≥ (ms)
Peroneal nerve R.	50.2	54
Tibial nerve R.	51.2	54
H-reflex R.	33.0	34
H-reflex L.	32.8	34

Sensory Nerve Studies

Nerve	Onset Latency (ms)	Normal Onset Latency ≤ (ms)	Amp (μV)	Normal Amp ≥ (μV)
Sural nerve R.	3.8	4.0	21	11
Lat. fem. cut. R.	**NR**	3.6	**NR**	3–10
Lat. fem. cut. L.	3.5	3.6	10	3–10

EMG Data

Muscle	Insrt Activity	Fibs	Pos Waves	Fasc	Amp	Dur	Poly	Pattern
Lumbar paraspinal R.	Norm	None	None	None	Norm	Norm	None	Full
Tensor fasciae latae R.	Norm	None	None	None	Norm	Norm	None	Full
Biceps femoris, long head R.	Norm	None	None	None	Norm	Norm	None	Full
Tibialis anterior R.	Norm	None	None	None	Norm	Norm	None	Full
Gastrocnemius R.	Norm	None	None	None	Norm	Norm	None	Full

WHAT WERE THE EMG FINDINGS?

This test revealed normal motor and sensory conduction velocities, CMAP and SNAP amplitudes. The lateral femoral cutaneous SNAP was not elicited on the right. The opposite side was tested, and a small SNAP was obtained (Fig. 27-1).

Needle test of the right leg and paraspinal muscles was normal.

In summary, this EMG was normal, except for absent right lateral femoral cutaneous nerve SNAPs.

The patient was treated with a local steroid injection in the right lateral femoral cutaneous nerve with marked improvement.

DISCUSSION

It was concluded that this patient had neuropathy of the lateral femoral cutaneous nerve or meralgia paresthetica (MP; derived from *meros*: thigh, *algos*: pain). This condition is also called the Roth–Bernhardt syndrome.[1]

The lateral femoral cutaneous nerve (or lateral cutaneous nerve of the thigh) arises from the dorsal division of the ventral primary rami of L2 and L3 roots. It emerges from the lateral border of the psoas crossing the iliacus muscle and then passes under the lateral end of the inguinal ligament, through a small tunnel formed by a split in its lateral attachment of the anterior superior iliac spine[2]; there are many variations of this course.[3]

The lateral femoral cutaneous nerve could be compressed in several areas but is often idiopathic. It is frequently seen in diabetics.[1,2]

The term *meralgia paresthetica* is used not only for the idiopathic form of the neuropathy but also for those with compression or diabetes.

Other causes include neuromas, hematomas, surgery, pregnancy, obesity, injury, lacerations, surgical injury, and chronic compression by the sartorius muscle and by the tensor fasciae latae.[1–7]

It is also caused by compression from seat belts, wallets, guns, heavy keys, wearing "hip-hugger" trousers,[8] and soldiers wearing body armor.[9] In most patients, no cause is identifiable, but likely the nerve is compressed or kinked as it goes through the inguinal ligaments[4] (Fig. 27-2).

The symptoms consist of burning and a "funny feeling," accompanied by numbness in the lateral aspect of the thigh, as Sigmund Freud described in his own case.[10] There could be tenderness to palpation below the anterior superior iliac spine.

The diagnosis of MP is usually made clinically and by ruling out predisposing causes. The differential diagnosis includes L2 radiculopathy or plexopathies; MP could also be the initial manifestation of retroperitoneal tumors.[11]

Electromyographic studies should include measurement of the SNAPs of the lateral femoral cutaneous nerve[12,13] and are used to rule out other causes such as radiculopathies or plexopathies. Unfortunately, in our experience and that of others, the lateral femoral cutaneous SNAP is hard to obtain, even in normals and particularly in obese people; for this reason, one should always check the healthy side to make sure this is

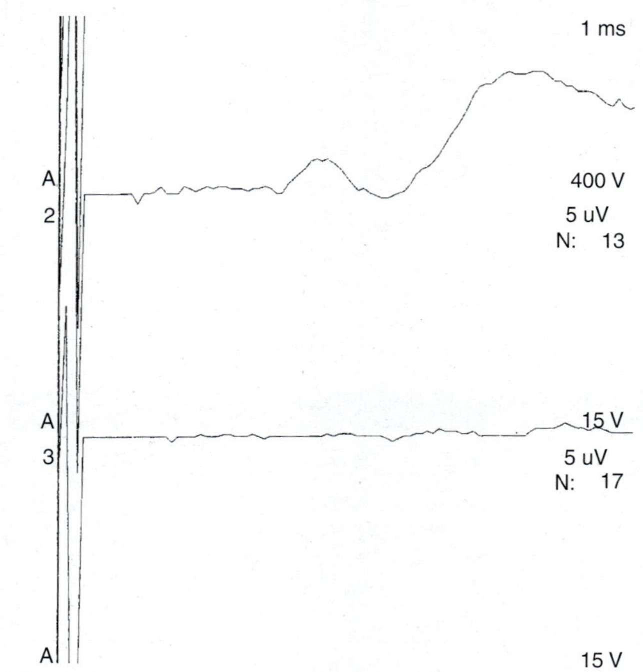

FIG. 27-1 An absent lateral femoral cutaneous SNAP in the right side (*bottom*) but present on the left (*top*) (10 μV/20 ms).

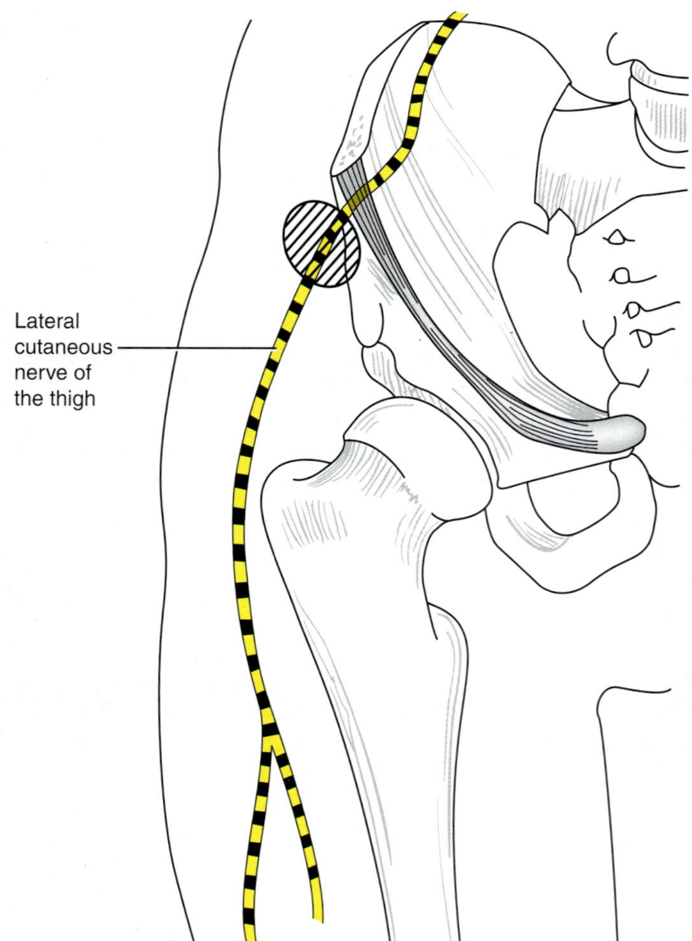

FIG. 27-2 Diagram of the lateral femoral cutaneous nerve and the location of its most common site of entrapment (*circle*).

present. If the SNAP is absent on the healthy side, then likely the absent SNAP in the affected nerve is also caused by technical difficulties, particularly when using surface stimulating and recording techniques.[1,13] In a recent report, however, a SNAP was obtained in the normal side in most patients with MP using needle recording electrodes.[14] Another study stressed the need to consider the variability of the course of the nerve when obtaining the SNAP.[15] Somatosensory-evoked responses with needle stimulation can be used in diagnosis.[16,17]

The prognosis is favorable. Patients respond to conservative management; local injections of corticosteroids and analgesics are of benefit.[1] Surgical decompression is sometimes necessary.[18,19]

SUMMARY

This man developed burning paresthesias in the thigh and was diagnosed as having MP. He was treated with corticosteroid injections with benefit.

IMPORTANT POINTS

- Meralgia paresthetica is a mononeuropathy of the lateral femoral cutaneous nerve.
- The disorder has many causes such as external compression, obesity, pregnancy, compression at the inguinal ligament, at the anterior superior iliac spine, the sartorius and tensor fasciae latae muscles, and neuromas.
- The disease is likely benign but occasionally may be a manifestation of a more severe disease, such as retroperitoneal tumors.
- Electrophysiologic studies are useful to rule out other conditions such as radiculopathy.
- An absent or low-amplitude SNAP in the affected side compared with the normal side is used for diagnosis, but this could be absent in normal people. Thus one should demonstrate its presence in the normal side first to make a diagnosis. If the SNAPs are absent in both sides, this could be technical; the diagnosis is based mostly on the history, clinical examination, and the absence of other abnormal findings on EMG.
- The treatment of meralgia paresthetica consists of removal of the cause of compression; local steroid injections are helpful.

REFERENCES

1. Dumitru D, Zwarts MJ. Lumbosacral plexopathies and proximal mononeuropathies. In: Dumitru D, Amato AA, Zwarts MJ, eds. *Electrodiagnostic Medicine*. 2nd ed. Philadelphia, PA: Hanley & Belfus; 2002:865–883.
2. Stewart JD. Lateral cutaneous nerve of the thigh. In: Stewart JD, ed. *Focal Peripheral Neuropathies*. 3rd ed. Philadelphia, PA: Lippincott Williams & Wilkins; 2000:475–481.
3. Boyce JR. Meralgia paresthetica and tight trousers. *JAMA*. 1984;251:1553.
4. Ecker AD, Woltman HW. Meralgia paresthetica: a report of one hundred and fifty cases. *JAMA*. 1938;110:1650–1652.
5. Ecker AD. Diagnosis of meralgia paresthetica. *JAMA*. 1985;253(7):976.
6. Ghent WR. Further studies on meralgia paresthetica. *Can Med Assoc J*. 1961;85:871–875.
7. Orton D. Meralgia paresthetica from a wallet. *JAMA*. 1984;252(24):3368.
8. Park JW, Kim DH, Hwang M, Bun HR. Meralgia paresthetica caused by hip huggers in a patient with aberrant course of the lateral femoral cutaneous nerve. *Muscle Nerve*. 2007;35(5):678–680.
9. Fargo MV, Konitzer LN. Meralgia paresthetica due to body armor wear in United States soldiers serving in Iraq: a case report and review of literature. *Mil Med*. 2007;172(6):663–665.
10. Schiller F. Sigmund Freud's meralgia paresthetica. *Neurology*. 1985;35:557–558.
11. Flowers RS. Meralgia paresthetica: a clue to retroperitoneal malignant tumor. *Am J Surg*. 1968;116:89–92.
12. Lagueny A, Deliac MM, Deliac P, Durandeau A. Diagnostic and prognostic value of electrophysiologic tests in meralgia paresthetica. *Muscle Nerve*. 1991;14:51–56.
13. Lysens R, Vandendriessche G, Van Mol Y, Rosselle N. The sensory conduction velocity in the cutaneous femoris lateralis nerve in normal adult subjects and in patients with complaints suggesting meralgia paresthetica. *Electromyogr Clin Neurophysiol*. 1981;21:505–510.
14. Seror P, Seror R. Meralgia paresthetica: clinical and electrophysiological diagnosis in 120 cases. *Muscle Nerve*. 2006;33:650–654.
15. Shin YB, Park JH, Kwon DR, et al. Variability in conduction of the lateral femoral cutaneous nerve. *Muscle Nerve*. 2006;33:645–649.
16. Seror P. Lateral femoral cutaneous nerve conduction *v* somatosensory evoked potentials for electrodiagnosis of meralgia paresthetica. *Am J Phys Med Rehabil*. 1999;78:313–316.
17. Po HL, Mei SN. Meralgia paresthetica: the diagnostic value of somatosensory-evoked potentials. *Arch Phys Med Rehabil*. 1991;73:70–72.
18. Harney D, Patijn J. Meralgia paresthetica: diagnosis and management strategies. *Pain Med*. 2007;8(8):669–677.
19. Coffey R, Gupta V. Meralgia paresthetica. In: *StatPearls (Internet)*. Treasure Island, FL: StatPearls Publishing; 2022.

28 CASE

A Man With Weakness and Fasciculations in the Lower Extremities

A 39-year-old black man presented with a 4-year history of pain across the lower back and legs with weakness and difficulty walking.

A previous EMG showed diffuse polyphasic motor unit potentials and fasciculations in the legs. A muscle biopsy of the right thigh showed neurogenic atrophy, and an MRI of the lumbosacral spine was reported as normal. He was referred for the evaluation for possible amyotrophic lateral sclerosis (ALS).

Past medical history was positive for traumatic fractures of the right shoulder and left foot.

He smoked 1½ packs of cigarettes per day but did not drink alcohol.

Review of systems revealed problems maintaining erections, some shortness of breath with exercise, and intermittent pain in the back and legs. He denied difficulty urinating.

Mentation and cranial nerve examination were unremarkable; in particular, there was no evidence of tongue atrophy or fasciculations. Strength in his upper extremities was normal. In the lower extremities there was 3–4/5 weakness in the foot dorsiflexors and evertors on the left leg with 5−/5 weakness of the glutei, iliopsoas, adductors, quadriceps, and hamstrings; the right hip muscles were 5−/5, other muscles were normal. Reflexes were 2+ in the upper extremities, 1 at the knees and trace at the right ankle. The ankle reflexes were absent. There were no Babinski signs. A bulbocavernous reflex could not be elicited, but the rectal examination revealed normal sphincter tone. There were no pathologic reflexes. Sensory examination was entirely normal, including the perianal area. Scattered fasciculations were detected in the legs but not in the arms. The rest of the examination was normal.

Thyroid-stimulating hormone, C3, C4, and FANA, a complete metabolic panel, and protein electrophoresis were normal. Serum creatine kinase (CK) was 663 IU/L (normal, <210 IU/L). Erythrocyte sedimentation rate was normal. A chest x-ray was normal.

AN EMG TEST WAS PERFORMED

Motor Nerve Studies

Nerve and Site	Latency(ms)	Amplitude (mV)	Conduction Velocity (m/s)
Peroneal Nerve L.	**Normal ≤ 5.7**	**Normal ≥ 3**	**Normal ≥ 40**
Ankle	4.9	5	–
Fibular head	12.1	3	44
Tibial Nerve R.	**Normal ≤ 5.3**	**Normal ≥ 4**	**Normal ≥ 40**
Ankle	5.2	4	–
Pop. fossa	13.6	4	49

F-Wave and Tibial H-Reflex Studies

Nerve	Latency (ms)	Normal Latency ≤ (ms)
Peroneal nerve L.	52.7	54.0
Tibial nerve R.	53.8	54.0
H-reflex L.	**NR**	34.0
H-reflex R.	**NR**	34.0

Sensory Nerve Studies

Nerve	Onset Latency (ms)	Normal Onset Latency ≤ (ms)	Peak Latency (ms)	Normal Peak Latency ≤ (ms)	Amp (μV)	Normal Amp ≥ (μV)	Conduction Velocity (m/s)	Normal Conduction Velocity ≥ (m/s)
Sural nerve L.	3.3	3.5	3.8	4.0	15	11	42	40

EMG Data

Muscle	Insrt Activity	Fibs	Pos Waves	Fasc	Amp	Dur	Poly	Pattern
Deltoid L.	Norm	None	None	None	Norm	Norm	**Few**	Full
Biceps brachii L.	Norm	None	None	None	Norm	Norm	**Few**	Full
1st dorsal interosseous L.	Norm	None	None	**Few**	Norm	Norm	Norm	Full
Gluteus medius L.	Norm	None	None	**Few**	Norm	Norm	**Few**	Full
Rectus femoris L.	**Myok**	**Few**	None	None	Norm	Norm	Norm	**Red**
Tibialis anterior L.	**Myok**	None	None	**Few**	Norm	Norm	Norm	**Red**
Peroneus longus L.	**Myok**	None	None	**Few**	Norm	Norm	Norm	**Red**
Gastrocnemius L.	**Myok**	None	None	**Few**	Norm	Norm	Norm	**Red**

WHAT WERE THE EMG FINDINGS?

This test showed normal motor nerve conduction velocities and CMAP amplitudes and latencies. F-wave latencies and sural SNAP were normal. H-reflexes were absent bilaterally. The needle test showed prominent fasciculations and long-duration polyphasic motor unit potentials in the legs diffusely. The recruitment patterns appeared normal, except for the left rectus femoris muscle where motor unit recruitment was reduced; only rare fibrillations were seen in this muscle. Myokymic discharges were also seen in the legs. There were rare polyphasic motor unit potentials in the arm. The focal abnormalities and lack of diffuse denervation are against a motor neuron disease, such as spinal muscular atrophy or ALS; the lack of long tract signs is also against the latter.

WHAT IS THE DIFFERENTIAL DIAGNOSIS?

This patient presented with symptoms only in the lower extremities with weakness, fasciculations, and some sexual dysfunction. EMG abnormalities were prominent in the legs only, with large motor unit potentials and fasciculations suggesting a chronic lesion of the motor neurons; no prominent denervation was found. The upper extremity examination was essentially normal, except for rare polyphasic motor unit potentials, the cause of which was not clear.

He was previously considered to have a motor neuron disease. The lack of progression could suggest that he had a benign focal amyotrophy or monomelic amyotrophy. This is a condition that not only affects younger individuals causing nonprogressive or slowly progressive weakness and atrophy localized in an upper extremity,[1–3] but also occurs in the lower extremities.[4] The sexual dysfunction, however, would favor a spinal cord or cauda equina lesion, a tumor, or an inflammatory process, in spite of the normal sensory examination and normal rectal sphincter tone. The previous noncontrast MRI done to rule out disk disease was not available.

WHAT WILL BE THE NEXT DIAGNOSTIC TEST?

A repeat MRI of the lumbosacral spine that included the conus medullaris, with and without contrast, is very important in ruling out structural abnormalities. His MRI showed an enhancing mass in the T12–L1 area (Fig. 28-1).

The patient underwent surgery, which consisted of removal of a tumor attached to the filum terminale; the pathology was consistent with an ependymoma. This was a very cellular tumor with mature nuclei and mucinous degeneration; on EM the tumor showed multiple interdigitating processes filled with filaments (Fig. 28-2).

After surgery the patient had marked improvement of his symptoms but continued with mild weakness of the foot flexors on the left. His CK was normalized.

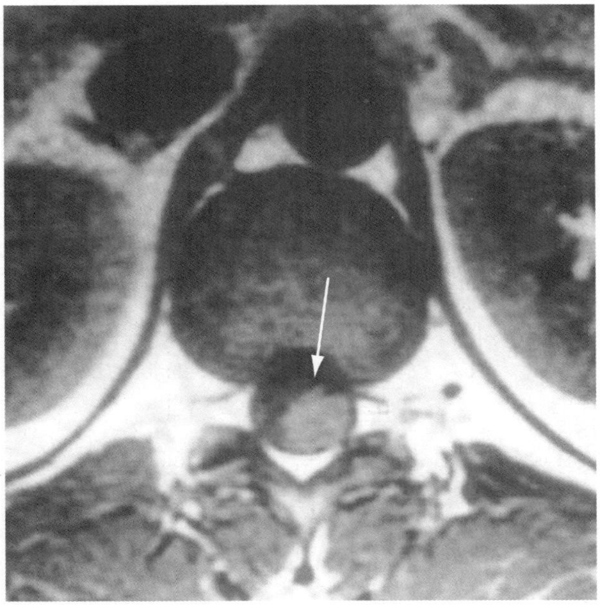

FIG. 28-1 MRI (axial view) showing a gadolinium-enhancing mass in the L1 area (*arrow*).

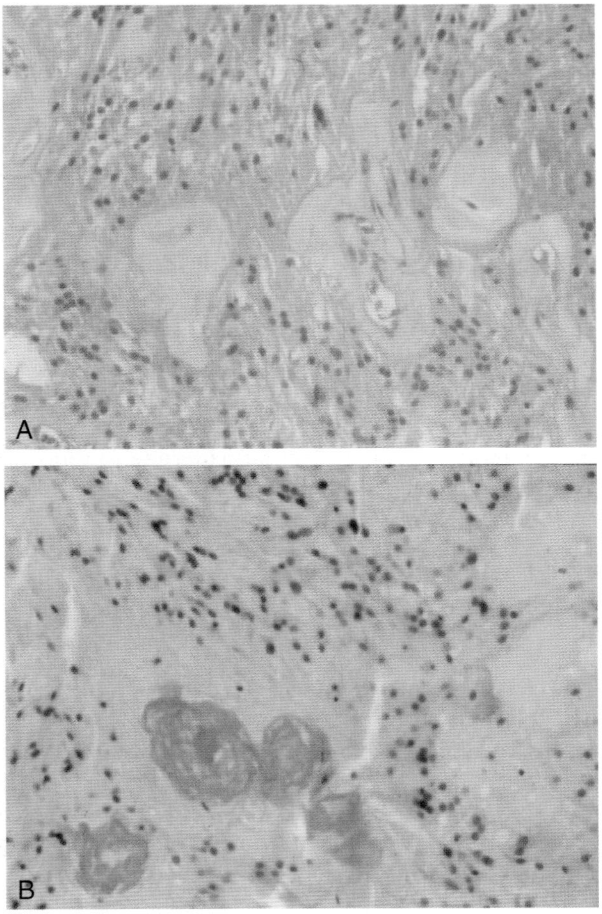

FIG. 28-2 **A**, Section of the tumor showing the ependymal cells with collars of mucinous material around blood vessels (H&E stain, ×200). **B**, Alcian blue stain showing positive-staining mucinous material in the perivascular area (×200).

DISCUSSION

This patient presented with an apparent motor neuron disorder with weakness and prominent fasciculations in the lower extremities. He, however, also had sexual dysfunction, which suggested a spinal cord process. A previous MRI was reported as normal. A repeat MRI with contrast demonstrated an enhancing tumor in the conus area. This was found to be an ependymoma, which was removed.

The patient had an elevated serum CK as typically seen in myopathies, but this can also occur in motor neuron disorders.[5,6] The cause of the elevation in those is not clear but could be caused by motor unit hyperactivity, such as muscle cramps and spasms, as in this case.

This case reinforces the notion that, although motor neuron disorders could begin in a focal fashion and even remain focal,[1–4] one should always aggressively search for a treatable cause, particularly in patients with unusual manifestations.

Imaging of the spine in patients with this presentation should always visualize the conus medullaris, which might not be included in studies for radiculopathy; particularly, one should always use contrast enhancement for the diagnosis of possible tumors in those.[7] Tumors of this area include ependymomas, meningiomas, and Schwannomas that are benign and could be removed.[8–10] Spinal metastasis or carcinomatosis could also have this presentation, but in those the prognosis is poor.[11–14]

Spinal cord ependymomas are usually cavitated or cystic lesions that are better visualized using contrast MRI. These benign tumors can be completely removed.[15]

SUMMARY

This patient with lower extremity weakness and an EMG that showed fasciculations only in the legs was referred for possible ALS. A previous noncontrasted MRI of the lumbosacral spine was reported as normal. He was found to have a lower motor neuron syndrome only in the legs from an ependymoma in the conus area.

IMPORTANT POINTS

- Patients presenting with prominent lower motor neuron signs in the lower extremities should have an MRI of the lumbosacral and lower thoracic spine including imaging of the conus using contrast. Benign focal amyotrophy could manifest in the legs, but one should always look carefully for other causes to explain the symptoms, particularly when there is urinary or sexual dysfunction.
- Tumors of the spinal cord and conus medullaris include ependymomas, neurofibromas, meningiomas, and metastasis.
- Elevation of serum CK can occur not only in motor neuron diseases but also in other disorders affecting the lower motor neurons.
- Ependymoma of the lower spinal cord can be successfully removed.

REFERENCES

1. Hirayama K. Juvenile non-progressive muscular atrophy localized in the hand and forearm: observations in 38 cases. *Rinsho Shinkeigaku*. 1972;12:313–324.
2. Hirayama K, Tomonaga M, Kitano K, et al. Focal cervical poliopathy causing juvenile muscular atrophy of distal upper extremity: a pathological study. *J Neurol Neurosurg Psychiatry*. 1987;50:285–290.
3. Riggs JE, Schochet SS Jr, Gutmann L, Rana PV. Benign focal amyotrophy: variant of chronic spinal muscular atrophy. *Arch Neurol*. 1984;41:678–679.
4. Prabhakar S, Chopra JS, Banerjee AK, et al. Wasted leg syndrome: a clinical, electrophysiological and histopathological study. *Clin Neurol Neurosurg*. 1981;83:19–28.
5. Rudnik-Schoneborn S, Lutzenrath S, Borkowska J, et al. Analysis of creatine kinase activity in 504 patients with proximal spinal muscular atrophy types I–III from the point of view of progression and severity. *Eur Neurol*. 1998;39(3):154–162.
6. Murray B. Mitzumoto H Amyotrophic lateral sclerosis. In: Katirji B, Kaminski HJ, Preston DC, Ruff RL, Shapiro BE, eds. *Neuromuscular Disorders in Clinical Practice*. Boston, MA: Butterworth-Heinemann; 2002:417–444.
7. Katirji B. Cauda equina Schwannoma misdiagnosed as focal motor neuron disease. *J Clin Neuromuscul Dis*. 2001;3(1):36–38.
8. Cervoni L, Celli P, Scarpinati M, Cantore G. Neurinomas of the cauda equina: clinical analysis of 40 surgical cases. *Acta Neurochir (Vienna)*. 1994;127(3–4):199–202.
9. Takemoto K, Matsumura Y, Hashimoto H, et al. MR imaging of intraspinal tumors—capability in histological differentiation and compartmentalization of extramedullary tumors. *Neuroradiology*. 1988;30(4):303–309.
10. Dillon WP, Norman D, Newton TH, et al. Intradural spinal cord lesions: Gd-DTPA-enhanced MR imaging. *Radiology*. 1989;170 (Pt 1):229–237.
11. Schuknecht B, Huber P, Buller B, Nadjmi M. Spinal leptomeningeal neoplastic diseases: evaluation by MR, myelography and CT myelogram. *Eur Neurol*. 1993;32:11–16.
12. Byrne TN. Spinal cord compression from epidural metastasis. *N Engl J Med*. 1992;327:614–619.
13. Kamholtz R, Sze G. Current imaging in spinal metastatic disease. *Semin Oncol*. 1991;18:158–169.
14. Heinz P, Weiner D, Friedman H, Tien R. Detection of cerebrospinal fluid metastasis: CT myelography or MR? *Am J Neuroradiol*. 1995;16(5):1147–1151.
15. Nakama S, Higashi T, Kimura A, et al. Double myxopapillary ependymoma of the cauda equina. *J Orthop Sci*. 2005;10(5): 543–545.

A Woman With Unilateral Facial Weakness

A 52-year-old woman presented with a 5-day history of pain in the left ear; she then had 3 days of decreased taste and facial weakness. She had no significant previous medical history. There was no history of diabetes. She drank alcohol socially.

The examination was normal except for weakness of the left orbicularis oculi, orbicularis oris, frontalis, and other left facial muscles. There was flattening of the left nasolabial fold (Fig. 29-1). She also had decreased taste in the anterior left tongue. Examination of the ear was normal. Other cranial nerves were completely normal. Strength, reflexes, coordination, and sensory examinations were unremarkable. There were no Babinski signs.

WHAT IS THE MOST LIKELY DIAGNOSIS?

The most likely diagnosis is acute idiopathic seventh nerve neuropathy, or Bell's palsy.

WHAT TESTS NEED TO BE DONE?

A complete metabolic panel was normal, including blood sugar and erythrocyte sedimentation rate.

AN EMG TEST WAS PERFORMED

Motor Nerve Studies

Nerve and Site	Latency(ms)	Amplitude (mV)	Conduction Velocity (m/s)
Ulnar Nerve R.	**Normal ≤ 3.6**	**Normal ≥ 8**	**Normal ≥ 50**
Wrist	3.4	9	–
Below elbow	7.0	9	62
Facial Nerve	**Normal ≤ 2.6**	**Normal ≥ 2.5[a]**	
Facial nerve L.	3.5	**0.80**	–
Facial nerve R.	3.3	4	–

[a]50% reduction in amplitude compared with the opposite side is considered abnormal, if similar, waveforms.

Blink Reflex

	Ipsilateral R1 Normal ≤ 13.0 (ms)	Ipsilateral R2 ≤ 40 (ms)	Contralateral R2 ≤ 41 (ms)
Blink reflex L.	**NR**	**NR**	38
Blink reflex R.	12.0	30	**NR**

R1, upper limits of normal side-to-side difference is 1.2 ms. R2, upper limits of normal side-to-side difference is 5 ms.

EMG Data

Muscle	Insrt Activity	Fibs	Pos Waves	Fasc	Amp	Dur	Poly	Pattern
Orb. oculi L.	Norm	None	None	None	Norm	Norm	**Few**	**Red**
Orb. oris L.	Norm	None	None	None	Norm	Norm	**Few**	**Red**
Masseter L.	Norm	None	None	None	Norm	Norm	**Few**	**Red**
Orb. oris R.	Norm	None	None	None	Norm	Norm	None	Norm

WHAT WERE THE EMG FINDINGS?

This test showed normal motor conduction tests of the right ulnar nerve. She had low-amplitude facial nerve CMAP on the left compared to the right.

When stimulating the right supraorbital nerve, the blink reflex R1 latency was 12 ms and the R2 latency was 30 ms. No R2 was recorded on the left; no R1 or R2 responses were obtained on the left when the left supraorbital nerve was stimulated, but an R2 was obtained on the right with a latency of 38 ms, which was normal.

Needle electromyography showed scattered polyphasic unit action potentials with reduced recruitment but no evidence of denervation in the left facial muscles.

She was diagnosed as having peripheral VII cranial neuropathy, or Bell's palsy, and received prednisone 40 mg daily and acyclovir 200 mg five times a day for 1 week with significant improvement.

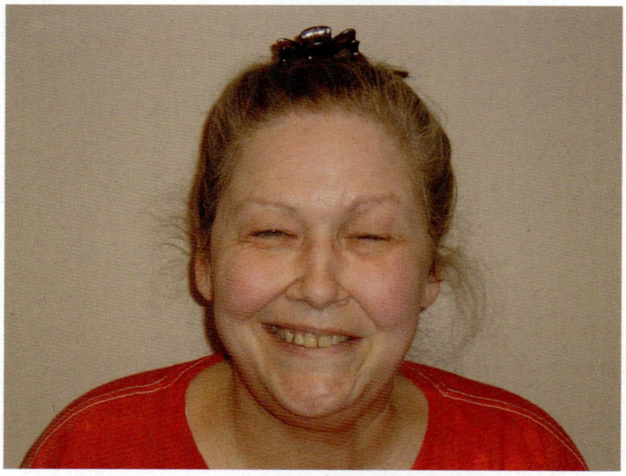

FIG. 29-1 The patient showing facial asymmetry from a left VII nerve palsy.

DISCUSSION

This patient had an idiopathic left VII nerve neuropathy, or Bell's palsy, manifesting with weakness and decreased taste.[1,2]

The VII cranial nerve, or facial nerve, is a sensorimotor nerve that innervates muscles of facial expression, the salivary and lacrimal glands, and the mucus membranes of the nasal and oral cavities.

The nerve also relays taste sensation to the anterior two-thirds of the tongue through the chorda tympani and provides tactile sensation in an area of the skin on the posterior external auditory canal and the tympanic and external acoustic membranes.

The motor fibers originate from the facial nucleus of the pons and exit in its ventral surface at the cerebellopontine angle, entering the temporal bone, from whence it exits the skull through the stylomastoid foramen (Fig. 29-2).

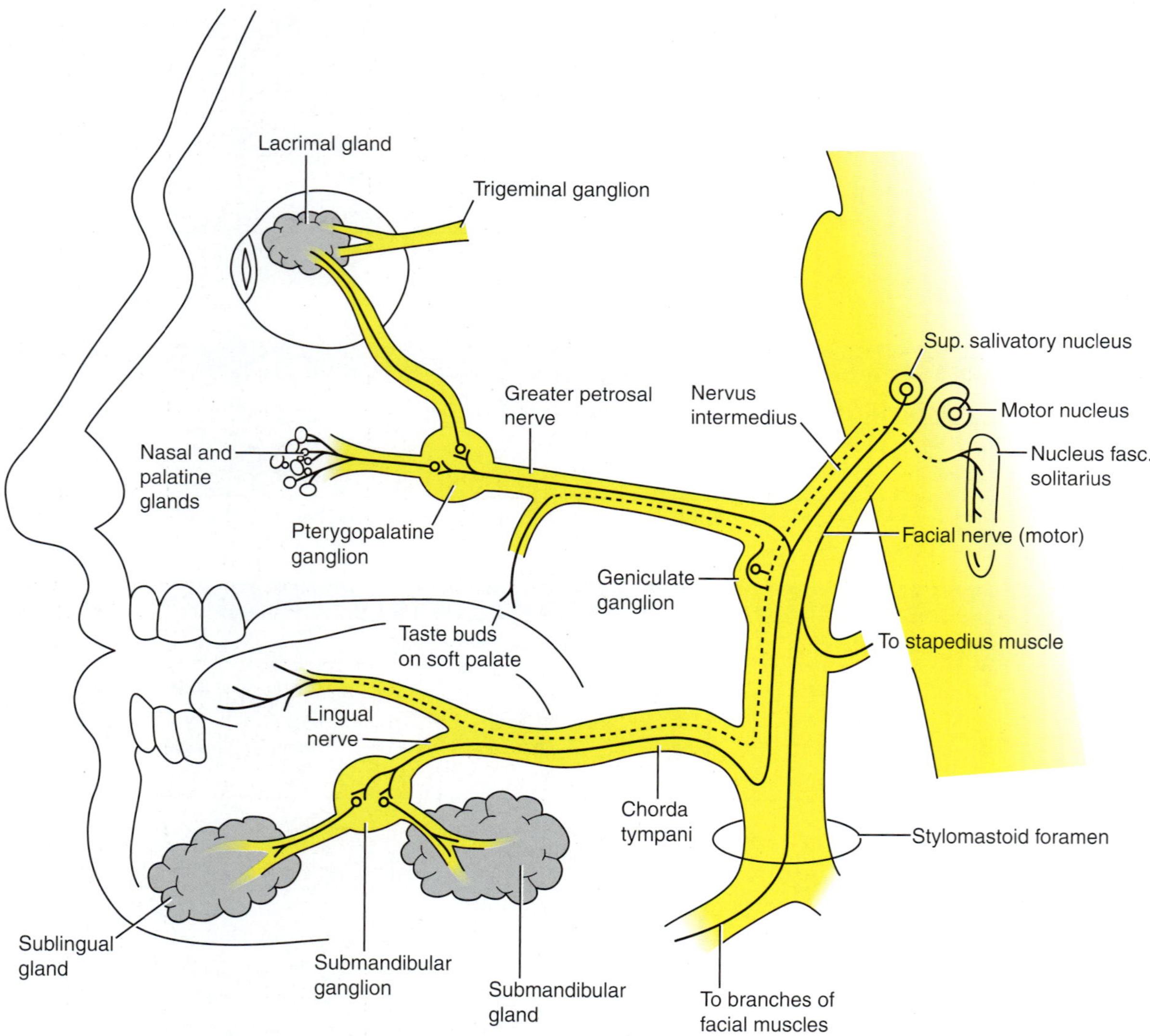

FIG. 29-2 Anatomy of the VII cranial nerve.

The facial muscles could be affected by lesions of the upper motor neuron of the opposite hemisphere and upper brainstem. Those usually spare the frontalis muscle that has bilateral innervation; these muscles are usually involved in Bell's palsy and cerebellopontine angle lesions. The peripheral nerve could also be affected at the temporal bone and after exiting the skull.

Idiopathic facial palsy (Bell's palsy) is the most common cause of a VII nerve dysfunction. Other causes include trauma, sarcoidosis, infections, and diabetes. Bell's palsy usually presents acutely with dull pain behind the ear, and then after 48–72 hours, patients develop weakness of the muscles of the hemiface. The lesion usually occurs in the proximal facial canal[1] with inflammation and demyelination; axonal degeneration may also occur.

The disease has a favorable prognosis, and most patients recover fully. The most common sequelae are persistent weakness and aberrant regeneration with synkinetic movements of the affected side when contracting other muscles (e.g., movements of the lips when blinking). Some patients may also develop hemifacial spasms and tearing when eating ("crocodile tears").[2]

Bell's palsy is caused by reactivation of herpes virus type I; this has been isolated from the geniculate ganglia at autopsy,[2] and the viral genome has been detected in the endoneurium of the VII nerve in 79% of patients.[3,4]

Herpes zoster infections in the geniculate ganglion produce facial palsy with vesicles in the external auditory canal with tinnitus and decreased hearing. This presentation is called the Ramsay Hunt syndrome.[5,6]

Recurrent facial neuropathy is more often seen in diabetics.[7] A bilateral VII nerve disease can be idiopathic, but can also be seen in a variety of conditions. It may appear acutely, as in the Guillain–Barré syndrome, or can also occur in the course of multiple sclerosis, during infections (particularly Lyme disease),[8] syphilis, leprosy, meningitis, and sarcoidosis.[9,10] Bell's palsy also occurs during pregnancy. The Melkersson–Rosenthal syndrome is a rare condition characterized by recurrent orofacial edema with tongue abnormalities and recurrent facial palsy.[11]

The diagnosis of facial palsy is based on clinical examination. EMG studies document diminished CMAP amplitudes in the affected side with a reduction of motor unit recruitment and later denervation potentials in severe cases.[12] The lack of motor unit action potentials during voluntary contractions or significant denervation with an absent ipsilateral R1 of the affected side indicates a poor prognosis.[13–15]

A study compared the CMAP between the normal and affected sides to estimate the degree of axonal damage and found that an amplitude of over 30% in the affected side suggests there will be a complete recovery. In those with CMAP amplitudes of 25% or less than the normal, there is a chance of some degree of permanent dysfunction.[16]

Imaging studies may document edema in the nerve or other abnormalities, like abnormal vessels.

The treatment of idiopathic facial palsy includes the use of steroids with acyclovir or vancyclovir and physical therapy.[17,18] There is no clear evidence that the addition of antivirals to prednisone (particularly if there are no vesicles or no indication of viral etiology).[19]

SUMMARY

This patient had Bell's palsy and had a complete recovery with steroids and acyclovir. She manifested pain in the ear, decreased taste, and weakness of the hemifacial muscles.

IMPORTANT POINTS

- Bell's palsy is a common acute neuropathy of the VII cranial nerve and is likely caused by a herpes virus infection.
- Electromyography has prognostic value; in particular, the blink reflex and CMAP amplitude measurement of both sides are important for the assessment of prognosis.
- The presence of denervation, a CMAP below 35% on the normal side, and the blink reflex missing an R1 in the affected side indicate a poorer prognosis.
- Sequelae of Bell's palsy include hemifacial spasms, synkinesias, and "crocodile tears."
- Recurrent Bell's palsy could be idiopathic and is seen in diabetes, sarcoidosis, and the Melkersson–Rosenthal syndrome.
- Bilateral Bell's palsy occurs in the Guillain–Barré syndrome, sarcoidosis, tuberculosis, Lyme disease, and syphilis.
- Acute Bell's palsy associated with vesicles in the ear, tinnitus, and decreased hearing is called the Ramsay Hunt syndrome and is usually caused by herpes zoster infections.
- Treatment for Bell's palsy consists of the use of steroids.

REFERENCES

1. Katusic SK, Beard CM, Wiederholt WC, et al. Incidence, clinical features and prognosis in Bell's palsy, Rochester, Minnesota, 1968–1982. *Ann Neurol.* 1986;20:622–627.
2. Hauser WA, Karnes WE, Annis J, Kurland LT. Incidence and prognosis of Bell's palsy in the population of Rochester, Minnesota. *Mayo Clin Proc.* 1971;46:258–264.
3. Adour KK, Bell DN, Hilsinger RL Jr. Herpes simplex virus in idiopathic facial paralysis (Bell's palsy). *JAMA.* 1975;233:527–530.
4. Adour KK, Bell FM, Hilsinger RL Jr, et al. The true nature of Bell's palsy: analysis of 1,000 consecutive patients. *Laryngoscope.* 1978;88:787–801.
5. Aitken RS, Brain RT. Facial palsy and infection with zoster virus. *Lancet.* 1933;1:19–22.
6. Harner SG, Heiny BA, Newell RC. Herpes zoster oticus. *Arch Otolaryngol.* 1970;92:632–635.
7. Johnson EW, Waylonis GW. Facial nerve conduction delay in patients with diabetes mellitus. *Arch Phys Med Rehabil.* 1964;45:131–139.
8. Kaiser R. Neuroborreliosis. *J Neurol.* 1998;245:247–255.
9. Colover J. Sarcoidosis with involvement of the nervous system. *Brain.* 1948;71:451–475.
10. Kline DG, Thomas PK. Disease of the seventh cranial nerve. In: Dyck PJ, Thomas PE, eds. *Peripheral Neuropathy.* 4th ed. Philadelphia, PA: WB Saunders; 2005:1219–1252.
11. Klaus SN, Brunsting LA. Melkersson-Rosenthal's syndrome (persistent swelling of the face, recurrent facial paralysis and lingua plicata). *Proc Staff Meet Mayo Clin.* 1959;34:365–370.

12. Alford BR. Electrodiagnostic studies in facial paralysis. *Arch Otolaryngol.* 1967;85:259–264.
13. Celik M, Forta H. Electrophysiological investigations and prognosis in idiopathic facial palsy. *Electromyogr Clin Neurophysiol.* 1997;37:311–315.
14. Kimura J. The blink reflex. In: Kimura J, ed. *Electrodiagnosis in Diseases of Nerve and Muscle: Principles and Practice.* 3rd ed. New York, NY: Oxford University Press; 2001:409–438.
15. de Bisschop G, de Bence G, Bence Y. Selection of the electrophysiological methods for diagnosis in facial palsy. In: Portman M, ed. *Facial Nerve.* New York, NY: Masson; 1984: 349–352.
16. May M, Blumenthal F, Kleins SR. Acute Bell's palsy: prognostic value of evoked electromyography, maximal stimulation, and other electrical tests. *Am J Otol.* 1983;5(1):1–7.
17. De Diego JI, Prim MP, De Sarria MJ, et al. Idiopathic facial paralysis: a randomized, prospective, and controlled study using single-dose prednisone vs acyclovir three times daily. *Laryngoscope.* 1998;108:573–575.
18. Hato N, Yomoda H, Kohno H, et al. Valacyclovir and prednisolone treatment for Bell's palsy: a multicenter randomized, placebo-controlled study. *Otol Neurotol.* 2007;28(3):408–413.
19. Somasundara D, Sullivan F. Management of Bell's palsy. *Aust Prescr.* 2017;40(3):94–97.

CASE 30

A Diabetic Woman With Muscle Weakness and Ophthalmoplegia

A 44-year-old woman presented with worsening low back pain of 1 month's duration. She also complained of difficulty chewing and blurred vision for 1 week and diffuse weakness in the lower extremities. She denied headaches, vertigo, or other neurologic symptoms. Her medical history was remarkable for insulin-dependent diabetes for over 6 years. She did not smoke, drink alcohol, or use recreational drugs.

General physical examination was unremarkable. Neurologic examination revealed mild bilateral peripheral facial weakness and bilateral external rectus muscle weakness; other cranial nerves were normal (Fig. 30-1). She had 4/5 strength with tenderness to palpation in the proximal muscles of the lower extremities and back. Distal leg muscles were 5−/5. Reflexes were absent throughout. Vibration sense was absent in the ankles and decreased at the knees. Pain and touch sensation was decreased up to the ankles. The rest of the examination was unremarkable.

WHAT IS THE DIFFERENTIAL DIAGNOSES?

This diabetic patient developed bilateral VI and VII nerve palsies and had a polyneuropathy. The combination of findings can be present in central nervous system disorders such as multiple sclerosis. However, there was no evidence of long tract signs or other findings to suggest a central lesion, and the presentation appeared to involve only peripheral nerves. The findings on examination could suggest a diabetic polyneuropathy with cranial neuropathies.[1] Other possibilities include vasculitic neuropathy from connective tissue disorders such as Sjögren's and lupus,[2] but there was no evidence of asymmetric neuropathy in the limbs or other manifestations of those disorders. Leprosy could present with bilateral facial neuropathy but characteristically not with VI nerve palsies.[3] Lyme disease could also cause facial palsy and other cranial neuropathies.[4]

Tuberculosis and sarcoidosis can manifest with basilar meningitis and cranial nerve palsies, and those should be included in the differential diagnosis.[5,6] She also complained of back pain; this could be related to a lumbar disk disease as her other neurologic problems were caused by an inflammatory process in the lumbosacral nerves or roots. Another consideration is a nervous system lymphomatosis.

AN EMG TEST WAS PERFORMED

Motor Nerve Studies

Nerve and Site	Latency (ms)	Amplitude (mV)	Conduction Velocity (m/s)
Peroneal Nerve R.	**Normal ≤ 5.7**	**Normal ≥ 3**	**Normal ≥ 40**
Ankle	5.4	**2**	–
Fibular head	13.6	**2**	**37**
Knee	16.6	**1**	**33**
Nerve and Site	**Latency (ms)**	**Amplitude (mV)**	**Conduction Velocity (m/s)**
Tibial Nerve L.	**Normal ≤ 5.3**	**Normal ≥ 4**	**Normal ≥ 40**
Ankle	5.2	4	–
Pop. fossa	15.1	**3**	**39**
Nerve and Site	**Latency (ms)**	**Amplitude (mV)**	**Conduction Velocity (m/s)**
Median Nerve R.	**Normal ≤ 4.2**	**Normal ≥ 6**	**Normal ≥ 50**
Wrist	**8.1**	6	–
Elbow	13.2	6	**43**
Ulnar Nerve R.	**Normal ≤ 3.6**	**Normal ≥ 8**	**Normal ≥ 50**
Wrist	**3.8**	13	–
Below elbow	7.8	13	53
Median Nerve L.	**Normal ≤ 4.2**	**Normal ≥ 6**	**Normal ≥ 50**
Wrist	**5.5**	15	–
Elbow	9.9	15	50
Nerve and Site	**Latency (ms)**	**Amplitude (mV)**	**Conduction Velocity (m/s)**
Facial Nerve	**Normal ≤ 2.6**	**Normal ≥ 2.5**	
Facial nerve R.	**4.85**	2.5	–
Facial nerve L.	**4.45**	2.7	–

F-Wave and Tibial H-Reflex Studies

Nerve	Latency (ms)	Normal Latency ≤ (ms)
Peroneal nerve R.	**58.8**	54
Tibial nerve L.	**61**	54
Median nerve R.	**36.8**	30
Ulnar nerve R.	29.6	30
Median nerve L.	**31**	30
H-reflex R.	NR	34
H-reflex L.	NR	34

Sensory Nerve Studies

Nerve	Onset Latency (ms)	Normal Onset Latency ≤ (ms)	Peak Latency (ms)	Normal Peak Latency ≤ (ms)	Amp (μV)	Normal Amp ≥ (μV)	Conduction Velocity (m/s)	Normal Conduction Velocity ≥ (m/s)
Sural nerve R.	**NR**	3.5	**NR**	4.0	**NR**	11	**NR**	40
Median nerve R.	**NR**	2.6	**NR**	3.1	**NR**	20	**NR**	50
Ulnar nerve R.	2.4	2.6	2.9	3.1	**8**	13	50	50
Median nerve L.	**4.3**	2.6	**4.8**	3.1	**12**	20	**30**	50

EMG Data

Muscle	Insrt Activity	Fibs	Pos Waves	Fasc	Amp	Dur	Poly	Pattern
Deltoid R.	None	None	None	None	Norm	Norm	None	Full
Biceps brachii R.	None	None	None	None	Norm	Norm	None	Full
Flexor carpi radialis R.	None	None	None	None	Norm	Norm	None	Full
Abductor pollicis brevis R.	**Inc**	**2+**	**2+**	**None**	**Lg**	**Inc**	None	**Red**
First dorsal interosseous R.	None	None	None	None	**Lg**	**Inc**	None	**Red**
Abductor pollicis brevis L.	None	None	None	None	**Lg**	**Inc**	None	**Red**
First dorsal interosseous L.	None	None	None	None	**Lg**	**Inc**	None	**Red**
Vastus lateralis R.	None	None	None	None	**Lg**	**Inc**	None	**Red**
Tibialis anterior R.	None	None	None	None	**Lg**	**Inc**	None	**Red**
Gastrocnemius R.	None	None	None	None	**Lg**	**Inc**	None	**Red**
Tibialis anterior L.	None	None	None	None	**Lg**	**Inc**	None	**Red**
Gastrocnemius L.	None	None	None	None	**Lg**	**Inc**	None	**Red**
Orbicularis oculi R.	**Inc**	**1+**	**1+**	None	Norm	Norm	None	**Red**
Orbicularis oculi L.	**Inc**	**1+**	**1+**	None	Norm	Norm	None	**Red**

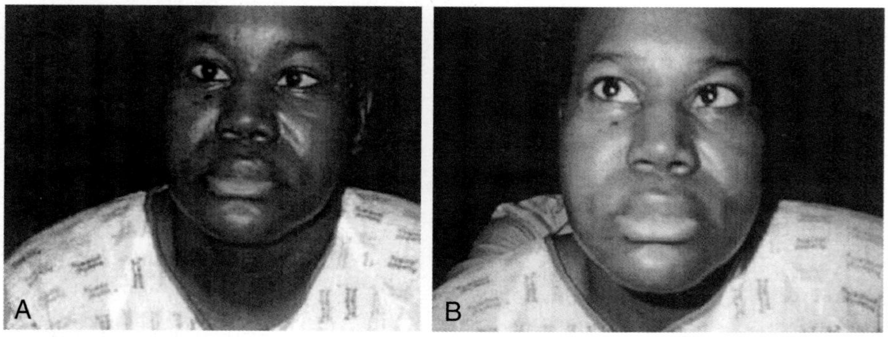

FIG. 30-1 The patient showing inward deviation of the left eye caused by external rectus weakness (A); there is also inability to smile from facial muscle weakness. Notice right external rectus muscle weakness on right lateral gaze (B).

WHAT WERE THE EMG FINDINGS?

The nerve conduction test demonstrated absent right median and sural SNAPs; the left median SNAP was of low amplitude, prolonged latency, and slow velocity; the right ulnar nerve SNAP was of low amplitude. Median nerve distal motor latency was prolonged, while the distal motor latency of the ulnar nerve was only mildly prolonged; median nerve conduction velocity of the right was below normal; and the tibial nerve had borderline CMAP amplitude and slow velocity. The right peroneal CMAP was of low amplitude, and the conduction velocity was slow. The facial nerves had only mildly decreased CMAP amplitudes and prolonged latencies compatible with bilateral facial neuropathies.

On the needle test, there were denervation potentials in the right adductor pollicis brevis muscle and the motor unit action potentials had increased amplitude, prolonged duration, and decreased recruitment. In the lower extremity, there was no denervation but there were also large motor unit potentials. Denervation potentials were also present in facial-innervated muscles bilaterally.

The electrophysiologic diagnosis was sensorimotor polyneuropathy with bilateral VI and VII nerves neuropathy and median neuropathy at the wrists, worse on the right.

WHAT SHOULD BE DONE NEXT?

The complete metabolic panel was normal except for glucose of 248 mg/dL (normal, <120 mg/dL). Liver function tests (LFTs) were normal. Serum creatine kinase was 273 IU/L (normal, <225 IU/L). Alanine transaminase was 44 mg/dL (normal, <40 mg/dL). Serum protein electrophoresis was normal. Spinal fluid had a white blood cell count of 93 and protein of 410 mg/dL (normal, <45 mg/dL). Sugar was 52 mg/dL (normal, >50 mg/dL). A CT scan of the head was normal. Cerebrospinal fluid was negative for AFB, fungus, and malignant cells. (All cells were lymphocytes.)

Thyroid studies, rapid plasma regain (RPR), anti-DNA studies, B_{12}, C3, and C4 complement were all normal. Fluorescent antinuclear antibody was positive at 1:60 with a homogenous pattern; erythrocyte sedimentation rate was normal. Angiotensin-converting enzyme was normal.

Chest x-rays demonstrated hilar lymphadenopathy.

WHAT IS THE DIFFERENTIAL DIAGNOSIS?

This patient had a polyneuropathy, likely from diabetes, and apparent carpal tunnel syndrome (CTS). There were no clinical or laboratory findings to suggest other common causes of polyneuropathy, although some cases of familial amyloidosis can manifest with bilateral facial palsy or CTS but not with ophthalmoplegia. Furthermore, she had elevated spinal fluid cells and increased protein. Thus, one needed to consider another cause for this, in addition to diabetic neuropathy. Syphilis could manifest with cranial nerve palsy, but her RPR test was negative.

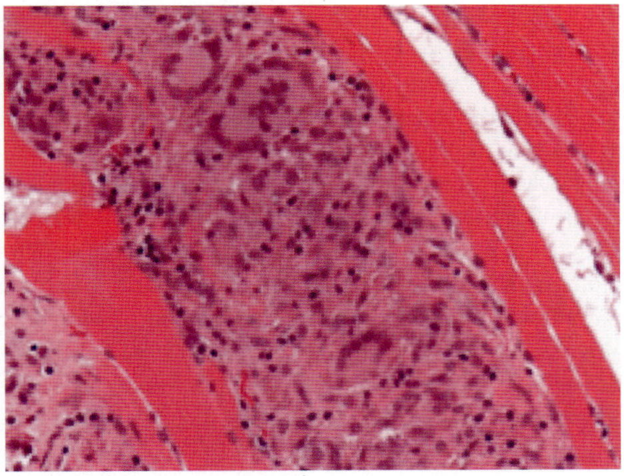

FIG. 30-2 Granuloma in muscle with lymphocytes, epithelioid cells, and giant cells (H&E stain, ×400).

Other inflammatory processes such as tuberculosis or sarcoidosis should be considered, particularly in light of the pulmonary lymphadenopathy.

WHAT SHOULD BE DONE NEXT?

Tuberculin and mumps skin tests were negative. Liver scan and abdominal ultrasound were normal. MRI was not available, but CT scan of the head was unremarkable.

A quadriceps muscle biopsy revealed a granulomatous myopathy (Fig. 30-2), mild neurogenic atrophy, and type II muscle fiber atrophy. AFB stains were negative.

The patient was diagnosed with sarcoidosis, and while carefully monitoring her diabetes mellitus, she was treated with corticosteroids and had marked improvement. For 10 years thereafter she was off steroids and asymptomatic.

DISCUSSION

This diabetic patient also had sarcoidosis affecting cranial nerves VI and VII likely from sarcoid meningitis without hydrocephalus or papilledema.

Sarcoidosis is a multisystem granulomatous disease of which 50% of patients have neurologic complications.[5] It manifests as a myopathy or a neuropathy, which includes polyneuropathy, mononeuritis, and cranial neuropathies, which are the most common manifestations,[6] among them optic neuropathy. Recurrent bilateral cranial VII nerve palsy is a characteristic manifestation of sarcoidosis.[7,8] Polyneuropathy is not frequently seen and occurs in only 14% of patients.[7,8] This is mainly sensorimotor but is occasionally a mononeuritis multiplex.[9–12] Other presentations include a purely sensory neuropathy,[7] a small fiber neuropathy,[9,13] and isolated Horner syndrome.[14] Radiculopathy and extramedullary granuloma with cauda equina syndrome are other manifestations.[7]

The diagnosis of sarcoidosis is based on x-rays showing interstitial fibrosis or enlarged mediastinal lymph nodes. Angiotensin-converting enzyme is usually elevated when the disease affects the lungs. A muscle biopsy is the best and least traumatic way to diagnose sarcoidosis to find the characteristic noncaseating granulomas; liver and lymph node biopsies are also useful. These have a central collection of epithelioid cells derived from macrophages. There are giant cells, which are conglomerates of epithelioid cells sharing the same cytoplasm with multiple nuclei.[15–17] Lymphocytes are not only seen predominantly in the center of the granuloma but are also found in the periphery.[18] Granulomas are seldom found in peripheral nerves, where they can be seen around blood vessels.[18] Nerve biopsies might show demyelination and axonal degeneration.[19] Vasculitis could be found in some cases.

The neuropathy in sarcoidosis could be caused by compression of the axons by the granuloma or damage of the vasa-nervorum neurons and by immuno-pathogenic mechanisms.

MRI of the brain can demonstrate meningeal enhancement (Fig. 30-3), while muscle MRI can sometimes show a star-shaped central lesion of decreased intensity and peripheral enhancement with gadolinium.[20,21] Gallium scans are helpful in locating the site of inflammation in systemic sarcoidosis and can be used to choose the site for muscle biopsy.[22]

The treatment of sarcoidosis, sarcoid neuropathy, and myopathy includes steroids[15,23] and immunosuppressant drugs.[24,25] Intravenous gamma globulin and anti–tumor necrosis factor (TNF)-α treatment is used in some cases of polyneuropathy.[26]

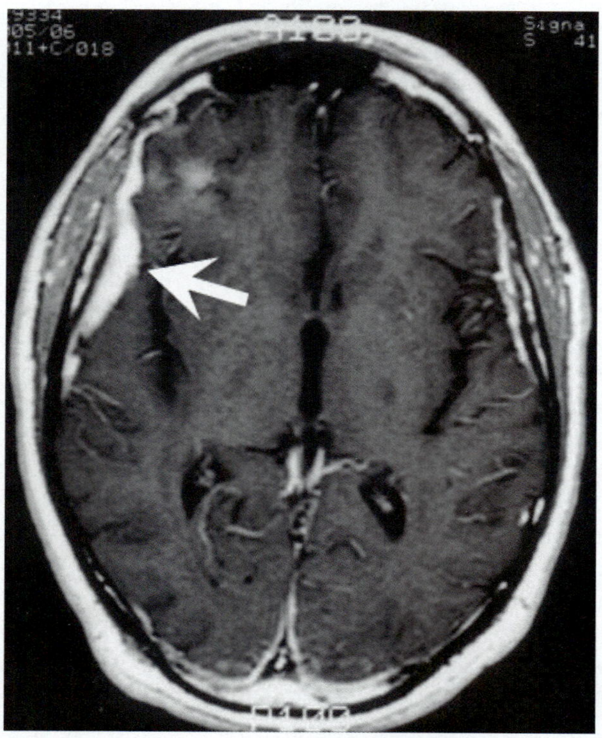

FIG. 30-3 Gadolinium enhancement of the meninges on MRI (*arrow*) in another patient with neurosarcoidosis.

SUMMARY

This diabetic patient developed bilateral cranial VI and VII nerve palsies and a polyneuropathy. She had increased cells and protein in the spinal fluid and was diagnosed with sarcoidosis by muscle biopsy; she responded well to steroids.

IMPORTANT POINTS

- Sarcoidosis can involve the central and peripheral nervous system and can manifest with bilateral facial and VI nerve palsies, optic nerve damage, polyneuropathy, radiculopathies, and a granulomatous myopathy.
- The diagnosis of sarcoidosis is based on abnormalities on chest x-ray and negative skin test for streptokinase, mumps, and tuberculosis. The spinal fluid in sarcoid meningitis usually shows increased cells and protein; the spinal fluid sugar may be decreased.
- The diagnosis of muscle sarcoidosis can be made on gadolinium scan and muscle MRI. In neurosarcoidosis, there is also enhancement of the meninges on cranial MRI.
- A muscle biopsy provides a sensitive and less traumatic tissue for biopsy.
- Sarcoidosis is treated with steroids and immunosuppressant drugs.

REFERENCES

1. Bird SJ, Burns MJ. Diabetic neuropathy. In: Katirji B, Kaminski HJ, Preston DC, Ruff RL, Shapiro BE, eds. *Neuromuscular Disorders in Clinical Practice*. Boston, MA: Butterworth-Heinemann; 2002:598–621.
2. Johnson RT, Richardson EP. The neurological manifestations of systemic lupus erythematosus: a clinical-pathological study of 24 cases and review of the literature. *Medicine*. 1968;47:337–369.
3. Said G. Leprous neuropathy. In: Mendell JR, Kissel JT, Cornblath DT, eds. *Diagnosis and Management of Peripheral Nerve Disorders*. New York, NY: Oxford University Press; 2001:551–564.
4. Kaiser R. Neuroborreliosis. *J Neurol*. 1998;245:247–255.
5. Seraci AP, Wulff EA, Simpson DM. Infections and granulomatous neuropathies. In: Katirji B, Kaminski HJ, Preston DC, Ruff RL, Shapiro BE, eds. *Neuromuscular Disorders in Clinical Practice*. Boston, MA: Butterworth-Heinemann; 2002:710–735.
6. Voortman M, Drent M, Baughman RP. Management of neurosarcoidosis: a clinical challenge. *Curr Opin Neurol*. 2019;32(3):475–483.
7. Stern BJ, Krumholz A, Johns C, et al. Sarcoidosis and its neurological manifestations. *Arch Neurol*. 1985;42:909–917.
8. Gainsborough N, Hall SM, Hughes RA, Leibowitz S. Sarcoid neuropathy. *J Neurol*. 1991;238:177–180.
9. Lower EE, Broderick JP, Brott TG, Baughman RP. Diagnosis and management of neurological sarcoidosis. *Arch Intern Med*. 1997;157:1864–1868.
10. Zuniga G, Ropper AH, Frank J. Sarcoid peripheral neuropathy. *Neurology*. 1991;41:1558–1561.
11. Wiederholt WC, Siekert RG. Neurological manifestations of sarcoidosis. *Neurology*. 1965;15:1147–1154.

12. Garg S, Wright A, Reichwein R, et al. Mononeuritis multiplex secondary to sarcoidosis. *Clin Neurol Neurosurg.* 2005;107(2):140–143.
13. Hoitsma E, Faber CG, van Kroonenburgh MJ, et al. Association of small fiber neuropathy with cardiac sympathetic dysfunction in sarcoidosis. *Sarcoidosis Vasc Diffuse Lung Dis.* 2005;22(1):43–50.
14. Cohen DM, Reinhardt RA. Systemic sarcoidosis presenting with Horner's syndrome and mandibular paresthesia. *Oral Surg Oral Med Oral Pathol.* 1982;53:577–581.
15. Kompf D, Neundorfer B, Kayser-Gatchalian C, et al. Mononeuritis multiplex in Boeck's sarcoidosis. *Nervenarzt.* 1976;47:687–689.
16. Banker BQ. Other inflammatory myopathies. In: Engel AG, Franzini-Armstrong C, eds. *Myology*. New York, NY: McGraw-Hill; 1994:1461–1486.
17. Silverstin A, Siltzbach LE. Muscle involvement in sarcoidosis: asymptomatic myositis and myopathy. *Arch Neurol.* 1969;21(3): 235–241.
18. Takanashi T, Suzuki Y, Yoshino Y, Nonaka I. Granulomatous myositis: pathologic re-evaluation by immunohistochemical analysis of infiltrating mononuclear cells. *J Neurol Sci.* 1997; 145(1):41–47.
19. Oh SJ. Sarcoid polyneuropathy: a histologically proved case. *Ann Neurol.* 1980;7:178–181.
20. Otake S. Sarcoidosis involving skeletal muscle: imaging findings and relative value of imaging procedures. *Am J Roentgenol.* 1994; 162:369–375.
21. Otake S, Imagumbai N, Suzuki M, Ohba S. MR imaging of muscular sarcoidosis after steroid therapy. *Eur Radiol.* 1998;8: 1651–1653.
22. Bekerman C, Szidon JP, Pinsky S. The role of gallium-67 in the clinical evaluation of sarcoidosis. *Semin Roentgenol.* 1985;20: 400–409.
23. Said G, Lacroix C. Sarcoid neuropathy. In: Dyck PJ, Thomas PK, eds. *Peripheral Neuropathy*. 4th ed. Philadelphia, PA: WB Saunders; 2005. 2115–2125.
24. Aqbogu BN, Stern BJ, Sewell C, Yang G. Therapeutic considerations in patients with refractory neurosarcoidosis. *Arch Neurol.* 1995;52:875–879.
25. Patel AV, Stickler DE, Tyor WR. Neurosarcoidosis. *Curr Treat Options Neurol.* 2007;9(3):161–168.
26. Tavee JO, Karwa K, Ahmed Z, Thompson N, et al. Sarcoidosis-associated small fiber neuropathy in a large cohort: clinical aspects and response to IVIG and anti-TNF alpha treatment. *Respir Med.* 2017;126:135–138.

31 CASE

A Man With a Dropped Head

A 64-year-old man developed weakness in his arms over 6 months. In the last 2 months, he noticed a tendency for his head to drop forward, and he had difficulty raising it when lying in bed. He also had mild difficulty swallowing.

Past medical history was remarkable for benign prostatic hypertrophy and mild hypertension.

Examination revealed normal mentation and cranial nerves. There was no tongue weakness, atrophy, or fasciculations. He had weakness of the neck extensors with a tendency for the neck to drop forward (Fig. 31-1). There were no neck flexor contractions when lying in lateral decubitus suggestive of dystonia causing head flexion. He had flattening of the right shoulder from muscle atrophy. Neck flexion strength was 4/5, extension was 3−/5. Strength was 4+/5 in the left shoulder; 3/5 in the right shoulder; 4+/5 in both biceps; 5/5 in the triceps, wrist flexors, and extensors; and 3/5 in hand muscles. There was bilateral interossei muscle atrophy. Hip flexors and extensors were 4+/5; quadriceps, hamstrings, and distal leg muscles were 4/5. Reflexes were 3+ in the upper extremities and 2+ in the lower extremities with a right Babinski sign. Sensory examination and coordination were normal. There was no rigidity. Fasciculations were noted in the right shoulder and interossei muscles.

WHAT IS THE DIFFERENTIAL DIAGNOSIS?

This patient presented with dropped head syndrome (DHS) caused by weakness of neck extensor muscles. DHS has many etiologies[1,2] (Table 31-1), and in patients with this presentation, one should always look for treatable causes, such as myasthenia gravis that is diagnosed with an edrophonium test (Fig. 31-2), measurement of acetylcholine receptor antibody titers, and, if negative, muscle-specific protein kinase antibodies and repetitive stimulation tests. Polymyositis should be considered, for which the patient is checked for elevated serum creatine kinase (CK) and the characteristic EMG and muscle biopsy. Other reversible causes include endocrine disorders and electrolyte abnormalities.

Amyotrophic lateral sclerosis (ALS) is another cause of DHS, and this is diagnosed by the presence of tongue and limb weakness, fasciculations, and long tract signs. There is also evidence of diffuse denervation and fasciculations and decreased motor unit recruitment with normal nerve conduction tests on EMG.

The presence of a Babinski sign in this person with head drop and the interossei muscle atrophy is against the diagnosis of myasthenia and polymyositis. There were also some fasciculations in the shoulder and interossei, suggesting that he had ALS.

Laboratory studies included serum CK, T4, thyroid-stimulating hormone, B_{12}, and fluorescent antinuclear antibody titers. A complete metabolic panel was normal.

AN EMG TEST WAS PERFORMED

Motor Nerve Studies

Nerve and Site	Latency (ms)	Amplitude (mV)	Conduction Velocity (m/s)
Median Nerve R.	**Normal ≤ 4.2**	**Normal ≥ 6**	**Normal ≥ 50**
Wrist	3.7	15	–
Elbow	8.3	15	53

Nerve and Site	Latency (ms)	Amplitude (mV)	Conduction Velocity (m/s)
Ulnar Nerve R.	**Normal ≤ 3.6**	**Normal ≥ 8**	**Normal ≥ 50**
Wrist	2.9	16	–
Below elbow	7.7	16	51
Above elbow	9.7	16	60

Nerve and Site	Latency (ms)	Amplitude (mV)	Conduction Velocity (m/s)
Peroneal Nerve R.	**Normal ≤ 5.7**	**Normal ≥ 3**	**Normal ≥ 40**
Ankle	4.9	8	–
Fibular head	10.9	8	48
Knee	12.3	7	43
Tibial Nerve R.	**Normal ≤ 5.3**	**Normal ≥ 4**	**Normal ≥ 40**
Ankle	3.4	16	–
Pop. fossa	11.9	13	45

F-Wave and Tibial H-Reflex Studies

Nerve	Latency (ms)	Normal Latency ≤ (ms)
Median nerve R.	27.2	30
Ulnar nerve R.	26.8	30
Peroneal nerve R.	53.0	54
Tibial nerve R.	51.2	54
H-reflex R.	33.8	34
H-reflex L.	33.4	34

Sensory Nerve Studies

Nerve	Onset Latency (ms)	Normal Onset Latency ≤ (ms)	Peak Latency (ms)	Normal Peak Latency ≤ (ms)	Amp (μV)	Normal Amp ≥ (μV)	Conduction Velocity (m/s)	Normal Conduction Velocity ≥ (m/s)
Median nerve R.	2.4	2.6	2.9	3.1	21	20	54	50
Ulnar nerve R.	2.2	2.6	2.7	3.1	13	13	55	50
Sural nerve R.	3.3	3.5	3.8	4.0	12	11	42	40

EMG Data

Muscle	Insrt Activity	Fibs	Pos Waves	Fasc	Amp	Dur	Poly	Pattern
Cervical paraspinals R.	**Inc**	None	None	**Few**	**Dec**	**Brief**	**Many**	Full
Tongue R.	Norm	None	None	None	Norm	Norm	None	Full
Infraspinatus R.	Norm	None	None	None	Norm	Norm	None	Full
Trapezius R.	Norm	None	None	None	Norm	Norm	None	Full
Deltoid R.	**Inc**	**1+**	**1+**	**Few**	**Variable/Lg**	**Inc**	**Many**	**Red**
Biceps brachii R.	**Inc**	**1+**	**1+**	**Few**	**Variable/Lg**	**Inc**	**Many**	Full
First dorsal interosseus R.	**Inc**	**1+**	**1+**	**Few**	**Variable/Lg**	**Inc**	None	**Red**
Thoracic paraspinal R.	**Inc**	**1+**	**1+**	**Few**	Norm	Norm	None	Full
Vastus lateralis R.	**Inc**	None	None	**Few**	**Lg**	**Inc**	None	**Red**
Tibialis anterior R.	**Inc**	None	**1+**	None	**Lg**	**Inc**	None	**Red**
Peroneus longus R.	Norm	None	None	**Few**	**Lg**	**Inc**	None	Full
Gastrocnemius R.	**Inc**	**1+**	**1+**	**Few**	**Lg**	**Inc**	None	Full

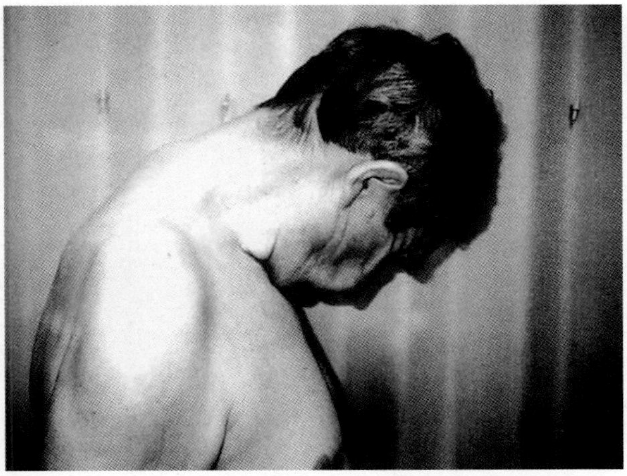

FIG. 31-1 Patient with head drop and some shoulder muscle wasting.

WHAT WERE THE EMG FINDINGS?

This study showed normal motor and sensory nerve conduction velocities, CMAPs and SNAPs amplitudes and latencies, and mildly prolonged F-wave and tibial H-reflex latencies. A repetitive stimulation test was not done.

There were denervation potentials and fasciculations with scattered large motor units and decreased recruitment in several muscles tested. There were also unstable motor units with amplitude variability.

The study was diagnostic of ALS based on clinical findings and the presence of denervation in three body segments: the arms, the legs, and the thoracic paraspinal muscles. Motor unit variability is seen in this disease. Nerve conduction tests were essentially normal; the mild prolongation of the proximal

TABLE 31-1 Conditions Associated With Cervical Paraspinal Muscle Weakness and Dropped Head Syndrome

Prominent, early paraspinal weakness in generalized processes
- Amyotrophic lateral sclerosis
- Myasthenia gravis
- Polymyositis/dermatomyositis

Isolated paraspinal muscle weakness
- Isolated neck extensor myopathy
- Bent spine syndrome
- Benign focal amyotrophy

Other diseases associated with paraspinal weakness or atrophy, or both
- Chronic inflammatory demyelinating polyneuropathy
- Eaton–Lambert myasthenic syndrome
- Inclusion body myositis
- Facioscapulohumeral dystrophy
- Nemaline myopathy
- Proximal myotonic myopathy
- Mitochondrial myopathy
- Acid maltase deficiency
- Carnitine deficiency
- Hypokalemic myopathy
- Hyperparathyroidism

Disorders that mimic dropped head syndrome
- Cervical dystonia (anterocollis), Parkinson disease
- Fixed skeletal deformities of the spine

From Narayanaswami P, Bertorini T. The dropped head syndrome. *J Clin Neuromuscul Dis.* 2000;2:106–112.

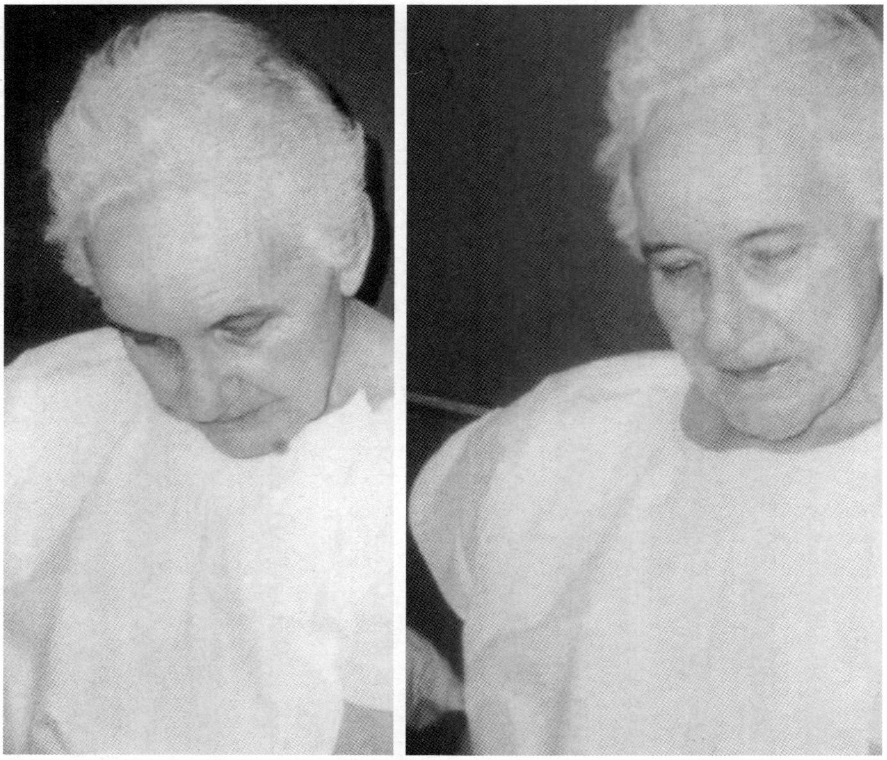

FIG. 31-2 Patient with myasthenia gravis showing head drop (*left*) with mild improvement after 8 mg of edrophonium IV (*right*).

responses could be secondary to a dropout of fast conduction axons.[3]

The patient later developed tongue atrophy and fasciculations. He became progressively weaker and had diffuse hyperreflexia.

DISCUSSION

This patient who presented with DHS from neck extensor muscle weakness was diagnosed to have ALS.

Lange et al. first described what was called "floppy head syndrome" in a report of 12 patients with weakness of the neck extensors.[4] The diagnoses included myasthenia gravis, motor neuron disease, polymyositis, and facioscapulohumeral dystrophy. In 1992 Suarez and Kelly[5] used the term "dropped head syndrome" for an inflammatory myopathy restricted to cervical paraspinal muscles.

DHS has many etiologies which include, among others, inclusion body myositis, proximal myotonic myopathy, and metabolic myopathies, such as acid maltase deficiency, mitochondrial disorders, and inflammatory neuropathies[2,6–12] or an isolated paraspinal myositis.[5,13] It can also be caused by electrolyte and endocrine abnormalities, such as hypokalemia, hyperparathyroidism, and hypothyroidism.[1,14] The workup in patients with DHS is listed in Table 31-2.

This patient had ALS, a progressive disorder that affects the upper and lower motor neurons. The upper motor neuron manifestations include spasticity, weakness, hyperreflexia, and Babinski signs. Patients could also have pseudobulbar symptoms and lower motor neuron signs, including weakness and atrophy, particularly of the tongue (Fig. 31-3), and fasciculations of the tongue but without sensory findings.

TABLE 31-2 Diagnostic Workup of Dropped Head Syndrome

Routine blood chemistry (including serum potassium, calcium, phosphate, and alkaline phosphatase)
Edrophonium (Tensilon) test
Serum creatine kinase
Serum acetylcholine receptor antibodies (MuSK antibodies if negative and suspecting myasthenia gravis) test
Serum lactic acid
Nerve conduction studies, repetitive nerve stimulation needle, electromyography, and single fiber electromyography
Muscle biopsy
MRI of the cervical spine

Most ALS cases are sporadic, but 10% of patients are familial and of these about 10%–20% have a mutation of the superoxide dismutase gene.[15,16] There are several other genetic defects, particularly of autosomal-recessive inheritance,[17] and in those with chromosome 17–linked frontotemporal dementia. The most common gene mutation in the European population is the *C9orf72* in chromosome 9 open reading frame. Actually, this can also be found in sporadic cases. Other genes have been reported in families. The SOD mutation is most common in Japan.[17] Other genetic mutations in familial ALS include TAR-DNA

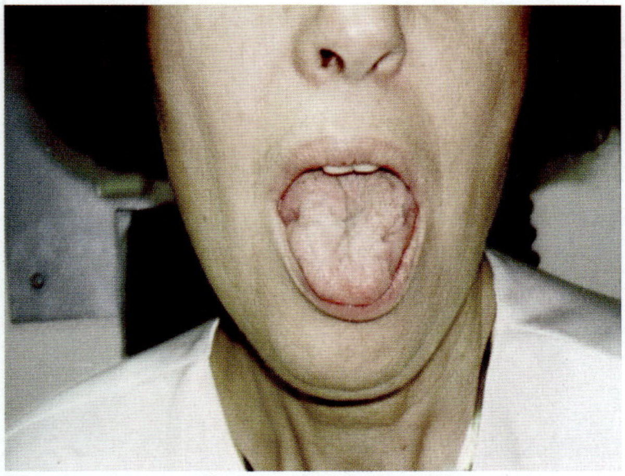

FIG. 31-3 Another patient with a motor neuron disease showing tongue atrophy.

binding protein (*TARBPT*) gene and the fused in sarcoma gene (*FUS*), the *FIG4* gene, the phosphoinositide phosphatase gene and the ANG gene.[18]

ALS was initially described by Charcot in 1874.[19] It is also called Charcot disease, but previous to this, in 1850, Aran reported patients with progressive muscular atrophy.[20] The term *motor neuron disease* was used by Brain in 1933[21] to include disorders of upper or lower motor neurons or both. The name "Lou Gehrig's disease" is used mostly in North America from the famous baseball player who died from the disease.

The diagnosis of ALS is made clinically and by electromyography studies documenting widespread denervation with fasciculations with normal nerve conduction tests, although the CMAPs could be of low amplitude.

Diagnostic criteria were initially proposed by a group of researchers in El Escorial,[22] and these were revised in 2000 (Table 31-3).[3] The Awaji criteria allow the use of EMG findings of fasciculations to support the diagnosis.[23]

Muscle biopsies characteristically show atrophic angular fibers, target fibers, and group atrophy. This test, seldom necessary in those with a diagnostic EMG, is sometimes done to rule out other diseases, such as inclusion myositis, or to document widespread denervation not proved on EMG. On autopsy, there is atrophy of the motor cortex and the ventral spinal roots with degeneration of the corticospinal tracts. There is also a loss of neurons of the motor cortex, the anterior horns of the spinal cord, and the motor brainstem nuclei. The extraocular muscles and the Onuf nuclei on the sacral spinal cord are usually spared. Microscopically, there are filamentous accumulations with axonal swelling, Bunina bodies, and ubiquitin-positive inclusions.[24]

During the evaluation of patients suspected of having ALS, one should always rule out other conditions that have similar presentations, such as spinocerebellar degenerations or multisystem atrophy; spinal cord disorders, such as spondylosis or tumors; disorders of the craniocervical junction; and also more benign motor neuron disorders, such as Kennedy disease. In a younger individual with an atypical presentation, other rare hereditary conditions affecting motor neurons, such as hexosaminidase A deficiency and polyglucosan body disease, should also be considered.

The differential diagnosis also includes disorders of neuromuscular transmission, particularly Eaton–Lambert syndrome,

TABLE 31-3 Revised Diagnostic Criteria for Amyotrophic Lateral Sclerosis

The diagnosis of ALS requires the presence of
- Evidence of LMN degeneration by clinical, electrophysiologic, or neuropathologic examination,
- Evidence of UMN degeneration by clinical examination, and
- Progressive spread of symptoms or signs within a region or to other regions,

Together with the absence of
- Electrophysiologic and pathologic evidence of other disease processes that might explain the signs of LMN and/or UMN degeneration and
- Neuroimaging evidence of other disease processes that might explain the observed clinical and electrophysiologic signs.

Diagnostic Categories

Clinically definite ALS and *clinically probable ALS* are terms used to describe these categories of clinical diagnostic certainty on clinical criteria alone:
- *Clinically definite ALS* is defined on clinical evidence alone by the presence of UMN, as well as LMN, signs, in the bulbar region and at least two spinal regions, or the presence of UMN and LMN signs in three spinal regions.
- *Clinically probable ALS* is defined on clinical evidence alone by UMN and LMN signs in at least two regions, with some UMN signs necessarily rostral to (above) the LMN signs.

The terms *clinically probable ALS laboratory–supported* and *clinically possible ALS* are used to describe these categories of clinical certainty on clinical laboratory studies and criteria or only clinical criteria:
- *Clinically probable ALS laboratory-supported* is defined when clinical signs of UMN and LMN dysfunction are in only one region, or when UMN signs alone are present in one region and LMN signs defined by EMG criteria are present in at least two regions, with a proper application of neuroimaging and clinical laboratory protocols to exclude other causes.
- *Clinically possible ALS* is defined when clinical signs of UMN and LMN dysfunction are found together in only one region or UMN signs are found alone in two or more regions, or LMN signs are found alone in two or more regions; or LMN signs are found rostral to UMN signs and the diagnosis of clinically probable ALS laboratory-supported cannot be proved by evidence on clinical grounds in conjunction with electrodiagnostic, neurophysiologic, neuroimaging, or clinical laboratory studies. Other diagnoses must have been excluded to accept a diagnosis of clinically possible ALS.
- *Clinically suspected ALS* may be suspected in many settings in which the diagnosis of ALS could not be regarded as sufficiently certain to include the patient in a research study. Hence, this category is deleted from the revised *El Escorial Criteria for the Diagnosis of ALS*.

ALS, Amyotrophic lateral sclerosis; *LMN*, lower motor neuron; *UMN*, upper motor neuron.

Adapted from Brooks BR, Miller RG, Swash M, Munsat TL, World Federation of Neurology Research Group on Motor Neuron Disorders. El Escorial revisited: revised criteria for the diagnosis of amyotrophic lateral sclerosis. *Amyotroph Lateral Scler Other Motor Neuron Disord*. 2000;1(5):293–299.

and also sometimes myasthenia gravis and myopathies such as inclusion body myositis, as discussed earlier, which are ruled out with proper electrophysiologic and histologic tests.

The reason for the topographic variability in ALS is unknown, but there are many theories concerning its etiology. These include excessive excitotoxicity caused by a defect of glutamine transporters, oxidative stress with free radical accumulation and neuronal damage caused by superoxide dismutase gain of function in those with the genetic defect causing this autosomal-dominant form of the disease,[25] and the transgenic mouse which is used as a disease model.[26] Oxidative stress could cause mitochondrial dysfunction leading to apoptotic neuronal cell death. A defect of DNA repair has also been proposed.[25] Another possible etiology is an autoimmune process. Infectious causes have not been found, even though patients who previously had poliomyelitis later develop a similar progressive weakness (postpolio amyotrophy). Rarely, HIV-infected patients can develop a motor neuron disorder.

Environmental factors could have a pathogenic role. For example, aluminum accumulation might damage the neuronal cytoskeleton, and, similarly, lead and mercury exposure could cause ALS-like symptoms.

Although the diagnosis of a motor neuron disease usually indicates a poor prognosis, it is variable and more severe in those with progressive bulbar palsy; whereas those with progressive lateral sclerosis or classic ALS, but with upper motor neuron–predominant symptoms, have a better prognosis.[27]

There is currently no cure for ALS. The glutamate antagonist riluzole slows the progression, particularly in the bulbar form of the disease. The drug is used in doses of 50 mg twice a day. It is eliminated in the liver, and its metabolism can be affected by other drugs. Side effects include dizziness, liver disease, neutropenia, and thrombocytopenia. Other drugs have not shown a demonstrable significant benefit.[26] Recently, a multicenter trial of minocycline, a drug with antiinflammatory and antiapoptic effects, experimentally, showed no benefits from this drug.[29] The antiapoptotic drug TCH346 was found not to be beneficial, despite promising preclinical results.[30] A whole genome analysis in sporadic ALS provided results suggesting increased frequency of predisposing genes that affect cytoskeletal regulation,[31] raising hope for novel therapies aimed to modify their effects. Experimental studies using gene therapy, ribonucleic acid interference, and stem cell therapy appear promising for future use.[32]

There is a report that lithium is beneficial in the progression of ALS[33] but this has not been confirmed. Edaravone given intravenously was beneficial[34] as was the oral preparation which is now been approved by the FDA. Sodium phenylbutyrate and taurursidiol is given to reduce endoplasmic reticulum stress and mitochondrial dysfunction. This was proven beneficial[35] and was also approved by the FDA. Masitinib could prolong survival.[36] Tofersen is an antisense oligonucleotide (AON) given intratecally to patients with the familial SOD mutations. This was found beneficial[37] and approved by the FDA. This mode of therapy is been tried in cases with the *C9orf72* mutations. Intrathecal stemm cell administration is been tried.[38]

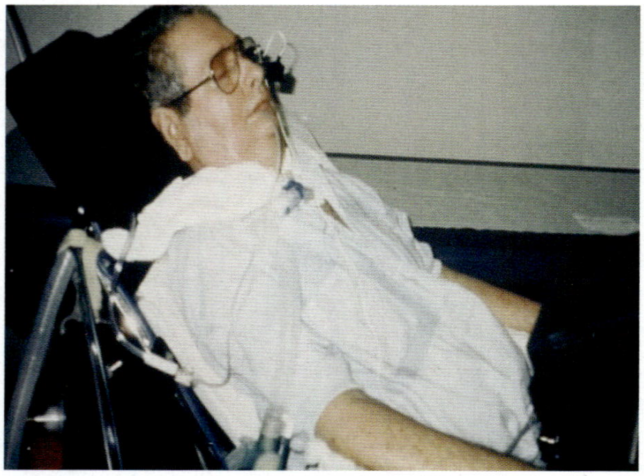

FIG. 31-4 A patient with advanced ALS using eye movement to activate a computer to communicate; he has written a book using this equipment. *ALS*, Amyotrophic lateral sclerosis.

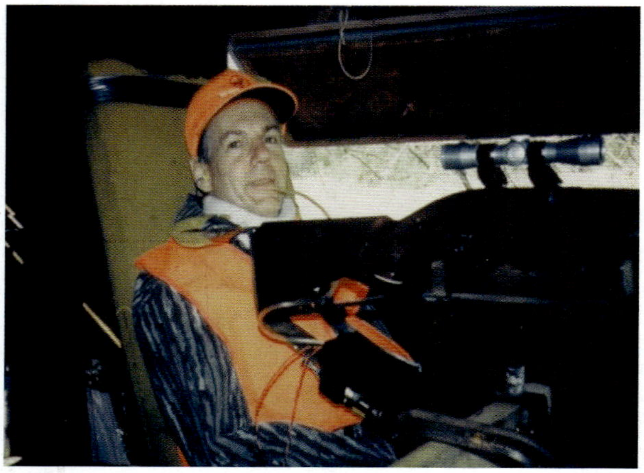

FIG. 31-5 Another patient using a mouthpiece to trigger a gun for deer hunting.

Patients' survival and quality of life improve with proper management, such as gastrostomy and respiratory assistance (Figs. 31-4 and 31-5); these prolong survival and there is a suggestion that the natural history of the disease has become slower because of comprehensive multidisciplinary approaches.[39]

Other symptomatic treatment is helpful, such as, in this patient, the use of neck support. Anticholinergic drugs are used to decrease sialorrhea. Antispasticity drugs and antidepressants help with pseudobulbar symptoms.[40,41]

SUMMARY

This patient presented with head drop, which was found to be caused by ALS.

There are multiple causes of dropped head syndrome that should be ruled out prior to diagnosing ALS.

IMPORTANT POINTS

- DHS can have multiple causes. The most important to recognize are Parkinson's features, dystonia, electrolyte and endocrine abnormalities, myasthenia, and polymyositis, which are treatable. Patients with ALS could also manifest with a dropped head.

- ALS is a slowly progressive disease, the cause of which is unclear. Electrophysiologic findings include normal nerve conduction tests. The CMAP amplitude could be low, and motor conduction velocities could be mildly slow. The SNAPs should be normal, and needle EMG will reveal denervation potentials and fasciculations with reduced recruitment motor units, which are frequently polyphasic.
- Electromyography findings that support the diagnosis of ALS should be found in at least three of the four central nervous system regions (bulbar, cervical, thoracic, or lumbosacral).
- Most ALS cases are sporadic, but about 10% are familial.
- The treatment of ALS is conservative; riluzole slows the progression, particularly in the bulbar form of the disease.

REFERENCES

1. Narayanaswami P, Bertorini TE. The dropped head syndrome. *J Clin Neuromuscul Dis*. 2000;2:106–112.
2. Rahim R, Gupta D, Bertorini TE, Le Doux MS. Dropped head presentation of mitochondrial myopathy. *J Clin Neuromuscul Dis*. 2003;5:108–114.
3. Brooks BR, Miller RG, Swash M, Munsat TL. World Federation of Neurology Research Group on Motor Neuron Disorders: El Escorial revisited: Revised criteria for the diagnosis of amyotrophic lateral sclerosis. *Amyotroph Lateral Scler Other Motor Neuron Disord*. 2000;1:293–299.
4. Lange DJ, Fetell MR, Lovelace RE, et al. The floppy head syndrome. *Ann Neurol*. 1986;20:133.
5. Suarez GA, Kelly Jr. JJ. The dropped head syndrome. *Neurology*. 1992;42:1625–1627.
6. Hoffman D, Gutmann L. The dropped head syndrome with chronic inflammatory demyelinating polyneuropathy. *Muscle Nerve*. 1994;17:808–810.
7. Massey JM. Acquired myasthenia gravis. *Neurol Clin*. 1997;15:577–595.
8. Dushay KM, Zibrak JD, Jensen WA. Myasthenia gravis presenting as isolated respiratory failure. *Chest*. 1990;97:232–234.
9. Hund E, Heckl R, Goebel HH, et al. Inclusion body myositis presenting with isolated erector spinae paresis. *Neurology*. 1995;45:993–994.
10. Evidente VGH, Cook A. Floppy head syndrome resulting from proximal myotonic muscular dystrophy. *Ann Neurol*. 1997;42:417.
11. Bleck TP. Dropped head syndrome. *Neurology*. 1993;43:846–847.
12. Katz JS, Wolfe GI, Burns DK, et al. Isolated neck extensor myopathy: A common cause of dropped head syndrome. *Neurology*. 1996;46(4):917–921.
13. Gaeta M, Mazziotti S, Toscano A, et al. "Dropped-head" syndrome due to isolated myositis of neck extensor muscles: MRI findings. *Skeletal Radiol*. 2006;35(2):110–112.
14. Askmark H, Olsson Y, Rossitti S. Treatable dropped head syndrome in hypothyroidism. *Neurology*. 2000;55:896–897.
15. Rosen DR, Siddique T, Patterson D, et al. Mutations in Cu/Zn superoxide dismutase gene are associated with familial amyotrophic lateral sclerosis. *Nature*. 1993;362:59–62.
16. Anderson PM. Genetic aspects of amyotrophic lateral sclerosis/motor neuron disease. In: Shaw P, Strong MJ, eds. *Motor Neuron Disorders*. Philadelphia: Butterworth-Heinemann; 2003:207–235.
17. Neusch C, Bahr M, Schneider-Gold C. Glia cells in amyotrophic lateral sclerosis: New clues to understanding an old disease? *Muscle Nerve*. 2007;35(6):712–724.
18. Zou ZY, Zhou ZR, Che CH, Liu CY, et al. Genetic epidemiology of amyotrophic lateral sclerosis: a systemic review and meta-analysis. *J Neurol Neurosurg Psychiatry. Jul*. 2017;88(7):540–549.
19. Charcot JM. De la Sclerose laterale amyotrophique. *Prog Med*. 1874;23:235–237. 24:341–342, and 29:453–455.
20. Aran FA. Recherches sur une maladie non encore decrite du système musculaire (atrophie musculaire progressive). *Arch Gen Med*. 1850;24:5–35.
21. Brain WR. *Diseases of the Nervous System*. London, England: Oxford University Press; 1933.
22. Brooks BR. El Escorial World Federation of Neurology, criteria for the diagnosis of amyotrophic lateral sclerosis. Subcommittee on motor neuron diseases of the World Federation of Neurology Research Group on Neuromuscular Disorders. El Escorial: Clinical limits of ALS workshop contribution. *J Neurol Sci*. 1994;24:96–107.
23. Cosa J, Swash M, de. Carvalho M. Awaji criteria for the diagnosis of amyotrophic lateral sclerosis: a systematic review. *Arch Neurol*. Nov. 2012;69(11):1410–1416.
24. Wharton SP, Ince PG. Pathology of motor neuron disorders. In: Shaw P, Strong MJ, eds. *Motor Neuron Disorders*. Philadelphia: Butterworth-Heinemann; 2003:17–49.
25. Shaw PJ, Kunch RW. Current concepts of the pathogenesis of ALS. In: Kunel RW, ed. *Motor Neuron Disease*. New York, NY: WB Saunders; 2002:37–75.
26. Gurney ME, Pu H, Chiu AY, et al. Motor neuron degeneration in mice that express a human Cu, Zn superoxide dismutase mutation. *Science*. 1994;264(5166):1772–1775.
27. Gordon PH, Cheng B, Katz IB, et al. The natural history of primary lateral sclerosis. *Neurology*. 2006;66:647–653.
28. de Carvalho M, Costa J, Swash M. Clinical trials in ALS: A review of the role of clinical and neurophysiological measurements. *Amyotroph Lateral Scler Other Motor Neuron Disord*. 2005;6(4):202–212.
29. Gordon PH, More DH, Florence JM, et al. Results of the phase III randomized corticoid trial of minocycline in ALS. *Neurology*. 2007;68(Suppl 1):A90.
30. Miller R, Bradley W, Cudkowicz M, et al. Phase II/III randomized trial of TCH346 in patients with ALS. *Neurology*. 2007;69:776–784.
31. Dunckley T, Huentelman MJ, Craig DW, et al. Whole-genome analysis of sporadic amyotrophic lateral sclerosis. *N Engl J Med*. 2007;357(8):775–778.
32. Federici T, Boulis NM. Gene-based treatment of motor neuron diseases. *Muscle Nerve*. 2006;33:302–323.
33. Fornai F, Longone P, Cafaro L, Kastsuichenka O, et al. Lithium delays progression of amyotrophic lateral sclerosis. *Proc Natl Acad Sci USA*. 2008;105(6):2052–2057.
34. Writing Group Edaravone (MCI-186) ALS 19 Study Group Safety and efficacy of edaravone in well defined patients with amyotrophic lateral sclerosis: a randomized, double-blind, placebo-controlled trial. *Lancet Neurol*. Jul. 2017;16(7):505–512.
35. Paganoni S, Mackln EA, Hendrix S, Berry JD, et al. Trial of Sodium Phenylbutyrate-Taurursodiol for Amyotrophic Lateral Sclerosis. *N Engl J Med*. Sep 3. 2020;383(10):919–930.
36. Mora J.S., Bradley W.G., Chaverri, D., Hernandez-Barral M., et al. Long-term survival analysis of masitinib in amyotrophic lateral sclerosis. Ther Adv Neurol Disord. Jul 19;14:17562864211030365. 2021.

37. Miller T, Cudkowicz M, Shaw PJ, Andersen PM, et al. Phase 1-2 Trial of Antisense Oligonucleotide Tofersen for SOD1 ALS. *N Engl J Med.* Sep 22. 2022;387(12):1099–1110.
38. Baloh RH, Glass JD, Swendsen CN. Stem cell transplantation for amyotrophic lateral sclerosis. *Curr Opin Neurol.* Oct. 2018;31(5):655–661.
39. Czaplinski A, Yen AA, Simpson EP, Appel SH. Slower disease progression and prolonged survival in contemporary patients with amyotrophic lateral sclerosis: Is the natural history of amyotrophic lateral sclerosis changing? *Arch Neurol.* 2006;63(8):1139–1143.
40. Anneser J, Borasio GD. Symptom control in amyotrophic lateral sclerosis. In: Shaw P, Strong MS, eds. *Motor Neuron Disorders.* Philadelphia: Butterworth-Heinemann; 2003:485–490.
41. Rosow L, Lomen-Hoerth C. Treatment and management of adult motor neuron disease. Chapter 12, 1248-1260. In: Bertorini TE, ed. *Treatment and Management of Neuromuscular disorders.* Elsevier; 2022.

A Man in the "Barrel"

A 37-year-old man presented with a 3-week history of difficulty with his right handgrip. He denied numbness, paresthesias, or leg weakness. He had some mild chronic neck pain, but his MRI of the spine was normal. Family history and past medical and social histories were noncontributory.

Mentation and cranial nerve examination were normal. There was atrophy of the right first dorsal interosseous muscle with weakness of the hand intrinsic muscles, but other muscles were normal. There were no fasciculations. Sensory examination and reflexes and the rest of the examination were normal.

WHAT IS THE DIFFERENTIAL DIAGNOSIS?

The atrophy and weakness in the hand muscles suggest a C8 radiculopathy or a lower trunk or medial cord plexus lesion. The lack of significant pain or sensory abnormalities is against these diagnoses. The lack of pain and normal MRI also ruled out other spinal diseases.

Other possibilities include a motor neuron disease and multifocal motor neuropathy (MMN), but in this disease, there is usually weakness with little atrophy. A mononeuritis multiplex could be considered, but it is hard to make this diagnosis when only one level is affected and, particularly, with the lack of sensory findings. Adult-onset myopathies with hand wasting such as debrancher enzyme deficiency and Welander muscular dystrophy are less likely possibilities, as they are usually symmetrical at onset.

AN EMG TEST WAS PERFORMED

Motor Nerve Studies

Nerve and Site	Latency (ms)	Amplitude (mV)	Conduction Velocity (m/s)
Median Nerve R.	**Normal ≤ 4.2**	**Normal ≥ 6**	**Normal ≥ 50**
Wrist	**5.5**	**2**	–
Elbow	10.3	**2**	51
Ulnar Nerve R.	**Normal ≤ 3.6**	**Normal ≥ 8**	**Normal ≥ 50**
Wrist	3.0	15	–
Below elbow	6.8	13	55
Above elbow	8.6	11	66
Axilla	10.8	11	55
Median Nerve L.	**Normal ≤ 4.2**	**Normal ≥ 6**	**Normal ≥ 50**
Wrist	3.7	15	–
Elbow	7.5	13	61

Nerve and Site	Latency (ms)	Amplitude (mV)	Conduction Velocity (m/s)
Peroneal Nerve R.	**Normal ≤ 5.7**	**Normal ≥ 3**	**Normal ≥ 40**
Ankle	4.2	4	–
Fibular head	10.3	3	47
Knee	12.1	3	56

F-Wave and Tibial H-Reflex Studies

Nerve	Latency (ms)	Normal Latency ≤ (ms)
Median nerve R.	**31.0**	30
Ulnar nerve R.	28.6	30
Median nerve L.	27.7	30
Peroneal nerve R.	47.8	54
H-reflex R.	30.3	34

Sensory Nerve Studies

Nerve	Onset Latency (ms)	Normal Onset Latency ≤ (ms)	Peak Latency (ms)	Normal Peak Latency ≤ (ms)	Amp (μV)	Normal Amp ≥ (μV)	Conduction Velocity (m/s)	Normal Conduction Velocity ≥ (m/s)
Median nerve R.	**2.8**	2.6	**3.3**	3.1	31	20	**46**	50
Ulnar nerve R.	2.3	2.6	2.8	3.1	16	13	52	50
Median nerve L.	**2.9**	2.6	**3.4**	3.1	31	20	**45**	50
Sural nerve R.	3.1	3.5	3.6	4.0	37	11	45	40

EMG Data

Muscle	Insrt Activity	Fibs	Pos Waves	Fasc	Amp	Dur	Poly	Pattern
Tongue	Norm	None	None	None	Norm	Norm	None	Full
Thoracic paraspinals R.	Norm	None	None	None	Norm	None	None	Full
Supraspinatus R.	Norm	None	None	None	Norm	Norm	None	Full
Deltoid R.	**CRD**	None	**1+**	None	Norm	Norm	None	Full
Biceps brachii R.	**Inc**	None	None	**Few**	**Lg**	**Inc**	None	Full
Flexor carpi radialis R.	**Inc**	**2+**	**2+**	None	**Lg**	**Inc**	None	Full
Flexor carpi ulnaris R.	**Inc**	**2+**	**2+**	**Few**	**Lg**	**Inc**	None	**Red**
Triceps R.	**Inc**	None	None	**Few**	**Lg**	**Inc**	None	**Red**
Extensor digitorum comm. R.	**Inc**	**2+**	**2+**	None	Norm	Norm	None	Full
Sternocleidomastoid R.	Norm	None	None	None	Norm	Norm	None	Full
Abductor poll. brevis R.	**Inc**	None	**2+**	None	**Lg**	**Inc**	None	**Red**
First dorsal interosseous R.	**Inc**	**2+**	**2+**	None	**Lg**	**Inc**	None	**Red**
Vastus lateralis R.	Norm	None	None	None	**Lg**	**Inc**	None	**Red**
Tibialis anterior R.	**Inc**	None	**1+**	None	**Lg**	**Inc**	None	Full
Peroneus longus R.	**Inc**	None	**1+**	None	Norm	Norm	None	Full
Gastrocnemius R.	**Inc**	None	**1+**	None	Norm	Norm	None	Full
Deltoid L.	Norm	None	None	None	Norm	Norm	None	Full
Biceps brachii L.	Norm	None	None	None	**Lg**	**Inc**	None	Full
Flexor carpi ulnaris L.	Norm	None	None	None	Norm	Norm	None	Full
Extensor digitorum comm. L.	Norm	None	None	None	Norm	Norm	None	Full
Abductor poll. brevis L.	**Inc**	None	**1+**	None	**Lg**	**Inc**	None	**Red**
First dorsal interosseous L.	**Inc**	None	**1+**	None	**Lg**	**Inc**	None	**Red**

WHAT WERE THE EMG FINDINGS?

The EMG and nerve conduction velocity study showed normal motor nerve conduction velocities of the ulnar, median, and peroneal nerves with normal distal latencies and F-responses. The CMAP amplitude was reduced only in the right median nerve that had a prolonged distal latency. Sensory-evoked responses were normal except for the median nerve SNAP latency and conduction velocity, which were mildly abnormal; this could be secondary to a mild carpal tunnel syndrome but did not explain the symptoms.

There were denervation potentials and reduced motor unit potentials with only a few fasciculations in several muscles innervated by various roots and nerves of the right arm; there was also denervation in the left arm and only rare denervation potentials in the legs but not in the paraspinal muscles or the tongue.

This test did not demonstrate a peripheral neuropathy, and there was no evidence of conduction block, although root stimulation to rule out a proximal block was not done. The findings were suggestive of a motor neuron disease, but the lack of bulbar involvement, minimal denervation in the legs, with normal findings in the tongue and thoracic paraspinal muscles were not sufficient for the definitive diagnosis of amyotrophic lateral sclerosis (ALS).

Complete metabolic panel, serum creatine kinase, protein electrophoresis, and IgG were normal. GM_1 antibody titers were not elevated; rapid plasma regain, B_{12}/folate, rheumatoid factor, and Lyme antibodies were all negative. A 24-hour arsenic and porphyrin test was normal. A thyroid profile was normal.

The MRI of the cervical spine was reviewed, and this, indeed, was normal.

A muscle biopsy of the left quadriceps showed scattered internalized nuclei and type II fiber predominance without angular atrophic fibers.

Cerebrospinal fluid study was normal.

WHAT IS THE MOST LIKELY DIAGNOSIS?

This patient presented with muscle weakness and atrophy of one distal upper extremity but with EMG evidence of denervation of both arms and some in the legs.

The asymmetric and distal weakness is against the diagnosis of a myopathy, particularly with the presence of fasciculations and scattered denervation with reduced motor unit recruitment on EMG. These findings suggest a peripheral nerve/motor neuron disorder. Cervical spondylosis should always be included in the differential diagnosis in a patient with this presentation, but in this case the cervical MRI was normal.

As discussed, neuropathies with similar presentation include MMN with conduction block,[1] but in this case, there was no evidence of conduction block or elevated levels of GM_1 antibodies. There is a multifocal axonal motor neuropathy without conduction blocks[2]; some of these patients have elevated GM_1 antibodies and might respond to IgG infusions like those with MMN. The slow progression, lack of pain, and lack of significant SNAP abnormalities are against a bilateral brachial plexopathy.[3]

Monomelic amyotrophy, or benign focal amyotrophy,[4] is a benign motor neuron disease that affects the upper extremities with very little progression. This is usually unilateral, usually affecting distal muscles and both arms, and can, rarely, be present in the legs. The disease progression in this case makes that diagnosis unlikely. The lack of family history and of prominent

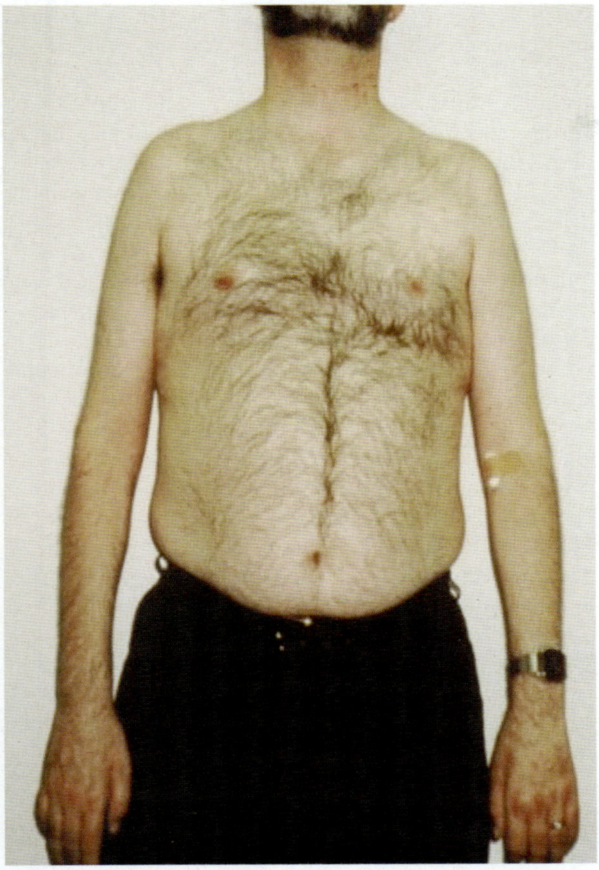

FIG. 32-1 Notice in this patient proximal and distal wasting with arm pronation. He could not raise his arms, but his legs were normal.

leg involvement is against the diagnosis of adult-onset familial spinal muscular atrophy but does not rule out progressive spinal muscular atrophy, a variant of ALS.[5] The lack of bulbar involvement is against Kennedy's disease.[6]

Because this patient presented initially with a purely lower motor neuron syndrome and the diagnosis was not clear, a trial of IgG infusions was given without benefit.

A follow-up neurologic evaluation 6 months later revealed the same findings except for more severe weakness of the interossei muscles bilaterally, and diffuse fasciculations were detected in the arms.

Over the next 2 years, he got progressively weaker in both upper extremities, mostly of the proximal muscles with inability to use his arms (Fig. 32-1), but cranial nerves remained normal.

The predominant involvement of the upper extremities and slow progression in this patient suggest brachial amyotrophic diplegia (BAD) presenting as "man in the barrel" syndrome (MBS).[7] Eight years later, he developed tongue atrophy, weakness in the legs, and hyperreflexia.

WHAT IS "MAN IN THE BARREL" SYNDROME?

MBS is characterized by significant arm weakness, mainly proximal, with normal strength of the lower extremities. This has multiple causes that include watershed infarcts between the middle and anterior cerebral arteries, as well as lacunar infarcts, cerebral metastasis, pontine lesions,[8] cervical spondylosis, brachial plexopathies,[9] myelopathies, and motor neuron disorders. HIV-infected patients may develop a motor neuron syndrome,[10] and recently a motor neuron disorder presenting as the MBS was reported in a human T-lymphotropic virus 1-positive patient.[11]

BAD is slowly progressive and affects initially and predominantly the upper extremities, sparing the bulbar and respiratory muscles. The most commonly affected areas are the territories of C5–C6 and C7 myotomes.[7]

The disease is likely a variant of ALS and has several names such as "flail arm" syndrome, "dangling arm" syndrome, bibrachial palsy, rhizomelic amyotrophy, orangutan sign, and "dead arm" sign. It is believed that up to 10% of patients with ALS may have this or similar presentations, with a survival time longer than those with classic ALS and a greater predominance of men.[12–14]

Because classic ALS may present initially with prominent arm symptoms,[15,16] the slow progression is the only way to make the diagnosis and assume a possible prognosis. The later bulbar involvement and leg weakness, as in this case, indicates that BAD is a variant of progressive spinal muscular atrophy or of ALS,[7,12,13] which progresses more slowly (see Case 31).

WHAT IS THE TREATMENT OF BRACHIAL AMYOTROPHIC DIPLEGIA?

There is no treatment for BAD. Bracing with slings and orthopedic devices may be helpful. Otherwise, we manage these patients as we do those with typical ALS.

SUMMARY

This patient had progressive weakness, atrophy, and fasciculations first in one arm. He later developed the inability to move his arms yet had normal lower extremity function. Electrophysiologically, he was found to have a motor neuron disorder.

He was diagnosed as having MBS from BAD. Later, weakness involved bulbar muscles and legs.

IMPORTANT POINTS

- The differential diagnosis of predominant upper extremity weakness should include cervical spondylosis or other causes of cord lesions, for which an MRI is very useful. Other diagnoses include MMN, multifocal motor axonal neuropathy, distal myopathies including Welander muscular dystrophy and debrancher enzyme deficiency, and more benign motor neuron disorders such as monomelic amyotrophy and, when proximal, BAD. The initial workup should include serum creatine kinase values, a detailed EMG, GM_1 antibodies, and MRI of the spine.
- Some motor neuron disorders such as benign focal amyotrophy, BAD, and progressive lateral sclerosis have a longer survival than classic ALS.

- BAD is a variant of ALS with predominant involvement of the upper extremities, presenting as MBS, which is also called "flail arm," "dead arm," "dangling arm," and orangutan sign.
- There is no cure for BAD.

REFERENCES

1. Pestronk A. Multifocal motor neuropathy: diagnosis and treatment. *Neurology*. 1998;51(Suppl 5):S22–S24.
2. Katz JS, Barohn RJ, Kojan S, et al. Axonal multifocal motor neuropathy without conduction block or other features of demyelination. *Neurology*. 2002;58:615–620.
3. Dumitru D. Brachial plexopathy and proximal mononeuropathies. In: Harper CM Jr, Thomas JE, eds. *Electrodiagnostic Medicine*. Philadelphia: Hanley & Belfus; 1995:585–642.
4. Gouri-Devi M, Suresh TG, Shankar SK. Monomelic amyotrophy. *Arch Neurol*. 1984;41:388–394.
5. Ross MA. Acquired neuromuscular diseases: acquired motor neuron disorders. *Neurol Clin*. 1997;15:481–500.
6. Kennedy WR, Alter M, Sung JH. Progressive proximal spinal and bulbar muscular atrophy of late onset: a sex-linked recessive trait. *Neurology*. 1998;4:583–593.
7. Katz JS, Wolfe GI, Anderson PB, et al. Brachial amyotrophic diplegia: a slowly progressive motor neuron disorder. *Neurology*. 1999;53:1071–1076.
8. Paulin M, de Seze J, Wyremblewski P, et al. Man-in-the-barrel syndrome caused by a pontine lesion. *Neurology*. 2005;64(10):1703.
9. Foncea N, Yurrebaso I, Gomez Beldarrain M, Garcia-Monco JC. Postoperative bilateral brachial plexopathy mimicking the "man-in-the-barrel" syndrome. *Neurologia*. 2002;17(7):388–390.
10. Brew BJ. The peripheral nerve complications of human immunodeficiency virus (HIV) infection. *Muscle Nerve*. 2003;28:542–552.
11. Vainstein G, Gordon CR, Gadoth N. HTLV-1 associated motor neuron disease mimicking "man-in-the barrel" syndrome. *J Neuromuscul Dis*. 2005;6(3):127–131.
12. Gamez J, Cervera C, Codina A. Atypical form of amyotrophic lateral sclerosis: a new term to define a previously well known form of ALS. *J Neurol Neurosurg Psychiatry*. 2000;68:118–119.
13. Hu MT, Ellis CM, Al-Chalabi A, et al. Flail arm syndrome: a distinctive variant of amyotrophic lateral sclerosis. *J Neurol Neurosurg Psychiatry*. 1998;65:950–951.
14. Pearlman S, Pourmand R. Evaluation of a patient presenting with progressive weakness and atrophy of the upper extremities: neuromuscular disease review. *Clin Neuromuscul Dis*. 2003;1:51–59.
15. Caroscio JT, Mulvihill MN, Sterling R, Abrams B. Amyotrophic lateral sclerosis: its natural history. *Neurol Clin*. 1987;5:1–8.
16. Gubbay SS, Kahana E, Zilber N, et al. Amyotrophic lateral sclerosis: a study of its presentation and prognosis. *J Neurol*. 1985;232:295–300.

A Man With a Long History of Muscle Weakness in One Arm

A 35-year-old man presented with complaints of pain in the left shoulder and neck. Over the next 4 years, he developed progressive proximal left arm weakness and marked atrophy of the left shoulder girdle. Despite several evaluations during the next 3 years, including a normal myelogram, the etiology for his weakness was unclear, but the symptoms did not spread.

He presented for a disability evaluation 12 years after the onset of symptoms, which had remained stable and did not progress. He denied previous neck or shoulder trauma. He had no bladder/bowel or sensory complaints, sexual dysfunction, or any history of diabetes, poliomyelitis, or surgery. He had occasional tingling in all of the fingers of the right hand with intermittent dull pain in his right forearm.

General examination showed a well-developed, well-nourished man in apparent good health. Mental status, cranial nerves, and sensory testing were normal.

Examination of the left upper extremity and shoulder girdle revealed a full range of passive motion with minimal shoulder tenderness at the extremes of abduction and external rotation. He had prominent atrophy in his left shoulder girdle (Fig. 33A-1). There was prominent left upper extremity proximal weakness; the deltoid and infraspinatus muscles were 2/5, the latissimus dorsi was 3/5, pectoralis, biceps, and brachioradialis 4/5, and triceps were 4+/5. The left wrist and hand had normal strength. His right arm and bilateral leg strength was normal.

Reflexes were brisk in the left upper extremity and were normal in the right upper extremity and both legs. Toes were downgoing. No pathologic reflexes or spasticity were noticed.

WHAT ARE THE DIFFERENTIAL DIAGNOSES?

This patient had a segmental disorder of the left upper extremity; the differential diagnosis includes a focal spinal cord lesion (such as a tumor, syringomyelia, or radiculopathy), but the lack of sensory findings, pain, or symptoms is against these. The lack of progression or spread is against a typical motor neuron disorder such as amyotrophic lateral sclerosis (ALS). Another possibility includes monomelic amyotrophy, a benign motor neuron disease.[1] This condition usually affects one arm more distally. Other possibilities that need to be considered are a motor neuropathy, such as multifocal motor neuropathy, and also a multifocal axonal neuropathy. These, however, usually affect distal muscles. The lack of sensory findings argues against other focal neuropathies or plexopathies.

AN EMG TEST WAS PERFORMED

Motor Nerve Studies

Nerve and Site	Latency(ms)	Amplitude (mV)	Conduction Velocity (m/s)
Median Nerve L.	**Normal ≤ 4.2**	**Normal ≥ 6**	**Normal ≥ 50**
Wrist	3.8	9	–
Elbow	8.2	9	52

This case was reported in Metcalf JC Jr, Wood JB, Bertorini TE. Benign focal amyotrophy: metrizamide CT evidence of cord atrophy. *Muscle Nerve*. 1987;10:338–345.

Motor Nerve Studies—cont'd

Nerve and Site	Latency (ms)	Amplitude (mV)	Conduction Velocity (m/s)
Ulnar Nerve L.	**Normal ≤ 3.6**	**Normal ≥ 8**	**Normal ≥ 50**
Wrist	3.4	10	–
Below elbow	8.0	10	52
Above elbow	10.0	9	60

Nerve and Site	Latency (ms)	Amplitude (mV)	Conduction Velocity (m/s)
Peroneal Nerve L.	**Normal ≤ 5.7**	**Normal ≥ 3**	**Normal ≥ 40**
Ankle	5.5	6	–
Fibular head	12.6	6	44

F-Wave and Tibial H-Reflex Studies

Nerve	Latency (ms)	Normal Latency ≤ (ms)
Median L.	30	30
Ulnar L.	29.8	30
Peroneal L.	52.3	54
H-reflex L.	33.6	34
H-reflex R.	33.9	34

Sensory Nerve Studies

Nerve	Onset Latency (ms)	Normal Onset Latency ≤ (ms)	Peak Latency (ms)	Normal Peak Latency ≤ (ms)	Amp (μV)	Normal Amp ≥ (μV)	Conduction Velocity (m/s)	Normal Conduction Velocity ≥ (m/s)
Median nerve L.	2.4	2.6	2.9	3.1	22	20	54	50
Ulnar nerve L.	2.2	2.6	2.7	3.1	13	13	54	50
Sural nerve L.	3.3	3.5	3.8	4.0	11	11	42	40

EMG Data

Muscle	Insrt Activity	Fib	Pos Waves	Fasc	Amp	Dur	Poly	Pattern
Deltoid L.	Norm	None	None	None	**Lg**	**Inc**	None	**Red**
Supraspinatus L.	Norm	None	None	None	**Lg**	**Inc**	None	**Red**
Biceps brachii L.	**CRD**	None	None	**Few**	**Lg**	**Inc**	None	**Red**
Triceps L.	**CRD**	None	None	**Few**	Norm	Norm	None	Full
Brachioradialis L.	**CRD**	None	None	**Few**	Norm	Norm	None	Full
Flexor carpi rad. L.	Norm	None	None	None	Norm	Norm	None	Full
Flexor carpi uln. L.	Norm	None	None	None	Norm	Norm	None	Full
Ext. dig. comm. L.	Norm	None	None	None	Norm	Norm	None	Full
First dorsal int. L.	Norm	None	None	None	Norm	Norm	None	Full
Vastus lat. L.	Norm	None	None	None	Norm	Norm	None	Full
Tibialis anterior L.	Norm	None	None	None	**Lg**	**Inc**	None	**Red**
Gastrocnemius L.	Norm	None	None	**Few**	Norm	Norm	None	Full

CRD, Complex repetitive discharges.

WHAT WERE THE EMG FINDINGS?

This test showed normal median, ulnar, and peroneal motor nerve conduction velocities, distal latencies, and CMAP amplitudes; F-responses and tibial H-reflexes were normal. There was chronic denervation and reinnervation with large motor unit action potentials and fasciculations in the C5–C6 myotomes of the right upper extremity, suggestive of a chronic focal motor neuron disorder; however, these can also be seen in plexus or nerve disorders. There were some fasciculations and large motor unit potentials in the right leg, but no evidence of active denervation.

The nerve conduction tests and EMG showed no evidence of conduction block or a diffuse motor neuron disease such as ALS, and although the presence of occasional large motor unit potentials and fasciculations in the legs could suggest a more diffuse process, no denervation potentials were seen to suggest ALS.

Initial laboratory studies including complete blood count, erythrocyte sedimentation rate, rapid plasma reagin, creatine phosphokinase, basic metabolic panel, urinalysis, and chest x-ray were normal.

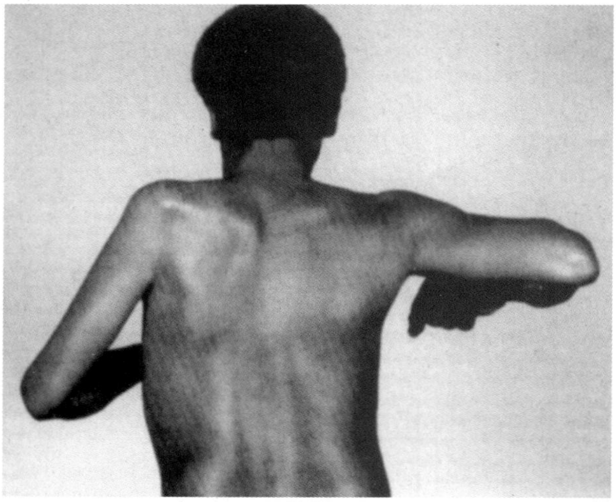

FIG. 33A-1 Posterior view of the patient at rest reveals marked atrophy of the left shoulder girdle and proximal left arm.

BASED ON THIS, WHAT OTHER TESTS SHOULD BE DONE?

Cervical spine imaging is the most important diagnostic test due to the focal neurologic deficit in this case.

A CT myelogram was performed following lumbar metrizamide insertion (190 mg/mL), 5 mL with 5-mm contiguous cuts from the base of the skull to the inferior border of the T1 vertebrae. The myelogram revealed anterolateral cord atrophy from the superior aspects of C3 to C7 (Fig. 33A-2A).

There was no evidence of mass effect, foraminal, or osseous abnormality, nor was there delayed filling to indicate a syrinx cavity on serial scans at 4, 8, and 12 hours postmetrizamide. The contour of the cord above and below the area of abnormality was normal (see Fig. 33A-2B).

Concurrently obtained cerebrospinal fluid revealed protein 28 mg/dL, glucose 68 mg/dL, and 2 lymphocytes.

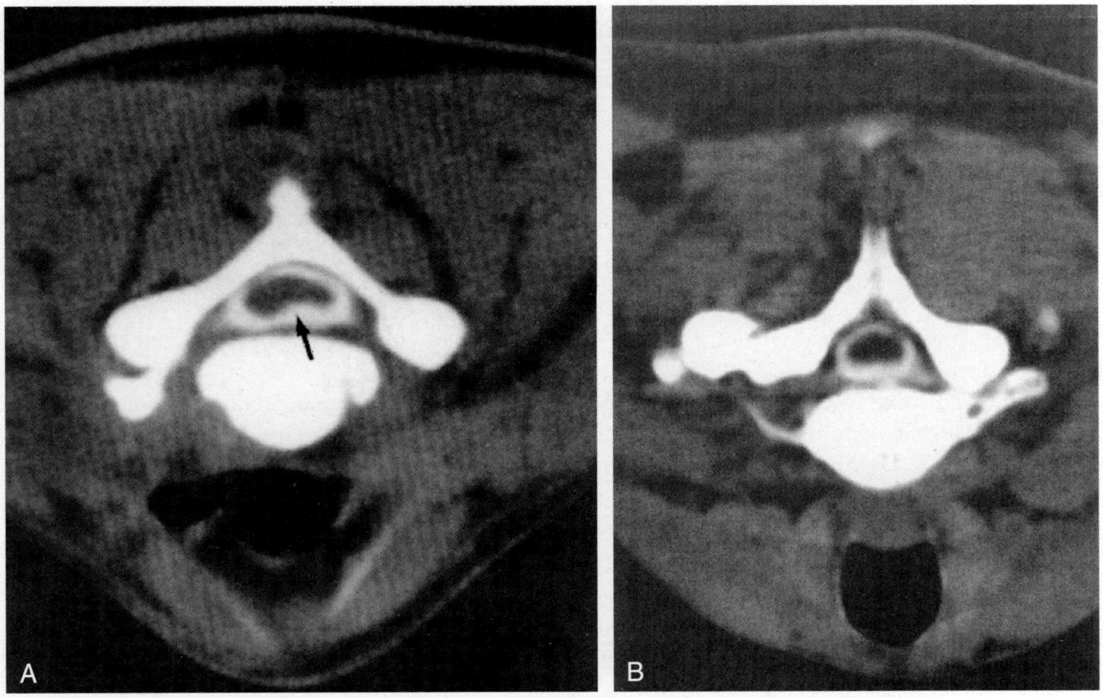

FIG. 33A-2 **A**, Anterolateral atrophy of the spinal cord at the level of C5 vertebral body on the left (*arrow*). **B**, Normal spinal canal and contents at the level of the C7 vertebral body.

A muscle biopsy of the right quadriceps was studied with a complete battery of histochemical stains on frozen sections[2]; this revealed mild neurogenic changes, characterized by occasional angular fibers. No fiber-type grouping or other pathologic abnormalities were present.

WHAT IS THE MOST LIKELY DIAGNOSIS?

This patient had a benign focal amyotrophy or monomelic amyotrophy with focal spinal cord atrophy. He had proximal upper extremity involvement rather than the more typical distal involvement seen in this disease.[3–5] The minor abnormalities in the leg could suggest that the process was more widespread, but it did not progress for over 10 years.

SUMMARY

This patient has a stable and nonprogressive atrophy and weakness in one upper extremity without sensory abnormalities. The EMG was consistent with a focal lower motor neuron disorder. He was diagnosed as having BFA or monomelic amyotrophy with radiologic evidence of focal spinal cord atrophy.

In a patient with this presentation, one should always rule out a structural spinal cord lesion. Monomelic amyotrophy is usually a benign condition that might be secondary to a previous trauma and is a slowly progressive or nonprogressive benign motor neuron disorder. The treatment is conservative.

For important points and references, see Case 33b.

33B CASE

A Young Man With Longstanding Weakness in Both Arms

A 29-year-old gentleman presented with a 10-year history of slowly progressive weakness.

Previous workup revealed some evidence of cervical spondylosis. EMG showed diffuse denervation in the arms and there were no cranial nerve problems. His main complaint was difficulty extending his fingers.

Neurological examination revealed normal mentation and cranial nerves. He had wasting and weakness, particularly in the distal muscles of both upper extremities with difficulty extending the fingers (Fig. 33B-1) and mild hand tremor. Manual muscle exam revealed that extension of the fingers of the right hand was 2.5/5 and the left hand 2.5/5, abduction of the fingers of the right hand and the left hand was 2.5/5, and flexion strength of the right thumb and the left thumb was 4.5/5. Reflexes were somewhat hyperactive in the leg at 3+; reflexes were 2+ in the upper extremities without pathological reflexes. Sensation was very normal.

WHAT TO DO NEXT?

An EMG was done. This showed normal sensory studies and normal nerve conduction velocities with low-amplitude ulnar responses. There was denervation in the lower myotomes with chronic changes and this was bilateral.

WHAT SHOULD BE DONE?

An MRI of the spine showed flattening of the cervical spinal cord with mild spondylosis and "snake eye" finding (Fig. 33B-2). No flexion contrast MRI was done. This could show dilatation of the cervical epidural space (Fig. 33B-3).

DIFFERENTIAL DIAGNOSIS

This patient could have cervical spine disorder such as cervical spondylosis affecting multiple roots, but the lack of pain and sensory deficits is somewhat against this. Other than tumor, other possibilities would be intermedullary tumor or syringomyelia. This produces wasting in the hands, but the patients usually have a cape anesthesia, which is similar to intermedullary tumors.

There are cases of multifocal motor neuropathy that are predominantly axonal. Although they do not have a noticeable conduction block, this condition should be taken into consideration when making a differential diagnosis because it is not present in the patient's case of Hirayama disease.

Spinal muscular atrophy of distal loss has been reported, and this is unusual; however, Welander muscular dystrophy affects mainly the upper extremities and should be considered in the differential diagnosis. Usually these patients have an elevated creatine kinase. Ulnar decompression was most likely not necessary in this patient who also had involvement of other muscles innervated by the ulnar nerve. If he had nerve conduction slowing at that time, HNPP should also be a consideration, although again there was no other nerve involvement.

SUMMARY

This patient had bilateral Hirayama disease based on the clinical and EMG findings and had "snake eye" findings on the MRI. He was treated conservatively.

DISCUSSION FOR CASES 33A AND 33B

Since the initial description by Hirayama in 1959 of a group of patients with juvenile muscular atrophy of a unilateral upper extremity, there have been several reports of similar cases given various descriptive terms, including benign focal amyotrophy (BFA) and monomelic amyotrophy.[1–4] Although the total number of reported cases is small, one study concluded this to be a benign focal atrophy which represented 11% of motor neuron diseases.[3] The condition appears to be a more benign form of motor neuron disease with a fairly distinct course. The differential diagnoses include juvenile spinal muscular atrophy,[5] ALS, late motor neuron degeneration after poliomyelitis,[6,7] syringomyelia,[8] radiculopathy or brachial plexopathy,[9] multifocal motor neuropathy,[10] and multifocal acquired motor axonopathy.[11] Juvenile spinal muscular atrophy is unlikely as this characteristically is bilateral and symmetrical involving arms and legs with atrophy. Weakness seen as a late sequela of poliomyelitis typically occurs several years after a polio attack and is progressive.[7] Syringomyelia usually includes sensory abnormalities, as well as characteristic CT and myelographic findings. Brachial neuritis often has severe pain, selective sensory involvement, and no fasciculations and does not progress. Multifocal motor neuropathy affects individual nerves, showing evidence of conduction block in nerve conduction tests. Multifocal axonal neuropathy also affects individual nerves, but no conduction block is demonstrated. Structural lesions, such as arteriovenous malformation, tumor, or a central herniated disk, can give rise to a variety of findings referable to the upper extremities and have characteristic radiologic findings.

Due to the selective involvement of predominantly one limb, most patients undergo imaging studies to rule out the presence of such a structural lesion. Previous case reports of BFA have

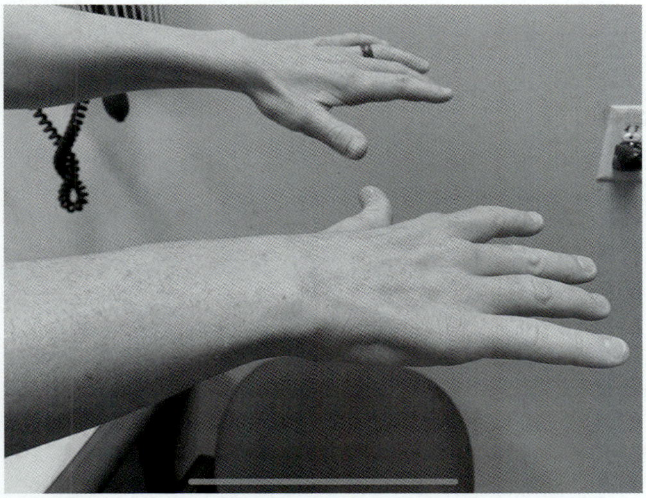

FIG. 33B-1 Patient's hands showing interossei muscle wasting and difficulty extending the fingers.

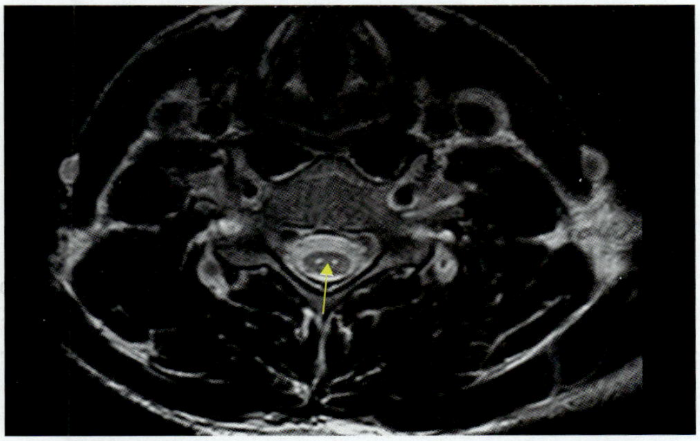

FIG. 33B-2 T2-weighted MRI image of the cervical spine showing "snake eyes "lesions (*arrow*)

shown normal radiologic studies,[12–14] although Mukai et al.[15] recently reported in the Japanese literature that their patients with distal and segmental muscular atrophy showed focal cord atrophy, as in Case 33A. The pathologic findings of typical motor neuron diseases include degeneration of large anterior horn cells in the spinal cord with resulting atrophy of the anterior roots, degeneration of the pyramidal tracts, and diffuse involvement of the anterolateral columns. Due to the benign nature of BFA, pathological findings are scarce, but this shows shrinkage and necrosis of the anterior horns.[14,16] MRI imaging, which was not available at the time that patient 33A was studied, provides less traumatic and more objective means to demonstrate cord atrophy and other features which could include the presence of "snake eyes" as well as shrinkage of the cord and dilatation of the epidural space and veins.[17–20]

We concluded that these patients had a syndrome consistent with BFA, although in this condition distal arm involvement is more characteristic. The limited monomelic involvement in Case 33A, age of onset, electrophysiologic findings, and clinical course are quite consistent with descriptions of the disorder.

Increased reflexes in atrophic denervated limbs have been reported and occur in up to 15% of patients. The hyperreflexia could suggest involvement of the upper motor neurons, but the lack of upper motor neuron signs is against that possibility. A bilateral presentation as in Case 33B is being reported.[21,22]

The radiologic finding on CT myelography showing a defect in the anterolateral cervical cord in Case 33A is consistent with cord atrophy. This defect could represent localized degeneration of anterior horn cells thought to be involved in the pathogenesis of the syndrome. Spinal cord atrophy has been documented by CT in cases of cervical spine trauma, spondylosis, and syringomyelia.[23-25]

MR imaging, which was not available at the time that patient 33A was studied, provides a less traumatic and more objective means of demonstrating localized spinal cord atrophy and rule out other focal diseases.

The etiology of BFA is unclear but has been postulated to be caused by immobilization of the neck after trauma.[26] This is supported by the findings that neck flexion flattens the cord and stretches its vessels, which could produce ischemia.[27] Alternatively, the dura and cord may be compressed against the body of the vertebrae during flexion.[28] Neck flexion has been reported to cause electrophysiologic dysfunction.[29] A recent study documented an anterior displacement of the dural sac with flattening of the cord during flexion, associated with engorgement of the epidural venous plexus by venography.[30] Rare familial cases have been reported,[31,32] one was associated with a mitochondrial DNA deletion.[33] There has also been an association with airway allergy, suggesting an autoimmune-mediated process in some patients.[34] A benign monomelic amyotrophy of the lower extremity has been reported.[35]

There is no specific therapy for this disease, although cervical collars may slow the progression in early cases.[36]

IMPORTANT POINTS

- Focal atrophy of muscles in a proximal upper extremity could be caused by a C5–C6 radiculopathy, upper trunk plexopathy, and/or a motor neuron disorder such as ALS, or by multifocal motor neuropathy and BFA or monomelic amyotrophy or Hirayama disease.
- Distal upper extremity weakness, atrophy and fasciculations, and the lack of sensory findings with a very slow progression are characteristic of BFA. This condition demonstrates that not all acquired motor neuron disorders have a grim prognosis.
- The EMG in patients with this presentation should include several myotomal levels, at least one upper and one lower extremity, and the opposite limb if a motor neuron disorder is suspected. Paraspinal muscles should also be studied. Needle testing should include muscles innervated by motor cranial nerves such as those of the tongue and, if necessary, thoracic paraspinals to rule out ALS.
- BFA is a nonprogressive, or slowly progressive motor neuron disorder that affects mainly young individuals with involvement of distal upper extremities but may manifest in the proximal arm and in the lower extremities and can be bilateral.
- Post-myelography CT scan or MRI may show segmental cord atrophy and dilatation of veins in the epidural space.

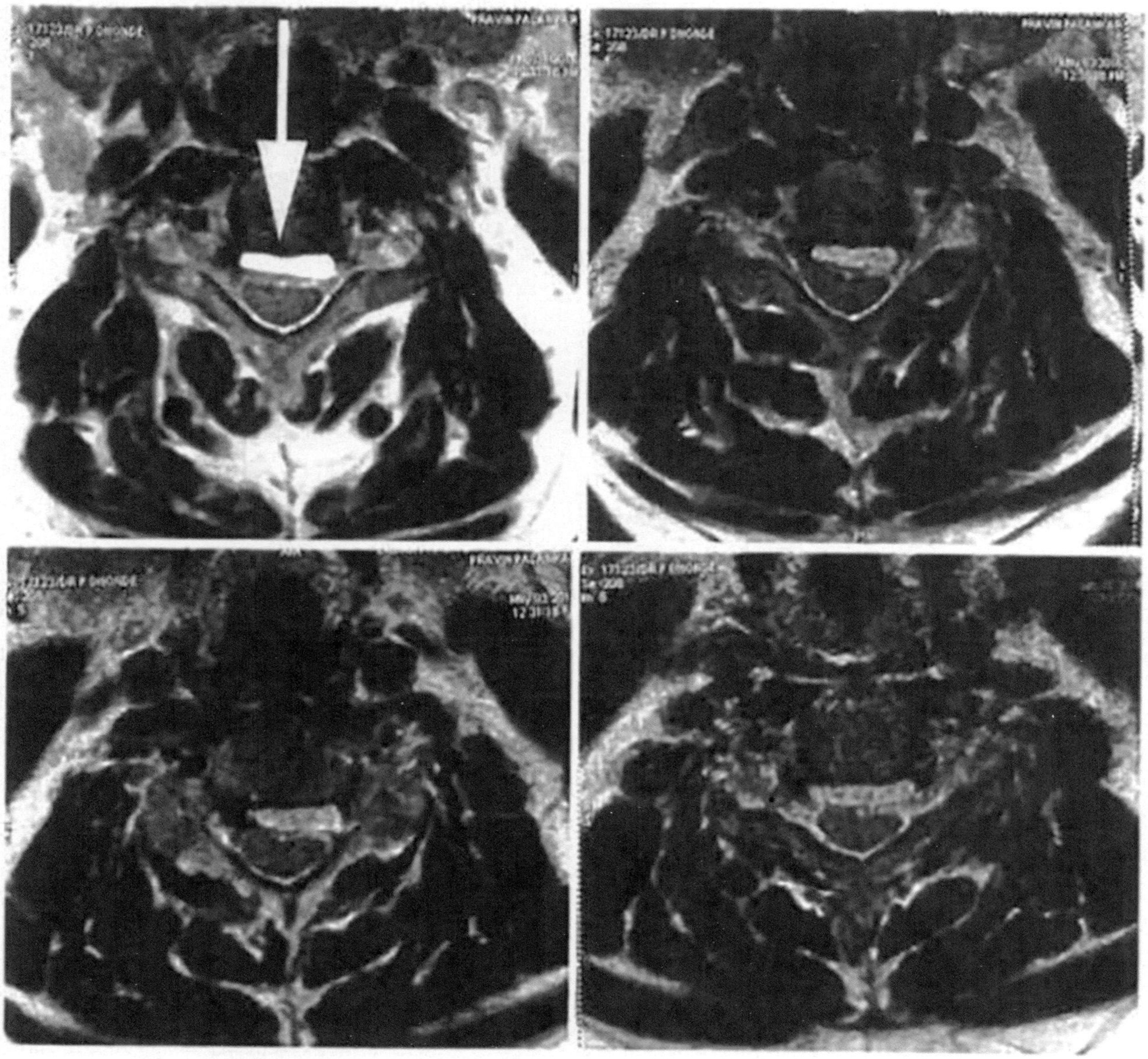

FIG. 33B-3 Dilatation of the cervical epidural space (*arrow*). (Reproduced with permission by Khadilkar SV, Yadav RS, Patel BA. *Neuromuscular Disorders: A Comprehensive Review With Illustrative Cases*. Springer; 2018.)

- Hirayama disease is thought to be caused by epidural venous distension of the cervical spine which can be diagnosed with flexion MRI with contrast. MRI findings in Hirayama disease can also show "snake eye" findings.
- The treatment of Hirayama disease is conservative and braces can help.

REFERENCES

1. Adornato BT, Engel WK, Kucera J, Bertorini TE. Benign focal amyotrophy. *Neurology*. 1978;28:399.
2. Gourie-Devi DM, Suresh TG, Shankar SK. Monomelic amyotrophy. *Arch Neurol*. 1984;41:388–394.
3. Hirayama K, Tsubaki T, Toyokura Y, Okinaka S. Juvenile muscular atrophy of unilateral upper extremity. *Neurology*. 1963;13:373–380.
4. Donofrio PD. AAEM a case report 28: monomelic amyotrophy. *Muscle Nerve*. 1994;17:1129–1134.
5. Pearce J, Harriman DGF. Chronic spinal muscular atrophy. *J Neurol Neurosurg Psychiatry*. 1966;29:509–520.
6. Campbell AM, Williams ER, Pearce J. Late motor neuron degeneration following poliomyelitis. *Neurology*. 1969;19: 1101–1106.
7. Mulder DW, Rosenbaum RA, Layton Jr DD. Late progression of poliomyelitis or form fruste of ALS? *Mayo Clin Proc*. 1972;47:756–761.
8. Finlayson AI. Syringomyelia and related conditions. In: Baker AB, Baker LH, eds. *Clinical Neurology*. New York, NY: Harper & Row; 1982:1–17.

9. Spillane JD. Localized neuritis of the shoulder girdle: a report of 46 cases in the MEF. *Lancet*. 1943;2:532.
10. Parry EG, Clarke S. Multifocal acquired demyelinating neuropathy masquerading as motor neuron disease. *Muscle Nerve*. 1988;11(2):103–107.
11. Katz JS, Barohn RJ, Kojan S, et al. Axonal multifocal motor neuropathy without conduction block or other features of demyelination. *Neurology*. 2002;58(4):615–620.
12. Riggs JE, Schochet SS, Gutmann L. Benign focal amyotrophy: variant of chronic spinal muscular atrophy. *Arch Neurol*. 1984;41:678–679.
13. Singh N, Sachdev KK, Susheela AK. Juvenile muscular atrophy localized to arms. *Arch Neurol*. 1980;37:297–299.
14. Sobue I, Saito N, Iida M, Ando K. Juvenile type of distal and segmental muscular atrophy of upper extremities. *Ann Neurol*. 1978;3:429–432.
15. Mukai E, Sobue I, Muto T, et al. Abnormal radiological findings in juvenile-type distal and segmental muscular atrophy of upper extremities. *Rinsho Shinkeigaku*. 1985;25:620–626.
16. Hirayama K. Juvenile muscular atrophy of distal upper extremity (Hirayama disease). *Internal Medicine*. 2000(4): 283–290.
17. Xu Haochong, Zhang Minghao Shao Fan, et al. "Snake-eyes" appearance on MRI occurs during the late stage of Hirayama disease and indicates poor prognosis. *Blomed Res Int*. 2019:9830243.
18. Lebouteux MV, Franques J, Guillevin R, et al. Revisiting the spectrum of lower motor neuron diseases with snake eyes appearance on magnetic resonance imaging. *Eur J Neurol*. 2014;21:1233–1241.
19. Mizuno J, Nakagawa H, Inoue T, et al. Clinicopathological study of "snake-eye appearance" in compressive myelopathy of the cervical spinal cord. *J Neurosurg*. 2003;99:162–168.
20. Kumar S, Mehta VK, Shukia R. Owl's eye sign: a rare neuroimaging finding in flail arm syndrome. *Neurology*.. 2015 Apr 7;84(14):1500.
21. Burton CV. The practical present and the anticipated future of CT. In: Post MJD, ed. *Computed Tomography of the Spine*. Baltimore, MD: Williams & Wilkins; 1984:227.
22. Haughton VM. Computed tomography of the spine. In: Spariro R, ed. *Myelography*. 4th ed. Chicago, IL: Yearbook Medical Publishers; 1984:653–656.
23. Borual DK, Sanyal S, Prakash A, et al. Bimelic symmetric Hirayama disease: spectrum of magnetic resonance imaging findings and comparative evaluation with classical monomelic amyotrophy and other motor neuron disease. *Iran J Neurol*. 2017;16:136–145.
24. Pradhan S, Brashon S. Bilateral symmetric form of Hirayama disease. *Neurology*.. 2009;72(24):2083–2089.
25. Quencher RM. The detection and characterization of posttraumatic spinal cord cysts. In: Latchaw R, ed. *CT of Head, Neck and Spine*. Chicago, IL: Yearbook Medical Publishers; 1985:707–714.
26. Paradiso S. Monomelic amyotrophy following trauma and immobilization in children. *Mucle Nerve*. 1997;20:425–430.
27. Breig A, Turnbull I, Hassler O. Effects of mechanical stresses on the spinal cord in cervical spondylosis: a study on fresh cadaver material. *J Neurosurg*. 1966;25(1):45–56.
28. Hirayama K, Tomonaga M, Kitano K, et al. Focal cervical poliopathy causing juvenile muscular atrophy of distal upper extremity: a pathological study. *J Neurol Neurosurg Psychiatry*. 1987;50(3):285–290.
29. Restuccia D, Rubino M, Valeriani M, et al. Cervical cord dysfunction during neck flexion in Hirayama's disease. *Neurology*. 2003;60(12):1980–1983.
30. Elseikh B, Wicklund M, Christoforides G, et al. Spinal angiography reveals functional venous engorgement in Hirayama's syndrome. *Neurology*. 2006;66(Suppl 2):A245.
31. Gucuyener K, Aysun S, Topaloglu H, et al. Monomelic amyotrophy in siblings. *Pediatr Neurol*. 1991;7(3):220–222.
32. Schlegel U, Jerusalem F, Tackmann W, et al. Benign juvenile focal muscular atrophy of upper extremities—a familial case. *J Neurol Sci*. 1987;80(2–3):351–353.
33. Fetoni V, Briem E, Carrara F, et al. Monomelic amyotrophy associated with the 7472insC mutation in the mtDN tRNASer(UCN) gene. *Neuromuscul Disord*. 2004;14(11):723–726.
34. Ochi H, Murai H, Osoegawa M, et al. Juvenile muscular atrophy of distal upper extremity associated with airway allergies: two cases successfully treated by plasma exchange. *J Neurol Sci*. 2003;206(1):109–114.
35. Munchau A, Rosenkranz T. Benign monomelic amyotrophy of the lower limb: case report and brief review of the literature. *Eur Neurol*. 2000;43(4):238–240.
36. Tokumaru Y, Hirayama K. A cervical collar therapy for non-progressive juvenile spinal muscular atrophy of the distal upper limb (Hirayama's disease). *Rinsho Shinkeigaku*. 1992;32(10): 1102–1106.

34 CASE

A Man With Progressive Leg Muscle Weakness 20 Years After an Acute Paralysis

A 54-year-old man presented initially at age 24 with an acute episode of right lower extremity weakness and urinary hesitancy. Examination at that time revealed right lower extremity weakness of 3/5 proximally and distally, decreased sensation over both feet, ankles, and right saddle area, absent right lower extremity reflexes, and diminished left ankle jerk. Atrophy was not documented. Cerebrospinal fluid was normal with protein 26 mg/dL (normal, 20–w40 mg/dL), glucose 77 mg/dL (normal, 40–60 mg/dL), 1 white cell/mm^3 (normal, 0–5 white cell/mm^3), and normal protein electrophoresis.

Electrodiagnostic studies were not performed at that time, and MRI was not availablew. He improved over 18 months but continued to have residual perianal and right foot numbness; he also required self-catheterization for 4 years followed by occasional bladder evacuation difficulties for years. Eight years after the initial episode, he developed "chronic fatigue syndrome" with a positive Epstein–Barr virus antibody, which resolved with acyclovir therapy.

Although he had mild residual right foot weakness, he remained physically active and played tennis several times a week until age 42, when he presented with progressive right lower extremity wasting and weakness. He denied back or leg pain or sexual dysfunction. The bladder symptoms had resolved.

Examination at the time revealed weakness and wasting of the right tibialis anterior (3/5), gastrocnemius, tibialis posterior and peronei (4/5). Upper and lower extremity reflexes were normal. Pinprick sensation was diminished over the left foot and perianal region. Plantar responses were flexor. Rectal tone was normal. Over the next 2 years, he developed weakness of the right quadriceps and hamstrings (4/5), ankle areflexia, and right knee hyporeflexia. The right leg was 4.5 cm smaller in circumference at mid-calf (Fig. 34-1).

The weakness increased over the next 6 years. Playing tennis became difficult as he tended to trip over his right foot. Limb measurements revealed a 1-cm decrease in right calf girth over 6 years. During 1 year prior to the present evaluation, he noted difficulty in standing on his left toes.

The following studies were unremarkable: blood counts, chemistries, creatine kinase, thyroid functions, vitamin B_{12}, folate, rheumatoid factor, serum protein electrophoresis and immunoelectrophoresis, ganglioside antibodies, antibodies to myelin-associated glycoprotein, Lyme antibodies, and cytomegalovirus antibodies. Cerebrospinal fluid examination was normal, with protein 28 mg/dL, glucose 69 mg/dL, and no cells. The IgG index was 0.4 (normal, 0.3–0.7) and myelin basic protein 0.7 ng/mL (normal, <0.5 ng/mL). The fluorescent antinuclear antibody test was weakly positive at 1:80. Epstein–Barr virus antibody (IgG) was positive. Poliovirus antibody titers were not measured.

WHAT IS THE DIFFERENTIAL DIAGNOSIS AND WHAT TESTS NEED TO BE DONE?

The progressive nature of the condition suggests a motor neuron disease, but the sensory changes and urinary symptoms are against this diagnosis. The slow progression and focal presentation make a mononeuritis multiplex unlikely, but a plexopathy is possible. Spinal canal diseases, such as a tumor and stenosis, or syringomyelia, are also considerations, and because the symptoms have always been localized to the spinal cord territory, a localized benign lesion such as a hemangioma or arteriovenous malformation with focal edema remains a possibility. Benign focal amyotrophy usually affects the upper extremities but can occur in the legs. This disorder, however, is not progressive.

An EMG could document the characteristics and distribution of the pathology and determine if there is a radiculopathy, a plexopathy, or a recent diffuse motor neuron disease.

AN EMG TEST WAS PERFORMED AT AGE 44

Motor Nerve Studies

Nerve and Site	Latency(ms)	Amplitude (mV)	Conduction Velocity (m/s)
Median Nerve R.	**Normal ≤ 4.2**	**Normal ≥ 6**	**Normal ≥ 50**
Wrist	3.5	7	–
Elbow	6.8	7	58
Ulnar Nerve R.	**Normal ≤ 3.6**	**Normal ≥ 8**	**Normal ≥ 50**
Wrist	3.3	9	–
Below elbow	6.7	9	60
Above elbow	8.5	9	67
Peroneal Nerve R.	**Normal ≤ 5.7**	**Normal ≥ 3**	**Normal ≥ 40**
Ankle	5.0	4	–
Fibular head	11.4	4	46
Knee	18.4	4	49

Motor Nerve Studies—cont'd

Nerve and Site	Latency (ms)	Amplitude (mV)	Conduction Velocity (m/s)
Tibial Nerve R.	**Normal ≤ 5.3**	**Normal ≥ 4**	**Normal ≥ 40**
Ankle	3.9	6	–
Pop. fossa	13.5	6	43

F-Wave and Tibial H-Reflex Studies

Nerve	Latency (ms)	Normal Latency ≤ (ms)
Median nerve R.	28.8	30
Ulnar nerve R.	29.2	30
Peroneal nerve R.	53.8	54
Tibial nerve R.	54.0	54
H-reflex R.	**NR**	34
H-reflex L.	**NR**	34

Sensory Nerve Studies

Nerve	Onset Latency (ms)	Normal Onset Latency ≤ (ms)	Peak Latency (ms)	Normal Peak Latency ≤ (ms)	Amp (μV)	Normal Amp ≥ (μV)	Conduction Velocity (m/s)	Normal Conduction Velocity ≥ (m/s)
Median nerve R.	2.4	2.6	2.9	3.1	21	20	54	50
Ulnar nerve R.	2.5	2.6	3.0	3.1	13	13	50	50
Sural nerve R.	3.2	3.5	3.7	4.0	12	11	44	40
Sural nerve L.	3.3	3.5	3.8	4.0	11	11	43	40

EMG Data

Muscle	Insrt Activity	Fibs	Pos Waves	Fasc	Amp	Dur	Poly	Pattern
Lumbar paraspinals R.	**Inc**	**1+**	**1+**	None	Norm	Norm	**Few**	Full
Iliopsoas R.	Norm	None	None	None	Norm	Norm	None	Full
Tensor fasciae latae R.	**Inc**	None	None	None	**Lg**	**Inc**	**Few**	Full
Vastus lateralis R.	**Inc**	None	None	None	**Lg**	**Inc**	**Few**	Full
Biceps femoris–long head R.	**Inc**	None	None	None	Norm	Norm	None	Full
Tibialis anterior R.	**Inc**	**2+**	**2+**	**Few**	**Lg**	**Inc**	**Few**	**Red**
Tibialis posterior R.	**Inc**	**2+**	**2+**	**Few**	**Lg**	**Inc**	**Few**	**Red**
Peroneus longus R.	**Inc**	**1+**	**1+**	**Few**	**Lg**	**Inc**	**Few**	**Red**
Gastrocnemius R.	**Inc**	**1+**	**1+**	**Few**	**Lg**	**Inc**	**Few**	**Red**
Tensor fasciae latae L.	Norm	None	None	None	Norm	Norm	None	Full
Tibialis anterior L.	Norm	None	None	None	**Lg**	**Inc**	**Few**	**Red**
Gastrocnemius L.	Norm	None	None	None	Norm	Norm	None	Full
Deltoid R.	Norm	None	None	None	Norm	Norm	None	Full
Biceps brachii R.	Norm	None	None	None	Norm	Norm	None	Full
Flexor carpi ulnaris R.	Norm	None	None	None	Norm	Norm	None	Full
Extensor dig. communis R.	Norm	None	None	None	Norm	Norm	None	Full
First dorsal interosseus R.	Norm	None	None	None	Norm	Norm	None	Full

WHAT WERE THE EMG FINDINGS?

Nerve conduction tests and EMG in the upper extremities and right arm and leg were normal except for absent tibial H-reflexes. Fibrillations and fasciculations (1–2+) were noted in the right gastrocnemius, tibialis anterior, posterior, and peroneus longus muscles with large motor unit potentials and with decreased recruitment during voluntary activity in these and other right leg muscles and in the left tibialis anterior. Positive sharp waves (2+) were present in the right lower lumbar paraspinal muscles. It appeared that his disease was limited mainly to the right L4–S1 levels. The absent H-reflex and mildly prolonged F-responses could be caused by a radiculopathy or plexopathy, but could also be caused by a decreased motor neuron pool and drop-out of fast-conducting axons. The normal SNAPs argue against a plexopathy, and paraspinal denervation localized the lesion to the root or proximally. The fasciculations suggest involvement of the motor neurons, although this sometimes can be seen in radiculopathies and neuropathies. Since there were fasciculations in more than one root territory, a spinal cord disorder, such as a tumor, vascular malformation, or stenosis, is a consideration.

WHAT WOULD YOU DO NEXT?

MRI of the thoracolumbar spine revealed an area of T2 hyperintensity within the conus medullaris, more prominent on the right, without enhancement or cord enlargement (Fig. 34-2). This remained unchanged on three scans between ages 42 and 54.

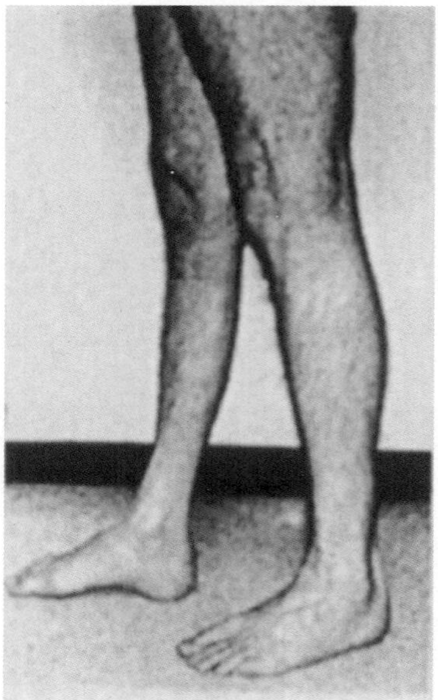

FIG. 34-1 Lateral view of the distal extremities showing wasting of the right lower extremity.

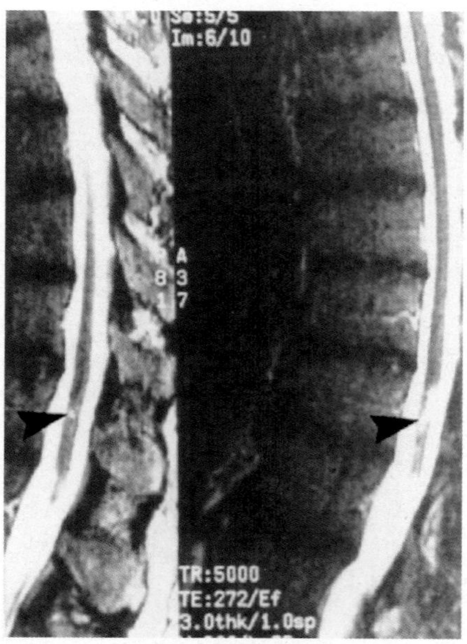

FIG. 34-2 MRI of the thoracolumbar spine performed with a 1.5T magnet revealed an area of T2 hyperintensity within the conus medullaris without mass effect; there was no contrast enhancement. This suggested an old insult, such as transverse myelitis (unchanged on serial scans between 1992, 1994, and 1998).

WHAT IS THE MOST LIKELY DIAGNOSIS?

This patient appears to have a progressive focal motor neuron disease which is secondary to a previous episode of myelopathy and thus similar to postpolio amyotrophy (PPA).[1]

He was treated with gentle exercise, physical therapy, and bracing.

DISCUSSION

This man initially had an acute myelopathic episode followed 20 years later by a progressive amyotrophy. The initial lumbosacral myelopathy or myelitis had an uncertain etiology. The T2 hyperintensity in the conus medullaris on MRI is suggestive of gliosis. Lack of contrast enhancement makes an intramedullary tumor unlikely.[2] Syringomyelia of the conus medullaris is usually associated with radiologic evidence of conus enlargement[3] and its characteristic cavity.[4,5]

He had mild, but definite, progression of motor deficits, but his sensory examination, sphincter function, and the T2 hyperintensity on MRI remained unchanged. His EMG revealed active denervation and reinnervation of the right L4–S1-innervated muscles and the left tibialis anterior, likely as a consequence of anterior horn cell loss 20 years after a partial insult from a myelopathy.

The development of slowly progressive weakness and wasting after a myelopathy in this patient resembles PPA.[1,6,7] PPA muscle biopsy often demonstrates a progressive increase in the number of angulated fibers with an eventual development of group atrophy.[8,9] Delayed weakness in patients with antecedent poliomyelitis may be due to an increase in metabolic demands to the surviving motor neuron pool,[6] or dysfunction of surviving motor neurons may cause a slow degeneration of terminal axons.[10,11] Reinnervation occurs by distal axonal sprouting from the remaining motor neurons. The increased territory, however, eventually overburdens these motor neurons, leading to apoptosis causing their death. Similar mechanisms may also be etiologic in this patient who developed delayed weakness after a previous insult to the anterior horn cells of the conus medullaris. Reports of delayed amyotrophy after trauma and immobilization[12] or radiation[13,14] support the possibility that delayed amyotrophy may occur as a consequence of diverse partial motor neuron insults. A progressive amyotrophy has been reported in a case where a spinal lipoma anchored the spinal cord.[15]

SUMMARY

This patient had a previous episode of acute paralysis, which in retrospect appeared to have been an acute myelitis of the conus medullaris. He later developed progressive weakness and fasciculations.

It is likely that the focal lesion of the spinal cord produced a secondary focal amyotrophy similar to PPA.

IMPORTANT POINTS

- The presence of active and chronic denervation associated with fasciculations in one limb suggests a motor neuron disorder, but it is not always indicative of amyotrophic lateral sclerosis and can have other causes.
- In a focal disorder with progressive weakness of one leg, an MRI with and without contrast of the lower spine, including the conus medullaris, should always be done or considered.
- A postmyelopathy progressive amyotrophy is likely related to progressive anterior horn cell disorder.
- In myelopathy and PPA, progressive motor neuron degeneration may be caused by progressive motor neuron loss, remodeling of motor neuron territory, and increased metabolic burden of surviving motor neurons.

This case was reported in Narayanaswami P, Bertorini T. Progressive amyotrophy as a late complication of myelopathy. J Neurol Sci. 2001;184:11–13

REFERENCES

1. Dalakas MC. The post-polio syndrome as an evolved clinical entity: definition and clinical description. *Ann NY Acad Sci.* 1995;753:68–80.
2. Mathew P, Todd NV. Diagnosis of intradural conus and cauda equina tumors. *Br J Hosp Med.* 1993;50(4):169–174.
3. Nassar SI, Correll JW, Housepian EM. Intramedullary cystic lesions of the conus medullaris. *J Neurol Neurosurg Psychiatry.* 1968;31:106–109.
4. Lee BCP, Zimmerman RD, Manning JJ, Deck MDF. MR imaging of syringomyelia and hydromyelia. *AJNR Am J Neuroradiol.* 1985;6:221–228.
5. Sherman JL, Barkovich AJ, Citrin CM. The MR appearance of syringomyelia: new observations. *Am J Roentgenol.* 1987;148(2): 381–391.
6. Jubelt B, Cashman NR. Neurological manifestations of post-polio syndrome. *Crit Rev Neurobiol.* 1987;3:199–220.
7. Trojan DA, Cashman NR. Post-poliomyelitis syndrome. *Muscle Nerve.* 2005;31(1):6–19.
8. Dalakas M, Illa I. Post-polio syndrome: concepts in clinical diagnosis, pathogenesis, and etiology. *Adv Neurol.* 1991;56:495–511.
9. Dalakas MC, Elder G, Hallett M, et al. A long-term follow-up study of patients with post-poliomyelitis neuromuscular symptoms. *N Engl J Med.* 1986;314(15):959–963.
10. Dalakas MC. Pathogenetic mechanisms of post-polio syndrome: morphological, electrophysiological, virological and immunological correlations. *Ann NY Acad Sci.* 1995;753: 167–185.
11. Dalakas MC. Why drugs fail in postpolio syndrome: lessons from another clinical trial. *Neurology.* 1999;53:1166–1167.
12. Paradiso G. Monomelic amyotrophy following trauma and immobilization in children. *Muscle Nerve.* 1997;20:425–430.
13. Jackson M. Post radiation monomelic amyotrophy. *J Neurol Neurosurg Psychiatry.* 1992;55:629.
14. Lamy C, Mas JL, Varet B, et al. Postradiation lower motor neuron syndrome presenting as monomelic amyotrophy. *J Neurol Neurosurg Psychiatry.* 1991;54:648–649.
15. Masjuan Vallejo J, Herrero Valverde AM, Martinez San Millán J, et al. Progressive amyotrophy of a limb as the presenting symptom of anchored spinal cord syndrome with lipoma. *Rev Neurol.* 2001;32(5):437–440.

35 CASE

A Man With One Large Calf

A 47-year-old man was referred because of weakness, tightness, and pain in the right calf for 5 years, becoming worse in the past 8 months.

Past medical history was unremarkable. He smoked one pack of cigarettes a day.

His neurologic examination was unremarkable except for a large right calf with a circumference 5 cm larger than the left side (Fig. 35-1) and an absent right ankle jerk. All other reflexes were normal, and there were no Babinski signs. Sensory examination, coordination, and the rest of the examination were normal.

WHAT IS THE DIFFERENTIAL DIAGNOSIS?

Although muscle enlargement is not uncommon in neuromuscular diseases, this is usually symmetric. A focal enlargement suggests several possibilities, such as a tumor, inflammation, a muscle infarct, parasitic infections, a muscle hernia, a ruptured tendon, or, rarely, a radiculopathy with partial denervation.

AN EMG TEST WAS PERFORMED

Motor Nerve Studies

Nerve and Site	Latency (ms)	Amplitude (mV)	Conduction Velocity (m/s)
Peroneal Nerve R.	**Normal ≤ 5.7**	**Normal ≥ 3**	**Normal ≥ 40**
Ankle	4.5	8	–
Knee	11.4	8	49

Motor Nerve Studies—cont'd

Tibial Nerve R.	Normal ≤ 5.3	Normal ≥ 4	Normal ≥ 40
Ankle	4.6	5	–
Pop. fossa	14.4	5	41

Motor Nerve Studies—cont'd

Nerve and Site	Latency (ms)	Amplitude (mV)	Conduction Velocity (m/s)
Tibial Nerve L.	**Normal ≤ 5.3**	**Normal ≥ 4**	**Normal ≥ 40**
Ankle	4.8	8	–
Pop. fossa	11.6	8	54

F-Wave and Tibial H-Reflex Studies

Nerve	Latency (ms)	Normal Latency ≤ (ms)
Peroneal nerve R.	51	54
Tibial nerve R.	53	54
Tibial nerve L.	50	54
H-reflex R.	**NR**	34
H-reflex L.	33.6	34

Sensory Nerve Studies

Nerve	Onset Latency (ms)	Normal Onset Latency ≤ (ms)	Peak Latency (ms)	Normal Peak Latency ≤ (ms)	Amp (µV)	Normal Amp ≥ (µV)	Conduction Velocity (m/s)	Normal Conduction Velocity ≥ (m/s)
Sural nerve R.	3.3	3.5	3.8	4.0	15	13	42	40
Superficial peroneal R.	3.2	3.5	3.7	4.0	13	10	43	40

EMG Data

Muscle	Insrt Activity	Fibs	Pos Waves	Fasc	Amp	Dur	Poly	Pattern
Lumbar paraspinal R.	Norm	None	None	None	Norm	Norm	None	Full
Tensor fasciae latae R.	**CRD**	**2+**	**2+**	**Many**	**Lg**	Norm	None	**Red**
Vastus lateralis R.	**Myok**	**2+**	**2+**	**Many**	**Lg**	Norm	None	**Red**
Deltoid R.	Norm	None	None	None	Norm	Norm	None	Full

EMG Data—cont'd

Muscle	Insrt Activity	Fibs	Pos Waves	Fasc	Amp	Dur	Poly	Pattern
Biceps brachii R.	Norm	None	None	None	Norm	Norm	None	Full
First dorsal int. R.	Norm	None	None	None	Norm	Norm	None	Full
Tibialis anterior R.	**Inc**	**2+**	**2+**	None	**Lg**	Norm	None	**Red**
Peroneus longus R.	Norm	None	None	None	Norm	Norm	None	Full
Gastrocnemius R.	**Myok**	2+	2+	**Few**	**Lg**	Norm	None	Full
Lumbar paraspinal L.	Norm	None	None	None	Norm	Norm	None	Full
Tensor fasciae latae L.	**Inc**	2+	2+	None	Norm	Norm	None	**Red**
Vastus lateralis L.	Norm	None	None	**Few**	Norm	Norm	None	Full
Tibialis anterior L.	**CRD**	None	None	None	**Lg**	Norm	None	Full
Gastrocnemius L.	**Myok**	None	None	None	**Lg**	Norm	None	Full

CRD, Complex repetitive charges.

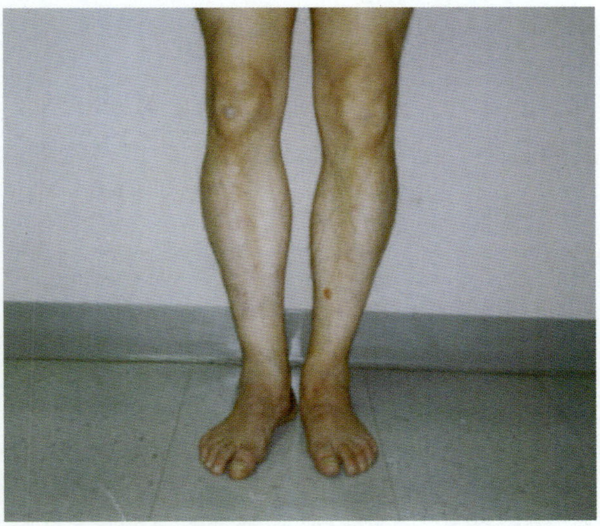

FIG. 35-1 Patient showing larger right calf.

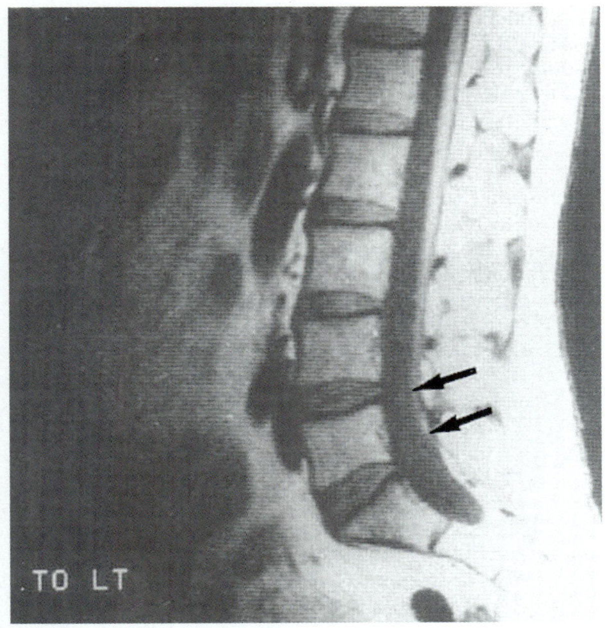

FIG. 35-2 T1-weighted MRI (sagittal view) of the lumbosacral spine showing the spinal cord placed as low as S1 (*arrows*).

WHAT WERE THE EMG FINDINGS?

This test showed normal nerve conduction tests, except for an absent right tibial nerve H-reflex. F-responses were normal in the peroneal and tibial nerves. Large motor unit potentials were present in both legs, but were more prominent on the right, particularly in the gastrocnemius muscle where the maximal amplitude was 8 mV. Fibrillation potentials (2+) and complex repetitive discharges (CRDs) were also present in the right gastrocnemius and tensor fasciae latae. Myokymic discharges with 3–4 potentials firing at a rate of 12–18 times per second were present in some areas in the gastrocnemius and vastus lateralis muscles. Occasional fasciculations were observed in both legs, mainly in the right tensor fasciae latae, gastrocnemius, and quadriceps muscles.

In summary, the EMG showed chronic and active denervation in the legs, with myokymia, fasciculations, and frequent CRDs. The EMG was normal in the arms.

The findings did not localize the lesion, and the abnormalities were not confined to a particular root. The presence of fasciculations could suggest a motor neuron disorder, but they were only present in the legs; fasciculations can also occur focally in root and in some peripheral nerve disorders. Myokymia frequently suggests a plexus lesion, but by itself it is nonlocalizing and occurs in other disorders. The nerve conduction tests were normal. The absent right H-reflex could be caused by lesions of the S1 root, lumbosacral plexus, or sciatic or tibial nerves.

WHAT WOULD BE THE NEXT TESTS?

A spinal MRI showed a cord that terminated lower than normal at the S1 vertebral level (Fig. 35-2). MR imaging of the legs revealed diffusely increased signal on T1-weighted images in the enlarged right calf muscle. A large area of increased signal was also seen in the T2-weighted images in the right calf (Fig. 35-3).

A muscle biopsy of the right calf showed numerous atrophic angular fibers, pyknotic nuclei, increased interstitial fat, and predominantly type I fiber hypertrophy and fiber splitting. Numerous fibers contained rimmed vacuoles, but no inclusion bodies or inflammation were seen; fiber-type grouping was evident in the ATPase staining (Fig. 35-4).

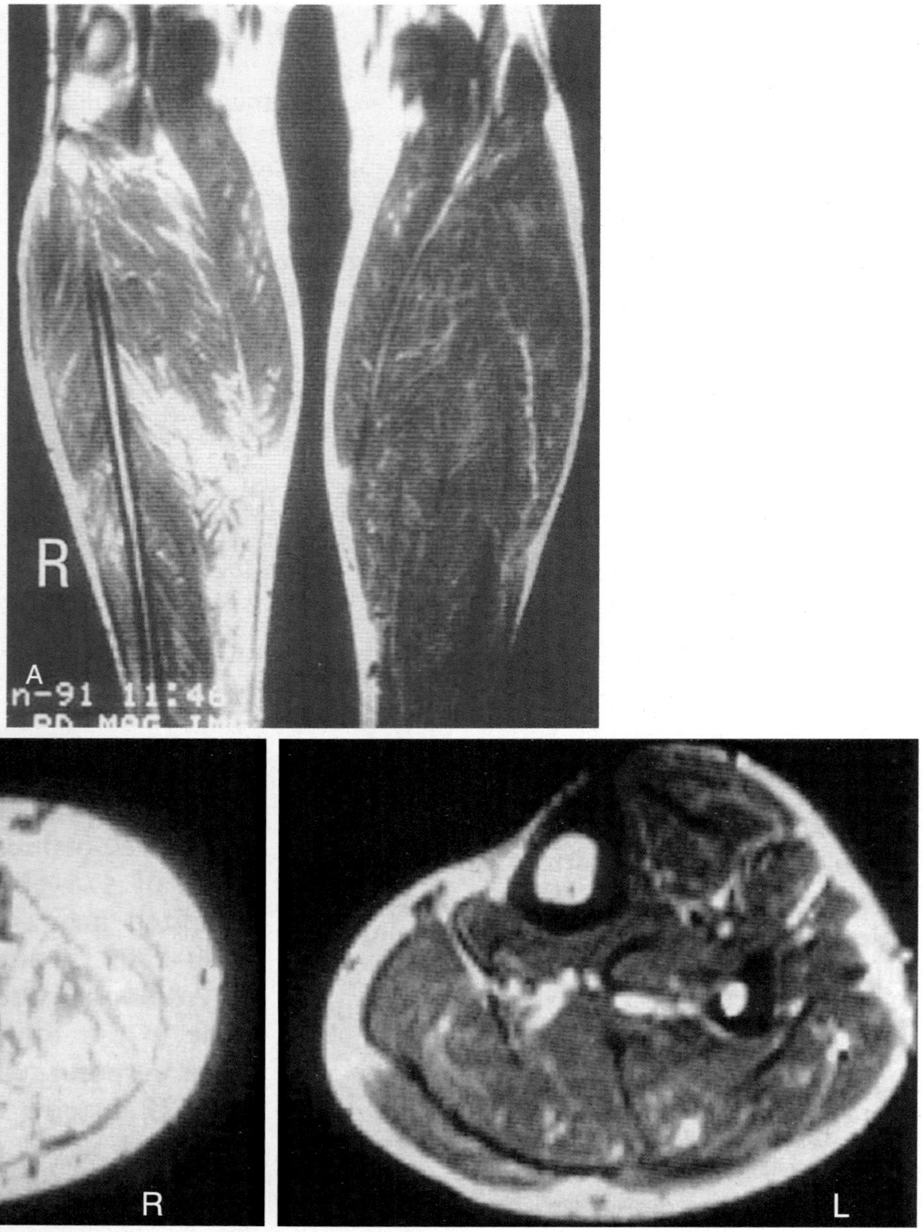

FIG. 35-3 **A**, T2-weighted MRI (coronal view) showing increased signal in right calf. **B**, T1-weighted MRI showing diffuse increased signal representing fat in the right calf.

DISCUSSION

It was concluded that in this patient the muscle hypertrophy, EMG, and biopsy findings were caused by a tethered cord. Surgery was offered, but the patient declined.

Muscle enlargement can be caused by true muscle hypertrophy but may also be due to infiltrates such as these from amyloid.[1,2] Inflammation causes enlargement in myositis[3] and in parasitic infections.[4] Myopathies can have compensatory hypertrophy and pseudohypertrophy.[5,6] Frequent diffuse spontaneous depolarization of muscle in myotonia and nerve in Isaacs syndrome also cause hypertrophy.[7] In radiculopathy and peripheral nerve lesion, hypertrophy is likely the result of frequent abnormal discharges, such as myokymic[8] or CRDs.[9–16]

This patient had neurogenic muscle fiber atrophy and hypertrophy. Exercise of healthy fibers induces hypertrophy of muscle fibers type II.[17] In animals, however, partial denervation and increased stretching of weak muscles cause type I fiber hypertrophy.[18,19] This mechanism could have played a role in the hypertrophy seen in this patient. It is also likely that the repetitive discharges and myokymia produced excessive work of both fiber types, resulting in hypertrophy. This is similar to the neuromuscular irritability seen in Isaacs syndrome,[7] in which muscle enlargement can be improved by phenytoin and similar drugs.

The correlation between the segmental hypertrophy and the presence of rimmed vacuoles seen in the muscle biopsy in this patient was unclear. Rimmed vacuoles are found in a variety of neuromuscular disorders.[20,21] The vacuoles may represent focal

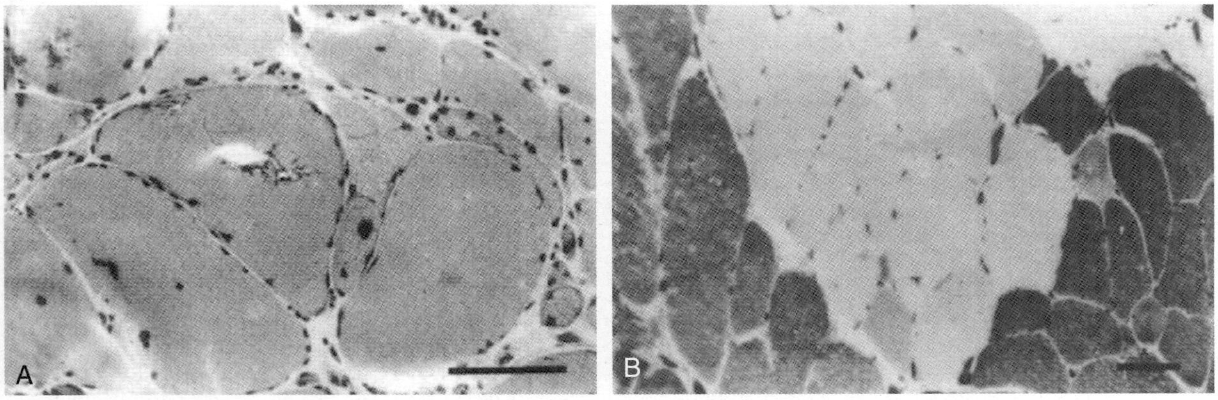

FIG. 35-4 **A**, A rimmed vacuole, muscle hypertrophy, and atrophy, right gastrocnemius muscle (modified trichrome stain, bar = 100 μm). **B**, Fiber-type groups are seen on the ATPase stain, bar = 100 μm.

muscle necrosis, distinct from that of muscular dystrophies, as postulated by Satoyoshi.[22] The focal myofibrillary degeneration in this patient could have been caused by excessive muscle activity, stretching, or work overload. In cases similar to this, rimmed vacuoles have been reported in neurogenic muscle hypertrophy with CRDs.[13]

The MRI findings on the T1 images of fatty infiltrates likely played a role in the calf enlargement, whereas the increased signal in the T2 images could represent focal fiber necrosis. Similar findings have been described in inflammatory myopathies,[23,24] in metabolic myopathies after exercise,[25] and in normal patients after excessive work.[26]

This patient had tethered cord syndrome, which can occur in children in association with other congenital anomalies. In adults the symptoms could be indolent and chronic[27] and may mimic multiple sclerosis or motor neuron disease,[28–31] producing weakness, but also sphincter disturbances. The syndrome causes stretching and ischemia of the cord and roots.[32] The MRI characteristics have been thoroughly described by Raghavan et al.[33] Early recognition is important because surgical intervention stops the progression of the neurologic deficits.[34,35]

SUMMARY

In conclusion, this patient has tethered cord syndrome with chronic anterior horn or root dysfunction, causing partial denervation and increased neuromuscular activity. Fiber hypertrophy and muscle fiber degeneration formed the rimmed vacuoles which corresponded to the increased signal seen in the T2 images on muscle MRI.

IMPORTANT POINTS

- Focal muscle enlargement can be caused by infections, edema, amyloidosis, parasites, myositis, infarcts, tumors, and partial denervation.
- Partial denervation causes neurogenic pseudohypertrophy with frequent spontaneous muscle activity manifested as myokymia and CRDs. Fatty infiltration may contribute to the enlargement.
- Rimmed vacuoles can be seen in inclusion body myositis, familial inclusion body myopathy, and other distal muscular dystrophies and oculopharyngeal dystrophy. In this case rimmed vacuoles were likely caused by focal myofiber degeneration, stretching, or work overload.
- Tethered cord syndrome can present with or without other congenital anomalies. It can manifest with weakness and sphincter disturbances, may mimic multiple sclerosis and motor neuron diseases, and it can cause partial chronic muscle denervation and hypertrophy.

This case was reported in Bertorini T, Woodhouse C, Horner L. Muscle hypertrophy secondary to the tethered cord syndrome. Muscle Nerve. 1994;17(3):31–35.

REFERENCES

1. Ringel SP, Claman HN. Amyloid-associated muscle pseudohypertrophy. *Arch Neurol.* 1982;39:413–417.
2. Whitaker JN, Hashimoto K, Quinones M. Skeletal muscle pseudohypertrophy in primary amyloidosis. *Neurology.* 1977;27:47–54.
3. Heffner RR Jr, Barron SA. Denervating changes in focal myositis, a benign inflammatory pseudotumor. *Arch Pathol Lab Med.* 1980;104:261–264.
4. Sawhney BB, Chopra JS, Banerji AK, Wahi PL. Pseudohypertrophic myopathy in cysticercosis. *Neurology.* 1976;26:270–272.
5. Dubowitz V, ed. *Muscle Disorders in Childhood.* London, England: WB Saunders; 1978:19–69.
6. Matsushita S, Ikeda S, Hanyu N, et al. Muscular pseudohypertrophy in an adult case with centronuclear myopathy. *Eur Neurol.* 1991;31(3):172–174.
7. Zisfein J, Sivak M, Aron AM, Bender AN. Isaacs syndrome with muscle hypertrophy reversed by phenytoin therapy. *Arch Neurol.* 1983;40:241–242.
8. Valenstein E, Watson RT, Parker JL. Myokymia, muscle hypertrophy and percussion "myotonia" in chronic recurrent polyneuropathy. *Neurology.* 1978;28:1130–1134.
9. Korczyn AD, Kuritzky A, Sandbank U. Muscle hypertrophy with neuropathy. *J Neurol Sci.* 1978;38:399–408.
10. Mielke U, Ricker K, Emser W, Boxler K. Unilateral calf enlargement following S1 radiculopathy. *Muscle Nerve.* 1982;5:434–438.

11. Montagna P, Martinelli P, Rasi F, et al. Muscular hypertrophy after chronic radiculopathy. *Arch Neurol.* 1984;41:397–398.
12. Nix WA, Butler IJ, Roontga S, et al. Persistent unilateral tibialis anterior muscle hypertrophy with complex repetitive discharges and myalgia: report of two unique cases and response to botulinum toxin. *Neurology.* 1992;42:602–606.
13. Nagasawa T, Sudo A, Fukumizu M, et al. Congenital monomelic neurogenic disorder with calf muscle hypertrophy. *Brain Dev.* 2003;25(8):571–573.
14. van de Warrenburg BP, Zwarts MJ, van Engelen BG. A swollen painless calf caused by neurogenic muscle (pseudo) hypertrophy. *Ned Tijdschr Geneeskd.* 2003;147(44):2183–2186.
15. Bernat JL, Ochoa JL. Muscle hypertrophy after partial denervation: a human case. *J Neurol Neurosurg Psychiatry.* 1978;41:719–725.
16. Bertorini TE, Igarashi M. Postpoliomyelitis muscle pseudohypertrophy. *Muscle Nerve.* 1985;8:644–649.
17. Dubowitz V, ed. *Muscle Biopsy: A Practical Approach.* 2nd ed. Philadelphia, PA: Bailliere Tindall; 1985.
18. Sarnat HB, Portnoy JM, Chi DY. Effects of denervation and tenotomy on the gastrocnemius muscle in the frog: a histologic and histochemical study. *Anat Rec.* 1977;187:335–346.
19. Sola OM, Christensen DL, Martin AW. Hypertrophy and hyperplasia of adult chicken anterior latissimus dorsi muscles following stretch with and without denervation. *Exp Neurol.* 1973;41:76–100.
20. Carpenter S, Karpati G, Wolfe L. Virus-like filaments and phospholipid accumulation in skeletal muscle: study of a histochemically distinct chronic myopathy. *Neurology.* 1970;20:889–903.
21. Fukuhara N, Kumamoto T, Tsubaki T. Rimmed vacuoles. *Acta Neuropathol.* 1980;51:229–235.
22. Satoyoshi E. Distal myopathy. *Tohoku J Exp Med.* 1990;161(S):1–19.
23. Fujino H, Kobayashi T, Goto I, Onitsuka H. Magnetic resonance imaging of the muscles in patients with polymyositis and dermatomyositis. *Muscle Nerve.* 1991;14:716–720.
24. Hernandez RJ, Keim DR, Sullivan DB, et al. Magnetic resonance imaging appearance of the muscles in childhood dermatomyositis. *J Pediatr.* 1990;117:546–550.
25. Fleckenstein JL, Peshock RM, Lewis SF, Haller RG. Magnetic resonance imaging of muscle injury and atrophy in glycolytic myopathies. *Muscle Nerve.* 1989;12:849–855.
26. Shellock FG, Fukunaga T, Mink JH, Edgerton VR. Acute effects of exercise on MR imaging of skeletal muscle: concentric vs eccentric actions. *Am J Roentgenol.* 1991;156:765–768.
27. Fitz CR, Harwood-Nash DC. The tethered conus. *Am J Roentgenol Radium Ther Nucl Med.* 1975;125:515–523.
28. Holtzman RNN, Stein BM, eds. *The Tethered Spinal Cord.* New York, NY: Thieme-Stratton; 1985:1–147.
29. Pang D. Tethered cord syndrome in adults. In: Holtzman RNN, Stein BM, eds. *The Tethered Spinal Cord.* New York, NY: Thieme-Stratton; 1985:99–115.
30. Salvati M, Orlando Ramundo E, Artico M, et al. The tethered cord syndrome in the adult: report of three cases and review of the literature. *Zentralbl Neurochir.* 1990;51:91–93.
31. Scatliff JH, Kendall BE, Kingsley DP, et al. Closed spinal dysraphism: analysis of clinical, radiological, and surgical findings in 104 consecutive patients. *Am J Roentgenol.* 1989;152:1049–1057.
32. Tani S, Yamada S, Knighton RS. Extensibility of the lumbar and sacral cord: pathophysiology of the tethered spinal cord in cats. *J Neurosurg.* 1987;66:116–123.
33. Raghavan N, Barkovich AJ, Edwards M, Norman D. MR imaging in the tethered spinal cord syndrome. *Am J Roentgenol.* 1989;152:843–852.
34. Huttmann S, Krauss J, Collmann H, et al. Surgical management of tethered spinal cord in adults: report of 54 cases. *J Neurosurg.* 2001;95:173–178.
35. Haro H, Komori H, Okawa A, et al. Long-term outcomes of surgical treatment for tethered cord syndrome. *J Spinal Disord Tech.* 2004;17:16–20.

A Man With Muscle Spasms and Elevated Serum Creatine Kinase

A 46-year-old, right-handed man presented with mild lower-extremity weakness of a year's duration. He is a house painter who developed low back and neck pain with progressive upper-extremity weakness after a fall at work about 3 months prior to our evaluation. He had progressive difficulty walking with falls at least once a day. He also had some numbness in all four extremities for about a year. He had no bulbar dysfunction or sphincter disturbances but had cramps and muscle spasms in all four extremities since early childhood. He also had a history of muscles "twitching." His family history was negative for neurologic illnesses. He had one healthy daughter.

The initial workup included normal complete blood count and routine chemistry profile including electrolytes, glucose, blood urea nitrogen creatinine, calcium, and phosphorus. Serum creatine kinase (CK) was elevated at 2573 IU/L (normal, 30–220 IU/L), lactate dehydrogenase 873 IU/L (normal, 0–250 IU/L), and aspartate transaminase 68 IU/L (normal, 0–40 IU/L). Erythrocyte sedimentation rate, serum protein electrophoresis, fluorescent antinuclear antibody, rheumatoid factor, thyroid function tests, B_{12}/folate, urine heavy metal screen, GM_1 ganglioside antibodies, and cerebrospinal fluid were normal/negative. An MRI of the cervical spine was normal.

The patient received a trial of gamma globulin infusions without benefit and was referred to us.

General physical examination was normal, and he had no organomegaly, gynecomastia, or testicular atrophy. He had normal mentation, and the cranial nerves were normal except for perioral fasciculations. No tongue atrophy or weakness was noted. He had moderate proximal weakness in all four extremities and bilateral hand weakness and mild interossei muscle wasting (Fig. 36-1). There was areflexia in all four limbs with diffuse scattered fasciculations. No Babinski signs were elicited. He had hypoesthesia to pinprick with diminished vibration sense in the hands and feet. Position sense was intact. Gait was somewhat slow and waddling, but it was not ataxic. The rest of the examination was normal.

WHAT IS THE DIFFERENTIAL DIAGNOSIS?

The diffuse weakness and fasciculations are suggestive of a motor neuron disease, but the lack of bulbar symptoms and long tract signs is against the diagnosis of amyotrophic lateral sclerosis (ALS). A lower motor neuron syndrome such as progressive spinal muscular atrophy and familial spinal muscular atrophy[1] should be considered, particularly as the patient has had cramps since childhood. A craniocervical junction disease or a cervical spondylosis is also a possibility, particularly because of the history of neck pain, but the distal sensory findings and fasciculations in the face are against these diagnoses, which were ruled out by the normal MRI.

The sensory complaints and findings with areflexia could also suggest a peripheral neuropathy such as chronic inflammatory demyelinating polyradiculoneuropathy, but fasciculations are not typical for this disease, particularly when present in the face. Limb fasciculations could be seen in multifocal motor neuropathy and sometimes in multifocal motor sensory neuropathy, or Lewis–Sumner syndrome,[2] but they do not occur in the face. The sensory complaints would favor the latter, but in those, the presentation is more asymmetric and multifocal. A hereditary polyneuropathy, such as Charcot–Marie–Tooth disease, is unlikely, due to the lack of a family history or high arches, the presence of facial fasciculations, and proximal weakness.

The lack of family history, bulbar signs, gynecomastia, or testicular atrophy are somewhat against the diagnosis of bulbospinal atrophy or Kennedy's disease, a condition in which there could be evidence of a mild sensory neuropathy and facial fasciculations; about 50% of these patients have an elevated CK as in this case.[3,4]

The elevation of CK could also suggest a myopathy, but the fasciculations and sensory findings make that diagnosis unlikely. Elevated CK can also occur in motor neuron disorders such as ALS and spinal muscular atrophy.[5]

AN EMG TEST WAS PERFORMED

Motor Nerve Studies

Nerve and Site	Latency(ms)	Amplitude (mV)	Conduction Velocity (m/s)
Peroneal Nerve R.	**Normal ≤ 5.7**	**Normal ≥ 3**	**Normal ≥ 40**
Ankle	4.2	4	–
Fibular head	13.5	3	44
Knee	15.1	3	**38**
Tibial Nerve L.	**Normal ≤ 5.3**	**Normal ≥ 4**	**Normal ≥ 40**
Ankle	3.9	4	–
Pop. fossa	15.2	4	43

Motor Nerve Studies—cont'd

Nerve and Site	Latency (ms)	Amplitude (mV)	Conduction Velocity (m/s)
Ulnar Nerve R.	**Normal ≤ 3.7**	**Normal ≥ 8**	**Normal ≥ 50**
Wrist	3.4	9	–
Below elbow	8.6	8	51
Above elbow	10.8	8	53

F-Wave and Tibial H-Reflex Studies

Nerve	Latency (ms)	Normal Latency ≤ (ms)
Peroneal nerve R.	54	54
Tibial nerve L.	53.9	54
Ulnar nerve R.	29.9	30
H-reflex R.	33.4	34
H-reflex L.	34	34

Sensory Nerve Studies

Nerve	Onset Latency (ms)	Normal Onset Latency ≤ (ms)	Peak Latency (ms)	Normal Peak Latency ≤ (ms)	Amp (μV)	Normal Amp ≥ (μV)	Conduction Velocity (m/s)	Normal Conduction Velocity ≥ (m/s)
Sural nerve R.	3.5	3.5	4.0	4.0	**7**	11	40	40
Sural nerve L.	3.4	3.5	3.9	4.0	**9**	11	41	40
Ulnar nerve R.	2.5	2.6	3.0	3.1	13	13	50	50

EMG Data

Muscle	Insrt Activity	Fibs	Pos Waves	Fasc	Amp	Dur	Poly	Pattern
Tongue	**CRD**	None	None	**Few**	Norm	Norm	None	Full
Deltoid R.	Norm	None	None	**Few**	Norm	Norm	None	Full
Biceps brachii R.	**CRD**	None	None	None	**Lg**	**Inc**	None	Full
Brachioradialis R.	Norm	None	None	None	Norm	Norm	None	Full
First dorsal interosseous R.	Norm	None	None	**Few**	**Lg**	**Inc**	None	Full
Tensor fasciae latae R.	Norm	None	None	None	Norm	Norm	None	Full
Vastus lateralis R.	Norm	None	None	**Few**	Norm	Norm	None	Full
Tibialis anterior R.	Norm	None	None	**Few**	**Lg**	**Inc**	None	**Red**
Gastrocnemius R.	**CRD**	None	None	None	Norm	Norm	None	**Red**
Vastus lateralis L.	Norm	None	None	**Few**	Norm	Norm	None	**Red**
Tibialis anterior L.	**CRD**	None	None	**Few**	**Lg**	**Inc**	None	**Red**
Gastrocnemius L.	Norm	None	None	**Few**	Norm	Norm	None	**Red**

CRD, Complex repetitive discharges.

WHAT WERE THE EMG FINDINGS?

The test showed a mild neuropathy with slowing of the right peroneal nerve conduction velocity across the knee and low-amplitude sural and borderline ulnar SNAP amplitudes. These findings are not suggestive of Charcot–Marie–Tooth disease type I.

There were fasciculations and high-frequency discharges, including in the tongue, which suggest a motor neuron disease. There were large motor unit action potentials with decreased recruitment in the limbs, which is against a myopathy despite the high serum CK. The combination of a mild neuropathy with bulbar findings is suggestive of Kennedy's disease.

WHAT OTHER TESTS COULD BE USEFUL?

A biopsy of the left gastrocnemius muscle showed atrophic angular fibers, group atrophy, and targets. There was also some necrosis with phagocytosis and minimal interstitial inflammation, but no perivascular inflammation (Fig. 36-2).

A sural nerve biopsy showed only mild dropout of myelinated fibers and some segmental demyelination.

WHAT SHOULD BE DONE NEXT?

In spite of the lack of systemic manifestations and of significant bulbar signs, except for fasciculations in the face and complex repetitive discharges in the tongue, Kennedy's disease was considered because of the combination of lower motor neuron signs with mild sensory nerve abnormalities.

DNA testing was done in lymphocytes and showed 42 cytosine-adenosine-guanine (CAG) repeats in the androgen receptor gene within the X chromosome (normal, 11–33).[6–8]

The patient did reasonably well, but 1 year later developed laryngeal spasms with choking and was treated with mexiletine 150 mg twice a day with moderate relief of these symptoms.

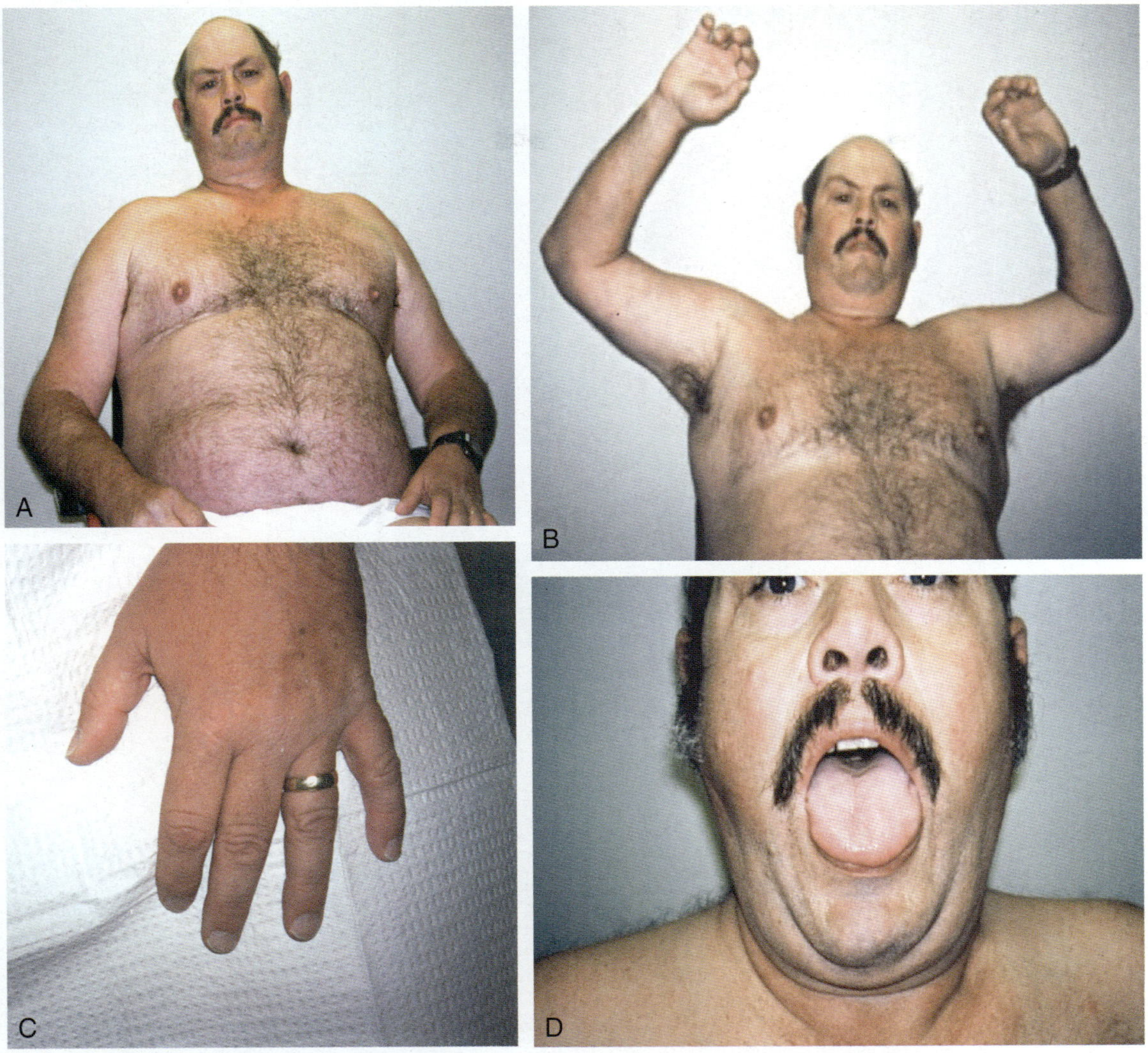

FIG. 36-1 **A and B**, The patient is obese, but without obvious gynecomastia. **C**, Mild interosseous muscle wasting. **D**, Notice lack of tongue atrophy.

WHAT IS KENNEDY'S DISEASE?

Bulbospinal muscular atrophy was initially described by William Kennedy and colleagues in 1968.[3] It is an X-linked recessive disease characterized by bulbar and predominantly proximal weakness with fasciculations, particularly in the face, and areflexia. Facial fasciculations are seen in 90% of the cases; some patients also have a hand tremor. Significant sensory symptoms are not common or mild.[3] Systemic manifestations include gynecomastia (Fig. 36-3), testicular atrophy, and impotence with an azoospermia; diabetes can also occur. Patients might not have these manifestations.

Motor nerve conductions in Kennedy's disease are usually normal, but the SNAPs are of low amplitude or are absent.[9,10] Serum CK is usually elevated, even in asymptomatic individuals.[11]

Muscle biopsies show atrophy and signs of denervation. Myopathic features are seen.[12] Nerve biopsies could show some demyelination, axonal atrophy, and a decreased number of myelinated fibers, as in this case.[13]

The disease is caused by increased CAG repeat expansions of the first exon of the androgen receptor gene,[6–8] and affected individuals usually have 40–52 repeats. The phenotype is variable and is not related to the number of expansions; the number of expansions, however, might be related to the age of onset.[14,15] The disease can rarely be seen in women.[12]

The androgen receptor is expressed in perikarya and nuclei of neurons and nonneural tissues such as testis and scrotal skin and muscle. Most likely the condition is caused by polyglutamine expansions, resulting in a toxic gain of function with aggregations of abnormal proteins causing degeneration of motor neurons.[16] Autopsy studies demonstrate nuclear accumulations of androgen receptor protein in motor neurons and other areas of the nervous system.[17–19] There is loss of motor neurons and of small neurons in the intermediate zone of the spinal gray matter. Posterior root ganglion neurons are relatively preserved, but there is a decreased number of large-diameter sensory axons.

Kennedy's disease has no cure, and the treatment is only symptomatic. The progression, however, with therapy in this condition is promising. For example, insulin-like growth

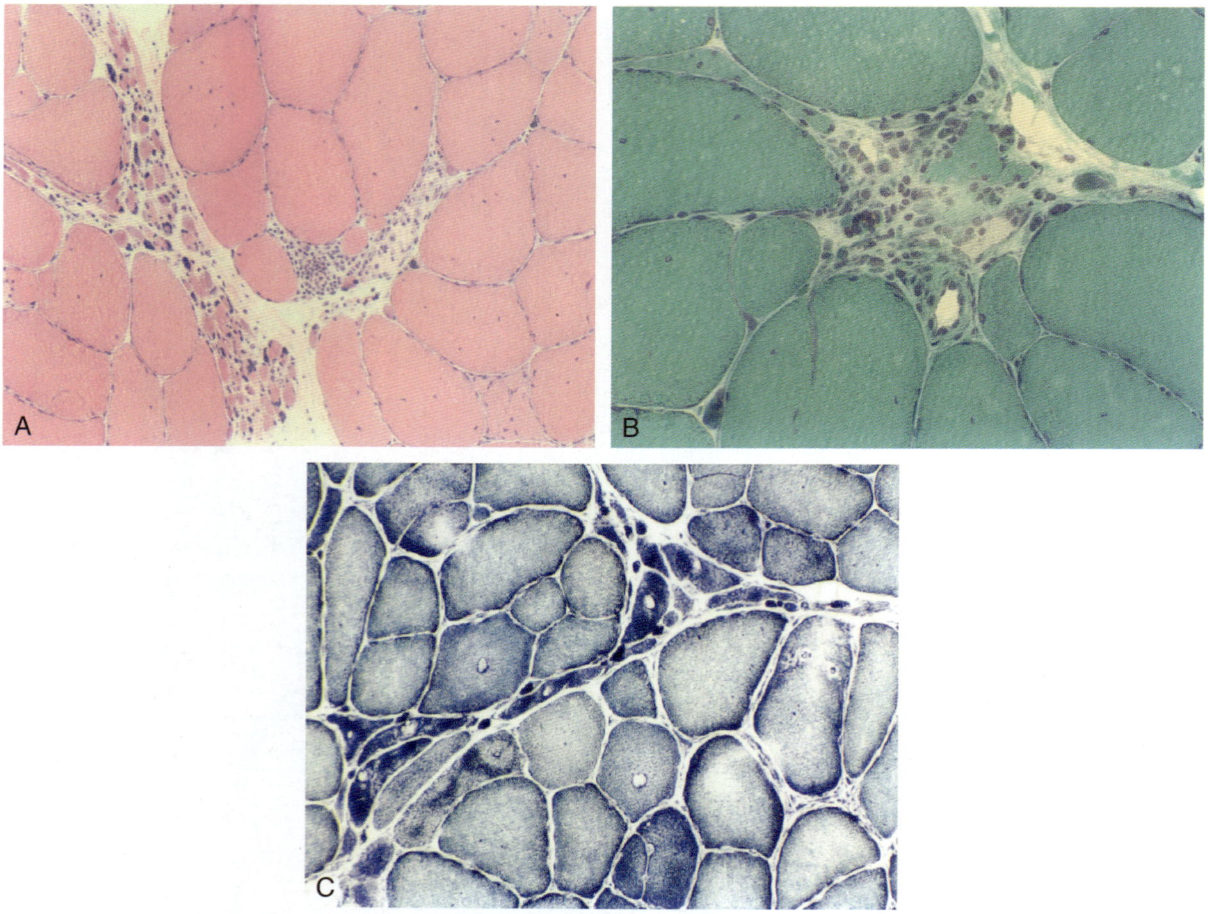

FIG. 36-2 **A**, Muscle biopsy showing group atrophy, pyknotic muscle, variation in fiber size, and mild inflammation (H&E stain, ×200). **B**, Necrotic fibers with phagocytosis and mild inflammation (trichrome stain, ×400). **C**, Atrophic fibers and target fibers (NADH-TR, ×400).

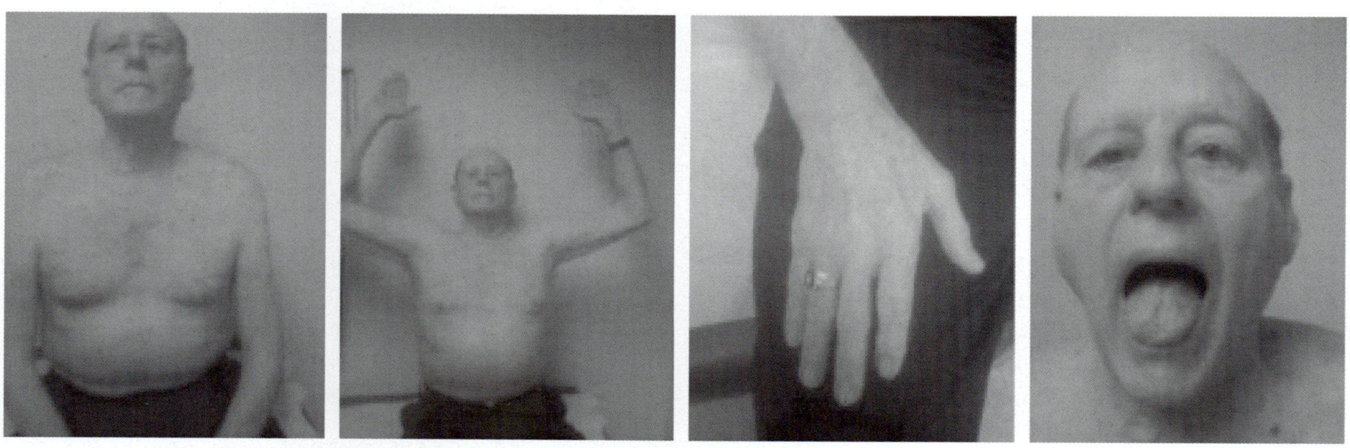

FIG. 36-3 Another patient with Kennedy's disease showing gynecomastia, tongue atrophy, and interossei muscle wasting.

factor ameliorates motor function in animal models.[20] Also, the gonadotrophic-releasing hormone, leuprorelin appears to improve motor function and there are some very mild benefits.[21]

This case emphasizes that Kennedy's disease can occur without systemic manifestation and should be ruled out in patients with a progressive lower motor neuron syndrome.

SUMMARY

This patient presented with an adult onset of weakness, cramps, and fasciculations. The cramps had been present since childhood. He had an elevated serum CK, and EMG showed diffuse fasciculations, high-frequency discharges, and low-amplitude SNAPs.

Although he did not have systemic manifestations or a positive family history, he did have increased CAG repeat expansion of the androgen receptor gene, characteristic of Kennedy's disease.

IMPORTANT POINTS

- Muscle weakness, cramps with fasciculations (particularly in the face) and areflexia, low-amplitude SNAPs, and an elevation of CK suggest Kennedy's disease, even in the absence of systemic manifestations. Therefore this condition should be ruled out in patients with lower motor neuron syndromes, even without a family history of systemic manifestations.
- CK levels are increased in myopathies but can also occur in motor neuron disorders and some neuropathies.
- Kennedy's disease is caused by increased CAG repeat expansions of the androgen receptor gene.
- The disease is caused by polyglutamine accumulation which leads to deposits of abnormal proteins in motor neurons.
- Kennedy's disease has no cure and the treatment is only symptomatic. Sodium channel blockers, such as mexiletine, are helpful for the muscle spasms and cramps.

REFERENCES

1. Rudnik-Schöheborn S, De Visser M, Zerres K. Spinal muscular atrophies. In: Engel AG, Franzini-Armstrong C, eds. *Myology*. 3rd ed. New York, NY: McGraw-Hill; 2004:1845–1864.
2. Lewis RA, Sumner AJ, Brown MJ, Asbury AK. Multifocal demyelinating neuropathy with persistent conduction block. *Neurology*. 1982;32(9):958–964.
3. Kennedy WR, Alter M, Sung JH. Progressive proximal spinal and bulbar muscular atrophy of late onset: a sex linked recessive trait. *Neurology*. 1968;18:671–680.
4. Papapetropoulos T, Panayiotopoulos CP. X-linked spinal and bulbar muscular atrophy of late onset (Kennedy-Stefanis disease?). *Eur Neurol*. 1981;20:485–488.
5. Rudnik-Schöneborn S, Lutzenrath S, Borkowska J, et al. Analysis of creatine kinase activity in 504 patients with proximal spinal muscular atrophy types I–III from the point of view of progression and severity. *Eur Neurol*. 1998;39(3):154–162.
6. La Spada AR, Wilson EM, Lubahn DB, et al. Androgen receptor gene mutations in X-linked spinal and bulbar muscular atrophy. *Nature*. 1991;352:77–79.
7. Fischbeck KH, Ionasescu V, Ritter AW, et al. Localization of the gene for X-linked spinal muscular atrophy. *Neurology*. 1986;36:1595–1598.
8. Fischbeck KH, Souders D, La Spada A. A candidate gene for X-linked spinal muscular atrophy. *Adv Neurol*. 1991;56: 209–213.
9. Olney RK, Aminoff MJ, So YT. Clinical and electrodiagnostic features of X-linked recessive bulbospinal neuronopathy. *Neurology*. 1991;41(6):823–828.
10. Meriggioli MN, Rowin J, Sanders DB. Distinguishing clinical and electrodiagnostic features of X-linked bulbospinal neuronopathy. *Muscle Nerve*. 1999;22:1693–1697.
11. Sorenson EJ, Klein CJ. Elevated creatine kinase and transaminases in asymptomatic SBMA. *Amyotroph Lateral Scler*. 2007;8(1): 62–64.
12. Manzano R, Soraru G, Grunseich C, Fratta P, Zuccaro E. Beyond motor neurons: expanding the clinical spectrum in Kennedy's disease. *J Neurol Neurosurg Psychiatry*. 2018;89(8):808–812.
13. Amato AA, Prior TW, Barohn RJ, et al. Kennedy's disease: a clinicopathologic correlation with mutations in the androgen receptor gene. *Neurology*. 1993;43:791–794.
14. Igarashi S, Tanno Y, Onodera O, et al. Strong correlation between the number of CAG repeats in androgen receptor genes and the clinical onset of features of spinal and bulbar muscular atrophy. *Neurology*. 1992;42:2300–2302.
15. La Spada AR, Roling DB, Harding AE, et al. Meiotic stability and geotype-phenotype correlation of trinucleotide repeat in X-linked spinal and bulbar muscular atrophy. *Nat Genet*. 1991;2:301–304.
16. Abel A, Taye AA, Fischbeck KH, Merry DE. Truncated androgen receptor gene with an expanded CAG repeat causes phenotypic changes in transgenic mice. *Am J Hum Genet*. 1998;63:A319.
17. Ordway JM, Tallaksen-Greene S, Gutekunst CA, et al. Ectopically expressed CAG repeats cause intranuclear inclusions and a progressive late-onset neurological phenotype in the mouse. *Cell*. 1997;91:753–763.
18. Li M, Miwa S, Kobayashi Y, et al. Nuclear inclusions of the androgen receptor protein in spinal and bulbar muscular atrophy. *Ann Neurol*. 1998;44:249–254.
19. Lieberman AP, Fischbeck KH. Triplet repeat expansion in neuromuscular disease. *Muscle Nerve*. 2000;23:843–850.
20. Darrington RS, Butler R, Leigh PN, et al. Ligand-dependent aggregation of polyglutamine-expanded androgen receptor in neuronal cells. *Neuro Report*. 2002;13(16):2117–2120.
21. Arnold FJ, Merry DE. Molecular mechanisms and therapeutics for SBMA/Kennedy's disease. *Neurotherapeutics*. 2019;16(4): 928–947.

37 CASE

A Man With Muscle Twitching and Poor Balance

A 37-year-old man presented with a 2-year history of loss of balance and weakness. He also had muscle cramps, twitching, and difficulty in speaking. Previous workup showed a normal magnetic resonance imaging (MRI) of the brain and visual, auditory, and somatosensory-evoked responses. He also had normal spinal fluid studies, HIV and human T-lymphotropic virus 1 titers, complete blood count, and chemistry profile. He was referred for a possible motor neuron disease.

Past medical history was unremarkable. His father and paternal uncle were diagnosed with possible multiple sclerosis (MS) as they had weakness and ataxia. The patient did not smoke or drink and had not been exposed to toxins.

Neurologic examination revealed normal mental status with a score of 30/30 on the mini-mental state examination. He was mildly dysarthric. Visual fields were normal. There was mild limitation of the medial and lateral gaze and upward gaze. At times, he had a tendency to squint while looking forward (Fig. 37-1). He had fasciculations in the face. Other cranial nerves were normal, including facial strength. The tongue appeared normal and showed no atrophy or weakness. Gag reflex and jaw jerk were increased. Although he complained of weakness, his muscle strength was normal on testing. Reflexes were hyperactive with positive Hoffmann signs bilaterally, but no Babinski signs. There were scattered muscle fasciculations in the limbs without atrophy. Vibration sense was diminished in the toes, but position sense, pain, and touch sensation were normal. He had difficulty with tandem gait. The finger-to-nose test was normal, but the heel-to-shin test was poorly done.

AN EMG TEST WAS PERFORMED

MOTOR NERVE STUDIES

Nerve and Site	Latency (ms)	Amplitude (mV)	Conduction Velocity (m/s)
Peroneal Nerve L.	**Normal ≤ 5.7**	**Normal ≥ 3**	**Normal ≥ 40**
Ankle	4.6	12	–
Fibular head	10.9	11	49
Knee	12.9	11	50
Tibial Nerve L.	**Normal ≤ 5.3**	**Normal ≥ 4**	**Normal ≥ 40**
Ankle	3.4	17	–
Pop. fossa	11.9	16	48

Nerve and Site	Latency (ms)	Amplitude (mV)	Conduction Velocity (m/s)
Ulnar Nerve R.	**Normal ≤ 3.6**	**Normal ≥ 8**	**Normal ≥ 50**
Wrist	2.9	12	–
Below elbow	6.1	12	61
Above elbow	8.1	12	60

F-Wave and Tibial H-Reflex Studies

Nerve	Latency (ms)	Normal Latency ≤ (ms)
Peroneal nerve R.	47.4	54
Tibial nerve L.	50.1	54
Ulnar nerve R.	26.3	30
H-reflex R.	30.3	34

Sensory Nerve Studies

Nerve	Onset Latency (ms)	Normal Onset Latency ≤ (ms)	Peak Latency (ms)	Normal Peak Latency ≤ (ms)	Amp (μV)	Normal Amp ≥ (μV)	Conduction Velocity (m/s)	Normal Conduction Velocity ≥ (m/s)
Sural nerve R.	3.5	3.5	4.0	4.0	12	11	40	40
Ulnar nerve R.	2.6	2.6	3.1	3.1	13	13	50	50

EMG Data

Muscle	Insrt Activity	Fibs	Pos Waves	Fasc	Amp	Dur	Poly	Pattern
Tongue	Norm	None	None	None	Norm	Norm	None	Full
Masseter R.	Norm	None	None	**Few**	**Lg**	**Inc**	None	Full
Deltoid R.	Norm	None	None	**Few**	**Lg**	**Inc**	None	Full
Biceps brachii R.	Norm	None	None	None	**Lg**	**Inc**	**Few**	Full
1st dorsal interosseous R.	Norm	None	None	None	**Lg**	**Inc**	None	**Red**
Vastus lateralis R.	Norm	None	None	**Few**	**Lg**	**Inc**	None	**Red**
Tibialis anterior R.	Norm	None	None	None	Norm	Norm	None	Full
Gastrocnemius R.	Norm	None	None	None	Norm	Norm	**Few**	Full
Tibialis anterior L.	Norm	None	None	None	Norm	Norm	None	Full
Gastrocnemius L.	Norm	None	None	None	Norm	Norm	None	Full

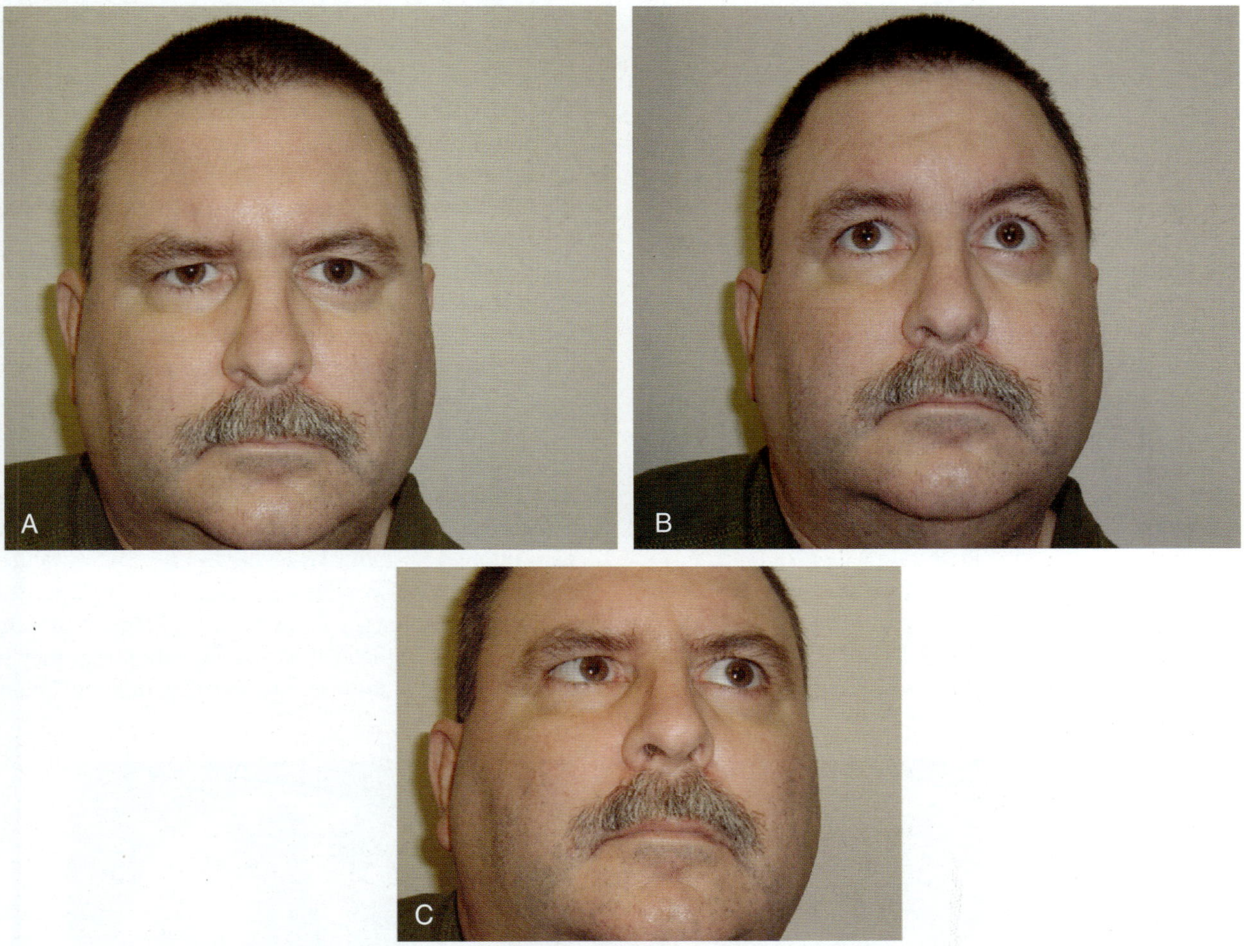

FIG. 37-1 **A**, The patient looking straight with a tendency to squint. Notice the limitation of upward gaze **(B)** and lateral gaze **(C)**.

WHAT WERE THE EMG FINDINGS?

The electrophysiologic studies revealed normal motor and sensory nerve conduction velocities, latencies, and amplitudes of the compound muscle action potentials and sensory nerve action potential (SNAPs). There were large motor unit potentials with decreased recruitment in the lower extremities, with fasciculations but no denervation potentials. Scattered fasciculations without denervation were also seen on the face but not in the tongue. The findings seemed to indicate a mild chronic motor neuron disorder.

WHAT IS THE DIFFERENTIAL DIAGNOSIS?

This patient was initially referred for fasciculations and weakness. He has a positive family history of "possible MS," but likely that diagnosis was incorrect as, although there is an increased incidence of MS in families, autosomal dominant inheritance is rare. Furthermore, the fasciculations in the face and limbs are unusual for this disease. Fasciculations, however, not only occur in motor neuron diseases but also can sometimes be seen in neuropathies; localized limb fasciculations are seen in radiculopathy. They are seen diffusely in a number of other diseases, including multifocal motor neuropathy, some spinocerebellar degenerations, Kennedy's disease, Jakob–Creutzfeldt syndrome, and debrancher enzyme deficiency. This patient's presentation with fasciculations and hyperreflexia with scattered large motor unit potentials on electromyography suggests a relatively benign chronic motor neuron syndrome. The apparent autosomal dominant inheritance could suggest a hereditary amyotrophic lateral sclerosis (ALS) which is usually more rapidly progressive, but the extraocular abnormalities and leg ataxia indicate a more widespread disorder; furthermore, the lack of denervation potentials makes the diagnosis of ALS or similar diseases unlikely. Facial fasciculations can be seen in Kennedy's syndrome[1] and Machado–Joseph spinocerebellar degeneration.[2] Patients with Kennedy's disease might have systemic manifestations, show SNAP abnormalities, and have elevated serum creatine kinase, which are not seen in this case. The mode of inheritance, ataxia, lack of tongue atrophy, and abnormalities of the extraocular movements are not characteristic of this disorder.

Multisystem degeneration might present with weakness, fasciculations, and tremor but without extraocular involvement or significant ataxia. Those, however, occur in spinocerebellar degenerations. The autosomal dominant inheritance, age of onset, hyperactive reflexes, lack of significant proprioceptive sensory deficits, up-going toes, scoliosis, fasciculations, and normal SNAPs rule out the possibility of a later-onset Friedreich's ataxia. An acquired autoimmune or toxic cause seems unlikely.

The history and findings in this patient are suggestive of an autosomal dominant spinocerebellar ataxia (SCA). The lack of atrophy on the initial MRI could be related to the recent onset of the disease. Of the SCAs, Machado–Joseph disease (MJD) is an important consideration in this case, particularly because of the facial fasciculations.

WHAT TESTS SHOULD BE DONE?

A repeated MRI showed cerebellar atrophy (Fig. 37-2). DNA tests for autosomal dominant spinocerebellar degenerations by protein catabolic rate amplification were performed in blood, and the patient had one allele with 27 CAG repeats and one with 78 (normal, <40), diagnostic of MJD or autosomal dominant SCA type 3.

DISCUSSION

The patient was diagnosed as having MJD, an autosomal dominant condition characterized by ataxia, spasticity, and hyperreflexia accompanied by abnormalities of ocular movements. Some patients might also have extrapyramidal signs. This spinocerebellar degeneration is caused by CAG repeat expansions, usually from 54 to 86, in chromosome 14q24.3–32.[3] This is the most common autosomal dominant ataxia.

Spinocerebellar degenerations are a group of disorders that manifest with ataxia and variable manifestations of nervous system dysfunction. The most widely recognized disorder and frequent ataxia is Friedreich's ataxia, which is relatively easy to diagnose because of its clinical manifestations with scoliosis, spinal cord and peripheral nerve involvement, and autosomal recessive inheritance. A carrier of mutation of the *FRDA* gene with a GAA trinucleotide repeat expansion causes a reduction in the protein ataxin.[4] Those with autosomal dominant SCA have more variable presentations, are therefore difficult to differentiate clinically, and are usually separated by their genetic defects[5] (Tables 37-1 and 37-2).

MJD (SCA3), also called Azorean disease, was described initially in three separate famwilies with different presentations in the Azores,[6–8] but later it became apparent that they had the same disease.[9] It is now recognized that different phenotypes

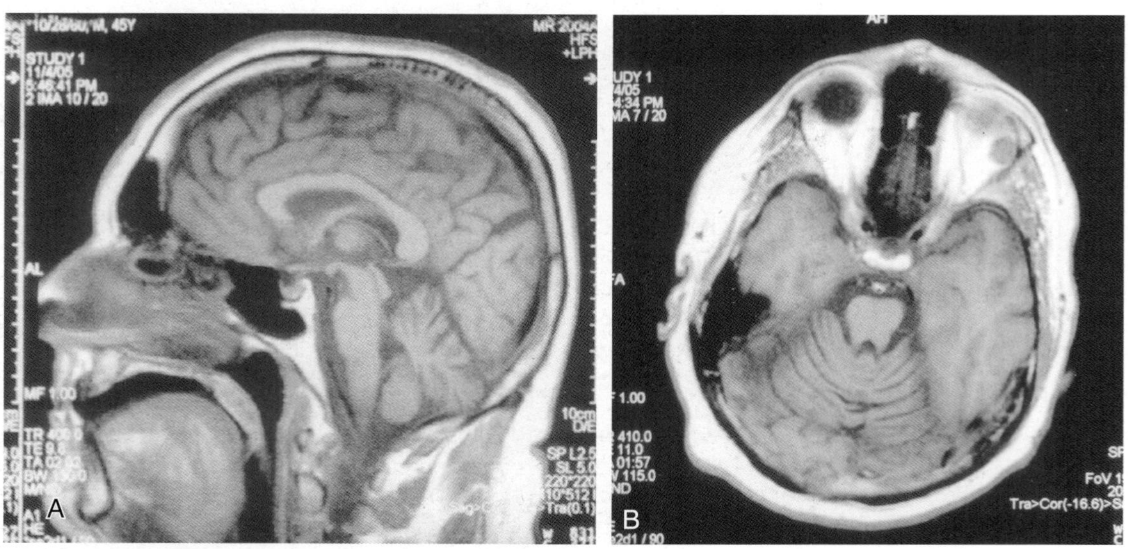

FIG. 37-2 **A,** T1-weighted MRI of brain (sagittal view); notice cerebellar atrophy. **B,** MRI showing atrophy with prominent folia (axial view). *MRI,* Magnetic resonance imaging.

TABLE 37-1 Typical Clinical Findings in Spinocerebellar Ataxia (SCA) Subtypes

Disease Name	Mean Age at Onset in Years (Range)	Characteristic Signs	CT or MRI Findings
SCA1	37 (4–74)	Ataxia, dysarthria, nystagmus, slow saccades, ophthalmoplegia, spasticity, PNP, executive dysfunction Increase in PMCT and CMCT	OPCA
SCA2	32 (1–65)	Ataxia, dysarthria, slow saccades, hyporeflexia, titubation, dementia, (rarely) parkinsonism	OPCA + spinal atrophy, some cortical atrophy
SCA3 (Machado–Joseph disease)	36 (5–70)	Ataxia, dysarthria, nystagmus, lid retraction, diplopia, faciolingual fasciculation, dystonia, parkinsonism, restless legs, temperature discrimination; onset <35 years with ataxia + spasticity, onset >45 years with ataxia + PNP	OPCA (mild), 4th ventricle enlarged
SCA4	(19–72)	Ataxia, dysarthria, sensory axonal neuropathy, pyramidal signs	CA
SCA5	30 (10–68)	"Pure" ataxia, dysarthria, normal life expectancy; (rarely) hyperreflexia	CA
SCA6	52 (30–71)	"Pure" ataxia, dysarthria, nystagmus, normal life expectancy (commonly), diplopia (rare and mild), PNP, pyramidal signs Negative family history owing to late onset	CA
SCA7	35 (0–70)	Ataxia, dysarthria, visual loss owing to pigmentary retinopathy, slow saccades, pyramidal signs	OPCA
SCA8	40 (1–73)	Ataxia, dysarthria, nystagmus, tremor	CA
SCA9	40 (1–73)	Ataxia, dysarthria, nystagmus, tremor	CA
SCA10	36 (26–45)	Ataxia, dysarthria, nystagmus, epilepsy	CA
SCA11	25 (15–43)	"Pure" ataxia, dysarthria, nystagmus, normal life expectancy, (rarely) hyperreflexia	CA
SCA12	35 (8–55)	Ataxia, nystagmus, tremor, bradykinesia, hyperreflexia	CA + cerebral atrophy
SCA13	Childhood (<1–45)	Ataxia, dysarthria, nystagmus, hyperreflexia, mental + motor retardation, slow progression	OPCA
SCA14	27 (12–42)	Ataxia (slow progression) ± head tremor or myoclonus (early onset)	CA (vermis)
SCA15	26 (10–50)	"Pure" ataxia, dysarthria, nystagmus, normal life expectancy; some patients with hyperreflexia	CA (vermis)
SCA16	40 (20–66)	"Pure" ataxia, dysarthria, nystagmus, normal life expectancy; some patients with head tremor	CA
SCA17	33 (6–48)	Ataxia, dysarthria, nystagmus with dementia, slow saccades or epilepsy, hyperreflexia, akinesia, dystonia, chorea, psychosis, mutism	CA, some general atrophy
SCA18	15 (12–25)	Ataxia, dysarthria, nystagmus, sensory-motor axonal neuropathy, Babinski sign	CA
SCA19	34 (11–45)	Mild ataxia, dysarthria, nystagmus, cognitive (some) impairment, myoclonus, tremor, hyporeflexia, cerebral atrophy, hyperreflexia	CA
SCA20	Not defined	Ataxia	CA
SCA21	18 (7–30)	Ataxia, dysarthria, akinesia, rigidity, postural and rest tremor, hyporeflexia, cognitive impairment	CA
SCA22	(10–46)	Ataxia, dysarthria, nystagmus, slow progression, hyporeflexia	CA
SCA25	(1–39)	Ataxia, dysarthria, nystagmus, sensory neuropathy	CA (for description of 26–40, see Reference 4)
DRPLA	30 (0–62)	Ataxia, onset <20 years with myoclonus, epilepsy; onset >20 years with choreoathetosis, dementia, psychosis	OPCA, cerebral white-matter lesions

CA, Cerebellar atrophy; *CMCT*, central motor conduction time; *DRPLA*, dentorubral pallidoluysian atrophy; *FGF*, fibroblast growth factor; *OPCA*, olivopontocerebellar atrophy; *PMCT*, peripheral motor conduction time; *PNP*, peripheral neuropathy.
Modified from Schols L, Bauer P, Schmidt T, et al. Autosomal dominant cerebellar ataxia: clinical features, genetics, and pathogenesis. *Lancet Neurol.* 2004;3:297.

occur even in the same family. Since the initial description, the disease has been reported in different parts of the world.

MJD (SCA3), usually starts at the age of 20–39, but can begin as early as 6 years and sometimes presents as late as in the 70s.[10] Four different presentations have been recognized.[11,12] *Type 1* has an early onset, at about 25 years, characterized by dysarthria, an akinetic-rigid syndrome, spasticity, and ataxia, and can be rapidly progressive. *Type 2* usually starts at around the age of 40 and progresses slowly; these patients have prominent cerebellar and pyramidal tract symptoms and signs of ophthalmoplegia.

TABLE 37-2 Genetics of Spinocerebellar Ataxia (SCA)

Disease Name	Gene, Gene-Product	Locus
SCA1	SCA1, ataxin 1	6p23
SCA2	SCA2, ataxin 2	12q24
SCA3	MJD, ataxin-3	14q24.3–q31
SCA4	–	16q22,1
SCA5	Beta 2 spectrin, SPTBN2	11p111–q11
SCA6	SCA6, CACNA1A	19p13
SCA7	SCA7, ataxin 7	3p21,1–p12
SCA8	ATXN8	13q21
SCA9	Not assigned	–
SCA10	SCA10, ataxin 10	22q13
SCA11	–	15q14–q21.3
SCA12	SCA12	5q31–q33
SCA13	–	19q13.3–q13.4
SCA14	PRKCY	19q13.4qter
SCA15	–	3p24.2-ptr
SCA16	TPR1	8q22.1–q24.1
SCA17	TBP, TATA-box binding protein	6q27
SCA18	–	7q22–q32
SCA19	KCNP3 (allelic to PSCA22)	1p21–q21
SCA20	–	Reserved
SCA21	TMEMP	1p3633
SCA22	–	1p21–q23
SCA23	–	20p
SCA24	P36 (ATX)	p36 (AR)
SCA25	426	2p15–21
SCA26	See Reference 5	
DRPLA	DRPLA, atrophin-1	12p13.31

DRPLA, Dentorubral pallidoluysian atrophy.
Modified with permission from Schols L, Bauer P, Schmidt T, et al. Autosomal dominant cerebellar ataxia: clinical features, genetics, and pathogenesis. *Lancet Neurol.* 2004;3:293. Article to site 227–237 and 237–249.

Peripheral nerve findings are minimal. It is the most common form, and this patient appeared to have this type. *Type 3* starts late, at the age of 50, with cerebellar and ophthalmoplegic findings, prominent wasting, and peripheral neuropathy. *Type 4* has a later-onset disease with prominent parkinsonism which responds to levodopa. These patients also have ataxia and distal atrophy.

Pathologic findings in SCA3 include degeneration and gliosis of the globus pallidus, subthalamic and oculomotor nuclei, the pontocerebellar tract, and Clarke's columns,[10] with lesser damage of the substantia nigra, hypoglossus, ambiguous, trigeminal, and vestibular nuclei, and the anterior horns. Intranuclear inclusions can be seen.[12–14]

The phenotype variability and the age of onset are likely related to the length of the repeats.[15] The size of the normal allele might also have a contributory effect. MJD is a polyglutamine disease; the diseased protein is called *ataxin-3*, a ubiquitin-binding protein that binds chains of ubiquitin to other proteins. Normally, this ubiquitination of proteins allows them to be delivered to the proteosome for degradation. The genetic defect causes accumulation and misfolding of proteins and inclusions.[15] Disruption of axonal transport in polyglutamine diseases could lead to cell death.[16–18]

There is no treatment for SCA3, although symptomatic management of the spasticity is helpful, and muscle cramps can be treated with muscle relaxants and antiarrhythmics.[19]

Experimental studies in cell cultures, using ribonucleic acid interference, are being used to neutralize messenger RNA, and to slow the production of the abnormal proteins caused by the defective gene.[20] This technique has been successfully applied to a transgenic mouse with SCA1.[21] It is very encouraging to know that there are new therapies for these unusual disorder, for example, omaveloxolone compound improves mitochondrial function and shows significant clinical benefit in Friedreich's ataxia[22] and has been recently approved by the FDA.

SUMMARY

This young man presented with an abnormal gait, weakness, fasciculations, and hyperreflexia and was initially thought to have a motor neuron disease. His limitation of gaze and ataxia raised the suspicion for a spinocerebellar degeneration.

DNA testing proved that he had SCA3 from increased CAG repeats in chromosome.[14] He had a history of "familial MS," which most likely represented the same disorder.

IMPORTANT POINTS

- A neurologic disorder in several members of a family likely represents an inherited disease rather than an autoimmune disorder (such as MS), although autoimmune disorders can sometimes occur in families.
- Muscle fasciculations can be seen not only in ALS but also in many other disorders such as multisystem degeneration, Jacob–Creutzfeldt disease, Kennedy's disease, radiculopathies, neuropathies, debrancher enzyme deficiency, and spinocerebellar degenerations such as MJD.
- SCA3 is an autosomal dominant disorder often characterized by ataxia, hyperreflexia, and ophthalmoplegia.
- SCA3 is caused by increased CAG repeat expansions in chromosome 14q. The CAG repeats encode glutamine; thus, the disorder is a polyglutamine disease. The protein is called ataxin-3, a ubiquitin-binding protein.
- There is no cure for MJD, only palliative treatment.

REFERENCES

1. Kennedy WR, Alter M, Sung JH. Progressive proximal spinal and bulbar muscular atrophy of late onset: A sex-linked recessive trait. *Neurology*. 1968;18(7):671–680.
2. Lopes-Cendes I, Silveira I, Maciel P, et al. Limits of clinical assessment in the accurate diagnosis of Machado-Joseph disease. *Arch Neurol*. 1996;53(11):1168–1174.
3. Kawaguchi Y, Okamoto T, Taniwaki M, et al. CAG expansions in a novel gene for Machado-Joseph disease at chromosome 14q32.1. *Nat Genet*. 1994;8:221–228.

4. Opal P., Zoghbi H.Y. The spinocerebellar ataxias. UpToDate July 2022.
5. Subramony SH, Filla A. Autosomal dominant spino-cerebellar ataxias ad infinitum? *Neurology*. 2001;56:287–289.
6. Nakano KK, Dawson DM, Spence A. Machado disease: A hereditary ataxia in Portuguese emigrants to Massachusetts. *Neurology*. 1972;22(1):49–55.
7. Woods BT, Schaumburg HH. Nigro-spino-dentatal degeneration with nuclear opthalmoplegia: a unique and partially treatable clinico-pathological entity. *J Neurol Sci*. 1972;17:149–166.
8. Rosenberg RN, Nyhan WL, Bay C, Shore P. Autosomal dominant striatonigral degeneration: A clinical, pathologic, and biochemical study of a new genetic disorder. *Neurology*. 1976;26(8):703–714.
9. Romanul FC, Fowler HL, Radvany J, et al. Azorean disease of the nervous system. *N Engl J Med*. 1977;296:1505–1508.
10. Rosenberg RN. Joseph disease. In: Kark P, Rosenberg RN, Schut LJ, eds. *The Inherited Ataxias: Biochemical, Viral, and Pathological Studies*. New York, NY: Raven Press; 1978:33–57.
11. Pulst SM, Perlman SL. Hereditary ataxias. In: Pulst SM, ed. *Neurogenetics, Contemporary Neurology Series*. New York, NY: Oxford University Press; 2000:231–263.
12. Matilla T, McCall A, Subramony SH, et al. Molecular and clinical correlations in spinocerebellar ataxia type 3 and Machado-Joseph disease. *Ann Neurol*. 1995;38:68–72.
13. Durr A, Stevanin G, Cancel G, et al. Spinocerebellar ataxia 3 and Machado-Joseph disease: Clinical, molecular, and neuropathologic features. *Ann Neurol*. 1996;39:490–499.
14. Paulson HL, Perez MK, Trottier Y, et al. Intranuclear inclusions of expanded polyglutamine protein in spinocerebellar ataxia type 3. *Neuron*. 1997;19:333–344.
15. Maruyama H, Nakamura S, Matsuyaina Z, et al. Molecular features of the CAG repeats and clinical manifestations of Machado-Joseph disease. *Hum Mol Genet*. 1995;4:807–812.
16. Gadoth N, Slogotora J, Merims D. Correlation between clinical and molecular genetic analysis in Machado-Joseph disease. *Neurology*. 1996;46(Suppl):A329.
17. Ikeda H, Yamaguchi M, Sugai S, et al. Expanded polyglutamine in the Machado-Joseph disease protein includes cell death in vitro and in viro. *Nat Genet*. 1996;13:196–202.
18. Gunawardena S, Goldstein LS. Polyglutamine diseases and transport problems: Deadly traffic jams on neuronal highways. *Arch Neurol*. 2005;62(1):46–51.
19. Kanai K, Kuwabara S, Arai K, et al. Muscle cramp in Machado-Joseph disease: Altered motor axonal excitability properties and mexiletine treatment. *Brain*. 2003;126(Pt 4):965–973.
20. Davidson BL, Paulson HL. Molecular medicine for the brain: Silencing of disease genes with RNA interference. *Lancet Neurol*. 2004;3(3):145–149.
21. Xia H, Mao Q, Eliason SL, et al. RNAi suppresses polyglutamine-induced neurodegeneration in a model of spinocerebellar ataxia. *Nat Med*. 2004;10(8):816–820.
22. Lynch D.R., Chin, M.P., Delatycki M.B., et al. Safety and Efficacy of Omaveloxolone in Friedreich Ataxia (MOXIe Study). *Ann Neurol*. 89(2):212-225. https://doi.org/10.1002/ana.25934. Epub.2020 Nov 5.

38 CASE

A Floppy Child

A 4-month-old boy was referred for valuation of weakness. He was born after a normal pregnancy and delivery at term, with Apgar scores of 7 and 8 at 1 and 5 minutes, respectively. He presented as a floppy baby with generalized weakness. He was able to suck and swallow but with some difficulty.

His family history was contributory for a maternal female cousin who was floppy and died shortly after birth.

Examination revealed a baby lying in a froglike position (Fig. 38-1). His head circumference was normal at 41 cm, and he had no evidence of ptosis or ophthalmoplegia. The pupils were normal. There were fasciculations in the tongue and diffuse muscle atrophy. Reflexes were absent throughout, and he had profound hypotonia. No Babinski signs were present. He smiled normally and cried when he was pinched. There was no visceromegaly, and the rest of the examination was normal.

WHAT IS THE DIFFERENTIAL DIAGNOSIS?

This patient manifested as a floppy infant, a syndrome that has many causes (Table 38-1 and Fig. 38-2). The absent reflexes are against a central nervous system disorder, and the lack of ophthalmoplegia and ptosis is against a defect of neuromuscular transmission. The presence of tongue fasciculations and the apparent autosomal-recessive inheritance suggest spinal muscular atrophy (SMA).

A complete metabolic panel, complete blood count, serum creatine phosphokinase, and thyroid-stimulating hormone were normal.

WHAT SHOULD BE THE NEXT TEST?

With this clinical presentation, lymphocyte DNA analysis to detect deletions of chromosome 5q, typical of SMA, is important and should be the first diagnostic test when there is a positive family history. An EMG is, however, particularly useful to rule out other causes, and it was done in this case, as DNA testing was not available at that time. A muscle biopsy could also be used to rule out other causes.

AN EMG TEST WAS PERFORMED

Motor Nerve Studies

Nerve and Site	Latency (ms)	Amplitude (mV)	Conduction Velocity (m/s)
Median Nerve R.	**Normal ≤ 1.6**	**Normal ≥ 5**	**Normal ≥ 35**
Wrist	2.2	**1.5**	–
Elbow	3.8	**1.5**	50

Sensory Nerve Studies

Nerve	Peak Latency Normal ≤ 2.0–2.9 (ms)	Amplitude Normal ≥ 20–70 (μV)
Median nerve R.	2.2	24

EMG Data

Nerve	Insrt Activity	Fibs	Pos Waves	Fasc	Amp	Dur	Poly	Pattern
Deltoid R.	**Inc**	**2+**	**2+**	**Few**	Norm	Norm	None	**Red**
Biceps brachii R.	**Inc**	**1+**	**1+**	None	**Lg**	**Inc**	None	**Red**
Vastus lateralis R.	Norm	None	None	**Few**	Norm	Norm	None	**Red**
Gastrocnemius R.	**Inc**	None	None	**Few**	**Lg**	**Inc**	None	**Red**
Vastus lateralis L.	**Inc**	**1+**	**1+**	None	**Lg**	**Inc**	None	**Red**

WHAT WERE THE EMG FINDINGS?

This study showed normal median motor conduction velocity and latency with mildly decreased CMAP amplitudes. The median nerve SNAP was normal.

There were diffuse fasciculations with denervation potentials. Some motor unit potentials appeared large, were fast-firing, and appeared to have low recruitment, although this was hard to assess. These findings indicated a diffuse lower motor neuron disease and were compatible with the diagnosis of SMA.

WHAT IS THE NEXT TEST?

DNA studies should be done, and there are several techniques, and the most useful is multiplex-ligation–dependent probe amplification (MLPA) but this was not available at the time this

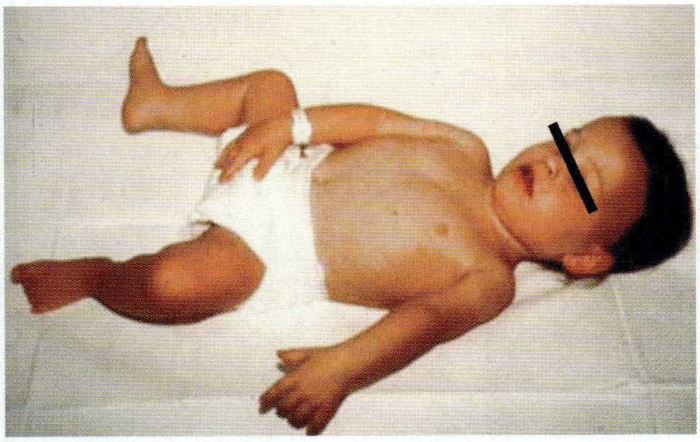

FIG. 38-1 Patient with SMA type I; notice normal facial expression, froglike position. *SMA*, Spinal muscular atrophy.

TABLE 38-1 Causes of Floppy Infants

Central nerve system disorders
Cerebral palsy
Mental retardation
Mixed (central and peripheral)
Metachromatic leukodystrophy and other lipidosis
Neuroaxonal atrophy
Giant axonal neuropathy
Fukuyama-type congenital muscular dystrophy
Anterior horn cell disease
Infantile spinal muscular atrophy
Neuropathies
Charcot–Marie–Tooth disease, particularly types 3 and 4
Diseases of the neuromuscular junction
Congenital myasthenic syndromes
Infantile botulism
Neonatal transient autoimmune myasthenia gravis
Myopathies
Infantile metabolic myopathies (e.g., acid maltase deficiencies or Pompe disease, infantile phosphorylase deficiency)
Congenital muscular dystrophy
Other congenital myopathies (e.g., central core disease, myotubular myopathy, nemaline myopathy)
Congenital myotonic dystrophy
Myopathy from electrolyte and endocrine abnormalities

Reprinted with permission from Pearn J. Autosomal dominant spinal muscular atrophy: a clinical and genetic study. *J Neurol Sci.* 1978;38:263–275.

case was studied; a biopsy of the left thigh showed muscle fiber atrophy with most atrophic fibers in groups. Atrophic fibers were of both types, and many stained dark with nonspecific esterase. Large type I fibers were also seen (Fig. 38-3).

It was concluded that this child had infantile SMA.

DISCUSSION

Infantile SMA is a progressive, hereditary disease characterized by generalized weakness, atrophy, hyporeflexia, and hypotonia. The condition is autosomal-recessive in most cases, although autosomal-dominant inheritance and sporadic cases have been reported.[1] The adult form is most frequently autosomal-dominant.[2]

SMA was described initially by Werdnig in 1891[3] and 2 years later by Hoffmann.[4] Kugelberg and Welander later described the more benign, or juvenile, type.[5]

The disease affects approximately 1/11,000 newborns. There are different presentations of SMA (Table 38-2):

Type I, the most severe infantile form, starts at birth or can be detected at 1 month of age. Characteristically, the child lies in a froglike position and has a bell-shaped chest and tongue fasciculations. There is paradoxical breathing, hyporeflexia, and hypotonia. Patients usually die by the age of 2 years.

Type II, or intermediate form, starts at about 8 months. Patients may be able to sit independently (Fig. 38-4A) and develop contractures; 50% of those have fasciculations. The biopsy could show fiber-type grouping and group atrophy (Fig. 38-4B).

Type III, or Kugelberg–Welander disease, may also start in early childhood, usually by 15 years, and these patients are able to walk on their own. This form is divided into two subtypes. *Type IIIA* has its onset during the first 3 years of life; these children walk with difficulty (Fig. 38-5). Fifty percent are wheelchair-bound by 14 years after onset. In *Type IIIB*, weakness appears between the ages of 3 and 30. Clinically, this subtype resembles Becker's dystrophy[5,6] (Fig. 38-6), but SMA patients usually have weakness of the iliopsoas, quadriceps, and adductor muscles, whereas the gluteus maximus is strong, unlike those with Becker's dystrophy in whom the iliopsoas and quadriceps are stronger, and the glutei are weaker. There is an early weakness of the triceps muscle and evidence of fasciculations. These patients may also have elevated serum creatine kinase but not as high as in muscular dystrophy.

Type IV is usually of adult onset and slowly progressive, and the prognosis is more benign.

The genetic defect in SMA was identified in 1990 in chromosome 5 at 5q11.2–13.3.[7,8] by Judy Melkins. Several deletions and microsatellite markers in this area of 5q can be detected in patients with SMA. The SMN (survival motor neuron) gene has two copies, a *telomeric* (in the tip of the chromosome) and a *centromeric* (in the center). The *SMN1* gene is in the telomeric region, and there is an almost identical centromeric gene (*SMN2*) that differs only in one nucleic acid. The Bonobo monkeys and humans are the only mammals that have these genes.

Deletions of the telomeric copy of the *SMN1* gene are specific for SMA, whereas deletions of the other gene are also detected in the normal population.

Ninety-five percent of patients with SMA type I have mutations of the *SMN1* gene[9]; the defect is a single nucleotide mutation in exon 7. The severity of the disease can be modulated by the number of the centromeric *SMN2* copies.[10] Normally due to differential splicing, the *SMN2* gene produces only 10% of full-length SMN protein (Fig. 38-7).

The SMN1 protein is ubiquitous and is present in nuclei and cytoplasm of several cells in the body in structures called *gems* (for geminis of the coiled bodies). Current evidence indicates that SMN1 is involved in RNA transcription. SMN1 is absent in SMA.

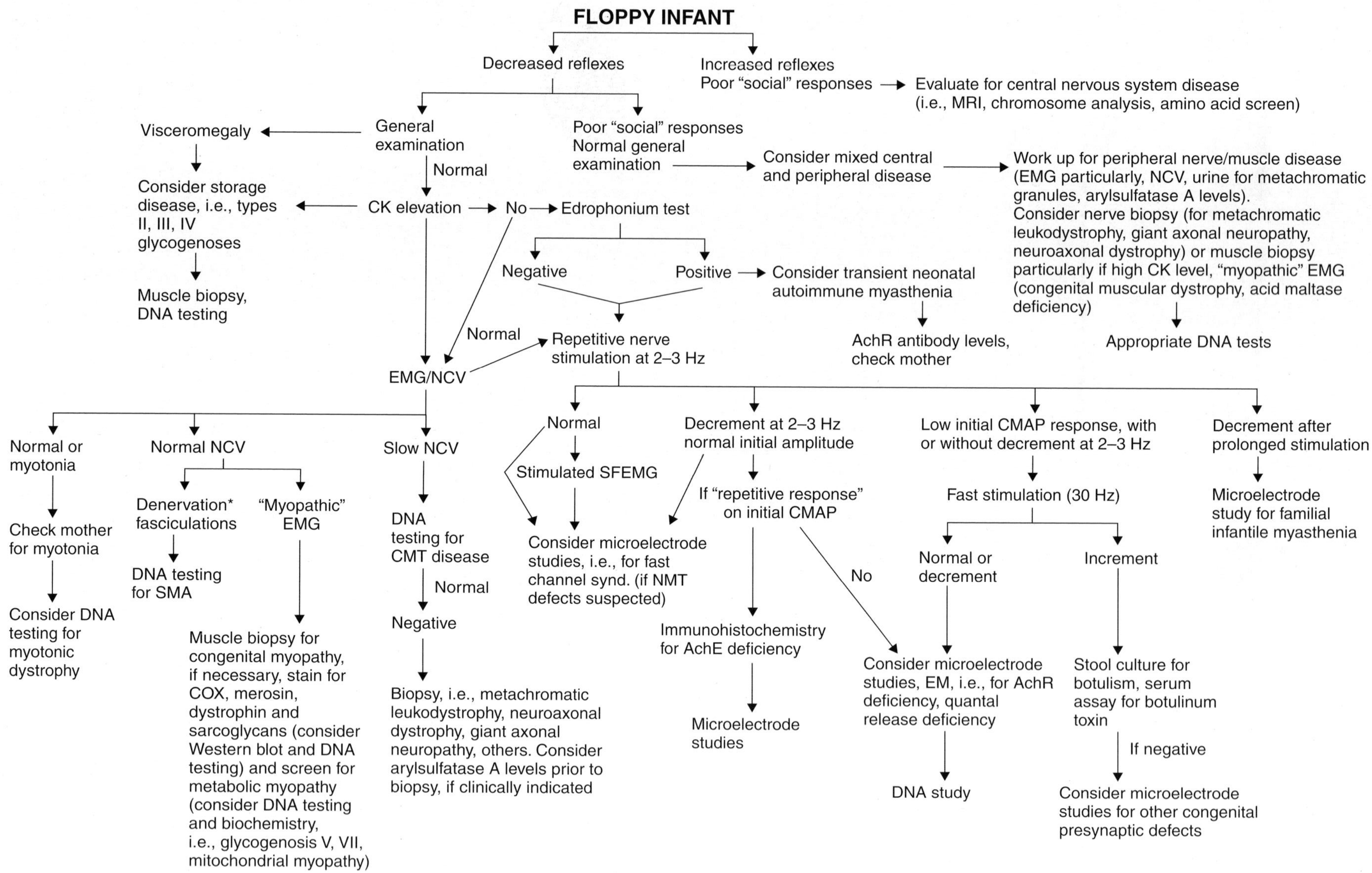

*If negative do histamine test for Riley-Day syndrome, consider DNA test.

FIG. 38-2 Diagram of the workup of floppy babies. *CK*, Creatine kinase; *COX*, cytochrome oxidase; *NCV*, nerve conduction velocity; *NMT*, neuromuscular transmission; *SFEMG*, single fiber electromyography.

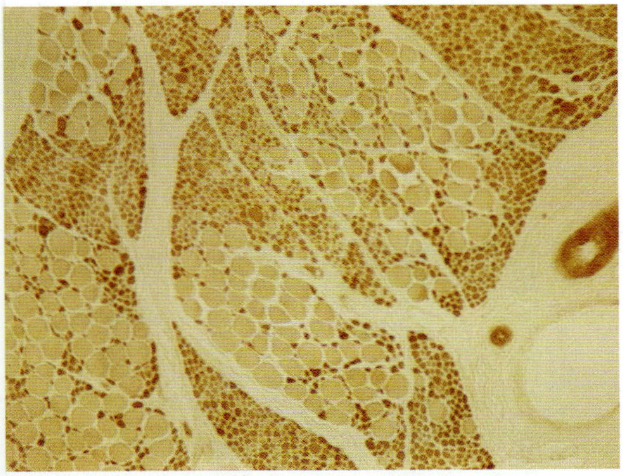

FIG. 38-3 Muscle biopsy showing group of atrophic fibers and some hypertrophic type I fibers. All atrophic fibers appear dark (ATPase stain, ×200).

TABLE 38-2 Classification of Proximal Spinal Muscular Atrophy Modified According to the International Spinal Muscular Atrophy (SMA) Consortium

SMA Type	Principal Symptoms	Definition	Genetics
I	Werdnig–Hoffmann disease Acute infantile SMA	Sitting not achieved Onset usually within the first 6 months Death usually in the first 2 years of life	Autosomal-recessive (~95% SMN1 deletions)
II	Chronic childhood SMA Arrested Werdnig–Hoffmann disease	Unaided sitting possible, walking not achieved Onset usually in the first year of life Survival > 90% by 10 years	Autosomal-recessive (~95% SMN1 deletions)
III	Kugelberg–Welander disease Juvenile SMA	Walking without aids achieved IIIa: onset ≤ 3 years IIIb: onset > 3 years Mild course, life span not markedly reduced	Autosomal-recessive (80%–90% SMN1 deletions), rarely autosomal-dominant mutations Excess of men
IV	Adult SMA	Onset > 30 years Variable severity, normal life span	Mostly sporadic Autosomal-dominant (gene defect unknown) Autosomal-recessive (extremely rare)

Data from Zerres K, Davies KE. 59th ENMC International Workshop: spinal muscular atrophies: recent progress and revised diagnostic criteria 17-19 April 1998, Soestduinen, The Netherlands. *Neuromuscul Disord.* 1999;9(4):272–278; Rudnik-Schöneborn S, de Vissen M, Zerres K. Spinal muscular atrophies. In: Engel AG, Franzini-Armstrong C, eds. *Myology.* 3rd ed. New York, NY: McGraw-Hill; 2004:1845–1865.

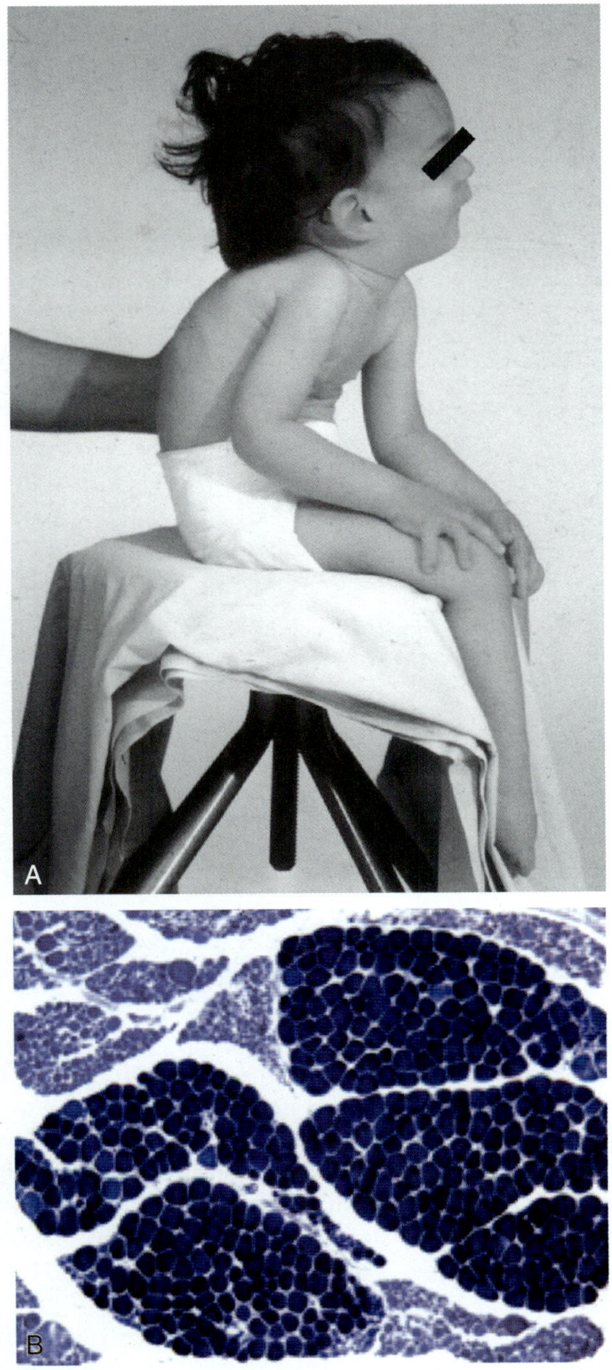

FIG. 38-4 A, Patient with SMA type II at 9 months of age; he needs assistance to sit. **B**, Muscle biopsy of this patient showing group of normal fibers, mainly type I, and many atrophic fibers (NADH-TR stain, ×200).

As the larger amount of SMN2 protein is associated with milder phenotypes, therapeutic strategies aim at increasing the production of SMN2 product size by up-regulating gene expression.

The antisense oligonucleotide Nusinersen targets the intronic splicing silencer N1 (ISS-N1) and is given intrathecally every four months and is beneficial.[11] There is newborn screening for early detection so that cases can be treated early.

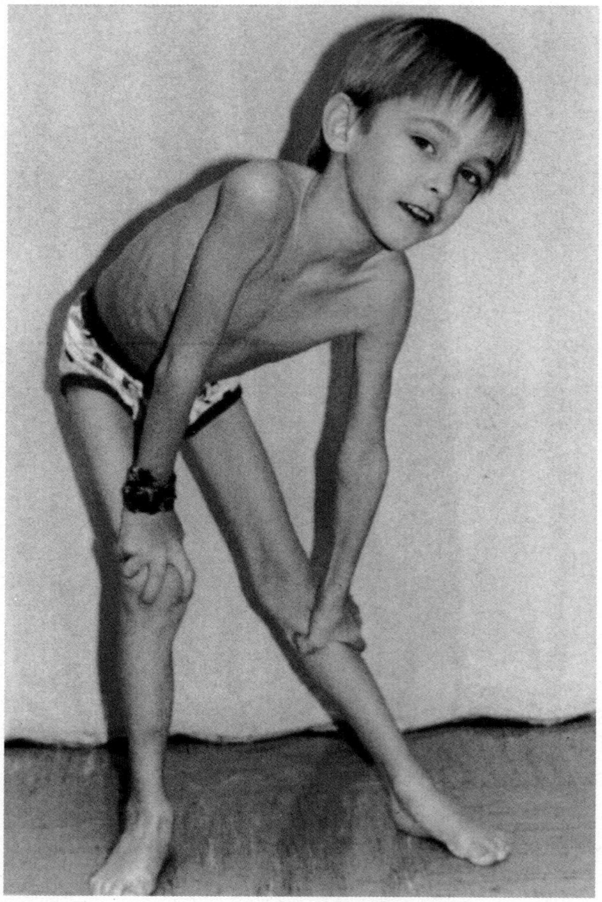

FIG. 38-5 Patient with SMA type IIIA performing Gowers maneuver to rise from floor; notice prominent muscle atrophy. *SMA*, Spinal muscular atrophy.

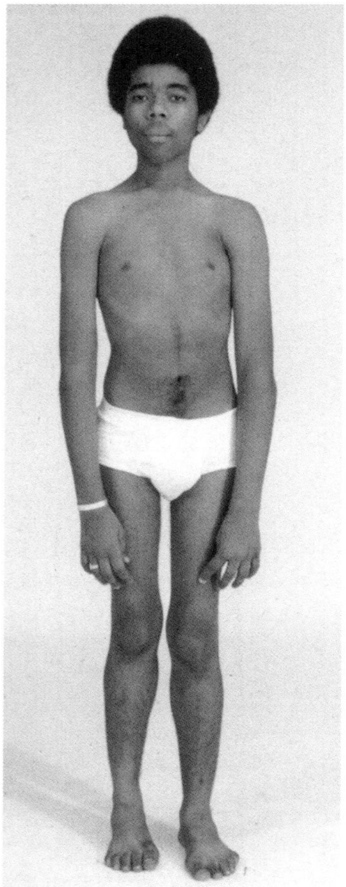

FIG. 38-6 Patient with SMA type IIIB; notice proximal atrophy with relatively large calves resembling those in Becker's dystrophy. *SMA*, Spinal muscular atrophy.

Nusinersen also improves the outcome in adults.[12,13] Because the effect decreases before the four months, there is a trial using higher doses.[14] Gene replacement therapy, Zolgensma is given intravenously at a single dose; this therapy is beneficial and has been approved as treatment in children.[15]

Risdiplam is a new oral splicing modifier that increases the inclusion of exon 7 and this is given orally and is also beneficial.[16]

The outcomes of this disorder have been greatly improving with early treatment.[17] Guidelines for diagnosis and management for adults and children have been published.[18,19]

Current treatment of SMA also consists of respiratory assistance, percutaneous endoscopic gastrostomy (PEG) tube feedings, and bracing, depending on the clinical manifestations.[1]

SUMMARY

This child presented as a floppy baby and was found to have SMA with characteristic EMG and muscle biopsy findings. DNA testing was not available.

The DNA mutation causing SMA is located in chromosome 5q and expresses the *SMN* gene.

The treatment of SMA is conservative.

IMPORTANT POINTS

- The floppy infant syndrome has many causes. The most common are central neurologic disorders, usually suggested by the presence of normal reflexes, and other neurologic findings.
- SMA can manifest as floppy infant syndrome and is characterized by hypotonia, areflexia, fasciculations, and denervation on EMG with normal nerve conduction tests. There are also patients with more benign phenotypes.
- SMA is caused by mutation of chromosome 5q of the SMN gene. This gene has two copies, telomeric *(SMN1)* and centromeric *(SMN2)*. Deletions of the telomeric copy of the gene are specific for the disease. In less severe forms of the disease, there is an increased number of *SMN2* copies.
- *SMN1* produces a 38 kDa protein that is ubiquitous. The lack of production of this protein is pathogenic.
- The best diagnosis of SMA is by genetic testing. DNA mutations are detected in 90% of cases, and EMG and biopsy might not be necessary as DNA tests are informative in most cases. EMG shows characteristic findings of a motor neuron disorder; the muscle biopsy shows round atrophic fibers, group atrophy, and hypertrophy of type I fibers.
- There is no cure for SMA; however, there are several new treatments which include the ASO Nusinersen which is

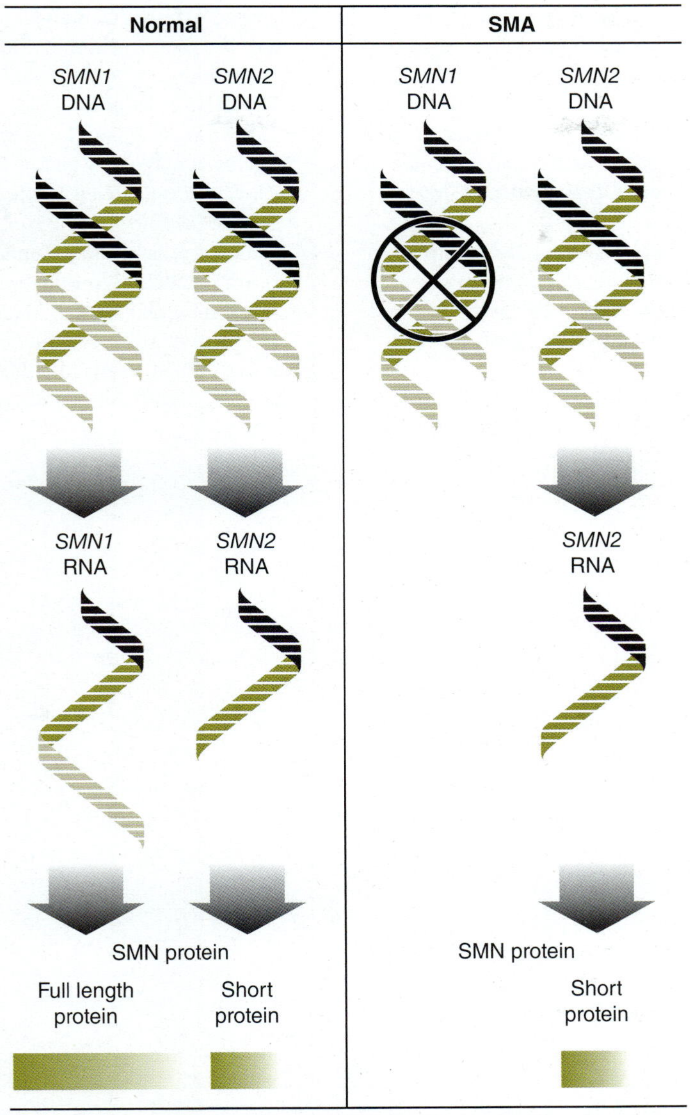

FIG. 38-7 Drawing of *SMN1* and *SMN2* genes in a normal person (*left*) and in a patient with SMA (*right*); notice that SMN protein is produced from *SMN2* but not *SMN1*. *SMA*, Spinal muscular atrophy.

given intrathecally every four months, and Risdiplam is an SMN2 splice modifier given orally and gene replacement therapy given intravenously. PEG tube feeding and respiratory assistance are beneficial.

REFERENCES

1. Rudnik-Schöneborn S, de Vissen M, Zerres K. Spinal muscular atrophies. In: Engel AG, Franzini-Armstrong C, eds. *Myology*. 3rd ed. New York, NY: McGraw-Hill; 2004:1845–1865.
2. Pearn J. Autosomal dominant spinal muscular atrophy: a clinical and genetic study. *J Neurol Sci*. 1978;38:263–275.
3. Werdnig G. Zwei fruhinfantile hereditare Falle von progressiven Muselatrophie unter dem Bilde der Dystrophie, aber auf neurotischer Grundlage. *Arch Psychiatric*. 1891;22:437–481.
4. Hoffmann J. Uber chronische spinal Musakelatrophiie im Kindeasalter, auf familiarer Basis. *Dtsch Z Nervenheilk*. 1893;3:427–470.
5. Kugelberg E, Welander L. Heredofamilial juvenile muscular atrophy simulating muscular dystrophy. *AMA Arch Neurol Psychiatry*. 1956;75(5):500–509.
6. Zerres K, Rudnick-Schoneborn S. Natural history in proximal spinal muscular atrophy: clinical analysis of 445 patients and suggestions for a modification of existing classifications. *Arch Neurol*. 1995;52:518–523.
7. Brzustowicz LM, Lehner T, Castilla LH, et al. Genetic mapping of chronic childhood-onset spinal muscular atrophy to chromosome 5q11.2–13.3. *Nature*. 1990;344:540–541.
8. Melki J, Abdelhak S, Sheth P, et al. Gene for chronic spinal muscular atrophies maps to chromosome 5q. *Nature*. 1990;344:767–768.
9. Hahnen E, Forkert R, Marke C, et al. Molecular analysis of candidate genes in chromosome 5q13 in autosomal recessive spinal muscular atrophy: evidence of homozygous deletions of the SMN gene in unaffected individuals. *Hum Mol Genet*. 1995;4(10):1927–1933.
10. Coovert DD, Le TT, McAndrew PE, et al. The survival motor neuron protein in spinal muscular atrophy. *Hum Mol Genet*. 1997;6:1205–1214.
11. Finkel RS, Mercuri E, Darras BT, Connolly AM. Nusinersen versus sham control in infantile-onset spinal muscular atrophy. *N Engl J Med*. 2017;377(18):1723–1732.

12. Walter MC, Wenninger S, Thiele S, Stauber J, et al. Safety and treatment effects of nusinersen in longstanding adult 5q-SMA type 3—a prospective observational study. *J Neuromuscul Dis.* 2019;6(4):453–465.
13. Bertorini TE, Knickerboker J, Metter J, et al. Clinical findings and segmental bioimpedance studies in adults with spinal muscular atrophy receiving intrathecal Nusinersen therapy. *Muscle Nerve.* 2019;65:21.
14. Finkel R.S., Mitchell-Sweeney N., Foster P., Son L. *Escalating Doses and Randomization Controlled Study of Nusinersen in Patients With Spinal Muscular Atrophy a Study Designed of Phase 2-3 PEVOTE (232M 203) Study to Explore High Doses of Nusinersen AAN Annual Meeting*; 2020.
15. Mendell JR, Al-Zaidy S, Shell WD, Arnold LR, et al. Single dose gene replace therapy for spinal muscular atrophy. *New Engl J Med.* 2017;377(18):1713–1722.
16. Markti T, Fisher G, Ramdas S, et al. Risdiplam: an investigational survival motor neuron 2 (SMN2) splicing modifier for spinal muscular atrophy (SMA). *Expert Opin Investig Drugs.* 2022;31(5):451–461.
17. Govoni A., Gagliardi D., Comi G., Cort S. *Time is Motor Neuron: Therapeutic Window and Its Correlation with Pathogenetic Mechanisms in Spinal Muscular Atrophy. Mol Neurobiol.* 2018;55(8):6307–6318.
18. Glascock J, Sampson J, Connolly AM, Darras BT, et al. Revised recommendations for the treatment of infants diagnosed with spinal muscular atrophy via newborn screening who have 4 copies of SMN2. *J Neuromuscul Dis.* 2020;7(2):97–100.
19. Rad N, Cai H, Weiss MD. Management of spinal muscular atrophy in the adult population. *Muscle Nerve.* 2022;65(5): 498–507.

A Man With Acute Areflexic Paralysis and Central Nervous System Symptoms

A 43-year-old man presented initially to an ophthalmologist complaining of double vision for 3 weeks. Ten days later, he developed numbness and weakness in both upper extremities which then progressed to his right lower extremity; 5 days afterward he presented to the emergency room because his symptoms had worsened. He denied bowel or bladder dysfunction, headache, neck pain or trauma, diarrhea, or respiratory infection.

Past medical history was significant for a 2-year history of intermittent hand tingling which had been diagnosed as carpal tunnel syndrome, but the surgical release of the median nerve failed to provide relief. One year prior to the presentation, he had bilateral foot tingling which lasted 1 week. For the past 2 years, he had intermittent shocklike sensations going down his back upon flexing the neck. He had medication-controlled hypertension and mild diabetes mellitus controlled by diet.

Social history revealed 2-pack-a-day cigarette smoking, but he denied alcohol abuse. He is a woodworker and denied any exposure to toxins.

Family history was significant for Guillain–Barré syndrome (GBS) in his father and breast cancer in his mother.

Neurologic examination showed normal mental function, pupils, and visual fields. There was mild diplopia on right lateral gaze and mild peripheral bilateral facial weakness. Strength was 4/5 in the upper extremities and 3/5 in both lower extremities. Reflexes were 1+ in the upper extremities, trace at the knees, and absent at the ankles; plantar reflexes were mute. Sensory examination revealed mildly decreased pinprick and vibration senses to the ankles. Coordination was preserved. He was unable to walk. The rest of the examination was normal.

WHAT IS THE DIFFERENTIAL DIAGNOSIS?

This patient presented with an acute diffuse paralytic illness that progressed in 4 days. He had diminished reflexes and mild sensory abnormalities that were out of proportion to the weakness. The lack of a cord sensory level or sphincter disturbance argued against a myelopathy. The diminished reflexes and sensory findings suggested an acute neuropathy, and for this reason the differential diagnosis in cases like this should include arsenic poisoning and porphyria, suggested by his father's similar illness. There was no other history or clinical findings to suggest either disease, and the cranial nerve abnormalities argued against both arsenic poisoning and porphyria. The most likely diagnosis would be an acute inflammatory demyelinating polyradiculoneuropathy (AIDP) or GBS. Tests for Lyme and HIV should also be done. The absence of fever was against a diagnosis of diphtheria. West Nile virus and COVID-19 had yet to be seen in the United States at the time of his presentation; also, weakness in that disease is usually asymmetric.

Extraocular weakness occurs in GBS and its variants but can also suggest a primary central nervous system condition such as multiple sclerosis (MS). The history of a Lhermitte's sign and the episodic sensory and motor symptoms are also suggestive of MS. The sign, however, occurs not only in MS but also in patients with cervical spondylosis, spinal cord lesions, and demyelinating disease of peripheral nerves. The lack of long tract signs or urologic symptoms lowered the probability of MS.

AN EMG TEST WAS PERFORMED

Motor Nerve Studies

Nerve and Site	Latency (ms)	Amplitude (mV)	Conduction Velocity (m/s)
Peroneal Nerve R.	**Normal ≤ 5.7**	**Normal ≥ 3**	**Normal ≥ 40**
Ankle	**8.9**	**0.8**	–
Fibular head	21.2	**0.5**	**29**
Knee	22.7	**0.4**	56
Tibial Nerve L.	**Normal ≤ 5.3**	**Normal ≥ 4**	**Normal ≥ 40**
Ankle	**9.1**	**1**	–
Pop. fossa	27.4	**0.3**	**26**
Median Nerve R.	**Normal ≤ 4.2**	**Normal ≥ 6**	**Normal ≥ 50**
Wrist	**7.5**	**4**	–
Elbow	13.2	**3**	**48**
Ulnar Nerve R.	**Normal ≤ 3.6**	**Normal ≥ 8**	**Normal ≥ 50**
Wrist	**5.4**	**3**	–
Below elbow	10.5	**1**	**47**
Above elbow	16.1	**1**	**21**

Nerve and Site	Latency (ms)	Amplitude (mV)	Conduction Velocity (m/s)
Facial Nerve R. Side-to-side comparison	**6.2**	**2**	–

F-Wave and Tibial H-Reflex Studies

Nerve	Latency (ms)	Normal Latency ≤ (ms)
Peroneal nerve R.	**NR**	54
Tibial nerve L.	**NR**	54
Median nerve R.	**43.1**	30
Ulnar nerve R.	**39.1**	30
H-reflex R.	**NR**	34
H-reflex L.	**NR**	34

NR, No response.

Sensory Nerve Studies

Nerve	Latency (ms)	Normal Latency ≤ (ms)	Amp (μV)	Normal Amp ≥ (μV)
Sural nerve R.	**NR**	4.0	**NR**	11
Median nerve R.	**NR**	3.1	**NR**	20
Ulnar nerve R.	**NR**	3.1	**NR**	13

EMG Data

Muscle	Insrt Activity	Fibs	Pos Waves	Fasc	Amp	Dur	Poly	Pattern
Biceps brachii R.	Norm	None	None	None	Norm	Norm	None	Full
Flexor carpi ulnaris R.	Norm	None	None	None	Norm	Norm	None	Full
First dorsal interosseus R.	Norm	None	None	None	Norm	Norm	None	**Red**
Vastus lateralis R.	Norm	None	None	None	Norm	Norm	None	**Red**
Tibialis anterior R.	Norm	None	None	None	Norm	Norm	**Few**	**Red**
Gastrocnemius R.	Norm	None	None	None	Norm	Norm	None	**Red**

WHAT WERE THE EMG FINDINGS?

The nerve conduction study demonstrated low-amplitude CMAPs consistent with axonal degeneration. The prolonged distal motor latencies (150% of normal) were out of proportion to the low-amplitude CMAP and indicated demyelination. There was also significant conduction slowing in some nerves, and in the ulnar nerve, there was focal slowing at the elbow. The F-waves were prolonged or absent, and the H-reflexes were absent. These findings were also compatible with demyelination.[1]

The absent SNAPs may be secondary to axonal degeneration or from demyelination with severe temporal dispersion. This can sometimes be seen in GBS in which the SNAPs could also be normal. Normal leg SNAP associated with absent upper extremity SNAPs is more characteristic, however.

Needle EMG did not demonstrate denervation potentials but rather reduced motor unit recruitment in most muscles.

The combination of findings indicated the involvement of motor and sensory axons, with demyelination and axonal degeneration. These findings are not characteristic of acute motor sensory axonal neuropathy, as there was more evidence of demyelination than a primary axonal degeneration. Thus it was concluded that the patient had AIDP or GBS.

WHAT ADDITIONAL TESTS SHOULD BE DONE?

A 24-hour urine study for heavy metals and porphyrins was negative. A complete blood count revealed mild leucocytosis (white blood cell count, 13.7) with a normal differential. Liver function tests and electrolytes were normal. The erythrocyte sedimentation rate, rapid plasma reagin, fluorescent antinuclear antibody, rheumatoid factor, angiotensin-converting enzyme, C3, C4, complement B_{12}, fatty acid, glycosylated hemoglobin, T4, thyroid-stimulating hormone, and serum immunoelectrophoresis were normal. Antibodies for HIV, human T-lymphotropic virus 1, antinuclear double-stranded DNA, single-stranded A DNA, single-stranded B DNA, SM antibody, and antineutrophil cytoplasmic antibody measurements were negative. West Nile antibody measurements were not available during this time; Lyme antibody, *Campylobacter jejuni*, and GQ1b were negative. A tuberculin skin test was negative. (See Fig. 40-1 for the differential diagnosis and work-up of patients with acute active paralysis.)

The cerebrospinal fluid (CSF) on admission showed 300 white cells/mL[3] (92% lymphocytes); protein was 426 mg/dL (normal, 20–40 mg/dL), and glucose was normal. Gram stain, cultures, cytology, and cryptococcal antigen were negative. Oligoclonal bands were present, and the IgG index was elevated at 59.2 (normal, <0.70). Three days later, CSF had a 143 white blood cell count, a protein of 580 mg/dL, and normal glucose.

The increased number of cells was out of proportion for the diagnosis of GBS,[1,2] and for this reason other conditions, such as lymphoma, Lyme, HIV, and other infections, need to be ruled out.

WHAT OTHER TESTS ARE IMPORTANT?

Cervical MRI was normal. MRI of the lumbar spine revealed diffuse nerve root enhancement. Head MRI showed multiple enhancing white matter lesions, mostly periventricular, with "Dawson's fingers" highly suggestive of MS (Fig. 39-1).

The somatosensory-evoked responses were absent on the right median nerve. Visual evoked potential tests revealed a low-voltage P100 wave with a prolonged latency on the right. The left brainstem auditory-evoked responses (BAERs) were absent, and the right BAERs had a delayed V-wave latency with preserved III–V-wave latencies. The evoked-response findings were consistent with central, and also likely peripheral, demyelination.

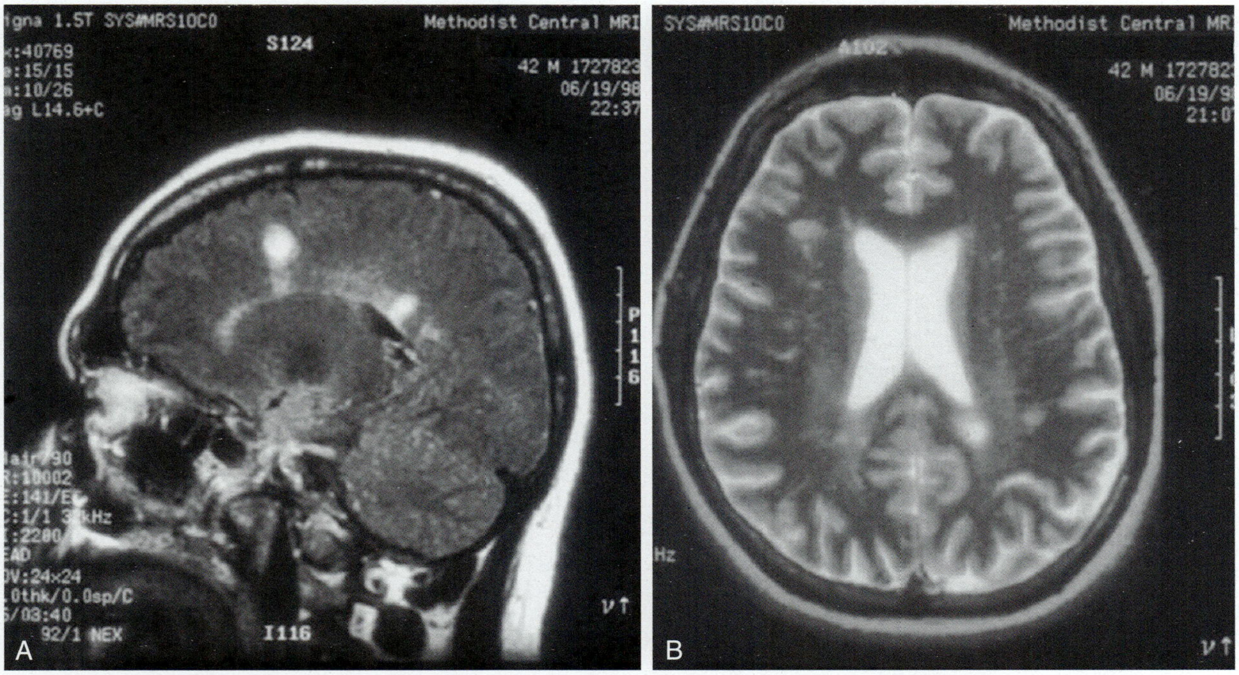

FIG. 39-1 A, Head MRI, sagittal view: FLAIR pericallosal plaques, or "Dawson's fingers." **B**, Head MRI; T2-weighted image also showing white matter lesions.

The patient was treated with IV IgG infusions 500 mg/kg per day for 4 days. This was followed by methylprednisolone 250 mg IV every 6 hours for 3 days; this treatment is not beneficial in GBS but was given because of the patient's history and MRI findings compatible with MS. He was then started on prednisone 80 mg per day, which was tapered off over 6 weeks. After 3 weeks in the rehabilitation unit the patient was able to ambulate with a walker. Motor strength recovered to 5/5 proximally and 4+/5 distally in the upper extremities and 4/5 proximally and 3/5 distally in the lower extremities. He recovered completely after 6 months and has been asymptomatic on β-interferon therapy for 6 years.

DISCUSSION

This man had acute peripheral neuropathy superimposed on central nervous system demyelination. The spinal fluid pleocytosis is not typical for GBS (Table 39-1) or MS, but no other cause was found. Table 39-2 lists the differential diagnoses of GBS and Fig. 39-2 shows the World Health Organization guidelines for the diagnosis.

The association of central and peripheral demyelination in the same patient is unusual, but central demyelination has been reported in chronic inflammatory demyelinating polyneuropathy (CIDP),[3] and patients with MS can also have peripheral demyelination.[4–6]

Typically, GBS presents as a monophasic illness characterized by ascending flaccid weakness with accompanying areflexia. Ophthalmoplegia is seen in the Miller Fisher variant of GBS, and it has been suggested that this variant in some patients is caused primarily by a brainstem inflammatory process.[7] Clinicopathologic studies, however, have demonstrated isolated peripheral demyelination with retrograde chromatolysis.[8,9] The presentation of this case was not characteristic of the Miller Fisher variant. Patients with otherwise classic GBS can also develop ophthalmoplegia, and hyperreflexia has been reported in patients with the motor variant of GBS following *C. jejuni* infection,[10–13] but the absence of long tract signs in those patients does not suggest central nervous system involvement. As in this case, however, demyelinating plaques characteristic of MS have also been reported in GBS.[14,15]

The occurrence of GBS in members of the same family is unusual, but it has been reported[16,17] and it may indicate a genetic predisposition as it has been associated with some human leukocyte antigen types,[17,18] as it happens in MS.[19]

The exact pathogenesis of GBS is not clear, but this occurs frequently after an infectious process, not only with *C. jejuni* but also with other organisms. This is likely secondary to an autoimmune process in which there is a molecular mimicry, and the peripheral nerve gangliosides are the target antigens.[20,21] We are not certain if the association of central and peripheral demyelination in this case is coincidental or caused by an autoimmune attack to similar peripheral and central nervous system antigens.

Classic GBS was first described in 1960.[22] The condition, which has an incidence of 1–2 per 100,000, manifests by an acute ascending paralysis with areflexia and frequent bulbar muscle involvement and active inflammatory demyelinating polyneuropathy. Patients have mild sensory complaints, relatively mild sensory findings, and could have dysautonomia. The spinal fluid shows the classic elevated protein with normal or mildly elevated cell numbers (albuminocytologic disassociation).[22] Electrophysiologic findings in GBS demonstrate demyelination, but there could also be secondary axonal degeneration.

TABLE 39-1 Diagnostic Criteria for Typical Guillain–Barré Syndrome

Clinical Features
Features required for the diagnosis
Progressive weakness in both arms and legs
Areflexia
Features strongly supporting the diagnosis
Progression of symptoms over days to 4 weeks
Relative symmetry of symptoms
Mild sensory symptoms or signs
Cranial nerve involvement, especially facial diplegia
Recovery beginning 2–4 weeks after progression ceases
Autonomic dysfunction
Absence of fever at the onset
Features making the diagnosis doubtful
Sensory level
Marked, persistent asymmetry of symptoms or signs
Severe and persistent bladder or bowel dysfunction
Features excluding the diagnosis
Diagnosis of botulism, myasthenia gravis, poliomyelitis, or toxic neuropathy
Abnormal porphyrin metabolism
Recent diphtheria
Laboratory Criteria
Elevated cerebrospinal fluid protein concentration with fewer than 10 cells/mm^3
Electrophysiologic Criteria (Any 3 or 4 Criteria)
Reduction of conduction velocity of two or more motor nerves
<80% LLN, if amplitude > 80% of LLN; <70% of LLN, if amplitude < 80% of LLN
Prolonged distal latencies in two or more motor nerves
>125% of ULN, if amplitude > 80% of LLN; >150% of ULN, if amplitude < 80%
Absent or prolonged minimum F-waves in two or more motor nerves
>120% of ULN, if amplitude > 80% of LLN; >150% of ULN, if amplitude is < 80% of LLN
Conduction block or abnormal temporal dispersion (>20% drop in amplitude, or >25% change in duration between proximal and distal sites) in one or more motor nerves

LLN, Lower limit of normal; *ULN*, upper limit of normal.
Reprinted with permission from Asbury AK, Cornblath DR. Assessment of current diagnostic criteria for Guillain-Barré syndrome. *Ann Neurol.* 1990;27(Suppl):S21–S24.

TABLE 39-2 Differential Diagnosis of AIDP-GBS

* Brain Stem Stroke
* Myelopathy-Myelitis
- Polyneuropathies—critical illness myopathy—HIV, Lyme's West Nile infection, polio infections
* Porphyria—heavy metals (arsenic intoxication) vasculitic neuropathy
- Neuromuscular junction disorder, botulism, myasthenia gravis, organophosphate poisoning
- Myopathies, hypokalemia, periodic paralysis
* Hypophosphatemia
* Myositis, critical illness myopathy
* Rhabdomyolysis from metabolic myopathy or toxic

An early finding is the absence or delayed F-responses and H-reflexes. Pathologic studies show patchy demyelination and inflammation.

There are several variants of GBS or AIDP. Among others, these include acute motor sensory neuropathy, acute motor axonal neuropathy, Miller Fisher syndrome, acute sensory neuropathy, and acute dysautonomic neuropathy. Overlap of these also occurs.[21] The treatment of GBS consists of plasmapheresis or gamma globulin infusions[21] (see Table 40-2). Because the findings suggest MS, he also received steroids, which are beneficial in MS but not GBS.

Concerning the central nervous system involvement, it is known that the adhesion molecules like neurofascins NF186 and NF155 cluster sodium channels at the nodes and paranodes of Ranvier in peripheral and central nervous systems and NF155 are expressed at the paranodal loops of oligodendrocytes and Schwan cells [23,24] that act as a ligand of the contactin-associated protein 1 essential for saltatory conduction.[25] Antibodies to these proteins cause central and peripheral demyelination and have occurred in 0.52% of multiple sclerosis cases, whereas 2.8% tested with CIDP in Japan had central demyelination.[26]

SUMMARY

This patient had evidence of central nervous system demyelination with an abnormal MRI, presence of oligoclonal bands in the spinal fluid, and abnormal evoked responses.

He presented with an acute ascending paralysis and showed evidence of peripheral motor and sensory degeneration. The CSF lymphocytic pleocytosis is unusual for GBS unless these occur in HIV-infected patients, but can sometimes be seen with acute MS attacks.

His peripheral nerve disorder was monophasic, and he recovered with IgG infusions and steroids.

IMPORTANT POINTS

- GBS presents with an acute ascending paralysis. The differential diagnosis includes myelopathy, motor neuron disease, disorders of neuromuscular transmission, myopathies, and other acute neuropathies, including porphyria, arsenic poisoning, and HIV-induced polyradiculoneuropathy.
- GBS is a motor neuropathy; however, sensory complaints and mild sensory findings may be present.
- GBS is a primary demyelinating disease but can also be associated with axonal degeneration, as demonstrated by EMG. There is also a primarily axonal form of GBS.
- Significantly elevated spinal fluid cells are not characteristic of GBS; therefore other conditions such as HIV, sarcoidosis, West Nile, Lyme, polio, and other infections, as well as lymphoma, should be ruled out.
- GBS is treated with plasma exchange or IgG infusions.
- Central demyelination can be seen with GBS, but the association may be coincidental.

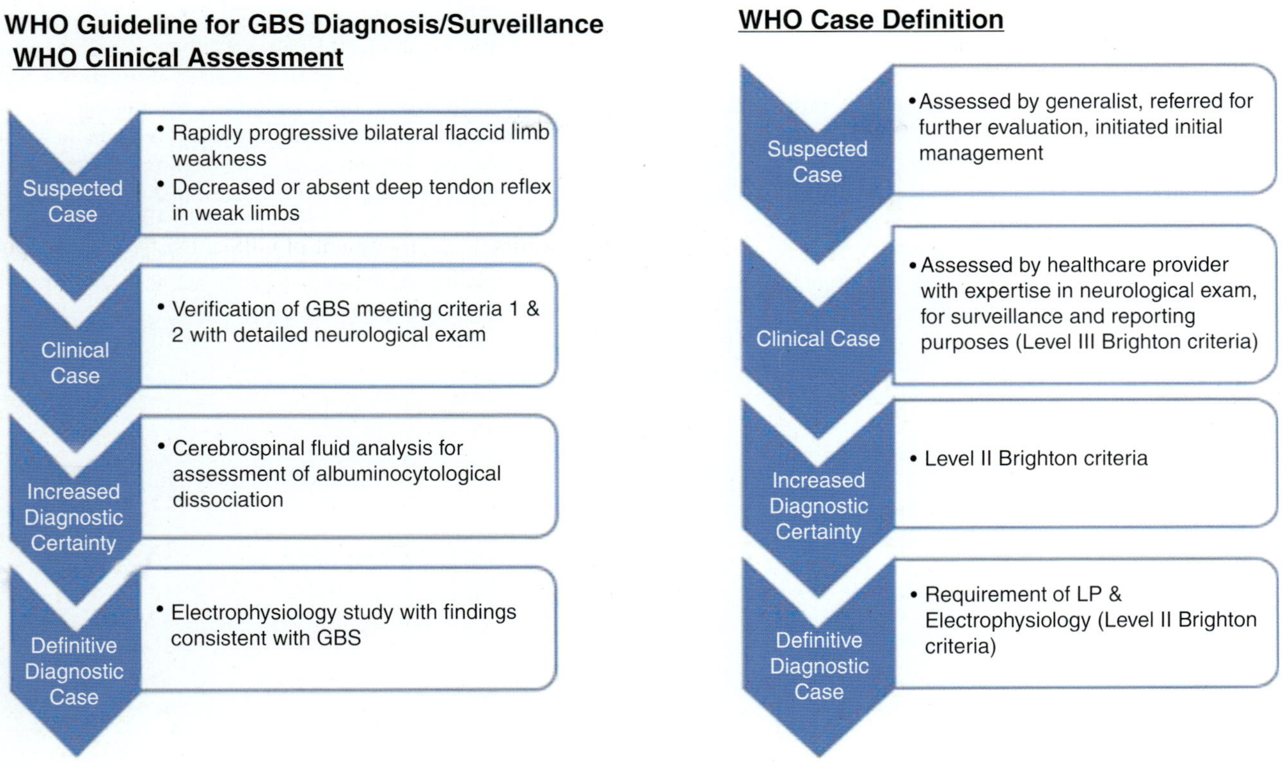

FIG. 39-2 WHO guideline for GBS diagnosis/surveillance. *GBS*, Guillain–Barré syndrome; *LP*, Lumbar puncture; *WHO*, World Health Organization.

REFERENCES

1. Oh SJ. Nerve conduction velocity tests: their clinical applications. In: Bertorini TE, ed. *Clinical Evaluation and Diagnostic Tests in Neuromuscular Disorders*. Boston, MA: Butterworth-Heinemann; 2002:141–207.
2. Asbury AK, Cornblath DR. Assessment of current diagnostic criteria for Guillain-Barré syndrome. *Ann Neurol*. 1990;27(Suppl): S21–S24.
3. Mendell JR, Kolkin S, Kissel JT, et al. Evidence for central nervous system demyelination in chronic inflammatory demyelinating polyradiculoneuropathy. *Neurology*. 1987;37(8):1291–1294.
4. Pareyson D, Ciano C, Fiacchino F, et al. Combined central and peripheral acute demyelination. *Ital J Neurol Sci*. 1993; 14(1):83–86.
5. Forester C, Lascelles RG. Association between polyneuritis and multiple sclerosis. *J Neurol Neurosurg Psychiatry*. 1979;42(9): 864–866.
6. Lassmann H, Budka H, Schnaberth G. Inflammatory demyelinating polyradiculitis in a patient with multiple sclerosis. *Arch Neurol*. 1981;38(2):99–102.
7. Al-Din A, Anderson M, Bickerstaff E, et al. Brainstem encephalitis and the syndrome of Miller Fisher: a clinical study. *Brain*. 1982;105:481–495.
8. Maier H, Schmidbauer M, Pfausler B, et al. Central nervous system pathology in patients with the Guillain-Barré syndrome. *Brain*. 1997;120:451–464.
9. Phillips M, Stewart S, Anderson J. Neuropathological findings in Miller Fisher syndrome. *J Neurol Neurosurg Psychiatry*. 1984;47:492–495.
10. Yuki N, Hirata K. Preserved tendon reflexes on *Campylobacter* neuropathy. *Ann Neurol*. 1998;43:546–547.
11. Kuwabara S, Ogawara K, Koga M, et al. Hyperreflexia in Guillain-Barré syndrome: relation with acute motor axonal neuropathy and anti-GM1 antibody. *J Neurol Neurosurg Psychiatry*. 1999;67: 180–184.
12. Susuki K, Atsumi M, Koga M, et al. Acute facial diplegia and hyperreflexia: a Guillain-Barré syndrome variant. *Neurology*. 2004;62(5):825–827.
13. Oshima Y, Mitsui T, Yoshino H, et al. Central motor conduction in patients with anti-ganglioside antibody associated neuropathy syndromes and hyperreflexia. *J Neurol Neurosurg Psychiatry*. 2002;73(5):568–573.
14. Best PV. Acute polyradiculoneuritis associated with demyelinated plaques in the central nervous system: report of a case. *Acta Neuropathol (Berl)*. 1985;67(3–4):230–234.
15. Capello E, Roccatagliata L, Schenone A, et al. Acute axonal form of Guillain-Barré syndrome in a multiple sclerosis patient: chance association or linked disorders? *Eur J Neurol*. 2000;7(2):223–225.
16. Bar-Joseph G, Etzioni A, Hemli J, Gershoni-Baruch R. Guillain-Barré syndrome in three siblings less than 2 years old. *Arch Dis Childhood*. 1991;66:1078–1079.
17. Davidson DLW, O'Sullivan AF, Morley KD. HLA antigens in familial Guillain-Barré syndrome. *J Neurol Neurosurg Psychiatry*. 1991;55:508–509.
18. Wilmshurst JM, Pohl KRE, Vaughan RW, Hughes RAC. Familial Guillain-Barré syndrome. *Eur J Neurol*. 1999;6:499–503.
19. International Multiple Sclerosis Genetics Consortium Risk alleles for multiple sclerosis identified by a genome-wide study. *N Engl J Med*. 2007;357(9):851–862.
20. Yuki N. Ganglioside mimicry and peripheral nerve disease. *Muscle Nerve*. 2007;35:691–711.
21. Bertorini TE, Narayanswami P. Autoimmune neuropathies. *Compr Ther*. 2003;29:194–209.

22. Guillain G, Barré JA, Strohl PA. Sur un syndrome de vacliculo-neurite auer hyperalkuminose du liquide cephalorachindren sans reaction cellulaire. Remarques sur les characters clinques et graphigues der reflex tendineux. *Bull Soc Med Hosp Paris.* 1916;40:1462–1470.
23. Davis JQ, Lambert S, Bennett V. Molecular composition of the node of Ranvier: identification of ankyrin-binding cell adhesion molecules neurofascin (mucin+/third FNIII domain −) and NrCAM at nodal axon segments. *J Cell Biol.* 1996;135(5):1355–1367.
24. Stathopoulos P, Alexopoulos H, Dalakas MC. Autoimmune antigenic targets at the node of Ranvier in demyelinating disorders. *Nat Rev Neurol.* 2015;11(3):143–156. https://doi.org/10.1038/nrneurol.2014.260.
25. Kadoya M, Kaida K, Koike H, et al. IgG4 anti-neurofascin155 antibodies in chronic inflammatory demyelinating polyradiculoneuropathy: clinical significance and diagnostic utility of a conventional assay. *J Neuroimmunol.* 2016;301: 16–22. https://doi.org/10.1016/j.neuroim.2016.10.013. Epub 2016 Nov 9.
26. Kira JI, Yamasaki R, Ogata H. Antineurofascin autoantibody and demyelination. *Neurochem Int.* 2019;130:104360. https://doi.org/10.1016/j.neuint.2018.12.011.

A Man With Acute Muscle Weakness and Respiratory Failure

A 28-year-old man entered the hospital because of leg weakness which had developed 1 week following some flu-like symptoms. He had been almost unable to walk for 2 days. He became progressively short of breath and had to be intubated in the emergency room because of severe respiratory insufficiency.

Past medical history was unremarkable. He did not smoke or drink.

On examination he was alert and followed commands well while on respiratory assistance; his vital capacity was about 800 mL. Pupils, disks, and extraocular movements were normal. There was a mild bilateral facial weakness but no ptosis, and he had abundant oral secretions. He could not raise his arms above the head or his left leg off the bed. He had weakness of 3−/5 in proximal and distal muscles of the arm and 2+/5 in proximal and distal muscles of the legs. He was areflexic. There was diminished vibration sense in his toes, but pinprick and position senses were normal. There were no Babinski signs.

A complete blood count, serum creatine kinase (CK), and metabolic panel were normal.

Spinal fluid showed normal opening pressure. Protein was 85 mg/dL (normal, <45 mg/dL). There were 120 cells, 80% lymphocytes. Cytology was negative. Glucose was 58 mg/dL (normal, >50 mg/dL). Serum protein electrophoresis was normal.

WHAT IS THE DIFFERENTIAL DIAGNOSIS?

The differential diagnosis of any patient who presents with acute progressive quadriparesis should always include a myelopathy, particularly at a high cervical level. The lack of sensory levels and Babinski signs are against this possibility. Other possibilities include periodic paralysis and disorders of neuromuscular transmission; myositis or rhabdomyolysis are unlikely because of the areflexia, normal serum CK and spinal fluid findings (Fig. 40-1).

The presentation was typical of acute inflammatory demyelinating polyneuropathy (AIDP), or Guillain–Barré syndrome (GBS). Other neuropathies, such as porphyria or arsenic poisoning, are less likely because of the facial weakness and the spinal fluid findings. His acute polyneuropathy with increased cells in the spinal fluid suggests HIV-associated AIDP. Other causes of increased cells in the spinal fluid should be considered, such as Lyme disease and a polio-like paralysis caused by the West Nile virus; however, the patient was not febrile.

WHAT TESTS SHOULD BE DONE?

His blood chemistry profile was normal. A urine test for porphyrins was negative. Arsenic levels were not elevated. Thyroid profile was normal. HIV tests were positive; rapid plasma regain was negative. Hepatitis serology was negative. Lyme and West Nile titers were not tested.

AN EMG TEST WAS PERFORMED

Motor Nerve Studies

Nerve and Site	Latency(ms)	Amplitude (mV)	Conduction Velocity (m/s)
Peroneal Nerve R.	**Normal ≤ 5.7**	**Normal ≥ 3**	**Normal ≥ 40**
Ankle	**7.1**	8	–
Fibular head	14.8	5	**36**
Knee	17.3	5	**34**
Nerve and Site	**Latency (ms)**	**Amplitude (mV)**	**Conduction Velocity (m/s)**
Tibial Nerve L.	**Normal ≤ 5.3**	**Normal ≥ 4**	**Normal ≥ 40**
Ankle	**6.4**	7	–
Knee	16.5	4	**38**
Nerve and Site	**Latency (ms)**	**Amplitude (mV)**	**Conduction Velocity (m/s)**
Median Nerve R.	**Normal ≤ 4.2**	**Normal ≥ 6**	**Normal ≥ 50**
Wrist	**4.9**	9	–
Elbow	11.1	7	**44**
Ulnar Nerve R.	**Normal ≤ 3.6**	**Normal ≥ 8**	**Normal ≥ 50**
Wrist	**4.4**	12	–
Below elbow	10.4	9	**42**
Above elbow	14.2	9	**41**

F-Wave and Tibial H-Reflex Studies

Nerve	Latency (ms)	Normal Latency ≤ (ms)	Persistence (%)
Peroneal nerve R.	**77.5**	54	**20**
Tibial nerve L.	**68.2**	54	**60**
Median nerve R.	**45.5**	30	**20**
Ulnar nerve R.	**47.6**	30	**40**
H-reflex R.	**NR**	34	–
H-reflex L.	**NR**	34	–

Sensory Nerve Studies

Nerve	Onset Latency (ms)	Normal Onset Latency ≤ (ms)	Peak Latency (ms)	Normal Peak Latency ≤ (ms)	Amp (μV)	Normal Amp ≥ (μV)	Conduction Velocity (m/s)	Normal Conduction Velocity ≥ (m/s)
Sural nerve R.	3.5	3.5	4.0	4.0	**5**	11	40	40
Superficial peroneal R.	**NR**	4.0	**NR**	**4.0**	**NR**	**8–10**	**NR**	40
Median nerve R.	**2.8**	2.6	**3.3**	3.1	**13**	20	**46**	50
Ulnar nerve R.	2.6	2.6	3.1	3.1	**6**	13	50	50

EMG Data

Muscle	Insrt Activity	Fibs	Pos Waves	Fasc	Amp	Dur	Poly	Pattern
Deltoid R.	Norm	None	None	None	Norm	Norm	None	**Red**
Biceps brachii R.	Norm	None	None	None	Norm	Norm	None	**Red**
Triceps R.	Norm	None	None	None	Norm	Norm	None	**Red**
Extensor digitorum com. R.	Norm	None	None	None	Norm	Norm	None	**Red**
Flexor carpi ulnaris R.	Norm	None	None	None	Norm	Norm	None	**Red**
Flexor carpi radialis R.	Norm	None	None	None	Norm	Norm	None	**Red**
First dorsal interosseous R.	Norm	None	None	None	Norm	Norm	None	**Red**
Tensor fasciae latae R.	Norm	None	None	None	Norm	Norm	None	**Red**
Vastus lateralis R.	Norm	None	None	None	Norm	Norm	None	**Red**
Tibialis anterior R.	Norm	None	None	None	Norm	Norm	None	**Red**
Peroneus longus R.	Norm	None	None	None	Norm	Norm	None	**Red**
Gastrocnemius R.	Norm	None	None	None	Norm	Norm	None	**Red**

WHAT WERE THE EMG FINDINGS?

The nerve conduction study showed predominantly demyelination with prolonged distal motor latencies, slow conduction velocities with normal CMAP amplitudes, no H-reflexes, and prolonged F-waves with reduced F-wave persistence in the legs. The superficial peroneal SNAP was absent, and the other SNAPs were of low amplitude indicating sensory fiber involvement.

The needle test showed no spontaneous potentials and normal motor unit action potential size and shape, but there was decreased motor unit recruitment. This EMG is compatible with AIDP.

The man was diagnosed as having HIV-associated AIDP and was treated with IV gamma globulin infusions 500 mg daily for 4 days. Steady improvement was seen. The weakness improved, and after 4 weeks he was able to ambulate with help.

DISCUSSION

This patient's presentation was characteristic of AIDP, but the increased cells in the spinal fluid suggested that this was associated with HIV infection, which was confirmed. He was treated with gamma globulin infusions with marked improvement.

HIV-infected patients can develop several types of neuropathies (Table 40-1). Those that occur early during seroconversion and when CD4 counts are over 500 cells include AIDP with a clinical presentation and EMG findings identical to classic GBS[1] in non-HIV patients.[2] The pathology is similar to AIDP. The cells present in the sural nerves are also similar in both groups, but there are more CD4 cells than CD8 in classic GBS, whereas there are fewer CD4 cells in HIV-positive patients. The response to IgG infusions and plasma exchange is similar. (Table 40-2 lists the treatment/management of GBS.)

HIV-infected patients may also develop mononeuropathies, such as facial palsy and brachial neuritis or a sensory neuropathy[2]; the trigeminal nerve is affected less frequently. Other causes of neuropathies in these patients should always be considered and ruled out. These include herpes zoster and hepatitis C, as well as lymphomatous infiltrations of nerves. Some patients may also develop syphilitic infections.

Chronic inflammatory demyelinating polyneuropathy (CIDP) can also be seen in early HIV patients,[1] and their presentation and diagnostic studies are similar to classic idiopathic CIDP.[3] There is an increased number of cells in the cerebrospinal fluid. Pathologically, those with HIV show more obvious inflammation, particularly by CD8 lymphocytes,[4,5] and there is more axonal loss than in non-HIV patients.[5] They usually respond well to plasma exchange or IgG infusions and to corticosteroids, unlike GBS, which should be used carefully because of the risk of opportunistic infections. The prophylactic use of cotrimoxazole is usually recommended. Highly active antiretroviral therapy is also useful.[6]

Patients having moderately advanced HIV infections may develop two forms of mononeuritis multiplex: one appears to be immune-mediated, and the other is caused by vasculitis.[7] The clinical presentations are similar to non-HIV patients,[8] and

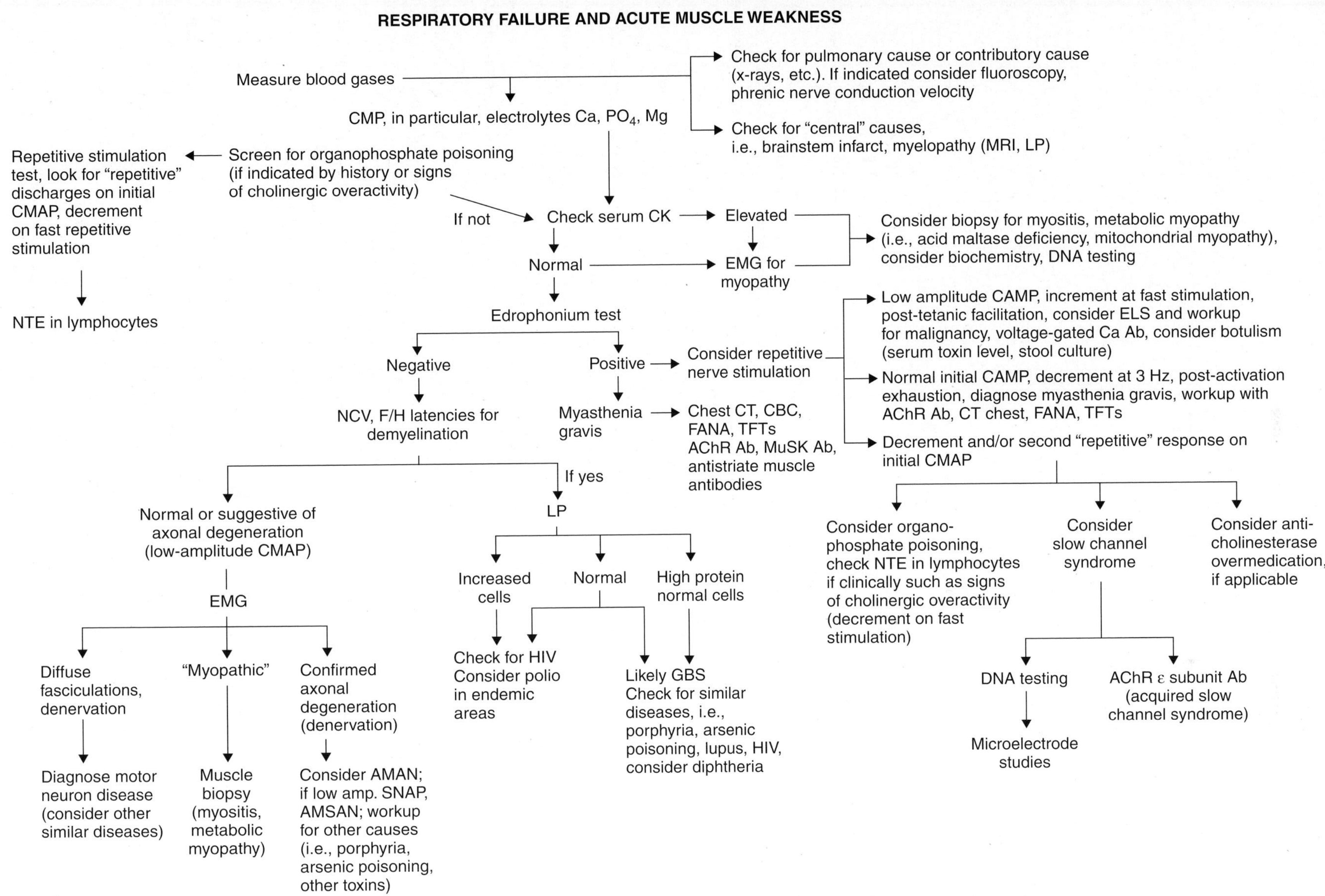

FIG. 40-1 Pathways for the evaluation of patients with respiratory failure and acute muscle weakness. *Ab*, Antibody; *AChR*, acetylcholine receptor; *AMAN*, acute motor axonal neuropathy; *AMSAN*, acute motor sensory axonal neuropathy; *Ca*, calcium; *ELS*, Eaton–Lambert syndrome; *F/H*, F-waves/H-reflex; *FANA*, fluorescent antinuclear antibody; *GBS*, Guillain–Barré syndrome; *Mg*, magnesium; *MuSK*, muscle-specific kinase; *LP*, lumbar puncture; *NCV*, nerve conduction velocity; *NTE*, neurotoxic esterase; PO_4, phosphate; *TFT*, thyroid function test.

TABLE 40-1 Classification of Peripheral Nerve Complications in HIV Disease

Early HIV Disease
Seroconversion-related neuropathies
Guillain–Barré syndrome
Mononeuropathies
Moderately Advanced HIV Disease
Chronic inflammatory demyelinating polyneuropathy
Mononeuritis multiplex
Diffuse infiltrative lymphocytosis syndrome
Syphilitic polyradiculopathy
Hepatitis C infection–related neuropathy
Human T-lymphotropic virus infection type I–related neuropathy
Motor neuron disease syndrome
Advanced HIV Disease
Distal symmetrical sensory polyneuropathy
Autonomic neuropathy
HIV-related lumbosacral polyradiculopathy
Cytomegalovirus infection–related polyradiculopathy
Cytomegalovirus infection mononeuritis multiplex
Medication-Related Neuropathy
Antiretroviral drugs: didanosine, stavudine, and zalcitabine
Other drugs: ethambutol, HMG CoA reductase inhibitors, isoniazid, paclitaxel (Taxol), thalidomide, vinblastine, and vincristine

Reprinted with permission from Brew BJ. The peripheral nerve complications of human immunodeficiency virus (HIV) infection. *Muscle Nerve*. 2003;28:542–552.

TABLE 40-2 Therapeutic Plan for Patients With Guillain–Barré Syndrome

Admit the patient to the hospital for observation until there is clinical improvement, as recurrence after improvement is unusual, but could occur. Observation then could be done in a rehabilitation unit.
Determine the forced vital capacity every 6 h. Place on cardiac monitor.
Place patient in intensive care unit if vital capacity is below 2 L, or if there is cardiac arrhythmia or autonomic dysfunction.
Diagnostic studies should be done upon admission.
Placement of nasogastric tube if patient has swallowing difficulties.
Elective intubation for vital capacity below 1 L.
Respiratory assistance if there is poor arterial oxygen saturation.
Plasmapheresis as soon as the diagnosis is suspected (while diagnostic workup is being done). Treatment includes 2–3 L/day for 3 days, then every other day for 2 days. If relapse occurs, another trial for 3 days can be done.
Alternatively, infusions of gamma globulin 400 mg/kg/day for 5 days over 6–8 h, or 1 g/kg/day for 2 days in infusions from 10 to 12 h.
Elastic stockings.
Subcutaneous heparin or Lovenox every 12 h.
Analgesia for muscle pains, which are not uncommon.
Physical therapy. Plan transfer to rehabilitation unit when stable.
Emotional support.

EMG demonstrates evidence of a multifocal neuropathy. Nerve biopsies might show a perivascular inflammatory infiltrate or a necrotizing vasculitis.[8] The treatment consists of immunotherapy, such as IgG infusions.[9]

HIV-infected patients may also develop neuropathies caused by diffuse infiltrative lymphocytosis[10] and hepatitis C.[11] Lumbosacral cytomegalic virus infection[12] and syphilitic polyradiculopathy can also occur.[13]

Those with more advanced HIV infection develop a distal symmetric sensory-motor neuropathy.[14] GBS overlap, however, has been reported in an advanced HIV patient.[15] Finally, clinicians should keep in mind that drugs used to treat HIV, as well as malnourishment, can cause a neuropathy.

SUMMARY

This patient developed quadriparesis, had increased cells in the spinal fluid, and was diagnosed with AIDP. He was found to be HIV-positive. He responded well to gamma globulin infusions.

Patients with HIV can present with an acute polyneuropathy that is indistinguishable from GBS except for elevated cells in the spinal fluid.

IMPORTANT POINTS

- The differential diagnosis in patients with acute quadriparesis includes, among others, myelopathy, defects of neuromuscular transmission, and neuropathies such as GBS, HIV-associated polyradiculoneuropathy, porphyria or arsenic poisoning, and myopathies such as from hypokalemia, myositis, and rhabdomyolysis.
- The spinal fluid of patients with GBS usually shows albuminocytologic dissociation and an increased number of cells and should raise the suspicion of an infection, not only from HIV but also from other infections, such as Lyme disease and West Nile virus.
- HIV infection causes AIDP identical to that seen in patients not infected with GBS, and such cases respond similarly to plasma exchange or IgG infusions.
- HIV patients might develop several neuropathies, such as GBS, CIDP, mononeuritis multiplex, radiculopathies, and a diffuse sensory-motor neuropathy. Other neuromuscular manifestations include polymyositis and inclusion body myositis, a mitochondrial myopathy caused by drugs, and a cachectic myopathy.
- Neuropathies or radiculopathies seen in HIV patients can also be caused by infections, such as syphilis, cytomegalovirus, and hepatitis C, or antiviral drugs.

REFERENCES

1. Cornblath DR, McArthur JC, Kennedy PG, et al. Inflammatory demyelinating peripheral neuropathies associated with human T-cell lymphotropic virus type III infection. *Ann Neurol.* 1987;21:32–40.
2. Piette AM, Tusseau F, Vignon D, et al. Acute neuropathy coincident with seroconversion for anti-LAV/HTLV-III. *Lancet.* 1986;1:852.
3. Brew BJ. The peripheral nerve complications of human immunodeficiency virus (HIV) infection. *Muscle Nerve.* 2003;28:542–552.
4. Cornblath DR, Griffin DE, Welch D, et al. Quantitative analysis of endoneurial T-cells in human sural nerve biopsies. *J Neuroimmunol.* 1990;26(2):113–118.

5. Griffin JW, Crawford TO, McArthur JC. Peripheral neuropathies associated with HIV infection. In: Gendelman HE, Lipton SA, Epstein L, Swindells S, eds. *The Neurology of AIDS*. New York, NY: Chapman & Hall; 1998:275–278.
6. Markus R, Brew BJ. HIV-1 peripheral neuropathy and combination antiretroviral therapy. *Lancet*. 1998;352(9144):1906–1907.
7. Fuller GN, Jacobs JM, Guiloff RJ. Nature and incidence of peripheral nerve syndromes in HIV infection. *J Neurol Neurosurg Psychiatry*. 1993;56:372–381.
8. Bradley WG, Verma A. Painful vasculitic neuropathy in HIV-1 infection: relief of pain with prednisone therapy. *Neurology*. 1996; 47:1446–1451.
9. Said G, Saimot AG, Lacroix C, Tardieu M. Peripheral nerve disease in HIV infected patients. In: Said G, Samot AG, Lacroix C, Tardieu M, eds. *Neurological Complications of HIV and AIDS*. Philadelphia, PA: WB Saunders; 1997:159.
10. Gherardi RK, Chretien F, Delfau-Larue M-H, et al. Neuropathy in diffuse infiltrative lymphocytosis syndrome. *Neurology*. 1998;50: 1041–1044.
11. Authier FJ, Pawlotsky JM, Viard JP, et al. High incidence of hepatitis C virus infection in patients with cryoglobulinemic neuropathy. *Ann Neurol*. 1993;34:749–750.
12. Cohen BA, McArthur JC, Grohman S, et al. Neurologic prognosis of cytomegalovirus polyradiculomyelopathy in AIDS. *Neurology*. 1993;43:493–499.
13. Brew BJ. Infective causes of peripheral neuropathy in advanced HIV disease. In: Brew BJ, ed. *HIV Neurology*. New York, NY: Oxford University Press; 2001:202–208.
14. Cornblath DR, McArthur JC. Predominantly sensory neuropathy in patients with AIDS and AIDS related complex. *Neurology*. 1988;38:794–796.
15. Hiraga A, Kuwabara S, Nakamaru A, et al. Fisher/Guillain-Barré overlap syndrome in advanced AIDS. *J Neurol Sci*. 2007;258(1–2): 148–150.

41 CASE

A Young Woman With Acute Onset of Clumsiness and Ophthalmoplegia

A 23-year-old woman came with a 2-day history of increased clumsiness and blurred vision; she had flu-like symptoms with diarrhea 2 weeks prior to her presentation. Past medical history and social history were unremarkable.

During examination, she was alert and had normal mentation. She had limitation of gaze in all directions with relative preservation of the right lateral rectus function (Fig. 41-1) and had bilateral ptosis with normal pupils, and mild bilateral facial weakness. She developed complete ophthalmoplegia after 2 days.

The patient had very mild proximal leg and foot dorsiflexor weakness but severe limb and truncal ataxia and difficulty walking. She was areflexic and had mildly decreased vibratory and position senses in the toes; pain and temperature sensations were normal. There were no Babinski signs, and the rest of the examination was normal.

WHAT IS THE MOST LIKELY DIAGNOSIS?

This young woman had an acute onset of ataxia and ophthalmoplegia and was areflexic but had normal mental function. Ophthalmoplegia and ptosis could suggest myasthenia gravis; however, in myasthenia, reflexes are present and patients are not ataxic. When in doubt, an edrophonium test could be important to rule out myasthenia. Another neuromuscular transmission defect that needs to be considered in these patients is botulism, which presents with ophthalmoplegia and areflexia, but such patients are usually severely weak, are not ataxic, and have dilated pupils. Ataxia and ophthalmoplegia occur in mitochondrial disease, but these are chronic conditions. The lack of long tract signs and normal mental status makes a brainstem disorder unlikely. Ataxia, ophthalmoplegia, and areflexia suggest the Miller Fisher syndrome (MFS), a variant of Guillain–Barré syndrome (GBS). Brainstem encephalitis has a similar presentation, and some believe that MFS is caused by an inflammation of the brainstem. Wernicke's encephalopathy presents acutely in alcoholics with ataxia, areflexia, and ophthalmoplegia, but these patients have altered mental status. Multiple sclerosis presents with ophthalmoplegia, although it is usually intermittent; patients can be ataxic but are not areflexic and usually have long tract signs. Rarely, patients with classic GBS might also develop ophthalmoplegia, but this patient had only very mild weakness.

WHAT TESTS SHOULD BE DONE?

Although there was no clinical evidence to suggest a disease of the brainstem, the pupils were spared, and there was no nystagmus, an MRI was done to rule out a central nervous system (CNS) disease in this patient. Her MRI was normal.

AN EMG TEST WAS PERFORMED

Motor Nerve Studies

Nerve and Site	Latency(ms)	Amplitude (mV)	Conduction Velocity (m/s)
Peroneal Nerve R.	**Normal ≤ 5.7**	**Normal ≥ 3**	**Normal ≥ 40**
Ankle	3.7	9	–
Fibular head	8.4	9	60
Knee	10.0	9	63

Nerve and Site	Latency (ms)	Amplitude (mV)	Conduction Velocity (m/s)
Tibial Nerve L.	**Normal ≤ 5.3**	**Normal ≥ 4**	**Normal ≥ 40**
Ankle	3.1	23	–
Pop. fossa	9.2	20	54

Nerve and Site	Latency (ms)	Amplitude (mV)	Conduction Velocity (m/s)
Ulnar Nerve R.	**Normal ≤ 3.6**	**Normal ≥ 8**	**Normal ≥ 50**
Wrist	2.9	18	–
Below elbow	6.7	18	61
Above elbow	9.7	18	60

F-Wave and Tibial H-Reflex Studies

Nerve	Latency (ms)	Normal Latency ≤ (ms)
Peroneal nerve R.	54.0	54
Tibial nerve L.	53.8	54
Ulnar nerve R.	30.0	30
H-reflex R.	**NR**	34
H-reflex L.	**NR**	34

Sensory Nerve Studies

Nerve	Onset Latency (ms)	Normal Onset Latency ≤ (ms)	Peak Latency (ms)	Normal Peak Latency ≤ (ms)	Amp (μV)	Normal Amp ≥ (μV)	Conduction Velocity (m/s)	Normal Conduction Velocity ≥ (m/s)
Sural nerve R.	3.4	3.5	3.9	4.0	**5**	11	41	40
Superficial peroneal R.	**NR**	3.5	**NR**	4.0	**NR**	8–10	**NR**	40
Ulnar nerve R.	2.4	2.6	2.9	3.1	**10**	13	50	50

Repetitive Stimulation Test

Ulnar nerve R.—normal
Facial nerve R.—normal

EMG Data

Muscle	Insrt Activity	Fibs	Pos Waves	Fasc	Amp	Dur	Poly	Pattern
Deltoid R.	Norm	None	None	None	Norm	Norm	None	Full
Biceps brachii R.	Norm	None	None	None	Norm	Norm	None	Full
Triceps R.	Norm	None	None	None	Norm	Norm	None	Full
Brachioradialis R.	Norm	None	None	None	Norm	Norm	None	Full
First dorsal interosseus R.	Norm	None	None	None	Norm	Norm	None	Full
Tensor fasciae latae R.	Norm	None	None	None	Norm	Norm	None	Full
Tibialis anterior R.	Norm	None	None	None	Norm	Norm	None	**Red**
Gastrocnemius R.	Norm	None	None	None	Norm	Norm	None	Full

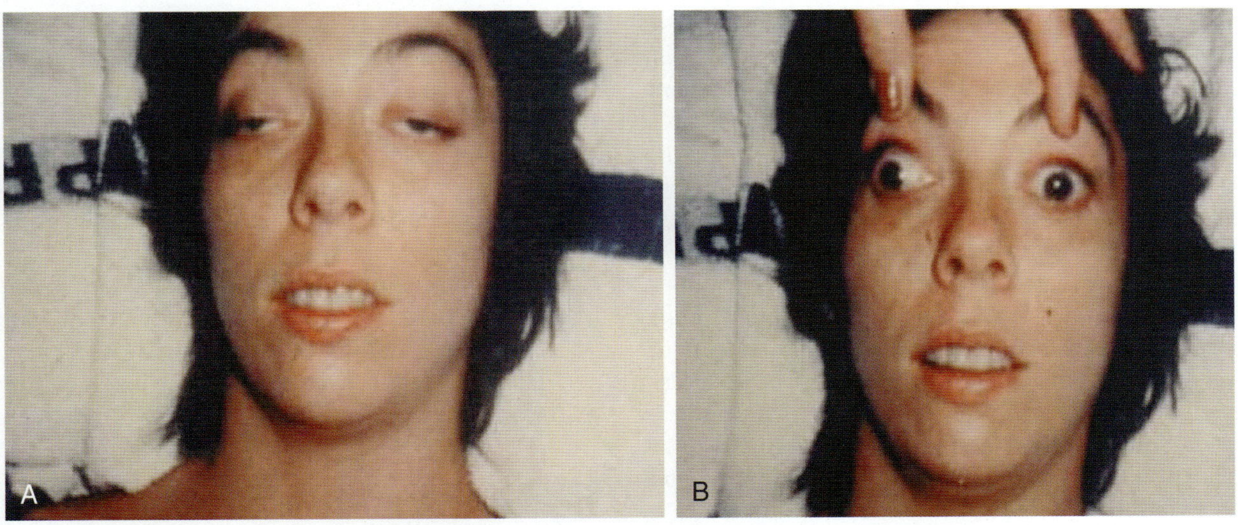

FIG. 41-1 The patient showing bilateral ptosis (**A**) and ophthalmoplegia with relative preservation of the right external rectus function (**B**) resembling intranuclear ophthalmoplegia. There was also limitation of upward and downward gaze.

WHAT WERE THE EMG FINDINGS?

The EMG showed normal motor conduction velocities, latencies, and CMAP amplitudes; F-responses were also normal. There were, however, no H-reflexes and the sural and ulnar SNAPs were of low amplitude, and there was no superficial peroneal SNAP. Repetitive stimulation tests and needle electromyography were essentially normal, except for a mildly decreased motor unit recruitment only in the tibialis anterior muscle. These electrophysiologic findings indicate a primary involvement of large sensory axons.

WHAT OTHER TESTS WOULD BE DONE?

An edrophonium test was negative. GQ1b antibodies were not measured, as this test was not available when this patient was seen.

Spinal fluid showed a protein of 60 mg/dL with 12 lymphocytes. Glucose was normal. A complete metabolic panel, fluorescent antinuclear antibody titer, and thyroid studies were normal. HIV serology was negative.

DISCUSSION

This patient was diagnosed to have the MFS variant of GBS. The condition, initially reported by Fisher in 1956, is characterized by ophthalmoplegia, ataxia, and areflexia.[1] The syndrome accounts for about 5% of cases of GBS, and some patients with generalized weakness and features of GBS also have ophthalmoplegia.

In MFS, ophthalmoplegia is the first symptom, and it could be asymmetric, affecting mainly the 6th nerve, evolving to complete ophthalmoplegia with ptosis. The pupils are usually preserved, although, rarely, patients might have pupillary abnormalities. They might also have distal paresthesias or dysphagia; some have mild weakness, as in this case. Reflexes are usually absent.[2]

MFS could be confused with a brainstem lesion, such as an infarct or encephalitis, and this has raised the theory that Miller Fisher is a brainstem disease. The electrodiagnostic studies, however, indicate a neuropathy showing absent or low-amplitude SNAPs and absent H-reflexes.

There is considerable debate regarding the peripheral versus central pathology in MFS, and it is of interest that Bickerstaff and Cloake reported in 1951 a disorder characterized by an acute ophthalmoplegia. They concluded that this was a mesencephalitis or rhombencephalitis.[3] They later expanded their observations to describe clinical features of drowsiness and cerebrospinal fluid pleocytosis; they also demonstrated CNS pathology.[4,5]

In his initial report, Miller Fisher also considered the possibility of CNS involvement but concluded that the manifestations were of peripheral nerve origin.[1] Some cases of MFS, however, also appear to have CNS involvement clinically or by MRI.[6,7] The proposed central origin of the clinical findings of classic MFS was opposed by Ropper,[8] and indeed, in most cases there is no clinical or other evidence of CNS disease. To muddy the waters further, the characteristic presence of GQ1b antibodies that occurs in MFS[9,10] might be seen in Bickerstaff encephalitis, although less frequently.[11,12] Some propose a spectrum of these disorders and call it *anti-GQ1b antibody syndrome*.[11,13] A good compromise would be a consideration that only some cases of MFS have CNS pathology, and when this is clearly demonstrated clinically or by imaging studies, the term *Bickerstaff encephalitis* could be used.

Spinal fluid protein in MFS is usually elevated, and, as discussed, patients frequently have antibodies against the ganglioside GQ1b in the serum. These antibodies could be pathogenic, and the extraocular muscle involvement can be explained by the fact that the perinodal areas of nerves to those muscles are enriched with these gangliosides. Although cranial nerve II has the richest GQ1b content, this is usually spared. Patients with clinical GBS associated with ophthalmoplegia might also have raised titers of these antibodies.[14]

MFS may be preceded by *Campylobacter jejuni* (CJ) or other infections; the association with CJ infection could represent an autoimmune molecular mimicry, as CJ has epitopes similar to GQ1b.[15]

MFS is one of several Guillain–Barré variants, which include a pure sensory variant, a pure dysautonomic variant, and a purely motor variant, and some patients have motor and sensory variants.[14] Others might develop a limited or regional involvement, affecting the oropharyngeal, cervical, and brachial muscles. These could have elevation of GT1a antibodies, and some patients might also develop arm and leg weakness.[16] A case of GBS, Miller Fisher overlap syndrome was reported after a COVID-19 case.[17]

The treatment of MFS is similar to that of GBS, which includes supportive care, immunotherapy with gamma globulin infusions,[18] or plasma exchange.[14] This therapy has also been beneficial in patients with apparent Bickerstaff encephalitis.[19] The prognosis of MFS is usually benign.

SUMMARY

This woman presented with ophthalmoplegia, ataxia, and areflexia and had electrodiagnostic features compatible with the Miller Fisher variant of GBS; she responded well with plasma exchange.

IMPORTANT POINTS

- MFS is a variant of GBS. The disease affects mainly sensory nerves, and the ataxia is a sensory ataxia due to a severe proprioceptive fiber dysfunction.
- MFS patients frequently have elevated antibodies against GQ1b ganglioside.
- The involvement of the extraocular muscles in MFS could be related to an overexpression of GQ1b ganglioside in the extraocular nerves.
- MFS can be associated with CJ infections, and the disorder could be caused by molecular mimicry from similarities between CJ epitopes and GQ1b gangliosides.
- Treatment of MFS consists of plasmapheresis or IgG infusions.
- The prognosis is good.

REFERENCES

1. Fisher CM. An unusual variant of acute idiopathic polyneuritis (syndrome of ophthalmoplegia, ataxia and areflexia). *N Engl J Med.* 1956;255:57–65.
2. Albers JW, Kelly JJ Jr. Acquired inflammatory demyelinating polyneuropathies: clinical and electrodiagnostic features. *Muscle Nerve.* 1989;12:435–451.
3. Bickerstaff ER, Cloake PC. Mesencephalitis and rhombencephalitis. *Br Med J.* 1951;4723:77–81.
4. Bickerstaff ER. Brainstem encephalitis: further observations on a grave syndrome with benign prognosis. *Br Med J.* 1957;1(5032): 1384–1387.
5. Al-Din AN, Anderson M, Bickerstaff ER, Harvey I. Brainstem encephalitis and the syndrome of Miller Fisher: a clinical study. *Brain.* 1982;105:481–495.

6. Barontini F, Sita D. The nosological position of Fisher's syndrome (ophthalmoplegia, ataxia and areflexia). *J Neurol*. 1983;229:33–44.
7. Meienberg O, Ryffel E. Supranuclear eye movement disorders in Fisher's syndrome of ophthalmoplegia, ataxia and areflexia. *Arch Neurol*. 1983;40:402–405.
8. Ropper AH. The CNS in Guillain-Barré syndrome. *Arch Neurol*. 1983;40:397–398.
9. Willison HJ, Veitch J, Paterson G, Kennedy PG. Miller Fisher syndrome is associated with serum antibodies to GQ1b ganglioside. *J Neurol Neurosurg Psychiatry*. 1993;56:204–206.
10. Yuki N, Sato S, Tsuji S, et al. Frequent presence of anti GQ1b antibody in Fisher's syndrome. *Neurology*. 1993;43:414–417.
11. Odaka M, Yuki N, Hirata K. Anti-GQ1b IgG antibody syndrome: clinical and immunological range. *J Neurol Neurosurg Psychiatry*. 2001;70:50–55.
12. Winer JB. Bickerstaff's encephalitis and the Miller Fisher syndrome. *J Neurol Neurosurg Psychiatry*. 2001;71:433–435.
13. Lo YL. Clinical and immunological spectrum of the Miller Fisher syndrome. *Muscle Nerve*. 2007;36(5):615–627.
14. Bertorini T, Narayanaswami P. Autoimmune neuropathies. *Comp Ther*. 2003;29:194–209.
15. Yuki N. Molecular mimicry between gangliosides and lipopolysaccharides of *Campylobacter jejuni* isolated from patients with Guillain-Barré syndrome and Miller Fisher syndrome. *J Infect Dis*. 1997;176:S150–S153.
16. Nagashima T, Koga M, Odaka M, et al. Clinical correlates of serum anti-GT1a IgG antibodies. *J Neurol Sci*. 2004;219(1–2):139–145.
17. Mohammadi SM, Abdi R, Karimi Z, Mortazavi F. Guillain-Barre/Miller Fisher overlap syndrome in a patient after coronavirus disease-2019 infection: a case report. *J Med Case Rep*. 2022;16(1):63. https://doi.org/10.1186/s13256-021-03245-y.
18. Mori M, Kuwabara S, Fukutake T, Hattori T. Intravenous immunoglobulin therapy for Miller Fisher syndrome. *Neurology*. 2007;68(14):1144–1146.
19. Ozawa T, Onodera O, Inuzuka T, et al. Efficacy of early plasmapheresis in Bickerstaff's encephalitis. *Inter Med*. 1998;37:986–989.

42 CASE

A Woman With Seafood Poisoning in Catfish Country

A 49-year-old woman developed nausea, vomiting, and diarrhea 4 hours after she ate at a local Memphis restaurant. Her dinner consisted of a salad and broiled grouper. She remained nauseated the next day, but diarrhea stopped, and she had no fever. Two days later, she developed burning of the lips, tongue, fingers, and toes and pain in the teeth. She had a sensation of burning in the limbs when exposed to cold temperatures, and both drinking and washing her hands with fresh and warm tap water produced a burning sensation. The patient received ciprofloxacin and cimetidine for 3 days without help, and both were discontinued. She was placed on gabapentin 300 mg three times a day for 3 days with minimal improvement. Other symptoms included muscle aches, hypersomnia, increased sensitivity to light, and watery eyes, but no headaches.

She had a history of hepatitis A 15 years before without sequelae. Family history was noncontributory. The patient drank alcohol occasionally and stated that drinking wine made her symptoms worse.

Physical examination revealed normal vital signs and general physical examination, except that her distal limbs felt cold to the examiner. She had normal pulses. Mentation and cranial nerves were also normal. Muscle strength and reflexes were normal and symmetrical. There were no pathologic reflexes. Sensory examination was unremarkable, except that she described aching and burning sensations when the examiner touched her with a cold tuning fork. Gait and coordination were normal, and there was no myotonia.

AN EMG TEST WAS PERFORMED

Motor Nerve Studies

Nerve and Site	Latency (ms)	Amplitude (mV)	Conduction Velocity (m/s)
Peroneal Nerve R.	**Normal ≤ 5.7**	**Normal ≥ 3**	**Normal ≥ 40**
Ankle	4.2	11	–
Fibular head	9.8	10	47
Knee	11.7	10	47

F-Wave and Tibial H-Reflex Studies

Nerve	Latency (ms)	Normal Latency ≤ (ms)
Peroneal nerve R.	45	54
H-reflex R.	32	34

Sensory Nerve Studies

Nerve	Peak Latency (ms)	Normal Peak Latency ≤ (ms)	Amp (µV)	Normal Amp ≥ (µV)
Sural nerve R.	3.8	4	32	13

Sympathetic Skin Response

Rt. hand—normal
Rt. foot—normal

EMG Data

Muscle	Insrt Activity	Fibs	Pos Waves	Fasc	Amp	Dur	Poly	Pattern
Vastus lateralis R.	Norm	None	None	None	Norm	Norm	None	Full
Tibialis anterior R.	Norm	None	None	None	Norm	Norm	None	Full
Gastrocnemius R.	Norm	None	None	None	Norm	Norm	None	Full

WHAT WERE THE EMG FINDINGS?

The nerve conduction tests and needle EMG were normal in the arm and leg including the sympathetic skin responses.

Complete blood count and chemistry profile, including liver enzymes, serum creatine kinase, and erythrocyte sedimentation rate, were normal.

WHAT IS THE MOST LIKELY DIAGNOSIS?

This patient presented with a history of paresthesias with burning sensations and paradoxical sensations to cold and heat after a gastrointestinal illness which occurred 4 hours after the ingestion of seafood, suggesting seafood poisoning.

The initial gastrointestinal symptoms could have been caused by a bacterial infection such as *Salmonella* or *Escherichia coli*. She, however, never had fever, and her gastrointestinal symptoms disappeared, while her neurologic symptoms persisted, which is not characteristic of these infections.

Botulism could also present with gastrointestinal symptoms, but this produces paralysis and ophthalmoplegia, and patients are usually constipated.

Scombroid fish poisoning is caused by eating tuna and mackerel that are infested with *Proteus morganii* bacteria containing high levels of histamine and a substance called *saurine*. The symptoms include coryza, flushing, headaches, and dry mouth.[1] This patient had none of these symptoms; rather, her presentation suggested ciguatera poisoning. She was treated with intravenous mannitol 25% with marked improvement.

WHAT IS CIGUATERA POISONING?

Ciguatera is the most common fish poisoning in the world; it is caused by certain strains of a *Benthic dinoflagellate* which was initially isolated in the Gambier Islands and is called *Gambierdiscus toxicus*. The incidence of the disease is about 25,000 cases annually, which is higher in warmer climates, particularly in the Caribbean. The poison is acquired by eating tropical or subtropical fish, such as barracuda, eels, mackerel, amberjack, snapper, and grouper.

The name ciguatera comes from *Turbo pica*, a marine snail called "*cigua*" in Spanish. The term was later applied to poisoning by fish.

Common symptoms include abdominal pain, diarrhea, vomiting, myalgia, paradoxical reversal of temperature sensations, paresthesias, mood disorders, ataxia, dental pain, tremors, stiffness, and increased salivation. These start 20 minutes to over 24 hours after the ingestion of contaminated fish. Patients might also develop fatigue, flaccidity, skin rash, and autonomic dysfunctions, such as hypertension, brachycardia or tachycardia, and orthostatic hypotension.[2–4] Rarely, they develop a polyneuropathy[5] or a myositis.[6] Cigua toxins activate voltage-sensitive sodium channels, causing hyperparalyzation-shifts and spontaneous repetitive nerve discharges. Excessive activation of small myelinated and unmyelinated fibers could cause the symptoms.[7–9]

Electrophysiologic tests in ciguatera poisoning could be normal or could show slowing of motor and sensory conduction velocities.[10]

The diagnosis is purely clinical, although an enzyme-linked immunosorbent assay (ELISA) test[11] can be done in serum; this is not commercially available.

The treatment of ciguatera poisoning consists of infusions, 1 g/kg, of 25% mannitol intravenously over 3–6 hours.[12,13] Benefits in more chronic cases have also been reported.[14] For maximum benefit the treatment should be given within 72 hours of toxin ingestion.[15] A recent report indicated that mannitol is not superior to normal saline infusions.[16] Other treatments include antihistaminics, sodium channel blockers, and gabapentin.[17]

The prognosis of ciguatera poisoning is usually good, although the disease can last for months. Fatalities are rare but do occur.[18]

Food poisoning such as this could be an important public health problem, particularly as the contaminated fish are not identified and because the toxin is heat-resistant and not eliminated by common cooking. It is recommended that fish poisoning should be reported to the public health services. For further information, one can refer online to http://www.csfan.fda.gov.

WHAT ARE OTHER INGESTIBLE SEAFOOD TOXINS?

Maitotoxin is another toxin that can produce symptoms similar to ciguatera; it comes from a dinoflagellate present in the gut of sturgeon that causes increased calcium accumulation in nerves and endocrine glands. Prominent muscle spasms also occur.[18] *Palytoxins* are also biotoxins from tropical fish that can cause muscle spasms, seizures, and elevated serum creatine kinase levels.

Another important toxin that was unlikely in this case is *tetrodotoxin*, caused by ingestion of puffer-fish, producing paresthesias and paralysis which could be lethal. In that condition the poison blocks sodium channels.[19,20] (The recent novel by Robin Cook, *Crisis*, provides an entertaining reading on tetrodotoxin poisoning and of concierge medicine.)

Shellfish poisoning by molluscs, such as mussels infected by the dinoflagellate that causes "red tides,"[21] produces paresthesias and reverse cold/hot temperature sensations but can also cause ataxia and other neurologic symptoms. *Amnestic shellfish poisoning* is caused by cultured blue mussels that contain the *domoic* toxin, a glutamate antagonist similar to *kainic* acid. It usually causes muscle cramps and diarrhea, and, later, neuropathy, seizures, and memory loss.[22] Similar contaminations have been reported in crabs and clams. *Hallucinating mullet poisoning* from ingesting that contaminated fish causes delirium and hallucinations. This poison is likely a variant of ciguatera.

Clupeotoxin is another toxin present in contaminated herring and anchovies. It causes headaches, convulsions, and even coma.[23] A more severe *paralytic shellfish poisoning* that develops within hours of ingestion of shellfish[24] is caused by a mixture of toxins including *saxitoxins* that block voltage-dependent sodium channels in nerve and muscle; its symptoms include paresthesias, dysphagia, weakness, and respiratory failure.

A lipid-soluble toxin, called *carchatoxin*, which infects sharks' flesh, has similar symptoms to ciguatera but could be much more severe and even lethal.[20]

SOME HISTORICAL ASPECTS OF SEAFOOD POISONING

It appears that Egyptians knew that puffer-fish could be poisonous, as a puffer-fish drawing is shown in a tomb of the Fifth Dynasty during 2500 BCE. Knowledge of poisoning by eating puffer-fish was introduced to Western Civilization by Kaempfer in the *History of Japan* in 1727.[24] Puffer-fish is a delicacy in Japan where the fish is prepared by expert cooks in licensed restaurants; these cooks are able to carefully remove the liver and roe which are highly toxic.

The awareness of symptoms that appear to be ciguatera poisoning is also described during the T'ang Dynasty in CE 618–907, and sailors with the explorer Fernandez de Quiroz, who became sick after eating pargo (red snapper) in 1600, likely had ciguatera poisoning.[23]

The great explorer Captain James Cook (Fig. 42-1) traveled extensively in the South Pacific,[25] and during his second journey in the HMS Resolution, he apparently ate a piece of puffer-fish

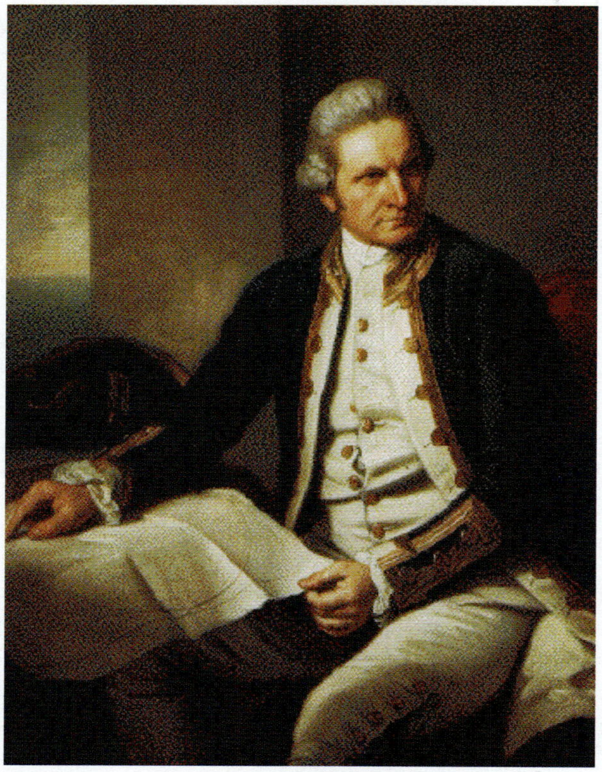

FIG. 42-1 The explorer Captain James Cook. Copyright © National Maritime Museum, London.

liver and became acutely ill in New Caledonia in 1774. During this voyage, he also reported more episodes of sea poisoning from eating two other types of fish.[26] He described paradoxical sensations from seafood poisoning as follows:

> *We found ourselves seized with an extraordinary weakness and numbness all over our limbs attended with numbness of sensation like to that caused by exposing one's hands and feet to a fire after having been pinched much by frost. I had almost lost the sense of feeling; nor could I distinguish between light and heavy bodies, of such as I had the strength to move, a quart pot full of water and feather being the same in my hand.*[23]

SUMMARY

This patient presented with an acute gastrointestinal illness followed by the neurologic symptoms, paresthesias, abnormal taste, and paradoxical perception of heat and cold. The symptoms are characteristic of ciguatera poisoning. These occurred shortly after she ate grouper. She was treated initially with gabapentin and then with a mannitol infusion with marked improvement.

IMPORTANT POINTS

- The diagnosis of ciguatera poisoning is made clinically in persons who develop gastrointestinal and neurologic symptoms shortly after eating seafood. The neurologic symptoms are characterized by paradoxical sensations, metallic taste, lassitude, tooth pain, and paresthesias.
- Ciguatera poisoning is the most common seafood poisoning in the world. The disease is caused by cigua toxins that activate voltage-gated sodium channels in nerves. The toxin is produced by dinoflagellate-infected fish, including grouper, barracuda, and snapper.
- The diagnosis is made clinically, especially by the history. The toxins can be detected by ELISA, but this test is not commercially available.
- There is currently no method to prevent the disease.
- The treatment of ciguatera poisoning consists of intravenous infusions of mannitol or saline solutions. The symptoms improve with sodium channel blockers, gabapentin, or other pain modulators.
- The prognosis is usually good in ciguatera poisoning, but fatalities can occur.

REFERENCES

1. Sims JK. A theoretical discourse of the pharmacology of toxic marine ingestions. *Ann Emerg Med.* 1987;16(9):1006–1015.
2. Levine DZ. Ciguatera: current concepts. *J Am Osteopath Assoc.* 1995;95(3):193–198.
3. Bagnis R. Concerning a fatal case of ciguatera poisoning in the Tuamotu Islands. *Clin Toxicol.* 1970;3:579–583.
4. Rakita RM. Ciguatera poisoning. *J Travel Med.* 1995;2:252–254.
5. Sozzi G, Marotta P, Aldeghi D, et al. Polyneuropathy secondary to ciguatoxin poisoning. *Ital J Neurol Sci.* 1988;9:491–495.
6. Stommel EW, Jenkyn LR, Parsonnet J. Another case of polymyositis after ciguatera toxin exposure. *Arch Neurol.* 1993;50:571.
7. Cameron J, Capra MF. The basis of the paradoxical disturbance of temperature perception in ciguatera poisoning. *J Toxicol Clin Toxicol.* 1993;31:571–579.
8. Cameron J, Flowers AE, Capra MF. Modification of the peripheral nerve disturbance in ciguatera poisoning in rats with lidocaine. *Muscle Nerve.* 1993;16:782–786.
9. Bidard JN, Vijverberg HP, Frelin C, et al. Ciguatoxin is a novel type of Na+ channel toxin. *J Biol Chem.* 1984;259:8353–8357.
10. Cameron J, Flowers AE, Capra MF. Electrophysiological studies on ciguatera poisoning in man (Part II). *J Neurol Sci.* 1991;101(1):93–97.
11. Fleming LE, Baden DG, Ayyar RA, et al. A pilot study of a new ELISA test for ciguatoxin in humans. *Bull Soc Pathol Exot.* 1992;85:508–509.
12. Palafox NA, Jain LG, Pinano AZ, et al. Successful treatment of ciguatera fish poisoning with intravenous mannitol. *JAMA.* 1988;259:2740–2742.
13. Palafox NA. Review of the clinical use of intravenous mannitol with ciguatera fish poisoning from 1988 to 1992. *Bull Soc Pathol Exot.* 1992;85:423–424.
14. Blythe DG, De Sylva DP, Fleming LE, et al. Clinical experience with i.v. Mannitol in the treatment of ciguatera. *Bull Soc Pathol Exot.* 1991;85:425–426.
15. Friedman MA, Fernandez M, Backer LC, Dickey RW, et al. An updated review of ciguatera fish poisoning: clinical, environmental, epidemiological, environmental, and public health management. *Mar Drugs.* 2017;15(3):72. https://doi.org/10.3390/md15030072.

16. Schnorf H, Taurarii M, Cundy T. Ciguatera fish poisoning: a double-blind randomized trial of mannitol therapy. *Neurology.* 2002;58(6):873–880.
17. Perez CM, Vasquez PA, Perret CF. Treatment of ciguatera poisoning with gabapentin. *N Engl J Med.* 2001;344(9):692–693.
18. Bagnis R, Kuberski T, Laugier S. Clinical observations on 3,009 cases of ciguatera (fish poisoning) in the South Pacific. *Am J Trop Med Hyg.* 1979;28:1067–1073.
19. Lewis RJ. Ciguatera (fish poisoning). In: Williamson JA, Fenner PF, Burnett JW, Rifkin J, eds. *Venomous and Poisonous Marine Animals: A Medical and Biological Handbook.* Sydney, Australia: New South Wales University Press; 1996:347–353.
20. Fenner P, Lewis R. Ciguatera (fish poisoning). In: Rose MR, Griggs RC, eds. *Channelopathies of the Nervous System.* Oxford, England: Butterworth-Heinemann; 2001:295–307.
21. Hughes JM, Merson MH. Current concepts of fish and shellfish poisoning. *N Eng J Med.* 1976;295(20):1117–1120.
22. Teitelbaum J, Zatorre RJ, Carpenter S, et al. Neurologic sequelae of domoic acid intoxication due to the ingestion of contaminated mussels. *N Engl J Med.* 1990;322(25):1781–1787.
23. Mills AR, Passmore R. Pelagic paralysis. *Lancet.* 1988;1(8578): 161–164.
24. Halstead BW. *Poisonous and Venomous Marine Animals of the World.* Princeton, NJ: Darwin Press; 1988.
25. Martin D. *Farther Than Any Man: The Rise and Fall of Captain James Cook.* New York, NY: Washington Square Press; 2001.
26. Doherty MJ. Captain Cook on poison fish. *Neurology.* 2005;65: 1788–1791.

43 CASE

A Woman With a Kingly Disease

A 34-year-old woman was admitted to the hospital with nausea, vomiting, abdominal pain, and a weight loss of 3 weeks' duration. She developed weakness of the lower extremities associated with tingling at the tips of her toes 2 days prior to evaluation. She lost all feeling in the lower extremities on the day of admission, and this gradually progressed upward to the chest. She did not have incontinence of urine or stools.

Past medical history was remarkable for a traumatic brain injury with resultant bifrontal partial lobectomy, which left her with a severe craniofacial deformity and a left eye prosthesis.

Review of systems was negative for headache, neck pain, and problems swallowing or speaking. She had no fever, chills, cough, chest pain, or shortness of breath but had abdominal pain, nausea, and vomiting a few minutes after eating for the last week. Family history was noncontributory.

She was alert, awake, and oriented. There were frontal cranial deformities. Cranial nerve examination revealed the right pupil to be normal and reactive to light and accommodation; there was a left-side eye prosthesis; extraocular movements were intact on the right; there was no facial, palate, or tongue weakness. Strength in the upper extremities was 4/5 proximally and 4−/5 distally bilaterally, and both lower extremities were 0/5. Reflexes were absent all over. There were no Babinski signs. Sensory examination revealed loss of pinprick sensation to the waist and loss of vibration and position senses in both legs in the feet and ankles.

Cervical and thoracic MRI were normal. In the hospital, she received IV fluids and metoclopramide HCl. Five days after admission her arms weakened, and she became quadriparetic, reportedly became confused and disoriented, and developed respiratory failure. She was intubated and transferred to the ICU.

WHAT IS THE DIFFERENTIAL DIAGNOSIS?

The differential diagnosis of a patient with acute paralysis includes myelopathy, which could be suggested in this patient because of the confusing sensory findings, but there were no Babinski signs or incontinence, and her spinal MRI was negative. The sensory findings are against a motor neuron disease such as polio or amyotrophic lateral sclerosis.

Disturbance of a neuromuscular transmission, particularly botulism, could present acutely but usually causes large pupils. This patient's pupil was normal. The sensory findings, areflexia, and lack of extraocular involvement were all against myasthenia gravis. There were no cholinergic signs to suggest organophosphate poisoning. Myopathies, such as those that cause rhabdomyolysis, like metabolic disorders or from toxins, as well as polymyositis and infectious myositis, are also unlikely because of the areflexia and the sensory findings. In summary, this patient appeared to have a rapidly progressive acute polyneuropathy, such as Guillain–Barré syndrome (GBS), and the differential diagnosis also includes porphyria, as well as arsenic intoxication (Fig. 43-1).

WHAT TESTS SHOULD BE DONE?

Laboratory studies revealed a white blood count of 18.7 thou/mm^3 (normal, 5–10 thou/mm^3), hematocrit 30.3% (normal, 40%–54%), mean corpuscular volume 73 fL (normal, 80–95 fL), hemoglobin 9.5 g/dL (normal, 14–18 g/dL); chemistries were within normal limits. Serum creatine kinase was 50 IU/L; L-lactate dehydrogenase, 810 IU/L; liver function tests were normal except for mildly elevated alkaline phosphatase at 196 IU/L (normal, 39–117 IU/L); erythrocyte sedimentation rate was 28 (normal, <30). No infectious process was found. HIV antibody and hepatitis screenings were negative. Serum immunofixation electrophoresis revealed increased polyclonal IgG. Quantitative immunoglobulins were within normal limits. She received IgG infusions 2 g/kg over 4 days.

AN EMG TEST WAS PERFORMED

Motor Nerve Studies

Nerve and Site	Latency(ms)	Amplitude (mV)	Conduction Velocity (m/s)
Peroneal Nerve L.	**Normal ≤ 5.7**	**Normal ≥ 3**	**Normal ≥ 40**
Ankle	4.1	**2**	–
Fibular head	10.9	**2**	41
Knee	13.0	**2**	50
Tibial Nerve L.	**Normal ≤ 5.3**	**Normal ≥ 4**	**Normal ≥ 40**
Ankle	4.1	6	–
Pop. fossa	13.4	6	40
Median Nerve L.	**Normal ≤ 4.2**	**Normal ≥ 6**	**Normal ≥ 50**
Wrist	3.5	6	–
Elbow	6.9	6	53

Motor Nerve Studies—cont'd

Ulnar Nerve L.	Normal ≤ 3.6	Normal ≥ 8	Normal ≥ 50
Wrist	2.6	10	–
Below elbow	5.6	10	60
Above elbow	7.5	10	63
Axilla	9.6	10	67
Median Nerve R.	**Normal ≤ 4.2**	**Normal ≥ 6**	**Normal ≥ 50**
Wrist	3.7	**5**	–
Elbow	7.4	**5**	50

Nerve and Site	Latency (ms)	Amplitude (mV)	Conduction Velocity (m/s)
Ulnar Nerve R.	**Normal ≤ 3.6**	**Normal ≥ 8**	**Normal ≥ 50**
Wrist	2.7	**6**	–
Below elbow	5.7	**6**	60
Above elbow	7.5	**6**	67

Motor Nerve Studies—cont'd

Peroneal Nerve R.	Normal ≤ 5.7	Normal ≥ 3	Normal ≥ 40
Ankle	4.0	3	–
Fibular head	11.0	**2**	41
Knee	13.2	**2**	45

F-Wave and Tibial H-Reflex Studies

Nerve	Latency (ms)	Normal Latency ≤ (ms)
Peroneal nerve L.	**NR**	54
Tibial nerve L.	51.1	54
Median nerve L.	24.3	30
Ulnar nerve L.	25.5	30
Median nerve R.	25.4	30
Ulnar nerve R.	25.5	30
Peroneal nerve R.	46.6	54
H-reflex L.	**NR**	34
H-reflex R.	**NR**	34

NR, No response.

Sensory Nerve Studies

Nerve	Onset Latency (ms)	Normal Onset Latency ≤ (ms)	Peak Latency (ms)	Normal Peak Latency ≤ (ms)	Amp (μV)	Normal Amp ≥ (μV)	Conduction Velocity (m/s)	Normal Conduction Velocity ≥ (m/s)
Sural nerve L.	**3.7**	3.5	**4.2**	4.0	**3**	11	**38**	40
Ulnar nerve L.	2.2	2.6	2.7	3.1	14	13	55	50
Median nerve L.	2.6	2.6	3.1	3.1	21	20	50	50
Median palmar L.	0.8	1.0	1.3	1.5	40	30	86	50
Ulnar nerve R.	1.9	2.6	2.4	3.1	**8**	13	63	50
Median nerve R.	2.4	2.6	2.9	3.1	**15**	20	54	50

EMG Data

Muscle	Insrt Activity	Fibs	Pos Waves	Fasc	Amp	Dur	Poly	Pattern
Vastus lateralis R.	**Inc**	**2+**	**2+**	None	[a]	[a]	None	**Absent**
Tibialis anterior R.	**Inc**	**2+**	**2+**	None	[a]	[a]	None	**Absent**
Gastrocnemius R.	**Inc**	**2+**	**2+**	None	[a]	[a]	None	**Absent**
Deltoid R.	Norm	None	None	None	Norm	Norm	None	Full
Biceps brachii R.	Norm	None	None	None	Norm	Norm	None	**Red**
Flexor carpi radialis R.	Norm	None	None	None	Norm	Norm	None	**Red**
First dorsal interosseous R.	**Inc**	None	None	None	Norm	Norm	None	**Red**
Vastus lateralis L.	**Inc**	**2+**	**2+**	None	[a]	[a]	None	**Absent**
Tibialis anterior L.	**Inc**	**1+**	**1+**	None	[a]	[a]	None	**Absent**
Deltoid L.	Norm	None	None	None	Norm	Norm	None	Full
Biceps brachii L.	Norm	None	None	None	Norm	Norm	None	**Red**
Flexor carpi radialis L.	Norm	None	None	None	Norm	Norm	None	**Red**
First dorsal interosseus L.	**Inc**	None	None	None	Norm	Norm	None	**Red**
Gastrocnemius L.	**Inc**	**2+**	**2+**	None	[a]	[a]	None	**Absent**

[a]No motor units were recruited.

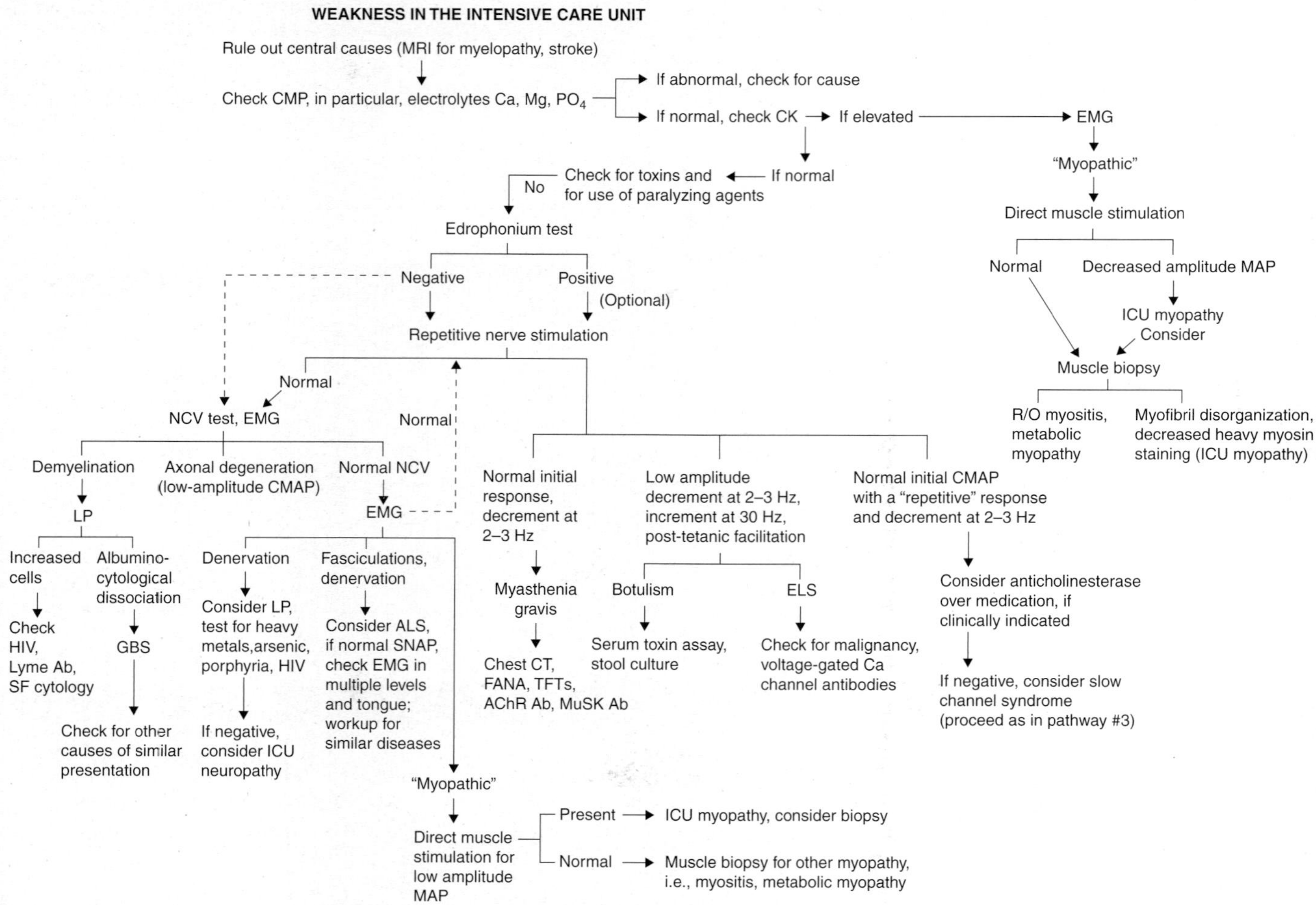

FIG. 43-1 Diagram of workup of patients who develop weakness in the intensive care unit. *Ab*, Antibody; *AChR*, acetylcholine receptor; *ALS*, amyotrophic lateral sclerosis; *Ca*, calcium; *CK*, creatine kinase; *ELS*, Eaton–Lambert syndrome; *FANA*, fluorescent antinuclear antibody; *GBS*, Guillain-Barré syndrome; *ICU*, intensive care unit; *LP*, lumbar puncture; *Mg*, magnesium; *MuSK*, muscle-specific kinase; *NCV*, nerve conduction velocity; *NTE*, neurotoxic esterase; PO_4, phosphate; *R/O*, rule out; *SF*, spinal fluid; *TFT*, thyroid function test.

WHAT WERE THE EMG FINDINGS?

Nerve conduction velocities, CMAPs, latencies, and amplitudes were normal in the upper and lower extremities, except for low-amplitude peroneal, right median, and ulnar CMAPs. She had absent H-reflexes and low-amplitude SNAPs of the sural nerve and right ulnar nerve. F-responses were normal in latency and persistence, except for the peroneal nerve on the left, where no response could be obtained. H-reflexes were absent.

Needle electromyography showed denervation potentials in both lower extremities. There was markedly reduced motor unit action potentials recruitment in both upper and lower extremities.

In summary, this electromyographic study reveals a predominantly axonal, mainly motor neuropathy in spite of the fairly normal amplitude of most CMAPs. She had low amplitude of some SNAPs and denervation potentials. There were no prolonged distal latencies, decreased persistence, prolonged F-waves, nerve conduction slowing, conduction block, or temporal dispersion.

Arsenic poisoning, porphyria, and acute severe vasculitic neuropathy are considerations. The EMG findings are against classic GBS; however, an axonal form is a possibility to be considered. The gastrointestinal symptoms and abdominal pain suggest porphyria.

WHAT WOULD BE DONE NEXT?

Cryoglobulins and hepatitis profile were normal. A lumbar puncture showed no cells and a protein of 45 mg/dL with normal sugar. A 24-hour urine test was negative for arsenic. Her urine appeared normal initially but became a dark tan color with light exposure (Fig. 43-2). A 24-hour urine porphyrin test showed aminolevulinic acid (ALA) of 8.7 (normal, <5), porphobilinogen of 16 μG (normal, <2 μG), uroporphyrins high at 458 (normal, <45), coproporphyrins high at 373 μG/24 hours (normal, <110 μG/24 hours).

Red cell porphyrin levels were high at 282 μg/dL (normal, 16–60 μg/dL). Coproporphyrin I in stool was 1200 μg/24 hours (normal, 0–495 μg/24 hours), coproporphyrin III was 1800 μg/

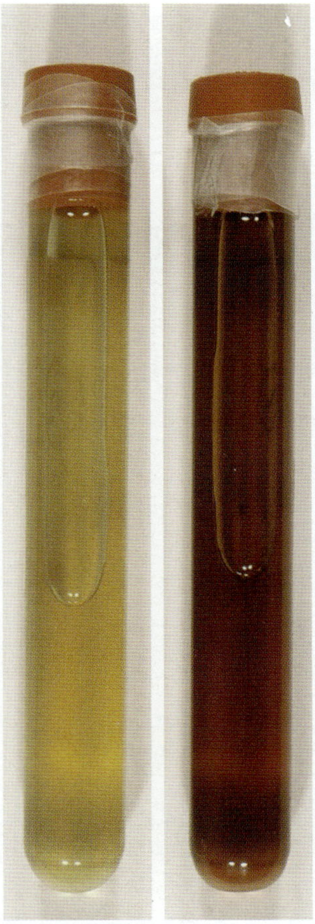

FIG. 43-2 Urine of patient immediately after voiding (*left*) and after 1 hour of exposure to light (*right*); notice the characteristic port-wine color.

24 hours (normal, 0–399 µg/24 hours), and protoporphyrin was 800 µg/24 hours (normal, 0–1499 µg/24 hours). Coproporphyrinogen oxidase level was not measured.

BASED ON THE FINDINGS, WHAT IS THE MOST LIKELY DIAGNOSIS?

The elevation of urine coproporphyrins and uroporphyrins indicates the patient has coproporphyria. She received 300 g of glucose a day, was properly hydrated, and received 4 daily treatments of hematin 3 g/kg. The patient recovered slowly and was transferred to a rehabilitation hospital.

DISCUSSION

This patient has a form of hepatic porphyria. Porphyrias are a group of metabolic disorders affecting the synthesis of heme, an oxygen carrier essential for aerobic metabolism and adenosine triphosphate production. These disorders are of either erythropoietic or hepatic origin, depending on the site of the enzymatic defect. Hepatic porphyrias can cause neurologic disorders, particularly peripheral neuropathies, psychosis, and autonomic dysfunction.

The term *porphyria* comes from the Greek *porphuros*, which means purple, to describe the color of urine.[1] (Table 43-1 indicates the different enzyme deficiencies and the laboratory findings in the various hepatic porphyrias.)

The synthesis of heme starts with the production of δ ALA by the combination of coenzyme A and glycine in a reaction that is catalyzed by the enzyme ALA synthetase. This is the rate-limiting step of heme formation due to a feedback inhibition. ALA synthetase is inhibited by heme concentration in the liver and also by pyridoxine deficiency. Feedback inhibition does not occur in red cells.

Heme is required for the synthesis for several proteins, particularly the cytochrome P450, and acute attacks of porphyria are associated with an increased production of heme products. Upon activation of the P450 system, for example, by P450-inducing drugs or hormones, heme is incorporated into the hepatic cytochromes, depleting its reservoir, and increasing ALA synthetase activity with excretion of porphyrins and attacks of porphyria. These also occur with ingestion of hexachlorobenzene and with lead intoxication, causing neurologic manifestations. The pathway is activated during increased heme synthesis. Patients with porphyria, thus, overproduce the precursors which are neurotoxic and excreted in urine and feces. Oxidation of these products gives the urine the characteristic port-wine color.

The excretion of the various products determines the diagnosis of different porphyrias. The enzymatic pathway of heme synthesis and its defects are shown in Fig. 43-3.

It is important to recognize that many subjects who have enzymatic defects that cause porphyria never develop the disease.

The neurologic manifestations of the hepatic porphyrias include a predominantly motor neuropathy, psychosis, anxiety, abdominal pain, and autonomic dysfunction.[1,2] The weakness could be asymmetric and sometimes affect the arms more than the legs. A sensory deficit in the anterior chest (bathing trunk) can be seen. Some patients develop the syndrome of inappropriate antidiuretic hormone (SIADH).[3–5]

The clinical characteristic of the neuropathy is similar in the various hepatic porphyrias; pathologically there is axonal degeneration with secondary demyelination.[2] Electrophysiologic tests show low-amplitude motor action potentials and SNAPs with evidence of denervation.[6,7]

The hepatic porphyrias are as follows:

- *ALA dehydratase deficiency* is the only autosomal recessive disease presenting in infancy with weakness caused by a defect in chromosome 9.[1,8,9]
- *Acute intermittent porphyria*, the most common form of porphyria, is caused by a partial deficiency of porphobilinogen deaminase. The disease has an autosomal dominant inheritance caused by a defect in the short arm of chromosome 11.[10] This disease causes increased ALA and coproporphyrins in the urine but not in the feces.
- *Hereditary coproporphyria* is caused by the deficiency of coproporphyrinogen oxidase from a defect in chromosome 3.[11,12] This is a very rare condition.
- *Variegate porphyria* is also an autosomal dominant disease, in which the attacks of weakness occur with only a 50% deficiency of protoporphyrinogen oxidase. This is a rare

TABLE 43-1 Predominant Patterns of Heme Precursors in Urine and Feces in Patients With Porphyric Neuropathies

Diseases	Gene Derivative	Enzyme Deficiency	Urine[a]	Feces[b]
ALA dehydratase deficiency	9q34	ALA dehydratase	ALA coproporphyrins	None
ALA intermittent porphyria	11q23	Porphobilinogen deaminase	ALA porphobilinogen uroporphyrins	None
Hereditary coproporphyrins	3q12	Coproporphyrinogen oxidase	ALA porphobilinogen uroporphyrins coproporphyrins	Increased coproporphyrins over protoporphyrins
Variegate porphyria	1q21–23	Protoporphyrinogen oxidase	ALA porphobilinogen uroporphyrins coproporphyrins	Increased protoporphyrins over coproporphyrins

[a]Auto-oxidation products are common in the urine and result in confusing profiles that may vary.
[b]Fecal porphyrins provide the best differential clue for the diagnosis of variegate porphyria and hereditary coproporphyria.
ALA, Aminolevulinic acid.
Modified with permission from Albers JW, Fink JK. Porphyric neuropathy. *Muscle Nerve.* 2004;30:419.

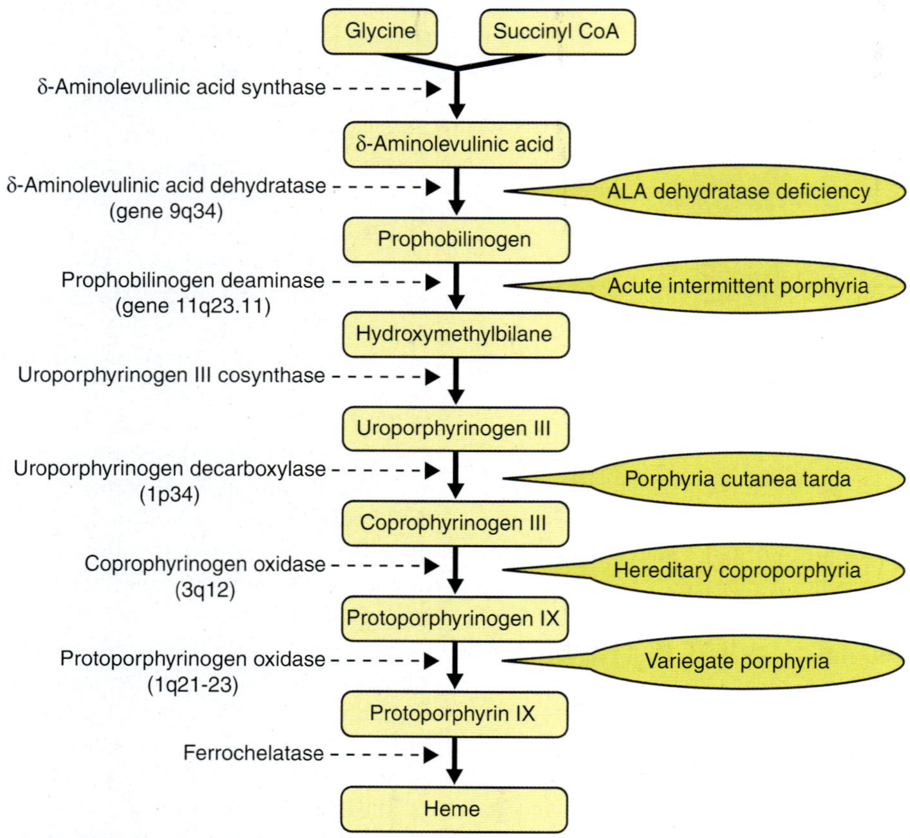

FIGURE 43-3 Pathway of heme synthesis, the diseases associated with enzyme deficiencies (*right*), and their genetic defects (*left*).

autosomal dominant condition that occurs mainly in South Africa and European countries.[13] The genetic defect is located in chromosome 1q21–23.

Historically, George William Fredrick, King of England from 1760 to 1811 (Fig. 43-4), had episodes of madness, abdominal pain, constipation, weakness, and dark urine, likely caused by porphyria.[14–16] (The film *The Madness of King George* shows the history of the king and his attacks.)

The illness (the "royal malady") can be traced to several members of the family of Mary, Queen of Scots. It had been suspected that King George signed the Stamp Act provoking the American Revolution during a porphyric attack.

Another important historical note: the legends of vampires may have arisen from individuals with cutaneous porphyria having severe photosensitivity and increased fragility of the skin with bullae and hypertrichosis. From these the affected person developed an aversion to light and only went out at nighttime.[2] There is no evidence, however, that the most famous vampire, Count Dracula Vlad (the "Impaler") Tepez of Walenchia, suffered from porphyria.

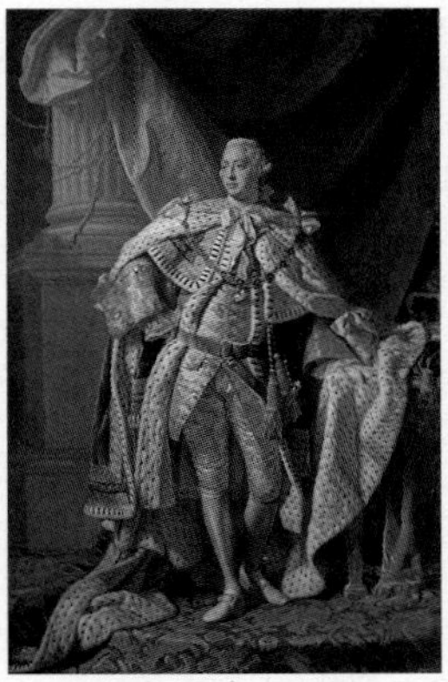

FIG. 43-4 King George III reigned in England from 1760 to 1820 and had porphyria.

WHAT IS THE TREATMENT OF PORPHYRIA?

The management of porphyria consists in avoiding drugs that might precipitate attacks, particularly those that induce the P450 system[17–19] (Table 43-2).

The treatment includes proper hydration and adequate carbohydrate intake of about 300–500 grams of glucose per day.[19,20] Hematin decreases the production of porphyrins due to feedback inhibition, and this can be used in doses of 1–4 mg/kg a day for 4 days to 2 weeks.[21,22]

Patients should also be observed and treated properly if they develop SIADH. Management, otherwise, consists of physical therapy, management of dysautonomia, and respiratory assistance, if necessary, similar to GBS. The number of attacks can be reduced by using Givosiran, a small interferon RNA molecule targeting ALA synthetase that is given subcutaneously every month[23] and also elimination of precipitating factors.

TABLE 43-2 Examples of Medications and Substances Reported to Be Potentially Safe, Potentially Unsafe, and Unsafe for Use in Patients With Hepatic Porphyria

Potentially Safe[a]	Potentially Unsafe	Unsafe
Acetaminophen	Agents including cytochrome P450	Alcohol
Acyclovir	Alkylating agents	Barbiturates
Amantadine	Chloroquine	Calcium channel blockers
Aspirin	Clonidine	Carbamazepine
Atropine	Erythromycin	Chloramphenicol
Beta blockers	Estrogens	Chlorpropamide
Bromides	Hydralazine	Clonazepam
Chloral hydrate	Ketamine	Danazol
Chlorpromazine	Lidocaine	Dapsone
Cimetidine	Methyldopa	Ergots
Colchicine	Nalidixic acid	Felbamate
Dopamine	Nortriptyline	Griseofulvin
Fentanyl	Pentazocine	Halothane
Gabapentin	Phenoxybenzamine	Ketamine
Glucocorticoids	Rifampin	Meprobamate
Haloperidol	Spironolactone	Phenytoin
Insulin	Theophylline	Primidone
Narcotic analgesics		Progestins
Neostigmine		Succinimide
Penicillin		Sulfonamides
Phenothiazine		Theophylline
Procaine		Tolazamide
Propofol		Tolbutamide
Propranolol		Tranquilizers
Reserpine		Trimethadione
Serotonin reuptake inhibitors		Valproic acid
Streptomycin		
Tetracycline		
Vitamins		

[a]Numerous medications are reported to precipitate acute attacks of porphyria, and all medications should be used with caution, weighing the potential risk/benefit ratio, considering alternative treatment choices, and consulting current sources of drug information.
From Albers JW, Fink JK. Porphyric neuropathy. *Muscle Nerve*. 2004; 30:419.

SUMMARY

This patient presented with acute paralysis resembling GBS; electrophysiologic tests revealed an axonal neuropathy. She was diagnosed as having coproporphyria, which was treated, and she recovered slowly. Porphyria should be considered in the diagnosis of an acute paralytic illness.

IMPORTANT POINTS

- The porphyrias are hereditary disorders of the metabolism of heme. Patients with hepatic porphyrias may have attacks of paralysis, psychosis, and abdominal pain (some also have skin lesions). These attacks are precipitated by stress, hormones, or drugs that induce the P450 system. The metabolic blockade inhibits the production of heme, which is important in the oxidative metabolism and adenosine triphosphate synthesis.
- The paralysis in porphyria is caused by an axonal neuropathy with secondary demyelination, resembling GBS. The neuropathy can be asymmetric, sometimes with more severe weakness in the arms.
- The diagnosis of porphyria is made by measurement of porphyrins in urine and feces.
- The treatment consists of avoidance of drugs that can precipitate an attack, along with proper hydration, carbohydrate intake, and hematin (heme) infusions.

REFERENCES

1. Albers JW. Porphyric neuropathy. In: Mendell JR, Kissel JT, Cornblath DR, eds. *Diagnosis and Management of Peripheral Nerve Disorders*. New York, NY: Oxford University Press; 2001: 344–366.
2. Albers JW, Fink JK. Porphyric neuropathy. *Muscle Nerve*. 2004;30: 410–422.
3. Becker DM, Kramer S. The neurological manifestations of porphyria: a review. *Medicine (Baltimore)*. 1977;56:411–423.
4. Hierons R. Acute intermittent porphyria. *Postgrad Med J*. 1967;43: 605–608.
5. Sorenson EJ, Albers JW. Neurological manifestations of porphyria. In: Aminoff MH, Boller F, Swaab DF, eds. *Handbook of*

Clinical Neurology. vol 70. Amsterdam, Netherlands: Elsevier; 1998:299–312.
6. Albers JW, Robertson WC Jr, Daube JR. Electrodiagnostic findings in acute porphyric neuropathy. *Muscle Nerve*. 1978;1: 292–296.
7. Flugel KA, Druschky KF. Electromyogram and nerve conduction in patients with acute intermittent porphyria. *J Neurol*. 1977;214: 267–279.
8. Adams A. *Update on Porphyria: Blood Line, Acute Porphyria, Drug Information*. Available from: http://www.dotpharmacy.com/uporphy.html.
9. Sassa S, Kappas A. Molecular aspects of the inherited porphyrias. *J Intern Med*. 2000;247:169–178.
10. Kauppinen R, Mustajoki S, Pihlaja H, et al. Acute intermittent porphyria in Finland: 19 mutations in the porphobilinogen deaminase gene. *Hum Mol Genet*. 1995;4:215–222.
11. Grandchamp B, Lamoril J, Puy H. Molecular abnormalities of coproporphyrinogen oxidase in patients with hereditary coproporphyria. *J Bioenerg Biomembr*. 1995;27:215–219.
12. Cacheux V, Martasek P, Fougerousse F, et al. Localization of the human coproporphyrinogen oxidase gene to chromosome band 3q12. *Hum Genet*. 1994;94:557–559.
13. Kirsch RE, Meissner PN, Hift RJ. Variegate porphyria. *Semin Liver Dis*. 1998;18:33–41.
14. MacAlpine I, Hunter R. The "insanity" of King George 3d: a classic case of porphyria. *Br Med J*. 1966;5479:65–71.
15. MacAlpine I, Hunter R, Rimington C. Porphyria in the royal houses of Stuart, Hanover, and Prussia: a follow-up study of George 3d's illness. *Br Med J*. 1968;1:7–18.
16. MacAlpine I, Hunter R, Rimington C. Royal malady. *Br Med J*. 1968;1:705–706.
17. Elder G. Welsh Medicines Information Center. *Acute Porphyrias: Drugs That Are Considered to be Safe for Use in the Acute Porphyrias*. Available from: http://www.ukmi.nhs.uk.
18. Laiwah AC, McColl KE. Management of attacks of acute porphyria. *Drugs*. 1987;34:604–616.
19. Moore MR, McColl KE. Therapy of the acute porphyrias. *Clin Biochem*. 1989;22:181–188.
20. Ellefson RD. Porphyrinogens, porphyrins, and the porphyrias. *Mayo Clin Proc*. 1982;57:454–458.
21. Lamon JM, Frykholm BC, Hess RA, Tschudy DP. Hematin therapy for acute porphyria. *Medicine (Baltimore)*. 1979;58:252–269.
22. McColl KE, Moore MR, Thompson GG, Goldberg A. Treatment with haematin in acute hepatic porphyria. *QJ Med*. 1981;50: 161–174.
23. Zhao L, Wang X, Zhang X, Liu X, et al. Therapeutic strategies for acute intermittent porphyria. *Intractable Rare Dis Res*. 2020;9(4):205–216. https://doi.org/10.5582/irdr.2020.03089.

A Myasthenic Woman With Persistent Weakness

An 80-year-old woman was admitted to another hospital because of acute respiratory failure from myasthenia gravis (MG), diagnosed 2 years before with a positive edrophonium test and elevated acetylcholine receptor antibody titers. She was treated with corticosteroids early with improvement. However, her condition had deteriorated recently after a respiratory infection. She was intubated and maintained on methylprednisolone 60 mg every 6 hours and pyridostigmine 60 mg every 4 hours. She was transferred after 10 days because of a lack of improvement.

Past medical history included hypertension and a mastectomy secondary to carcinoma of the breast.

On examination the patient was intubated and on respiratory assistance. She was afebrile; blood pressure and pulse were normal. She was alert, and her cranial nerves were normal without ptosis or ophthalmoplegia. There was prominent drooling. Muscle strength showed neck flexors 2+/5, shoulders 3/5, biceps and triceps 4/5, grip 4/5, hand 4/5, iliopsoas 3−/5, and quadriceps 4/5. No clear fatigue was detected on repetitive testing. Reflexes were 1+ at the brachioradialis and ankles, trace at the knees and biceps, and 2+ at the triceps equally in both sides; she had normal sensory examination. There were no Babinski signs.

An edrophonium test produced no obvious improvement.

She received plasma exchange for 5 consecutive days without significant benefit.

WHAT IS THE DIFFERENTIAL DIAGNOSIS?

This patient had been properly diagnosed with MG. She then developed severe weakness, was intubated, and received high doses of corticosteroids. She was transferred for evaluation and plasma exchanges because of a lack of improvement.

The causes of weakness in the ICU are outlined in Table 44-1 (see Fig. 43-1 in Case 43 for the workup of patients who develop weakness in the ICU). The generalized weakness, in this case, suggests that she was in a myasthenic crisis or that she was overmedicated with pyridostigmine which might explain the drooling. The dose, however, was low, and she did not improve when it was discontinued afterward. Edrophonium produced no improvement.

The decreased reflexes could suggest another disorder or neuromuscular transmission, such as Eaton–Lambert myasthenic syndrome or botulism, but she had excessive salivation and no pupillary abnormalities, and the diagnosis of MG was well documented. The lack of long tract signs and fasciculations was against amyotrophic lateral sclerosis; the presence of reflexes was against Guillain–Barré syndrome and similar neuropathies, including critical illness polyneuropathy (CIP).[1] There was no history of exposure, and she did not have muscle spasms or increased sweating to suggest organophosphate poisoning.

Myopathies appear to be a good possibility; among them, polymyositis, inclusion body myositis, and acid maltase deficiency can present with acute respiratory failure. Other possibilities include electrolyte imbalance and hypophosphatemia. Finally, critical illness myopathy (CIM) should be considered because she had been intubated and received high doses of corticosteroids. Although she did not receive paralyzing agents, MG itself could have caused weakness and predisposed her to CIM, which can also occur in patients on corticosteroids who are not receiving paralyzing agents.[2]

WHAT OTHER TESTS SHOULD BE DONE?

Serum creatine kinase (CK) was 260 IU/L (normal, 80–200 IU/L); a complete blood chemistry profile and complete blood count were normal, except the hematocrit was 28% (normal, 35%–45%).

AN EMG TEST WAS PERFORMED

Motor Nerve Studies

Nerve and Site	Latency (ms)	Amplitude (mV)	Conduction Velocity (m/s)
Peroneal Nerve R.	**Normal ≤ 5.7**	**Normal ≥ 3**	**Normal ≥ 40**
Ankle	4.9	**0.7**	–
Fibular head	11.3	**0.7**	41
Peroneal Nerve R.*	**Normal ≤ 4.6**	**Normal ≥ 3**	**Normal ≥ 40**
Fibular head	**11.0**	**0.8***	–
Knee	**13.3**	**0.8***	43
Tibial Nerve L.	**Normal ≤ 5.3**	**Normal ≥ 4**	**Normal ≥ 40**
Ankle	5.3	**2**	–
Pop. fossa	17.9	**2**	41
Ulnar Nerve R.	**Normal ≤ 3.6**	**Normal ≥ 8**	**Normal ≥ 50**
Wrist	3.4	**5**	–
Below elbow	6.4	**5**	53
Above elbow	8.4	**5**	60

*Needle recording at tibialis ant. muscle. The amplitude was equal during nerve and muscle stimulation.

Motor Nerve Studies—cont'd

Nerve and Site	Latency (ms)	Amplitude (mV)	Conduction Velocity (m/s)
Median Nerve R.	**Normal ≤ 4.2**	**Normal ≥ 6**	**Normal ≥ 50**
Wrist	3.1	**1**	–
Elbow	7.5	**1**	58

F-Wave Studies

Nerve	Latency (ms)	Normal Latency ≤ (ms)
Peroneal nerve R.	53.6	54
Tibial nerve L.	52.8	54
Ulnar nerve R.	28.9	30
Median nerve R.	29.2	30

Sensory Nerve Studies

Nerve	Onset Latency (ms)	Normal Onset Latency ≤ (ms)	Peak Latency (ms)	Normal Peak Latency ≤ (ms)	Amp (μV)	Normal Amp ≥ (μV)	Conduction Velocity (m/s)	Normal Conduction Velocity ≥ (m/s)
Sural nerve R.	3.3	3.5	3.8	4.0	15	11	42	40
Ulnar nerve R.	2.2	2.6	2.7	3.1	14	13	55	50
Median nerve R.	2.5	2.6	3.0	3.1	23	20	52	50

Repetitive stimulation R. ulnar nerve was normal.

EMG Data

Muscle	Insrt Activity	Fibs	Pos Waves	Fasc	Amp	Dur	Poly	Pattern
Deltoid R.	Norm	None	None	None	**Red**	**Brief**	**Many**	Full
Biceps brachii R.	Norm	None	None	None	**Red**	**Brief**	**Many**	Full
Triceps R.	Norm	None	None	None	**Red**	**Brief**	**Few**	Full
First dorsal interosseous R.	Norm	None	None	None	Norm	Norm	None	Full
Iliopsoas R.	Norm	None	None	None	**Red**	**Brief**	**Few**	Full
Tensor fasciae latae R.	Norm	None	None	None	**Red**	**Brief**	**Few**	Full
Tibialis anterior R.*	Norm	None	None	None	Norm	Norm	None	Full
Gastrocnemius R.	Norm	None	None	None	Norm	Norm	None	Full

TABLE 44-1 Causes of Paralysis and Respiratory Failure Encountered in the Intensive Care Unit

Myelopathies
Amyotrophic lateral sclerosis and other motor neuron disorders
Myasthenia gravis and, rarely, Eaton–Lambert myasthenic syndrome and other myasthenic syndromes
Persistent pharmacological paralysis
Tick paralysis
Botulism
Organophosphate poisoning
Guillain–Barré syndrome
Toxic, vasculitic neuropathies (rarely)
Chronic inflammatory demyelinating polyneuropathy (rarely)
Porphyria
Critical illness neuropathy
Inflammatory myopathies
Toxic myopathies and other causes of rhabdomyolysis
Critical illness myopathy
Acid maltase deficiency
Muscular dystrophies, congenital myopathy, and mitochondrial myopathy
Endocrine and electrolyte imbalance

WHAT WERE THE EMG FINDINGS?

The test showed low-amplitude compound muscle action potentials (CMAPs) but normal sensory nerve action potentials (SNAPs), conduction velocities, latencies, and F-responses. H-reflexes were not tested. The needle test showed no denervation potentials but brief polyphasic motor unit action potentials in several muscles.

A repetitive stimulation test was normal. The CMAPs in the tibialis anterior muscle were of almost identical low amplitude during nerve and direct muscle stimulation, indicating a primary muscle disorder. In neuropathies the CMAPs examined with direct muscle stimulation are larger than those obtained with nerve stimulation[2,3] (Table 44-2).

WHAT SHOULD BE DONE?

A muscle biopsy of the quadriceps muscle showed a type II fiber smallness and patchy decreased staining on the ATPase; on the NADH-TR stain, there were moth-eaten fibers and pale centers. No necrosis, vasculitis, or inflammation was seen. Electromicroscopy showed fibers with disorganization of myofibrils and loss of thick filaments (Fig. 44-1).

TABLE 44-2 Electrophysiological Features Typical of the Neuromuscular Disorders That Develop in the Setting of Critical Illness

	Critical Illness Myopathy	Persistent Pharmacological Paralysis	Critical Illness Polyneuropathy
Nerve Conduction Studies			
SNAP amplitude	NL (occasionally ↓)	NL	↓ To absent
CMAP amplitude	↓ To absent	↓ To absent	↓ To absent
Repetitive nerve stimulation	NL	Decremental CMAP response	NL
Needle Electromyographic Studies			
Spontaneous activity	None to prominent	None	Usually; often prominent
MUP morphology	↓ Amplitude and duration	↓ Amplitude and duration	Normal (early): ↑ amplitude, duration, and polyphasia (later, after collateral sprouting)
MUP recruitment	Early full	Early full	Decreased
Direct muscle stimulation	Absent or ↑	Normal	Normal

CMAP, Compound muscle action potential; *MUP*, motor unit potential; *NL*, normal; *SNAP*, sensory nerve action potential; ↑, increased; ↓, decreased.

Modified from Bird SJ. Myopathies and disorders of neuromuscular transmission. In: Brown WF, Bolton CF, Aminoff MJ, eds. *Neuromuscular Function and Disease: Basic, Clinical and Electrodiagnostic Aspects*. Vol 2. Philadelphia, PA: *WB* Saunders; 2002:1509.

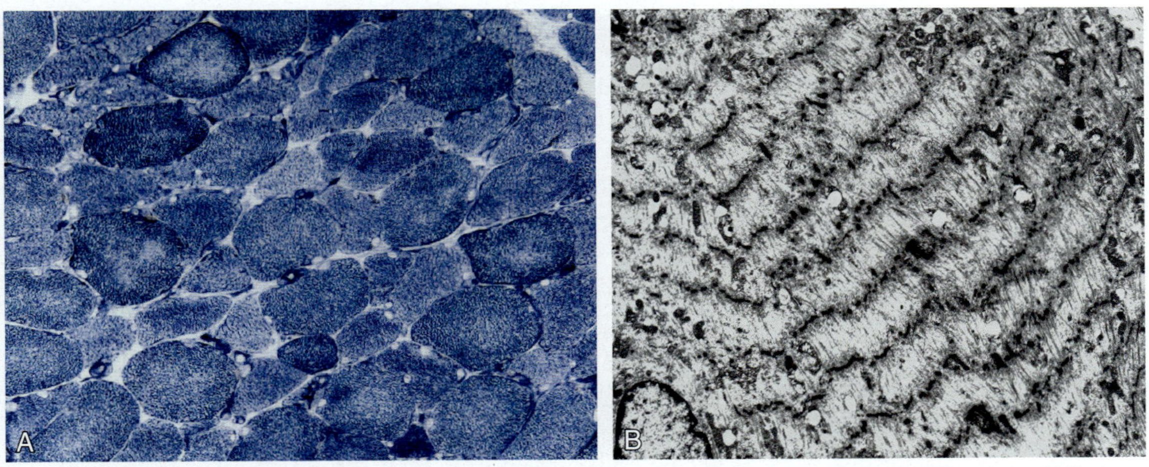

FIG. 44-1 A, Muscle biopsy showing muscle fiber atrophy and pale centers (NADH-TR stain, ×200). **B**, Electromicroscopy showing lack of thick filaments (×12,000).

It was concluded that this patient had CIM. Corticosteroids were tapered, and she showed some improvement but later developed sepsis and cardiac arrest and died; no autopsy was performed.

DISCUSSION

This patient developed weakness in the ICU. This can be caused by the primary disease that brought the patient to the ICU, such as in this case, MG, or the paralysis could be a complication of the treatment. ICU patients can develop prolonged weakness from immobilization with the use of paralyzing agents. In those the weakness improves upon removal of these medications, although the improvement could be delayed. They have normal serum CK values, and electrophysiologic testing shows evidence of decremental responses on repetitive nerve stimulation test.[4,5] CIP also develops in ICU causing severe weakness, and this is secondary to sepsis or systemic inflammatory response and is associated with severe axonal degeneration,[6] which is documented on EMG. (For diagnostic criteria of CIP, see Table 44-3.)

TABLE 44-3 Diagnostic Criteria for Critical Illness Polyneuropathy

1. The patient is critically ill (sepsis and multiple organ failure, systemic inflammatory response syndrome)
2. Difficulty weaning patient from ventilator after non-neuromuscular causes such as heart and lung disease have been excluded
3. Possible limb weakness
4. Electrophysiologic evidence of axonal motor and sensory polyneuropathy

These diagnostic criteria are now well established, but in certain circumstances, other acute axonal polyneuropathies, such as those due to thiamin deficiency, porphyria, etc., should be excluded.

Reprinted with permission from Bolton CF. Neuromuscular manifestations of critical illness. *Muscle Nerve*. 2005;32:148.

CIM, also called acute necrotizing myopathy of the intensive care, thick filament myopathy, and acute quadriplegic myopathy, was first reported in 1977 in a patient treated for status asthmaticus[7] and later in other similar cases.[8,9] It can also be seen in patients with other causes of respiratory failure, including MG,[10] as in this case. CIM occurs particularly in those receiving a total dose of at least 1 g of corticosteroids but sometimes also after lower doses.

CIM is characterized by proximal weakness and could have a mildly elevated CK. This helps to differentiate from rhabdomyolysis caused by infection or pharmacologic agents, in which the CK is much higher and there is prominent muscle fiber necrosis. Risk factors for CIM include the use of neuromuscular blocking agents and corticosteroids. This myopathy has been reported in 7% of patients undergoing liver transplantation.[11] In some, sepsis and the systemic inflammatory response may also play a role,[12] and patients could have both CIM and CIP.

The typical presentation of CIM is that of a patient who receives steroids in addition to neuromuscular blocking agents and is usually also septic. The weakness occurs fairly acutely, though it might be only mild in some, while others are severely affected and unable to be weaned off the ventilator.[13]

Electrophysiologic studies show normal SNAPs, decreased CMAP amplitude during direct muscle and nerve stimulation, and normal repetitive stimulation tests (see Table 44-2). Fibrillation potentials could sometimes be seen, and the motor unit potentials are of low amplitudes and duration.[14] (For diagnostic criteria of CIM, see Table 44-4.)

TABLE 44-4 Diagnostic Criteria of Critical Illness Myopathy[a]

Major Diagnostic Features	Supportive Features
1. Sensory nerve action potential amplitudes >80% of lower limit of normal in 2 or more nerves	1. Compound muscle action potential amplitudes <80% of lower limit of normal in 2 or more nerves without conduction block
2. Needle EMG with short-duration, low-amplitude motor unit potentials with early or normal full recruitment, with or without fibrillation potentials	2. Elevated serum muscle/cardiac enzymes, assessed in the first week of illness
3. Absence of a decremental response on repetitive nerve stimulation	3. Demonstration of muscle inexcitability
4. Muscle histopathologic findings of myopathy with myosin loss	–

[a]Definitive diagnosis includes all four major features; probable diagnosis with three major and at least one supportive feature; possible diagnosis with major features 1 and 3 or 2 and 3 and at least one supportive feature.

Modified with permission from Lacomis D, Zochodne DW, Bird SJ. Critical illness myopathy. *Muscle Nerve*. 2000;23(12):1785–1788.

The most characteristic finding on muscle biopsy is the presence of pale areas seen on the ATPase and oxidative stains with disrupted myofibrillary network; there is also type II muscle fiber atrophy, and the atrophic fibers might appear eosinophilic on the H&E stain. Electromicroscopy shows myofiber disorganization with preservation of the Z-bands and absent myosin thick filaments.[15,16] These findings are characteristic but are not pathognomonic and can be seen in other conditions.

The possible pathogenesis of CIM includes myotoxicity from steroids, altered calcium homeostasis which causes a reduction of myosin filaments and other structural proteins, increased sodium channel inactivation, and decreased muscle excitability[2] (Fig. 44-2).

Treatment consists of tapering corticosteroids and aggressive physical therapy. The condition usually improves after 1–3 months, when properly managed. Intensive insulin therapy and treatment of sepsis reduce the chances of developing CIM and CIP.[17]

SUMMARY

This elderly woman with MG developed a myasthenic crisis that was treated with steroids and she was intubated. She then developed a myopathy and was found to have CIM.

IMPORTANT POINTS

- Weakness in ICU can have many causes, including, among others, toxic myopathies, acid maltase deficiency, polymyositis, and other acquired myopathies with rhabdomyolysis; also Guillain–Barré syndrome, porphyria or toxic neuropathies, MG, and amyotrophic lateral sclerosis. The causes of weakness that develop while patients are in the ICU also include CIP and CIM. In some, the weakness is caused by the prolonged use of neuromuscular blocking agents.
- In CIP, there is evidence of axonal degeneration and low-amplitude CMAPs during nerve stimulation and fairly normal CMAPs amplitude upon direct muscle stimulation. There are denervation potentials on the EMG. In CIM, there is more proximal weakness, and there is a lack of significant denervation on EMG. There are brief polyphasic motor unit potentials, and the serum CK is mildly elevated. Nerve stimulation and direct muscle stimulation produce similar CMAP amplitudes.
- In paralysis from prolonged neuromuscular blockade, routine EMG is essentially normal, although the repetitive stimulation test could show a decremental response.
- CIM is usually associated with the use of high doses of corticosteroids with paralyzing drugs and often during sepsis. Patients with MG receiving steroids could also develop this myopathy.
- In CIM the muscle biopsy characterizes fiber atrophy by pale areas in the muscle fibers on ATPase stain, with disorganization of myofilaments on electromicroscopy.
- The treatment consists of tapering or discontinuation of corticosteroids and aggressive physical therapy.

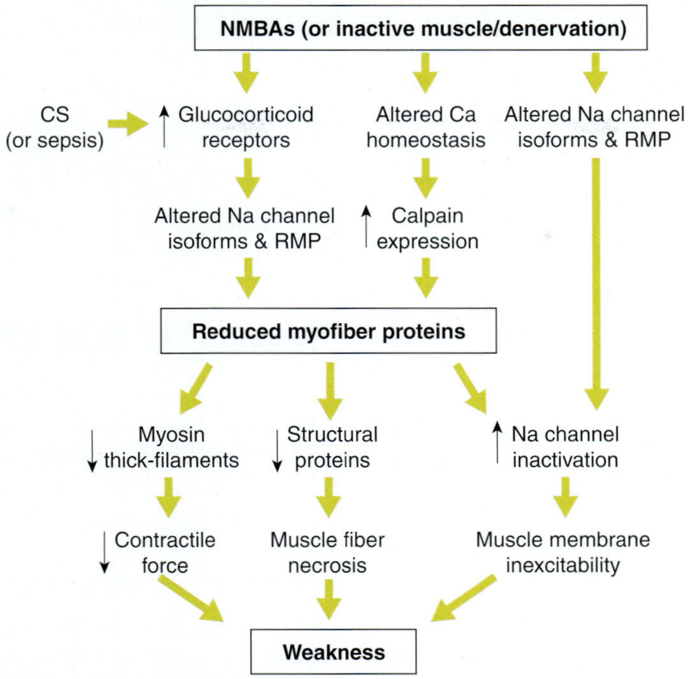

FIG. 44-2 Diagram of the possible pathogenesis of critical illness myopathy. *Ca*, Calcium; *CS*, corticosteroids; *Na*, sodium; *NMBAs*, neuromuscular blocking agents; *RMP*, resting membrane potential. From Bird SJ. Myopathies and disorders of neuromuscular transmission. In: Brown WF, Bolton CF, Aminoff MJ, eds. *Neuromuscular Function and Disease: Basic, Clinical and Electrodiagnostic Aspects*. Vol 2. Philadelphia, PA: *WB* Saunders; 2002.

REFERENCES

1. Green DM. Weakness in the ICU: Guillain-Barré syndrome, myasthenia gravis, and critical illness polyneuropathy/myopathy. *Neurologist*. 2005;11(6):338–347.
2. Bird SJ. Myopathies and disorders of neuromuscular transmission. In: Brown WF, Bolton CF, Aminoff MJ, eds. *Neuromuscular Function and Disease: Basic, Clinical and Electrodiagnostic Aspects*. vol 2. Boston, MA: WB Saunders; 2002.
3. Rich MM, Bird SJ, Raps EC, et al. Direct muscle stimulation in acute quadriplegic myopathy. *Muscle Nerve*. 1977;20:665–673.
4. Barohn RJ, Jackson CE, Rogers SJ, et al. Prolonged paralysis due to nondepolarizing neuromuscular blocking agents and corticosteroids. *Muscle Nerve*. 1994;17:647–654.
5. Bird SJ, Rich MM. Neuromuscular complications of critical illness. *Neurologist*. 2000;6:2–11.
6. Bolton CF. Electrophysiologic studies of critically ill patients. *Muscle Nerve*. 1987;10:129–135.
7. MacFarlane IA, Rosenthal FD. Severe myopathy after status asthmaticus. *Lancet*. 1977;2:615.
8. Bachmann P, Gaussorgues P, Piperno D, et al. Acute myopathy after status asthmaticus. *Presse Med*. 1987;16:1486.
9. Lacomis D, Smith TW, Chad DA. Acute myopathy and neuropathy in status asthmaticus: case report and literature review. *Muscle Nerve*. 1993;16:84–90.
10. Panegyres PK, Squier M, Mills KR, Newsom-Davis J. Acute myopathy associated with large parenteral dose of corticosteroid in myasthenia gravis. *J Neurol Neurosurg Psychiatry*. 1993;56:702–704.
11. Campellone JV, Lacomis D, Kramer DJ, et al. Acute myopathy after liver transplantation. *Neurology*. 1998;50:46–53.
12. Bolton CF. Neuromuscular complications of sepsis. *Intensive Care Med*. 1993;19(Suppl):S58–S63.
13. Bolton CF. Neuromuscular manifestations of critical illness. *Muscle Nerve*. 2005;32:140–163.
14. Lacomis D, Zochodne DW, Bird SJ. Critical illness myopathy. *Muscle Nerve*. 2000;23:1785–1788.
15. Danon MJ, Carpenter S. Myopathy with thick filament (myosin) loss following prolonged paralysis with vecuronium during steroid treatment. *Muscle Nerve*. 1991;14:1131–1139.
16. al-Lozi MT, Pestronk A, Yee WC, et al. Rapidly evolving myopathy with myosin-deficient muscle fibers. *Ann Neurol*. 1994;35:273–279.
17. Bird SJ. Diagnosis and management of critical illness polyneuropathy and critical illness myopathy. *Curr Treat Options Neurol*. 2007;9(2):85–92.

45 CASE

A Woman With COVID-19 Infection and Quadriparesis

A 36-year-old 8-month pregnant female presented to the hospital with severe weakness and fever for 2 days. She was diagnosed having COVID-19 infection.

She underwent an emergency cesarean section and was intubated in the prone position; this situation lasted for over 6 weeks. The patient was extubated and improved, and she had generalized weakness, more severe in the right upper extremity.

Examination revealed normal mentation and cranial nerves. There was profound weakness; this was more severe in the lower extremities, more distally than proximally, and in the proximal right arm. She was areflexic. Sensory examination showed decreased vibration sense in the toes. She had decreased pinprick in the right upper extremity, particularly in the outer aspect of the forearm and the second and third digits.

WHAT IS THE MOST LIKELY DIAGNOSIS?

This patient appears to have had an ICU neuropathy and possible myopathy. She also appears to have a compression of the brachial plexus, likely from positioning during intubation.

WHAT IS THE NEXT STEP?

An EMG showed a sensorimotor neuropathy with denervation potentials, mainly in the distal muscles, and small polyphasic motor units in the proximal muscles. There was also denervation mainly in muscles innervated by the right upper trunk and of the brachial plexus.

WHAT IS THE MOST LIKELY DIAGNOSIS?

It was concluded that this patient had an ICU neuropathy and myopathy as well as a plexopathy due to stretching or compression based on the clinical and EMG findings.

Critical illness polyneuropathy (CIP) is a generalized paralyzing condition with a high incidence of mortality.[1] Sepsis, trauma and burns, and viral infections invoke a severe systemic response or systemic inflammatory response and as many as 70% of patients with systemic inflammatory response and multiorgan dysfunction may develop clinical, electrophysiological, and histopathological evidence of peripheral nerve dysfunction.[2] CIP usually is recognized as severe when there is an

Motor Nerve Conduction Studies

Nerve/Sites	Muscle	Latency ms	Ref. ms	Amplitude mV	Ref. mV	Velocity m/s	Ref. m/s
R Median-APB Wrist	APB	4.5	≤4.40	3.7	4.0	49	
R Ulnar-ADM Wrist	ADM	3.1	≤3.3.0	4.6	26.0	61	
L Peroneal-EDB Ankle	EDB	4.9	≤6.50	2.9	≥2.0		
Fib head	EDB			5.3		44	≥44.0
Pop fossa	EDB			5.0		43	≥44..0
L Tibial-AH							
Ankle	AH	***NR***	≤5.80	***NR***	≥4.0		
Pop fossa	AH	***NR***		***NR***			≥41.0

F-Wave Studies

Nerve	Flat ms	Ref. ms	M Lat ms
R Median-APB	50	≤31.0	3.8
R Ulnar-ADM	.51	≤320	3.2
L Peroneal-EDB	NR	≤56.0	NR
L Tibial-AH	NR	≤56.0	NR

Sensory Nerve Studies

Nerve/Sites	Rec. Site	Peak Lat ms	Ref. ms	Amp V	Ref. V	Segments
R Median Wrist	Dig II	NR	≤3.5	NR	≥20.0	Wrist- Dig II
Ulnar Wrist	Dig V	NR	≤3.1	NR	≥17.0	Wrist - Dig V
L Sural Calf	Ankle	NR	≤4.4	NR	≥6.0.	Calf - Ankle

EMG Summary

			Spontaneous				MUAP			Recruitment	
Muscle	Nerve	Roots	IA	Fib	PSW	Fasc	Dur.	Amp	PPP	Pattern	Effort
R. Deltoid	Axillary	C5-C6	Normal	1+	1+2+	None	Decr.	Normal	Normal	Reduced	Normal
R. Biceps brachii	Musculocutaneous	C5-C6	Incr.	1+	2+	None	Normal	Normal	Normal	Reduced	Normal
R. Iliopsoas	Femoral	L2-L3	Normal	None	None	None	Decr.	Normal	Normal	Normal	Normal
R. Quadriceps	Femoral	L2-L4	Incr.	1+	1+	None	Normal	Decr.	Normal	Normal	Normal
R. Tibialis anterior	Deep peroneal (Fibular)	L4-L5	Normal	None	None	None	Normal	Normal	Normal	Normal	Normal
R. Gastrocnemius (Medial head)	Tibial	S1-S2	Incr.	1+	1+	None	Sl. Incr.	Sl.Incr.	Normal	Reduced	Normal
L. Tibialis anterior	Deep peroneal (Fibular)	L4-L5	Incr.	1+	1+	None	Sl. Incr.	Sl.Incr.	Normal	Reduced	Normal
L. Gastrocnemius (Medial head)	Tibial	51-82	Incr.	1+	1+	None	Sl. Incr.	Sl. Incr.	Normal	Reduced	Normal

existing encephalopathy with a sepsis response. The severity of the neuropathy increases with time in the ICU, and hyperglycemia and hypoalbuminemia are contributors. This is a symmetric neuropathy that causes limb weakness and difficulty weaning off the ventilator. Patients have atrophy, areflexia, and decreased distal sensation. It may resemble an axonal type of Guillain–Barré syndrome (GBS) with which sometimes this is confused.[3] Some drugs, such as corticosteroids, neuromuscular blocking agents, and drugs such as aminoglycoside and magnesium, increase the incidence. Nerve conduction studies typically show low amplitude of motor and sensory compound action potentials. The compound muscle action potentials decline early, whereas sensory nerve action potential decline occurs later. The EMG may also show evidence of denervation. Needle EMG of the diaphragm helps to establish a diagnosis in patients who have difficulty weaning from the ventilator. This diagnosis should be differentiated from critical illness myopathy (CIM) and paralysis from prolonged use of neuromuscular junction blockades. The lack of facial weakness and electrophysiological studies as well as normal spinal fluid protein differentiates this condition from GBS. Patients should be treated aggressively with physical therapy and range-of-motion movements.

CIM could be associated with CIP, which sometimes is named critical illness myopathy–neuropathy.[4] This usually affects patients who are exposed to high-dose corticosteroids in combination with a nondepolarizing neuromuscular junction blocker, and can occur in people with asthma who receive high doses of IV corticosteroids, and occurs in 7% of organ transplant patients.[5,6] The main clinical features include flaccid muscle weakness that occurs after the onset of critical illness and symmetrically in proximal more than distal muscles. The pathogenesis is uncertain, although triggering factors are recognized, especially with corticosteroids and neuromuscular blocking agents.

This patient had a combination of features of both CIP and CIM, and brachial plexopathy, but more aggressive tests like biopsy and histology were not done.

She developed complications of COVID-19 infection, and with the increasing number of COVID-19 infections, there are neurological complications. This infection affects many organs including respiratory failure. Neuromuscular complications include clinical illness neuropathy and myopathy, rhabdomyolysis, GBS, and Miller Fisher syndrome.[7–12] This can occur not only after the onset of the systemic illness but at presentation also. About 19% to 35% of patients with COVID-19 infections suffer from myalgias and high CK,[9] and some have COVID-related myositis or rhabdomyolysis, which suggests that SARS-COV2 may cause a viral myositis.[13]

Any patient with an acute paralytic illness should be tested for SARS-COVID-19 infection, and lymphopenia or thrombocytopenia should prompt immediate suspicion for the diagnosis. The AANEM has published guidelines for the performance of electrodiagnostic studies in patients with COVID-19 infection emphasizing prescreening, scheduling and coordinating the need to study and potentially change management, and the use of protective equipment.[14]

Special care should be given to patients with neuropathies and disorders of neuromuscular transmission.[15]

Vaccinations are very valuable to decrease the incidence of infection, but there are also complications due to vaccines, such as GBS, Miller Fisher syndrome, and myelitis, although these are rare.[16]

The management of these patients includes aggressive respiratory management. Patients with neuromuscular disorders are at increased risk of complications due to impaired respiratory capacity.

In addition to vaccines for COVID-19, there are several medications that appear to be useful during the infection, particularly monoclonal antibodies, convalescent plasma, baricitinib, remdesivir, and nirmatrelvir as well as dexamethasone.

Prompt physical therapy and management of complications are necessary.

SUMMARY

We concluded that this patient has COVID-19–induced respiratory failure and ICU neuropathy and myopathy in addition to a compressive plexopathy.

IMPORTANT POINTS

- Prolonged ICU stay with intubation can cause ICU neuropathy and myopathy.
- SARS-COVID-19 infection can predispose patients to acute paralysis.
- Paralytic illness in patients treated on a respirator could also predispose patients to compression, particularly in those with prolonged positioning if no proper protection with padding is applied.
- The prognosis of ICU polyneuropathy is poor; patients can recover, but this could be very slow.
- There are several new drugs that appear to be beneficial in patients with COVID-19 infection.
- COVID-19 vaccinations are very useful and rarely cause complications.

REFERENCES

1. Dellinger RP, Carlet JM, Masur H, Gerlach H, et al. Surviving Sepsis Campaign guideline for management of severe sepsis and septic shock. *Crit Care Med*. 2004;32(3):858–873. https://doi.org/10.1097/01.ccm.0000117317.18092.e4.
2. Bolton CF, Young GB, Zochodne DW. The neurological complications of sepsis. *Ann Neurol*. 1993;33:94–100.
3. Bertorini TE, Finder JD, Bassan BA. Perioperative management in patients with neuromuscular disorders. Chapter 10. In: Bertorini TE, ed. *Neuromuscular Disorders: Treatment and Management*. 2nd ed. Amsterdam, Netherlands: Elsevier; 2022:206–224.
4. Latronico N, Fenzi F, Recupero D, et al. Critical illness myopathy and neuropathy. *Lancet*. 1996;347:1579–1582.
5. Lacomis D, Guilliant MJ, Van Cou A, et al. Acute myopathy of intensive care: clinical, EMG, and pathological aspects. *Ann Neurol*. 1996;40:645–654.
6. Perea M, Picon M, Miro O, et al. Acute quadriplegic myopathy with loss of thick (myosin) filaments following heart transplantation. *J Heart Lung Transplant*. 2001;20:1136–1141.
7. Zivkovic S, Linden PR. Liver transplantation. In: Biller J, ed. *Interface of Neurology and Internal Medicine*. Philadelphia, PA: Lippincott Williams & Wilkins; 2008:290–294.
8. Ahmad I, Rathor FA. Neurological manifestations and complications of COVID-19: a literature review. *J Clin Neurosci*. 2020;77:8–12. https://doi.org/10.1016/j.jocn.2020.05.017.
9. Guidon AC, Amato AA. COVID-19 and neuromuscular disorders. *Neurology*. 2020;94(22):959–969. https://doi.org/10.1212/WNL0000000000009566.
10. Dalakas MC. Guillain-Barré syndrome: the first documented COVID-19-triggered autoimmune neurologic disease: more to come with myositis in the offing. *Neurol Neuroimmunol Neuroinflamm*. 2020;7(5):e781. https://doi.org/10.1212/NXI.0000000000000781.
11. Reyes-Bueno JA, Trujillo Lg, Urbaneja P, Ciano-Peterson NL, et al. Miller-Fisher syndrome after SARS-CoV-2 infection. *Eur J Neurol*. 2020;9:1759–1761. https://doi.org/10.1111/ene.14383.
12. Toscano G, Palmerini F, Ravaglia S, Ruiz L, et al. Guillain-Barre syndrome associated with SARS-CoV-2. *N Engl J Med*. 2020;382(26):2574–2576. https://doi.org/10.1056/NEJMc200919191.
13. Manzano GS, Woods JK, Amato AA. COVID-19–associated myopathy caused by type I interferonopathy. *N Engl J Med*. 2020;383:2389–2390. https://doi.org/10.1056/NEJMc2031085. Pub ahead of print. FMID: 33216474.
14. Desai U, Kassardjian CD, Toro Del D, Gleveckas-Martens N, et al. Guidance for resumption of routine electrodiagnostic testing during the COVID-19 pandemic. *Muscle Nerve*. 2020;62(2):176–181. https://doi.org/10.1002/mus.26990.
15. International MG/COVID-19 Working Group Jacob S, Muppidi S, Guidon A, et al. Guidance for the management of myasthenia gravis (MG) and Lambert-Eaton myasthenic syndrome (LEMS) during the COVID-19 pandemic. *J Neurol Sci*. 2020;412:116803. https://doi.org/10.1016/j.jns.2020.116803.
16. Siddiqi AR, Khan T, Tahir MJ, et al. Miller Fisher syndrome after COVID-19 vaccination: case report and review of literature. *Medicine (Baltimore)*. 2022;10(20):e29333.

A Man With Neck Pain and Numbness in the Hands

A 69-year-old man came with a 3-month history of numbness and tingling primarily in the hands and only some mild numbness in the bottom of his feet and toes. The hand tingling got worse when he made a fist; he also noticed that he lost his grip when he played golf. He denied nocturnal pain or numbness. He had neck pain for a long time with limitation of movements and had been told this was from osteoarthritis.

Past medical history was remarkable for kidney stones, hemorrhoidectomy, a fistula repair, and right hip replacement. He is a retired executive who did not smoke or drink.

Examination revealed normal cranial nerves and mentation. Muscle strength and tone were normal and symmetrical. Reflexes were normal, and there were no pathologic reflexes. Sensory examination was normal except for decreased vibration and position senses and two-point discrimination in the fingers and toes. Phalen test was negative, and he had no Tinel's sign at the wrist. There was mild limitation of neck movements in all directions. The Romberg test was negative. There were no Babinski signs, and the rest of the examination was normal.

WHAT IS THE MOST LIKELY DIAGNOSIS?

This patient presented with numbness and tingling in the hands and feet, which was somewhat more prominent in the hands. A polyneuropathy was a consideration, and this could be associated with carpal tunnel syndrome as suggested by his hand symptoms; there was, however, no clinical finding of carpal tunnel syndrome.

Common causes of neuropathy should be evaluated first. These include diabetes, thyroid disease, and B_{12} deficiency which could cause prominent hand symptoms. He was on no medications nor had he been exposed to toxins.

Because the patient had cervical osteoarthritis, it was also possible that cervical spondylosis produced the symptoms, but these were also present in the legs, and there was no evidence of long tract involvement to explain the leg symptoms. The patient also needed to be worked up for conditions that cause neck stiffness, including rheumatoid arthritis.

WHAT TESTS WERE DONE?

A complete metabolic panel was normal. Erythrocyte sedimentation rate was 4 mm/h (normal, <20 mm/h); mean corpuscular volume was 109 fL (normal, 80–100 fL); mean corpuscular hemoglobin was 36.1 pg (normal, 27–33 pg); red blood count was normal; hemoglobin was 14.5 g/dL (normal, 13.8–17.2 g/dL); hematocrit was 43.7% (normal, 41%–50%); B_{12} was 203 pg/mL (normal, 200–1100 pg/mL); and folate was 20.7 ng/mL (normal, ≥3.1 ng/mL). Thyroid-stimulating hormone, rheumatoid factor, and fluorescent antinuclear antibody test were normal.

MRI of the neck showed degenerative changes (Fig. 46-1), with narrowing of the neuroforamina of the right C5–C6 and C6–C7 without neural axis pathology.

AN EMG TEST WAS PERFORMED

Motor Nerve Studies

Nerve and Site	Latency (ms)	Amplitude (mV)	Conduction Velocity (m/s)
Peroneal Nerve R.	**Normal ≤ 5.7**	**Normal ≥ 3**	**Normal ≥ 40**
Ankle	4.1	8	–
Fibular head	11.1	8	44
Knee	13.1	7	45
Tibial Nerve R.	**Normal ≤ 5.3**	**Normal ≥ 4**	**Normal ≥ 40**
Ankle	4.6	17	–
Pop. fossa	14.5	14	46
Nerve and Site	**Latency (ms)**	**Amplitude (mV)**	**Conduction Velocity (m/s)**
Median Nerve R.	**Normal ≤ 4.2**	**Normal ≥ 6**	**Normal ≥ 50**
Wrist	3.5	15	–
Elbow	8.1	14	52

F-Wave and Tibial H-Reflex Studies

Nerve	Latency (ms)	Normal Latency ≤ (ms)
Peroneal nerve R.	52.7	54
Tibial nerve R.	54.0	54
Median nerve R.	28.4	30
H-reflex R.	33.8	34
H-reflex L.	34.0	34

Sensory Nerve Studies

Nerve	Onset Latency (ms)	Normal Onset Latency ≤ (ms)	Peak Latency (ms)	Normal Peak Latency ≤ (ms)	Amp (μV)	Normal Amp ≥ (μV)	Conduction Velocity (m/s)	Normal Conduction Velocity ≥ (m/s)
Sural nerve R.	3.5	3.5	4.0	4.0	14	11	40	40
Superficial peroneal R.	3.5	3.5	4.0	4.0	10	8–10	40	40
Median nerve R.	2.4	2.6	2.9	3.1	28	20	54	50
Median palmar R.	0.7	1.0	1.2	1.5	44	30	[a]	50
Median nerve L.	2.6	2.6	3.1	3.1	28	20	50	50
Median palmar L.	0.7	1.0	1.2	1.5	47	30	[a]	50

[a]Not calculated.

EMG Data

Muscle	Insrt Activity	Fibs	Pos Waves	Fasc	Amp	Dur	Poly	Pattern
Biceps brachii R.	Norm	None	None	None	Norm	Norm	None	Norm
Pronator quadratus R.	Norm	None	None	None	Norm	Norm	None	Norm
Extensor digitorum com. R.	Norm	None	None	None	Norm	Norm	None	Norm
Flexor carpi radialis R.	Norm	None	None	None	Norm	Norm	None	Norm
First dorsal interosseous R.	Norm	None	None	None	Norm	Norm	None	Norm
Tibialis anterior R.	Norm	None	None	None	Norm	Norm	None	Norm
Gastrocnemius R.	Norm	None	None	None	Norm	Norm	None	Norm

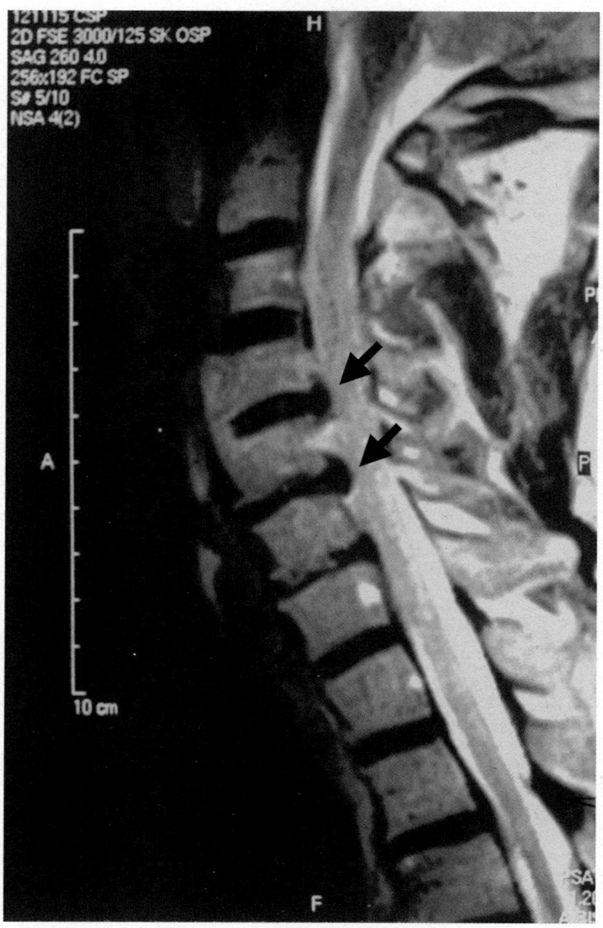

FIG. 46-1 MRI (sagittal view), T2-weighted image showing prominent bulging disk, particularly at C5–C6, without evidence of cord compression or demyelinating lesions (*arrows*).

WHAT WERE THE EMG FINDINGS?

Nerve conduction velocities were normal with normal CMAP amplitudes and latencies; there were borderline H-reflex latencies. No denervation potentials or other abnormalities were seen on EMG.

In conclusion, the test was essentially normal without electrophysiologic evidence of carpal tunnel syndrome, radiculopathy, or polyneuropathy, although it is possible that he had a neuropathy not detectable by these studies.

WHAT WOULD ONE DO NEXT?

The findings of predominantly proprioceptive deficit with normal routine electrophysiologic findings and elevated erythrocytes mean corpuscular volume make the diagnosis of pernicious anemia a good possibility, even with normal B_{12} levels. Homocysteine level was 121.7 μM/L (normal, 4–17 μM/L); methylmalonic acid level was 15.02 μM/L (normal, <0.41 μM/L); and antiparietal cell antibody titer was 35 (normal, <20). A repeat B_{12} was then done and was 144 pg/mL. Somatosensory-evoked response tests could have been useful, but this was not done.

SUMMARY

This patient presented with paresthesias and numbness mostly in the hands and had normal nerve conduction tests and EMG. He also had neck pain and cervical spondylosis. His workup initially revealed normal B_{12} levels. However, because the elevated mean corpuscular volume, homocysteine, and methylmalonic acid levels were measured and found to be elevated, the B_{12} test was repeated and was subnormal. He was diagnosed as having pernicious anemia and responded to replacement.

For further discussion, important points, and references, see Case 47.

CASE 47

A Woman With Peripheral Neuropathy and Frequent Falls

A 51-year-old woman was referred for peripheral neuropathy of unknown cause. Ten months prior to the presentation, she developed a tendency to fall backward, stumbling and hitting the wall when she got up in the morning. This got progressively worse. She also started complaining of burning and tingling paresthesias in the feet.

Her past medical history was positive for hypothyroidism, and she was receiving thyroid replacement. She smoked one pack of cigarettes daily but did not drink.

General physical examination, higher cortical function, and cranial nerves were normal. There was mild weakness of foot and toe dorsiflexors bilaterally. Reflexes were 2+ in the upper extremities and absent in the legs. She had a questionable Babinski sign on the right and a definitive one on the left. Muscle tone was mildly increased. There was decreased vibration sense in the fingers, toes, ankles, and knees and decreased pinprick, touch, and temperature sensations up to the knees. Position sense was markedly decreased in the toes and decreased in the ankles. Her gait was unsteady, and she had a positive Romberg test. Coordination and the rest of the examination were normal.

AN EMG TEST WAS PERFORMED

Motor Nerve Studies

Nerve and Site	Latency (ms)	Amplitude (mV)	Conduction Velocity (m/s)
Peroneal Nerve R.	**Normal ≤ 5.7**	**Normal ≥ 3**	**Normal ≥ 40**
Ankle	5.2	5	–
Fibular head	12.7	4	41
Knee	14.7	4	50
Tibial Nerve R.	**Normal ≤ 5.3**	**Normal ≥ 4**	**Normal ≥ 40**
Ankle	4.9	8	–
Pop. fossa	14.9	6	**38**
Median Nerve R.	**Normal ≤ 4.2**	**Normal ≥ 6**	**Normal ≥ 50**
Wrist	3.7	7	–
Elbow	8.0	7	55
Ulnar Nerve R.	**Normal ≤ 3.6**	**Normal ≥ 8**	**Normal ≥ 50**
Wrist	3.2	**6**	–
Below elbow	7.2	**5**	55
Above elbow	9.2	**5**	60

F-Wave and Tibial H-Reflex Studies

Nerve	Latency (ms)	Normal Latency ≤ (ms)
Peroneal nerve R.	**57.8**	54
Tibial nerve R.	**NR**	54
Median nerve R.	**31.2**	30
Ulnar nerve R.	**32.0**	30
H-reflex R.	**NR**	34
H-reflex L.	**NR**	34

Sensory Nerve Studies

Nerve	Onset Latency (ms)	Normal Onset Latency ≤ (ms)	Peak Latency (ms)	Normal Peak Latency ≤ (ms)	Amp (μV)	Normal Amp ≥ (μV)	Conduction Velocity (m/s)	Normal Conduction Velocity ≥ (m/s)
Sural nerve R.	3.1	3.5	3.6	4.0	**10**	11	45	40
Superficial peroneal R.	3.4	3.5	3.9	4.0	**6**	8–10	41	40
Median nerve R.	**2.7**	2.6	**3.2**	3.1	21	20	**48**	50
Ulnar nerve R.	2.0	2.6	2.5	3.1	**12**	13	60	50
Median nerve L.	**2.7**	2.6	**3.2**	3.1	25	20	50	50
Medial plantar R.	**NR**	3.2	**NR**	3.7	**NR**	10	**NR**	40
Lateral plantar R.	**NR**	3.2	**NR**	3.7	**NR**	8	**NR**	40
Medial plantar L.	**NR**	3.2	**NR**	3.7	**NR**	10	**NR**	40
Lateral plantar L.	**NR**	3.2	**NR**	3.7	**NR**	8	**NR**	40

EMG Data

Muscle	Insrt Activity	Fibs	Pos Waves	Fasc	Amp	Dur	Poly	Pattern
Vastus lateralis R.	Norm	None	None	None	Norm	Norm	None	Norm
Tibialis anterior R.	Norm	None	None	None	Norm	Norm	None	Norm
Gastrocnemius R.	Norm	None	None	None	Norm	Norm	None	Norm
Abductor hallucis longus R.	Norm	None	None	None	Norm	Norm	None	Norm
Tibialis anterior L.	Norm	None	None	None	Norm	Norm	None	Norm
Gastrocnemius L.	Norm	None	None	None	Norm	Norm	None	Norm
First dorsal interosseous L.	Norm	None	None	None	Norm	Norm	None	Norm

WHAT WERE THE EMG FINDINGS?

This study demonstrated normal motor conduction tests, except borderline low tibial nerve conduction velocity with a low-amplitude ulnar CMAP. There was an absent tibial nerve plantar SNAP and a borderline prolonged median nerve SNAP latency. Sural and superficial peroneal SNAPs were of low amplitude; H-reflexes were absent. Needle examination was normal.

These findings indicate a predominantly sensory polyneuropathy.

Other tests included a normal thyroid-stimulating hormone level and thyroxine level. Hemoglobin was 10.4 mg/dL (normal, 13.8–17.2 mg/dL); hematocrit was 35.6% (normal, 41%–80%); mean corpuscular volume (MCV) was 101.4 fL (normal, 80–100 fL); mean corpuscular hemoglobin was 34 pg (normal, 27–33 pg); and white blood cells and platelets were normal.

WHAT OTHER TEST SHOULD BE ORDERED?

A fasting blood sugar, anti–myelin-associated glycoprotein (MAG) antibodies, sulfatide, Hu-antibodies, fluorescent antinuclear antibody, Sjögren's associated antibodies, and immunoelectrophoresis were normal. B_{12} was normal at 323 pg/mm (normal, 200–1000 pg/mm). Serum folate was normal and antinuclear antibody tests were negative. Spinal fluid was normal, except protein was 60 mg/dL (normal, <50 mg/dL).

MRI of the cervical spine was normal.

WHAT IS THE DIFFERENTIAL DIAGNOSIS?

This patient appeared to have a predominantly sensory neuropathy, and the differential diagnosis included diabetes, cobalamin deficiency, and hypothyroidism, but she had normal thyroid tests and B_{12} levels. Other possibilities, such as thiamine deficiency, pyridostigmine intoxication, alcohol- or drug-induced neuropathy, and copper deficiency were not compatible with her history. There was no evidence of demyelination on nerve conduction tests which would suggest a chronic distal demyelinating neuropathy, which in some cases can be associated with MAG antibodies.[1] These and her immunoelectrophoresis were normal. The presence of a Babinski sign was atypical, although some patients with neuropathy, such as chronic inflammatory demyelinating polyradiculoneuropathy (CIDP), might have central demyelination.[2] An elevated spinal fluid protein, as was hers, is seen in CIDP; in this the values are usually higher, but she lacked proximal weakness, areflexia, and evidence of demyelination on the EMG for classic CIDP.

The predominant large fiber involvement was against an isolated microangiopathic vasculitic neuropathy, but this could not be ruled out without a nerve biopsy.

WHAT WOULD YOU DO NEXT?

Although the patient's normal B_{12} was against the diagnosis of pernicious anemia (PA), the high MCV prompted the measurement of homocysteine and methylmalonic acid levels. Homocysteine was 29.5 μM/L (normal, <9 μM/L), and methylmalonic acid was 2244 μM/L (normal, 60–250 μM/L). Parietal cell antibody titers were 54 (normal, <20). These findings were diagnostic of PA.

A Schilling test was done, and stage 1 cobalamin excretion was 0 (normal, >10%). Stage 2 showed excretion of only 1% of administered dose, indicating also an abnormal intestinal absorption of B_{12} from prolonged cobalamin deficiency, caused by chronic PA. This could occur in several conditions, while some others can cause misleading levels. Most likely, she had PA and belongs to the group of patients who have a normal B_{12} level in standard tests. It has been reported that about 5%–10% of PA patients have levels between 200 and 300, and less than 1% might have levels over 300.[3]

WHAT IS THE IMPORTANCE OF COBALAMIN DEFICIENCY?

Cobalamin is a compound of four pyrrole rings and central cobalt ion. In humans, there are two cobalamin-dependent enzymatic reactions[3]:

Reaction I is the conversion of methylmalonyl-coenzyme A (CoA) from methylmalonic acid to succinyl-CoA, using adenosyl-cobalamin as a cofactor, and thus a deficiency of cobalamin causes increased methylmalonyl-CoA and methylmalonic acid (Fig. 47-1). Succinyl-CoA is an important enzyme of intermediate metabolism.

Reaction II consists of the synthesis of methionine from homocysteine and tetrahydrofolate (from folic acid) using methylcobalamin (Cbl) as a cofactor. Methionine and tetrahydrofolate are used for DNA synthesis, and methionine is converted to *S*-adenosyl-methionine, which is used for methylation reactions in the central nervous system. In cobalamin or folate deficiencies the underutilized homocysteine is elevated.

These reactions explain the rise of both methylmalonic acid and homocysteine in PA, and when this disease is suspected, these should be tested even in patients with normal B_{12} levels, particularly when the erythrocyte MCV is high.

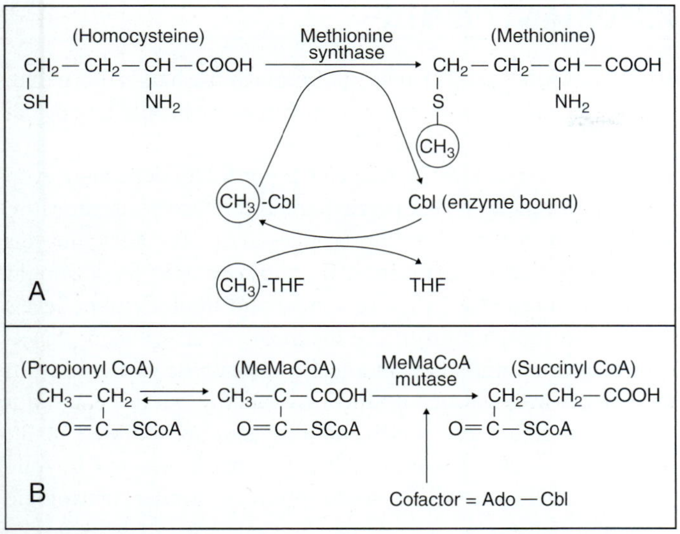

FIG. 47-1 A, Cofactor activity of methylcobalamin (CH3-Cbl) in methionine synthesis. THF = tetrahydrofolate. **B,** Cofactor activity of adenosylcobalamin (Ado-Cbl) in succinyl-coenzyme A (CoA) synthesis. MeMaCoA = methylmalonyl-coenzyme A. Tefferi, A., Pruthi, RK. (1994) The Biochemical Basis of Cobalamin Deficiency. *Mayo Clinic Proceedings*, 69 (2), 181–186.

Cobalamin is an essential vitamin that is not synthesized in the human body and requires proper supplementation from meats and dairy products. It is absorbed and released in the stomach. The free vitamin then binds to haptocorrins ("R" binders). Later, in the duodenum, it is liberated by trypsin where it binds to the intrinsic factor produced by the parietal cells of the stomach. This factor is necessary for the absorption of the vitamin in the distal ileum.

WHAT IS THE SCHILLING TEST?

The Schilling test is used to diagnose the site of the disorder causing cobalamin deficiency. In *stage 1* the patient is given radioactively labeled cobalamin. If there is a deficiency of B_{12}, the excretion of the percentage of administered B_{12} in a 24-hour urine collection is low.

In *stage 2* the test is repeated, but the patient is also given intrinsic factor. An abnormal test indicates poor absorption of the vitamin. This could have several causes. One could be bacterial overgrowth, and for this reason, a *stage 3* of the Schilling test could be done, by repeating stage 1 after antibiotic therapy.[3]

It is noteworthy that a chronic B_{12} deficiency might also cause a dysfunction of the ileum producing abnormalities in stage 2[3]. (Table 47-1)

An important test in PA is the measurement of antiparietal cell antibodies, which are elevated in 85% of patients.[4,5]

SUMMARY

This patient had a neuropathy with a Babinski sign. Workup revealed macrocytosis with normal B_{12} levels. She had elevated homocysteine and methylmalonic acid levels and an abnormal Schilling test. She responded to parenteral vitamin B_{12} supplementation.

TABLE 47-1 Cobalamin (Cbl) Absorption and Transport

Step	Clinical Significance
In many foods, Cbl is bound to proteins. When food enters the stomach, acid facilitates the even release of Cbl. The presence of food also stimulates the secretion of IF, a glycoprotein produced by gastric parietal cells. However, in conditions of low pH, unbound Cbl preferentially attaches to salivary haptocorrin (formerly referred to as "R" binder) rather than to IF.	If gastric production of acid is reduced, Cbl absorption from food may be impaired, even when IF is present. However, unbound Cbl supplemental vitamin preparations will still be absorbed normally. A decrease in serum Cbl levels has been demonstrated after 3–4 years of omeprazole therapy, and it has been suggested that serum Cbl levels be measured in patients undergoing prolonged treatment with proton pump inhibitors.
In the neutral pH of the duodenum, IF displaces the salivary haptocorrin with the aid of pancreatic enzymes.	Patients with pancreatic insufficiency may have reduced Cbl absorption although they rarely become Cbl-deficient.
The IF-Cbl complex passes through the small intestine and is taken up by receptor-mediated endocytosis in the terminal ileum.	Bacterial overgrown of fish tapeworm infestation may cause Cbl deficiency because of competition for Cbl in the intestine before the IF-Cbl complex reaches the terminal ileum.
Cbl is released from the complex and binds either to the TC II protein or to serum haptocorrins (formerly referred to as TC I and TC III). TC II, which accounts for only 10%–30% of the measurable serum Cbl level, is the physiologically important transport protein.	Congenital TC II deficiency may cause megaloblastic anemia despite normal serum Cbl levels. In some patients with myeloproliferative disorders or liver disease, levels of serum haptocorrins may increase, leading to increases in the measured serum Cbl level.
An active enterohepatic circulation conserves the vitamin. Once Cbl reenters the gut in the bile, IF is again necessary for reabsorption.	Compared with patients with pernicious anemia, strict vegetarians (who produce IF normally) retain more Cbl from the enterohepatic circulation and therefore take much longer (10–20 years) to become Cbl-deficient.

IF, Intrinsic factor; *TC*, transcobalamin.

DISCUSSION (CASES 46 AND 47)

The patient from Case 47 presented with weakness and positive Babinski signs with evidence of a polyneuropathy and signs of combined degeneration of the spinal cord. The patient from Case 46 had hand numbness, which is another initial presentation of the disease also likely from early spinal cord disease. Both cases were diagnosed as having PA.

PA is an acquired disease caused by antibodies against parietal cells resulting in a deficiency of the intrinsic factor, impairing B_{12} absorption and resulting in its deficiency. Patients complain of paresthesias, particularly in the hands with minimal or no weakness. There could be hyporeflexia or areflexia with Babinski signs; some have spasticity and hyperreflexia. Joint position and vibratory senses are abnormal, and later, patients might manifest with a psychiatric disorder[6–11]; rarely, there is also optic atrophy.

In PA there is a macrocytic anemia and hypersegmented neutrophils, and to diagnose B_{12} deficiency, there should be a study of the blood smear for the presence of these and of large red cells with an increased MCV. B_{12} levels should be measured, although this might not be diagnostic, particularly when the levels are borderline. Measurements of methylmalonic acid and homocysteine levels are very important. The Schilling test is also still useful.

EMG studies could show evidence of peripheral neuropathy with slowing of conduction velocities and abnormal SNAPs. Somatosensory-evoked responses (SSERs) are usually abnormal.[12,13]

Sural nerve biopsies show axonal degeneration; autopsy studies reveal degeneration of the posterior columns and corticospinal tracts, hence the name *combined degeneration of the spinal cord*.

The most common cause of B_{12} deficiency is PA from antibodies against the parietal cells, blocking the production of the "intrinsic factor."[5] As discussed, other causes include poor absorption from intestinal infections, steatorrhea, iliac and gastric resections, dietary deficiencies, particularly in strict vegetarians, and tapeworm infestations.[8,10,13,14] (Table 47-1 outlines the steps of cobalamin absorption and the explanation for the deficiency.) Patients with HIV infections appear to be predisposed to this disease. The abuse or recurrent use of nitrous oxide, particularly by dentists, could cause combined degeneration of the spinal cord because nitrous oxide oxidizes B_{12}, converting the vitamin to its inactive trivalent state.[15] There are also genetic disorders that cause B_{12} deficiency, such as a defect of methionine synthetase.

It is important to remember that the neurologic manifestations of PA can be present even without evidence of anemia or macrocytosis.[16]

The association of B_{12} deficiency with a neurologic disorder was first reported in the 1880s.[8] The term *subacute combined degeneration of the spinal cord* was later used based on the pathologic findings of demyelination of posterior columns and corticospinal tracts[9]; this can sometimes be seen on MRI, and the brain MRI could show lesions that resembled MS. In this disease the demyelination is limited. There is also evidence of peripheral nerve involvement.[10,11]

PA was a major cause of illness and death in the last century until Minor and Whipple demonstrated that the daily intake of 100–200 g of beef liver could reverse this anemia. Later, in an elegant study, William Castle was able to demonstrate that gastric acid contained an *intrinsic factor* required to absorb the *extrinsic factor*, or B_{12}. The vitamin was isolated in 1948.[8]

The treatment of B_{12} deficiency consists of the use of intramuscular injections of 1000 mg of B_{12} daily for 5 days, then weekly for 1 month, and then monthly.

IMPORTANT POINTS

- B_{12} deficiency could cause numbness in the hands more than the feet, and routine nerve conduction tests could be normal initially.
- Elevated red cell MCV suggests B_{12} or folate deficiency even with normal B_{12} levels, particularly if they are borderline low.
- In patients with a clinical presentation or laboratory findings suggestive of B_{12} deficiency, B_{12} and folic acid levels should be measured. Methylmalonic acid and homocysteine levels are also most useful in the diagnosis, even when B_{12} levels are normal, and they should be measured, particularly in patients with elevated erythrocyte MCV.
- Homocysteine and methylmalonic acid are elevated in B_{12} deficiency, whereas only homocysteine is elevated in folic acid deficiency, which could produce similar neurologic manifestations.
- The symptoms of PA include paresthesias and numbness; the examination shows proprioceptive deficits, hyporeflexia or areflexia, and Babinski signs. Patients may also develop neuropsychiatric dysfunction and optic atrophy.
- Motor nerve conduction velocities are normal in PA, but the SNAPs could be of low amplitude or absent, and the SSER could be absent, slow, or of low amplitude.
- Eighty-five percent of patients with PA have antiparietal cell antibodies, causing deficiency of the intrinsic factor.
- Nerve biopsy shows axonal degeneration, and autopsy studies show combined degeneration in the spinal cord.
- The treatment consists of parental B_{12} supplementation.

REFERENCES

1. Katz JS, Saperstein DS, Gronseth G, et al. Distal acquired demyelinating symmetric neuropathy. *Neurology*. 2000;54:615–620.
2. Mendell JR, Kolkin S, Kissel JT, et al. Evidence for central nervous system demyelination in chronic inflammatory demyelinating polyradiculoneuropathy. *Neurology*. 1987;37(8):1291–1294.
3. Snow CF. Laboratory diagnosis of vitamin B_{12} and folate deficiency: a guide for the primary care physician. *Arch Intern Med*. 1999;159:1289–1298.
4. Veldek TE, Abels J, Anders GJ, et al. A family study of pernicious anemia by an immunologic method. *J Lab Clin Med*. 1964;84:177–187.
5. Chanarin I, Metz J. Diagnosis of cobalamin deficiency: the old and the new. *Br J Haematol*. 1997;97:695–700.
6. Healton EB, Savage DG, Brust JC, et al. Neurologic aspects of cobalamin deficiency. *Medicine*. 1991;70:229–245.
7. Cox-Klazinga M, Endtz LJ. Peripheral nerve involvement in pernicious anemia. *J Neurol Sci*. 1980;45:367–371.
8. Toh BH, van Driel IR, Gleeson PA. Pernicious anemia. *N Engl J Med*. 1997;337(20):1441–1448.
9. Victor M, Lear AA. Subacute combined degeneration of the spinal cord: current concepts of the disease process: value of serum vitamin B-12 determinations in clarifying some of the common clinical problems. *Am J Med*. 1956;20:896–911.
10. Pruthi RK, Tefferi A. Pernicious anemia revisited. *Mayo Clin Proc*. 1994;69:144–150.
11. Fine EJ, Hallett M. Neurophysiological study of subacute combined degeneration. *J Neurol Sci*. 1980;45:331–336.

12. Fine EJ, Soria E, Paroski MW, et al. The neurophysiological profile of vitamin B12 deficiency. *Muscle Nerve*. 1990;13:158–164.
13. Best CN. Subacute combined degeneration of the spinal cord after extensive resection of ileum in Crohn's disease. *Br Med J*. 1959;2:862–864.
14. Holloway KL, Alberico AM. Postoperative myeloneuropathy: a preventable complication in patients with B12 deficiency. *J Neurosurg*. 1990;72(5):732–736.
15. Layzer RB. Myeloneuropathy after prolonged exposure to nitrous oxide. *Lancet*. 1978;2(8102):1227–1230.
16. Lindenbaum J, Healton EB, Savage DG, et al. Neuropsychiatric disorders caused by cobalamin deficiency in the absence of anemia or macrocytosis. *N Engl J Med*. 1988;318:1720–1728.

48 CASE

A Woman With Progressive Four Limb Paresthesias

A 58-year-old woman was evaluated for progressive four limb paresthesias and difficulty with gait and balance. Six months before the evaluation, she noticed numbness, tingling, and burning sensations in both legs and more recently developed numbness and tingling in both hands. She also had gait difficulty and loss of balance, which worsened in the last month to the point that she was unable to walk without support. She also had mild weakness in her legs.

Her medical history included hypertension, diabetes, chronic obstructive pulmonary disease, anemia, obstructive sleep apnea, depression, restless leg syndrome, coronary artery disease, cardiomyopathy, internal cardiac defibrillator placement for polymorphic ventricular tachycardia, and gastric bypass surgery for obesity.

Her medications included bronchodilators, carvedilol, alprazolam, citalopram, ropinirole, and zinc sulfate.

The family history was noncontributory.

She was a remote smoker and did not drink alcohol or use any illicit drugs.

Examination revealed a normal mental status and speech. Cranial nerve examination was essentially unremarkable. Motor exam showed normal strength in the upper extremities; hip flexion was 4/5 bilaterally, whereas the remaining lower extremity muscle groups had normal strength. Muscle stretch reflexes were normal and symmetric, except for decreased ankle reflexes bilaterally. She had a positive Babinski sign on the right. There was decreased light touch and pain sensation to the level of the knee, markedly decreased vibration and proprioception sensation in the toes, and decreased vibration sensation in the ankles and knees bilaterally. Coordination was intact on the finger-to-nose and heel-to-shin maneuvers with eyes open but was impaired with eyes closed. Gait was wide base and she had a positive Romberg sign.

WHAT IS THE DIFFERENTIAL DIAGNOSIS?

This patient had an apparent myelopathy and neuropathy. She also had bariatric surgery and can have many complications that should be considered[1] (Table 48-1). This patient could have combined degeneration of the spinal cord, from B_{12} deficiency, a condition that affects the posterior columns and corticospinal tracts, and the patient may also have a neuropathy.[2] Folate deficiency may also present with combined degeneration of the spinal cord. Syphilis is unlikely as patients with tabes dorsalis do not have evidence of corticospinal tract involvement; they usually have pupillary irregularities. HIV infections produce a vacuolar myelopathy which occurs in late stages of AIDS. In typical cases, a slowly progressive spastic paraparesis can be seen. The upper extremities are usually normal. Multiple sclerosis is another possibility; although she is somewhat old for this condition, it may present in this manner. Devic disease should be a consideration in a patient presenting with a myelopathy, either with or without optic nerve involvement.

Other possibilities include Sjögren syndrome,[3] lupus,[4] and a paraneoplastic syndrome.[5] HTLV-1 is more common in other countries, but not in the United States, and this is slowly progressive in myelopathy, and patients may also have a mild neuropathy.[6] Neurosarcoidosis can present with spinal cord dysfunction.

Another possibility is copper deficiency myelopathy,[5] which can also have this presentation.

WHAT TESTS SHOULD BE DONE?

An MRI was not done in this case. B_{12}, methylmalonic acid levels, and folic acid levels were normal. HSTLV-1 was normal. Serum vitamin B_1 level was 4.8 µg/dL. The alpha-tocopherol level was 18.7 (normal 5.5–18). The serum zinc level was 881 which was normal. The copper level was undetectable. RPR was negative as well as HTLV-1 and HIV.

EMG showed a mild neuropathy.

DISCUSSION

It was concluded that this patient has copper deficiency myeloneuropathy, and she was treated with copper supplementation.

Copper is an essential trace metal and is a component of many key metalloenzymes, and many proteins are involved in the structure and function of the CNS.

Copper absorption in humans most likely occurs in the stomach and proximal duodenum.[7] Its deficiency can be divided into two categories, inherited and acquired. Menkes disease is an X-linked inherited copper deficiency, which is associated with mutations in the *ATP7A* gene. This encodes a P-type adenosine triphosphatase (MNK) that has multiple copper-binding motifs near its amino terminus.[8] Loss of function of this protein causes failure of copper transfer across the gastrointestinal tract and blood–brain barrier with resultant copper deficiency and its neurologic disturbances. Because of copper's ubiquitous distribution and low daily requirement, acquired copper deficiency is rare.[9] In humans, populations at the highest risk are elderly people who have a history of gastrointestinal surgery (including gastroplasty, gastrectomy, and small bowel resection), excessive zinc ingestion, malabsorption states, renal and liver disease, and prolonged total parenteral nutrition[10]; however, often the cause is unknown. An elevated serum zinc level in either excessive zinc ingestion or absence of exogenous ingestion is commonly seen.[11]

Zinc is known to cause upregulation of metallothionein production in the enterocyte, which effectively decreases intestinal absorption of copper.[12]

An ataxic myelopathy resulting from copper deficiency has been documented in ruminant animals, known as swayback.[13,14] The neurologic manifestations of acquired copper deficiency in humans have been increasingly recognized in the last decade. The most common manifestation is myelopathy as well as an associated peripheral neuropathy. Its symptoms include sensory ataxia, spastic gait, and acral paresthesias. An isolated peripheral neuropathy, CNS demyelination, and optic neuritis have also been reported to be associated with copper deficiency.[13] Other associated abnormalities include anemia and leukopenia. The anemia may be microcytic, macrocytic, or normocytic. Thrombocytopenia and resulting pancytopenia are relatively rare[15–18] (Table 48-2).

EMG/NCV usually shows a varying degree of axonal peripheral neuropathy. Nerve biopsy demonstrates the evidence of axonal degeneration. Brain MRI findings are generally nonspecific, including mild lacunar atrophy. However, manifestations on brain MRI do occur in patients with copper deficiency myelopathy and cerebrospinal fluid studies, including oligoclonal bands, myelin basic protein, and IgG index, are negative or within normal limits.[13,16] The most consistent findings on MRI of the spine are abnormal cord signal with two hyperintensities in the posterior column in both the cervical and thoracic levels (Fig. 48-1). This occurs in 44% of patients with copper deficiency myeloneuropathy.[7]

Oral copper supplementation is generally the preferred route of supplementation despite a suspected absorption defect. A treatment protocol for copper deficiency myeloneuropathy has been proposed[19] that includes a short period of replacement with high oral doses of copper (e.g., 6 mg/day for 1 week followed by 4 mg/day for 1 week) followed by long-term supplementation with 2 mg/day oral copper to maintain normal serum levels. Prompt recognition of copper deficiency and then supplementing with copper may prevent further neurologic injury.[19]

During the clinical course, this patient received oral copper 6 mg daily and zinc supplementation was discontinued. The neurologic symptoms gradually improved and at the time of reevaluation her serum copper level was normal up to 0.98 mg/mL. After 4 months, she no longer had symptoms, and the copper was then tapered.

TABLE 48-1 Complications of Bariatric Surgery

Encephalopathy
Behavioral abnormalities
Seizures
Cranial nerve palsies
Ataxia
Myelopathy
Plexopathies
Peripheral neuropathy
Mononeuropathies
Carpal tunnel syndrome
Meralgia paresthetica
Compartment syndromes
Myopathy
Myotonia

TABLE 48-2 Clinical, Physical, and Laboratory Findings in Copper Deficiency Myeloneuropathy

Sensory ataxia
Polyneuropathy
Myelopathy
Anemia and leukopenia
Lower serum copper and ceruloplasmin levels
Elevated serum zinc levels
Axonal peripheral neuropathy on nerve conduction studies and electromyography
T2 hyperintensity in the posterior column in the cervical and thoracic spine on MRI

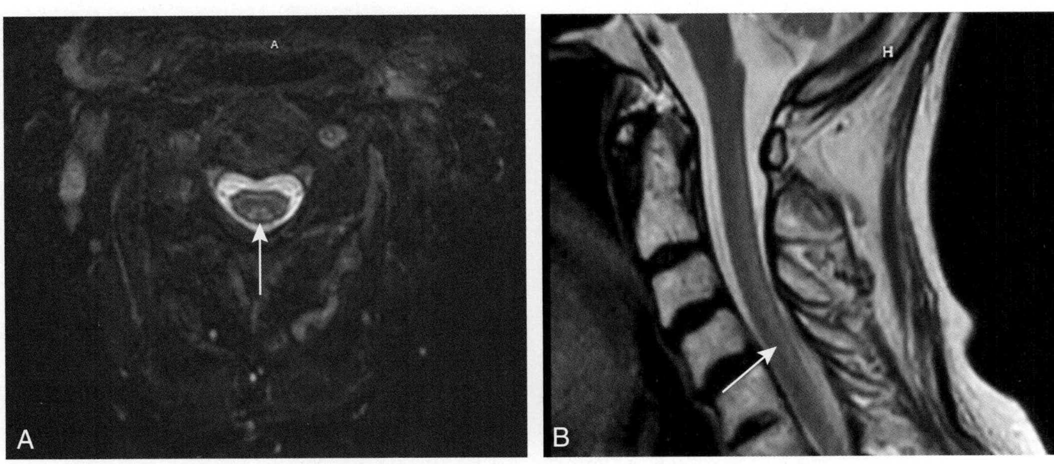

FIG. 48-1 **A**, MRI of the cervical spine, T2 image showing increased signal in posterior columns. **B**, Sagittal view MRI showing an area of increased signal—for another patient with copper deficiency.

SUMMARY

A woman developed a myeloneuropathy after gastric bypass surgery and zinc supplementation. This was found to be caused by copper deficiency, as she improved with copper supplementation.

KEY POINTS

1. Copper deficiency can cause a myeloneuropathy which closely resembles combined degeneration of the spinal cord caused by B_{12} deficiency. This can be seen after gastric bypass surgery, particularly in patients receiving excessive zinc supplementation.
2. Clinical findings that should raise suspicion for copper deficiency include sensory ataxia, spastic gait, and acral paresthesias.
3. Serum copper, ceruloplasmin, and zinc testing should be part of the diagnostic workup in myeloneuropathy.
4. Early recognition and copper supplementation can improve symptoms.

This case was reported as Chai Y, Bertorini T. A female with progressive four limb paresthesias and gait difficulty. J Clin Neuromusc Dis. 2016;11(4):191–197.

REFERENCES

1. Berger JR. The neurological complications of bariatric surgery. *Arch Neurol.* 2004;61:1185–1189.
2. Oh R, Brown DL. Vitamin B12 deficiency. *Am Fam Physician.* 2003;67:979–986.
3. Williams CS, Butler E, Román GC. Treatment of myelopathy in Sjögren syndrome with a combination of prednisone and cyclophosphamide. *Arch Neurol.* 2001;58:815–819.
4. Greenberg BM. The neurologic manifestations of systemic lupus erythematosus. *Neurologist.* 2009;15:115–121.
5. Schleper B, Smerenburg HJ. Copper deficiency associated myelopathy in a 46 year old woman. *J Neurol.* 2001;248:705–706.
6. Stacy A, Rudnicki SA, Dalmau J. Paraneoplastic syndromes of the spinal cord, nerve, and muscle. *Muscle Nerve.* 2000;23: 1800–1818.
7. Kumar N, Gross JB Jr, Ahlskiog JE. Copper deficiency myelopathy produces a clinical picture like subacute combined degermation. *Neurology.* 2004;63:33–39.
8. Mercer JF, Livingston J, Hall B, et al. Isolation of a partial candidate gene for Menkes disease by positional cloning. *Nat Genet.* 1993;3: 20–25.
9. Williams DM. Copper deficiency in humans. *Semin Hematol.* 1983; 20:118–128.
10. Karpel JT, Peden VH. Copper deficiency in long-term parenteral nutrition. *J Pediatr.* 1972;80:32–36.
11. Spain RI, Leist TP, De Sousa EA. When metals compete: a case of copper-deficiency myeloneuropathy and anemia. *Nat Clin Pract Neurol.* 2009;59:106–111.
12. Kumar N, McEvoy KM, Ahiskog JE. Myelopathy due to copper deficiency following gastrointestinal surgery. *Arch Neurol.* 2003; 60:1782–1785.
13. Kumar N. Copper deficiency myelopathy (human swayback). *Mayo Clin Proc.* 2006;81:1371–1384.
14. Prodan CI, Holland NR, Wisdom PJ, et al. CNS demyelination associated with copper deficiency and hyperzincemia. *Neurology.* 2002;59:1453–1456.
15. Gyorly EJ, Chan H. Copper deficiency and microcytic anemia resulting from prolonged ingestion of over-the-counter zinc. *Am J Gastroenterol.* 1992;87:1054–1055.
16. Fohrman MP, Hermann V, Masidonski P, et al. Pancytopenia after removal of copper from total parenteral nutrition. *J Parenter Enternal Nutr.* 2000;24:361–366.
17. Gregg XT, Reddy V, Prchal JT. Copper deficiency masquerading as myelodysplastic syndrome. *Blood.* 2002;100:1493–1495.
18. Greenberg SA, Brienberg HR. A neurological and hematological syndrome associated with zinc excess and copper deficiency. *J Neurol.* 2004;251:111–114.
19. Kelkar P, Chang S, Muley SA. Response to oral supplementation in copper deficiency myeloneuropathy. *J Clin Neuromuscul Dis.* 2008;10:1–3.

An Elderly Woman With Frequent Falls and Abnormal MRI

An 87-year-old woman presented with a 4-year history of progressive leg weakness with incontinence and frequent falls. She also had nighttime spasms.

The patient's past history is unremarkable.

She has a son and a nephew who have leg weakness. It was thought the disease was familial. The nephew was initially thought to have Schilder disease.

A previous MRI of the patient was suggestive of multiple sclerosis.

Physical examination revealed normal mentation and cranial nerves. She had moderate weakness in the lower extremities with increased reflexes and Babinski signs were present. She had absent vibration sense in the legs, and diminished position sense in the toes and feet. She had decreased pinprick up to the mid-calf.

WHAT IS THE DIFFERENTIAL DIAGNOSIS?

This patient has evidence of spinal cord dysfunction and an apparent neuropathy. The differential diagnoses are large, including spinal cord mass or compression in a patient with neuropathy which could be caused by diabetes. Pernicious anemia is also a consideration as well as primary progressive MS. Other possibilities include familial spastic paraparesis and copper deficiency. She had no history of headaches to suggest cerebral autosomal dominant arteriopathy with subcortical infarcts and leukoencephalopathy (CADASIL) or weakness to suggest a muscular dystrophy which sometimes is accompanied by MRI abnormalities. Human immunodeficiency virus (HIV) and human T-lymphocytic virus (HTLV) type1 should also be a consideration.

WHAT TO DO NEXT?

Blood chemistry profile, hemoglobin A1C, and B_{12}/folate were normal.

An EMG showed evidence of an axonal neuropathy and mild sensorimotor axonal neuropathy.

An MRI of the head showed diffuse white matter changes without enhancement (Fig. 49-1), and there was spinal cord atrophy.

It was found that the patient had no B_{12} deficiency, and the diagnosis of MS was unlikely. We measured very long chain fatty acids (VLCFAs), which were elevated (docosanoic acid, C22:0 was 2200 and 2.50 [normal, 42.9–112.7], tetracosanoic acid, C24:0 was 200 [normal, 35.6–101.6], and hexacosanoic acid, C26:0 was 7.4 [normal, 0.31–0.81] and the ratio of C24/C22 was 3.3 [normal up to 7.6–0.988] and the ratio of C26:0–C22:0 was 1.5 [normal, 0.049–00118]). It was concluded that this patient had increased levels of VLCFAs. Her son was later tested for the ABCD gene and he had a mutation of this gene. The patient declined DNA testing.

DISCUSSION

It was concluded that this patient had adrenoleukodystrophy due to the elevation of very high fatty acids. No DNA testing was done.

Adrenomyeloneuropathy and adrenoleukodystrophy are the most common peroxisomal disorders with an incidence of 1:14, 700 with a different clinical presentation of the same X-linked genetic mutation with little correlation between the mutations and the phenotype.[1] The disorders are characterized by accumulation of saturated VLCFAs in the brain.[2]

The genetic cause is a mutated gene that encodes the ABCD1 protein, which is a member of the ABC-transported family that functions by transporting VLCAs into the peroxisome, where they undergo beta oxidation.[3]

The childhood form with the effects manifests early: children over age 4–8 years have attention deficit disorder, behavioral disorders, progressive cortical blindness, paraparesis, and seizures accompanied by adrenal insufficiency.[1] The pathological findings of the brains in these patients show intense inflammatory demyelination beginning in the occipital lobes. They do not have a neuropathy.

Adrenal myeloneuropathy is a variant presenting in adults with progressive spastic paraparesis with large fiber sensory loss and sphincter disturbances without inflammatory changes affecting the corticospinal tract, dorsal columns, and peripheral nerves.[4,5] This usually affects males at ages 20s–30s and affects about 50% of the females who start having symptoms during postmenopausal time. There are about500 mutations of the ABCD gene. Approximately 80% of the cases develop adrenal insufficiency.

The pathophysiology consists of the accumulation of cholesterol and VLCFAs in the nervous system.[6] There is also an accumulation of this in the adrenal glands. This accumulation triggers oxidative stress, apoptosis, and inflammation.

The diagnosis of adrenoneuromyelopathy is difficult unless there is a clear family history and/or other causes of myelopathy or myeloneuropathy have been considered and ruled out. These patients are often misdiagnosed with multiple sclerosis and the differential diagnoses include vitamin B_{12} and folate deficiencies, copper accumulation, primary lateral sclerosis,

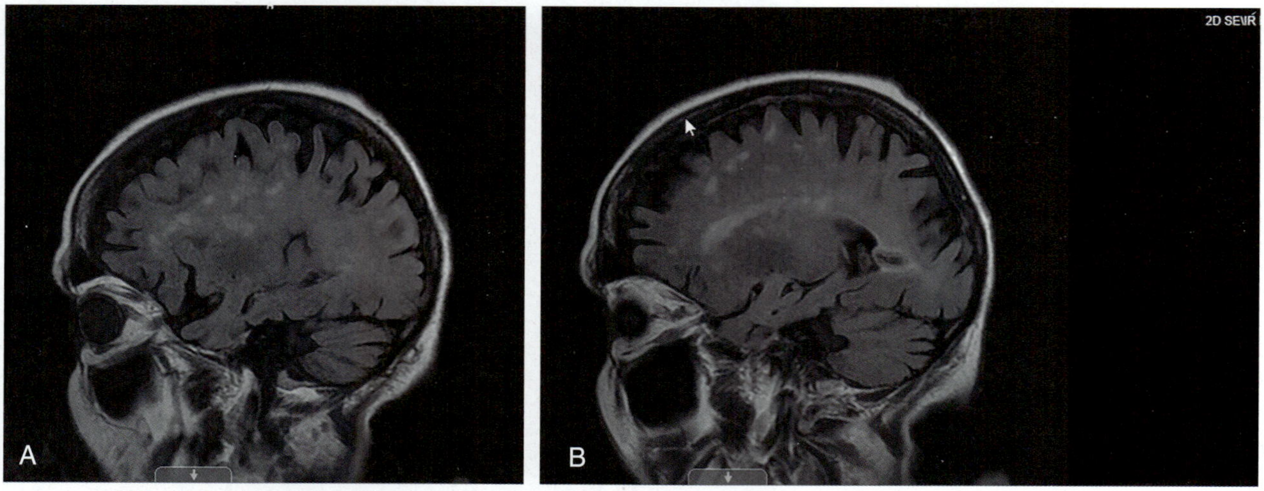

FIG. 49-1 A and B, Sagittal views of T2-weighted flair images of the brain in Case 49. Notice the diffuse increased signal in the white matter.

HTLV-1, and familial spastic paraparesis. The final diagnosis is made by genetic testing as well as measuring the VLCFAs which show elevation of C26 and increased ratios of C24.0 and C26.0–C22.0. The female carriers could have elevation of VLCAs, but false-negative tests occur. DNA sequencing, obviously, is more important.[1,2]

The treatment in adults is conservative although those with adrenal insufficiency receive corticosteroids. In the past diets to reduce VLCFAs have been tried including Lorenzo's oil, about which a movie was made, and this is a combination of 4:1 erucic acid and oleic acid (glyceryl trioleate and glyceryl trierucate). This has not been demonstrated to be beneficial in clinical trials, but there is a suggestion that it will slow the progression.[5,7]

Childhood screening allows clinicians to treat children early[2] with hemopoietic stem cell therapy[8] and gene therapy.[6]

SUMMARY

An elderly woman who presented with frequent falls had a myelopathy and a neuropathy with diffuse white matter changes on MRI. She had increased VLCFAs, and her son had an ABCD gene mutation. She has been diagnosed as a manifest carrier of adrenomyeloneuropathy.

IMPORTANT POINTS

- Whenever there are diffuse white matter changes on the brain MRI, several other disorders should be ruled out including adrenoleukodystrophy, CADASIL, small vessel disease, and some cases of muscular dystrophy prior to assuming the patient has multiple sclerosis.
- Adrenoleukodystrophy manifests as a myelopathy and peripheral neuropathy showing diffuse white matter changes on the MRI. It is X-linked recessive disorder and could manifest in females with a milder phenotype.
- Adrenoleukodystrophy and adrenoneuromyelopathy are disorders caused by the ABCD1 gene mutation which causes the accumulation of VLCFAs in the brain, spinal cord, and adrenal glands. The diagnosis is made by measuring VLCFAs in blood and DNA testing.
- In adults the treatment is symptomatic. Stem cell treatment therapy and gene therapy are promising in children.
- The MRI on these patients may have white matter changes similar to those in MS.

REFERENCES

1. Turk BR, Theda C, Fatemi A, Moser AB. X-linked adrenoleukodystrophy: pathology, pathophysiology, diagnostic testing, newborn screening and therapies. *Int J Dev Neurosci*. 2020;80(9):52–72. https://doi.org/10.1002/jdn.10003. Epub 2020 Jan 26.
2. Moser AB, Jones RO, Hubbard WC, et al. Newborn screening for X-linked adrenoleukodystrophy. *In J Neonatal Screen*. 2016; 2(4):15.
3. Igarashi M, Schaumburg HH, Powers J, Kishmoto Y, et al. Fatty acid abnormality in adrenoleukodystrophy. *J Neurochem*. 1976;26(4): 851–860.
4. Griffin JW, Gorn E, Schaumburg H, Engel WK, Loriaux L. Adrenomyeloneuropathy: a probable variant of adrenoleukodystrophy. I. Clinical and endocrinologic. *Neurology*. 1977;27(12):1107–1113.
5. Moser HW, Ramond GV, Dubey P. Adrenoleukodystrophy: new approaches to a neurodegenerative disease. *JAMA*. 2005;294(24): 3131–3134.
6. Raymond GV, Moser AB, Fateini A. X-linked adrenoleukodystrophy. In: Haines JL, Korf BR, Morton CC, Seidman CE, Seidman JG, Smith DR, eds. *GeneReviews (Internet)*. Vol. 58. Seattle, WA: University of Washington; 2018:17.6.1–17.6.23.
7. Motley W, Chaudry V, Lloyd TE Treatment and management of hereditary neuropathies. In: Bertorini TE, ed. *Neuromuscular Disorders: Treatment and Management*. Amsterdam, Netherlands: Elsevier; 2022. 2nd ed.
8. Eichler F, Duncan C, Musolino PL, Orchard PJ, DeOliveira S, et al. Hematopoietic stem-cell gene therapy for cerebral adrenoleukodystrophy. *N Engl J Med*. 2017;377(17):1630–1638.

A Man With Weakness in the Legs

A 36-year-old patient was referred for evaluation of progressive weakness in the legs and feet numbness for 4 years.

Past medical history and family history were noncontributory. He did not smoke or drink.

Examination revealed normal mentation and cranial nerves. He was able to walk on his heels and toes. Muscle strength was 5/5 in the neck, and arms proximally, 4/5 in the hand muscles; hip flexion, extension, and adduction were 4/5; leg flexion and extension were 5−/5; the foot extensors, dorsiflexors, and evertors were 3/5; flexors were 4/5. Reflexes were trace at the knees and triceps and absent elsewhere. Toes were down-going. There was absent vibration sense in the toes and decreased in the ankles and fingers. Position sense was decreased in the toes. He had decreased pinprick, touch, and temperature sensations to 16 cm above both ankles and up to the wrists in the upper extremities. Romberg test and gait were normal. The rest of the neurologic examination was normal, and there was no visceromegaly, nerve hypertrophy, or high arches. No muscle atrophy was noted.

WHAT IS THE DIFFERENTIAL DIAGNOSIS?

This patient, with a negative family history, developed a polyneuropathy with proximal and distal weakness, areflexia, and prominent sensory loss of large fibers, but also small fibers (decreased pain and temperature sensations). Common causes of polyneuropathies to be considered include diabetes, thyroid disease, toxins, HIV infections, monoclonal gammopathy, and B_{12} deficiency. He was not an alcoholic and had not been exposed to toxins. A familial neuropathy, such as Charcot–Marie–Tooth disease, is a possibility, but his neuropathy was recently acquired. He had no family history and did not have high arches. Small fiber involvement is not typical but can occur in this disorder. A chronic inflammatory demyelinating polyneuropathy (CIDP) is a consideration because, although patients with CIDP usually have mostly large fiber involvement, pain and temperature sensory deficits can also be present. CIDP associated with a monoclonal gammopathy and with AIDS is also a consideration. He did not have a history of a connective tissue disease, and the slow progression is against a vasculitic neuropathy. Porphyric neuropathy is unlikely because this usually presents with intermittent attacks and affects mainly motor axons.

Laboratory studies included a normal erythrocyte sedimentation rate; complete metabolic panel, complete blood count, B_{12}/folate, HIV, immunoelectrophoresis, thyroid-stimulating hormone, and fluorescent antinuclear antibody were all normal.

AN EMG TEST WAS PERFORMED

Motor Nerve Studies

Nerve and Site	Latency (ms)	Amplitude (mV)	Conduction Velocity (m/s)
Peroneal Nerve R.	**Normal ≤ 5.7**	**Normal ≥ 3**	**Normal ≥ 40**
Ankle	**8.8**	3	–
Fibular head	27.2	**0.9**	**17**
Knee	29.9	**0.9**	**25**
Tibial Nerve L.	**Normal ≤ 5.3**	**Normal ≥ 4**	**Normal ≥ 50**
Ankle	**14.7**	**1**	–
Pop. fossa	47.9	**0.5**	**13**
Median Nerve R.	**Normal ≤ 4.2**	**Normal ≥ 6**	**Normal ≥ 50**
Wrist	**7.4**	8	–
Elbow	19.0	**3**	**20**
Axilla	22.1	**3**	**42**
Ulnar Nerve R.	**Normal ≤ 3.6**	**Normal ≥ 8**	**Normal ≥ 50**
Wrist	**6.3**	8	–
Below elbow	17.0	**3**	**19**
Above elbow	21.9	**3**	**24**

F-Wave and Tibial H-Reflex Studies

Nerve	Latency (ms)	Normal Latency ≤ (ms)
Peroneal nerve R.	**79.6**	54
Tibial nerve L.	**NR**	54
Median nerve R.	**55.7**	30
Ulnar nerve R.	**42.4**	30
H-reflex R.	**NR**	34
H-reflex L.	**NR**	34

Sensory Nerve Studies

Nerve	Latency (ms)	Normal Latency ≤ (ms)	Amp (μV)	Normal Amp ≥ (μV)
Sural nerve R.	**NR**	4.0	**NR**	11
Median nerve R.	**NR**	3.1	**NR**	20
Ulnar nerve R.	**NR**	3.1	**NR**	13

EMG Data

Muscle	Insrt Activity	Fibs	Pos Waves	Fasc	Amp	Dur	Poly	Pattern
Deltoid R.	**Inc**	None	None	None	**Lg**	**Inc**	None	Full
Biceps brachii R.	Norm	None	None	None	Norm	Norm	None	Full
Brachioradialis R.	**Inc**	None	**1+**	None	**Lg**	**Inc**	None	Full
Flexor carpi radialis R.	**Inc**	None	**1+**	None	**Lg**	**Inc**	None	Full
Flexor carpi ulnaris R.	**Inc**	None	**1+**	None	**Lg**	**Inc**	None	Full
First dorsal interosseous R.	**Inc**	None	**1+**	None	**Lg**	**Inc**	None	Full
Tensor fasciae latae R.	**Inc**	None	None	None	**Lg**	**Inc**	None	Full
Vastus lateralis R.	Norm	None	None	None	**Lg**	**Inc**	None	Full
Tibialis anterior R.	**Inc**	None	None	None	**Lg**	**Inc**	None	Full
Gastrocnemius R.	**Inc**	None	**1+**	None	**Lg**	**Inc**	None	Full
Vastus lateralis L.	Norm	None	None	None	**Lg**	**Inc**	None	Full
Tibialis anterior L.	**Inc**	None	**1+**	None	**Lg**	**Inc**	None	Full
Gastrocnemius L.	**Inc**	None	**1+**	None	**Lg**	**Inc**	None	Full

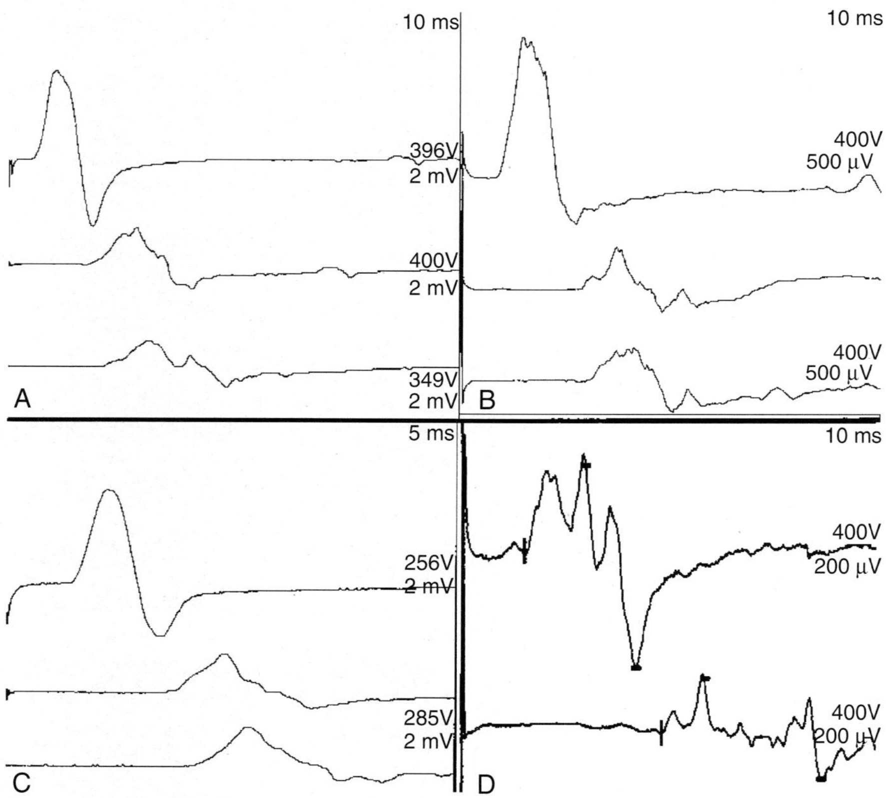

FIG. 50-1 A, Right ulnar motor nerve conduction test showing temporal dispersion and drop in amplitude of the CMAP from proximal stimulation sites: elbow and above the elbow (lower two tracings) compared with wrist stimulation (top tracing) (2 mV/10 ms). **B**, Motor nerve conduction test of the right peroneal nerve showing temporal dispersion of the CMAP at knee and above knee stimulation sites (bottom two tracings), compared with ankle stimulation (top tracing) (500 μV/10 ms). **C**, Nerve conduction tests of the right median nerve showing low-amplitude CMAP, with temporal dispersion from elbow and above elbow stimulation (bottom two tracings) compared with wrist stimulation (top tracing) (2 mV/5 ms). **D**, Left tibial nerve conduction test showing low-amplitude CMAP with temporal dispersion at ankle (top tracing) and knee stimulation (bottom tracing) (200 μV/10 ms).

WHAT WERE THE EMG FINDINGS?

This test showed marked slowing of motor nerve conduction velocities with temporal dispersion and partial conduction block (Fig. 50-1). The F-responses and distal motor latencies were prolonged. H-reflexes and SNAPs were absent.

Needle test showed mild chronic denervation with reinnervation because of the presence of large motor unit action potentials, but the findings were out of proportion to the significant conduction slowing. It was concluded that he had a predominantly demyelinating neuropathy. The nonuniform slowing and temporal dispersion indicate that the neuropathy was acquired rather than hereditary. The absent SNAPs could be secondary to either demyelination or axonal degeneration.

A lumbar puncture showed a protein of 76 mg/dL (normal, <40 mg/dL) without cells and was otherwise normal.

WHAT IS THE DIFFERENTIAL DIAGNOSIS?

Acquired demyelinating neuropathies have many causes. This patient did not have a gammopathy, nor was he diabetic. He was HIV-negative. He had no history of hepatitis, and his liver function tests were normal. He had no thyroid disease or history of small bowel disorder or connective tissue disorder. The symmetrical presentation and prominent demyelination are also against vasculitis.

He was diagnosed as having CIDP and was treated with monthly IgG infusions of 2 g/kg for 3 months. After this, he became asymptomatic for 1 year without treatment.

For discussion and important points, see Case 52.

SUMMARY

This patient had a progressive neuropathy with slow nerve conduction velocities and temporal dispersion. He also had elevated protein in spinal fluid. He was diagnosed as having CIDP, and he responded well to IgG infusions.

51 CASE

An Elderly Woman With Asymmetric Weakness and a Monoclonal Gammopathy

A 70-year-old woman was evaluated for a 1-year history of weakness and numbness that manifested initially in the legs and in the left hand and for the last 6 weeks also in the right hand. She developed mild bilateral footdrop in the last month.

Past medical history included mild glucose intolerance for which she took glyburide for several months. She had had two C-sections, appendectomy, hemorrhoidectomy, and three ear surgeries, as she also had a chronic history of left otitis and mastoiditis for which she received antibiotics periodically and had hearing loss on the left.

General physical examination revealed mild splenomegaly. Mentation and cranial nerves were normal, except for decreased hearing in the left ear. Facial muscle strength was normal. She had weakness of finger extensors of both hands, with significant weakness of the interosseous and thenar muscles on the left. Neck and proximal upper extremity muscles were normal. She had moderate proximal leg weakness of 3+/5, foot dorsiflexors, evertors, and toe extensors 3− bilaterally. Foot flexors were minimally weak. She was areflexic and had no pathologic reflexes.

Vibration sense was absent in the toes and decreased in the fingers and ankles; position sense was minimally decreased in the toes. Pinprick, temperature, and touch sensations were decreased up to the ankles, all symmetrically. Reflexes were absent throughout. No fasciculations were seen. There were no Babinski signs. Romberg's test was negative; coordination and gait were normal.

WHAT IS THE DIFFERENTIAL DIAGNOSIS?

This woman had progressive, asymmetric weakness with more severe involvement of the left upper extremity. A spinal canal disease causing a C8 radiculopathy could explain the hand findings, but not her generalized areflexia and weakness with sensory deficits in the legs, unless she had two disorders. Because of the sensory findings, a motor neuron disorder is also unlikely. The asymmetric presentation could suggest a vasculitic neuropathy, but the slow progression is somewhat unusual for this. She could have a polyneuropathy such as from diabetes, with a superimposed radiculopathy or a left brachial plexus lesion. Her neuropathy could also have other causes, such as being associated with a monoclonal gammopathy or a connective tissue disease. Thyroid disease and B_{12} deficiency neuropathy do not present with prominent weakness, unless there is evidence of combined degeneration of the spinal cord in the latter. Acquired demyelinating inflammatory neuropathies are usually symmetrical, but sometimes patients might have an asymmetric presentation and could have predominant involvement of the upper extremities.[1] The chronic recurrent infections could suggest a secondary amyloidosis, but her degree of weakness was out of proportion to the sensory findings, which are more prominent in amyloidosis. A multifocal motor and sensory neuropathy, or Lewis–Sumner syndrome, is a possibility, particularly with the more prominent manifestations in the left hand. This condition is multifocal and affects mainly the upper extremities,[2] however, and she also had symmetrical leg findings. Distal demyelinating neuropathy associated with a monoclonal gammopathy occurs in elderly persons, mainly in men, and is more symmetrical.

AN EMG TEST WAS PERFORMED

Motor Nerve Studies

Nerve and Site	Latency (ms)	Amplitude (mV)	Conduction Velocity (m/s)
Peroneal Nerve L.	**Normal ≤ 5.7**	**Normal ≥ 3**	**Normal ≥ 40**
Ankle	**25.5**	**0.1**	–
Fibular head	38.5	**0.1**	**19**
Knee	42.0	**0.1**	**24**
Tibial Nerve L.	**Normal ≤ 5.3**	**Normal ≥ 4**	**Normal ≥ 40**
Ankle	**13.1**	**0.3**	–
Pop. fossa	36.1	**0.3**	**16**
Tibial Nerve R.	**Normal ≤ 5.3**	**Normal ≥ 4**	**Normal ≥ 40**
Ankle	**22.2**	**0.2**	–
Pop. fossa	59.2	**0.2**	**10**
Median Nerve L.	**Normal ≤ 4.2**	**Normal ≥ 6**	**Normal ≥ 50**
Wrist	**8.5**	**4**	–
Elbow	16.6	**3**	**23**
Ulnar Nerve L.	**Normal ≤ 3.6**	**Normal ≥ 8**	**Normal ≥ 50**
Wrist	**5.8**	**3**	–
Below elbow	14.0	**0.4**	**15**
Above elbow	23.2	**0.4**	**13**
Median Nerve R.	**Normal ≤ 4.2**	**Normal ≥ 6**	**Normal ≥ 50**
Wrist	**8.0**	**5**	–
Elbow	**NR**	**NR**	–

Motor Nerve Studies—cont'd

Nerve and Site	Latency (ms)	Amplitude (mV)	Conduction Velocity (m/s)
Ulnar Nerve R.	**Normal ≤ 3.6**	**Normal ≥ 8**	**Normal ≥ 50**
Wrist	**8.2**	**1.6**	–
Below elbow	25.2	**0.2**	**9**
Above elbow	NR	**NR**	**NR**

F-Wave and Tibial H-Reflex Studies

Nerve	Latency (ms)	Normal Latency ≤ (ms)
Peroneal nerve L.	**NR**	54
Tibial nerve R.	**71.2**	54
Tibial nerve L.	**69.9**	54
Median nerve L.	**43.5**	30

F-Wave and Tibial H-Reflex Studies—cont'd

Nerve	Latency (ms)	Normal Latency ≤ (ms)
Ulnar nerve L.	**41.5**	54
Median nerve R.	**44.2**	30
Ulnar nerve R.	**42.4**	30
H-reflex L.	**NR**	34
H-reflex R.	**NR**	34

Sensory Nerve Studies

Nerve	Latency (ms)	Normal Latency ≤ (ms)	Amp (μV)	Normal Amp ≥ (μV)
Sural nerve L.	**NR**	4.0	**NR**	11
Median nerve L.	**NR**	3.1	**NR**	20
Ulnar nerve L.	**NR**	3.1	**NR**	13

EMG Data

Muscle	Insrt Activity	Fibs	Pos Waves	Fasc	Amp	Dur	Poly	Pattern
Biceps brachii R.	Norm	None	None	None	**Lg**	**Inc**	None	Full
Flexor carpi ulnaris R.	**Inc**	**3+**	**3+**	None	**Lg**	**Inc**	**Many**	**Red**
First dorsal interosseus R.	**Inc**	**3+**	**3+**	None	**Lg**	**Inc**	None	**Red**
Vastus lateralis R.	Norm	None	None	None	**Lg**	**Inc**	**Few**	**Red**
Tibialis anterior R.	**Inc**	**3+**	**3+**	None	**Lg**	**Inc**	**Few**	**Red**
Peroneus longus R.	**Inc**	**2+**	**2+**	None	**Lg**	**Inc**	None	**Red**
Gastrocnemius R.	**Inc**	**3+**	**3+**	None	**Lg**	**Inc**	None	**Red**

What Were The EMG Findings?

The motor nerve conduction velocities were very slow, and the distal latencies were markedly prolonged even in nerves in which the amplitude was not significantly decreased. There was also evidence of temporal dispersion and conduction blocks, particularly in both ulnar and median nerves (Fig. 51-1). SNAPs were absent. The F-responses were prolonged.

The needle test showed denervation potentials and large motor unit potentials with decreased motor unit recruitment diffusely. Thus she had a demyelinating neuropathy and also had axonal degeneration.

WHAT OTHER STUDIES NEED TO BE DONE?

Complete metabolic panel and erythrocyte sedimentation rate were normal; fluorescent antinuclear antibody test was positive at 1:40, speckled pattern. Serum immunoelectrophoresis showed an IgG monoclonal gammopathy with κ light chains. Hepatitis profile and bone survey were normal. Bone marrow biopsy showed an increased number of normal-appearing non-monoclonal plasma cells; GMI ganglioside antibodies were not elevated. She had mild hepatomegaly and splenomegaly on abdominal ultrasound, and a liver biopsy was normal. Alkaline phosphatase was elevated at 250 mg/dL (normal, <140 mg/dL). Skeletal survey showed no bone lesions.

Cerebrospinal fluid protein was 146 mg/dL (normal, <40 mg/dL); there were no cells, and the test was otherwise normal. Nerve biopsy showed segmental demyelination, axonal degeneration, and large axons without myelin. No inflammation was seen.

The patient was treated initially with prednisone, without improvement, and developed significant side effects. She later received azathioprine 100 mg/day, which was considered therapeutic based on her white blood count and mean corpuscular volume values and also monthly gamma globulin infusions with marked improvement.

Four years later, she became weaker and developed severe anemia; a bone marrow aspirate showed small cell lymphoma. She was treated with chlorambucil and IgG infusions.

For further discussion, important points, and references, see Case 52.

SUMMARY

This elderly woman presented with a polyneuropathy with more pronounced findings in the left upper extremity. She had electrophysiologic, spinal fluid, and biopsy findings consistent with chronic inflammatory demyelinating polyradiculoneuropathy. She also had an IgG gammopathy. She responded to immunotherapy but later developed a small cell lymphoma.

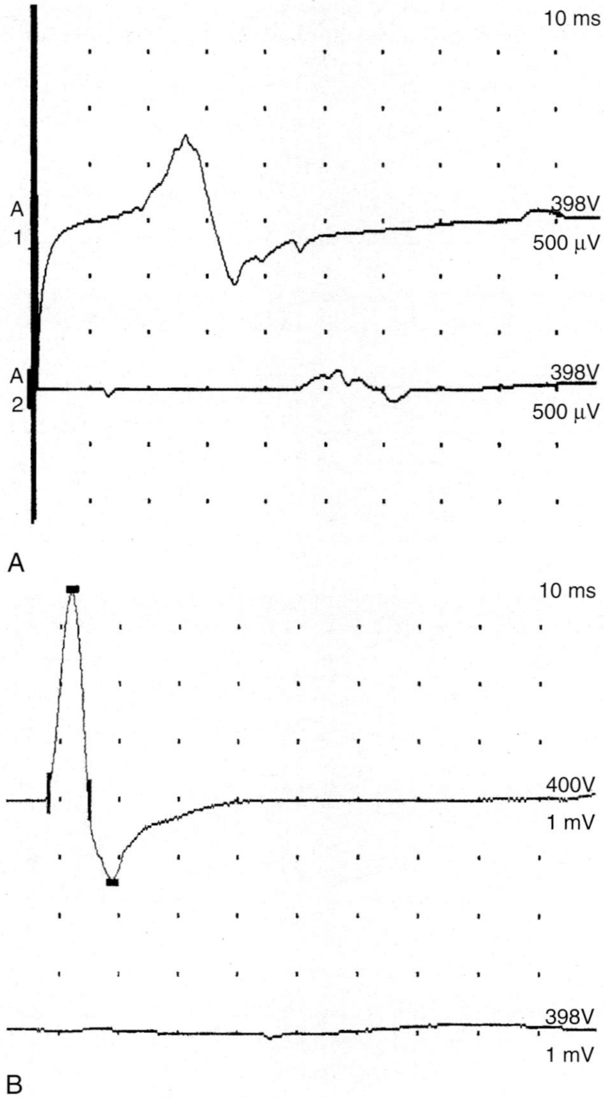

FIG. 51-1 **A**, Right ulnar nerve conduction tests showing partial conduction block and temporal dispersion of the CMAP from proximal stimulation sites at wrist (**A1**) and elbow (**A2**) (500 μV/10 ms). **B**, Complete conduction block in the right median nerve; notice the CMAP from wrist stimulation (*top*); no response from proximal elbow stimulation (*bottom*) (1 mV/10 ms).

A Man With Progressive Weakness and Fasciculations

A 37-year-old man presented with a 1-year history of progressive weakness in the upper and lower extremities, difficulties raising his arms above his head, and difficulty combing his hair. He was unable to walk upstairs or arise up from a toilet. He had no sensory complaints or difficulty swallowing.

Past medical history was negative. He smoked occasionally and drank alcohol on weekends. He was referred with a diagnosis of a motor neuron disease. Family history was negative for neurologic disorders.

Examination showed normal mentation and cranial nerves. He was unable to raise his arms above his shoulders and to walk unassisted (Fig. 52-1). No significant wasting was noted, except for the first dorsal interosseous muscles (see Fig. 52-1B). He also had high foot arches (see Fig. 52-1C). Motor examination revealed normal neck muscles; deltoids were 2+/5; biceps and triceps were 4/5; wrist and hand muscles, 3−/5; iliopsoas, 2/5; gluteus, 3/5; quadriceps, 3/5; and hamstrings, 2/5. Foot dorsiflexors and evertors were 2/5; flexors were 5. He was hyporeflexic all over and had diffuse fasciculations. Sensory examination to pinprick, touch, temperature, vibration, and position was normal. There were no Babinski signs or nerve hypertrophy.

WHAT IS THE DIFFERENTIAL DIAGNOSIS?

This man had a recent onset of progressive symmetrical arm and leg weakness and fasciculations, but minimal atrophy. The fact that he has high arches raises the possibility of Charcot–Marie–Tooth (CMT) disease; however, the weakness was of recent onset and involved prominently proximal muscles. He had no sensory complaints, but patients with CMT may have only mild sensory deficits. It is also possible that the patient has familial spinal muscular atrophy and also some distal dystrophies which can present with high arches; but again, his weakness was of recent onset and was proximal as well as distal. It is indeed possible that high arches or hammertoes are not related and that he has two different conditions or that the weakness has been more long-standing than he reports. There are also reported cases of hereditary neuropathy that develop chronic inflammatory demyelinating polyradiculoneuropathy (CIDP).

Weakness with fasciculations and hyporeflexia could suggest a progressive spinal muscular atrophy. Amyotrophic lateral sclerosis is unlikely because he had no long tract signs, and no bulbar signs to suggest either this or Kennedy disease.

Multifocal motor neuropathy (MMN) presents with weakness, fasciculations, and little atrophy, but in this condition the weakness affects mainly the upper extremities,[1,2] and it is asymmetric in the territory of individual nerves.[3–5] Multifocal-acquired motor axonopathy (MAMA) has a similar presentation but without conduction blocks. Lewis–Sumner syndrome is also similar, but patients also have sensory deficits.[6]

Symmetrical weakness affecting the upper and lower extremities occurs in CIDP, a disease in which there is large sensory fiber loss. There are, however, cases of a purely motor CIDP.[7]

He was not exposed to toxins or medications that affect the peripheral nerves.

WHAT WOULD ONE DO NEXT?

The workup included a complete metabolic panel, serum creatine kinase test, and thyroid studies that were normal, and an EMG was ordered.

AN EMG TEST WAS PERFORMED

Motor Nerve Studies

Nerve and Site	Latency (ms)	Amplitude (mV)	Conduction Velocity (m/s)
Peroneal Nerve R.	**Normal ≤ 5.7**	**Normal ≥ 3**	**Normal ≥ 40**
Ankle	**7.8**	**1.9**	–
Fibular head	18.0	**1.3**	**37**
Knee	19.9	**1.3**	47
Tibial Nerve R.	**Normal ≤ 5.3**	**Normal ≥ 4**	**Normal ≥ 40**
Ankle	**6.2**	**1.8**	–
Pop. fossa	20.2	**1.2**	**37**
Peroneal Nerve L.	**Normal ≤ 5.7**	**Normal ≥ 3**	**Normal ≥ 40**
Ankle	**12.1**	**0.6**	–
Fibular head	25.1	**0.3**	**24**
Knee	27.3	**0.3**	41
Median Nerve R.	**Normal ≤ 4.2**	**Normal ≥ 6**	**Normal ≥ 50**
Wrist	**9.9**	**1.9**	–
Elbow	14.8	**1.0**	51
Ulnar Nerve R.	**Normal ≤ 3.6**	**Normal ≥ 8**	**Normal ≥ 50**
Wrist	**5.0**	**4.4**	–
Below elbow	10.0	**2.9**	**45**
Above elbow	13.4	**2.3**	**35**
Axilla	16.8	**2.1**	**46**
Erb's point	24.6	**0.4**	**27**

Motor Nerve Studies—cont'd

Nerve and Site	Latency (ms)	Amplitude (mV)	Conduction Velocity (m/s)
Ulnar Nerve L.	**Normal ≤ 3.6**	**Normal ≥ 8**	**Normal ≥ 50**
Wrist	**7.0**	**2.1**	–
Below elbow	13.8	**0.9**	**35**
Above elbow	19.1	**0.3**	**23**
Axilla	21.5	**0.4**	69
Erb's point	24.8	**0.5**	61
Musculocutaneous Nerve R.			
Axilla	**7.4**	4.5	–
Erb's point	13.0	**0.5**	**21**

F-Wave and Tibial H-Reflex Studies

Nerve	Latency (ms)	Normal Latency(ms)
Peroneal nerve R.	**62.7**	54
Tibial nerve R.	**83.0**	54
Peroneal nerve L.	**NR**	54
Median nerve R.	**NR**	30
Ulnar nerve R.	**45.9**	30
H-reflex R.	**NR**	34
H-reflex L.	**NR**	34

Sensory Nerve Studies

Nerve	Onset Latency (ms)	Normal Latency (ms)	Peak Latency (ms)	Normal Peak Latency (ms)	Amp (mV)	Normal Amp ≥ (mV)	Conduction Velocity (m/s)	Normal Conduction Velocity ≥ (m/s)
Sural nerve R.	3.3	3.5	3.8	4.0	20	11	42	40
Median nerve R.	**3.3**	2.6	**3.8**	3.1	**16**	20	**39**	50
Ulnar nerve R.	2.2	2.6	2.7	3.1	18	13	55	50
Ulnar nerve L.	2.3	2.6	2.8	3.1	20	13	52	50

EMG Data

Muscle	Insrt Activity	Fibs	Pos Waves	Fasc	Amp	Dur	Poly	Pattern
Sternocleido. R.	Norm	None	None	None	Norm	Norm	None	Full
Thoracic paraspinals R.	**Inc**	**1+**	**1+**	None	Norm	Norm	None	Full
Lumbar paraspinals R.	Norm	None	None	None	Norm	Norm	None	Full
Deltoid R.	**Inc**	**2+**	**2+**	None	**Lg**	**Inc**	None	**Red**
Biceps brachii R.	**Inc**	**2+**	**2+**	**Few**	**Lg**	**Inc**	**Few**	**Red**
Flexor carpi radialis R.	**CRD**	**2+**	**2+**	None	**Lg**	**Inc**	None	**Red**
Flexor carpi ulnaris R.	**CRD**	**2+**	**2+**	**Few**	**Lg**	**Inc**	None	**Red**
1st dorsal interosseous R.	**Inc**	**2+**	**2+**	**Few**	**Lg**	**Inc**	None	**Red**
Vastus lateralis R.	**Inc**	**2+**	**2+**	**Few**	**Lg**	**Inc**	None	**Red**
Tibialis anterior R.	**Inc**	**1+**	**1+**	None	**Lg**	**Inc**	None	**Red**
Extensor hallucis longus R.	**Inc**	**2+**	**2+**	None	**Lg**	**Inc**	None	**Red**
Gastrocnemius R.	**Inc**	**2+**	**2+**	None	**Lg**	**Inc**	None	**Red**

WHAT WERE THE EMG FINDINGS?

The nerve conduction velocity (NCV) test showed all the features of demyelinating neuropathy with velocity slowing, temporal dispersion of the compound muscle action potentials, prolonged distal latencies and F-responses, and no H-reflexes. He also had evidence of partial conduction blocks (Fig. 52-2).

All the SNAPs were normal except for the median nerve that had prolonged latency, slow conduction velocity, and mildly decreased amplitude suggesting a mild median neuropathy at the wrist.

The needle tests showed diffuse denervation, indicating axonal degeneration, and there were also diffuse fasciculations.

Based on these findings, the differential diagnosis includes diseases that affect large myelinated fibers, such as CIDP, as well as CIDP associated with a monoclonal gammopathy of uncertain significance (MGUS), and with HIV. In these diseases, some diffuse or axonal degeneration can be seen. The lack of uniform slowing and the presence of conduction block are against a hereditary demyelinating neuropathy, such as CMT type 1, although this can be seen in CMT type X. Myelin-associated glycoprotein (MAG) neuropathy usually has distal numbness and weakness and is usually seen in older patients.

This patient had no exposure to drugs that cause a demyelinating neuropathy, such as amiodarone, nor did he have a history of weight loss or lymph node enlargement to suggest lymphoma. He was not a diabetic.

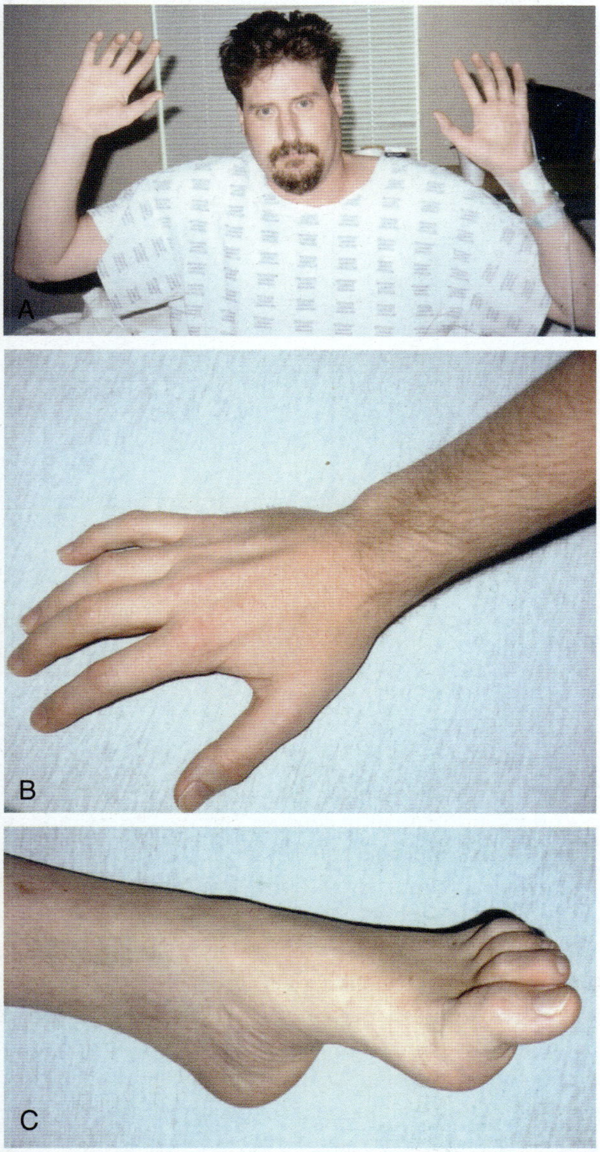

FIG. 52-1 **A**, Notice the patient in this case who is unable to raise his arms. **B**, Notice interosseous muscle wasting. **C**, Notice high arch and hammertoes in this patient.

Vasculitis is usually asymmetric, as in mononeuritis multiplex, but can sometimes present with a diffuse sensorimotor neuropathy. Conduction block can also be seen due to focal edema.[8] The diffuse symmetrical weakness with only motor involvement, along with the signs of demyelination seen on nerve conduction tests, makes that diagnosis unlikely.

WHAT OTHER TESTS SHOULD BE DONE?

Immunoelectrophoresis, erythrocyte sedimentation rate, fluorescent antinuclear antibody test, and HIV titers were normal. IgM GM_1 ganglioside antibody titers were 1:12,800, and the IgG was 1:3200 (normal, <1:800).

A muscle biopsy showed atrophic angular fibers and targets indicating denervation. A sural nerve biopsy was completely normal. A lumbar puncture showed spinal fluid with an elevated protein of 119 mg/dL (normal, <40 mg/dL) with no cells; the test was otherwise normal.

WHAT WOULD YOU DO NEXT?

The patient was started initially on prednisone 60 mg by mouth per day with a marked worsening of symptoms, so this was discontinued. He received IgG infusions in doses of 2 g/kg with marked improvement. This was repeated monthly, but, as he later deteriorated, cyclophosphamide was added in doses of 200 mg daily, orally, with which he improved and stabilized (Fig. 52-3). Because of the patient's high arches, DNA tests for demyelinating CMT types 1 and X were done, and these were negative.

SUMMARY

This man with progressive, diffuse muscle weakness and fasciculations was initially diagnosed as having a motor neuron disease. He had a demyelinating neuropathy with slowing and multifocal conduction block, which are features of a motor CIDP. He had an elevation of serum GM_1 antibodies and of spinal fluid protein; he worsened with steroids and responded to immunotherapy with IgG infusions and cyclophosphamide.

DISCUSSION (CASES 50–52)

Cases 50 and *51* had CIDP, a disease characterized by proximal and distal weakness, areflexia, and prominent large fiber sensory loss. They also had typical abnormal NCV tests, demonstrating conduction slowing, temporal dispersion, prolongation of distal latencies and F-responses, and conduction block,[9] although this can also be seen in vasculitis.[10] *Cases 50* and *51* also had some small fiber involvement, and all three also had axonal degeneration with reinnervation. All of these findings could occur in CIDP. *Cases 50* and *52* had no evidence of another disease associated with CIDP, but *Case 51* had a monoclonal gammopathy.

CIDP is an autoimmune disease with an incidence of between 0.81 and 1.9 per 100,000 population with a prevalence of 1–7.7 per 100,000[11,12] and constitutes 5%–20% of all neuropathies seen in referral centers.[13] Its presentation could be acute, slowly progressive, or recurrent. Patients present with weakness and areflexia but may also have a gait disturbance with paresthesias and numbness in the hands and feet. Weakness is usually symmetrical, but there could be asymmetry, as in *Case 51*. Muscle atrophy is not seen initially but might appear later. Cranial nerve involvement is rarely seen, affecting the extraocular, face, and bulbar muscles.[14,15] There could also be evidence of autonomic dysfunction,[16] and about 25% of the cases have disorder of micturition. Central demyelination can occur.[14]

Historically, Harris and Newcomb[17] initially reported a hypertrophic neuropathy with a recurrent course which could have been a case of CIDP, and later, Austin[18] reviewed the literature and reported two patients with a symmetrical motor neuropathy with a fluctuating course; some responded to steroids.

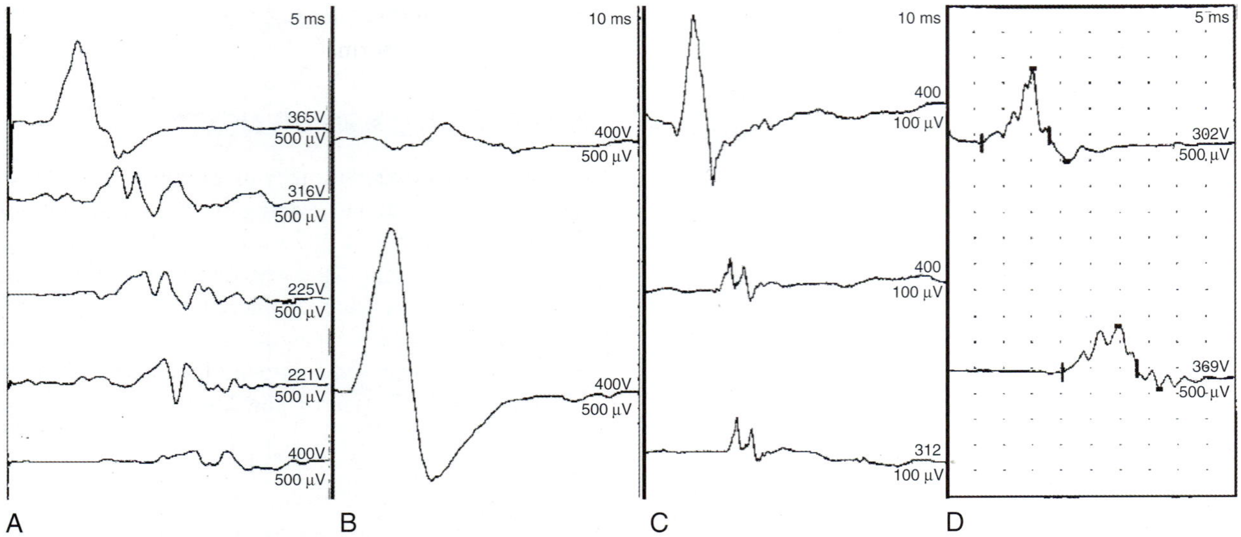

FIG. 52-2 **A**, Left ulnar nerve showing low-amplitude CMAP obtained from wrist stimulation *(top tracing)* and temporal dispersion of the CMAP from proximal stimulation sites: at the elbow, arm, axilla, and Erb's point *(lower four tracings, top to bottom)* (500 μV/5 ms). **B**, Musculocutaneous CMAP from axilla *(lower tracing)* and at Erb's point stimulation; top tracing shows conduction block (500 μV/10 ms). **C**, Left peroneal NCV tests showing low-amplitude CMAP with partial conduction block (100 μV/10 ms). **D**, Right median NCV test showing low-amplitude CMAPs and temporal dispersion (500 μV/5 ms). *CMAP*, Compound muscle action potential; *NCV*, nerve conduction velocity.

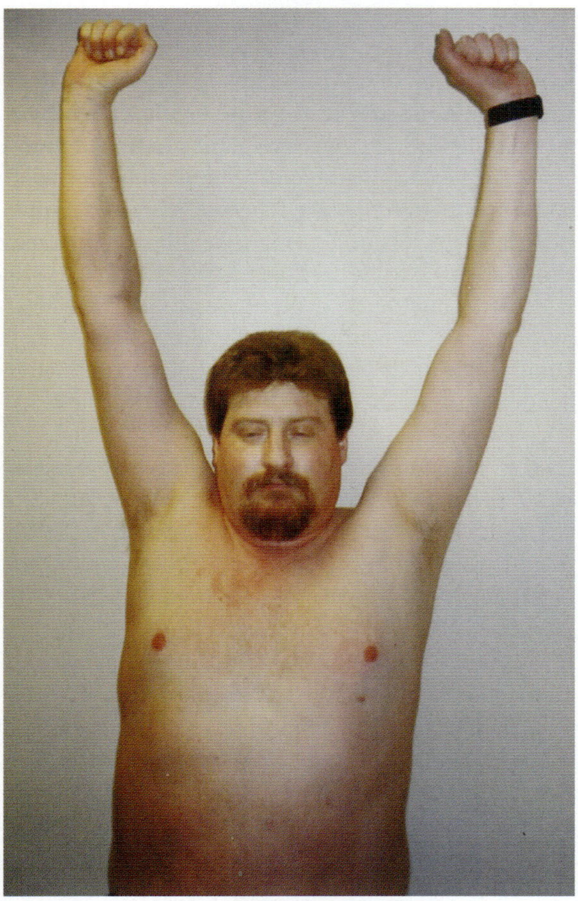

FIG. 52-3 The patient after treatment.

Adams and colleagues[19] reported a recurrent MMN with hypertrophic nerves and also noticed steroid responsiveness, while Hinman and Magee documented a predominantly motor disorder resembling Guillain–Barré syndrome (GBS), but of a more chronic or fluctuating course.[20] Similar observations were made by Thomas and colleagues.[21] Dyck and collaborators performed detailed studies and used the term *chronic inflammatory polyradiculoneuropathy*[22] by delineating its natural course and the clinical, electrodiagnostic, and spinal fluid findings. These authors described the pathologic features and documented the steroid responsiveness. Because of the evidence of demyelination, in addition to edema and inflammatory infiltrates, they later used the term *chronic inflammatory demyelinating polyradiculoneuropathy*.[23] This name is somewhat misleading, because inflammation is not seen often on nerve biopsies, likely because of its patchy nature, and because, in some cases, there is also axonal degeneration, although this could be secondary. Perhaps the name chronic autoimmune demyelinating polyradiculoneuropathy would be more accurate.

The differential diagnosis includes other demyelinating neuropathies, and particularly an identical presentation seen in HIV-infected patients, but those usually have an increased number of cells in the spinal fluid. CIDP also occurs in patients with MGUS, and in those with osteosclerotic myeloma. It can also be seen in association with lymphoma, melanoma, hepatitis, inflammatory bowel disease, nephrotic syndrome, and sarcoidosis, and, rarely, in Lyme disease and connective tissue disorders.[14,15] CIDP has also been reported in patients with CMT[24] and diabetes.[25]

The progression is variable; it can occur in different ages, although rarely in children.[26]

The clinical spectrum includes a purely motor variant[27,28] as in *Case 52*. There is also a purely sensory CIDP,[29,30] and, more recently, a sensory radiculoneuropathy has also been reported.[30,31] MMN[5] and multifocal motor sensory neuropathy[6] have asymmetric presentations with conduction blocks, as well as symptoms and findings related to individual nerves, as discussed later.

Workup in CIDP should include tests to rule out other demyelinating neuropathies and other associated diseases as discussed earlier, particularly HIV, hepatitis, Lyme, diabetes, vasculitis, and sarcoidosis. Immunoelectrophoresis should always be done. Older patients, mainly men, can present with a distal predominantly sensory demyelinating neuropathy having IgM monoclonals and MAG antibodies.[32]

Electrophysiologic studies in CIDP show slow NCVs and other demyelinating features such as conduction block, temporal dispersion, and prolongation of distal latency and proximal response. Needle EMG could be fairly normal or it could demonstrate signs of axonal degeneration which implies a less favorable prognosis. Several diagnostic criteria based on clinical and laboratory studies have been proposed for CIDP (Tables 52-1–52-3).[14,33–37] These could help in research but not necessarily in the clinical care of individual patients. Recently,

TABLE 52-1 Sets of Diagnostic Criteria for Chronic Inflammatory Demyelinating Polyneuropathy

	Barohn et al.	AAN Ad Hoc Subcommittee	Saperstein et al.	INCAT Group
Mandatory Clinical Features				
Pattern of clinical involvement	Symmetrical, proximal, and distal weakness	Motor and/or sensory dysfunction involving more than one limb	Major: symmetric, proximal, and distal weakness Minor: exclusively distal weakness or sensory loss	Motor and sensory dysfunction in more than one extremity; significant disability in arm or leg function
Reflexes	Areflexia or hyporeflexia	Areflexia or hyporeflexia	Areflexia or hyporeflexia	Areflexia or hyporeflexia
Time course	2 months	2 months	At least 2 months	≥2 months: stable or worsening
Laboratory Features				
Electrodiagnostic studies	Motor conduction velocity reduced <70% of LLN nerve	3 or 4 abnormal criteria, CD or TD in 1 or more nerves, slow NCV in 2 or more nerves, absent or prolonged F-waves, prolonged DL in 2 or more nerves	2 of 4 AAN criteria for CB in at least 1 motor nerve	Partial CB or TD in 2 or more nerves; reduced NCV, significantly prolonged DL, absent or significantly prolonged minimum F-latency in 1 other nerve. If no CB, at least a combination of abnormal DL, prolonged F-wave latency or reduced NCV in 3 motor nerves, or electrodiagnostic abnormalities indicating demyelination in 2 nerves and histological evidence of demyelination
CSF studies	CSF protein> 45 mg/dL	Mandatory: cell count <10/mm³; negative VDRL Supportive: elevated protein	Mandatory: protein > 45 mg/dL Supportive: cell count <10/mm³	Supportive but not mandatory
Nerve biopsy	Predominant features of demyelination and perivascular inflammation	Unequivocal evidence of demyelination and remyelination	Predominant features of demyelination inflammation (not required)	Supportive but not mandatory
Requirements for Diagnostic Category				
Definite	Clinical, electrodiagnostic, CSF, and biopsy	Clinical, electrodiagnostic, CSF, and biopsy	Clinical major, electrodiagnostic and CSF (biopsy supportive but not mandatory)	Clinical and electrodiagnostic
Probable	Clinical and 2 out of 3 laboratory features	Clinical, electrodiagnostic, CSF, and biopsy	Clinical major, electrodiagnostic of CSF (biopsy supportive but not mandatory)	–
Possible	Clinical and 1 out of 3 laboratory features	Clinical and electrodiagnostic	Clinical major and 1 out of 3; clinical minor and 2 out of 3	–

ANN, American Academy of Neurology; *CB*, conduction block; *CSF*, cerebrospinal fluid; *DL*, distal latency; *INCAT Group*, Inflammatory Cause and Treatment Group; *LLN*, lower limits of normalcy; *NCV*, nerve conduction velocity; *TD*, temporal dispersion.

Data from Barohn RJ, Kissel JT, Warmolts JR, et al. Chronic inflammatory demyelinating polyradiculoneuropathy: clinical characteristic, course, and recommendations for diagnostic criteria. *Arch Neurol.* 1989;46:878–884; Research criteria for diagnosis of chronic inflammatory demyelinating polyneuropathy (CIDP). Report from an Ad Hoc subcommittee of the American Academy of Neurology AIDS Task Force. *Neurology.* 1991;41:617–618; Saperstein DS, Katz JS, Amato AA, Barohn RJ. Clinical spectrum of chronic acquired demyelinating polyneuropathies. *Muscle Nerve.* 2001;24:311–324; Hughes R, Bensa S, Willison H, et al. Randomized controlled trial of intravenous immunoglobulin vs oral prednisolone in chronic inflammatory demyelinating polyradiculoneuropathy. *Ann Neurol.* 2001;50:195–201.

TABLE 52-2 American Academy of Electrodiagnostic Medicine Proposed Criteria for Partial Conduction Block

	Minimal Temporal Dispersion (Duration Increased by 30% or Less)				Moderate Temporal Dispersion (Duration Increased by 30%–60%)	
	Definite Partial Conduction Block		*Probable Partial Conduction Block*		*Probable Partial Conduction Block*	
Nerve Segment (Proximal/Distal)	**Amplitude Reduction (%)**	**Area Reduction (%)**	**Amplitude Reduction (%)**	**Area Reduction (%)**	**Amplitude Reduction (%)**	**Area Reduction (%)**
Median						
Forearm (E/W)	>50	>40	40–49	30–39	>50	>40
Arm (AX/E)	>50	>40	40–49	30–39	>50	>40
Proximal (EP/AX)	[a]	[a]	>40	>30	>50	>40
Ulnar						
Forearm (BE/W)	>50	>40	40–49	30–39	>50	>40
Across elbow (AE/BE)	>50	>40	40–49	30–39	>50	>40
Arm (AX/AE)	>50	>40	40–49	30–39	>50	>40
Proximal (EP/AX)	[a]	[a]	>40	>30	>50	>40
Radial						
Forearm (E/DF)	[a]	[a]	>50	>40	>60	>50
Arm (AX/E)	[a]	[a]	>50	>40	>60	>50
Proximal (EP/AX)	[a]	[a]	>50	>40	>60	>50
Peroneal						
Leg (BF/ankle)	>60	>50	50–59	40–49	>60	>50
Across FH (AF/BF)	>50	>40	40–49	30–39	>50	>40
Thigh (SN/AF)	[a]	[a]	>50	>40	>60	>50
Tibial						
Leg (knee/ankle)	>60	>50	50–59	40–49	>60	>50
Thigh (SN/knee)	[a]	[a]	>50	>40	>60	>50

[a]Not accepted. The original source can be consulted for the reason that definitive conduction block is not accepted for these segments.
AE, Above elbow; *AF*, above fibular head; *AX*, axilla; *BE*, below elbow; *BF*, below fibular head; *DF*, distal forearm; *E*, elbow; *EP*, Erb's point; *FH*, fibular head; *SN*, sciatic notch; *W*, wrist.
Reprinted with permission from Olney RK. Consensus criteria for the diagnosis of partial conduction block. *Muscle Nerve*. 1999;22(Suppl 8): S225–S229.

Magda and colleagues[37,38] found that the sensitivity of reported research criteria varied from 40% to 70%, based on a retrospective observation of clinical definitive CIDP cases, and proposed less stringent criteria, particularly in those related to electrodiagnostic tests. Contrast root enhancement on MRI occurs in CIDP.[39] The European Federation of Neurological Societies and the Peripheral Nerve Society have suggested a set of diagnostic criteria that included a response to treatment and MRI evidence of enhancement of the lumbosacral roots as supporting criteria[40,41] (Fig. 52-4).

Pathologically, in CIDP, there is a polyradiculoneuropathy involving motor and sensory fibers with segmental demyelination, and there could be inflammatory infiltrates. Axonal degeneration and endoneurial edema can also be seen.

Concerning the pathogenesis, there is evidence of activated CD4 and CD8 lymphocytes in nerve specimens[15] and disruption of the nerve–blood barrier, with downregulation of tight junction proteins having elevated levels of adhesion molecules, chemokines, and matrix metalloproteinases. A humoral-mediated mechanism is supported by the possible role of autoantibodies in the pathogenesis, as well as the presence of the immunoglobulins and complements in peripheral nerves and oligoclonal bands in the spinal fluid[9,41] (Fig. 52-5).

Serum IgG from affected patients causes conduction block in experimental animals.[41] Also some patients develop the disease after a recent immunization or after a *Campylobacter jejuni* infection. The target antigens include myelin protein PMP 22, protein zero, connexin, gangliosides, and glycolipids. A molecular mimicry similar to GBS is most likely the main pathogenetic mechanism.[41]

The nodes of Ranvier and paranodal areas have proteins that are important targets of antibodies in GBS and CIDP. The term "nodopathies" has been proposed for cases associated with these antibodies which correlate to axonal degeneration or transitory conduction failure[42] and the axonal form of GBS has been associated with antibodies against gangliosides at the node.[43,44]

TABLE 52.3 European Academy of Neurology and Peripheral Nerve Society Nerve Conduction Criteria for CIDP

One of the Following of Motor Nerve Conduction Tests
a. Prolonged distal latency of 50% or over in two nerves
b. Reduced conduction velocity of 30% or over in two nerves
c. Prolonged F latencies of 20% or over in two nerves
d. Absent F responses in two nerves plus one or more demyelination criteria in one or more nerves
Criteria Regarding Conduction Block
30% or more reduction in proximal CMAP amplitude relative to distal CMAP peak amplitude of 20% or more in two nerves or in one nerve plus one or more demyelination criteria except absent F waves in one or more other nerves
Abnormal temporal dispersion of 30% duration increase of the ratio proximal to distal CMAP peak of two or more nerves
Prolonged distal CMAP duration in one or more nerves plus demyelination criteria in one or more nerves
Sensory Studies (One Criteria Necessary)
a. Prolonged distal latency or reduced velocity.
b. Recued SNAP amplitude
c. Slow nerve conduction
d. One or more equal abnormals in two nerves

From Van den Bergh, PYK, et al. *Eur J Neurology* 2021; 28(11) 3556–3581.

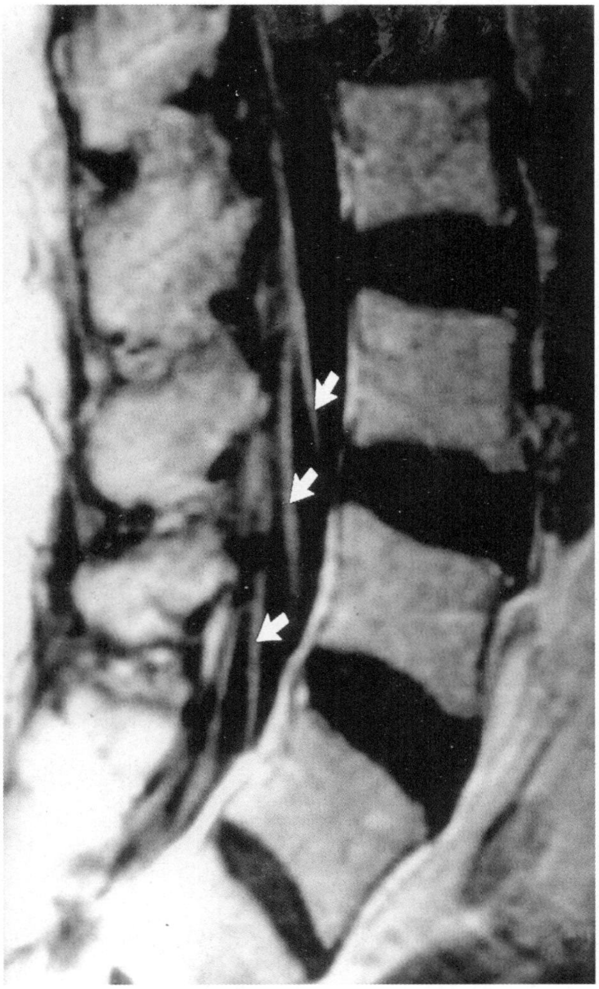

FIG. 52-4 Gadolinium enhancement of lumbosacral roots (*arrows*) in another case of CIDP.

The adhesion molecules such as neurofascin (NF155 and NF186) are targets to antibodies (see Fig. 52-5). Other important proteins in the node are gliomedin sodium channels and Ankyrin G. In the juxta paranode proteins are the transient glycoprotein-1 the contactin-associated protein and the potassium channels.[44,45] The nodes are very important in the generation of the nerve action potentials because of the high content of sodium channels and alteration of these structures can lead to blockage of conduction,[46] and some cases of CIDP have demonstratable antibodies against adhesion molecules.[47] Neurofascin is expressed in the paranodal loops of Schwann cells and oligodendrocytes in the CNS, and antibodies against these proteins can cause abnormalities in central and peripheral nervous systems.[44] Antibody binding to paranodal proteins can lead to detachment of Schwann cell loops of the paranodes and could explain CIDP with cranial nerve involvement.[47,48] There is a report of a CIDP case with a painful neuropathy.[49] These do not respond as well to standard therapy.

Case 51 has characteristics of CIDP with a more severe involvement in the left upper extremity. The diffuse findings, however, favor this disease rather than Lewis–Sumner syndrome.[50] She also had a monoclonal gammopathy and an endocrinopathy (diabetes) and visceromegaly. She thus had features of POEMS (polyneuropathy, organomegaly, endocrinopathy, monoclonal gammopathy, and skin changes) but did not have skin abnormalities. She had no evidence of osteosclerotic myeloma, which is frequently, but not always, associated with POEMS syndrome.[51]

This woman was diagnosed as having MGUS,[52] as a detailed workup initially failed to reveal a malignancy or increased population of monoclonal plasma cells in the bone marrow. She later developed a lymphoma supporting the notion that MGUS is not always benign, and that patients can later develop a malignant plasma cell disorder and lymphoma.[53,54] It is also possible that her azathioprine therapy played a role in the development of the lymphoma.[55]

Cases of CIDP associated with MGUS (CIDP/MGUS) are not much different clinically from those individuals who have the idiopathic disease, except that those with CIDP/MGUS are older and have somewhat more sensory symptoms.

The MGUS in CIDP could be IgG, IgA, or IgM. Some with IgM monoclonals have antibodies against MAG and manifest with a more distal demyelinating (distal acquired demyelinating symmetrical [DADS]) neuropathy (discussed in *Case 51*) which is less responsive to treatment.[32] The treatment of CIDP/MGUS is similar to those without a gammopathy.[18]

Case 52 presented with symmetrical distal, but also proximal, weakness with hyporeflexia and normal sensory examination. He had electrophysiologic evidence of motor conduction blocks, normal sensory studies, and sural nerve biopsy. His EMG showed denervation potentials, fasciculations, large motor units, and decreased motor unit recruitment. Cerebrospinal fluid protein and serum GM_1 antibodies were elevated.

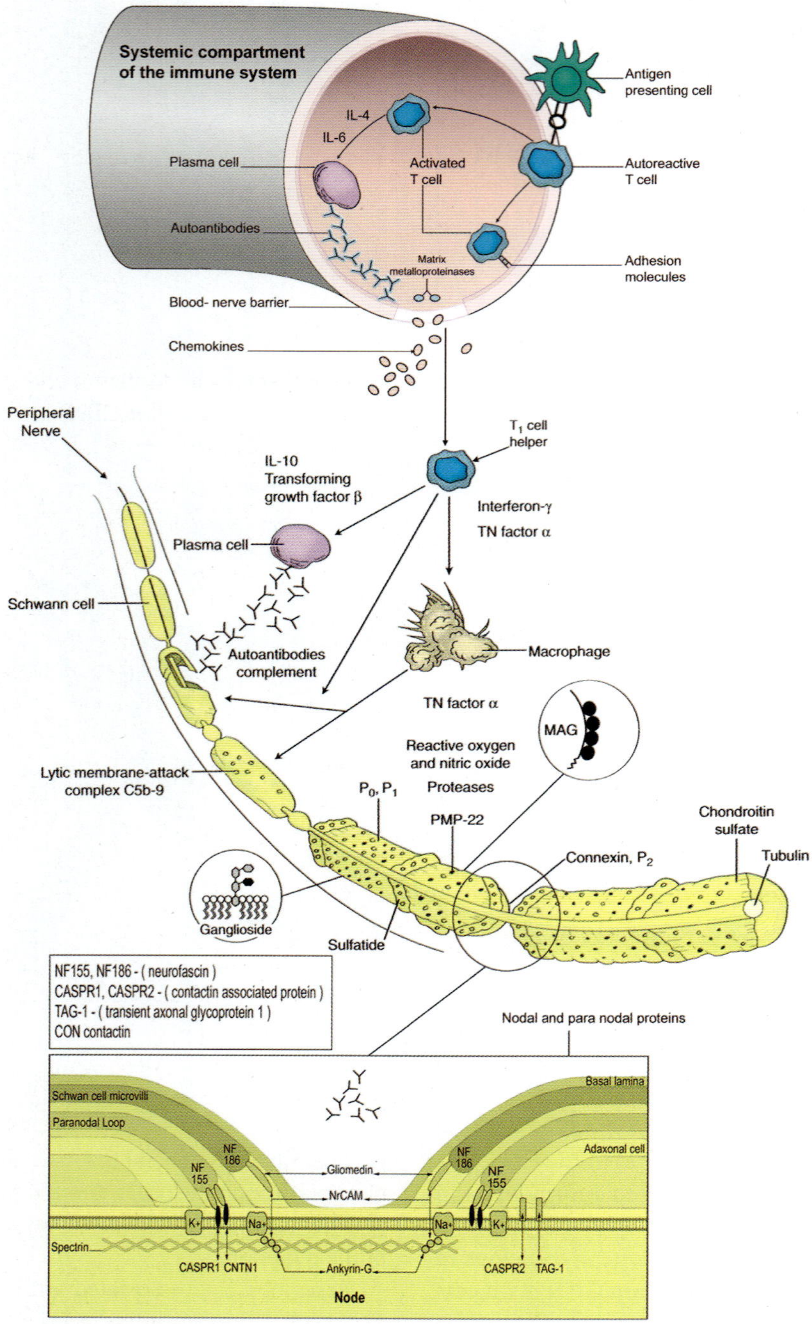

FIG. 52-5 Pathogenesis of CIDP. In summary: In the systemic compartment the antigen presenting cell activate T lymphocytes which penetrate the blood brain barrier with the help of adhesion molecules, and also releases chemokines and matrix metalloproteinase. There is also activation of plasma cells that secret antibodies that cross the blood nerve barrier. Then T helper cells activate macrophages to invade and destroy myelin, and also activate plasma cells to produce antibodies that mediate demyelination. At the bottom, there is representation of proteins of the node of Ranvier and paranodal areas, and these proteins are the target not for antibodies.

His relatively rapid progression, diffuse, symmetric weakness, hyporeflexia, and increased CSF protein were diagnostic of CIDP, and, as in this case, a "pure motor" variant has been described.[28] This constituted 10% of the series of Gorson, Allam, and Ropper.[27] A low titer GM_1 antibody elevation may be seen in 10%–30% of patients with CIDP.[44]

This patient demonstrated the difficulty in syndromic classification of acquired demyelinating neuropathies. The literature is confusing with reports that vary in presentation from classic CIDP, MMN, and the Lewis–Sumner syndrome, or multifocal motor sensory neuropathy (MMSN). In their initial description, Lewis and colleagues[6] reported five patients with chronic asymmetric weakness but with sensory deficits and conduction blocks. In that disease, there could also be evidence of nerve conduction slowing. The disease is similar to MMN, except for the sensory findings and better response to steroids.[56]

MMN affects motor nerves in an asymmetric fashion predominantly in the upper extremities and is usually associated with elevated GM_1 antibodies. The condition usually does not respond to steroids; in fact, steroids could actually worsen the symptoms.

There is also a reported purely axonal variant, or MAMA, and some of these patients had an elevation of GM_1 antibodies and responded to immunotherapy.[57] It is possible that in such cases the blocks were missed if proximal nerve or root stimulations were not done.

In *Case 52* the prominent fasciculations, high GM_1 antibody titer, and lack of response to corticosteroids, but therapeutic response to cyclophosphamide, are features of MMN,[3,4] but he also had prominent nerve conduction slowing.

The relationship between MMN and CIDP is being debated, as some suggest that MMN is a variant of CIDP,[7] while others believe these are separate entities.[50] Lewis et al. also suggested that MMSN is a variant of CIDP,[6] and Van den Berg-Vos and colleagues[58] reported six patients with an asymmetric sensorimotor neuropathy distinguishable from MMN and CIDP and suggested the name *multifocal inflammatory demyelinating neuropathy*. To try to clarify the issues, Dyck pointed out that it is more important to distinguish patients by pathophysiologic processes than by clinical distinction.[57,59] The report by Oh and colleagues of pathologic evidence of inflammatory demyelinating polyneuropathy in a patient with an MMN presentation underscores this point.[60]

The treatment of these autoimmune neuropathies includes IgG infusions, plasma exchange, and immunotherapy. Prednisone is useful; those with a purely motor presentation, such as MMN, however, should not be treated with steroids but with other immunosuppressants because prednisone could worsen the symptoms,[9] as occurred with *Case 52*. Rituximab has been reported beneficial in MMN.[50] A recent pilot study found that rituximab reduced the IgG requirements in some, but not in the majority of patients with autoimmune neuropathies.[61]

In cases that do not respond to monthly IVIG infusion, 500 mg/kg weekly could be prescribed and subcutaneous IgG could also be used and this may provide more steady IgG levels.[62] Belimumab is an antibody against B cell stimulator and appears to be a promising therapy as well as the complement inhibitors and the Fc receptor antagonist and these are undergoing therapeutic trails. The proteasome inhibitor bortezomib has been reported to help refractory cases.[63] The European Academy of Neurology and The Peripheral Nerve Society reported guidelines for the diagnosis and treatment of CIDP.[64]

IMPORTANT POINTS

- Causes of demyelinating neuropathy include, among others, CIDP, HIV, MGUS-associated neuropathy, diabetes, amiodarone therapy, CMT, and, in older persons, MAG-associated distal demyelinating neuropathy.
- Features of demyelination include conduction slowing, temporal dispersion, conduction blocks, prolonged distal latencies, prolonged F-responses, and absent H-reflexes.
- Acquired demyelinating neuropathies are associated with multifocal slowing, temporal dispersion, and conduction block, whereas uniform slowing is seen in most hereditary demyelinating neuropathies.
- CIDP usually progresses slowly and is of recent onset, affecting motor nerves and large sensory nerve fibers. There could also be some small fiber involvement. Patients have electrophysiologic evidence of demyelination and increased protein in spinal fluid.
- CIDP could have a purely motor or sensory presentation.
- Gadolinium enhancement of lumbosacral roots can help in the diagnosis of CIDP.
- Nerve biopsy shows demyelination associated with endoneurial edema and inflammation, but these could be absent.
- Diagnostic criteria for CIDP are useful for research but have limited value in individual patients, and should be considered when there is a high level of clinical suspicion.
- CIDP patients might have an IgG, IgA, or IgM monoclonal gammopathy. These are indistinguishable from classic CIDP, but patients with IgM MGUS may have a more indolent progressive disorder, but not respond as well to immunotherapy.
- Some patients with IgM monoclonal gammopathy have a predominantly distal demyelinating polyneuropathy (DADS) with antibodies against MAG.
- Although the course of MGUS neuropathy is usually benign, patients may later develop a malignancy.
- Corticosteroids are helpful in patients with CIDP with or without MGUS. Those with MMN and with motor CIDP may worsen with this therapy. The reason for this is unclear. These patients respond to other immunotherapeutic agents and gamma globulin infusions.
- Patients with gammopathies and CIDP should be treated similarly to classic CIDP.

REFERENCES

1. Nobile-Orazio E, Cappellari A, Priori A. Multifocal motor neuropathy: current concepts and controversies. *Muscle Nerve.* 2005;31(6):663–680.
2. Parry GJ, Sumner A. Multifocal motor neuropathy in peripheral neuropathy: new concepts and treatments. *Neurol Clin.* 1992;10(3): 671–682.
3. Kornberg AJ, Pestronk A. Chronic motor neuropathies: diagnosis, therapy and pathogenesis. *Ann Neurol.* 1995;37(Suppl 1):S43–S50.
4. Gorson KC, Ropper AH, Weinberg DH. Upper limb predominant, multifocal chronic inflammatory demyelinating polyneuropathy. *Muscle Nerve.* 1999;22:758–765.
5. Lewis RA. Chronic inflammatory demyelinating polyneuropathy and other immune-mediated demyelinating neuropathies. *Semin Neurol.* 2005;25(2):217–228.
6. Lewis RA, Sumner AJ, Brown MJ, Asbury AK. Multifocal demyelinating neuropathy with persistent conduction block. *Neurology.* 1982;32:958–964.
7. Krendel DA, Costigan DA. Multifocal motor neuropathy or CIDP? *Ann Neurol.* 1993;34(5):750–751.
8. Bertorini TE, Narayanaswami P. Autoimmune neuropathies. *Compr Ther.* 2003;29:194–209.
9. Barohn RJ, Kissel JT, Warmolts JR, et al. Chronic inflammatory demyelinating polyradiculoneuropathy: clinical characteristic,

course, and recommendations for diagnostic criteria. *Arch Neurol.* 1989;46:878–884.
10. Ropert A, Metral S. Conduction block in neuropathies with necrotizing vasculitis. *Muscle Nerve.* 1990;13:102–105.
11. McLeod JG, Pollard JD, Macaskill P, et al. Prevalence of chronic inflammatory demyelinating polyneuropathy in New South Wales, Australia. *Ann Neurol.* 1999;46:910–913.
12. Lunn MP, Manji H, Choudhary PP, et al. Chronic inflammatory demyelinating polyradiculoneuropathy: a prevalence study in southeast England. *J Neurol Neurosurg Psychiatry.* 1999;66: 667–680.
13. Latov N, Gorson KC, Brannagan 3rd TH, et al. Diagnosis and treatment of chronic immune-mediated neuropathies. *J Clin Neuromuscul Dis.* 2006;7:141–157.
14. Hahn FA, Hartung JP, Dyck PJ. Chronic inflammatory demyelinating polyradiculoneuropathy. In: Dyck PJ, Thomas I, eds. *Peripheral Neuropathy.* 4th ed. Philadelphia, PA: Elsevier-Saunders; 2002:2221–2252.
15. Simons Z. Chronic inflammatory demyelinating polyradiculoneuropathy. In: Bromberg M, Smith AG, eds. *Handbook of Peripheral Neuropathy.* Boca Raton, FL: Taylor & Francis; 2005:127–159.
16. Stamboulis E, Katsaros N, Koutsis G, et al. Clinical and subclinical autonomic dysfunction in chronic inflammatory demyelinating polyradiculoneuropathy. *Muscle Nerve.* 2006;33(1):78–84.
17. Harris W, Newcomb WD. A case of relapsing interstitial hypertrophic polyneuritis. *Brain.* 1929;52:108–116.
18. Austin JH. Recurrent polyneuropathies and their corticosteroid treatment; with a five-year observation of a placebo-controlled case treated with corticotrophin, cortisone, and prednisone. *Brain.* 1958;81:157–192.
19. Adams RD, Asbury AK, Michelsen JJ. Multifocal pseudohypertropic neuropathy. *Trans Am Neurol Assoc.* 1965;90:30–33.
20. Hinman RC, Magee KR. Guillain-Barré syndrome with slow progressive onset and persistent elevation of spinal fluid protein. *Ann Intern Med.* 1967;67(5):1007–1012.
21. Thomas PK, Lascelles RG, Hallpike JF, Hewer RL. Recurrent and chronic relapsing Guillain-Barré polyneuritis. *Brain.* 1969;92(3): 589–606.
22. Dyck PJ, Lais AC, Ohta M, et al. Chronic inflammatory polyradiculoneuropathy. *Mayo Clin Proc.* 1975;50(11):621–637.
23. Dyck PJ, Pineda A, Swanson C, et al. The Mayo Clinic experience with plasma exchange in chronic inflammatory-demyelinating polyneuropathy (CIDP). *Prog Clin Biol Res.* 1982;106:197–204.
24. Ginsberg L, Malik O, Kenton AR, et al. Coexistent hereditary and inflammatory neuropathy. *Brain.* 2004;127(pt1):193–202.
25. Uncini A, De Angelis MV, Di Muzio A, et al. Chronic inflammatory demyelinating polyneuropathy in diabetics: motor conductions are important in the differential diagnosis with diabetic polyneuropathy. *Clin Neurophysiol.* 1999;110(4): 705–711.
26. Connolly AM. Chronic inflammatory demyelinating polyneuropathy in childhood. *Pediatr Neurol.* 2001;24(3):177–182.
27. Gorson KC, Allam G, Ropper AH. Chronic inflammatory demyelinating polyneuropathy: clinical features and response to treatment in 67 consecutive patients with and without a monoclonal gammopathy. *Neurology.* 1997;48:321–328.
28. Sabatelli M, Madia F, Mignogna T, et al. Pure motor chronic inflammatory demyelinating neuropathy. *J Neurol.* 2001;248(9): 772–777.
29. Oh SJ, Joy JL, Kuruoglu R. Chronic sensory demyelinating neuropathy: chronic inflammatory demyelinating polyneuropathy presenting as a pure sensory neuropathy. *J Neurol Neurosurg Psychiatry.* 1992;55(8):677–680.
30. Cross D, Chiappa KH, Patel S, Gomwok S. Acquired pure sensory demyelinating polyneuropathy. A chronic inflammatory polyneuropathy variant. *Ann Neurol.* 1992;32:28–30.
31. Ikeda S, Koike H, Nishi R, Kawagashira Y, et al. Clinicopathological characteristics of subtypes of chronic inflammatory demyelinating polyradiculoneuropathy. *J Neurol Neurosurg Psychiatry.* 2019;90(9): 988–996.
32. Kaku DA, England JD, Sumner AJ. Distal accentuation of conduction slowing in polyneuropathy associated with antibodies to myelin-associated glycoprotein and sulphated glucuronyl paragloboside. *Brain.* 1994;117:941–947.
33. Research criteria for diagnosis of chronic inflammatory demyelinating polyneuropathy (CIDP) Report from an Ad Hoc Subcommittee of the American Academy of Neurology AIDS Task Force. *Neurology.* 1991;41:617–618.
34. Saperstein DS, Katz JS, Amato AA, Barohn RJ. Clinical spectrum of chronic acquired demyelinating polyneuropathies. *Muscle Nerve.* 2001;24:311–324.
35. Hughes R, Bensa S, Willison H, et al. Randomized controlled trial of intravenous immunoglobulin vs oral prednisolone in chronic inflammatory demyelinating polyradiculoneuropathy. *Ann Neurol.* 2001;50:195–201.
36. Latov N. Diagnosis of CIDP. *Neurology.* 2002;59(Suppl 6):S2–S6.
37. Sander HW, Latov N. Research criteria for defining patients with CIDP. *Neurology.* 2003;60(Suppl 3):S8–S15.
38. Magda P, Latov N, Brannagan 3rd TH, et al. Comparison of electrodiagnostic abnormalities and criteria in a cohort of patients with chronic inflammatory demyelinating polyneuropathy. *Arch Neurol.* 2003;60(12):1755–1759.
39. Bertorini T, Halford H, Lawrence J, et al. Contrast-enhanced magnetic resonance imaging of the lumbosacral roots in the dysimmune inflammatory polyneuropathies. *J Neuroimaging.* 1995;5(1):9–15.
40. European Federation of Neurological Societies/Peripheral Nerve Society European Federation of Neurological Societies/ Peripheral Nerve Society Guideline on management of chronic inflammatory demyelinating polyradiculoneuropathy: report of a Joint task force of the European Federation of Neurological Societies and the Peripheral Nerve Society. *J Peripher Nerv Syst.* 2005;10:220–228.
41. Koller H, Kieseier BC, Jander S, Hartung HP. Chronic inflammatory demyelinating polyneuropathy. *N Engl J Med.* 2005;352(13):1343–1356.
42. Uncini A, Susuki K, Yuki N. Nodo-paranodopathy: beyond the demyelinating and axonal classification in anti-ganglioside antibody-mediated neuropathies. *Clinical Neurophysiology.* 2013;124(10):1928–1931.
43. Goodfellow JA, Willison HJ. Antiganglioside, antiganglioside-complex, and antiglycolipid-complex antibodies in immune-mediated neuropathies. *Curr Opin Neurol.* 2016;29(5):572–580.
44. Abassi El, Soliman M, Leng MH, Englad SJ. Treatment and management of autoimmune neuropathies, chapter 15. In: Bertorini TE, ed. *Neuromuscular Disorders: Treatment and Management.* Amsterdam, Netherlands: Elsevier; 2022:312–344. 2nd ed.
45. Susuki K. Node of Ranvier disruption as a cause of neurological diseases. *ASN Neuro.* 2013;5(3):209–219.

46. Dalakas MC, Rakocevic G, Salajegheh M, et al. Placebo-controlled trial of rituximab in IgM anti–myelin-associated glycoprotein antibody demyelinating neuropathy. *Ann Neurol.* 2009;65(3):286–293.
47. Delmont F, Manso C, Querol L, Cortese A, et al. Autoantibodies to nodal isoforms of neurofascin and chronic inflammatory demyelinating polyneuropathy. *Brain.* 2017;140(7):851–858.
48. Ogata H, Yamasaki R, Hiwatashi A, Oka N, et al. Characterization of IgG4 anti-neurofascin 155 antibody-positive polyneuropathy. *Ann Clin Transl Neurol.* 2015;2(10):960–971.
49. Doppler K, Appeltshauser L, Villmann C, Martin C, et al. Auto-antibodies to contactin associated protein I (CASPR) in two patients with painful inflammatory neuropathy. *Brain.* 2016;139(Pt 10):2617–2630.
50. Ruegg SJ, Steek AJ. Rituximab stabilized multifocal motor neuropathy increasingly less responsive to IVIg. *Neurology.* 2004;63:2178–2179.
51. Soubrier MJ, Dubost JJ, Sauvezie BJ. POEMS syndrome: a study of 25 cases and a review of the literature. *Am J Med.* 1994;94: 543–553.
52. Kyle RA. "Benign" monoclonal gammopathy after 20 to 35 years of follow-up. *Mayo Clin Proc.* 1993;68(1):26–36.
53. Eurelings M, Lokhorst HM, Kalmijn S, et al. Malignant transformation in polyneuropathy associated with monoclonal gammopathy. *Neurology.* 2005;64(12):1079–2084.
54. Blade J. Clinical practice: monoclonal gammopathy of undetermined significance. *N Engl J Med.* 2006;35(26): 2765–2770.
55. Patel P, Moazzam N, Potti A, Mehdi SA. Azathioprine induced Hodgkin's lymphoma: a case report and review of literature. *Am J Clin Oncol.* 2005;28(4):427–428.
56. Saperstein DS, Amato AA, Wolfe GI, et al. Multifocal acquired demyelinating sensory and motor neuropathy: the Lewis-Sumner syndrome. Muscle Nerve. 1999;22(5):560–566.
57. Katz JS, Barohn RJ, Kojan S, et al. Axonal multifocal motor neuropathy without conduction block or other features of demyelination. *Neurology.* 2002;58(4):615–620.
58. Van den Berg-Vos RM, Van den Berg LH, Franssen H, et al. Multifocal inflammatory demyelinating neuropathy: a distinct clinical entity? *Neurology.* 2000;54:26–32.
59. Dyck PJ. Atypical varieties of chronic inflammatory demyelinating motor neuropathies. *Lancet.* 2000;355:1293–1294.
60. Oh SJ, Claussen GC, Odabasi Z, Palmer CP. Multifocal demyelinating motor neuropathy: pathologic evidence of "inflammatory demyelinating polyradiculoneuropathy". *Neurology.* 1995;45:1828–1832.
61. Gorson KC, Natarajan N, Ropper AH, Weinstein R. Rituximab treatment in patients with VIg-dependent immune polyneuropathy: a prospective pilot trial. *Muscle Nerve.* 2007;35(1):66–69.
62. van Schaik IN, Bril V, van Geloven N, Hartung HP, et al. Subcutaneous immunoglobulin for maintenance treatment in chronic inflammatory demyelinating polyneuropathy (PATH); a randomized, double-blind, placebo-controlled, phase 3 trial. *Lancet Neurol.* 2018;17(1):35–46.
63. Pitarokoili K, Yoon MS, Kroger Reinacher-Schick A, et al. Severe refractory CIDP: a case series of 10 patients treated with bortezomib. *J Neurol.* 2017;64(9):2010–2020.
64. Van Den Bergh PYK, van Doom PA, Hadden RDM, et al. European Academy of Neurology/Peripheral Nerve Society guideline on diagnosis and treatment of chronic inflammatory demyelinating polyradiculoneuropathy: Report of a joint Task Force-Second revision. *J Peripher Nerve Syst.* 2021;26(3): 242–268.

53 CASE

A Man With Diabetic Polyneuropathy Who Developed Rapidly Progressive Weakness

A 53-year-old obese, insulin-dependent, hypertensive diabetic man presented initially with a diabetic polyneuropathy characterized by numbness and burning paresthesias in the feet. His examination at that time was remarkable only for absent ankle reflexes, absent vibration sense in the toes and ankles, and decreased pinprick to the mid-calf and wrists. His electrodiagnostic tests showed borderline slow peroneal motor conduction velocities, mildly prolonged median distal motor latency, and absent sural SNAPs and H-reflexes. Median and ulnar nerve conduction velocities, CMAPs, and SNAPs were normal. The needle EMG showed scattered large motor unit potentials in the distal legs. He was treated with ibuprofen and amitriptyline.

He presented 2 years later with a 5-week history of progressive weakness in the lower extremities causing significant difficulty walking; he also had mild weakness in the upper extremities. His numbness had progressed to the distal shins.

Past medical history included back surgery for disk disease and polycythemia secondary to fluoxymesterone, given for impotence; this was discontinued 4 years prior to this presentation. Later, he had a penile implant.

The patient stopped using alcohol and tobacco 2 years previously after a myocardial infarction and coronary bypass surgery. Family history was noncontributory. Review of systems revealed excessive daytime sleepiness, snoring, and some jerking movements in the legs at night.

Physical examination revealed normal mentation and cranial nerves. Upper extremity strength was 4+/5 in the shoulder muscles, biceps, and triceps, and 3+/5 in the finger extensors, flexors, and hand muscles. Lower extremity strength was 3−/5 in the hips and 4/5 in the quadriceps and hamstrings; foot extensors were 2/5; foot dorsiflexors and evertors were 4/5. He was areflexic throughout. He had decreased touch and pain sensations to the distal shins and wrists. Vibration sense was absent in the toes and ankles and decreased in the knees and fingers. Position sense was absent in the toes and decreased in the ankles. Romberg test was negative. Coordination was normal. There were no Babinski signs. The rest of the examination was normal.

WHAT TESTS WERE DONE?

The chemistry profile was normal except for sugar of 249 mg/dL (normal, <110 mg/dL); he had normal serum immunoelectrophoresis, HIV, fluorescent antinuclear antibody test, erythrocyte sedimentation rate, B_{12} angiotensin-converting enzyme, and thyroid-stimulating hormone.

WHAT IS THE DIFFERENTIAL DIAGNOSIS?

This diabetic man had rapidly progressive weakness, and although this could be related to diabetic polyneuropathy, it also included proximal muscles. A superimposed myopathy, such as polymyositis, is a consideration, but the areflexia, particularly of the proximal reflexes and the prominent proprioceptive sensory deficit, suggests the weakness was secondary to a neuropathy. The rapidly progressive weakness with proprioceptive deficit is also against a motor neuron disorder. He could have had hypothyroidism causing a neuropathy in addition to his diabetic neuropathy. B_{12} deficiency might present with numbness, some weakness, and areflexia, but there could also be evidence of long tract signs. Other possibilities include a subacute form of inflammatory demyelinating polyneuropathy, a vasculitic neuropathy, sarcoidosis, HIV- or monoclonal gammopathy–associated demyelinating neuropathy, and a neuropathy associated with lymphoma.

He also appeared to have had sleep apnea.

AN EMG TEST WAS PERFORMED

Motor Nerve Studies

Nerve and Site	Latency (ms)	Amplitude (mV)	Conduction Velocity (m/s)
Peroneal Nerve R.	**Normal ≤ 5.7**	**Normal ≥ 3**	**Normal ≥ 40**
Ankle	**NR**	**NR**	**NR**
Fibular head	**NR**	**NR**	**NR**
Knee	**NR**	**NR**	**NR**
Tibial Nerve R.	**Normal ≤ 5.3**	**Normal ≥ 4**	**Normal ≥ 40**
Ankle	**21.8**	**0.15 μV**	–
Pop. fossa	**NR**	**NR**	–
Median Nerve R.[a]	**Normal ≤ 4.2**	**Normal ≥ 6**	**Normal ≥ 50**
Wrist	**12.4**	7	–
Elbow	27.2	**3**	**17**
Ulnar Nerve R.	**Normal ≤ 3.6**	**Normal ≥ 8**	**Normal ≥ 50**
Wrist	**6.8**	**5**	–
Below elbow	31.6	**1**	**9**
Above elbow	**NR**	**NR**	–

Motor Nerve Studies—cont'd

Median Nerve L.[a]	Normal ≤ 4.2	Normal ≥ 6	Normal ≥ 50
Wrist	**14.6**	**1.6**	–
Below elbow	32.4	**0.6**	**12**

[a]Dispersion noted on proximal CMAP.

F-Wave and Tibial H-Reflex Studies

Nerve	Latency (ms)	Normal Latency ≤ (ms)
Peroneal nerve R.	**NR**	54
Tibial nerve R.	**NR**	54
Median nerve R.	**NR**	30
Ulnar nerve R.	**NR**	30
Median nerve L.	**NR**	30
H-reflex R.	**NR**	34
H-reflex L.	**NR**	34

Sensory Nerve Studies

Nerve	Latency (ms)	Normal Latency ≤ (ms)	Amp (μV)	Normal Amp ≤ (μV)
Sural nerve R.	**NR**	4.0	**NR**	11
Sural nerve L.	**NR**	4.0	**NR**	11
Median nerve R.	**NR**	3.1	**NR**	20
Ulnar nerve R.	**NR**	3.1	**NR**	13
Median nerve L.	**NR**	3.1	**NR**	20

EMG Data

Muscle	Insrt Activity	Fibs	Pos Waves	Fasc	Amp	Dur	Poly	Pattern
Tensor fasciae latae R.	Norm	None	None	None	**Lg**	**Inc**	None	Full
Vastus lateralis R.	**Inc**	None	**1+**	None	**Lg**	**Inc**	None	**Red**
Tibialis anterior R.	**Inc**	None	**1+**	None	**Lg**	**Inc**	None	**Red**
Peroneus longus R.	**Inc**	None	**1+**	None	**Lg**	**Inc**	None	**Red**
Gastrocnemius R.	**Inc**	None	**1+**	None	**Lg**	**Inc**	None	**Red**
Tibialis anterior L.	**Inc**	None	**1+**	None	**Lg**	**Inc**	None	**Red**
Gastrocnemius L.	**Inc**	None	None	None	**Lg**	**Inc**	None	**Red**
Biceps brachii R.	**Inc**	None	**1+**	None	**Lg**	**Inc**	None	Full
Flexor carpi ulnaris R.	**Inc**	None	**1+**	None	**Lg**	**Inc**	None	Full
First dorsal interosseus R.	**Inc**	**1+**	**1+**	None	**Lg**	**Inc**	None	**Red**

WHAT WERE THE EMG FINDINGS?

This test showed profound slowing of motor nerve conduction velocities, including the arms, with normal CMAP amplitudes of the right median nerve, and also mildly decreased amplitude of the right ulnar nerve CMAP. The CMAP was of reduced amplitude in the left median nerve; this was not recordable in the peroneal nerve and was of very low amplitude in the tibial nerve. Motor distal latencies were prolonged. H-reflexes and F-responses were absent. There was also evidence of conduction block and temporal dispersion of the CMAPs. SNAPs were absent. The needle test showed denervation potentials, indicating also axonal degeneration with large motor unit action potentials indicating reinnervation.

It was concluded that he had an acquired demyelinating neuropathy, in addition to a diabetic polyneuropathy, with chronic and active axonal degeneration.

WHAT IS THE MOST LIKELY DIAGNOSIS?

This patient with a diabetic polyneuropathy developed a recent onset of diffuse weakness with an inability to walk. The degree of weakness, sensory deficits, and areflexia indicated a large fiber polyneuropathy. This type of presentation is unusual for diabetics, as they usually have a slowly progressive predominantly distal weakness, accompanied by significant small fiber dysfunctions, such as painful burning paresthesias and numbness. Other neuropathies should be considered; these include a neuropathy with monoclonal gammopathy, amyloidosis and polyneuropathy, organomegaly, endocrinopathy, monoclonal gammopathy, and skin changes (POEMS) as well as those caused by drugs or exposure to toxins, and vasculitis. Vasculitic neuropathy is usually asymmetric, but it can manifest as a diffuse polyneuropathy in some cases.[1]

A familial neuropathy, such as Charcot–Marie–Tooth disease type I, is unlikely, as his symptoms were of recent onset and there was partial conduction block and temporal dispersion on EMG not seen in that disease.[2] A demyelinating inflammatory neuropathy can also be seen in patients with lymphoma, HIV, sarcoidosis, hepatitis, and monoclonal gammopathy. He had no evidence of these.

He appears to have all the features of a chronic inflammatory demyelinating polyneuropathy (CIDP), except that the symptoms were less than the characteristic time of progression of this disease, which is over 2 months. However, some patients can have a shorter course, and a subacute form has been reported.[3]

WHAT SHOULD BE DONE NEXT?

A nerve biopsy was done, and although this is not absolutely necessary in suspected CIDP, it helps in the diagnosis. This showed segmental demyelination with short internodes; there was no evidence of inflammation and only rare axonal degeneration. Large axons without myelin or with thin myelin were present; there were some "onion bulbs," indicating chronic demyelination. The unmyelinated axons were not severely affected. The vessels had thick walls with duplication of the basal lamina as is commonly seen in diabetes (Fig. 53-1).

A lumbar puncture revealed a protein of 157 mg/dL (normal, 20–40 mg/dL), glucose of 121 mg/dL (normal, 40–60 mg/dL), and 3 lymphocytes/mm^3 (normal, <5 lymphocytes/mm^3). Immunoelectrophoresis and HIV tests were normal.

WHAT IS THE BEST TREATMENT FOR THIS PATIENT?

He was treated with plasmapheresis rather than steroid therapy because of his diabetes. This resulted in significant improvement. Five weeks later, he returned with increasing weakness and received 2 g/kg of intravenous gamma globulin with marked improvement.

After this, he underwent a polysomnographic test that showed evidence of obstructive sleep apnea (Fig. 53-2). He was given continuous positive airway pressure (CPAP) equipment to use at night which resulted in significant improvement of his daytime sleepiness.

DISCUSSION

This patient with diabetic neuropathy developed a subacute demyelinating autoimmune polyneuropathy confirmed by

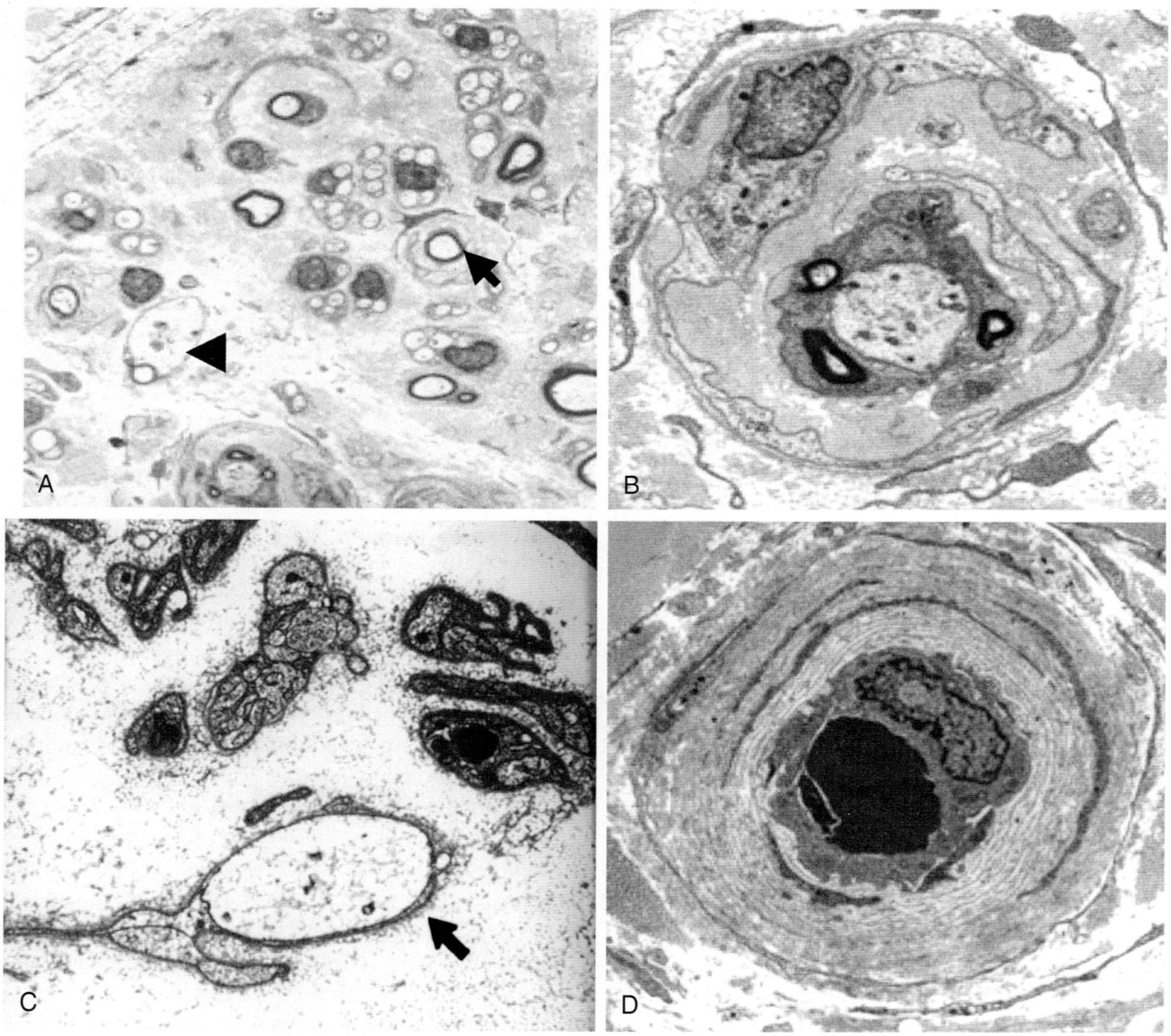

FIG. 53-1 **A**, Electromicroscopy of sural nerve showing axons without myelin (*arrowhead*) and an "onion bulb" (*arrow*); there is a decreased number of myelinated axons (×5900). **B**, An axon without myelin and several sprouting small myelinated axons (×9315). **C**, Large axon without myelin (*arrow*) (×9315). **D**, A vessel with duplication of basal lamina (×9315).

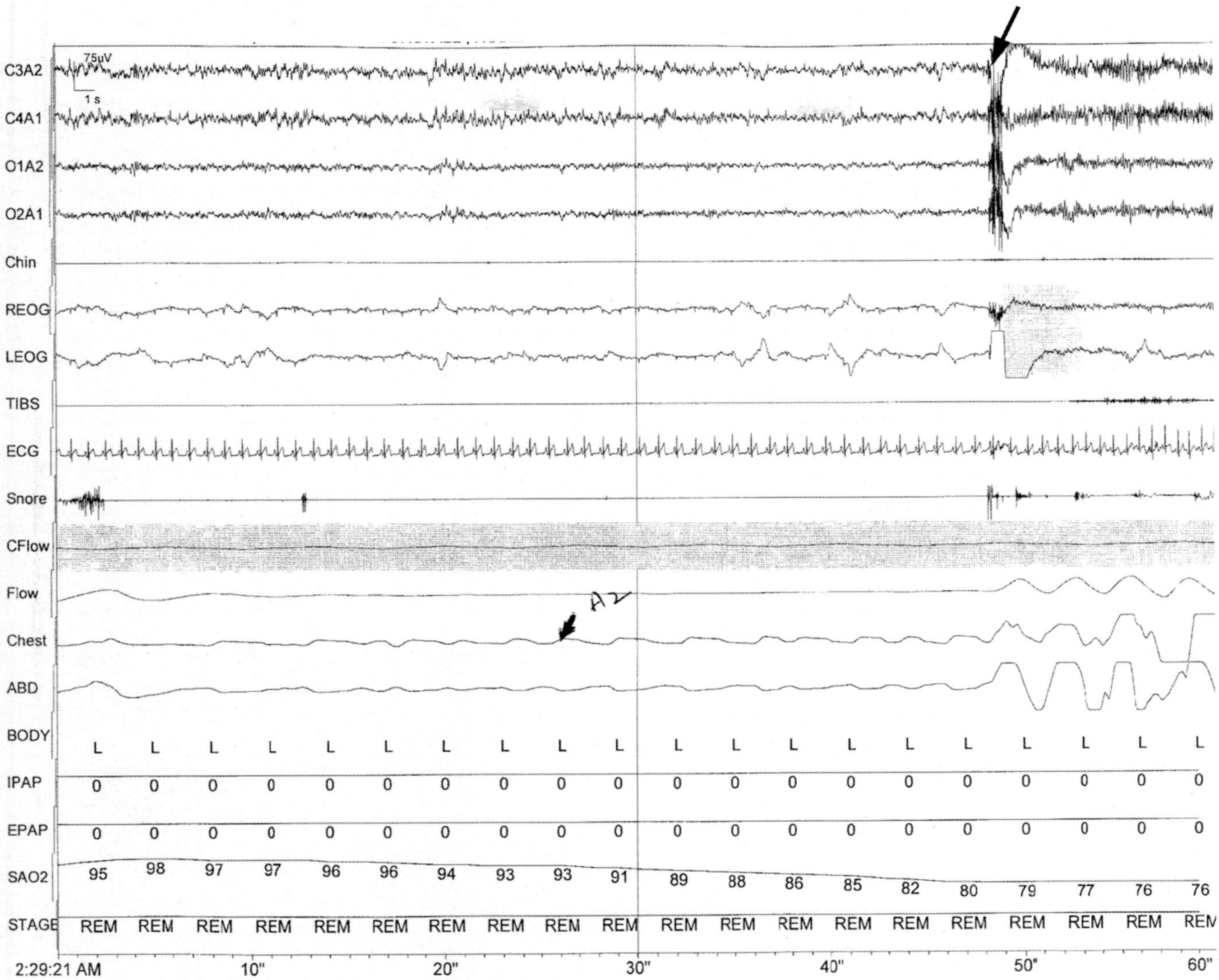

FIG. 53-2 Long episode of apnea causing awakening (*arrow*) and no airflow through the nose in channel titled "flow." There are continued respiratory efforts in the chest and abdominal muscles as demonstrated by the *lower arrow*. The event occurred in stage 3 rapid eye movements (REM); note rapid eye movements on channels right electrooculogram (REOG) and left electrooculogram (LEOG).

electrophysiologic studies. The elevated spinal fluid protein can occur in diabetic peripheral neuropathy and autoimmune neuropathies. Inflammation on nerve biopsy is seen in only 20% of patients with CIDP and does not differentiate between these disorders[4]; this was not present in his biopsy.

CIDP is a chronic and often recurrent condition characterized by proximal and distal weakness with deficits of the large fiber modalities of vibration and proprioception and having relative preservation of the small fiber modalities of pain and temperature. Nerve conduction studies showed evidence of prominent demyelination.

As in this patient, those with diabetic polyneuropathy can also develop CIDP,[4,5] and some postulate that diabetics are more predisposed to develop the disease. A determination that a diabetic also has CIDP should be based on the clinical manifestation, the electrophysiologic findings, and, particularly, the response to immunotherapy.

In a group of 64 patients with CIDP, Molenaar and colleagues found that the sural nerve biopsy did not aid in the diagnosis.[6] In another study, Stewart and colleagues also found that biopsy was not useful for the differentiation of CIDP from diabetic neuropathy when CIDP occurs in diabetes.[7] However, one study reported that nerve biopsy had a sensitivity of 80% for the diagnosis of CIDP in diabetes.[8] Another study reported the usefulness of immunoreactivity of the sural nerve to matrix metalloproteinase-9 for diagnosis.[9]

Enhancement of the lumbosacral roots can also help to differentiate CIDP from diabetic neuropathy,[10] although this was not available when this patient was studied.

The diagnosis of a subacute autoimmune demyelinating polyneuropathy in this patient was based on the clinical, electrophysiologic, and pathologic findings[11,12] and particularly his response to plasmapheresis and later gamma globulin infusions.

As in nondiabetics, CIDP in diabetes needs to be differentiated from other demyelinating neuropathies, such as those from monoclonal gammopathy, HIV, lymphoma, sarcoidosis, and familial neuropathies.

Autoimmune neuropathies in diabetics usually respond to immunotherapy,[13] particularly IgG infusions,[14–16] and it is important that the clinician recognize the possible complications of this treatment when choosing IgG therapy.[17] The brand of IgG should be chosen after consideration of the patient's clinical condition and the cost. In large patients, fluid overload is a consideration. In diabetics, glucose-containing products could increase blood glucose; therefore these patients require close monitoring. Glucose-containing products may also predispose patients to thromboembolic diseases. Sucrose-containing products do not increase blood glucose but can increase the risk of thromboembolic complications from increased osmolality. Those that contain glycine appear to be the safest but are much more expensive. Subcutaneous IgG could be considered. A recent report documented that the overall outcome is poorer in diabetics with CIDP than those with the idiopathic form.[18]

SUMMARY

This diabetic patient was diagnosed and treated for a subacute autoimmune demyelinating polyneuropathy with an excellent response to treatment, initially with plasmapheresis and later IgG infusions. The patient also had obstructive sleep apnea and was treated with a CPAP.

IMPORTANT POINTS

- The development of proximal and distal weakness from a demyelinating neuropathy in a diabetic should raise the possibility of superimposed autoimmune etiology.
- Nerve biopsy could be useful in documenting significant demyelination and in determining the presence of inflammation to diagnose CIDP, but the absence of inflammation does not rule this out.
- Evidence of lumbosacral root enhancement on MRI may be helpful in determining if a diabetic has CIDP.
- When CIDP is suspected in a diabetic, based on the clinical presentation and electrophysiologic findings, the patient should receive immunotherapy.
- Treatment in these patients includes immunosuppressant drugs, plasma exchange or immunoglobulin therapy, steroids (which should be given with caution and close monitoring), and proper treatment of diabetes.
- When choosing a brand, clinicians ordering IgG therapy should take into consideration the patient's condition and the cost.

REFERENCES

1. Bertorini T, Narayanaswami P. Autoimmune neuropathies. *Compr Ther*. 2003;29(4):194–209.
2. Bertorini T, Narayanaswami P, Rashed H. Charcot-Marie-Tooth disease (hereditary motor sensory neuropathies) and hereditary sensory and autonomic neuropathies. *Neurologist*. 2004;10(6):327–337.
3. Oh SJ, Kurokawa K, de Almeida DF, et al. Subacute inflammatory demyelinating polyneuropathy. *Neurology*. 2003;61(11):1507–1512.
4. Gorson KC, Ropper AH, Adelman LS, Weinberg DH. Influence of diabetes mellitus on chronic inflammatory demyelinating polyneuropathy. *Muscle Nerve*. 2000;23(1):37–43.
5. Sharma KR, Cross J, Farronay O, et al. Demyelinating neuropathy in diabetes mellitus. *Arch Neurol*. 2002;59(5):758–765.
6. Molenaar DS, Vermeulen M, de Haan R. Diagnostic value of sural nerve biopsy in chronic inflammatory demyelinating polyneuropathy. *J Neurol Neurosurg Psychiatry*. 1998;64(1):84–89.
7. Stewart JD, McKelvey R, Durcan L, et al. Chronic inflammatory demyelinating polyneuropathy (CIDP) in diabetics. *J Neurol Sci*. 1996;142(1–2):59–64.
8. Haq RU, Fries TJ, Pendlebury WW, et al. Chronic inflammatory demyelinating polyradiculoneuropathy: a study of proposed electrodiagnostic and histologic criteria. *Arch Neurol*. 2000;57(12):1745–1750.
9. Jann S, Bramerio MA, Beretta S, et al. Diagnostic value of sural nerve matrix metalloproteinase-9 in diabetic patients with CIDP. *Neurology*. 2003;61(11):1607–1610.
10. Bertorini T, Halford H, Lawrence J, et al. Contrast-enhanced magnetic resonance imaging of the lumbosacral roots in dysimmune inflammatory polyneuropathies. *J Neuroimaging*. 1995;5(1):9–15.
11. Uncini A, De Angelis MV, Di Muzio A, et al. Chronic inflammatory demyelinating polyneuropathy in diabetics: motor conductions are important in the differential diagnosis with diabetic polyneuropathy. *Clin Neurophysiol*. 1999;110(4):705–711.
12. Saperstein DS, Katz JS, Amato AA, et al. Clinical spectrum of chronic acquired demyelinating polyneuropathies. *Muscle Nerve*. 2001;24(3):311–324.
13. Munch C, Anagnostou P, Meyer R, Haas J. Rituximab in chronic inflammatory demyelinating polyneuropathy associated with diabetes mellitus. *J Neurol Sci*. 2007;256(1–2):100–102.
14. Berger AR, Bradley WG, Brannagan TH, et al. Guidelines for the diagnosis and treatment of chronic inflammatory demyelinating polyneuropathy. *J Peripher Nerv Syst*. 2003;8(4):282–284.
15. Dalakas MC. Intravenous immunoglobulin in autoimmune neuromuscular diseases. *JAMA*. 2004;291(19):2367–2375.
16. Wiles CM, Brown P, Chapel H, et al. Intravenous immunoglobulin in neurological disease: a specialist review. *J Neurol Neurosurg Psychiatry*. 2002;72(4):440–448.
17. Bertorini TE, Nance A, Horner LH, et al. Complications of intravenous gamma-globulin in neuromuscular and other diseases. *Muscle Nerve*. 1996;19(3):388–391.
18. Kalita J, Misara UK, Yadav RK. A comparative study of chronic inflammatory demyelinating polyradiculoneuropathy with and without diabetes mellitus. *Eur J Neurol*. 2007;14(6):638–643.

An Older Man With Leg Numbness

A 65-year-old man presented with a 1-year history of slowly progressive numbness in the feet and hands, without weakness.

Past medical history was noncontributory, except for a history of hyperlipidemia treated with statins. He did not smoke or drink.

Neurologic examination revealed normal mentation and cranial nerves. Motor examination was intact except for 4/5 weakness of both feet and toe dorsiflexors and foot evertors. There was no atrophy. Reflexes were 1+ in the upper extremities and absent in the lower extremities. There were no pathologic reflexes. Sensory examination showed decreased pinprick and touch sensation to the mid-calf, absent vibration sense in the toes, and decreased in the fingers and ankles; position sense was decreased in the toes. There were no fasciculations, Babinski signs, or nerve hypertrophy. He had a normal gait and coordination. Romberg test was negative.

WHAT ARE THE MOST LIKELY DIAGNOSTIC POSSIBILITIES?

This patient had sensorimotor polyneuropathy. He did not have diabetes or hypothyroidism by history, although these should be considered. Both hyperlipidemia[1] and the statin family of cholesterol-lowering agents have been reported to be associated with a peripheral neuropathy.[2] He denied exposure to alcohol or toxins or excessive use of vitamins.

WHAT SHOULD THE WORKUP INCLUDE?

Initial workup, including fasting blood sugar, glycosylated hemoglobin, complete metabolic panel, lipid profile, B_{12}/folate levels, and thyroid function tests, and a complete blood count were all normal.

AN EMG TEST WAS PERFORMED

Motor Nerve Studies

Nerve and Site	Latency (ms)	Amplitude (mV)	Conduction Velocity (m/s)
Peroneal Nerve L.[a]	**Normal ≤ 5.7**	**Normal ≥ 3**	**Normal ≥ 40**
Ankle	**16.4**	**1.3**	–
Fibular head	**41.7**	**0.9**	**12**
Knee	**46.7**	**0.6**	**18**

Motor Nerve Studies—cont'd

Tibial Nerve R.[b]	Normal ≤ 5.3	Normal ≥ 4	Normal ≥ 40
Ankle	**15.8**	**0.9**	–
Pop. fossa	**32.7**	**0.3**	**25**

[a]Terminal latency index: 0.402 ms; normal: 0.386–0.406 ms.
[b]Terminal latency index: 0.253 ms; normal: 0.420–0.447 ms.

Motor Nerve Studies—cont'd

Nerve and Site	Latency (ms)	Amplitude (mV)	Conduction Velocity (m/s)
Ulnar Nerve L.[c]	**Normal ≤ 3.6**	**Normal ≥ 8**	**Normal ≥ 50**
Wrist	**5.3**	10	–
Below elbow	**11.1**	10	**34**
Above elbow	**14.9**	8	**32**
Median Nerve L.[d]	**Normal ≤ 4.2**	**Normal ≥ 6**	**Normal ≥ 50**
Wrist	**8.7**	11	–
Elbow	**13.8**	9	**43**
Axilla	**15.0**	9	58

[c]Terminal latency index: 0.377 ms; normal: 0.396–0.414 ms.
[d]Terminal latency index: 0.183 ms; normal: 0.343–0.353 ms.

Motor Nerve Studies—cont'd

Nerve and Site	Latency (ms)	Amplitude (mV)	Conduction Velocity (m/s)
Tibial Nerve L.[e]	**Normal ≤ 5.3**	**Normal ≥ 4**	**Normal ≥ 40**
Ankle	**15.5**	**0.1**	–
Pop. fossa	**40.3**	**0.1**	**17**
Peroneal Nerve R.[f]	**Normal ≤ 5.7**	**Normal ≥ 3**	**Normal ≥ 40**
Ankle	**12.7**	**1**	–
Fibular head	**34.4**	**1**	**14**
Knee	**37.6**	**1**	**27**

[e]Terminal latency index: 0.374 ms; normal: 0.420–0.447 ms.
[f]Terminal latency index: 0.448 ms; normal: 0.386–0.406 ms.

F-Wave and Tibial H-Reflex Studies

Nerve	Latency (ms)	Normal Latency ≤ (ms)
Peroneal nerve L.	**NR**	54
Tibial nerve L.	**NR**	54
Ulnar nerve L.	**40.7**	30
Median nerve L.	**39.4**	30
H-reflex L.	**NR**	34
H-reflex R.	**NR**	34

Sensory Nerve Studies

Sural nerve L.	NR
Ulnar nerve L.	**NR**

EMG Data

Muscle	Insrt Activity	Fibs	Pos Wave	Fasc	Amp	Dur	Poly	Pattern
Deltoid L.	Norm	None	None	None	Norm	Norm	None	Full
Biceps brachii L.	Norm	None	None	None	Norm	Norm	None	Full
Abd. pollicis brevis L.	Norm	None	None	None	**Lg**	**Inc**	None	**Red**
Vastus lateralis L.	Norm	None	None	None	**Lg**	**Inc**	None	Full
Tibialis anterior L.	**Inc**	None	None	None	**Lg**	**Inc**	None	**Red**
Peroneus longus L.	**Inc**	None	None	None	**Lg**	**Inc**	None	**Red**
Gastrocnemius L.	**Inc**	None	None	None	**Lg**	**Inc**	None	**Red**
Biceps—long head L.	Norm	None	None	None	Norm	**Inc**	None	**Red**
Vastus lateralis R.	**Inc**	None	None	None	Inc	**Inc**	None	Full
Biceps—long head R.	Norm	None	None	None	Norm	**Inc**	None	Full
Tibialis anterior R.	**Inc**	None	None	None	**Lg**	**Inc**	None	**Red**
Peroneus longus R.	**Inc**	None	None	None	**Lg**	**Inc**	None	**Red**
Gastrocnemius R.	**Inc**	**1+**	**1+**	None	Norm	**Inc**	None	**Red**

WHAT WERE THE EMG FINDINGS?

The EMG test showed evidence of demyelination with conduction velocity below 80% of normal in the ulnar nerve that had an amplitude greater than 80% of normal; the median nerve was also slow. In the legs the CMAP amplitudes were below 50% of normal, and the slowing was below 70% of normal. Distal motor latencies were prolonged (over 150% of normal) in the tibial and peroneal nerves with CMAP amplitudes below 80% of normal. The motor distal latencies were over 120% of normal in the median and ulnar nerves with amplitudes over 80% of normal, fulfilling demyelination criteria.[3] Also, the H-reflexes were absent, and the F-responses were prolonged in the median and ulnar nerves and absent in the peroneal and tibial nerves. Ulnar and sural SNAPs were absent.

These findings are consistent with demyelination without conduction blocks, except for the tibial nerve. Temporal dispersion was present only in the tibial nerve. The absent SNAPs may have been caused by axonal degeneration or severe demyelination.

The terminal latency indices (TLIs) were decreased in tibial, ulnar, and median nerves, indicating a disproportionate distal demyelination in these nerves. This index is used to demonstrate prominent demyelination in patients with a peripheral neuropathy in the distal segments relative to proximal segments. A low index indicates disproportionally distal demyelination.[4]

The needle test demonstrated denervation with large motor unit potentials of decreased recruitment, mainly in distal muscles indicating axonal degeneration and reinnervation.

WHAT IS THE DIFFERENTIAL DIAGNOSIS?

Chronic inflammatory demyelinating polyneuropathy (CIDP) should be considered in this patient's diagnosis, but the decreased pain sensation and predominantly distal numbness, with only mild and mainly distal weakness, are not characteristic.[5] The demyelination is against the diagnosis of most toxic neuropathies. However, some, such as amiodarone toxicity and arsenic poisoning, can cause axonal degeneration and demyelination.

Familial neuropathies, such as Charcot–Marie–Tooth disease, can occasionally manifest in older people. This patient lacked both family history and clinical findings, such as high arches or hammertoes, and had more sensory than motor deficits.

The clinical features suggest that this patient had a distal acquired demyelinating symmetrical neuropathy (DADS).[6] DADS typically manifests with clinical and electrophysiologic evidence of distal demyelination, for which calculation of the TLIs is useful.[7–9] In this patient, there was evidence of proximal and distal demyelination, and the TLI was abnormal in some, but not all, nerves. This indicated a more distal disease.

DADS can be an autoimmune disorder, similar to CIDP, and have a favorable response to immunotherapy. On the other hand, it can be associated with an IgM monoclonal gammopathy with antibodies against myelin-associated glycoprotein (MAG)[10,11] with a poor response to immunotherapy.

WHAT OTHER LABORATORY TESTS SHOULD BE DONE?

Other laboratory studies should include immunoelectrophoresis for monoclonal gammopathy. Measurement of MAG antibodies is useful, particularly in those with an IgM monoclonal gammopathy. A 24-hour urine collection for arsenic and a nerve biopsy should also be considered.

WHAT WERE THE RESULTS OF THE TESTS?

Immunoelectrophoresis by immunofixation demonstrated normal IgG and IgA proteins; there was an IgM λ light chain spike; IgM levels were 618 mg/dL (normal, 40–345 mg/dL). Urinary arsenic levels were not measured. Spinal fluid protein was 53 mg/dL (normal, <45 mg/dL). MAG antibody titers were at 1:204,800 (normal, <1:400).

A gastrocnemius muscle biopsy showed scattered esterase-positive atrophic muscle fibers, fiber-type grouping, and rare scattered necrotic muscle fibers (Fig. 54A-1).

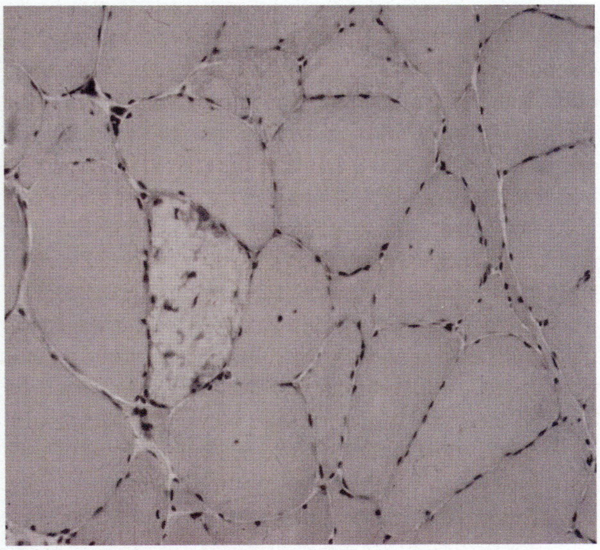

FIG. 54A-1 Muscle biopsy showing a necrotic fiber and scattered atrophic fibers (H&E stain, ×400).

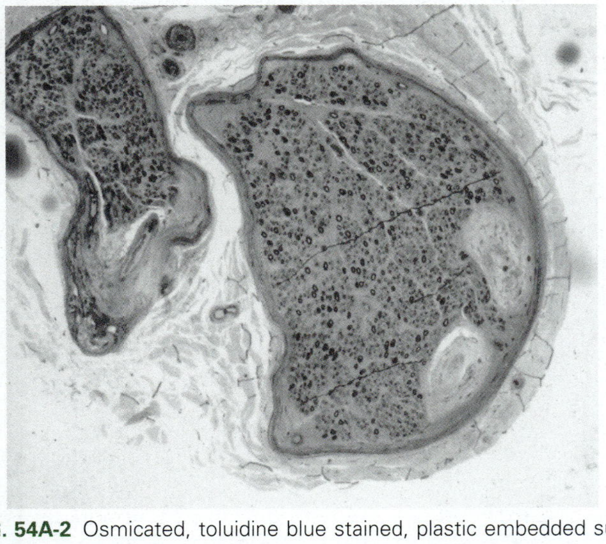

FIG. 54A-2 Osmicated, toluidine blue stained, plastic embedded sural nerve biopsy showing Renaut bodies, mild decreased number of myelinated fibers (×400).

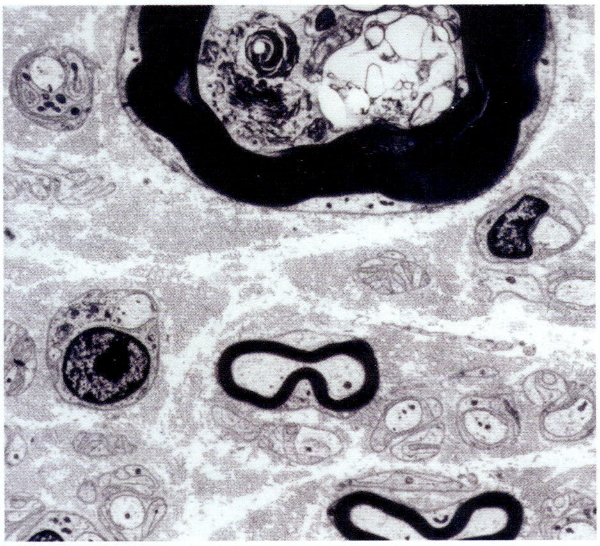

FIG. 54A-3 Nerve biopsy showing a degenerating axon on electromicroscopy (×6000).

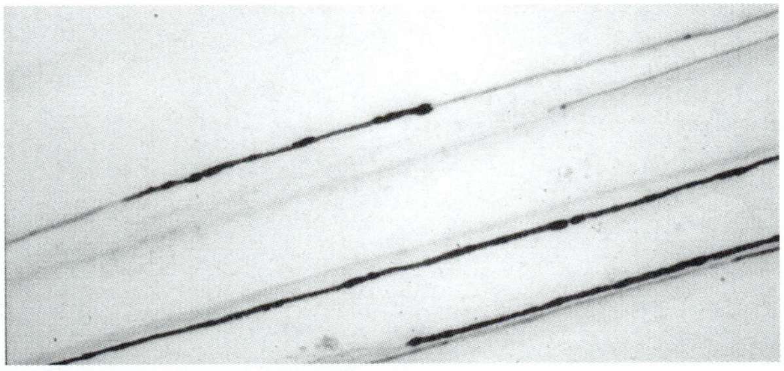

FIG. 54A-4 Teased nerve preparation showing paranodal swelling and segmental demyelination (×100).

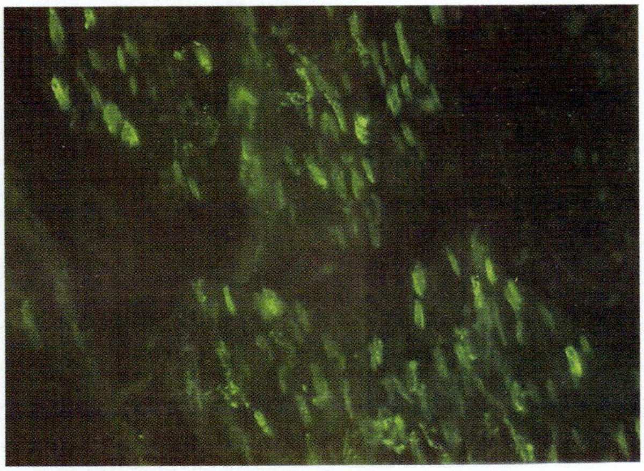

FIG. 54A-5 Immunofluorescence for IgM showing marked fluorescence of myelinated axons (×400).

A sural nerve biopsy showed mixed demyelinating and axonal neuropathy and a decreased number of myelinated axons. There were also Renaut bodies (Fig. 54A-2), flat unmyelinated axons, and degenerating myelinated fibers (Fig. 54A-3). Teased nerve preparation showed moderate segmental demyelination (Fig. 54A-4) and immunofluorescence deposits of IgM were seen in myelinated fibers (Fig. 54A-5). Widely spaced myelin lamella was not obvious on the electromicroscopy.

A bone marrow biopsy and bone survey were normal.

SUMMARY

This elderly man had slowly progressive sensorimotor neuropathy, an IgM monoclonal gammopathy, and antibodies against MAG. Electrophysiologic testing demonstrated a demyelinating neuropathy with secondary axonal damage. MAG-associated neuropathy is a predominantly distal demyelinating neuropathy that occurs more frequently in older men. These patients should be treated only if they have a severe and progressive weakness.

For further discussion, important points, and references, see Case 54B.

An Elderly Man With a Peripheral Neuropathy Like His Sister

A 70-year-old diabetic man was referred for weakness and numbness in the hand and feet. The patient limped due to quadricep muscle injury years before, while he was in the Armed Forces.

Past medical history includes successful lumbar laminectomy for back pain in the past; otherwise, the history was unremarkable.

The patient did not smoke or drink.

Family history revealed that his mother had macroglobulinemia and a sister has a peripheral neuropathy.

His previous EMG showed evidence of a peripheral neuropathy, "suggestive of a familial neuropathy."

On physical examination, vital signs are normal. Mentation and cranial nerves are normal. There is atrophy of the right quadriceps muscles with a surgical scar. Strength testing showed mild weakness in the interossei muscles of the hands and dorsiflexor weakness. Reflexes were 1+ in the arms, and absent in the legs. There is a glove/stocking sensory deficit and decreased pinprick in the right ulnar nerve distribution. The pinprick deficit was up to the mid-calf, whereas vibration sense deficit included the knees.

AN EMG TEST WAS PERFORMED

Nerve conduction Peroneal R.

Ankle	NR ms	NR mV	RI–ankle	m/s
Fibular head	NR ms	NR mV	Ankle–fibular head	m/s

Peroneal R.

Fibula (head)	12.0 ms	0.5 mV	Fibula (head) Popliteal fossa	24.1 m/s
Popliteal fossa	15.1 ms	0.5 mV		m/s

Tibial L.

Ankle	NR ms	NR mV	Ankle–popliteal fossa	m/s
Popliteal fossa	NR ms	NR mV		m/s

Median R.[a]

Wrist	19.1 ms	3.8 mV	APB–wrist	m/s
Elbow	32.5 ms	1.3 mV	Wrist–elbow	16.4 m/s

[a]T<1=0.22.

Ulnar R.[a]

Wrist	13.6 ms	1.3 mV	ADM–wrist	m/s
Below elbow	34.7 ms	1.6 mV	Wrist–below elbow	10.6 m/s
Above elbow	45.3 ms	1.1 mV	Below elbow–above elbow	11.3 m/s

[a]T<1=0.44.

Median L.[a]

Wrist	19.1 ms	1.2 mV	APB–wrist	m/s
Elbow	37.1 ms	1.1 mV	Wrist–below	12.5 m/s

[a]T<1=0.29.

Ulnar L.[a]

Wrist	12.4 ms	1.3 mV	ADM–wrist	m/s
Below elbow	30.3 ms	0.4 mV	Wrist–below elbow	11.7 m/s
Above elbow	56.9 ms	0.3 mV	Below elbow–above elbow	11.3 m/s

[a]T<1=0.46.

F-Wave Studies

Nerve	M-Latency	F-Latency
Median R.	19.8	39.5
Ulnar R.	13.7	
Median L.	32.7	64.7
Ulnar L.	19.0	

Sensory Nerve Conduction

Nerve and Site	Peak Latency (ms)	Amplitude (μV)	Segment	Latency Difference	Distance	Conduction Velocity
Median R.: Wrist	NR	NR	Index–wrist	ms	mm	m/s
Ulnar R.: Wrist	NR	NR		ms	mm	m/s
Median L.: Wrist	NR	NR	Index–wrist	ms	mm	m/s
Ulnar L.: Wrist	NR	NR		ms	mm	m/s

Needle EMG Examination

	Insertional	Spontaneous Activity		Volitional MUAPs					Max Volitional Activity		
Muscle	Insertional	Fibs	+Wave	Fasc	Duration	Amplitude	Poly	Config	Recruitment	Amplitude	Pattern	Effort
Tibialis anterior R.	Increased	None	+1	None	Sl. Incr.	Sl. Incr.	None	Normal	Normal	Normal	Full	Max.
Gatrocnemius R.	Normal	None	None	None	Normal	Normal	None	Normal	Normal	Normal	Full	Max.
First dorsal interosseous R.	Normal	None	None	None	Sl. Incr.	Sl. Incr.	None	Normal	Normal	Normal	Full	Max.
Vastus medialis L.	Normal	None	None	None	Sl. Incr.	Sl. Incr.	None	Normal	Normal	Normal	Full	Max.
Tibialis anterior L.	Normal	None	None	None	Sl. Incr.	Sl. Incr.	None	Normal	Normal	Normal	Full	Max.
Gastrocnemius L.	Increased	+2	+2	None	Normal	Normal	None	Normal	Normal	Normal	Full	Max.

WHAT ARE THE DIFFERENTIAL DIAGNOSES?

The differential diagnosis in this patient is a peripheral neuropathy; it could be diabetic. Other possibilities include amyloidosis and MAG-associated neuropathy. The family history is puzzling and important and that could suggest Charcot–Marie–Tooth disease. Chronic inflammatory demyelinating polyneuropathy (CIDP) is another possibility. Other acquired neuropathies like toxic or amyloidosis should also be considered.

WHAT TESTS DO WE DO?

EMG showed evidence of a demyelinating and axonal sensorimotor polyneuropathy. There was proximal and distal demyelination in the ulnar nerve, whereas in the median nerve the demyelination was more distal.

Routine blood tests were normal. Hemoglobin A1C was 6.9. B_{12} and TSH were normal. Immunoelectrophoresis showed an IgM monoclonal gammopathy, and the MAG antibodies were markedly elevated, 7360 (normal, <200).

No nerve biopsy or lumbar puncture was done.

It was also found from his sister that the patient also has a MAG neuropathy and responded well to rituximab. The patient is being treated with rituximab monthly with significant improvement.

SUMMARY

The patient is an older diabetic man with a neuropathy with distal and proximal demyelination, somewhat more distal demyelination, and his sister had a similar condition, and they both responded well to rituximab treatment.

DISCUSSION (CASES 54A AND 54B)

Patient 54A had chronic demyelinating neuropathy with somewhat more distal features (DADS) associated with an IgM monoclonal gammopathy and elevated MAG antibodies. He had no evidence of myeloma or other myeloproliferative disorder. DADS is a predominantly distal sensory demyelinating neuropathy most often seen in elderly men. The presentation is typically subacute to chronic with numbness, mild weakness, occasional gait ataxia and tremor, and, rarely, pain and dysautonomia.[11]

The Renaut bodies in the nerve biopsy in this case are usually a nonspecific finding; however, the IgM deposits are characteristic of DADS with MAG antibodies.[12–14] The atrophy and grouping seen on the muscle biopsy are compatible with chronic, axonal generation with reinnervation. The cause of the scattered muscle necrosis was not clear.

Usually, DADS associated with MAG has a relatively slow progression. It does not respond to steroids, IgG infusion, or plasma exchange. Those with progressive disability could be treated with cyclophosphamide or rituximab, which are somewhat effective in this disorder.[15] Patients with DADS without a monoclonal gammopathy or MAG respond better to immunotherapy. Patient 54A declined therapy and has been stable for several years.

WHAT ARE MONOCLONAL GAMMOPATHIES?

Monoclonal proteins (M-proteins) originate from plasma cells of monoclonal lineage. The heavy chain can be IgG, IgM, IgA, IgD, or IgE, and the light chains are either λ or κ. The M-proteins are described by their constituent heavy and light chains.

Some plasma cells produce only light chains, which are eliminated in the urine as Bence Jones protein.

The abnormal protein can arise from malignant cells such as multiple myeloma, lymphomas, or leukemia and is also associated with primary (nonfamilial) amyloidosis.

When a monoclonal gammopathy is not associated with another disease, it is usually called *monoclonal gammopathy of undetermined significance* (MGUS). MGUS has an incidence of about 1% after the age of 50 years, and this increases with age. MGUS is not always benign, as patients can later develop malignancy. Twenty-two percent of patients with MGUS later developed a hematologic malignancy or amyloidosis.[16] Polyneuropathy occurs in MGUS patients, and usually, the neuropathies in patients with IgM MGUS have clinical characteristics different from those with other gammopathies.[17]

DADS is more commonly associated with an IgM MGUS, while CIDP can be associated with an IgG or IgA MGUS, and those patients with IgG or IgA CIDP-MGUS are clinically similar to CIDP without a gammopathy.[18]

OTHER CONDITIONS ASSOCIATED WITH MONOCLONAL GAMMOPATHIES

Multiple myeloma is the most common malignancy associated with a monoclonal gammopathy. The most frequent neuromuscular manifestation of multiple myeloma is nerve root damage, but a mild distal symmetrical axonal sensorimotor neuropathy can also occur. A monoclonal gammopathy is detected in 90% of cases, often with κ light chains.[19]

Osteosclerotic myeloma is a form of localized myeloma that occurs in 3% of myeloma cases and is often associated with an IgG with λ light chain gammopathy. Some patients develop POEMS syndrome (also called Crow-Fukase syndrome).[20] Surgical resection of the tumor and/or radiation and chemotherapy are used in the treatment.[21,22]

Waldenström's macroglobulinemia is associated with IgM gammopathy in older patients, and 40%–50% have peripheral neuropathy. MAG antibodies have been rarely reported in this disease.[23]

Primary systemic amyloidosis is a monoclonal gammopathy seen in 90% of patients who have λ light chains in the serum or urine. Primary systemic amyloidosis causes a predominantly distal symmetrical sensory or sensorimotor neuropathy and can manifest as heart and renal failure.[17] The response to therapy is poor, but in disabled patients, immunotherapy may be of some benefit.

Cryoglobulinemia is a condition that manifests with a painful symmetric or asymmetric polyneuropathy and vasculitic purpura. Type I cryoglobulinemia has a monoclonal protein associated with plasmacytosis. Type II can have both a monoclonal and a polyclonal IgG M protein. Type III has a polyclonal gammopathy that may be associated with a chronic inflammatory disease or a connective tissue disorder. Types II and III are called "mixed" cryoglobulinemia and are often associated with hepatitis C.[24]

Other monoclonal gammopathies with polyneuropathy can be seen in cancer, lymphoma, and leukemia.

In about 50%–70% of patients with DADS and monoclonal gammopathy, the M protein reacts to MAG, which is a 110-kD glycoprotein that constitutes 1% of peripheral nerve myelin.[14,25] MAG antibodies react with the carbohydrate moiety shared by the proteins MAG P zero protein and sulfate glucuronyl carbohydrate epitopes of sulfate-3-glucuronyl paragloboside and sulfate-3-glucuronyl-*N*-acetyl lactosaminyl paragloboside,[26] and other gangliosides and sulfatides present in peripheral nerve myelin and axons.[26] Fifteen percent of patients with MAG antibodies do not have a monoclonal gammopathy.

Case 54B had a monoclonal gammopathy and diabetes. Most likely his neuropathy's recent onset was related to monoclonal gammopathy and MAG. The history of his sister and his mother who had macroglobulinemia indicates that there is a genetic predisposition for these disorders. Classical MAG-associated neuropathy presents with distal demyelination, prominent sensory deficit, and some weakness; however, more severe diffuse weakness could be present and cases may resemble CIDP rather than the typical distal demyelination and occurs in the elderly, particularly as his sister was much younger with the onset of symptoms.

Although DADS neuropathy is characteristically a more distal sensory neuropathy, some patients have diffuse weakness which may progress to a presentation similar to CIDP. Some patients may have IgM-κ antibodies and these are called DADSM. Those DADS that do not have an M protein are considered idiopathic DADS.

Most cases of MAG-associated neuropathy are idiopathic[27] and there are some reported cases associated with anti–TNF-α therapy.[28]

Case 54B is particularly interesting as his MAG neuropathy appears to be hereditary. This is very rare but monoclonal gammopathy can be hereditary[29,30] and also occurs with peripheral neuropathy.[31,32] Familial predisposition is also seen in macroglobulinemia.[33]

Immunomodulator medications have been used in these patients, and the response is usually not satisfactory, but in some cases like in Case 54A which may be slowly progressive, and did not require therapy. On the other hand, it appears that rituximab is useful in those with significant progression. A genetic profile was not done in the bone marrow on our patients; however, the occurrence of the MYD88 is seen in 88% of patients with MAG-associated polyneuropathy and is used in B cell–driven disease and in those with MAG neuropathy.[34] Venetoclax with rituximab is useful in cases of ibrutinib-resistant malignancy like with chronic lymphocytic leukemia and helped in the polyneuropathy with anti-MAG antibodies.[35]

IMPORTANT POINTS

- Five percent of patients with a monoclonal gammopathy have a neuropathy. Patients with demyelinating neuropathy should be worked up for a gammopathy, and those with an IgM gammopathy frequently have antibodies against MAG.
- Monoclonal gammopathy associated with a neuropathy can be seen in a variety of conditions, such as multiple myeloma, osteosclerotic myeloma, and other malignancies, macroglobulinemia, primary systemic amyloidosis, and cryoglobulinemia.
- DADS can have not only sensory but also motor problems and can be associated with IgM gammopathy with antibodies against MAG and occurring only in men and those without a gammopathy respond better.
- More prominent distal demyelination can be determined by calculating the terminal latency index.
- MAG-positive neuropathy could manifest with diffuse motor sensory neuropathy, but not necessarily distal sensory demyelination. In some cases the disorder may not progress significantly.
- MAG is a 110-kD glycoprotein that makes up 1% of peripheral nerve myelin.
- MAG-positive neuropathy can occur in families, and they could have a monoclonal IgM gammopathy.
- In some cases the disorder may not progress significantly.
- MAG neuropathy patients are not always associated with monoclonal gammopathy, and these patients may respond better to immunotherapy, particularly rituximab and those who have a myelopathy.[36,37]

REFERENCES

1. Kaufman M. Triglycerides and neuropathy. *Neurology*. 1995;45(11): 2119–2120.
2. Backes JM, Howard PA. Association of HMG-CoA reductase inhibitors with neuropathy. *Ann Pharmacoth*. 2003;37:274–278.

3. Saperstein DS, Katz JS, Amato AA, Barohn RJ. Clinical spectrum of chronic acquired demyelinating polyneuropathies. *Muscle Nerve*. 2001;24(3):311–324.
4. Shahani BT, Young RR, Potts F, Maccabee P. Terminal latency index (TLI) and late response studies in motor neuron disease (MND), peripheral neuropathies and entrapment syndrome studies. *Acta Neurol Scand*. 1979;73(Suppl):60 118.
5. Bertorini T, Narayanaswami P. Autoimmune neuropathies. *Compr Ther*. 2003;29(4):194–209.
6. Katz JS, Saperstein DS, Gronseth GS, et al. Distal acquired demyelinating symmetric neuropathy. *Neurology*. 2000;54: 615–620.
7. Kaku DA, England JD, Sumner AJ. Distal accentuation of conduction slowing in polyneuropathy associated with antibodies to myelin-associated glycoprotein and sulphated glucuronyl paragloboside. *Brain*. 1994;117:941–947.
8. Maisonobe T, Chassande B, Verin M, et al. Chronic dysimmune demyelinating polyneuropathy: a clinical and electrophysiological study of 93 patients. *J Neurol Neurosurg Psychiatry*. 1996;61(1): 36–42.
9. Lupu VD, Mora CA, Dambrosia J, et al. Terminal latency index in neuropathy with antibodies against myelin-associated glycoproteins. *Muscle Nerve*. 2007;35(2):196–202.
10. Gosselin S, Kyle RA, Dyck PJ. Neuropathy associated with monoclonal gammopathy of undetermined significance. *Ann Neurol*. 1991;30:54–61.
11. Mendell JR, Sahenk Z, Whitaker JN, et al. Polyneuropathy with IgM monoclonal gammopathy: studies on the pathogenic role of anti-myelin associated glycoprotein antibody. *Ann Neurol*. 1985;17:243–254.
12. Chassande B, Leger JM, Ben Younes-Chennoufi A, et al. Peripheral neuropathy associated with IgM monoclonal gammopathy: correlations between M-protein antibody activity and clinical/electrophysiological features in 40 cases. *Muscle Nerve*. 1998;21:55–62.
13. Kissel JT, Mendell JR. Neuropathies associated with monoclonal gammopathies. *Neuromuscul Disord*. 1995;6(11):3–18.
14. Braun PE, Frail DE, Latov N. Myelin-associated glycoprotein is the antigen for a monoclonal IgM in polyneuropathy. *J Neurochem*. 1982;39(5):1261–1265.
15. Renaud S, Gregor M, Fuhr P, et al. Rituximab in the treatment of polyneuropathy associated with anti-MAG antibodies. *Muscle Nerve*. 2003;27(5):611–615.
16. Kyle RA. "Benign" monoclonal gammopathy after 20 to 35 years of follow up. *Mayo Clin Proc*. 1993;68:26–36.
17. Bouch EP, Smith BE. Peripheral neuropathies associated with monoclonal proteins. *Med Clin North Am*. 1993;77:125–139.
18. Suarez GA, Kelly JJ Jr. Polyneuropathy associated with monoclonal gammopathy of undetermined significance: further evidence that IgM-MGUS neuropathies are different than IgG-MGUS. *Neurology*. 1993;43(7):1304–1308.
19. Kelly JJ, Kyle RA, Miles JM, et al. The spectrum of peripheral neuropathy in myeloma. *Neurology*. 1981;31:24–31.
20. Nakanishi T, Sobue I, Toyokura Y, et al. The Crow Fukase syndrome: a study of 102 cases in Japan. *Neurology*. 1984;34:702–710.
21. Kelly JJ, Kyle RA, Miles JM, et al. Osteosclerotic myeloma and peripheral neuropathy. *Neurology*. 1983;33:202–210.
22. Soubrier MH, Dubost JJ, Sauvezie BJ. POEMS syndrome: a study of 25 cases and a review of the literature. French Study Group on POEMS Syndrome. *Am J Med*. 1994;97:543–553.
23. Nobile-Orazio E, Marmiroli P, Baldini L, et al. Peripheral neuropathy in macroglobulinemia: incidence and antigen-specificity of M proteins. *Neurology*. 1987;37:1506–1514.
24. Agnello V, Romain PL. Mixed cryoglobulinemia secondary to hepatitis C virus infection. *Rheum Dis Clin North Am*. 1996; 22:1–21.
25. Latov N, Sherman WH, Nemni R, et al. Plasma-cell dyscrasia and peripheral neuropathy with monoclonal antibody to peripheral-nerve myelin. *N Engl J Med*. 1980;303(11):618–621.
26. Griffin JW. Antiglycolipid antibodies and peripheral neuropathies: links to pathogenesis. *Prog Brain Res*. 1999;101:313–323.
27. Nobile-Orazio E, Meucci N, Baldini L, Di Troia A, Scarlato G. Long-term prognosis of neuropathy associated with anti-MAG IgM M-proteins and its relationship to immune therapies. *Brain*. 2000;123:710–717.
28. McGinty RN, McNamera B, Moore H. DADS neuropathy associated with anti-TNF-α therapy. *BMJ Case Rep*. 2015 Nov. 25;2015; :bcr2015211781. https://doi.org/10.1136/bcr-2015-211781.
29. Greenberg AJ, Fajkumar V, Vachon CM. Familial monoclonal gammopathy of undetermined significance and multiple myeloma: epidemiology, risk factors and biologic characteristics. *Blood*. 2017;119(23):5359–5366.
30. Hemminki K. Forsti A, Sundquist K, et al. Familial associations of monoclonal gammopathy of unknown significance with autoimmune diseases. *Leukemia*. 2016;30(8):1766–1769. https://doi.org/10.1038/leu.2016.43. Epub 2016 Feb 29.
31. Latov N. Neuropathy, heredity, and monoclonal gammopathy Editorial. *Arch Neurol*. 2000;57(5):641–642.
32. Steck AJ. Anti-MAG neuropathy: from biology to clinical management. *Neuroimmunol*. 2021;361:577725. https://doi.org/10.1016/j.neuroim.2021.5777725.
33. Kapoor P, Paludo J, Ansell S. Waldenstrom macroglobulinemia: familial predisposition and the role of genomics in prognosis and treatment selection. *Curr Treat Options Oncol*. 2016;17(3):16. https://doi.org/10.1007/s11864-016-0391-7.
34. Castellani F, Visentin A, Campagnolo M, Salvalaggio A, et al. The Bruton tyrosine kinase inhibitor ibrutinib improves anti-MAG antibody polyneuropathy. *Neurol Neuroimmunol Neuroinflamm*. 2020;7(4):e720. https://doi.org/10.1212/NXI.0000000000000720. Print.
35. Briani C, Visentin A, Castellani F, et al. The BCL2 inhibitor venetoclax plus rituximab is active in MYD88 wild-type polyneuropathy with anti-MAG antibodies. *Neurol Neuroimmunol Neuroinflamm*. 2020;9(4):e1181. https://doi.org/10.1212/NXI.00000000000001181. Print 2022 Jul.
36. Kyle RA, Greipp PR. Amyloidosis (AL): clinical and laboratory features in 229 cases. *Mayo Clin Proc*. 1983;58:665–683.
37. Vos JM, Notermans NC, D'Sa S, Lunn MP, et al. High prevalence of the MYD88 L265P mutation in IgM anti-MAG paraprotein-associated peripheral neuropathy. *J Neurol Neurosurg Psychiatry*. 2018;89(9):1007–1009. https://doi.org/10.1136/jnnp-2017-316689.

A Man With Progressive Lower Extremity Weakness and Monoclonal Gammopathy

A 47-year-old man was evaluated for progressive ascending weakness in his lower extremities for 3–4 months becoming wheelchair bound within 4 months of onset of symptoms. He had mild paresthesias in his extremities.

Diabetes was diagnosed within the same period, and he was started on pioglitazone and later switched to glimepiride without any improvement of neurologic symptoms despite good glycemic control. There was no other significant medical history, and the family history was also unremarkable. He denied smoking, alcohol, or illicit drug use.

He was referred to us by his primary care physician with the above symptoms and after a quadriceps muscle biopsy reported to show nonspecific findings.

Neurological examination revealed a normal mental status. Cranial nerves were normal. He did not have tongue atrophy or fasciculation. Neck flexion and extension strength were normal. He had 5/5 strength in upper extremities and normal tone and no atrophy, and strength in lower extremities was 3/5 both proximally and distally. There was mild distal muscle atrophy. No fasciculations were seen. He had decreased stretch reflexes in upper and lower extremities, and plantar reflexes were downgoing bilaterally.

Sensory examination revealed absent vibration sense in the toes, diminished in ankles, and position sense impairment in feet. Pinprick sensation was mildly decreased up to the ankles. There was no sensory deficit in the upper extremities. Coordination was intact on finger-to-nose and heel-to-shin testing. Gait was not tested given his significant weakness in the legs. He was wheelchair-bound. His vital signs were normal and general exam was unremarkable including normal cardiac exam and lung auscultation. There were no skin lesions or nail abnormalities. No visceromegaly was appreciated.

WHAT IS THE DIFFERENTIAL DIAGNOSIS AND WHAT SHOULD BE THE INITIAL WORKUP?

This patient had a history of progressive lower extremity weakness, making him wheelchair-bound within 4 months. He also had mild paresthesias and examination revealed sensory deficits in the feet.

Absent reflexes and down-going plantar reflexes reflect a lower motor neuron or peripheral nerve lesion, making myelopathy less likely. With lower extremity weakness progressing distally to proximally and distal symmetric sensory deficit, a motor sensory neuropathy is likely and potential etiologies to be considered include:

1. metabolic: diabetes, hypothyroidism, and uremia;
2. toxic;
3. nutritional: B_{12} deficiency;
4. infectious: human immunodeficiency virus–related or hepatitis C–related neuropathy;
5. inflammatory or autoimmune: rheumatoid arthritis, small vessel vasculitis neuropathy, systemic lupus erythematosus, and sarcoidosis;
6. chronic inflammatory demyelination polyneuropathy (CIDP);
7. paraneoplastic disorders; and
8. paraproteinemia: primary amyloidosis, cryoglobulinemia, POEMS syndrome, monoclonal gammopathy of undetermined significance (MGUS).

Diabetes mellitus is the most common cause of metabolic polyneuropathy. Other metabolic causes include uremia, hypothyroidism, hepatic failure, acromegaly, and porphyria. In diabetic neuropathy, there may be sensory and motor symptoms and autonomic involvement. Patients usually complain of paresthesias in distal extremities and may experience some pain. Symptoms are usually symmetric and may progress proximally. Patients may develop progressive distal motor weakness and with autonomic involvement may present with erectile dysfunction, abnormalities in gastrointestinal motility, orthostatic hypotension, arrhythmias, and sudomotor syndromes.[1]

The progression of the disease is usually slow. The rapid onset of symptoms in our patient urged us to investigate further. He had normal renal function, thyroid panel, and liver enzymes making other metabolic disorders less likely. He did not have any gastrointestinal symptoms or psychiatric signs or symptoms suggestive of porphyria and his general examination did not show signs of acromegaly.

The patient has no history of use of medication besides pioglitazone and glimepiride. There were no Mees' lines or other signs indicative of heavy metal toxicity on exam. He gave no history of any toxin exposure and hence toxin-induced neuropathy was highly unlikely. He was not an alcoholic, and initial lab studies showed normal levels of serum thiamine, B_{12}, and folate. He tested negative for human immunodeficiency virus, hepatitis C, and Lyme disease. He had negative antinuclear antibody, perinuclear antineutrophilic cytoplasmic antibodies, and rheumatoid factor ruling out a connective tissue disorder.

A chest x-ray did not show a mass lesion or hilar lymphadenopathy, and serum angiotensin-converting enzyme was negative, suggestive of a diagnosis other than sarcoidosis.

WHAT OTHER TESTS SHOULD BE DONE?

As further workup, an lumbar puncture(LP) was performed, and cerebrospinal fluid analysis was remarkable for elevated protein of 425 mg/dL. Cerebrospinal fluid (CSF) white blood count was 6, leukocyte per mm, and other parameters were normal.

Serum protein electrophoresis showed an elevated gamma fraction and immunofixation showed immunoglobulin (Ig), lambda monoclonal protein reactive with light chain antisera. A 24-hour urine study was negative for M protein.

Nerve conduction studies showed absent motor responses in lower extremities. Right median motor studies showed a prolonged distal latency (125% of upper limit of normal), a normal amplitude, and slow conduction velocity (not 70%–80% of lower limit of normal). The right ulnar nerve motor studies showed prolonged distal latency (125% of upper limit of normal), normal amplitude, and slow conduction velocity 42.3 m/s (not 70%–80% of lower limit of normal). F waves for both right median and right ulnar nerves were prolonged (>120%–150% of upper limit of normal). The right peroneal compound muscle action potential (CMAP) could not be obtained. The left peroneal nerve had a slow velocity, low amplitude, and slow conduction velocity.

Sensory nerve action potentials were of low amplitude in the upper and lower extremities. Needle electromyogram (EMG) was normal in the upper extremities but showed denervation potentials in both lower extremities proximally and distally along with reduced motor unit recruitment.

These findings were consistent with peripheral neuropathy with demyelinating and axonal features without fulfilling all formal EMG criteria for primary demyelination such as CIDP.

WHAT IS THE DIFFERENTIAL DIAGNOSIS NOW?

Given the evidence of monoclonal gammopathy, CSF albumin cytologic dissociation, and EMG findings, the differential diagnoses were narrowed down to a peripheral neuropathy associated with monoclonal gammopathy. This includes MGUS-associated neuropathy, POEMS syndrome, multiple myeloma (MM), and primary amyloidosis.

MGUS is a disorder characterized by a serum monoclonal protein (<30 g/L) without hematological abnormalities of end-organ damage (hypercalcemia, renal failure, and bone lesions).[2] Although IgG is the most frequent paraprotein found in MGUS, peripheral neuropathy is more prevalent in patients with the IgM subtype.[3] The paraproteins are usually kappa light chains. The neuropathy of IgM MGUS usually occurs in older men and is a slowly progressive, distal, symmetric, and sensorimotor polyneuropathy. Patients may have prominent tremors and ataxia. Nerve conduction studies may show mixed features of demyelination and axonal degeneration. An overlap exists between the different subtypes of MGUS; however, there is more pronounced sensory loss and ataxia in IgM subtype than IgA and IgG and greater demyelination is found in IgM MGUS on nerve conduction studies.[4]

Approximately 50% of patients with IgM MGUS and polyneuropathy also have antibodies against myelin-associated glycoprotein. These patients are typically males in the sixth to ninth decades, presenting with slowly progressive, distal, and predominantly sensory neuropathy (DADS). Mild distal weakness may develop later in the course. The neuropathy is primarily demyelinating in nature as seen on electrodiagnostic studies and nerve biopsies. Vibration and proprioception sensations are affected more than pain and temperature resulting in sensory ataxia. Patients may respond to immunotherapy[5]; although rituximab is useful, some progress so slowly that they do not need therapy.

Neuropathy in IgA and IgG MGUS is less prevalent and could have features of CIDP, sensory, motor, or mixed neuropathy with electrophysiological features of axonal degeneration, demyelination or both. It usually has a more rapid progression than IgM MGUS and patients may have more motor weakness affecting both proximal and distal muscles.[6,7] CIDP associated with MGUS is usually clinically and electrodiagnostically indistinguishable from idiopathic CIDP. It typically occurs in the IgA and IgG subtypes and is usually more responsive to immunotherapy than IgM MGUS neuropathy.[3,8,9] The Peripheral Nerve Society has suggested a set of diagnostic criteria that includes enhancement of lumbosacral roots on MRI as supporting evidence of CIDP.[10]

This patient had clinical features that resemble CIDP; however, he does not fulfill the diagnostic criteria for definite CIDP. It is to be noted that about two-thirds of patients diagnosed with CIDP do not meet the electrodiagnostic criteria for this disorder.[11] He was treated with azathioprine and intravenous immunoglobulin (IVIG) and did not respond to the treatment.

POEMS syndrome, or Crow-Fukase syndrome,[12] or Takatsuki syndrome[13] is also a condition associated with *polyneuropathy, organomegaly, endocrinopathy, M protein, and skin changes*, hence, the acronym POEMS. It is associated with an osteosclerotic form of myeloma and features a predominantly demyelinating sensorimotor polyneuropathy along with greatly elevated protein in CSF and a monoclonal Ig spike in the blood. The paraproteins are lambda light chains. Clinically patients are in their fifth to seventh decades and have progressive and severe sensory symptoms and motor weakness. Elevated levels of vascular endothelial growth factor (VEGF) and tumor necrosis factor alpha are present.[14]

MM is a malignant disorder characterized by a monoclonal gammopathy with serum protein >30 g/L. The paraproteins are IgG in 50% of the cases[15] and kappa light chains. MM is associated with plasma cell proliferation in the bone marrow with the invasion of adjacent bone, resulting in destructive lesions and organ damage such as hypercalcemia, anemia, and renal insufficiency are other features of the disease.[15] The most common neurological manifestation of MM is radiculopathy because of nerve root compression from lytic bone lesions, plasmacytomas, or pathologic features; however, patients may also develop peripheral neuropathies. The neuropathy is usually axonal but may have demyelinating features.[16] It is usually symmetric and distal and could be sensory or sensorimotor manifesting as paresthesias/dysesthesias, numbness, and tingling in hands and feet. Treatment of the underlying MM usually does not improve the neuropathy and in fact may worsen it.[3]

Primary AL amyloidosis is a systemic disorder affecting multiple organ systems including the peripheral nerves. Approximately 17% of patients with primary amyloidosis have peripheral neuropathy and this may be the presenting feature of the disease. An M spike is present in serum and/or urine, usually consisting of IgG with lambda light chain more common than kappa.[17,18] The neuropathy is usually distal, symmetrical, and progressive affecting lower extremities before the upper extremities. It may be sensory or both sensory and motor and is frequently painful because of involvement of small-diameter sensory fibers. Autonomic dysfunction is common, resulting in postural hypotension, impotence, and bladder dysfunction. Approximately 25% of patients developed carpal tunnel syndrome because of accumulation of amyloid into the flexor retinaculum.[17,18]

Electrodiagnostic findings are those of an axonal sensorimotor peripheral neuropathy with sensory fibers affected more severely than motor axons.[17] The diagnosis is confirmed by the presence of congophilic amyloid deposits in tissues such as bone marrow, fat, rectal mucosa, or nerve.[18,19]

WHAT SHOULD BE THE NEXT DIAGNOSTIC TEST?

To differentiate MGUS neuropathy from neuropathy associated with myeloma, particularly osteosclerotic myeloma, the patient underwent a full osseous survey that revealed an expansile lytic lesion involving the left pelvis in the medial left supra-acetabulum. This case emphasizes the need to do a bone survey x-ray in patients who have CIDP and MGUS.

MRI of the pelvis showed abnormal enhancement and marrow replacement involving the left acetabulum and portions of the left ischemia and ilium with abnormality also affecting the obturator internus, obturator externus, and gluteus minimus muscles on the left (Fig. 55-1).

MRI of the lumbosacral spine with contrast revealed no bone lesions; however, there was enhancement of the nerve roots within the lumbosacral thecal sac (Fig. 55-2).

The patient underwent needle biopsy of the left acetabular lesion that revealed sheets of plasmacytoid cells suspicious for a plasma cell myeloma. The tumor was monoclonal for lambda light chains. A bone marrow biopsy and aspiration were obtained that were negative for atypical plasma cells. MM is ruled out without evidence of end-organ damage. Congo Red staining of bone marrow and subcutaneous fat aspirate were negative for amyloid, ruling out systemic amyloidosis. A sural nerve biopsy showed nonspecific findings but was negative for amyloid.

WHAT WAS THE FINAL DIAGNOSIS?

The patient presented with a subacute progressive lower extremity weakness and paresthesias. His neurological examination showed a mixed sensorimotor peripheral neuropathy. Most of his lab tests were within normal limits; however, CSF protein was significantly elevated and serum immunofixation showed a lambda light chain IgA spike. EMG/NCV study was consistent with a sensorimotor polyneuropathy with demyelinating and axonal features. MRI of the L spine showed enhancement of the nerve roots indicative of inflammatory demyelinating polyradiculoneuropathy.

MRI of the pelvis showed a bony lesion that was consistent with plasmacytoma on biopsy. He had recently been diagnosed with diabetes. Although our patient did not have visceromegaly or skin changes at presentation, he fulfilled the criteria for a diagnosis of POEMS syndrome, polyneuropathy, monoclonal plasma cell proliferation disorder, sclerotic bone lesion, and diabetes (endocrinopathy).

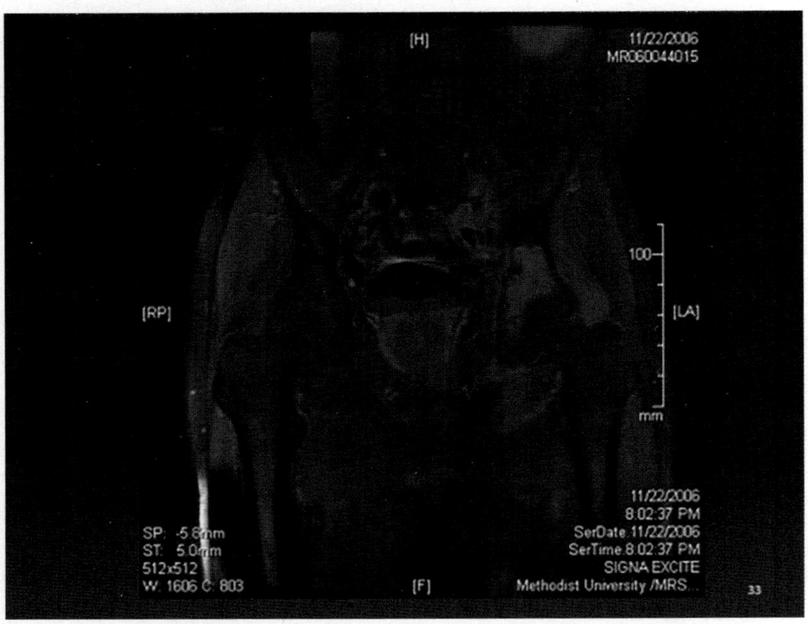

FIG. 55-1 MRI of the pelvis with contrast, axial view. Abnormal enhancement involving the left acetabulum.

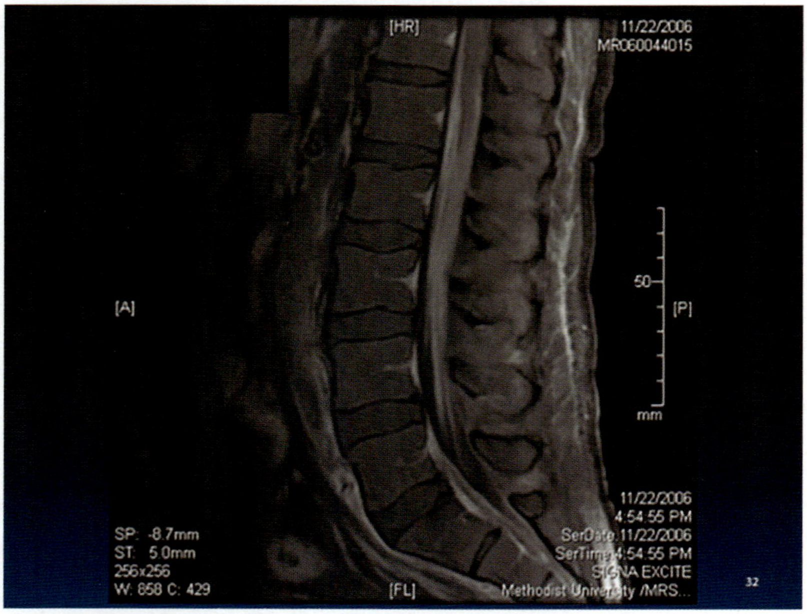

FIG. 55-2 MRI of the lumbosacral spine without contrast, sagittal view. Nerve root enhancement.

WHAT IS POEMS SYNDROME?

POEMS syndrome is a rare disorder characterized by clonal proliferation of plasma cells, monoclonal protein in the blood and associated polyneuropathy, organomegaly, endocrinopathy, and skin lesions as specified in the acronym.[20] Not all the features in the acronym are necessary to make the diagnosis. There are other important features of this syndrome that are not included in the acronym (Table 55-1).[21]

It was previously thought that this condition was more prevalent in people of Japanese descent[12,13] but more recent reports include cases from Europe and other countries.[22–24] The median age of onset is around 50 years and there is a slightly higher prevalence in men.

There is evidence by elevated serum monoclonal protein on immunofixation. The M protein is usually IgG or IgA and predominantly lambda light chain. Polyneuropathy may be the presenting feature of the syndrome and typically is an ascending, processing, and sensorimotor demyelinating polyneuropathy accompanied by pain and hyperesthesia in some patients. Muscular weakness is usually more prominent than sensory disturbance and distal lower extremities are affected more severely than upper extremities.[25,26] Papilledema may be present, [27] skin manifestations are variable and include hyperpigmentation, hemangioma, hypertrichosis, scleronomic changes, clubbing, and white nails.[28]

Solitary or multiple osteosclerosis lesions occur in approximately 95% of patients, although osteolytic or mixed lesions could also be present. Patients may develop thrombocytosis or erythrocytosis resulting in an increased risk of arterial and/or serious thrombosis.[29] Strokes may complicate the disease course in 10% of cases.[30]

Approximately 85% of patients develop endocrinopathies, most commonly hypogonadism, followed by thyroid dysfunction, diabetes, and adrenal insufficiency, and many patients suffer from multiple endocrinopathies.[31] Pulmonary features

TABLE 55-1 Major and Minor Criteria for Diagnosis of POEMS Syndrome

Mandatory Major Criteria symptoms/Signs	Minor Criteria	Other
Polyneuropathy	Organomegaly	Clubbing
Monoclonal plasma cell proliferative disorder	Extravascular volume overload	Weight loss
Other major criteria hypertension/ (one required)	Endocrinopathy	Pulmonary restrictive lung disease
Castleman disease	Skin changes (hyperpigmentation, hypertrichosis)	Hyperhidrosis
Sclerotic bone lesions	Papilledema	Low B_{12} values
VEGF elevation	Thrombocytosis/ polycythemia	Thrombotic diatheses

Diagnosis of POEMS syndrome is confirmed when both of the mandatory major criteria, one of the other major criteria, and one of the minor criteria are present. *VEGF*, Vascular endothelial growth factor.

of this syndrome include restrictive lung disease, pulmonary hypertension, and impaired carbon monoxide diffusion capacity.[28] Bone marrow biopsies show megakaryocyte hyperplasia and clonal plasma cells, 90% are lambda chains.[31]

Histologic features of dermis are variable and include vascular abnormalities with largely dilated blood vessels and complex anastomotic vessels.[32]

Nerve biopsies show segmental demyelination, axonal denegation, variable degrees of endoneurial fibrosis, and abnormal endoneurial vessels characterized by a thickened basal lamina and hypertrophies of endothelial cells.[33]

Serum levels of VEGF are elevated in patients with POEMS syndrome, correlating with activity of disease.[34,35] Other proinflammatory cytokines are also found to be elevated including tumor necrosis factor alpha, interleukin (IL)-6, and IL-1β; however, VEGF is a more specific marker and one of the other major diagnostic criteria for POEMS syndrome. VEGF selectively binds to endothelial cells and mediates endothelial cell proliferation and migration. Its expression can be introduced by hypoxia and so in ischemic tissues and tumors, hypoxia-induced VEGF promotes angiogenesis and neovascularization with resultant leaking vessels and edema. VEGF affects the blood–brain barrier by increasing vascular permeability with subsequent nerve damage secondary to increased endoneurial edema.[35] This is the proposed pathogenesis of polyneuropathy produced in this syndrome.

A recent study found markedly elevated serum levels of IL-12 along with elevated VEGF in patients with untreated POEMS syndrome, suggesting IL-12 to be an active participant in the pathogenesis of POEMS syndrome.[36] The study also showed that changes of serum IL-12 levels with treatment correlated well with the clinical course of patients. These findings advocate that IL-12 can be used as a biomarker of disease activity and a target for treatment. The exact mechanisms of this role in disease and overproduction remain unclear.

In POEMS syndrome, nerve conduction studies show a reduction in amplitudes of compound muscle action potentials, lower conduction velocities, prolonged distal latencies, and prolonged F waves.[37] Both CIDP and POEMS syndrome cause a demyelinating neuropathy and their electrodiagnostic tests are similar.[38] Electrophysiological features that may differentiate POEMS syndrome from CIDP include more marked reduction of motor nerve conduction velocities in the intermediate nerve segments than distal severe axonal loss, more severe CMAP in lower extremities than upper extremities, and lesser frequency of conduction block and temporal dispersion.[37,39]

As in this case, there have been other published patient cases reporting contrast enhancement of nerve roots on MRI in POEMS syndrome, although this is not commonly seen.[40]

POEMS may also be associated with plasma cell variant of Castleman disease (angiofollicular lymph node hyperplasia). Castleman disease is characterized by lymphoid hyperplasia and follicular capillary proliferation which could be involving a single lymph node or multiple nodes.[41]

The usual clinical course of POEMS syndrome is chronic with median survival rates of approximately 14 years.[42,43] Features that may shorten survival include the presence of fingernail clubbing, effusion, ascites, respiratory symptoms, and associated Castleman disease.[41] Lower VEGF levels may predict a better response to treatment.

There are no randomized clinical trials on treatment of POEMS syndrome and the treatment strategies are based on a large number of case reports and case series. Treatment should primarily target the underlying plasma cell disorder and then control VEGF production and levels.

In patients with a solitary plasmacytoma, without bone marrow involvement on biopsy, radiation therapy is recommended as the first-line therapy. If the disease does not stabilize despite radiation after 6–12 months, systemic therapy should be considered. In patients with bone marrow involvement and diffuse sclerotic lesions, systemic therapy is indicated.[44] The conventional treatments for demyelinating neuropathy such as steroids, intravenous Ig, and plasma exchange have proven to be minimally effective. Alkylating agents with or without corticosteroids are effective in some patients.[45,46]

High-dose chemotherapy along with peripheral blood stem cell transplant has shown to be an effective treatment[47] but relapses have been reported.[48] Other treatments that hold promise include thalidomide,[38] lenalidomide,[49] bevacizumab,[50] and bortezomib[51] all of which have antiplasmin cell effect and anti-VEGF and anti–tumor necrosis factor effects.[48] Peripheral neuropathy is the major dose-limiting complication of thalidomide and bortezomib. Lenalidomide is less neurotoxic. Further large studies are needed to determine the safety and efficacy of these drugs.[52]

Peripheral neuropathy may improve over the course of 6–36 months in patients who responded to systemic therapy.[21]

This patient was treated with radiation of the bone lesion and bone marrow transplant with high doses of melphalan. The neuropathy was stable and he still has had distal weakness for the last 10 years.

SUMMARY

A man presented with polyneuropathy with demyelinating and axonal features with elevated spinal fluid protein and contrast enhancement of the cauda equina roots on MRI. The patient was found to have a monoclonal gammopathy and was diagnosed as having osteosclerotic myeloma of the spine where he did not have all the features of POEMS syndrome. He responded well to bone marrow stem cell transplant.

IMPORTANT POINTS

- Patients with diabetes with rapidly progressively neuropathy should be evaluated for other causes of neuropathy.
- CIDP patients could have MGUS (monoclonal gammopathy of with undetermined significance).
- Patients with MGUS should be evaluated for the presence of localized myeloma with a bone survey and bone marrow biopsies.
- Patients with POEMS syndrome may present without all the clinical manifestations and may only present with diabetes.
- POEMS disorders may not respond to initial immunotherapy and may respond to bone marrow, stem cell transplant, and chemotherapy.

This case was reported as a case review: Mansoor S, Bertorini T. J Clin Neuromuscul Disord. 2013;14(4):194–203.

REFERENCES

1. Sullivan K, Feldman E. New developments in diabetic neuropathy. *Curr Opin Neurol.* 2005;18:586–590.
2. Kyle R. Monoclonal gammopathy of undetermined significance: natural history of 241 cases. *Ann J Med.* 1978;64:814–826.
3. Silberman J, Lonial S. Review of peripheral neuropathy in plasma cell disorders. *Hematol Oncol.* 2008;26:55–65.

4. Suarez GA, Kelly JJ. Polyneuropathy associated with monoclonal gammopathy of unknown significance: further evidence that IgM-MGUS neuropathies are different from IgG-MGUS. *Neurology*. 1993;43:1304–1308.
5. Nobile-Orazio E. Paraproteinemia related neuropathies. *Haematologic*. 2007;92(s2):62–64.
6. Ramchandren S, Lewis R. Monoclonal gammopathies and neuropathy. *Curr Opin Neurol*. 2008;22:480–485.
7. Hadden R, Nobile-Orazio E, Somer CL, et al. European Federation of Neurological Societies/Peripheral Nerve Society Guideline on management of paraproteinemic demyelinating neuropathies. Report of a Joint Task Force of the European Federation of Neurological Society and the Peripheral Nerve Society—first revision. *J Peripher Nerv Syst*. 2012;15:185–195.
8. Gertz MA. Managing monoclonal gammopathy-associated neuropathy. *Leuk Lymphoma*. 2006;47:785–786.
9. Saperstein DS, Kaz JS, Amata ASA, et al. Clinical spectrum of chronic acquired demyelinating polyneuropathies. *Muscle Nerve*. 2001;24:311–324.
10. European Federation of Neurological Societies/Peripheral Nerve Society European Federation of Neurological Societies/ Peripheral Nerve Society Guideline on management of chronic inflammatory demyelinating polyradiculoneuropathy. Report of a Joint Task Force of The European Federation of Neurological Societies and the Peripheral Nerve Society. *J Peripher Nerve Syst*. 2005;10:220–228.
11. Bromberg MB. Comparison of electrodiagnostic criteria for primary demyelination in chronic polyneuropathy. *Muscle Nerve*. 1991;14:968–976.
12. Nakanishi T, Sobue I, Toyokura Y, et al. The Crow-Fukase syndrome: a study of 102 cases in Japan. *Neurology*. 1984;34:712–720.
13. Takatsuki K, Sanada I. Plasma cell dyscrasia with polyneuropathy and endocrine disorder: clinical and laboratory features of 109 reported cases. *Jpn J Clin Oncol*. 1983;13:543–555.
14. Arimura K. Increased vascular endothelial growth factor (VEGF) is causative in Crow-Fukase syndrome (in Japanese). *Rinsbo Shinkeigaku*. 1999;39:84–85.
15. The international Myeloma Working Group Criteria for the classification of monoclonal gammopathies, multiple myeloma and related disorders: a report of the International Myeloma Working Group. *Br J Haematol*. 2003;121:749–757.
16. Ropper AH, Gorson KC. Current concepts: neuropathies associated with paraproteinemia. *N Engl J Med*. 1998;338:1601–6707.
17. Simmons Z, Specht CS. The neuromuscular manifestations of amyloidosis. *J Clin Neuromuscular Dis*. 2010;11:145–157.
18. Rosenzweig M, Landau H. Light chain (AL) amyloidosis: update on diagnosis and management. *J Hemtol Oncol*. 2011;4:47.
19. Kyle RA, Kelly JJ, Dyck PJ. Amyloidosis and neuropathy. In: Dyck PJ, Thomas PK, eds. *Peripheral Neuropathy*. 4th ed. Philadelphia, PA: Elsevier Saunders; 2005:2427–2451.
20. Bardwick PA, Zvaifler NH, Gill GN, et al. Plasma cell dyscrasia with polyneuropathy, organomegaly, endocrinopathy, M protein and skin changes: the POEMS syndrome: report on two cases and a review of the literature. *Medicine*. 1980;59:311–322.
21. Dispenzieri A. POEMS syndrome: 2011 update on diagnosis, risk-stratification, and management. *Am J Hematol*. 2011;86:591–601.
22. Singh D, Wadhwa J, Kumar L, et al. POEMS syndrome: experience with fourteen cases. *Leuk Lymphoma*. 2003;44:1749–1752.
23. Soubrir M, Dubost J, Sauvezie B. POEMS syndrome: a study of 25 cases and a review of the literature. French Study Group on POEMS Syndrome. *Am J Med*. 1994;97:543–553.
24. Zhang B, Song X, Liang B, et al. The clinical study of POEMS syndrome in China. *Neuro Endocrinol Lett*. 2010;31:229–237.
25. Kulkarni G, Mahadevan A, Taly A, et al. Clinicopathological profile of polyneuropathy, organomegaly, endocrinopathy, M protein and skin changes (POEMS) syndrome. *J Clin Neurosci*. 2011;18:356–360.
26. Min J, Hong Y, Lee K. Electrophysiological features of patients with POEMS syndrome. *Clin Neurophysiol*. 2005;116:965–968.
27. Koushik M, Pulido J, Abreu R, et al. Ocular findings in patients with polyneuropathy, organomegaly, endocrinopathy, monoclonal gammopathy, and skin changes syndrome. *Ophthalmology*. 2011; 118:778–782.
28. Barte S, Mouawad R, Choquet S, et al. Skin manifestations and vascular endothelial growth factor levels in POEMS syndrome: impact of autologous hematopoietic stem cell transplantation. *Arch Dermatol*. 2010;146:615–623.
29. Lesprit P, Authier F, Gherardi R, et al. Acute arterial obliteration: a new feature of the POEMS syndrome. *Medicine*. 1996;75:226–232.
30. Dupont S, Dispenzieri A, Mauermann M, et al. Cerebral infarction in POEMS syndrome: incidence, risk factors and imaging characteristics. *Neurology*. 2009;73:1308–1312.
31. Ghandi G, Basti R, Dispenzieri A, et al. Endocrinopathy in POEMS syndrome: the Mayo Clinic experience. *Mayo Clin Proc*. 2007;82:836–842.
32. Ishikawa O, Niheu Y, Ishikawa H. The skin changes of POEMS syndrome. *Br J Haematol*. 1987;117:523–526.
33. Subue G, Doyu M, Watanabe M, et al. Extensive demyelinating changes in the peripheral nerves of Crow-Fukase syndrome: a pathological study of one autopsied case. *Acta Neuropathol*. 1992;84:171–177.
34. Keddie S, Foldes D, Caimari F, et al. Clinical characteristics, risk factors and outcomes of POEMS syndrome: a longitudinal cohort study. *Neurology*. 2020;95(3):e268–e279.
35. Scarlato M, Previtali S, Carpo M, et al. Polyneuropathy in POEMS syndrome: role of angiogenic factors in the pathogenesis. *Brain*. 2005;128(pt 8):1911–1920.
36. Kanai K, Sawai S, Sogawa K, et al. Markedly upregulated serum interleukin-12 as novel biomarker in POEMS syndrome. *Neurology*. 2012;79:575–582.
37. Mauermann M, Sorenson E, Dispenzieri A, et al. Uniform demyelination and more severe axonal loss distinguish POEMS syndrome from CIDP. *J Neurol Neurosurg Psychiatry*. 2012;83: 480–486.
38. Kuwahara S, Misawa S, Kanai K, et al. Thalidomide reduces serum VEGF levels and improves peripheral neuropathy in POEMS syndrome. *J Neurol Neurosurg Psychiatry*. 2008;79:1255–1257.
39. Sung J, Kuwabara S, Ogawara K, et al. Patterns of nerve conduction abnormalities in POEMS syndrome. *Muscle Nerve*. 2002;26:189–193.
40. Ng AWY, Yuen KK, Tung SY, et al. Peripheral neuropathy: clinical diagnosis of POEMS syndrome and treatment with radiotherapy. *J HK Coll Radiol*. 2007;10:66–69.
41. Brown W, Lewis J, Filippa D, et al. The management of unicentric and multicentric Castleman's disease: a report of 16 cases and a review of the literature. *Cancer*. 1999;85:706–717.
42. Dispenzieri A, Kyle R, Lacy M, et al. POEMS syndrome: definitions and long-term outcome. *Blood*. 2003;101:2496–2506.
43. Khouri J, Nakashima M, Wong S Update on the diagnosis and treatment of POEMS (polyneuropathy, organomegaly, endocrinopathy, monoclonal gammopathy, and skin changes) syndrome: a review. *JAMA Oncol*. 2021;9:1383–1391.

44. Kuwabara S, Dispenzieri A, Arimura K, et al. Treatment for POEMS (polyneuropathy, organomegaly, endocrinopathy, M protein, and skin changes) syndrome. *Cochrane Database Syst Rev*. 2008;4:CD006828.
45. Dispenzieri A. POEMS syndrome. *Hematology Am Soc Hematol Educ Program*. 2005;1:360–367.
46. Li J, Zhang W, Jiao L, et al. Combination of melphalan and dexamethasone for patients with newly diagnosed POEMS syndrome. *Blood*. 2011;117:6445–6449.
47. Jaccard A, Royer B, Bordessoule D, et al. High dose therapy and autologous blood stem cell transplantation in POEMS syndrome. *Blood*. 2002;99:3057–3059.
48. Imai N, Taguchi J, Yagi N, et al. Relapse of polyneuropathy, organomegaly, endocrinopathy, M protein and skin changes (POEMS) syndrome without increased level of vascular endothelial growth factor following successful autologous peripheral blood stem cell transplantation. *Neuromuscul Disord*. 2009;19:363–365.
49. Dispenzieri A, Klein C, Mauermann M. Lenalidomide therapy in a patient with POEMS syndrome. *Blood*. 2007;110:1075–1076.
50. Badros A, Porter N, Zimrin A. Bevacizumab therapy for POEMS syndrome. *Blood*. 2005;106:1135.
51. Kaygusuz I, Tezcn H, Cetiner M, et al. Bortezomib: a new therapeutic option for POEMS syndrome. *Eur J Haematol*. 2010;84:175–177.
52. Dispenzieri A. How I treat POEMS syndrome. *Blood*. 2012;119:5650–5658.

56 CASE

A Woman With a Neuropathy and Symptoms of a Central Nervous System Disease

A 34-year-old woman presented initially to another center with a 4-month history of numbness of the right hemibody which developed after a fall at work. Two months later, she developed weakness in her right side, more in the leg than the arm. A year later, she experienced weakness of the left hemibody and burning sensations in the arms.

Family history and past medical history were negative. She did not smoke or drink alcohol and was on no medications.

She was examined then by a neurologist who reported decreased pain and temperature sensations in the right hemibody. Brain MRI revealed multiple areas of increased signal in the periventricular white matter of the left hemisphere consistent with multiple sclerosis (MS). She improved after 2 weeks of corticosteroid therapy and was then referred to us complaining of headache, right-sided weakness, and numbness with a burning sensation in all extremities for 3 months.

Mentation, cranial nerves, and strength were normal; there was no muscle atrophy. Reflexes were absent in the lower extremities, 1+ in the arms. She had patchy decreased sensation to vibration and pain in the right arm and leg and decreased sensation to vibration in the toes. There was no nerve hypertrophy, fasciculations, myotonia, hammertoes, or Babinski signs. Coordination was normal.

WHAT IS THE DIFFERENTIAL DIAGNOSIS?

The history and previous MRI suggest that the patient has a central demyelinating disease such as MS, which sometimes might also present with a neuropathy. It is also possible that the patient has MS and a neuropathy caused by another condition, such as diabetes or B_{12} deficiency. Other diseases with central and peripheral demyelination include rare forms of Charcot–Marie–Tooth (CMT) disease, particularly CMT type X,[1] HIV infection, metachromatic leukodystrophy, and adrenoleukodystrophy, but this usually occurs only in men. There are cases of mitochondrial encephalogastrointestinal neuropathy that can be confused with chronic inflammatory demyelinating polyradiculoneuropathy (CIDP) initially and later show central nervous system (CNS) demyelination.[2]

AN EMG TEST WAS PERFORMED

Motor Nerve Studies

Nerve and Site	Latency (ms)	Amplitude (mV)	Conduction Velocity (m/s)
Median Nerve R.	**Normal ≤ 4.2**	**Normal ≥ 6**	**Normal ≥ 50**
Wrist	**9.5**	**4.2**	–
Elbow	14.2	**3.6**	**29**
Ulnar Nerve R.	**Normal ≤ 3.6**	**Normal ≥ 8**	**Normal ≥ 50**
Wrist	**6.2**	**6.6**	–
Below elbow	12.2	**6.0**	**28**
Above elbow	16.8	**5.7**	**24**

Motor Nerve Studies—cont'd

Nerve and Site	Latency (ms)	Amplitude (mV)	Conduction Velocity (m/s)
Median Nerve L.	**Normal ≤ 4.2**	**Normal ≥ 6**	**Normal ≥ 50**
Wrist	**9.1**	**5**	–
Elbow	13.8	**5**	**47**
Ulnar Nerve L.	**Normal ≤ 3.6**	**Normal ≥ 8**	**Normal ≥ 50**
Wrist	**5.6**	**7**	–
Below elbow	11.6	**6**	**29**
Above elbow	16.2	**6**	**25**
Nerve and Site	**Latency (ms)**	**Amplitude (mV)**	**Conduction Velocity (m/s)**
Peroneal Nerve R.	**Normal ≤ 5.7**	**Normal ≥ 3**	**Normal ≥ 40**
Ankle	**11.6**	**0.2**	–
Fibular head	23.4	**0.2**	**30**
Knee	26.4	**0.2**	**33**

F-Wave and Tibial H-Reflex Studies

Nerve	Latency (ms)	Normal Latency ≤ (ms)
Median nerve R.	**NR**	30
Ulnar nerve R.	**NR**	30
Median nerve L.	**NR**	30
Ulnar nerve L.	**NR**	30
Peroneal nerve R.	**NR**	54
H-reflex R.	**NR**	34
H-reflex L.	**NR**	34

Sensory Nerve Studies

Nerve	Onset Latency (ms)	Normal Onset Latency ≤ (ms)	Peak Latency (ms)	Normal Peak Latency ≤ (ms)	Amp (μV)	Normal Amp ≥ (μV)	Conduction Velocity (m/s)	Normal Conduction Velocity ≥ (m/s)
Median nerve R.	**NR**	2.6	**NR**	3.1	**NR**	20	**NR**	50
Ulnar nerve R.	**2.8**	2.6	**3.3**	3.1	**6**	13	**43**	50
Sural nerve R.	**NR**	3.5	**NR**	4.0	**NR**	11	**NR**	40
Sural nerve L.	**NR**	3.5	**NR**	4.0	**NR**	11	**NR**	40

EMG Data

Muscle	Insrt Activity	Fibs	Pos Waves	Fasc	Amp	Dur	Poly	Pattern
Deltoid R.	None	None	None	None	**Lg**	**Inc**	None	Full
Biceps brachii R.	None	None	None	None	**Lg**	**Inc**	None	Full
Flexor carpi ulnaris R.	None	None	None	None	Norm	Norm	None	Full
First dorsal interosseous R.	None	None	None	None	**Lg**	**Inc**	None	**Red**
Tensor fasciae latae R.	None	None	None	None	**Lg**	**Inc**	None	Full
Vastus lateralis R.	None	None	None	None	**Lg**	**Inc**	None	Full
Tibialis anterior R.	None	None	None	None	**Lg**	**Inc**	None	**Red**
Gastrocnemius R.	None	None	None	None	**Lg**	**Inc**	None	Full
Tibialis anterior L.	None	None	None	None	**Lg**	**Inc**	None	**Red**
Gastrocnemius L.	None	None	None	None	Norm	Norm	None	Full

WHAT WERE THE EMG FINDINGS?

This test showed slow motor conduction velocities in arms and legs with prolonged distal motor latencies without evidence of conduction block or temporal dispersion (Fig. 56-1). There was also an absence of F-responses and H-reflexes and low-amplitude or absent SNAPs. This is characteristic of a demyelinating neuropathy, likely hereditary because of the uniform slowing.[3,4] The needle test showed no active denervation but large motor unit potentials with reduced recruitment in some muscles, indicating chronic axonal dropout with reinnervation.

These results indicated a demyelinating neuropathy. She also appeared to have MS, a diagnosis that should be confirmed. Central and peripheral demyelination also occurs in CIDP, but as this patient's neuropathy did not appear to be acquired, the possibility of CMT type 1 had to be considered.

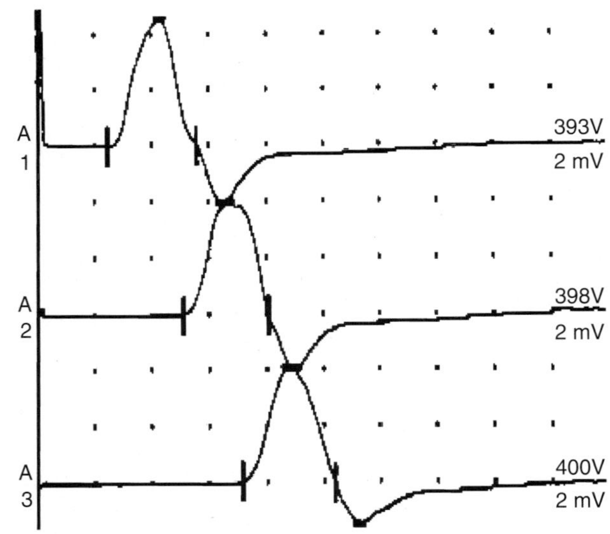

FIG. 56-1 Nerve conduction test showing uniform slowing of the ulnar nerve CMAP without changes of CMAP and without temporal dispersion.

WHAT OTHER TESTS SHOULD BE DONE?

Laboratory tests showed normal chemistry profile and a vitamin B_{12} level of 236 pg/mL (normal, 250–2200 pg/mL). Homocysteine and methylmalonic acid levels and thyroid function tests were normal. The cerebrospinal fluid studies' protein level was 68 mg/dL (normal, 15–45 mg/dL) and IgG level of 7.1 mg/dL (normal, 1.5–5.5 mg/dL), although the IgG index was 0.6 (normal, 0.3–0.7). Two oligoclonal bands were seen in the g region that were not present in serum. Glucose level was 63 mg/dL, with no cells; cultures were negative. HIV, syphilis, and Lyme serologies and antinuclear antibody titers were negative.

A repeated MRI showed an increased signal in the periventricular white matter which did not enhance with gadolinium (Fig. 56-2).

Visual-evoked potentials were normal. Brainstem auditory evoked response showed five well-formed major positive peaks present on the left side. Wave I could not be identified and wave V latency was prolonged on the right side. Median nerve somatosensory-evoked responses showed poorly identified Erb's point and P/N13 waves, and the latencies of N19 and P22 were prolonged bilaterally. These findings suggest central and peripheral demyelination.

WHAT SHOULD BE DONE NEXT?

Molecular genetic testing was done using Southern blot with pulse-field gel electrophoresis. This identified the presence of a peripheral myelin protein gene duplication characteristic of CMT type 1A.

During the next year, her right-sided body numbness was no longer present, but she still had numbness in her hands and feet with weakness in both legs. She received monthly B_{12} injections without clinical changes.

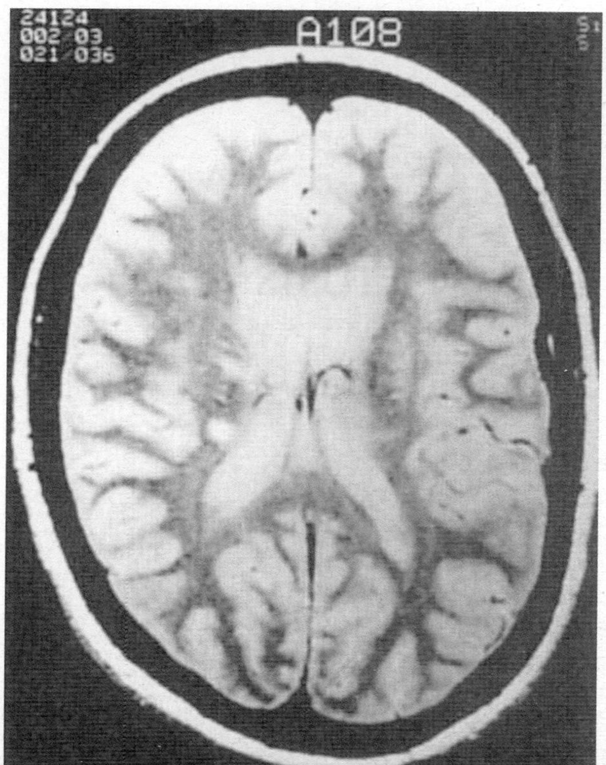

FIG. 56-2 MRI of the brain showing periventricular white matter changes, T2-weighted image.

DISCUSSION

This patient has a hereditary neuropathy of the CMT type 1A, as she had confirmed peripheral myelin protein 22 (*PMP22*) gene duplication mutation characteristic of this disease.[5–7] Based on clinical, MRI, and cerebrospinal fluid findings, she also definitively had MS. She also had mildly decreased vitamin B_{12} levels. B_{12} therapy did not alleviate her symptoms; therefore low vitamin B_{12} likely did not cause her condition.

MS is an autoimmune disease of the CNS, but patients with MS can also have peripheral nerve involvement,[8] presenting sometimes as chronic demyelinating or hypertrophic neuropathy.[9–12] Furthermore, demyelination has been found in sural nerve biopsy of some patients with MS, suggesting that a similar autoimmune mechanism affects peripheral and CNSs.[13,14] This is supported by both CNS and peripheral nervous system demyelination in guinea pigs with relapsing experimental allergic encephalitis, an animal model of MS.[15] It is also of interest that central demyelination can be seen in some cases of CIDP, suggesting common pathogenic mechanisms.[16,17]

The coexistence of MS and peripheral neuropathy in this case appears to be coincidental and not due to a disease causing both central and peripheral demyelination. The chance of the two diseases occurring simultaneously is 2.1% of the population,[7] based on their individual prevalences.[4,18] Although the probability of this occurrence is very low, it should remain a consideration in patients with this presentation.

This case demonstrates that a demyelinating peripheral neuropathy in a patient with MS is not necessarily autoimmune. Other causes, which would require different management and genetic counseling if hereditary, should be excluded.

Central demyelination can occur in CMT type X, likely not from autoimmune mechanisms but from a defect of the gap junction protein connexin 32.[1]

SUMMARY

This patient had symptoms and electrophysiologic, cerebrospinal fluid, and MRI findings diagnostic of MS. She also had a demyelinating neuropathy which proved to be CMT type 1A. The association appears to be coincidental.

IMPORTANT POINTS

- The association of peripheral and cerebral demyelination is not necessarily autoimmune.
- The presence of uniform slowing during various levels in motor conduction tests is characteristic of a familial neuropathy, such as CMT type 1A, rather than an acquired demyelinating neuropathy.

- Peripheral neuropathies can occur in MS, but when both conditions are present in one patient, other causes must be ruled out, such as vitamin deficiency and hereditary neuropathies.
- CMT type 1A is usually caused by a duplication of the *PMP22* gene in chromosome 17.

This case was reported by Almasaddi M, Bertorini TE, Seltzer WK. Demyelinating neuropathy in a patient with multiple sclerosis and genotypical HMSN-1. Neuromuscul Disord. 1998;8:27–89.

REFERENCES

1. Taylor RA, Simon EM, Marks HG, Scherer SS. The CNS phenotype of X-linked Charcot-Marie-Tooth disease: more than a peripheral problem. *Neurology*. 2003;61(11):1475–1478.
2. Bedlack RS, Vu T, Hammans S, et al. MNGIE neuropathy: five cases mimicking chronic inflammatory demyelinating polyneuropathy. *Muscle Nerve*. 2004;29(3):364–368.
3. Lewis RA, Sumner AJ. Electrodiagnostic distinctions between chronic acquired and familial demyelinative neuropathies. *Neurology*. 1982;32(6):592–596.
4. Dyck PJ, Chance P, Lebo R, Carney JA. Hereditary motor and sensory neuropathies. In: Dyck PJ, Thomas PK, Griffin JW, eds. *Peripheral Neuropathy*. Philadelphia, PA: WB Saunders; 1993:1094–1136.
5. Ionasescu VV. Charcot-Marie-Tooth neuropathies: from clinical description to molecular genetics. *Muscle Nerve*. 1995;18:267–275.
6. Roa BB, Garcia CA, Suter U, et al. Charcot-Marie-Tooth disease type 1A: association with a spontaneous point mutation in the PMP22 gene. *N Engl J Med*. 1993;329:96–101.
7. Bertorini T, Narayamaswami P, Rashed H. Charcot-Marie-Tooth disease (hereditary motor sensory neuropathies) and hereditary sensory and autonomic neuropathies. *Neurologist*. 2004;10(6):327–337.
8. Hasson J, Terry RD, Zimmerman HM. Peripheral neuropathy in multiple sclerosis. *Neurology*. 1958;8:503–510.
9. Anlar O, Tombul T, Kisli M. Peripheral sensory and motor abnormalities in patients with multiple sclerosis. *Electromyogr Clin Neurophysiol*. 2003;43(6):349–351.
10. Rosenberg NL, Bourdette D. Hypertrophic neuropathy and multiple sclerosis. *Neurology*. 1983;33:1361–1364.
11. Schoene WC, Carpenter S, Behan PO, Geschwind N. "Onion bulb" formations in the central and peripheral nervous system in association with multiple sclerosis and hypertrophic polyneuropathy. *Brain*. 1977;100:755–773.
12. Roy YI, Alexander CB, Oh SJ. Multiple sclerosis and hypertrophic demyelinating peripheral neuropathy. *Muscle Nerve*. 1983;6:312–316.
13. Pollock M, Calder C, Allpress S. Peripheral nerve abnormality in multiple sclerosis. *Ann Neurol*. 1977;2:41–48.
14. Kira J, Yamasaki R, Ogata H. Anti-neurofascin autoantibody and demyelination. *Neurochem Int*. 2019;130:104360. https://doi.org/10.1016/j.neuint.2018.12.011.
15. Madrid RE, Wisniewski HM. Peripheral nervous system pathology in relapsing experimental allergic encephalomyelitis. *J Neurocytol*. 1978;7:265–281.
16. Mendel JR, Kolkin S, Kissel JT, et al. Evidence for central nervous system demyelination in chronic inflammatory demyelinating polyradiculoneuropathy. *Neurology*. 1987;37:1291–1294.
17. Thomas PK, Walker RW, Rudge P, et al. Chronic demyelinating peripheral neuropathy associated with multifocal central nervous system demyelination. *Brain*. 1987;110:53–76.
18. Herndon RM, Rudick RA. Multiple sclerosis and related conditions. In: Joynt RJ, ed. *Clinical Neurology*. Vol. 3. Philadelphia, PA: JB Lippincott; 1993:3.

A Man With Progressive Weakness After a Gastroplasty

A 62-year-old man had gastroplasty for obesity 10 years previously. He presented with progressive weakness in his arms and legs with numbness in his feet for more than 2 months and in his hands for 1 month; he was treated with vitamin supplementation without improvement.

Past medical history included a right ulnar neuropathy at the elbow from trauma. He had a prostatic hypertrophy and a history of anemia from mild myelodysplastic syndrome, diagnosed by bone marrow aspiration, and received weekly erythropoietin infusions. He did not smoke or drink.

Mentation and cranial nerves were normal. There was symmetrical proximal leg weakness of 4/5 in the glutei and iliopsoas, 4+/5 in the quadriceps, 4/5 in the hamstrings and tibialis anterior, and 4+/5 in the peroneal and gastrocnemius. The intrinsic ulnar muscles were wasted and weak in the right hand with 3−/5; neck muscles were normal. Shoulder muscles were 5−/5 in both upper extremities; other muscles were normal. He was areflexic. Sensory examination revealed diminished vibration and position senses in the toes and decreased pinprick sensation to the mid-calf and in the right ulnar nerve distribution. There were no Babinski signs. Coordination and gait were normal. Romberg test was negative. The rest of the examination was normal.

WHAT IS THE DIFFERENTIAL DIAGNOSIS?

This patient had a motor sensory polyneuropathy. He had symmetrical areflexia and proximal and distal weakness suggestive of a demyelinating neuropathy, but the small fibers were also affected. He also had a remote ulnar neuropathy. The possibility of an autoimmune neuropathy, such as chronic inflammatory demyelinating polyradiculoneuropathy, had to be considered,[1] as did, because of his age, a distal acquired demyelinating symmetrical neuropathy, which in some persons could be associated with myelin-associated glycoprotein antibodies, but the proximal weakness was against this possibility.[2] He could also have a nutritional neuropathy associated with the bariatric surgery.[3] The cause of this could include B_{12}/folate and thiamine deficiencies. He was not diabetic. Finally, he could have a myeloproliferative disorder causing his neuropathy.

AN EMG TEST WAS PERFORMED

Motor Nerve Studies

Nerve and Site	Latency (ms)	Amplitude (mV)	Conduction Velocity (m/s)
Peroneal Nerve R.	**Normal ≤ 5.7**	**Normal ≥ 3**	**Normal ≥ 40**
Ankle	**6.2**	**1**	–
Fibular head	13.2	**1**[a]	**36**
Knee	16.6	**1**[a]	**36**
Tibial Nerve L.	**Normal ≤ 5.3**	**Normal ≥ 4**	**Normal ≥ 40**
Ankle	**5.9**	**1.2**	–
Pop. fossa	15.5	**1.2**[a]	**37**

[a]Dispersion of waveforms.

Motor Nerve Studies—cont'd

Nerve and Site	Latency (ms)	Amplitude (mV)	Conduction Velocity (m/s)
Ulnar Nerve R.	**Normal ≤ 3.6**	**Normal ≥ 8**	**Normal ≥ 50**
Wrist	3.4	**7.8**	–
Below elbow	7.7	**6.9**[b]	**48**
Above elbow	10.2	**5.3**[b]	**48**
Median Nerve R.	**Normal ≤ 4.2**	**Normal ≥ 6**	**Normal ≥ 50**
Wrist	4.2	10	–
Elbow	8.5	10	**47**

[b]Dispersion of waveforms.

F-Wave and Tibial H-Reflex Studies

Nerve	Latency (ms)	Normal Latency ≤ (ms)
Peroneal nerve R.	**55.7**	54
Tibial nerve L.	**56.8**	54
Ulnar nerve R.	**32.8**	30
Median nerve R.	**33.2**	30
H-reflex R.	**NR**	34
H-reflex L.	**NR**	34

Sensory Nerve Studies

Nerve	Onset Latency (ms)	Normal Onset Latency ≤ (ms)	Peak Latency (ms)	Normal Peak Latency ≤ (ms)	Amp (μV)	Normal Amp ≥ (μV)	Conduction Velocity (m/s)	Normal Conduction Velocity ≥ (m/s)
Sural nerve R.	**3.8**	3.5	**4.2**	4.0	**6**	11	**38**	40
Ulnar nerve R.	**2.7**	2.6	3.2	3.1	**8**	13	**49**	50
Median nerve R.	**2.7**	2.6	3.3	3.1	**15**	20	**49**	50
Ulnar dorsal cutaneous R.	**1.5**	1.7	1.9	2.2	5	13	**48**	50

EMG Data

Muscle	Insrt Activity	Fibs	Pos Waves	Fasc	Amp	Dur	Poly	Pattern
Deltoid R.	Norm	None	None	None	Norm	Norm	None	Full
Biceps brachii R.	Norm	None	None	None	Norm	Norm	None	Full
Brachioradialis R.	Norm	None	None	None	Norm	Norm	None	Full
Adductor pollicis brevis R.	Norm	None	None	None	Norm	Norm	None	Full
First dorsal interosseous R.	**Inc**	None	**1+**	None	Norm	Norm	None	**Red**
Tensor fasciae latae R.	Norm	None	None	None	Norm	Norm	None	Full
Vastus lateralis R.	Norm	None	None	None	Norm	Norm	None	Full
Tibialis anterior R.	**Inc**	None	**1+**	None	Norm	Norm	None	**Red**
Gastrocnemius R.	**Inc**	None	None	None	Norm	Norm	None	**Red**
Tibialis anterior L.	**Inc**	None	None	None	Norm	Norm	None	**Red**
Gastrocnemius L.	**Inc**	None	**1+**	None	Norm	Norm	None	**Red**

WHAT WERE THE EMG FINDINGS?

The test showed a mild demyelinating neuropathy affecting motor and sensory axons, with some dispersion of the CMAPs, although without evidence of conduction blocks. H-reflexes were absent, and F-responses were prolonged. The peroneal and ulnar CMAPs had low amplitude and mildly prolonged latencies. There was also evidence of axonal degeneration because of the denervation potentials in the legs; he also appeared to have an old ulnar neuropathy at the elbow.

WHAT SHOULD BE DONE NEXT?

White blood count was 3700/mm^3; platelets, hematocrit, and hemoglobin were normal; serum iron and chemistry profile were normal; mean corpuscular volume was 100 fL (normal, 80–100 fL); fluorescent antinuclear antibodies and folate were normal; B_{12} was 1450 pg/mL (normal, >211 pg/mL); homocysteine was 7.3 nmol/L (normal, 0–13 nmol/L) and methylmalonic acid was 0.08 μmol/L (normal, <41 mmol/L). Myelin-associated glycoprotein antibody titers were not elevated, and immunoelectrophoresis was normal. Hepatitis and HIV antibodies were negative. Anti-SSA and SSB (Sjögren syndrome antibodies) were normal; α-tocopherol was 10 mg/L (normal, 2.4–20 mg/L); gamma-tocopherol was 0.7 mg/L (normal, 0.2–4.6 mg/L); and vitamin B_1 was 4.4 mg/dL (normal, 0.8–2.8 mg/dL).

The patient underwent a lumbar puncture which showed spinal fluid of 56 mg/dL (normal, <45 mg/dL) and four lymphocytes.

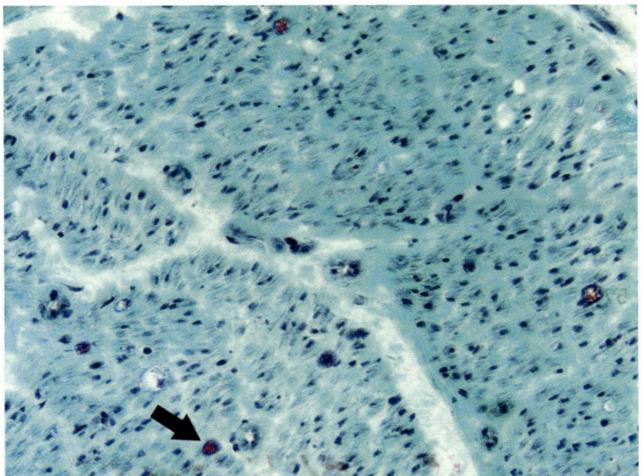

FIG. 57-1 Sural nerve biopsy showing markedly decreased number of myelinated axons (*arrow*) (modified trichrome stain, ×400).

Sural nerve biopsy showed a markedly decreased number of myelinated axons (Fig. 57-1). There was also evidence of subperineural edema (Fig. 57-2). Teased nerve preparation showed axonal degeneration with some segmental demyelination (Fig. 57-3). Frequent lymphocytes were present in the interstitial area (Fig. 57-4).

WHAT SHOULD BE DONE NEXT?

Because the patient did not improve after aggressive parenteral vitamin therapy he was given prednisone 1 mg/kg and IgG infusions, with marked improvement.

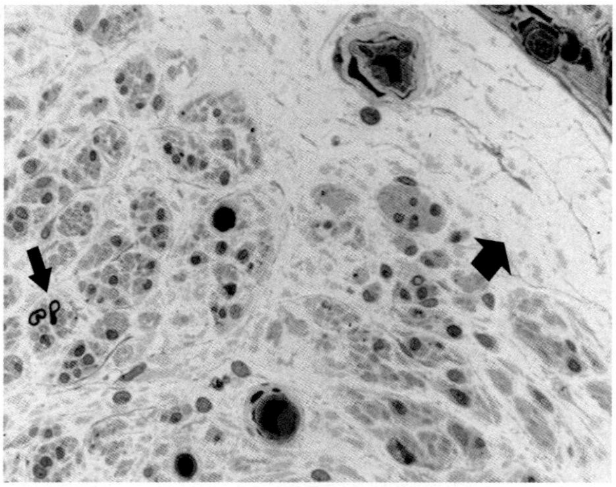

FIG. 57-2 Osmicated section of sural nerve, plastic-embedded stained with toluidine blue; notice interstitial and subperineural edema (*thick arrow*) and only a few myelinated axons (*arrow*) (×400).

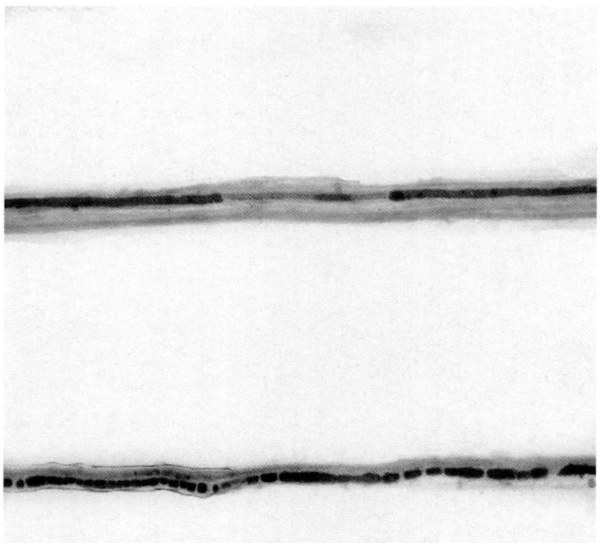

FIG. 57-3 Teased nerve preparation showing an axon with segmental demyelination (*top*) and one with axonal degeneration (*bottom*) (×100).

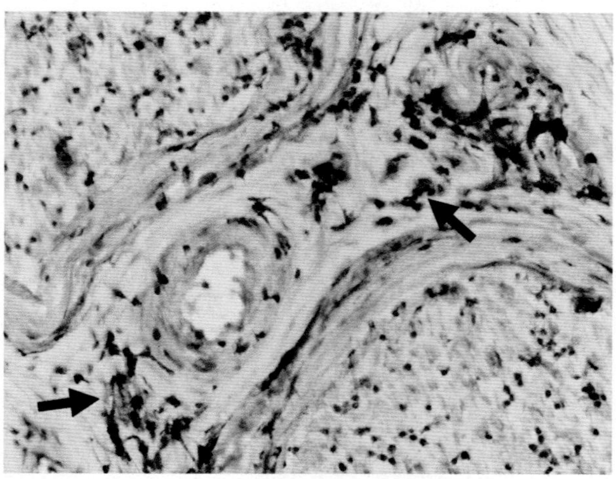

FIG. 57-4 Immunoperoxidase stain showing CD45 positive cells in the interstitial and perivascular areas (*arrows*) (×200).

DISCUSSION

This patient had bariatric surgery for obesity and developed a peripheral neuropathy, demonstrated on EMG and biopsy findings to be demyelinating with axonal degeneration and with evidence of inflammation. He did not respond to vitamin therapy.

Bariatric surgery has many complications, including those related to surgery, such as infections, pneumonia, and bleeding. Neurologic complications include peripheral neuropathy and polyradiculoneuropathy, meralgia paresthetica, and other mononeuropathies; some patients develop proximal weakness with a myotonic syndrome. Optic neuropathy, myelopathy, and Wernicke–Korsakoff psychosis also occur[4–11].

The peripheral neuropathy frequently improves with vitamin supplementation.[12] The myelopathy could develop after several years and is associated with decreased B_{12} or copper levels.[11] We recently observed a patient with Wernicke–Korsakoff psychosis who improved with only intravenous vitamin supplementation, while another patient with profound axonal neuropathy who did not respond to this therapy improved only after reoperation to correct the bypass.

Thaisetthawatkul and colleagues[13] noticed that peripheral neuropathy occurred more frequently in patients undergoing bariatric surgery than in those undergoing routine abdominal surgery. They reported that bariatric surgery patients frequently had a predominantly sensory neuropathy. Some had elevated spinal fluid protein with electrophysiologic evidence of demyelination, while some had a mononeuropathy and others, radiculoplexoneuropathy; pathologically, the neuropathy was predominantly axonal with perivascular inflammatory cells. In one case these were prominent in the endoneurium and epineurium.

This patient had inflammatory cells in the perineural and perivascular area with endomysial edema, axonal degeneration, and demyelinating features on nerve biopsy without clear vasculitis. An autoimmune etiology along with malnutrition was postulated as a cause of his neuropathy. He responded well to immunotherapy.

It is difficult to determine in what way autoimmune disorder is triggered by malnutrition or by gastroplasty. Similarly to this presentation, patients with diabetes can also develop a microvasculitic neuropathy for which the etiology is not clear.[14,15]

It was concluded that, whereas some patients with complications from bariatric surgery improve with intravenous vitamin therapy, those with an autoimmune process respond to immunotherapy.

SUMMARY

This patient presented with a peripheral neuropathy after bariatric surgery. He did not respond to vitamin therapy and was assumed to be autoimmune. He respond with the addition of prednisone and gamma globulin infusions.

IMPORTANT POINTS

- Bariatric surgery is associated with several neurologic complications which include a predominantly sensory neuropathy, mononeuropathy, myelopathy, and Wernicke–Korsakoff syndrome.

- The peripheral neuropathy after bariatric surgery usually responds to vitamin therapy.
- Some patients might develop an autoimmune neuropathy that may respond to immunotherapy.

REFERENCES

1. Bertorini TE, Narayanaswami P. Autoimmune neuropathies. *Compr Ther.* 2003;29(4):194–209.
2. Chassande B, Leger JM, Younes-Chennoufi AB, et al. Peripheral neuropathy associated with IgM monoclonal gammopathy: correlations between M-protein antibody activity and clinical/electrophysiological features in 40 cases. *Muscle Nerve.* 1998; 21(1):55–62.
3. Harwood SC, Chodoroff G, Ellenberg MR. Gastric partitioning complicated by peripheral neuropathy with lumbosacral plexopathy. *Arch Phys Med Rehabil.* 1987;68:310–312.
4. Berger JR. The neurological complications of bariatric surgery. *Arch Neurol.* 2004;61(8):1185–1189.
5. Koffman BM, Greenfield LJ, Ali II, Pirzada NA. Neurological complications after surgery for obesity. *Muscle Nerve.* 2006;33: 166–176.
6. Abarbanel JM, Berginer VM, Osimani A, et al. Neurologic complications after gastric restriction surgery for morbid obesity. *Neurology.* 1987;37:196–200.
7. Feit H, Glasberg M, Ireton C, et al. Peripheral neuropathy and starvation after gastric partitioning for morbid obesity. *Ann Intern Med.* 1982;96:453–455.
8. Maryniak O. Severe peripheral neuropathy following gastric bypass surgery for morbid obesity. *Can Med Assoc J.* 1984;131: 119–120.
9. MacGregor AM, Thoburn EK. Meralgia paresthetica following bariatric surgery. *Obes Surg.* 1999;9:364–368.
10. Cruz-Martinez A, Arpa J, Palau F. Peroneal neuropathy after weight loss. *J Peripher Nerv Syst.* 2000;5:101–105.
11. Juhasz-Pocsine K, Rudnicki SA, Archer RL, Harik SI. Neurological complications of gastric bypass surgery for morbid obesity. *Neurology.* 2007;68(21):1843–1850.
12. Bertorini TE, Finder JD, Bassam B. Perioperative management of patients with neuromuscular disorders. In: Bertorini TE, ed. *Neuromuscular Disorders: Treatment and Management.* Amsterdam, Netherlands: Elsevier; 2022:206–224. 2nd ed. Chapter 10.
13. Thaisetthawatkul P, Collazo-Clavell ML, Sarr MG, et al. A controlled study of peripheral neuropathy after bariatric surgery. *Neurology.* 2004;63(8):1462–1470.
14. Dyck PJB, Norell JE, Dyck PJ. Non-diabetic lumbosacral radiculoplexus neuropathy: natural history, outcome and comparison with the diabetic variety. *Brain.* 2001;124:1197–1207.
15. Dyck PJB, Norell JE, Dyck PJ. Microvasculitis and ischemia in diabetic lumbosacral radiculoplexus neuropathy. *Neurology.* 1999; 53:2113–2121.

58 CASE

A Diabetic Woman With Unilateral Proximal Leg Weakness and Pain

A 70-year-old woman with type II diabetes managed with oral agents had a 3-week history of weakness in the left lower extremity which developed a week after gallbladder surgery. She also had diffuse thigh pain, but no back pain, and was treated with physical therapy without improvement. The condition stabilized, but she continued to have some difficulty walking and had persistent discomfort.

Two months later, she developed progressive pain and weakness in the right lower extremity, and she had some occasional burning paresthesias in both feet. She was unable to walk for 2 weeks.

Past medical history included hypothyroidism treated with thyroid replacement and an L5 laminectomy 10 years previously for chronic back pain, radiating to the right leg; this pain disappeared after surgery.

Neurological examination showed normal mentation and cranial nerves. Upper extremity examination revealed normal strength, reflexes, and sensation bilaterally. She had weakness in the right hip flexors of 3+/5 and knee extensor of 2/5; thigh adductors were 3/5; and other muscles of the hip and leg were normal. In the left lower extremity, hip flexion and knee extension were 4/5 and knee flexion was normal; she also had 3+/5 weakness in adductors. Distal muscles were normal. Reflexes were normal in the upper extremities, absent in the knees, and trace at the ankles. Both adductor reflexes were absent. There were no Babinski signs. Straight leg raising and femoral stretch were negative. She had decreased vibration sense and two-point discrimination in the toes and decreased pain sensation up to the mid-calf level. She also had decreased pain in the anterior and lateral right thigh (Fig. 58-1). Coordination was normal and the rest of the examination was normal.

WHAT IS THE MOST LIKELY DIAGNOSIS FOR THIS PATIENT?

This patient had diabetes and a peripheral neuropathy. She also had prominent weakness in muscles innervated by L2–L4 roots bilaterally, with a mild distal sensory deficit that corresponds to a peripheral neuropathy, and had decreased pain sensation on the left thigh. The differential diagnosis included a lumbar canal disease such as disk disorder, but the lack of back pain is against this diagnosis. A diabetic lumbosacral radiculoplexus neuropathy, as well as a systemic vasculitis, are considerations. Plexopathy from a tumor should be ruled out. The motor deficit, including muscles innervated not only by the femoral nerve but also by the obturator nerve, is against a femoral neuropathy.

WHAT WILL BE THE NEXT DIAGNOSTIC TESTS?

Basic blood work was normal, except for an elevated glycosylated hemoglobin of 9.2 ml/dl (normal, <6.4 mm/dL) and blood sugar of 240 mg/dL (normal, 65–120 mg/dL). Erythrocyte sedimentation rate and antineutrophil cytoplasmic antibody and fluorescent antinuclear antibody titers were normal.

AN EMG TEST WAS PERFORMED

Motor Nerve Studies

Nerve and Site	Latency (ms)	Amplitude (mV)	Conduction Velocity (m/s)
Peroneal Nerve R.	**Normal ≤ 5.7**	**Normal ≥ 3**	**Normal ≥ 40**
Ankle	5.5	5	–
Fibular head	13.2	5	**34**
Knee	15.1	5	**39**
Tibial Nerve L.	**Normal ≤ 5.3**	**Normal ≥ 4**	**Normal ≥ 40**
Ankle	5.0	4	–
Pop. fossa	15.0	4	**37**

Nerve and Site	Latency (ms)	Amplitude (mV)	Conduction Velocity (m/s)
Ulnar Nerve R.	**Normal ≤ 3.6**	**Normal ≥ 8**	**Normal ≥ 50**
Wrist	3.4	19	–
Below elbow	7.1	18	50
Above elbow	9.2	17	57

F-Wave and Tibial H-Reflex Studies

Nerve	Latency (ms)	Normal Latency ≤ (ms)
Peroneal nerve R.	48.3	54
Tibial nerve L.	52.2	54
Ulnar nerve R.	28.2	30
H-reflex R.	**NR**	34
H-reflex L.	**NR**	34

Sensory Nerve Studies

Nerve	Onset Latency (ms)	Normal Onset Latency ≤ (ms)	Peak Latency (ms)	Normal Peak Latency ≤ (ms)	Amp (μV)	Normal Amp ≥ (μV)	Conduction Velocity (m/s)	Normal Conduction Velocity ≥ (m/s)
Sural nerve R.	3.3	3.5	3.8	4.0	**10**	11	42	40
Saphenous nerve R.	**NR**	2.2	**NR**	2.7	**NR**	8	**NR**	40
Superficial peroneal R.	**NR**	3.5	**NR**	4.0	**NR**	8–11	**NR**	40
Ulnar nerve R.	2.3	2.6	2.8	3.1	13	13	52	50

Sympathetic Skin Response

R. hand—**absent**
R. foot—**absent**

EMG Data

Muscle	Insrt Activity	Fibs	Pos Waves	Fasc	Amp	Dur	Poly	Pattern
Lumbar paraspinal R.	**Inc**	**1+**	**1+**	None	Norm	Norm	None	Full
Iliopsoas R.	**Inc**	**2+**	**2+**	None	Norm	Norm	**Few**	**Red**
Tensor fasciae latae R.	**Inc**	**2+**	**2+**	None	Norm	Norm	**Few**	**Red**
Gluteus medius R.	Norm	None	None	None	Norm	Norm	**Few**	Full
Adductor longus R.	**Inc**	**2+**	**2+**	None	Norm	Norm	**Few**	**Red**
Vastus lateralis R.	**Inc**	**2+**	**2+**	None	Norm	Norm	**Few**	**Red**
Tibialis anterior R.	Norm	None	None	None	Norm	Norm	**Few**	**Red**
Peroneus longus R.	Norm	None	None	None	Norm	Norm	**Few**	**Red**
Gastrocnemius R.	Norm	None	None	None	Norm	Norm	**Few**	Full
First dorsal interosseus R.	Norm	None	None	None	Norm	Norm	**Few**	Full
Lumbar paraspinal L.	Norm	None	None	None	Norm	Norm	**Few**	Full
Adductor longus L.	**Inc**	**2+**	**2+**	None	Norm	Norm	**Few**	**Red**
Vastus lateralis L.	**Inc**	**2+**	**2+**	None	Norm	Norm	**Few**	Full
Tibialis anterior L.	Norm	None	None	None	Norm	Norm	**Few**	**Red**
Peroneus longus L.	Norm	None	None	None	Norm	Norm	None	**Red**
Gastrocnemius L.	Norm	None	None	None	Norm	Norm	None	Full

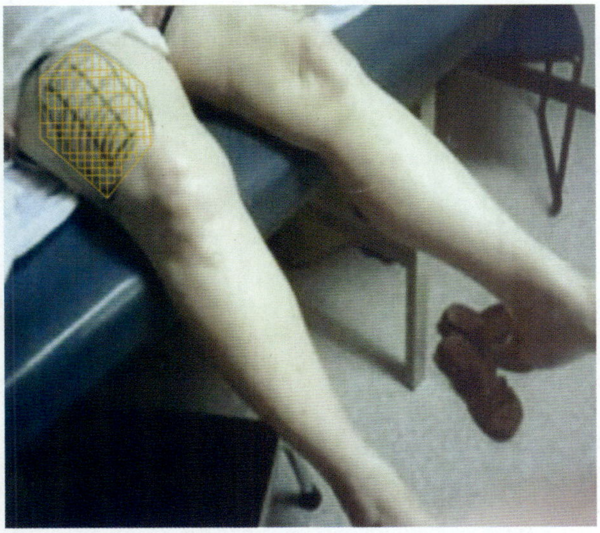

FIG. 58-1 Patient showing weakness of both knee extensors, worse on the right, and decreased sensation in shadowed area on the right thigh.

WHAT WERE THE EMG FINDINGS?

This test indicated a peripheral polyneuropathy with mildly slow motor nerve conduction velocities with normal CMAP amplitudes and distal latencies; there were no detectable superficial peroneal and saphenous nerve SNAPs, and she had a slightly low-amplitude sural SNAP. H-reflexes were absent, but F-responses were normal. She had denervation potentials with decreased motor unit recruitment in the L2–L5 innervated muscles in both legs and right paraspinal muscles and without denervation in the S1 innervated muscles and left lumbar paraspinals.

It was concluded that she had a polyneuropathy, likely from diabetes, and possibly a superimposed diabetic lumbosacral radiculoplexus neuropathy, bilaterally.

WHAT WOULD ONE DO NEXT?

An MRI of the spine was unremarkable. Lumbar puncture revealed an elevated protein of 81 mg/dL (normal, <40 mg/dL), but otherwise was normal.

A muscle and nerve biopsy to look for inflammation or vasculitis was considered but not done. She was diagnosed with a diabetic lumbosacral radiculoplexus neuropathy. It was opted to use corticosteroids, incorporating careful glucose monitoring with sliding-scale insulin therapy. This produced significant improvement, and the patient was soon able to ambulate; the pain markedly decreased.

WHAT IS DIABETIC LUMBOSACRAL RADICULOPLEXUS NEUROPATHY?

This form of neuropathy was initially described by Bruns,[1] but Garland and Taverner later reported it as a distinct entity[2] and termed the disease *diabetic amyotrophy*.[3] Other used names include diabetic femoral neuropathy,[4,5] proximal diabetic neuropathy,[6] femoral sciatic neuropathy,[7] diabetic polyradiculopathy,[8] the Bruns–Garland syndrome,[9–11] and diabetic polyradiculoneuropathy. These patients usually have more proximal muscle weakness in addition to a polyneuropathy.

The disease occurs in diabetics of 50 years of age or older, with symptoms such as anorexia, weight loss, and thigh pain, with mild-to-severe hip and thigh muscle weakness.[8–13] Patients might not have sensory deficits except for the characteristic findings of a polyneuropathy. A mild sensory loss, or hyperesthesias, in the thigh is seen in half of the cases.[8] The opposite leg can be affected during the same episode or later, even during recovery.[9] These symptoms can progress over days or months, but a symmetrical slowly progressive form has also been reported.[11] Most patients have elevated spinal fluid protein.[14,15]

In patients suspected of diabetic amyotrophy, other conditions, such as systemic vasculitis, demyelinating neuropathy, lumbar canal disease, and tumors involving the plexus, should be considered in the differential diagnosis. Motor neuron disease is unlikely because of the rapid onset and the pain.

This form of diabetic neuropathy can also occur in the upper extremities and is caused by a vasculopathy as multiple microinfarcts have been observed in peripheral nerves.[16] In a report of patients having painful lumbosacral radiculoplexopathy with elevated erythrocyte sedimentation rate, half were diabetic. Nerve biopsies showed axonal degeneration, and those with diabetes had evidence of a vasculopathy[17] with inflammatory infiltrates in the cutaneous nerves of the thigh.[17] Some patients with this condition also have evidence of a vasculitis.[18–21] A similar painful lumbosacral radiculoplexopathy has also been reported in nondiabetics.[22,23]

WHAT IS THE TREATMENT OF DIABETIC RADICULOPLEXUS NEUROPATHY?

Some patients improve spontaneously with good control of diabetes, and intravenous immunoglobulin infusions have been reported to be effective.[9,12,18] Others have reported dramatic response to corticosteroids,[19] but as the natural history frequently is one of slow improvements, it is hard to conclude definitively that the response is from the immunotherapy. Kifoyle and colleagues, however, in a retrospective study, compared the natural history of the disease in a group of patients treated with immunosuppressants and found that these patients had faster improvement.[24]

SUMMARY

This woman with type II diabetes had evidence of a peripheral neuropathy and a fairly rapid onset of weakness in the left lower extremity and later in the right lower extremity. She had a normal MRI of the spine, and an EMG showed a peripheral neuropathy and denervation, mainly in the muscles innervated by the upper lumbosacral roots and plexus. She was diagnosed with diabetic lumbosacral radiculoplexus neuropathy and treated with steroids with excellent response.

IMPORTANT POINTS

- Diabetic radiculoplexus neuropathy, or diabetic amyotrophy, manifests with unilateral and sometimes bilateral proximal muscle weakness and pain.
- Diabetic amyotrophy is believed to be caused by a vasculopathy, with evidence of inflammation in nerves suggesting an autoimmune etiology.
- EMG in a diabetic amyotrophy shows signs of denervation in the proximal muscles.
- Patients with a proximal diabetic neuropathy that is progressing should be treated with immunotherapy.

REFERENCES

1. Bruns L. Brunsh Veblr neuritscine Ldhmum gen bern diabetesmellitus. *Berl Kin Wochenschr*. 1890;27:509–515.
2. Garland H, Taverner D. Diabetic myelopathy. *Br Med J*. 1953;1:1405–1408.
3. Garland H. Diabetic amyotrophy. *Br Med J*. 1955;2:1287–1290.
4. Goodman LJ. Femoral neuropathy in relation to diabetes mellitus: report of 17 cases. *Diabetes*. 1954;3:266–273.
5. Coppack SW, Watkins PJ. The natural history of diabetic femoral neuropathy. *QJ Med*. 1991;79:307–313.
6. Asbury AK. Proximal diabetic neuropathy. *Ann Neurol*. 1977;2:179–180.
7. Gydell K, Skanse B. A rare type of femoral-sciatic neuropathy in diabetes mellitus. *Acta Med Scand*. 1956;155:463–468.
8. Bastron JA, Thomas JE. Diabetic polyradiculopathy: clinical and electromyographic findings in 105 patients. *Mayo Clin Proc*. 1981;56:725–732.
9. Barohn RJ, Sahenk Z, Warmolts JR, Mendell JR. The Bruns-Garland syndrome (diabetic amyotrophy): revisited 100 years later. *Arch Neurol*. 1991;48:1130–1135.
10. Pasnoor M, Dimachkie MM, Barohn RJ. Diabetic neuropathy. Part 2: Proximal and asymmetric phenotypes. *Neurol Clin*. 2013;31(2):447–462.
11. Diaz LA, Gupta V. Diabetic amyotrophy. In: *StatPearls [Internet]*. Treasure Island, FL: StatPearls Publishing; 2022. Last updated January 5, 2022.
12. Chokroverty S, Reyes MG, Rubino FA, et al. The syndrome of diabetic amyotrophy. *Ann Neurol*. 1977;2:181–194.
13. Locke S, Lawrence DG, Legg MA. Diabetic amyotrophy. *Am J Med*. 1963;35:775–785.

14. Leedman PJ, Davis S, Harrison LC. Diabetic amyotrophy: reassessment of the clinical spectrum. *Aust NZ J Med.* 1988;18: 768–773.
15. Pascoe MK, Low PA, Windebank AJ, Litchy WJ. Subacute diabetic proximal neuropathy. *Mayo Clin Proc.* 1997;72:1123–1132.
16. Raff MC, Sangalang V, Asbury AK. Ischemic mononeuropathy multiplex associated with diabetes mellitus. *Arch Neurol.* 1968; 18:487–499.
17. Said G, Goulon-Goeau C, Lacroix C, Moulonguet A. Nerve biopsy findings in different patterns of proximal diabetic neuropathy. *Ann Neurol.* 1994;35:559–569.
18. Kelkar P, Masood M, Parry GJ. Distinctive pathologic findings in proximal diabetic neuropathy (diabetic amyotrophy). *Neurology.* 2000;55:83–88.
19. Younger DS, Rosoklija G, Hays AP, et al. Diabetic peripheral neuropathy: a clinicopathologic and immunohistochemical analysis of sural nerve biopsies. *Muscle Nerve.* 1996;19:722–727.
20. Said G, Elgrably F, Lacroix C, et al. Painful proximal diabetic neuropathy: inflammatory nerve lesions and spontaneous favorable outcome. *Ann Neurol.* 1997;41:762–770.
21. Bradley WG, Chad D, Verghese JP, et al. Painful lumbosacral plexopathy with an elevated erythrocyte sedimentation rate: a treatable inflammatory syndrome. *Ann Neurol.* 1984;15: 457–464.
22. Said G, Thomas PK. Proximal diabetic neuropathy. In: Dyck PJ, Thomas PK, eds. *Diabetic Neuropathy.* 2nd ed. Philadelphia, PA: WB Saunders; 1999:474–480.
23. Hinchey JA, Preston DC, Logigian EL. Idiopathic lumbosacral neuropathy: a cause of persistent leg pain. *Muscle Nerve.* 1996;19(11):1484–1486.
24. Kifoyle D, Kelkar P, Parry GJ. Pulsed methylprednisolone is a safe and effective treatment for diabetic amyotrophy. *J Clin Neuromusc Dis.* 2003;4:168–170.

59 CASE

A Diabetic Man With Bilateral Arm Weakness

A 47-year-old left-handed diabetic man on oral antidiabetics developed pain in the right elbow down to the forearm. Two days later, he had numbness over the posterior aspect of the right forearm and in the first three digits of the right hand that became weak, and later he could not move his left wrist. He then developed weakness in both elbows and the shoulders. He also had numbness in both feet. He was seen by his local doctor, who performed a cervical spine MRI that was normal.

Past medical history was unremarkable. He did not drink alcohol or smoke and had not been exposed to drugs. Family history was noncontributory.

General physical examination, mentation, and cranial nerves were normal. There was wasting and weakness in both trapezii and right deltoids and biceps, with weakness of the triceps and intrinsic muscles bilaterally, more on the left than on the right with severe weakness of the wrist extensors/flexors worse on the left (Fig. 59-1). He had winging of the scapula more prominent on the right than on the left. Hand muscles were also weak. There were no fasciculations or myotonia. Strength in the lower extremities was normal. There was only a mild glove and stocking sensory deficit to all modalities to the midforearm and midleg. This was out of proportion to the weakness. There were no Babinski signs, and coordination and gait were normal.

WHAT IS THE DIFFERENTIAL DIAGNOSIS?

This patient's presentation of proximal and distal weakness of the arms could suggest a motor neuron disorder, but the sensory deficits, pain, and abrupt onset are against this diagnosis. Cervical spine diseases like spondylosis, ruptured disk, or tumor are a good possibility, but the previous normal MRI is against these. A bilateral brachial plexopathy is another consideration.

Due to the step-wise accumulation of deficits, he appeared to have a mononeuritis multiplex involving the upper extremities. This could be secondary to diabetes or a systemic vasculitis associated with a connective tissue disorder, or he could have nonsystemic vasculitis of the peripheral nerves. Other considerations are Lyme disease and HIV.

WHAT NEEDS TO BE DONE?

Erythrocyte sedimentation rate and a complete metabolic panel were normal, except for an elevated glucose of 242 mg/dL (normal, <110 mg/dL) and glycosylated hemoglobin of 8% (normal, <6%). Immunoelectrophoresis, fluorescent antinuclear antibody, antineutrophil cytoplasmic antibody, cryoglobulins, hepatitis profile, angiotensin-converting enzyme, Lyme serology, and HIV tests were all negative. Chest x-ray was normal.

AN EMG TEST WAS PERFORMED

Motor Nerve Studies

Nerve and Site	Latency (ms)	Amplitude (mV)	Conduction Velocity (m/s)
Peroneal Nerve R.	**Normal ≤ 5.7**	**Normal ≥ 3**	**Normal ≥ 40**
Ankle	5.4	**0.5**	–
Fibular head	21.2	**0.3**	**22**
Knee	23.2	**0.3**	**38**
Nerve and Site	**Latency (ms)**	**Amplitude (mV)**	**Conduction Velocity (m/s)**
Tibial Nerve L.	**Normal ≤ 5.3**	**Normal ≥ 4**	**Normal ≥ 40**
Ankle	**NR**	**NR**	–
Pop. fossa	**NR**	**NR**	**NR**
Nerve and Site	**Latency (ms)**	**Amplitude (mV)**	**Conduction Velocity (m/s)**
Median Nerve R.	**Normal ≤ 4.2**	**Normal ≥ 6**	**Normal ≥ 50**
Wrist	**6.0**	**0.2**	–
Elbow	**NR**	**NR**	**NR**
Ulnar Nerve R.	**Normal ≤ 3.6**	**Normal ≥ 8**	**Normal ≥ 50**
Wrist	**3.9**	**5**	–
Below elbow	11.2	**4**	**36**
Above elbow	14.9	**4**	**32**
Axilla	18.0	**4**	**45**

Side-by-Side Comparison

Nerve	Latency (ms)	Normal Latency ≤ (ms)	Amplitude (mV)
Accessory nerve L.	3.0	3.0	14
Accessory nerve R.	**4.2**	3.0	10

F-Wave and Tibial H-Reflex Studies

Nerve	Latency (ms)	Normal Latency ≤ (ms)
Peroneal nerve R.	**NR**	54
Median nerve R.	**NR**	30
Ulnar nerve R.	**35.7**	30
H-reflex R.	**44.9**	34
H-reflex L.	**43.7**	34

Sensory Nerve Studies

Nerve	Onset Latency (ms)	Normal Onset Latency ≤ (ms)	Peak Latency (ms)	Normal Peak Latency ≤ (ms)	Amp (μV)	Normal Amp ≥ (μV)	Conduction Velocity (m/s)	Normal Conduction Velocity ≥ (m/s)
Sural nerve R.	**NR**	3.5	**NR**	4.0	**NR**	11	**NR**	40
Median nerve R.	**NR**	2.6	**NR**	3.1	**NR**	20	**NR**	50
Ulnar nerve R.	**3.2**	2.6	**3.7**	3.1	**3**	13	**38**	50

EMG Data

Muscle	Insrt Activity	Fibs	Pos Waves	Fasc	Amp	Dur	Poly	Pattern
Cervical paraspinals L.	**CRD**	None	None	None	Norm	Norm	None	Full
Rhomboids L.	**Inc**	**2+**	**2+**	None	Norm	Norm	**Few**	Full
Supraspinatus L.	Norm	None	None	None	Norm	Norm	None	Full
Deltoid L.	Norm	None	None	None	**Lg**	**Inc**	None	Full
Biceps brachii L.	Norm	None	None	None	Norm	Norm	None	Full
Flexor carpi radialis L.	**Inc**	**3+**	**3+**	None	Norm	Norm	**Few**	**Red**
Triceps L.	**Inc**	**3+**	**3+**	None	–	–	–	**Absent**
Extensor indicis proprius L.	**Inc**	**3+**	**3+**	None	–	–	–	**Absent**
Brachioradialis L.	**Inc**	**3+**	**3+**	None	–	–	–	**Absent**
First dorsal interosseous L.	**Inc**	**2+**	**2+**	None	**Lg**	**Inc**	None	**Red**
Deltoid R.	**Inc**	**2+**	**2+**	None	**Lg**	**Inc**	**Few**	Full
Biceps brachii R.	Norm	None	None	None	Norm	Norm	None	**Red**
Brachioradialis R.	**Inc**	**2+**	**2+**	None	Norm	Norm	**Few**	**Red**
Flexor carpi radialis R.	**Inc**	**3+**	**3+**	None	Norm	Norm	**Many**	**Red**
Extensor digitorum communis R.	**Inc**	**2+**	**2+**	None	**Lg**	**Inc**	None	**Single unit**
First dorsal interosseus R.	**Inc**	None	**1+**	None	Norm	Norm	**Many**	Full
Vastus lateralis R.	Norm	None	None	None	**Lg**	**Inc**	**Many**	**Red**
Tibialis anterior R.	Norm	None	None	None	**Lg**	**Inc**	None	**Red**
Gastrocnemius R.	Norm	None	None	None	**Lg**	**Inc**	None	**Red**

WHAT WERE THE EMG FINDINGS?

This test showed low-amplitude CMAPs in multiple nerves; no response was obtained in some. The right ulnar nerve conduction velocity was slow with only mildly decreased CMAP amplitude; these findings indicated that there was axonal degeneration and demyelination. SNAPs were absent or of very low amplitude, which could be caused by either axonal degeneration or demyelination from severe temporal dispersion. The F-responses were prolonged or absent. The tibial H-reflexes were prolonged.

On the needle test, there were scattered large motor unit potentials and no denervation potentials in the lower extremities. In the upper extremities, there was diffuse denervation in muscles innervated by not only the median, radial, ulnar, and axillary nerves but also the rhomboids, and there were complex repetitive discharges in the cervical paraspinals. These findings indicate a polyradiculoneuropathy affecting mainly the upper extremities and a diffuse polyneuropathy, likely from diabetes.

A repeated MRI of the neck and brachial plexus, with and without contrast studying for swelling, edema, or infiltrates, was negative.

A quadriceps muscle biopsy showed atrophic angular fibers and duplication of the basal lamina of vessels without vasculitis.

A sural nerve biopsy showed a decreased number of myelinated fibers with some evidence of demyelination and axonal degeneration. There were also flattened unmyelinated axons. There was no inflammation or a focal decrease in the number of myelinated fibers to suggest vasculitis; there was duplication of the basal lamina as seen in diabetes.

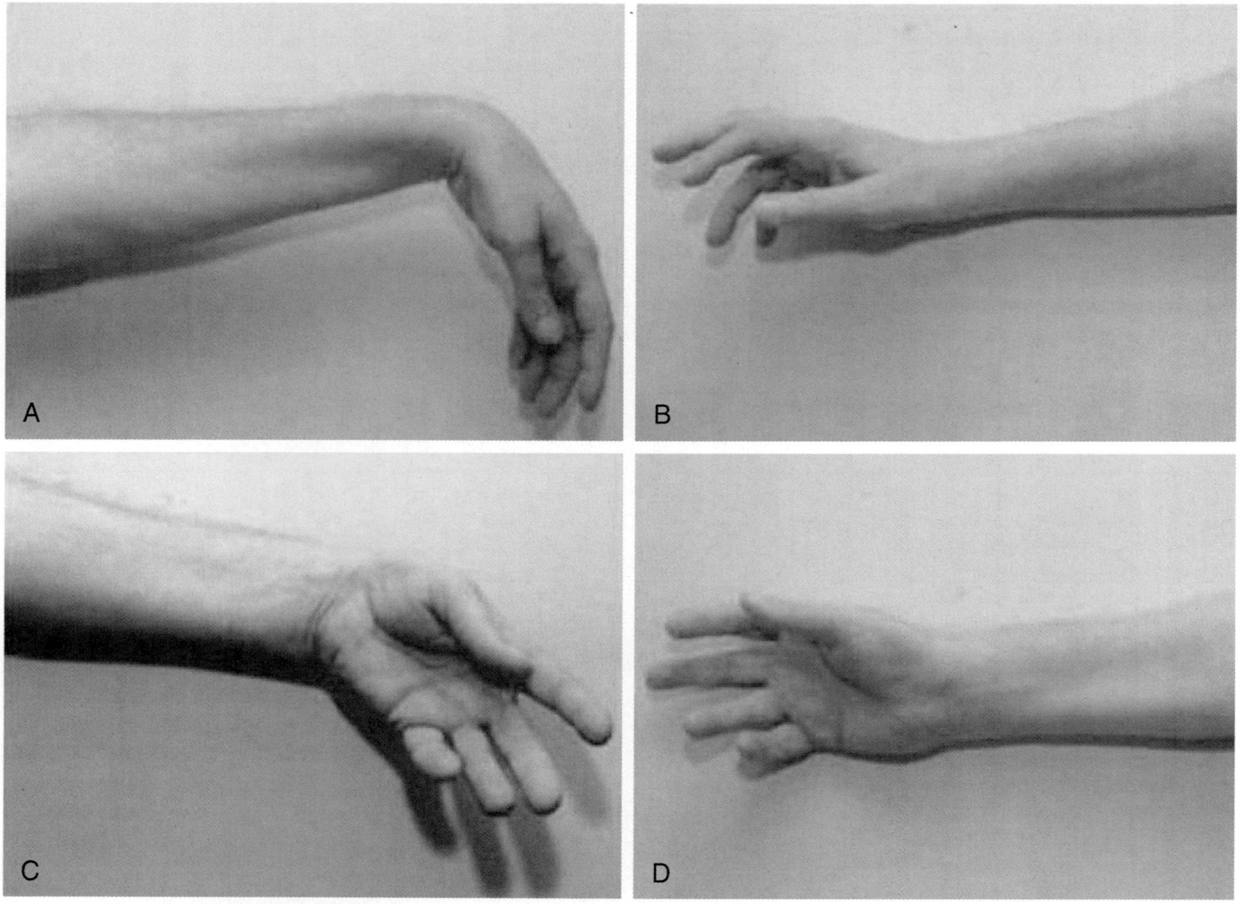

FIG. 59-1 A, Wrist drop in the left. **B**, Weakness of the finger extensors in the right. **C and D**, The patient showing difficulty flexing the digits of both hands.

Spinal fluid protein was 67 mg/dL (normal, <40 mg/dL), no cells, and normal IgG. Serum creatine kinase, immunofixation and thyroid profile, C3 and C4 complement, and rapid plasma reagin tests were all negative.

The patient was treated with cyclophosphamide 150 g daily and IgG infusions. He stabilized and improved slowly, but he continued to remain weak, particularly in the finger flexors and extensors.

DISCUSSION

This case presented with a rather rapid onset of weakness in one arm and then the other. The abrupt onset of upper extremity pain and wasting in proximal muscles was similar to brachial neuritis occurring in nondiabetic patients, but the weakness was also present in distal muscles. The condition seems to resemble the diabetic lumbosacral radiculoplexus neuropathy that occurs in the lower extremities.[1] The complex repetitive discharge denervation in the paraspinal muscles is in agreement with such a diagnosis; indeed, this syndrome has also been reported in the upper extremities.[2] The asymmetry was indicative of a mononeuritis multiplex, but the sensory deficits were not severe, and this case emphasized limited boundaries between these two conditions as both are caused by vasculopathies or vasculitis.[3–7] The vasculitis, however, could be missed in biopsies because of the patchy presentation.[8,9] It is interesting that autoimmune sensorimotor polyneuropathies might not stain positive for C5b-9 in vessels which could help in the diagnosis.[9] Vasculitic neuropathies are usually characterized by multiple painful sensory or sensorimotor mononeuropathies or mononeuropathy multiplex with acute or step-wise presentation in most cases.[9] Some consider lumbosacral radiculoplexus and neuralgic amyotrophy to be vasculitic of nonsystemic vasculitis neuropathies.[10,11]

The presence of vasculitis in patients with similar presentations suggests that corticosteroids and immunosuppressants could be useful in both radiculoplexus neuropathy and mononeuritis multiplex. The usual benign prognosis of proximal radiculoplexus neuropathy may cast doubt on this benefit, but rapid and severe progression, as in this case, and improvement noticed with the use of steroids in several cases,[10] serum neurofilament light chain levels correlate with disease activity,[12] both support the notion that these patients should be treated aggressively, particularly when the condition is progressing.

SUMMARY

This diabetic man developed severe weakness in both arms with pain and mild sensory deficits. There was more involvement of proximal muscles (radiculoplexus neuropathy) in addition to his polyneuropathy, but there was also a symmetric involvement of distal upper extremity muscles. He responded to immunotherapy.

IMPORTANT POINTS

- Diabetic amyotrophy and mononeuritis multiplex in diabetes are caused by a vasculopathy. This could be secondary to a microvasculitis.
- Diabetics with mononeuritis multiplex should be investigated for the possibility of other causes of systemic vasculitis.
- Diabetic radiculoplexoneuropathy can occur in the upper extremities.
- This form of diabetic mononeuritis multiplex, when progressing, should be treated with immunosuppressants and with aggressive pain control.

REFERENCES

1. Kelkar P, Parry GJ. Mononeuritis multiplex in diabetes mellitus: evidence for underlying immune pathogenesis. *J Neurol Neurosurg Psychiatry*. 2003;74(6):803–806.
2. Katz JS, Saperstein DS, Wolfe G, et al. Cervicobrachial involvement in diabetic radiculoplexopathy. *Muscle Nerve*. 2001;24(6):794–798.
3. Said G, Lacroix C, Lozeron P, et al. Inflammatory vasculopathy in multifocal diabetic neuropathy. *Brain*. 2003;126(Pt 2):376–385.
4. Kelkar P, Masood M, Parry GJ. Distinctive pathologic findings in proximal diabetic neuropathy (diabetic amyotrophy). *Neurology*. 2000;55(1):83–88.
5. Dyck PJ, Windebank AJ. Diabetic and nondiabetic lumbosacral radiculoplexus neuropathies: new insights into pathophysiology and treatment. *Muscle Nerve*. 2002;25(4):477–491.
6. Kilfoyle D, Kelkar P, Parry GJ. Pulsed methylprednisolone is a safe and effective treatment for diabetic amyotrophy. *J Clin Neuromusc Dis*. 2003;4:168–170.
7. Dyck PJ, Norell JE, Dyck PJ. Microvasculitis and ischemia in diabetic lumbosacral radiculoplexus neuropathy. *Neurology*. 1999; 53(9):2113–2121.
8. Bennett, DLH, Groves M, Blake J, Holton JL, et al. The use of nerve and muscle biopsy in the diagnosis of vasculitis: a 5 year retrospective study. *J Neurol Neurosurg Psychiatry*. 2008;79(12): 1376–1381.
9. Trikamji B, Pestronk A. Treatable, motor-sensory, axonal neuropathies with C5b-9 complement on endoneurial microvessels. *Muscle Nerve*. 2021;63(4):506–515.
10. Collins MP, Hadden RD. The nonsystemic vasculitic neuropathies. *Nat Rev Neurol*. 2017;13(5):302–316.
11. Barohn RJ, Sahenk Z, Warmolts JR, Mendell JR. The Bruns-Garland syndrome (diabetic amyotrophy): revisited 100 years later. *Arch Neurol*. 1991;48(11):1130–1135.
12. Bischof A, Manigold T, Barro C, Heijnen I, et al. Serum neurofilament light chain: a biomarker of neuronal injury in vasculitic neuropathy. *Ann Rheum Dis*. 2018;77(7):1093–1094.

60 CASE

A Diabetic Man With Acute Onset of Pain and Swelling in the Thigh

A 48-year-old insulin-dependent diabetic man presented with a 2-week history of pain and swelling in his right thigh muscle of acute onset.

Past medical history was negative. He had mild renal insufficiency with an elevated creatinine at 2.2 mg/dL (normal, 0.6–1.2 mg/dL).

Family history was not contributory.

Physical examination revealed marked edema, induration, and tenderness in the right thigh. There was evidence of diabetic retinopathy, but the cranial nerves were otherwise normal. Strength was normal, and reflexes were absent in the legs. He had a glove/stocking sensory deficit to all modalities. The remainder of the examination was unremarkable.

Blood sugar was 180 mg/dL (normal, <110 mg/dL). Glycosylated hemoglobin was 9% (normal, <6%); white blood cell count was 14,000 mm^3 with normal differential. Electrolytes were normal. Blood urea nitrogen was 60 mg/dL with a creatinine of 2.4 mg/24 hours. Erythrocyte sedimentation rate was 110 mm/h and serum creatine kinase was 400 IU/L (normal, 55–170 IU/L).

WHAT IS THE MOST LIKELY DIAGNOSIS?

The focal swelling in the leg in a patient with diabetes raises the possibilities of abscess, hematoma, venous thrombosis, fasciitis, osteomyelitis, tumor, and muscle infarct.[1–4]

WHAT WOULD ONE DO NEXT?

An MRI was done and was consistent with an infarction,[5] rather than an abscess, as there was marked edema of the vastus medialis muscle (Fig. 60-1).

A muscle biopsy of this area revealed marked necrosis with phagocytosis, hemorrhage, and edema (Fig. 60-2).

He recovered slowly over 1 month with only symptomatic treatment.

DISCUSSION

This man presented with pain and swelling of the thigh. An MRI of the area is useful in ruling out other conditions of similar presentation. MRI in this patient showed edema with increased signal in T2-weighted images. This presentation and the muscle biopsy showing necrosis, edema, and hemorrhage are consistent with the diagnosis of a muscle infarct.

Muscle infarctions or diabetic myonecrosis has been reported in over 100 cases, usually presenting in diabetics of various ages.[1] Both types of diabetes have been implicated, and patients also have evidence of other organ involvement by the disease.[1,6]

The clinical presentation, as in this case, consists of an acute onset of pain with tenderness, and a palpable mass with induration of surrounding tissue.[1,2] The pain is present at rest and is exacerbated by movements.[7] Strength is usually preserved.[8]

The most commonly involved muscles are the vastus lateralis, thigh adductors, and biceps femoris.[4,8,9]

The cause of diabetic muscle infarcts is unclear, although the pathogenesis is believed to be a thromboembolic event.[10,11] This, however, has not been clearly demonstrated.[6] Most likely, an initial ischemic event results in tissue swelling and muscle edema; this associates with increased pressure within the fascia and leads to further impairment of blood flow, resulting in infarct and necrosis.[1]

The treatment includes tight glycemic control, bed rest, physical therapy, and analgesics. Some perform surgery to remove the infarcted tissue, but the prognosis is no better than it is with medical treatment.[12] The symptoms usually disappear after weeks to months[1,2]; relapses occur, but the overall prognosis is benign. These patients, however, have an increased risk of death from vascular causes, such as myocardial infarction.[12]

SUMMARY

A diabetic man developed an acute onset of thigh swelling and pain. On MRI there was a T2-increased signal and gadolinium enhancement. The muscle biopsy showed necrosis, edema, and hemorrhage. He was diagnosed as having a diabetic muscle infarct.

IMPORTANT POINTS

- Unilateral leg swelling in a diabetic should suggest a muscle infarct; other possibilities include abscess, hematoma, osteomyelitis, venous thrombosis, and tumors.
- Diabetic muscle infarcts present as a painful mass, usually in the thigh, with edema and pain.
- The diagnosis is confirmed by MRI that shows the mass with high signal intensity in T2-weighted images and gadolinium enhancement. The test rules out other conditions such as an abscess or tumors.

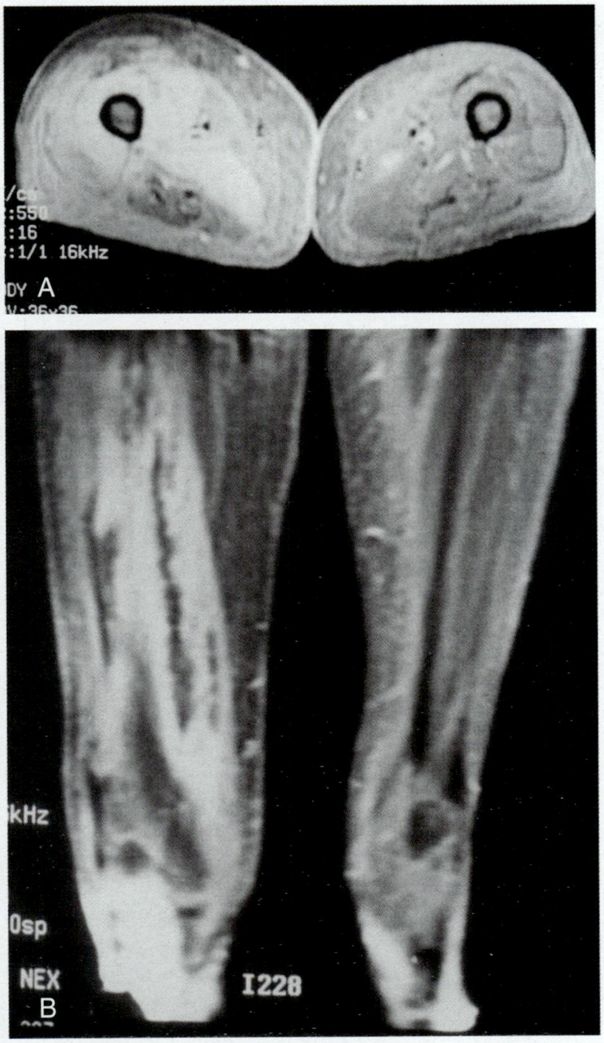

FIG. 60-1 A, MRI, T2-weighted image showing an area of increased signal in the right thigh. **B**, Gadolinium enhancement, T1-weighted MRI image showing enhancement of the right thigh.

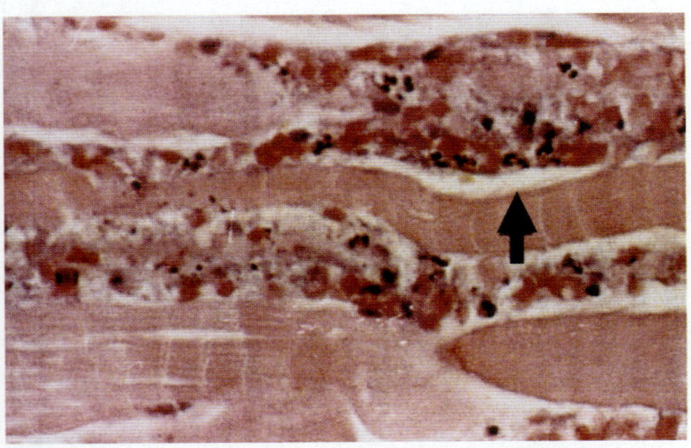

FIG. 60-2 Muscle biopsy showing necrosis and hemorrhage (*arrow*) (H&E stain, ×400).

- Biopsies of muscle infarcts show necrosis, hemorrhage, and edema.
- The etiology of diabetic infarcts is unclear but is thought to be caused by an initial ischemic event with edema and increased ischemia from fascial compression.
- Management is usually conservative.

REFERENCES

1. Trujillo-Santos AJ. Diabetic muscle infarction: an underdiagnosed complication of long-standing diabetes. *Diabetes Care*. 2003;26: 211–215.
2. Umpierrez GE, Stiles RG, Kleinbart J, et al. Diabetic muscle infarction. *Am J Med*. 1996;101:245–250.
3. Madhan KK, Symmans P, Te Strake L, et al. Diabetic muscle infarction in patients on dialysis. *Am J Kidney Dis*. 2000;35: 1212–1216.
4. Pedicelli A, Belli P, Fratino M, et al. Diabetic muscle infarction. *Am J Med*. 2001;111:671–672.
5. Aboulafia AJ, Monson DK, Kennon RE. Clinical and radiological aspects of idiopathic diabetic muscle infarction: rational approach to diagnosis and treatment. *J Bone Joint Surg Br*. 1999; 81:323–326.
6. Silbersein L, Britton KE, Marsh FP, et al. An unexpected cause of muscle pain in diabetes. *Ann Rheum Dis*. 2001;60:310–312.
7. Singer S, Rosenberg AE. A 54-year-old diabetic woman with pain and swelling of the leg. *N Engl J Med*. 1997;337:839–845.
8. Spengos K, Wohrle JC, Binder J, et al. Bilateral diabetic infarction of the anterior tibial muscle. *Diabetes Care*. 2000;23:699–701.
9. Miller JW, Fleckenstein J, Nodera H, et al. MRI in diabetic muscle infarction. *Neurology*. 2003;60:1019.
10. Chester CS, Banker BQ. Focal infarction of muscle in diabetes. *Diabetes Care*. 1986;9:623–630.
11. Horton WB, Taylor JS, Ragland TJ, Subauste AR. Diabetic muscle infarction: a systematic review. *BMJ Open Diabetes Res Care*. 2015;3(1):000082.
12. Kapur S, McKendry RJ. Treatment and outcomes of diabetic muscle infarction. *J Clin Rheumatol*. 2005;11(1):8–12.

61 CASE

A Uremic Man With Burning Feet

A 38-year-old man with a 2-year history of kidney failure caused by progressive glomerulonephritis requiring peritoneal dialysis presented with a 1-year history of numbness, tingling, and shooting pains in both feet and legs, associated with mild leg weakness and cramps. Review of systems revealed mild, nonspecific neck pain.

The patient denies a history of diabetes or of tobacco or alcohol use. Family history was noncontributory.

Examination revealed normal mental function, cranial nerves, and strength without evidence of muscle wasting or weakness. Biceps and triceps reflexes were normal, but brachioradialis and ankle reflexes were absent; they were trace in the knees. He had decreased vibration sense in the toes and decreased pain sensation up to the mid-calves. There was a mildly decreased pain sensation in the right ulnar nerve distribution in the hand. The rest of the examination was normal.

WHAT IS THE MOST LIKELY DIAGNOSIS?

This patient had a predominantly sensory neuropathy. The most likely diagnosis was a uremic polyneuropathy, although other common causes of neuropathy, such as diabetes, needed to be ruled out. Other possibilities included B_{12} deficiency, paraneoplastic neuropathy, amyloidosis, toxic neuropathies, and microangiopathic neuropathy. Pyridoxine intoxication or other toxic neuropathies caused by medications could have a similar presentation, but he had not taken excessive amounts of vitamins nor had he been exposed to toxins or medications that could cause neuropathies. Myelin-associated glycoprotein–associated neuropathy was unlikely because of his age and prominent small fiber involvement.

There was a suggestion of a right ulnar neuropathy.

WHAT TESTS SHOULD BE DONE?

Fasting blood sugar, glycosylated hemoglobin, erythrocyte sedimentation rate, immunoelectrophoresis, complete serum chemistry profile, and liver function tests were normal, except for blood urea of 60 mg/dL (normal, 24–49 mg/dL). Creatinine was 7.2 mg/dL (normal, 0.6–1.2 mg/dL).

AN EMG TEST WAS PERFORMED

Motor Nerve Studies

Nerve and Site	Latency (ms)	Amplitude (mV)	Conduction Velocity (m/s)
Median Nerve R.	**Normal ≤ 4.2**	**Normal ≥ 6**	**Normal ≥ 50**
Wrist	4.2	8	–
Elbow	9.2	8	50
Ulnar Nerve R.	**Normal ≤ 3.6**	**Normal ≥ 8**	**Normal ≥ 50**
Wrist	3.4	14	–
Below elbow	8.5	12	50
Above elbow	11.9	**8**	**35**
Axilla	14.5	**8**	51
Erb's point	18.1	**3**	69

Nerve and Site	Latency (ms)	Amplitude (mV)	Conduction Velocity (m/s)
Ulnar Nerve L.	**Normal ≤ 3.6**	**Normal ≥ 8**	**Normal ≥ 50**
Wrist	3.2	16	–
Below elbow	7.4	16	50
Above elbow	9.7	16	52
Peroneal Nerve R.	**Normal ≤ 5.7**	**Normal ≥ 3**	**Normal ≥ 40**
Ankle	4.8	**0.4**	–
Fibular head	15.8	**0.4**	**28**
Knee	18.9	**0.4**	**39**

Nerve and Site	Latency (ms)	Amplitude (mV)	Conduction Velocity (m/s)
Tibial Nerve R.	**Normal ≤ 5.3**	**Normal ≥ 4**	**Normal ≥ 40**
Ankle	5.0	**3**	–
Pop. fossa	16.6	**2**	**36**

F-Wave and Tibial H-Reflex Studies

Nerve	Latency (ms)	Normal Latency ≤ (ms)
Median nerve R.	**31.1**	30
Ulnar nerve R.	**39.1**	30
Ulnar nerve L.	**32.0**	30
Peroneal nerve R.	**NR**	54
Tibial nerve R.	**NR**	54
H-reflex R.	**40**	34
H-reflex L.	**39.9**	34

Sensory Nerve Studies

Nerve	Onset Latency (ms)	Normal Onset Latency ≤ (ms)	Peak Latency (ms)	Normal Peak Latency ≤ (ms)	Amp (μV)	Normal Amp ≥ (μV)	Conduction Velocity (m/s)	Normal Conduction Velocity ≥ (m/s)
Median nerve R.	2.6	2.6	3.1	3.1	23	20	50	50
Ulnar nerve R.	**3.2**	2.6	**3.7**	3.1	**4**	13	**38**	50
Sural nerve R.	**NR**	3.5	**NR**	4.0	**NR**	11	**NR**	40
Sural nerve L.	**NR**	3.5	**NR**	4.0	**NR**	11	**NR**	40

EMG Data

Muscle	Insrt Activity	Fibs	Pos Waves	Fasc	Amp	Dur	Poly	Pattern
Tibialis anterior R.	**Inc**	**1+**	**1+**	None	**Lg**	**Inc**	None	**Red**
Ext. hall. longus R.	**Inc**	**2+**	**2+**	None	**Lg**	**Inc**	None	**Red**
Gastrocnemius R.	**Inc**	None	**1+**	None	Norm	Norm	None	**Red**
Vastus lateralis R.	Norm	None	None	None	Norm	Norm	None	Full
Cervical paraspinals R.	Norm	None	None	None	Norm	Norm	None	Full
Deltoid R.	Norm	None	None	None	Norm	Norm	Few	Full
Triceps R.	Norm	None	None	None	Norm	Norm	None	Full
First dorsal interosseous R.	**Inc**	**1+**	**1+**	None	**Inc**	**Inc**	None	Full
Abductor poll. brevis R.	Norm	None	None	None	Norm	Norm	None	Full
Flexor carpi ulnaris R.	**Inc**	None	None	None	Norm	Norm	None	Full
Flexor carpi radialis R.	Norm	None	None	None	Norm	Norm	None	Full
First dorsal interosseous L.	**Inc**	None	None	None	Norm	Norm	None	Full

WHAT WERE THE EMG FINDINGS?

This test showed a normal right median motor nerve conduction velocity and borderline distal latency. The right ulnar nerve was normal from elbow to wrist but had decreased velocity with partial conduction block across the elbow with normal distal latency and amplitude. The left ulnar nerve was normal. The tibial and peroneal nerves had decreased CMAP amplitudes and conduction velocities; the sural SNAPs were absent. The median SNAP was normal, but the right digital ulnar was of low amplitude; the dorsal ulnar cutaneous nerve was not tested. Tibial and peroneal F-waves were not recordable. In the upper extremities the F-waves were mildly prolonged except for the right ulnar nerve, which was significantly prolonged. Tibial H-reflexes had prolonged latencies.

Needle electromyography showed denervation potentials with large motor unit potentials in the distal lower extremity muscles and in muscles innervated by the right ulnar nerve.

It was concluded that this patient had a predominant axonal sensory motor neuropathy with secondary demyelination that was most prominent in the legs. In addition, there was a right ulnar nerve entrapment at the elbow.

DISCUSSION

This case was diagnosed as having uremic polyneuropathy. He was treated with peritoneal dialysis at home and given a right elbow pad. He was also given 300 mg gabapentin three times a day with significant improvement of his leg pain. This drug should be given very carefully as it is eliminated through the kidneys. He later underwent a cadaveric kidney transplant with almost complete disappearance of the symptoms.

Uremic neuropathy is a sensorimotor symmetric polyneuropathy that affects predominantly the lower extremities and usually has a slow progression. The symptoms include cramps with painful paresthesias, although severe pain is unusual.[1] Some patients have restless legs syndrome. There are decreased vibratory, temperature, and pain sensation, and there can also be distal motor weakness and decreased reflexes.

Pathologically, uremic neuropathy shows evidence of axonal degeneration of myelinated axons with secondary demyelination[2]; there is also involvement of the unmyelinated fibers.[3]

Electrophysiologic findings indicate axonal damage and secondary demyelination, with decreased-amplitude CMAPs, mildly slow motor nerve conduction velocities, and signs of denervation on needle electromyography, particularly in the distal legs.[4–7] The sensory action potentials could be absent or of low amplitude.

There is a clear correlation between creatinine clearance and the degree of nerve conduction slowing.[8] A number of toxins have been associated with uremic neuropathy, and it has been postulated that it is caused by the accumulation of toxins of molecular weight 500–2000 D (middle molecular theory) (Fig. 61-1). These molecules are dialyzed more slowly than urea and creatine,[6–9] and the use of filters with high permeability to those proteins improves nerve conduction velocity.[10] There is also evidence that uremic nerves are in a chronically depolarized state prior to dialysis caused by hyperkalemia.[11]

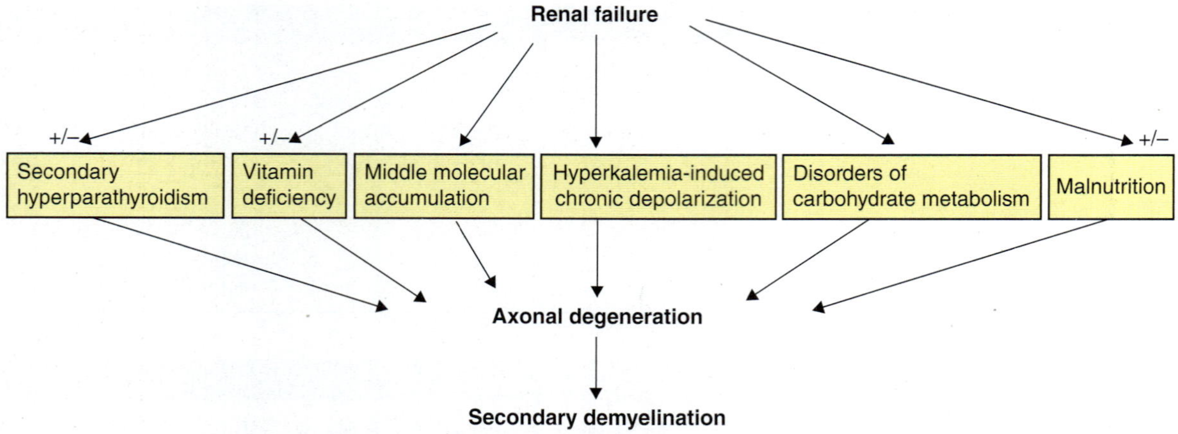

FIG. 61-1 Diagram of etiology of uremic polyneuropathy.

TABLE 61-1 Uremic Neuropathies

Type	Etiology
Polyneuropathy	Middle molecule toxins Miscellaneous (vitamin deficiency, malnutrition, secondary hyperparathyroidism, and abnormal carbohydrate metabolism), chronic hyperkalemia, causing a chronic depolarized state
Mononeuropathy	
Ischemic monomelic	Acute ischemia after shunt placement with or without diabetes mellitus with peripheral neuropathy and arteriosclerotic vascular disease
Steal syndrome	Reversal of arterial blood flow from shunt
Carpal tunnel syndrome	Dialysis amyloid (β-2-microglobulin) accumulation
Compressive neuropathies	Nerve compression (cachectic and bedridden patients)
Traumatic	Self-retaining retractors or surgical positioning (kidney transplant)

Other factors might play a pathogenic role, such as abnormalities of parathyroid hormones,[12] vitamin deficiency,[13] and malnutrition. Nerve entrapments can occur, and accumulation of β-2-microglobulin causes carpal tunnel syndrome.[14] Other entrapments and shunt-related neuropathies also occur in uremics as listed in Table 61-1 (see also Case 2).

Uremic polyneuropathy stabilizes or improves with hemodialysis and the use of zinc supplements.[15] Renal transplantation, however, is the best treatment and can yield complete resolution.[16] Pain is managed symptomatically with drugs commonly used to treat painful neuropathies.[17–19]

This case improved significantly after a cadaveric kidney transplantation, and after 2 years, he was no longer taking medications for pain control. His neurologic examination showed only decreased ankle reflexes and vibration sense in the toes. The ulnar neuropathy also improved.

SUMMARY

This patient developed distal paresthesias with numbness and weakness. His nerve conduction studies were consistent with a uremic sensorimotor polyneuropathy and had evidence of ulnar nerve entrapment at the elbow. His symptoms improved significantly with a kidney transplant.

IMPORTANT POINTS

- Uremic polyneuropathy is an axonal neuropathy with secondary demyelination.
- The symptoms of uremic neuropathy include distal numbness and paresthesias with mild distal weakness and areflexia.
- Electrophysiologic studies indicated low-amplitude motor and sensory action potential with some degree of demyelination. Denervation potentials could be seen in the distal legs.
- This polyneuropathy is believed to be caused by the accumulation of toxic middle-sized molecules (500–2000 D). Among others, important causes include a chronic depolarized state from hyperkalemia.
- Entrapment neuropathies are not unusual in uremics.
- Uremic neuropathy improves with dialysis and kidney transplantation.

REFERENCES

1. Laaksonen S, Metsarinne K, Voipio-Pulkki LM, Falck B. Neurophysiologic parameters and symptoms in chronic renal failure. *Muscle Nerve*. 2002;25(6):884–890.
2. Dyck PJ, Johnson WJ, Lambert EH, O'Brien PC. Segmental demyelination secondary to axonal degeneration in uremic neuropathy. *Mayo Clin Proc*. 1971;46(6):400–431.
3. Bassan BA, Bertorini TE. Neuromuscular manifestations of acquired metabolic, endocrine, or nutritional disorders. In: Bertorini T, ed. *Neuromuscular Disorders: Treatment and Management*. Amsterdam, Netherlands: Elsevier; 2022:528–553. 2nd ed. Chapter 21.

4. Bazzi C, Pagani C, Sorgato G, et al. Uremic polyneuropathy: a clinical and electrophysiological study in 135 short- and long-term hemodialyzed patients. *Clin Nephrol.* 1991;35(4):176–181.
5. Jurcic D, Bago J, Eljuga D, et al. Features of uremic neuropathy in long-term dialysis. *Coll Antropol.* 1998;22(1):119–125.
6. Nielsen VK. The peripheral nerve function in chronic renal failure: a survey. *Acta Med Scand Suppl.* 1976;573:1–32.
7. Babb AL, Ahmad S, Bergstrom J, Scribner BH. The middle molecule hypothesis in perspective. *Am J Kidney Dis.* 1981;1(1):46–50.
8. Milutinovic J, Babb AL, Eschbach JW, et al. Uremic neuropathy: evidence of middle molecule toxicity. *Artif Organs.* 1978;2(1):45–51.
9. Al-Hayk EA, Bertorini TE. Neuromuscular complications in uremics: a review. *Neurologist.* 2007;13:131–137.
10. Quellhorst E, Doht B, Schuenemann B. Hemofiltration: treatment of renal failure by ultrafiltration and substitution. *J Dial.* 1977;1(6):529–543.
11. Krishman AV, Kierman MC. Uremic neuropathy: clinical features and new pathophysiological insights. *Muscle Nerve.* 2007;35(3):273–290.
12. Di Giulio S, Chkoff N, Lhoste F, et al. Parathormone as a nerve poison in uremia. *N Engl J Med.* 1978;299(20):1134–1135.
13. Dobbelstein H, Korner WF, Mempel W, et al. Vitamin B-6 deficiency in uremia and its implications for the depression of immune responses. *Kidney Int.* 1974;5(3):233–239.
14. Kurer MH, Baillod RA, Madgwick JC. Musculoskeletal manifestations of amyloidosis: a review of 83 patients on haemodialysis for at least 10 years. *J Bone Joint Surg Br.* 1991;73(2):271–273.
15. Sprenger KB, Bundschu D, Lewis K, et al. Improvement of uremic neuropathy and hypogeusia by dialysate zinc supplementation: a double-blind study. *Kidney Int.* 1983;16(Suppl):S315–S318.
16. Bolton CF. Electrophysiologic changes in uremic neuropathy after successful renal transplantation. *Neurology.* 1976;26(2):152–161.
17. Wolfe GI, Barohn RJ. Painful peripheral neuropathy. *Curr Treat Options Neurol.* 2002;3:177–188.
18. Mendell JR, Sahenk Z. Clinical practice: painful sensory neuropathy. *N Engl J Med.* 2003;348(13):1243–1255.
19. Aljasam A, Hall L, Spicker M, Menkes DI. A practical approach to the treatment of painful polyneuropathy. In: Bertorini TE, ed. *Neuromuscular Disorders: Treatment and Management.* Amsterdam, Netherlands: Elsevier; 2022:118–142. 2nd ed. Chapter 6.

62A CASE

A Woman With Leg Numbness, Pain, Weakness, and Slow Nerve Conduction Velocities

A 41-year-old woman was referred by another neurologist because of leg pain with numbness and tingling in the feet for 4 years. In the last 2 years, she developed leg weakness and difficulty walking.

Her previous workup revealed EMG and nerve biopsy findings consistent with a demyelinating neuropathy with slow nerve conduction velocities. Spinal fluid protein was normal at 36 mg/dL. She had normal serum B_{12}, fasting blood sugar, glycosylated hemoglobin, immunoelectrophoresis, FANA, and thyroid function tests, and her HIV test was negative.

Past medical history was significant only for gallbladder surgery and appendectomy. Family history was negative.

The patient was infused with 2 g/kg of gamma globulin without benefit and was subsequently referred for evaluation.

Neurologic examination revealed normal mentation and cranial nerves. She had difficulty walking on heels or toes. Muscle strength in the upper extremities was normal except for 4/5 weakness in the hand interosseous muscles. In the lower extremities iliopsoas strength was 4+/5, glutei 4/5, quadriceps 5/5, tibialis anterior and peronei 4−/5, foot flexors and evertors 5/5, and toe extensors 4−/5. There was no evidence of muscle atrophy or fasciculations. Reflexes were absent throughout. Vibration sense was absent in the toes and ankles and diminished in the knees and fingers. Pinprick sensation was decreased up to the ankles. Two-point discrimination was abnormal in the fingers and toes. Position sense was decreased in the toes. Coordination was intact. There were no Babinski signs. She did not have visceromegaly, high arches (Fig. 62A-1), hammertoes, or nerve hypertrophy. No Mees lines were seen. The rest of the examination was normal.

WHAT IS THE DIFFERENTIAL DIAGNOSIS?

This patient had a polyneuropathy with a fairly recent onset of symptoms, a negative family history, lack of exposure to medications or toxins, and normal blood work for common causes of polyneuropathy.

She was previously diagnosed with a demyelinating polyneuropathy. The small nerve fiber involvement is not classical but can occur in those neuropathies. A presumptive diagnosis of chronic inflammatory demyelinating polyradiculoneuropathy (CIDP) was made initially, but she did not improve with IgG treatment. Other possibilities include a hereditary neuropathy, such as Charcot–Marie–Tooth (CMT) disease, although family history and stigmata were absent, she was not exposed to toxins and was not a diabetic.

AN EMG TEST WAS PERFORMED

Motor Nerve Studies

Nerve and Site	Latency (ms)	Amplitude (mV)	Conduction Velocity (m/s)
Peroneal Nerve R.	**Normal ≤ 5.7**	**Normal ≥ 3**	**Normal ≥ 40**
Ankle	**8.9**	**0.9**	–
Fibular head	21.6	**0.7**	**26**
Across knee	25.0	**0.6**	**16**

Nerve and Site	Latency (ms)	Amplitude (mV)	Conduction Velocity (m/s)
Tibial Nerve R.	**Normal ≤ 5.3**	**Normal ≥ 4**	**Normal ≥ 40**
Ankle	**10.7**	4	–
Pop. fossa	25.1	4	**29**

Nerve and Site	Latency (ms)	Amplitude (mV)	Conduction Velocity (m/s)
Tibial Nerve L.	**Normal ≤ 5.3**	**Normal ≥ 4**	**Normal ≥ 40**
Ankle	**9.6**	**2**	–
Pop. fossa	31.2	**1**	**29**
Median Nerve R.	**Normal ≤ 4.2**	**Normal ≥ 6**	**Normal ≥ 50**
Wrist	**7.9**	13	–
Elbow	16.8	10	**29**
Ulnar Nerve R.	**Normal ≤ 3.6**	**Normal ≥ 8**	**Normal ≥ 50**
Wrist	**6.1**	**6**	–
Below elbow	16.0	**6**	**23**
Above elbow	20.0	**6**	**30**
Axilla	26.6	**6**	**27**

F-Wave and Tibial H-Reflex Studies

Nerve	Latency (ms)	Normal Latency ≤ (ms)
Peroneal nerve R.	**87.4**	54
Tibial nerve R.	**61.0**	54
Tibial nerve L.	**NR**	54
Median nerve L.	**43.1**	30
Ulnar nerve L.	**47.3**	30
H-reflex R.	**46.5**	34
H-reflex L.	**45.3**	34

Sensory Nerve Studies

Sural nerve R.	**NR**
Median nerve R.	**NR**
Ulnar nerve R.	**NR**
Superficial peroneal R.	**NR**

EMG Data

Muscle	Insrt Activity	Fibs	Pos Waves	Fasc	Amp	Dur	Poly	Pattern
Vastus lateralis R.	Norm	None	None	None	**Lg**	**Inc**	None	Full
Tibialis anterior R.	Norm	None	None	None	**Lg**	**Inc**	None	**Red**
Gastrocnemius R.	Norm	None	None	None	**Lg**	**Inc**	None	Full

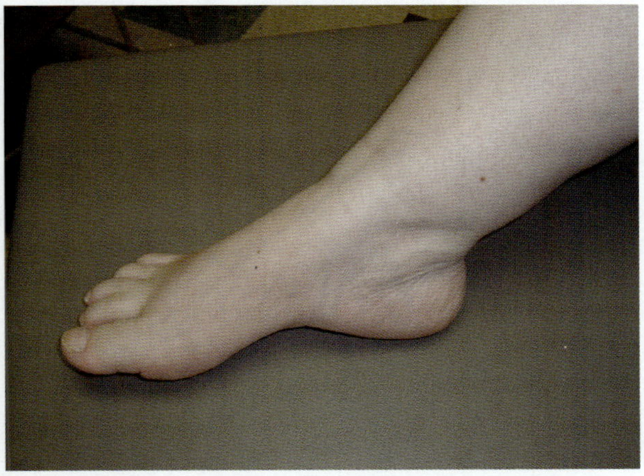

FIG. 62A-1 Foot of patient; notice that she had no high arch or hammertoes.

WHAT WERE THE EMG FINDINGS?

The distal motor latencies, F-waves, and tibial H-reflex latencies were prolonged, and the nerve conduction velocities were reduced to less than 80% of normal in nerves with normal amplitude CMAP and to less than 70% in those with low amplitude. These findings are consistent with a demyelinating neuropathy. The low-amplitude CMAPs in some nerves indicated axonal degeneration. The low-amplitude SNAPs could be explained by sensory nerve axonal degeneration but can also be caused by demyelination and temporal dispersion. The large motor unit action potentials without spontaneous activity are indicative of a chronic axonal loss with reinnervation. The peroneal nerve had decreased conduction velocity across the fibular head, suggesting a focal compression. The CMAPs had no temporal dispersion or conduction block; there were uniformly slow motor conduction velocities (Fig. 62A-2).

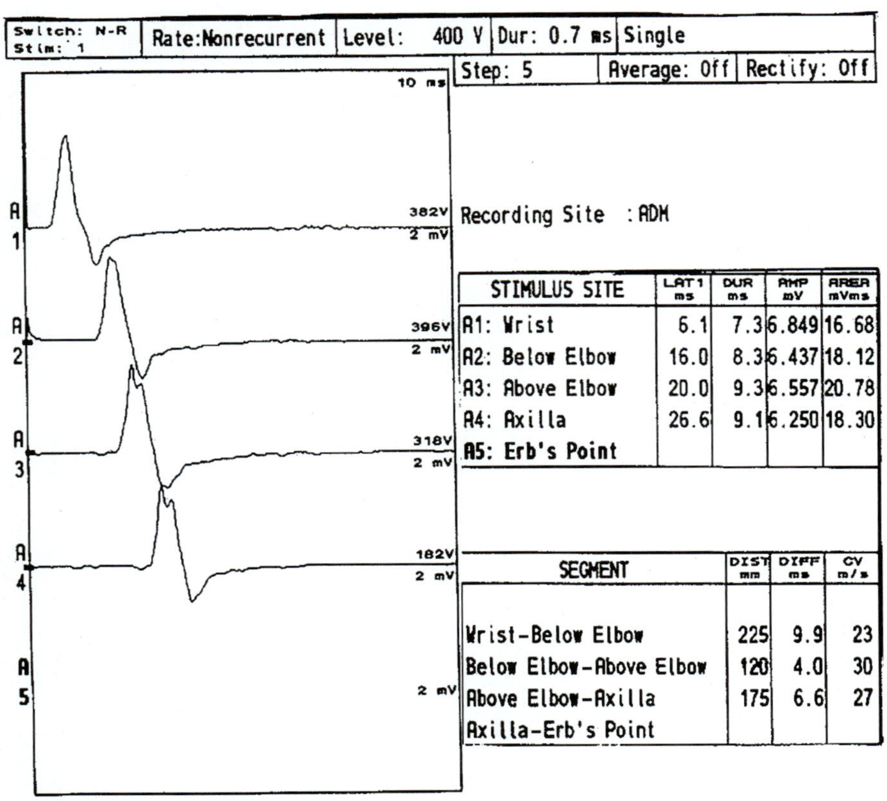

FIG. 62A-2 Ulnar motor nerve conduction test in patient showing a fairly uniform shape of CMAP without conduction block or temporal dispersion.

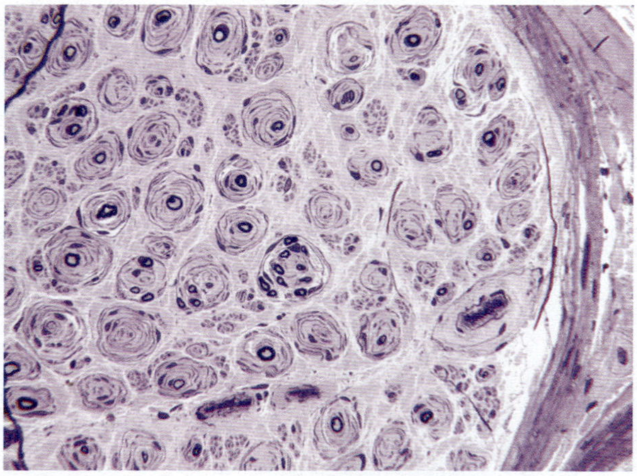

FIG. 62A-3 Plastic-embedded section osmicated and toluidine blue–stained sural nerve biopsy section showing increased connective tissue and decreased number of myelinated axons; the most prominent finding is the presence of "onion bulbs." There is also thickening of the vessel walls (×400).

The findings are suggestive of a hereditary demyelinating neuropathy, such as CMT type 1 (CMT1), rather than an acquired demyelinating neuropathy, such as CIDP, in which there are conduction blocks and nonuniform conduction slowing. Conduction blocks are also seen in multifocal motor neuropathy and multifocal motor and sensory neuropathy, in some hereditary neuropathies such as X-linked CMT disease (CMTX),[1] CMT1B and D, and in vasculitic neuropathy, but are not a characteristic finding in CMT1. In hereditary neuropathy with liability to pressure palsy (HNPP) the blocks occur in sites of entrapments.

WHAT SHOULD BE DONE NEXT?

The sural nerve biopsy was reviewed and showed a marked decrease in the number of myelinated fibers and frequent "onion bulbs" (Fig. 62A-3) without inflammation or axonal degeneration. These findings are consistent with a chronic demyelinating neuropathy such as CMT1. "Onion bulbs" and myelinated fiber loss can occur in other chronic neuropathies such as CIDP and diabetes but to a much lesser degree. Therefore DNA studies were performed and demonstrated a duplication of chromosome 17p in the *PMP22* gene, which is characteristic of CMT1A.

This case illustrates that if the clinical picture or EMG findings are consistent with CMT, DNA testing should be performed prior to an invasive test such as a nerve biopsy. If insurance companies refuse to cover DNA testing, then electrophysiologic studies of parents and children can document an autosomal-dominant pattern expected to be seen in CMT1A.

SUMMARY

This patient presented with symptoms of numbness and weakness and was found to have a demyelinating neuropathy. A familial neuropathy was suspected by uniform slowing of nerve conduction velocities, without temporal dispersion or lack of changes in the proximal, compared with the distal, fibers. Despite her not having the characteristics of high arches or hammertoes seen in CMT disease, she was proven to have CMT1A disease by DNA testing.

For further discussion, important points, and references, see Case 62B.

A Boy With Leg Weakness

A 17-year-old patient started walking on the sides of his feet and had a tendency for footdrop since the age of 8. He was the product of a normal pregnancy and delivery. Developmental milestones were normal. He had a healthy 5-year-old brother. His mother also had clumsiness, weakness, and tingling in the legs since she was a teenager.

Past medical history was unremarkable.

General physical examination, mentation, and cranial nerves were normal. There was thinning of the legs (Fig. 62B-1) with mild weakness in the hand interosseous muscles without significant atrophy and moderate bilateral weakness of the foot dorsiflexors and evertors with thinning of the anterior and posterior compartments. He had difficulty walking on his heels but could walk on his toes. Reflexes were 2+ in the upper extremities and knees but absent in the ankles. There were no pathologic reflexes. Sensory examination of proprioception, vibration, and pinprick sensation appeared grossly normal in the hands and legs except for vibration sense that was diminished in the toes and ankles. There was also decreased pinprick sensation in the toes. He had no scoliosis, high arches, hammertoes, or nerve hypertrophy. The rest of the examination was unremarkable.

WHAT IS THE DIFFERENTIAL DIAGNOSIS?

The distal weakness, absent ankle reflexes, and mild sensory deficit indicate a predominantly axonal neuropathy. A distal muscular dystrophy or distal spinal muscle atrophy is unlikely because of this deficit. He appeared to have an axonal polyneuropathy of childhood onset; the differential diagnosis of this is very limited.

The history of neuropathy in the mother suggests an autosomal-dominant disease, although an X-linked inheritance, such as in CMTX, is also a consideration. The preserved proximal reflexes and normal vibratory sense are against CMT type 1A (CMT1A), but not CMTX or CMT2, in which proximal reflexes could be present in younger patients. Other common causes of neuropathy, such as diabetes, are unlikely. The clinical presentation suggests the axonal variant or CMT2.

AN EMG TEST WAS PERFORMED

Motor Nerve Studies

Nerve and Site	Latency (ms)	Amplitude (mV)	Conduction Velocity (m/s)
Peroneal Nerve R.	**Normal ≤ 5.7**	**Normal ≥ 3**	**Normal ≥ 40**
Ankle	**NR**	**NR**	–
Fibular head	**NR**	**NR**	**NR**
Tibial Nerve L.	**Normal ≤ 5.3**	**Normal ≥ 4**	**Normal ≥ 40**
Ankle	**NR**	**NR**	–
Pop. Fossa	**NR**	**NR**	**NR**
Ulnar Nerve R.	**Normal ≤ 3.6**	**Normal ≥ 8**	**Normal ≥ 50**
Wrist	3.6	**7**	–
Below elbow	7.8	**7**	56
Above elbow	10.1	**7**	52
Nerve and Site	**Latency (ms)**	**Amplitude (mV)**	**Conduction Velocity (m/s)**
Peroneal Nerve R.[a]	**Normal ≤ 5.2**	**Normal ≥ 3**	**Normal ≥ 40**
Fibular head	**10.9**	4	–
Knee	13.1	3	46

[a]Recorded at tibialis anterior muscle.

F-Wave and Tibial H-Reflex Studies

Nerve	Latency (ms)	Normal Latency ≤ (ms)
Peroneal nerve R.	**NR**	54
Tibial nerve L.	**NR**	54
Ulnar nerve R.	29.8	30
H-reflex R.	**NR**	34
H-reflex L.	**NR**	34

Sensory Nerve Studies

Nerve	Onset Latency (ms)	Normal Onset Latency ≤ (ms)	Peak Latency (ms)	Normal Peak Latency ≤ (ms)	Amp (μV)	Normal Amp ≥ (μV)	Conduction Velocity (m/s)	Normal Conduction Velocity ≥ (m/s)
Sural nerve R.	**NR**	3.5	**NR**	4.0	**NR**	11	**NR**	40
Superficial peroneal R.	**NR**	3.5	**NR**	4.0	**NR**	8–10	**NR**	40
Ulnar nerve R.	2.4	2.6	2.9	3.1	**8**	13	50	50

EMG Data

Muscle	Insrt Activity	Fibs	Pos Waves	Fasc	Amp	Dur	Poly	Pattern
First dorsal interosseus L.	Norm	None	None	None	**Lg**	**Inc**	None	Full
Vastus lateralis L.	Norm	None	None	None	**Lg**	**Inc**	None	Full
Tibialis anterior L.	**Inc**	None	**1+**	None	**Lg**	**Inc**	None	**Red**
Gastrocnemius L.	**Inc**	None	**1+**	None	**Lg**	**Inc**	None	**Red**

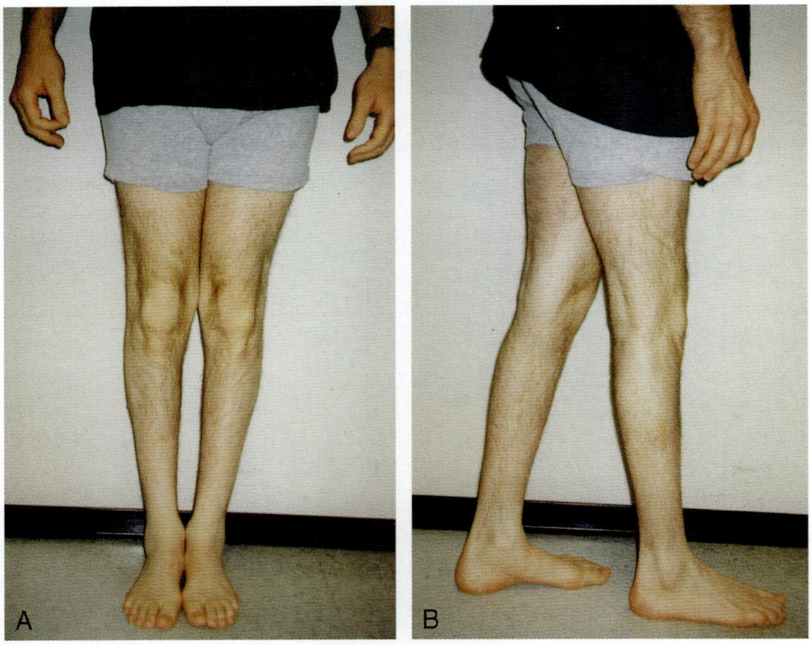

FIG. 62B-1 Patient showing minimal high arches **(A)** and leg atrophy **(B)**.

WHAT WERE THE EMG FINDINGS?

Ulnar motor nerve conduction velocity and distal latency were normal; the CMAP amplitude was borderline. There was no conduction block or temporal dispersion. Tibial and peroneal nerve conduction velocities could not be measured because of lack of measurable CMAPs recorded in the foot. The peroneal conduction velocity when recorded at the tibialis anterior muscle was normal. The ulnar SNAP was of low amplitude and had normal latency. Sural and superficial peroneal SNAPs were absent as were tibial nerve H-reflexes. The ulnar F-response had normal latency. Denervation potentials with large motor unit action potentials (MUAPs) with reduced recruitment were seen in the distal legs. Large MUAPs were seen in the first dorsal interosseous. These findings indicate a chronic motor and sensory axonal neuropathy.

The patient's mother was examined, and she had weakness distally in the limbs without high arches or hammertoes (Fig. 62B-2). She had trace knee reflexes, normal reflexes in the upper extremities, and absent ankle jerks. There was absent vibration sense in the toes and decreased in the ankles, and decreased pinprick up to the mid-calf. Her EMG study also showed an axonal neuropathy.

SUMMARY

This boy and his mother had a chronic axonal polyneuropathy; they were diagnosed as having CMT2 disease. No DNA testing was done.

DISCUSSION

Case 62A, who had a demyelinating neuropathy and no family history, was found to have CMT1A. Her late symptom onset and prominent paresthesias were somewhat unusual.

CMT disease was named after the initial descriptions by Charcot and Marie[1] and then by Tooth who called it *peroneal muscular atrophy*.[2] The condition has a prevalence of 36–49 per 100,000 population.[3] This neuropathy is usually subdivided into demyelinating (CMT1) or axonal (CMT2) forms, depending on the clinical and electrophysiologic findings (Table 62B-1 lists the different types of CMT diseases as well as hereditary sensory and autonomic, and hereditary motor neuropathies).

Charcot–Marie–Tooth Neuropathy Type 1

This autosomal-dominant disease with symptoms manifest in adolescence or early adulthood[4–6] is characterized by progressive weakness which initially involves the lower extremities, particularly the peroneal nerve-innervated muscles, and later spreads to the distal and proximal upper extremities. Patients often have high arches, hammertoes (Fig. 62B-3), and distal leg atrophy, so that the legs resemble inverted champagne bottles, or "stork" legs, but this could be absent as in *Case 62A*.

The neurologic examination usually reveals distal weakness and mild sensory abnormalities, which include predominantly loss of position and vibratory senses, with relative preservation of pain and temperature sensations until later in the disease. Nerve hypertrophy could also be present. Cranial nerve examination is usually normal, although sensorineural hearing loss may occur.

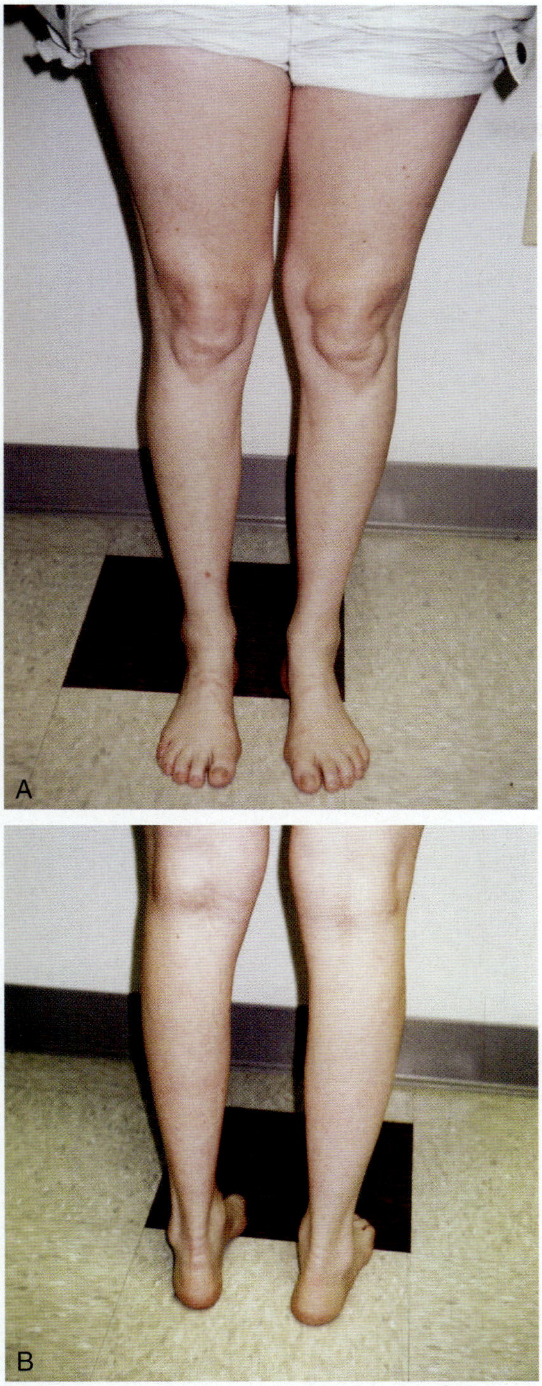

FIG. 6B-2 Mother of the patient B showing leg atrophy, anterior **(A)** and posterior **(B)** views.

Electrophysiologic studies of CMT1 show evidence of demyelination, with most patients having nerve conduction velocities of about 25% or less of the lower limits of normal[7] and with a usually uniform slowing in all nerve segments.[8] Sensory nerve action potentials can be of low amplitude or absent, and needle electromyography could show large motor units with little evidence of denervation potentials. Conventionally, demyelinating CMT is considered in those with upper extremity nerve conduction velocity below 38 m/s.[6] There are, however, families with intermediate forms of autosomal-dominant CMT, and those are described as dominant intermediate CMT (DICMT). Some have mutations in 19p12 or 10q24.

Histopathologic studies demonstrate a reduced number of myelinated fibers with many thinly myelinated axons and Schwann cell proliferation, prominent onion bulb formations,[9–11] and evidence of paranodal and segmental demyelination.

The disease has a very slow progression and usually does not affect survival, although some patients with a more severe phenotype become wheelchair-bound.

CMT1 is subdivided into various subtypes according to the genetic defect. Fig. 62B-4 is a diagram of peripheral nerve proteins affected in some hereditary and autoimmune neuropathies. Fig. 62B-5 shows a diagnostic algorithm for patients with Charcot–Marie–Tooth disease.

Charcot–Marie–Tooth Type 1A

This type is caused by duplication on the short arm of chromosome 17p11.2–12.[12,13] This duplication represents approximately 1 million base pairs, expanding 6 cM of genetic distance.[14] The gene product is the peripheral myelin protein 22, or *PMP22*.[15,16] Some cases appear de novo.

The disease is allelic to hereditary neuropathy with liability to form pressure palsies (HNPP) which is usually caused by gene deletions.[17] Some patients with CMT1A have point mutations.

Charcot–Marie–Tooth Type 1B

The genetic defect in this group has been located on chromosome 1. The protein defect in this type is human myelin protein zero (P_O or MPZ),[18] and the disease is linked to the Duffy blood type.[19] A mutation of Arg98 is associated with irregularly compacted myelin lamellae, whereas the Asp109Asn mutation is associated with thick myelin.[20] Patients with CMT1B usually have more severe clinical phenotype and histologic findings than those with CMT1A.

Charcot–Marie–Tooth Types 1C and 1D

Although CMT1C is conventionally considered as a group with unknown genetic abnormalities, some that are classified here are caused by a missense mutation on chromosome 10q21–22.[21] Most properly these patients should be classified as CMT1D. In some patients the 10q21–22 mutation can cause a phenotype of severe childhood demyelinating neuropathy, or Dejerine–Sottas disease (described as CMT3) (see Table 62B-1). The defective gene normally expresses the early growth response protein (EGR2), which is a transcription gene that binds a DNA regulating gene expression and possibly cell proliferation.[21,22] Recently, Street and colleagues[23] mapped the genetic defect in a group of patients with CMT1C to chromosome 16p13, identifying missense mutations in the *LITAF* gene (lipopolysaccharide-induced tumor necrosis factor) in three pedigrees. The *LITAF* or *SIMPLE* gene is a widely expressed gene that encodes a protein that may play a role in protein degradation pathways and a critical role in peripheral nerve function.

TABLE 62B-1 Hereditary Motor-Sensory Neuropathies Classification

Disease	Inheritance Pattern	Gene or Locus	Clinical Features
HMSN			
Demyelinating			Forearm NCV usually <38 m/s
CMT1	AD		Young adult onset, NCV 10–35 m/s
CMT1A		PMP22 (usually duplication)	Most common (70% of all CMT1)
			Mutations also cause CMT3
CMT1B		MPZ (P_0)	Mutations also cause CMT2 and CMT3
CMT1C		LITAF/SIMPLE	
CMT1D		EGR2	Broad clinical spectrum (also CMT3)
CMT1F		NEFL	DSS phenotype common
CMT1 plus		FBLN5	Macular degeneration; cutis laxa
CMT1		PMP2	Classic CMT1
SNCV/CMT1		ARHGEF10	Asymptomatic slowed NCVs
HNPP	AD	PMP22 (usually deletion)	Adult-onset episodic entrapment neuropathies, mild slowing (NCV 40–50 m/s)
CMT3			Severe, early-onset demyelinating
DSS	AD/X	CMT1 genes	Onset before age 3 years
	AR	PRX, MTMR2	
CHN	AD	PMP22, MPZ	Congenital onset
	AR	EGR2	AR-CHN, also known as CMT4E
CMT4	AR		Childhood onset, usually severe
CMT4A		GDAP1	Both axonal and demyelinating types
CMT4B1		MTMR2	Biopsy shows focally folded myelin
CMT4B2		SBF2/MTMR13	Same as above ± early-onset glaucoma
		SBF1/MTMR5	
CMT4C		SH3TC2	Scoliosis often severe, also axonal types
CMT4D		NDRG1	Dysmorphic features, deafness
CMT4E		EGR2	
CMT4F		PRX	DSS phenotype
CMT4G		HK1	
CMT4H		FGD4	
CMT4J		FIG4	
		SURF-1	
		CTDP1	
Slow NCV	AD	ARHGEF10	Asymptomatic NCV slowing
Intermediate			NCV 25–45 m/s
CMTX	X		
CMTX1		GJB1/Cx32	Similar to CMT1, but males more severely affected, CNS involvement common
CMTX2, Cowchuck syn		AIFM1	MR, deafness, axonal
CMTX5		PRPS1	Axonal CMT, deafness, optic atrophy
CMTX6		PDK3	Axonal CMT
CMTX		DRP2	Intermediate MCVs
CMTDI	AD		
DI-CMTA		10q24	
DI-CMTB		DNM2	Neutropenia
DI-CMTC		YARS	
DI-CMTD		MPZ	
DI-CMTE		IFN2	Focal segmental glomerulosclerosis
DI-CMTF		GNB4	
CMTRI	AR		
CMTR1A		GDAP1	
CMTR1B		KARS	
CMTR1C		PLEKHG5	
CMTR1D		COX6A1	
Axonal			NCV >38 m/s
CMT2	AD		Young adult onset

TABLE 62B-1 Hereditary Motor-Sensory Neuropathies Classification—cont'd

Disease	Inheritance Pattern	Gene or Locus	Clinical Features
CMT2A		MFN2 KIF1B (rare)	Most common; also HMSN V (optic atrophy), VI (spasticity), and early onset
CMT2B		RAB7	Severe sensory loss like HSAN-1
CMT2C		TRPV4	Vocal cord/diaphragm weakness
CMT2D		GARS	Arm > leg, motor predominant, similar to dHMN caused by BSCL2 mutations
CMT2E		NEFL	Allelic with CMT1E; variable phenotype
CMT2F		HSP27 (HSPB1)	Motor predominant
CMT2G		12q12–13.3	Proximal > distal weakness
CMT2H, K		GDAP1	Allelic with CMT4A
CMT2I, J		MPZ (P_0)	Cough, pain, autonomic/pupil, deafness
CMT2L		HSP22 (HSPB8)	Motor predominant, allelic with HMNIIa
CMTDIB, CMT2M		DNM2	Intermediate or CMT2; cataracts; ophthalmoplegia; ptosis
CMT2N		AARS	
CMT2P		LRSAM1	
CMT2Q		DHTKD1	
CMT2U		MARS	Late onset
CMT2V		NAGLU	Late onset painful sensory predominant
CMT2W		HARS	
CMT2Y		VCP	
CMT2Z		MORC2	Pyramidal signs
CMT2			
CMT2 with giant axons		DCAF8	Childhood onset
CMT2		TUBB3	
CMT2		DGAT2	
CMT2		JAG1	Vocal fold paralysis
SPG10, CMT2		KIF5A	
HMSNP		TFG	Proximal > distal
AR-CMT2	AR		
CMT2B1		LMNA	Also called CMT2B1 and CMT4C1
CMT2B2		MED25	
NMAN		HINT1	
CMT2R		TRIM2	
CMT2S		IGHMBP2	
CMT2T		HSJ1	
CMT2X		KIAA1840	
AR-CMT2	AR/AD	MME	Dominant mutations cause late onset
HSANs[a] and HMNs			
HSAN			Sensory (± autonomic) neuropathy
HSAN1A	AD	SPTLC1	Late onset, slowly progressive sensory axonal neuropathy ± SNHL, weakness
HSAN1B	AD	3p24-p22	Variant with cough, GERD, deafness
HSAN1C	AD	SPTLC2	
HSAN1D/SPG3A	AD	ATL1	
HSAN2A	AR	HSN2	Congenital sensory loss, acral mutilation
HSAN3	AR	IKBKAP	Severe dysautonomia, Ashkenazi Jews
HSAN4	AR	TRKA	Anhidrosis, acral mutilation, ± CNS
HSAN5	AR	NGFB	Congenital insensitivity to pain
HSAN6	AR	DST	Severe autonomic dysfunction, death by age 2
HSAN7	AD	SCN11A	Congenital insensitivity to pain, hyperhidrosis, GI dysfunction
HSAN8	AR	PRDM12	Congenital insensitivity to pain
HMN/dSMA			Distal wasting and weakness
HMNIIa	AD	HSPB8(HSP22)	Adult onset, allelic with CMT2L
HMNIIb	AD	HSP27(HSPB1)	Allelic with CMT2F
HMNVa	AD	GARS	Upper limb predominant

Continued

TABLE 62B-1 Hereditary Motor-Sensory Neuropathies Classification—cont'd

Disease	Inheritance Pattern	Gene or Locus	Clinical Features
HMNVb	AD	BSCL2	Allelic with SPG17/Silver syndrome
HMNVI	AR	IGHMBP2	Severe infantile respiratory distress/SMARD
HMNVIIa	AD	2q14	Adult onset, vocal cord paralysis
HMNVIIb	AD	DCTN1	Same as above
HMNX	X	Xq13.1-q21	
HMNJ	AR	9p21.1-p12	Childhood onset (Jerash type)
SBMA	X	Androgen receptor (CAG rpt)	Adult onset bulbar symptoms, proximal weakness, sensory neuronopathy, and gynecomastia

This table lists the inherited neuropathies that are generally considered to exclusively or predominantly affect the peripheral nerve, although as shown in the Clinical Features column, many of these diseases affect the CNS and other tissues. For the columns, in "Disease" column, name is usually abbreviated, full names below; inheritance pattern is listed as autosomal dominant (*AD*), autosomal recessive (*AR*), or X-linked (*X*); and for gene or locus, the affected gene(s) is listed if known; otherwise, the chromosomal locus is listed. In cases where the mutation is not a missense mutation, the type of mutation is listed in parentheses (duplication, deletion, or CAG repeat). The diseases are grouped according to phenotype: *HMSN*, hereditary motor and sensory neuropathy; *HS(A)N*, hereditary sensory and (± autonomic) neuropathy; *HMN*, hereditary motor neuropathy, also called dSMA (distal spinal muscular atrophy); *SBMA*, spinal bulbar and muscular atrophy. The HMSNs are further divided into demyelinating, axonal, and intermediate forms based on the usual range of nerve conduction velocity (*NCV*). *CHN*, Congenital hypomyelinating neuropathy; *CMT*, Charcot–Marie–Tooth disease; *CMTDI*, dominant intermediate CMT; *CNS*, central nervous system; *DSS*, Dejerine–Sottas disease; *GERD*, gastroesophageal reflux disease; *HNPP*, hereditary neuropathy with liability to form pressure palsies; *MCV*, motor conduction velocity; *MR*, mental retardation; *rpt*, repeat; *SMARD*, spinal muscular atrophy with respiratory distress; *SNHL*, sensorineural hearing loss; *SPG*, hereditary spastic paraplegia; *syn*, syndrome. From Motley W, Chaudry BA, Lloyd TE. Treatment and management of hereditary neuropathies. In: Bertorini TE, ed. Neuromuscular Disorders: Treatment and Management. 2nd ed. Amsterdam, Netherlands: Elsevier; 2022. Chapter 14.

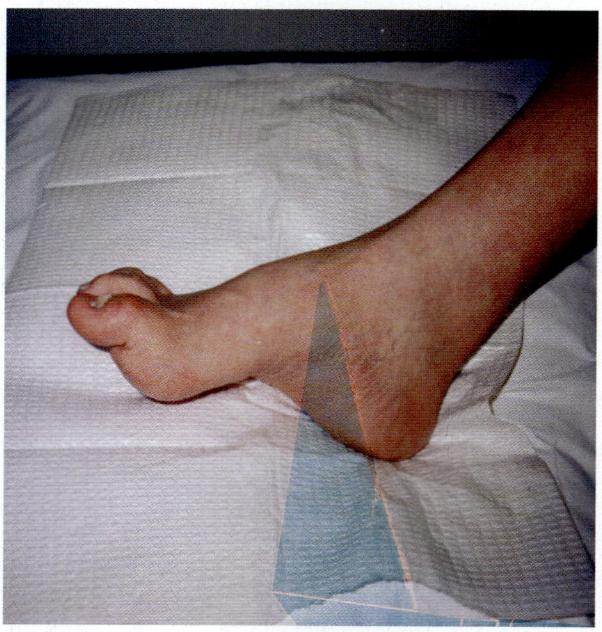

FIG. 62B-3 Foot of a patient with CMT1A. Notice high-arched foot and hammertoes. *CMT1A*, CMT type 1A.

Other Types of CMT Neuropathy

Patients with X-linked CMT (CMTX) are similar to those with CMT1A. Females are usually less affected. In some patients there could be nonuniform nerve conduction slowing. There could also be central demyelination. This disease is caused by mutations at Xq13–22, the gene that expresses connexin 32.[24–26]

Case 62B has a predominantly motor polyneuropathy and appears to have the axonal type of CMT2, **or hereditary motor and sensory neuropathy type 2 (HMSN2)**. This is a much less common condition than CMT1.

The distal weakness might involve the anterior as well as the posterior compartment with variable sensory loss, and the proximal reflexes are usually present or even hyperactive[27] until later in the disease.[28] Many cases could have a more severe neuropathy than CMT1. In some there could also be involvement of the diaphragm and vocal cords as well as the intercostal muscles. The disease can also manifest during infancy with respiratory dysfunction,[29] and in a child with no clear family history the disorder should be differentiated from the severe childhood demyelinating form, or CMT3, and from the autosomal-recessive form CMT4 (see Table 62B-1).

As in this case, the EMG in CMT2 shows normal or mildly slow conduction velocities with low-amplitude CMAPs and SNAPs. The disease is subdivided into various groups according to the genetic defects.

In some CMT2A the defect is located in the short arm of chromosome 1 at 1P33–36, which expresses kinesin family member protein 1B.[30] Most have mutations of mitofusin, whereas in CMT2B the genetic defect is located in the long arm of chromosome 3 at 3q13–22.[31,32] Another locus has been located at 19q13.3.[33]

Conventionally, those in which no genetic defect has been identified were classified as CMT2C; however, mutations in some of these patients include genes that express neurofilaments light chain, GARS, RAB7, MSP27 proteins,[34–36] and a defect of Xq24–26 (CMT2X)[37,38] (see Table 62B-1).

Pathologic studies of CMT2 demonstrate a dropout of axons, mainly of myelinated fibers with axonal atrophy and decreased myelin thickness. Occasionally, onion bulbs can be seen.

Currently, there is no cure for CMT disease. Bracing, physical therapy, and conservative management are necessary. Tendon releases and plantar fasciotomy seem to help.[39] Experimentally, an animal model of CMT1 improved with high

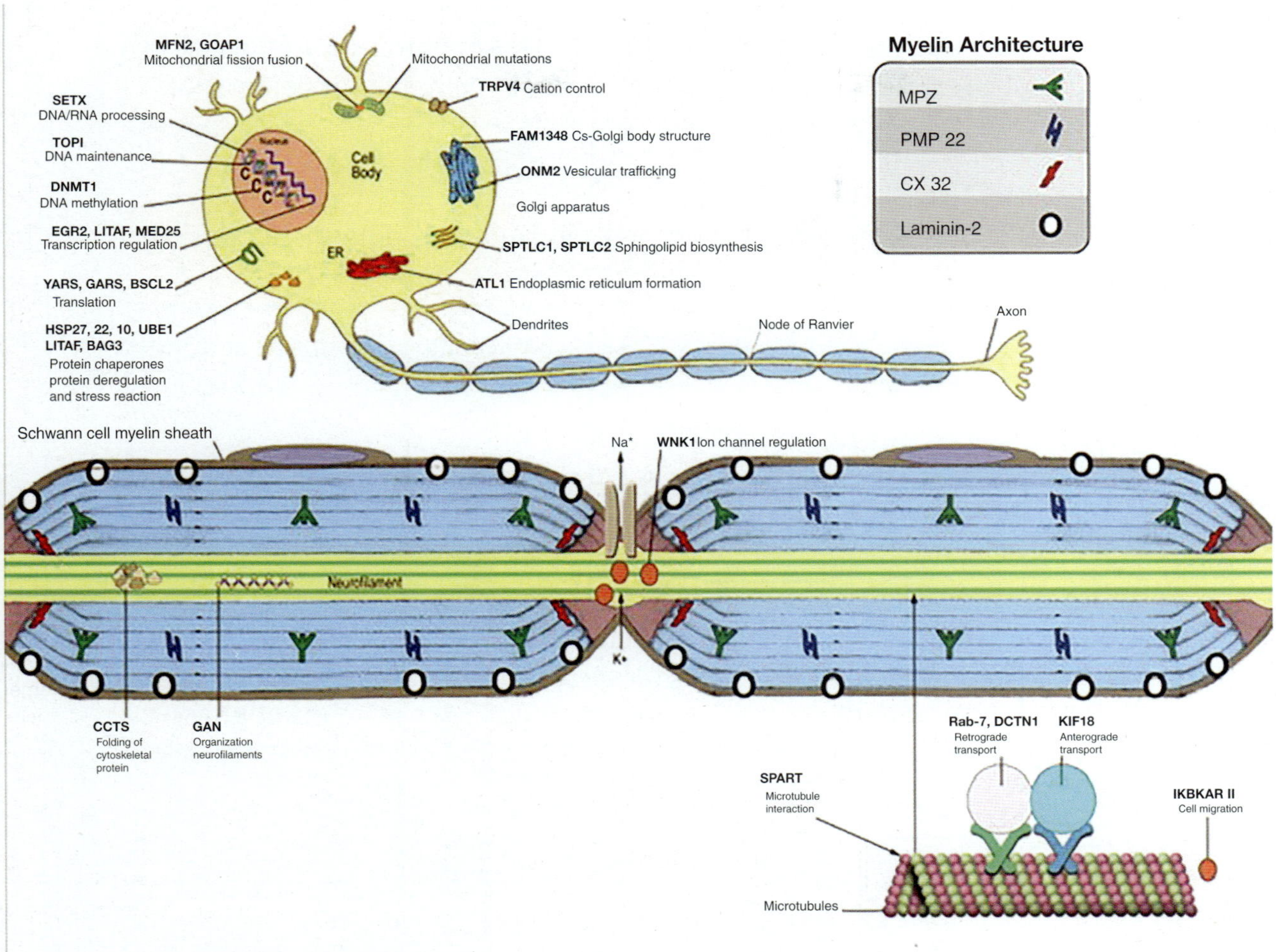

FIG. 62B-4 Diagram of the different proteins, gangliosides, and lipids associated with hereditary and autoimmune neuropathies.

doses of ascorbic acid, but this was not confirmed in a clinical trial.[40] Treadmill training is helpful.[41]

A double-blind placebo-controlled trial using Baclofen, naltrexone, and sorbitol was found to be beneficial in a controlled study.[42] Antisense oligonucleotide therapy to increase PMP22 has been beneficial in animal models[43] and CMT2D was generated by using the CRISPR/Cas9 and MiRNA; an allelic-specific delivery with a viral vector was beneficial.[44] Intrathecal gene therapy has been used in other animal models.[45]

IMPORTANT POINTS

- CMT disease can sometimes manifest with a very mild phenotype and without a positive family history.
- CMT1A disease is an autosomal-dominant disease caused by duplication in chromosome 17 of the gene that expresses myelin protein PMP22.
- CMT usually, but not always, presents with high arches, hammertoes, and atrophy in the legs.
- Electrophysiologic studies of CMT1 usually show uniform slowing of nerve conduction velocities without conduction block or temporal dispersion.
- Nerve biopsy in CMT1 shows onion bulb formation with demyelination and a decreased number of myelinated fibers.
- Conduction block and temporal dispersion occur in acquired neuropathies, such as CIDP or vasculitic neuropathy, and can be observed in some hereditary neuropathies, such as CMTX and HNPP (in sites of entrapment).
- CMT2 is an axonal neuropathy presenting with muscle weakness and variable sensory loss. Reflexes, particularly the proximal reflexes, are preserved until later. The condition has variable phenotypes but can be more severe than CMT1.
- Most cases of CMT are autosomal-dominant, although X-linked recessive cases have been reported.
- Some patients with CMT2 might present with diaphragmatic and vocal cord paralysis.
- In CMT2, motor nerve conduction velocities are normal or almost normal, but CMAPs, SNAPs, and amplitudes are decreased or absent. There is variable evidence of denervation on EMG.
- Nerve biopsy in CMT2 shows axonal atrophy and dropout of myelinated axons and only occasionally are there onion bulbs.
- Genetic testing is useful; however, tests for all recognized mutations are not commercially available.
- There is no cure for CMT; bracing, fasciotomy, and tendon releases can help. A combination of Baclofen, sorbitol, and naltrexone appears to help CMT1A.

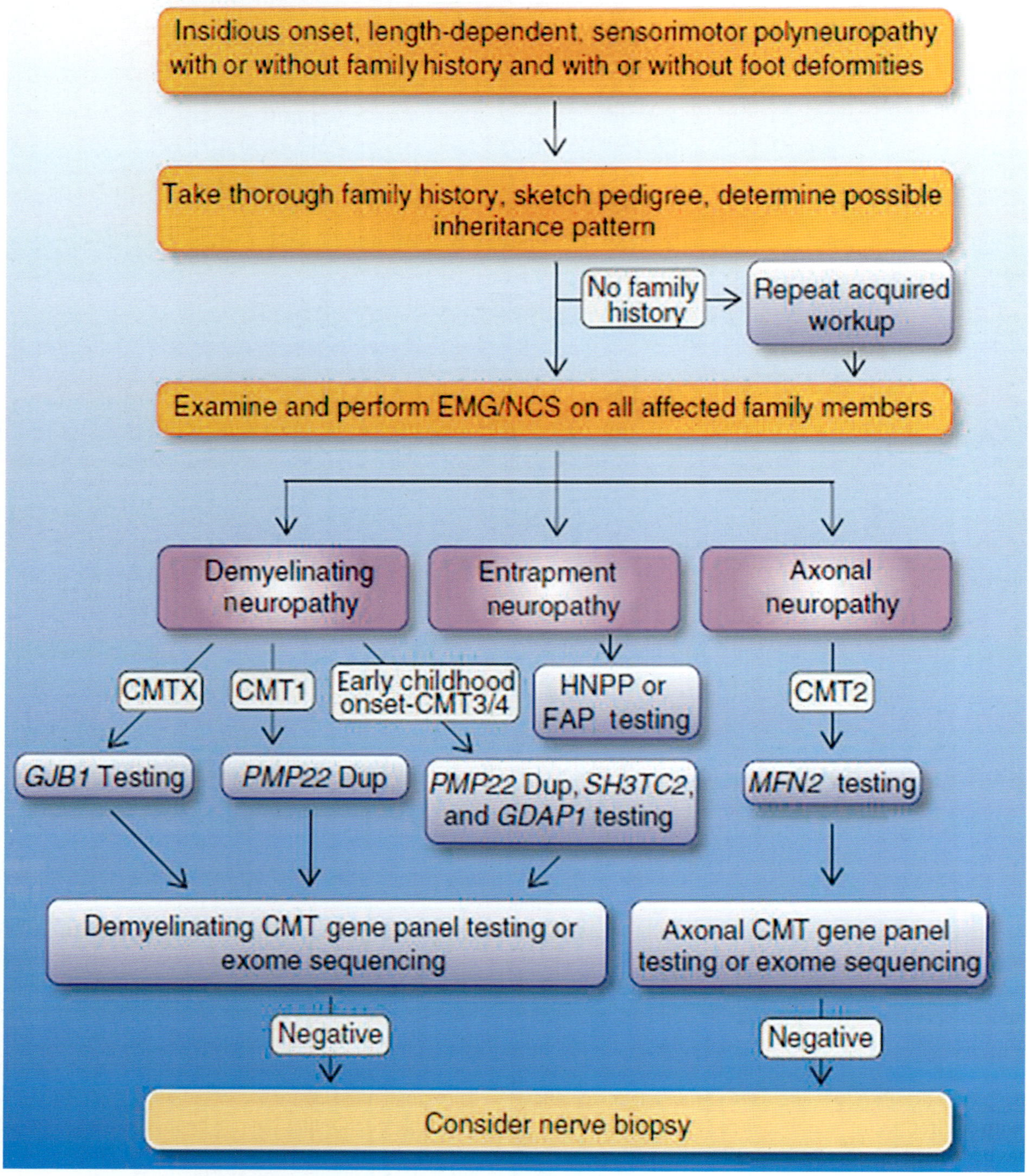

FIG. 62B-5 An algorithm used to diagnose in suspected cases of Charcot–Marie–Tooth Disease.

REFERENCES

1. Charcot J-M, Marie P. Sur une forme particuliere d'atrophie musculaire progressive souvent familial debutant par less pieds et less jambes et atteignant plus tard less mains. *Rev Med.* 1886;6:97–138.
2. Tooth HH. *The Peroneal Type of Progressive Muscular Atrophy.* London, England: HK Lewis; 1886:97–138.
3. Pareyson D. Charcot-Marie-Tooth disease and related neuropathies: molecular basis for distinction and diagnosis. *Muscle Nerve.* 1999;22: 1498–1509.
4. Dyck PJ. Inherited neuronal degeneration and atrophy affecting motor sensory and autonomic neurons. In: Dyck PJ, Thomas PK, Lambert EH, eds. *Peripheral Neuropathy.* Vol. 2. Philadelphia, PA: WB Saunders; 1970:825.
5. Davis CJ, Bradley WG, Madrid R. The peroneal muscular atrophy syndrome: clinical, genetic, electrophysiologic and nerve biopsy studies. *J Genet Hum.* 1978;26(4):311–349.
6. Harding AE, Thomas PK. The clinical feature of hereditary motor and sensory neuropathy types I and II. *Brain.* 1980;103:259–280.

7. Brust JC, Lovelace RE, Devi S. Clinical and electrophysiologic features of Charcot-Marie-Tooth syndrome. *Acta Neurol Scand Suppl*. 1976;68:1–142.
8. Kaku DA, Parry GJ, Malamut R, et al. Uniform slowing of conduction velocities in Charcot-Marie-Tooth polyneuropathy type 1. *Neurology*. 1993;43:2664–2667.
9. Mendell JR. Charcot-Marie-Tooth neuropathies and related disorders. *Semin Neurol*. 1998;18:41–47.
10. Dyck PJ, Gutrecht JA, Bastron JA, et al. Histologic and teased-fiber measurements of sural nerve disorders of lower motor and primary sensory neuron. *Mayo Clin Proc*. 1968;43:81–123.
11. Dyck PJ, Lambert EH. Lower motor and primary sensory neuron diseases with peroneal muscular atrophy, I: neurologic, genetic, and electrophysiologic findings in hereditary polyneuropathies. *Arch Neurol*. 1968;18(6):603–606.
12. Vance JM, Barker D, Yamaoka LH, et al. Localization of Charcot-Marie-Tooth disease type 1a (CMT1A) to chromosome 17p11.2. *Genomics*. 1991;9:623–628.
13. Raeymaekers P, Timmerman V, Nelis E, et al. Duplication in chromosome 17p11.2 in Charcot-Marie-Tooth neuropathy type 1a (CMT1a): the HMSN Collaborative Research Group. *Neuromuscul Disord*. 1991;1:93–97.
14. Raeymaekers P, Timmerman V, Nelis E, et al. Estimation of the size of chromosome 17p11.2 duplication in Charcot-Marie-tooth neuropathy. *J Med Genet*. 1992;29:5–11.
15. Editorial Dose response in Charcot-Marie-Tooth disease. *Nat Genet*. 1992;1:153–154.
16. Upadhyaya M, Roberts SH, Farnharm J, et al. Charcot-Marie-Tooth disease 1A (CMT1A) associated with a maternal duplication of chromosome 17p11.2–12. *Hum Genet*. 1993;91:392–394.
17. Bertorini TE, Narayanaswami P, Rashed H. Charcot-Marie-Tooth disease (hereditary motor sensory neuropathies) and hereditary sensory and autonomic neuropathies. *Neurologist*. 2004;10(6):327–337.
18. Hayasaka K, Himoro M, Sato W, et al. Charcot-Marie-Tooth neuropathy type 1B is associated with mutations of the myelin PO gene. *Nat Genet*. 1993;5:31–34.
19. Stebbins NB, Conneally PM. Linkage of dominantly inherited Charcot-Marie-Tooth neuropathy to the Duffy locus in an Indiana family. *Am J Hum Genet*. 1982;34:195A.
20. Lagueny A, Latour P, Vital A, et al. Peripheral myelin modification in CMT 1B correlates with MPZ gene mutations. *Neuromuscul Disord*. 1999;9:361–367.
21. Joseph LJ, Le Beau MM, Jamieson GA, et al. Molecular cloning, sequencing, and mapping of EGR2, a human early growth response gene encoding a protein with "zinc-binding finger" structure. *Proc Natl Acad Sci USA*. 1988;85:7164–7168.
22. Warner LE, Mancias P, Butler IJ, et al. Mutations in the early growth response 2 (EGR2) gene is associated with hereditary myelinopathies. *Nat Genet*. 1998;18:382–384.
23. Street VA, Bennett CL, Goldy JD, et al. Mutation of a putative protein degradation gene LITAF/SIMPLE in Charcot-Marie-Tooth disease 1C. *Neurology*. 2003;60(1):22–26.
24. Bergoffen J, Trofatter J, Pericak-Vance M, et al. Linkage localization of X-linked Charcot-Marie-Tooth disease. *Am J Hum Genet*. 1993; 52:312–318.
25. Erwin WG. A pedigree of sex-linked recessive peroneal atrophy. *J Hered*. 1944;35:24–26.
26. Hahn AF, Brown WF, Koopman WJ, Feasby TE. X-linked dominant hereditary motor and sensory neuropathy. *Brain*. 1990;113:1511–1525.
27. Bienfait HM, Baas F, Koelman JH, et al. Phenotype of Charcot-Marie-Tooth disease Type 2. *Neurology*. 2007;68(20):1658–1667.
28. Lupski JR, Garcia CA. Charcot-Marie-Tooth peripheral neuropathies and related disorders. In: Scriver CR, Beaudet AL, Sly WS, Valle D, eds. *The Metabolic and Molecular Bases of Inherited Disease*. 8th ed. New York, NY: McGraw-Hill; 2001: 5759–5788.
29. Davis CJF, Bradley WG, Madrid R. The peroneal muscular atrophy syndrome (clinical, genetic, electrophysiologic and nerve biopsy studies). *J Genet Hum*. 1978;26:311.
30. Mendell JR. Charcot-Marie-Tooth neuropathies and related disorders. *Semin Neurol*. 1998;18:41–47.
31. Hentati A, Lamy C, Melki J, et al. Clinical and genetic heterogeneity of Charcot-Marie-Tooth disease. *Genomic*. 1992;12(1): 155–157.
32. Kwon JM, Elliott JL, Yee W, et al. Assignment of a second Charcot-Marie-Tooth type II locus to chromosome 3q. *Am J Hum Genet*. 1995;57:853–858.
33. Leal A, Morera B, Del Valle G, et al. A second locus for an axonal form of autosomal recessive Charcot-Marie-Tooth disease maps to chromosome 19q13.3. *Am J Hum Genet*. 2001;68:269–274.
34. Klein CJ, Cunningham JM, Atkinson EJ, et al. The gene for HMSN2C maps to 12q23–24: a region of neuromuscular disorders. *Neurology*. 2003;60(7):1151–1156.
35. Ionasescu V, Searby C, Sheffield VC, et al. Autosomal dominant Charcot-Marie-Tooth axonal neuropathy mapped on chromosome 7p (CMT2D). *Hum Mol Genet*. 1996;5(9):1373–1375.
36. Nicholson GA. The dominantly inherited motor and sensory neuropathies: clinical and molecular advances. *Muscle Nerve*. 2006;33(50):589–597.
37. Priest JM, Fischbeck KH, Nouri N, Keats BJ. A locus for axonal motor sensory neuropathy with deafness and mental retardation maps to Xq24–26. *Genomics*. 1995;29:409–412.
38. Motley W, Chaudry BA, Lloyd TE. Treatment and management of hereditary neuropathies. In: Bertorini TE, ed. *Neuromuscular Disorders: Treatment and Management*. Amsterdam, Netherlands: Elsevier; 2022. 2nd ed. Chapter 14.
39. Warner WC. Orthopedic surgery in neuromuscular disorders. In: Bertorini TE, ed. *Neuromuscular Disorders: Treatment and Management*. Amsterdam, Netherlands: Elsevier; 2022. 2nd ed. Chapter 9.
40. Pareyson D, Reilly MM, Schenone A, Fabrizi GM, et al. Ascorbic acid in Charcot-Marie-Tooth disease type 1A (CMT-TRIAAL and CMT-TRAUK): a double-blind randomized trial. *Lancet Neurol*. 2011;10(4):320–328.
41. Mori L, Signori A, Prada V, Pareyson D, et al. Treadmill training in patients affected by Charcot-Marie-Tooth neuropathy: results of a multicenter, prospective, randomized, single-blind, controlled study. *Eur J Neurol*. 2020;27(2):280–287. https://doi.org/10.1111/ene.14074.
42. Attarian S, Young P, Brannagan TH, Adams D, et al. A double-blind, placebo-controlled, randomized trial of PXT3003 for the treatment of Charcot-Marie-Tooth type 1. *Orphanet J Rare Dis*. 2021;16(1):433.
43. Zhao HT, Damie S, Ikeda-Lee K, Kuntz S, et al. PMP22 antisense oligonucleotides reverse Charcot-Marie-Tooth disease type 1A features in rodent models. *J Clin Invest*. 2018;128(1):359–368. https://doi.org/10.1172/JCI96499. Epub 2017 Dec 4.
44. Morelli KH, Griffin LB, Pyne NK, Wallace LM, et al. Allele-specific RNA interference prevents neuropathy in Charcot-Marie-Tooth disease type 2D mouse models. *J Clin Invest*. 2019;129(12):5568–5583. https://doi.org/10.1172/JCI130600.
45. Lutz C, Pressa M, Davis C, Cook J, et al. Preclinical gene therapy in a mouse model of Charcot-Marie-Tooth disease type 4J. *Mol Genet Metab*. 2019;126(2):896–897.

63 CASE

A Man With Hand Weakness and Numbness After Skiing

A 45-year-old man had been in good health until right after he was snow skiing in Colorado, at which time he felt numb and weak in his hands; these symptoms progressed over the following week. He went to the emergency room where he had a CT scan of the head and an MRI, which were normal. He then had an EMG that showed a "polyneuropathy" and a lumbar puncture that showed elevated spinal fluid protein, and he received intravenous IgG treatment, but his hands remained numb and weak. He denied weakness in his legs. The patient was referred to us for evaluation.

Past medical history included numbness in the right calf 25 years before and a history of numbness in the ulnar nerve distribution 5 years before; both improved without treatment.

He was an attorney, drank alcohol on occasion, and did not smoke. Family history was noncontributory. His medications included allopurinol for hyperuricemia and simvastatin for mild hyperlipidemia.

Examination revealed mild weakness in the interosseous muscles of the hands but significant weakness in the abductor pollicis brevis (APB) muscles with mild atrophy of both thenar eminences. Other muscles of the upper and lower extremities were normal. Reflexes were 1+ in the upper extremities and knee and trace at the ankles. There was no nerve hypertrophy or fasciculations. Vibration sense was absent at the toes and diminished at the ankles; this was normal in the fingers. There was decreased pain and touch sensations up to the ankle on the right and 4–6 cm above the ankle on the left as well as diminished pain sensation in both median nerve distributions. He had positive Phalen and Tinel tests on the right median nerve at the wrist. He had no high arches. The rest of the examination was normal.

AN EMG TEST WAS PERFORMED

Motor Nerve Studies

Nerve and Site	Latency (ms)	Amplitude (mV)	Conduction Velocity (m/s)
Peroneal Nerve R.	**Normal ≤ 5.7**	**Normal ≥ 3**	**Normal ≥ 40**
Ankle	5.7	4	–
Fibular head	15.6	3	**36**
Knee	17.8	3	**39**

Motor Nerve Studies—cont'd

Nerve and Site	Latency (ms)	Amplitude (mV)	Conduction Velocity (m/s)
Tibial Nerve L.	**Normal ≤ 5.3**	**Normal ≥ 4**	**Normal ≥ 40**
Ankle	4.7	4	–
Pop. fossa	18.7	2	**33**
Median Nerve R.	**Normal ≤ 4.2**	**Normal ≥ 6**	**Normal ≥ 50**
Wrist	**5.2**	10	–
Elbow	11.0	9	**47**
Ulnar Nerve R.	**Normal ≤ 3.6**	**Normal ≥ 8**	**Normal ≥ 50**
Wrist	**4.1**	13	–
Below elbow	9.6	11	**47**
Above elbow	14.1	9	**27**
Axilla	17.7	8	**39**
Median Nerve L.	**Normal ≤ 4.2**	**Normal ≥ 6**	**Normal ≥ 40**
Wrist	**6.1**	7	–
Elbow	11.7	7	**43**

F-Wave and Tibial H-Reflex Studies

Nerve	Latency (ms)	Normal Latency ≤ (ms)
Peroneal nerve R.	**78.0**	54
Tibial nerve L.	**66.4**	54
Median nerve R.	**34.1**	30
Ulnar nerve R.	29.5	30
Median nerve L.	**36.0**	30
H-reflex R.	**45.2**	34
H-reflex L.	**46.7**	34

Sensory Nerve Studies

Nerve	Onset Latency (ms)	Normal Onset Latency ≤ (ms)	Peak Latency (ms)	Normal Peak Latency ≤ (ms)	Amp (μV)	Normal Amp ≥ (μV)	Conduction Velocity (m/s)	Normal Conduction Velocity ≥ (m/s)
Sural nerve R.	**NR**	3.5	**NR**	4.0	**NR**	11	**NR**	40
Superficial peroneal R.	**NR**	3.5	**NR**	10	**NR**	8–11	**NR**	40
Median nerve R.	**3.5**	2.6	**4.0**	3.1	**8**	20	**37**	50
Median nerve L.	**3.6**	2.6	**4.1**	3.1	**5**	13	**36**	50

EMG Data

Muscle	Insrt Activity	Fibs	Pos Waves	Fasc	Amp	Dur	Poly	Pattern
Biceps brachii R.	Norm	None	None	None	Norm	Norm	None	Full
Flexor carpi radialis R.	Norm	None	None	None	Norm	Norm	None	Full
Flexor carpi ulnaris R.	Norm	None	None	None	Norm	Norm	None	Full
First dorsal interosseous R.	Norm	None	None	None	**Lg**	**Inc**	None	**Red**
Abductor pollicis brevis R.	Norm	None	None	None	**Lg**	**Inc**	None	**Red**
Abductor pollicis brevis L.	Norm	None	None	None	**Lg**	**Inc**	None	**Red**
Vastus lateralis R.	Norm	None	None	None	**Lg**	**Inc**	None	Full
Tibialis anterior R.	Norm	None	None	None	**Lg**	**Inc**	None	**Red**
Gastrocnemius R.	Norm	None	None	None	Norm	Norm	None	Full

WHAT WERE THE EMG FINDINGS?

This test showed a diffuse polyneuropathy with mild slowing of motor conduction velocities, but there was also a significant slowing in areas of compression, such as the ulnar nerve across the elbow, and prolonged median distal motor latencies. Median nerve SNAPs were prolonged and of low amplitude.

There was also prolongation of the F-latencies in the left median tibial nerves and the right peroneal nerve. H-reflexes were also prolonged. There were large motor unit potentials, but no denervation in both APB nerves. Some large motor unit potentials were seen in the first dorsal interosseous muscle and leg muscles indicating a mild, chronic axonal involvement with reinnervation.

WHAT IS THE LIKELY DIAGNOSIS?

This patient presented with numbness in the hands in the distribution of the median nerves making the diagnosis a medial neuropathy, most likely from a carpal tunnel syndrome, which could have been aggravated by pressure during skiing and caused by acute compression. This was superimposed onto a sensorimotor polyneuropathy. Familial amyloidosis can present with carpal tunnel syndrome and diffuse polyneuropathy, but this is mainly an axonal sensorimotor polyneuropathy without other significant entrapments. He previously had symptoms in the ulnar nerve distribution and in the right leg that suggested a focal peripheral nerve involvement, although this was not documented. The presentation suggests the possibility of hereditary neuropathy with liability to pressure palsy (HNPP), despite the lack of family history.

Chronic inflammatory demyelinating polyradiculoneuropathy could also have been considered, but he had no generalized weakness or areflexia, and electrophysiologic tests showed no evidence of significant slowing on conduction studies, as this was prominent only at sites of entrapment.

Another possibility is an alcoholic neuropathy with superimposed carpal tunnel syndrome, but he did not drink much and had no history of progressive sensory complaints or leg weakness.

He could also have had a neuropathy associated with hyperlipidemia or caused by cholesterol-lowering agents, but these are predominantly sensory neuropathies without prominent entrapments.

WHAT WOULD BE THE NEXT TEST?

DNA testing for HNPP mutation revealed a deletion in one allele in the *PMP22* gene in chromosome 17, and it was concluded that this patient had HNPP.

SUMMARY

This patient developed bilateral median neuropathy at the wrist after snow skiing. He had electrophysiologic evidence of a polyneuropathy with significant slowing of the sites of entrapment. This was likely precipitated or aggravated by low temperature and compression from the skiing poles.

He was diagnosed as having HNPP by DNA testing in spite of a negative family history.

For further discussion, important points, and references, see Case 64.

64 CASE

A Man With Recurrent Foot Drop

A 44-year-old man presented with a 2-day history of tingling and weakness in the left leg. He had been seen 2 years previously for intermittent tingling and numbness in the hands. A detailed workup at that time indicated ulnar and median nerve entrapments at the elbows and wrists, respectively, which were treated conservatively. Two months prior to the current episode, he developed tingling in the right leg with some weakness which improved spontaneously. His past medical history was significant for foot drop as a child, for which he had to use crutches that produced muscle atrophy in his hands and pectoralis muscles, and these improved eventually. He was on paroxetine for depression. He smoked one pack of cigarettes per day and used to drink alcohol but quit 2 years ago.

General, mental, and cranial nerve examinations were normal. Motor examination revealed mild interossei muscle weakness in both hands. There was weakness on right foot dorsiflexion and eversion and ankle dorsiflexors and toe extensors on the left lower extremity. Reflexes were 2+ in both upper extremities and knees and 2 at the ankles. Sensory examination showed decreased pain sensation in a stocking-and-glove distribution and hypoesthesia in the left common peroneal nerve distribution with bilateral decrease in vibration sensation in the toes. There was thickening of the ulnar nerves. Cerebellar tests and the rest of the examination were normal.

WHAT IS THE DIFFERENTIAL DIAGNOSIS?

The patient had a polyneuropathy and right foot dorsiflexors, evertors, and toe dorsiflexion weakness.

Unilateral foot drop can be caused by disorders of the corticospinal tracts, as in multiple sclerosis, by compressive myelopathy, or by amyotrophic lateral sclerosis and other motor neuron diseases that are ruled out clinically. Besides those, the differential diagnosis includes an L5 radiculopathy, lumbosacral plexopathy, focal neuropathy of the peroneal division of the sciatic nerve, and the common or deep peroneal nerves, either as a mononeuropathy or as manifestations of mononeuritis multiplex (Tables 64-1 and 64-2).

Once the examination localizes the lesion, other studies, such as EMG and imaging, are helpful in ascertaining these findings (Table 64-3).

WHAT TESTS ARE INDICATED IN THIS CASE?

In this case, it was important to check for diabetes which could cause a polyneuropathy and mononeuritis multiplex. Complete blood count, basic metabolic panel, and glycosylated hemoglobin and liver function tests were normal. Vitamin B_{12}/folate levels were normal. Erythrocyte sedimentation rate and antinuclear antibody tests were negative. Serum immune electrophoresis was normal without evidence of monoclonal proteins. Cerebrospinal fluid studies showed no cells, and a total protein of 65 mg/dL; immunology (IgG index) was normal.

AN EMG TEST WAS PERFORMED

Motor Nerve Studies

Nerve and Site	Latency (ms)	Amplitude (mV)	Conduction Velocity (m/s)
Peroneal Nerve L.	**Normal ≤ 5.7**	**Normal ≥ 3**	**Normal ≥ 40**
Ankle	**9.1**	**0.78**	–
Fibular head	17.9	**0.62**	**35**
Knee	20.2	**0.12**	48
Tibial Nerve R.	**Normal ≤ 5.3**	**Normal ≥ 4**	**Normal ≥ 40**
Ankle	4.4	12	–
Pop. fossa	14.1	8	45
Median Nerve L.	**Normal ≤ 4.2**	**Normal ≥ 6**	**Normal ≥ 50**
Wrist	**5.7**	22	–
Elbow	10.2	21	54
Ulnar Nerve L.	**Normal ≤ 3.6**	**Normal ≥ 8**	**Normal ≥ 50**
Wrist	**3.7**	10	–
Below elbow	8.4	8	51
Above elbow	11.7	8	**36**
Axilla	14.2	**7**	58
Erb's point	17.5	**6**	67
Nerve and Site	**Latency (ms)**	**Amplitude (mV)**	**Conduction Velocity (m/s)**
Peroneal Nerve R.	**Normal ≤ 5.7**	**Normal ≥ 3**	**Normal ≥ 40**
Ankle	**6.8**	5	–
Fibular head	14.7	4	41
Knee	17.3	3	**35**

Motor Nerve Studies—cont'd

Ulnar Nerve R.	Normal ≤ 3.6	Normal ≥ 8	Normal ≥ 50
Wrist	3.6	11	–
Below elbow	8.3	9	**48**
Above elbow	10.9	8	**46**
Axilla	13.3	8	50
Erb's point	16.2	**6**	74

F-Wave and Tibial H-Reflex Studies

Nerve	Latency (ms)	Normal Latency ≤ (ms)
Peroneal nerve L.	**NR**	54
Tibial nerve L.	49.6	54
Median nerve L.	**32.6**	30
Ulnar nerve L.	**34.7**	30
Peroneal nerve R.	53.3	54
Ulnar nerve R.	**31.8**	30
H-reflex L.	**36.5**	34
H-reflex R.	**35.3**	34

Sensory Nerve Studies

Nerve	Onset Latency (ms)	Normal Onset Latency ≤ (ms)	Peak Latency (ms)	Normal Peak Latency ≤ (ms)	Amp (μV)	Normal Amp ≥ (μV)	Conduction Velocity (m/s)	Normal Conduction Velocity ≥ (m/s)
Sural nerve L.	**3.6**	3.5	**4.1**	4.0	**9**	11	40	40
Median nerve L.	**3.5**	2.6	**4.1**	3.1	**14**	20	**37**	50
Ulnar nerve L.	**3.9**	2.6	**3.5**	3.1	**9**	13	**31**	50

EMG Data

Muscle	Insrt Activity	Fibs	Pos Waves	Fasc	Amp	Dur	Poly	Pattern
Cervical paraspinals L.	Norm	None	None	None	Norm	Norm	None	Full
Biceps brachii L.	Norm	None	None	None	Norm	Norm	None	Full
Flexor carpi radialis L.	Norm	None	None	None	Norm	Norm	None	Full
Flexor carpi ulnaris L.	Norm	None	None	None	Norm	Norm	**Few**	Full
Brachioradialis L.	Norm	None	None	None	Norm	Norm	None	Full
Extensor digitorum communis L.	Norm	None	None	None	Norm	Norm	None	Full
Extensor carpi ulnaris L.	Norm	None	None	None	Norm	Norm	None	Full
Abductor pollicis brevis L.	Norm	None	None	None	**Lg**	**Inc**	None	Full
Abductor digiti minimi L.	Norm	None	None	None	**Lg**	**Inc**	None	Full
First dorsal interosseous L.	Norm	None	None	None	Norm	Norm	None	Full
Vastus lateralis L.	Norm	None	None	None	Norm	Norm	None	Full
Biceps femoris—short head L.	Norm	None	None	None	Norm	Norm	None	Full
Tibialis anterior L.	**Inc**	**1+**	**1+**	None	**Lg**	**Inc**	None	Red
Peroneus longus L.	**Inc**	**2+**	**2+**	None	**Lg**	**Inc**	None	Red
Gastrocnemius L.	Norm	None	None	Norm	Norm	Norm	None	Full

TABLE 64-1 Conditions That Can Cause Asymmetric Foot Drop

Lesions involving the corticospinal tract (stroke, multiple sclerosis, and myelopathies)
Motor neuron diseases (amyotrophic lateral sclerosis {ALS}, progressive spinal muscular atrophy)
Radiculopathies, particularly L5
Lumbosacral plexopathies
Mononeuropathies, particularly of the peroneal nerve but also the sciatic nerve

WHAT WERE THE EMG FINDINGS?

EMG and nerve conduction studies showed prolongation of distal motor latencies in some of the nerves with relatively preserved amplitudes, suggestive of a primary demyelination.

TABLE 64-2 Neuropathies That Could Cause Unilateral Peroneal Nerve Palsy

Peroneal nerve injury/trauma/compression, particularly in patients with an underlying polyneuropathy, that is, diabetic, uremic
Mononeuritis multiplex (vasculitis/idiopathic/diabetic)
HNPP
Lepromatous leprosy
Sarcoidosis
Vasculitis
MADSAM or the Lewis–Sumner syndrome
MAMA
Trauma
Tumors (i.e., neuromas)
Compressions

HNPP, Hereditary neuropathy with liability to pressure palsy; *MADSAM*, multifocal acquired demyelinating sensory and motor neuropathy; *MAMA*, multifocal acquired motor axonopathy.

TABLE 64-3 Neuromuscular Conditions Associated With Foot Drop, Clinical Findings, and Electrophysiologic Features

Conditions	Clinical Findings	Electrophysiologic Features
Motor neuron disease	Affect different muscles with fasciculations, bulbar muscle weakness could show long tract signs	Normal SNAPs and motor conduction tests, proximal latency; CMAPs could be of low amplitude, diffuse fibrillations, fasciculations.
L5 radiculopathy	Affect tibialis anterior Extensor hallucis Peronei muscles Tibialis posterior Gluteal muscles Tensor fasciae latae	SNAPs are normal, peroneal F latencies may be prolonged; EMG: paraspinal muscle may show denervation potentials, studies of the affected muscles are abnormal, normal motor conduction tests.
Lumbosacral plexopathy	Affect tibialis anterior Extensor hallucis Peronei muscles Tibialis posterior Tensor fasciae latae Gluteal, hamstring muscles	NCS: CMAPs of low amplitude, F latencies may be prolonged. Abnormal superficial peroneal SNAP while sural SNAP could be normal or abnormal. EMG: denervation in affected muscles, not paraspinal muscles. Poor recruitment of MUAPs and fibrillation potentials at rest in muscles supplied by the anterior rami of L5 spinal nerve.
Sciatic nerve (peroneal portion)	Affect tibialis anterior Extensor hallucis, extensor digitorum brevis, peronei muscles, and short head of biceps femoris	NCS: peroneal CMAPs may have a low amplitude or can be normal. F latencies may be prolonged. Abnormal superficial peroneal SNAP, while sural SNAP is usually normal. EMG: peroneal innervated muscles and the short head of biceps are abnormal. Other muscles such as glutei and paraspinals are normal.
Common peroneal nerve lesions	Affect tibialis anterior Extensor hallucis Peronei muscles Extensor digitorum brevis	NCS: peroneal CMAP may have a low amplitude or can be normal. Conduction block may be present at the knee, peroneal F latencies may be prolonged. Superficial peroneal SNAP can be abnormal. EMG: study of peronei muscles is abnormal with normal short head of biceps, hamstrings, and paraspinals.
Deep peroneal nerve lesions	Affect tibialis anterior Extensor hallucis Extensor digitorum brevis	NCS: peroneal CMAP may have a low amplitude. Conduction block may be present at the knee, peroneal F latencies may be prolonged, superficial peroneal SNAP is normal. EMG: study of the extensor hallucis muscle and tibialis anterior is abnormal while the peronei muscles are normal.

MUAPs, Motor unit action potentials; *NCS*, nerve conduction studies.

There was also peroneal nerve entrapment on the left side with some secondary axonal degeneration. There was slowing of the right ulnar nerve across and below the elbow and of the left ulnar nerve at the elbow. This picture was not suggestive of a length-dependent symmetrical neuropathy, since the tibial nerve conduction was completely normal with abnormal peroneal nerve conductions. The F-latency prolongation, seen in some nerves, was also suggestive of a mixed primary demyelinating process. The superficial peroneal nerve was not studied. The SNAPs of the other nerves were of low amplitude. The needle test showed denervation potentials in the left common peroneal nerve-innervated muscles. In conclusion, this patient had a demyelinating polyneuropathy with a superimposed peroneal neuropathy, with axonal degeneration. There was conduction slowing at sites of compression.

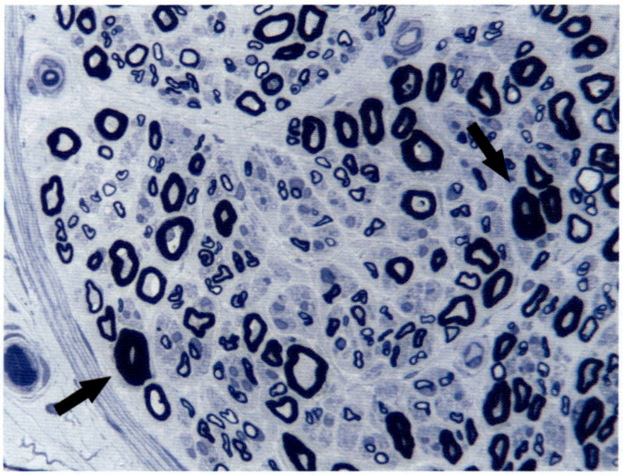

FIG. 64-1 Axons with thickened myelin (*arrows*) seen on the plastic embedded section (toluidine blue stain, ×400).

WHAT IS THE MOST LIKELY DIAGNOSIS?

This patient had acute onset of left foot drop from a common peroneal neuropathy. He had a similar episode and arm weakness as a child and episodes suggestive of compression neuropathies followed by spontaneous recovery. His EMG and nerve conduction studies were consistent with a polyneuropathy with prolongation or slowing *at sites of compression*, such as the median nerve at the wrist, ulnar nerve at the elbow, and peroneal nerve at the knee.

Given the very long recurrent history and the negative workup for vasculitis, DNA testing for hereditary neuropathy with liability to pressure palsy (HNPP) was done using Southern blot analysis and was reported as "inconclusive." For this reason a sural nerve biopsy was studied. The sample provided was not large enough for a teased nerve preparation, which would have shown the tomaculae characteristic of HNPP. There was, however, evidence of myelinated fiber dropout, and a few axons had thick myelin, which was highly suggestive of the disease (Fig. 64-1).

DNA testing was repeated after 1 year by restriction endonuclease digestion and Southern blot analysis on pulsed-field gel-electrophoresed genomic DNA on whole blood. This was significant for deletion in one allele in the peripheral myelin protein (*PMP22*) gene diagnostic of HNPP. The reason for the lack of diagnosis in the initial test is not clear, but likely an improved technology and better probes used allowed for a more definitive diagnosis. Another test used in detecting this disease is PCR amplification and automatic sequencing; this test, however, could also miss some deletions; thus, when the disease is strongly suspected, both tests need to be done if the results in one are inconclusive.

SUMMARY

This patient had recurrent entrapment neuropathies since childhood. His EMG and nerve conduction studies were consistent with a polyneuropathy and an acute common peroneal neuropathy. The polyneuropathy was mixed demyelinating and axonal with a slowing of conduction at sites of entrapment. He did not have a significant family history, although DNA testing confirmed the deletion in the *PMP22* gene. His sural nerve biopsy showed some axons with thickened myelin sheets. He was diagnosed as having HNPP.

DISCUSSION (CASES 63 AND 64)

Cases 63 and *64* have HNPP, a disease first described by De Jong in 1947 as a generalized demyelinating neuropathy, clinically characterized by recurrent painless focal neuropathies.[1] This is an autosomal-dominant disease with a high penetrance but variable expression. It has a prevalence of about 16 per 100,000,[2,3] but the condition is largely underrecognized.[4,5] The symptoms usually begin in the second or third decade, but occasionally the first episode occurs in childhood, and there is intrafamilial variability.[6] Persistent neurological deficits are uncommon. HNPP may be associated with pes cavus and hypo- or areflexia. Sometimes patients with a more severe phenotype, however, progress to a generalized neuropathy, similar to Charcot–Marie–Tooth disease type 1 (CMT1) (i.e., hereditary motor and sensory neuropathy type 1),[3] which is allelic, but this is rare.[7,8] Other manifestations of HNPP include diaphragmatic paralysis, laryngeal paralysis, weakness of muscles innervated by the spinal accessory nerve, or peroneal palsy after weight loss. Tarsal tunnel syndrome and radial nerve palsy also occur.[9–12]

Brachial neuritis is another manifestation of HNPP.[13] This usually presents with weakness of the shoulder girdle without pain (unlike the acquired form of brachial neuritis) but with electrophysiologic evidence of involvement of other nerves. The condition should be differentiated from hereditary neuralgic amyotrophy, which also causes recurrent brachial neuropathy, without pain, but it has dystrophic features and is caused by a different genetic defect.[14]

Careful electrophysiologic tests should be used to make a reliable diagnosis, even in asymptomatic patients, based on studies correlating clinical, electrophysiologic, and molecular genetic findings in families.[6,9,11] Segmental demyelination and remyelination are found in sural nerve biopsies; the most striking feature is the presence of focally thickened myelin sheaths in teased fiber preparations, referred to as tomaculae or "sausage-like" formations (Fig. 64-2) which are considered characteristic for HNPP.[6–9]

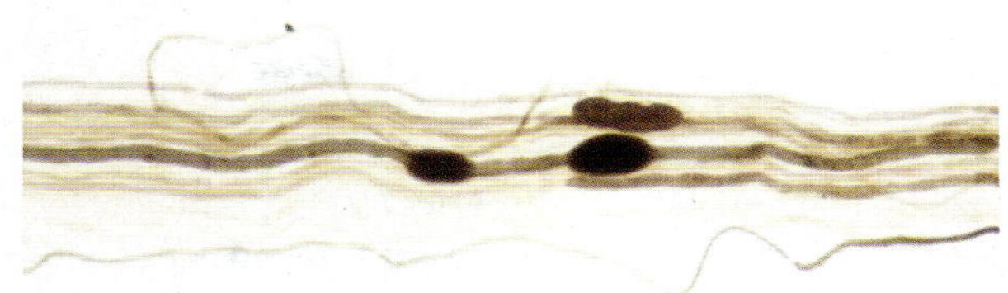

FIG. 64-2 Teased nerve preparation of a sural nerve biopsy from another patient showing the characteristic tomaculae (×400).

On EMG and nerve conduction studies HNPP has a distinctive background of sensorimotor polyneuropathy with superimposed entrapment neuropathies.[6,11,13,15] There is slowing of conduction velocity in most sensory nerves, less frequently distal motor nerve conduction velocity slowing, but with prominent slowing at sites of entrapment. In addition, the distal motor latencies could be prolonged, as are the F-wave latencies. Ultrasonography demonstrates multifocal increase of nerve cross areas.[16]

HNPP is usually caused by deletions in chromosome 17p11.2, which is present in 85% of patients.[3,10,12] A de novo event occurs in sporadic cases with HNPP[17] which are invariably of paternal origin and result from an unequal crossover in spermatogenesis.

The deleted gene in these patients is the *PMP22* gene, the same gene that is duplicated in CMT1A.[11,18] PMP22 is a transmembrane protein present in myelinated fibers of the peripheral nervous system and constitutes about 5% of its total protein content.[19] The exact function of *PMP22* is not known, but it is upregulated during developmental myelination, as well as during remyelination after peripheral nerve injury.[20]

The disease mechanism in HNPP is probably caused by a decrease in gene dose, whereas an increased dose causes CMT1A.[3,17] This produces a reduced expression of both messenger ribonucleic acid and the protein.[20,21] Some patients have deletions of smaller sizes (<1.5 Mb), although they still contain the *PMP22* gene.[22]

Several *PMP22* point mutations have been reported in HNPP.[23–26] The mutations are predicted to result in a premature termination of translation leading to a functional loss of one allele of the *PMP22* gene, similar to that caused by the HNPP deletion.[23,24,26]

There is presently no cure for HNPP. Patients presenting with focal entrapments should be treated conservatively. They should identify activities that cause symptoms, and they are usually advised to avoid leaning on their elbows or crossing their legs. Wrist splints can be worn at night. A padded wrist splint is considered better than one that is not padded. Orthotic devices can be used. Stabilization of the foot by triple arthrodesis can be done for cases with foot drop.

Physical therapy is of some help in a pressure palsy episode, but the "tincture of time" is often the best remedy.

Surgery for entrapments always increases the risk of nerve damage by manipulation and from lying still. Individuals with HNPP are at a much greater risk for this. Knowledge of patients' susceptibility to pressure palsies can help the surgical team obviate them by carefully positioning these patients.

If the foot drop is permanent, surgical treatment with tendon transfers may be considered. The transfer of the insertion of the tibialis posterior tendon to the dorsum of the foot can give good results. A two-tailed transfer of tibialis posterior to the extensor hallucis and digitorum tendons can be effective.

IMPORTANT POINTS

- Foot drop can be caused by disorders of the corticospinal tracts, the lower motor neuron, L5 root disease, lesions of the lumbosacral plexus, and sciatic neuropathy as well as by lesions of the common and deep peroneal nerves. They could be isolated or a manifestation of a mononeuritis multiplex, such as in diabetes, vasculitis, or HNPP. Clinical examination and electrophysiologic tests should help localize the lesion and determine if it affects the deep or common peroneal nerves or other regions. For example, in radiculopathy, there is paraspinal denervation; the peroneal nerve motor conduction tests and superficial peroneal SNAPs are normal. In plexopathies, peroneal conduction is normal; SNAPs could be of low amplitude and paraspinal muscles show no denervation. In sciatic neuropathy there could be involvement of other sciatic-innervated muscles, particularly the short head of the biceps. In common peroneal nerve lesions, there could be focal slowing or conduction block at the knee, or absent superficial peroneal SNAP, and there could be signs of denervation in muscles innervated by the superficial and deep peroneal nerves. In deep peroneal nerve lesions the superficial peroneal SNAP is normal and denervation is not seen in superficial peroneal-innervated muscles.
- HNPP might present with various phenotypes including polyneuropathy, entrapment neuropathies, such as carpal tunnel and tarsal tunnel syndromes, radial nerve palsy, and peroneal palsy. Some patients develop diaphragmatic paralysis with respiratory insufficiency. Other manifestations include a painless brachial neuropathy.
- Most cases of HNPP are caused by deletions of chromosome 17p11.2 from the gene that expresses the PMP22 protein, and the disease is allelic with CMT1A.
- Pathologic findings include demyelination and focal duplications on myelin resembling "sausages," or tomaculae.
- HNPP should be suspected in patients with slowing in multiple nerves in sites of entrapment.
- Currently, there is no cure for HNPP. Conservative management and sometimes surgical decompression are beneficial.

This case was reported in Gupta D, Bertorini TE. Clinical approach to a patient presenting with foot drop. J Clin Neuromuscul Dis. 2004;5(3):54–165.

REFERENCES

1. De Jong HGY. Over families met hereditaire disposite tot het optreden van neuritiden, gecocorrleered mit migraine. *Psychiatr Neurol Bull.* 1947;50:60–76.
2. Meretoja P, Silander K, Kalimo H, et al. Epidemiology of hereditary neuropathy with liability to pressure palsies (HNPP) in southwestern Finland. *Neuromuscul Disord.* 1997;7:529–532.
3. Nelis E, Van Broeckhoven C, De Jonghe P, et al. Estimation of the mutation frequencies in Charcot-Marie-Tooth disease type 1 and hereditary neuropathy with liability to pressure palsies: a European collaborative study. *Eur J Hum Genet.* 1996;4:25–33.
4. Kumar N, Muley S, Pakiam A, Parry GJ. Phenotypic variability leads to under-recognition of HNPP. *J Clin Neuromuscul Dis.* 2002;3:106–112.
5. Pareyson D, Scaioli V, Taroni F, et al. Phenotypic heterogeneity in hereditary neuropathy with liability to pressure palsies associated with chromosome 17p11.2–12 deletion. *Neurology.* 1996;46:1133–1137.
6. Karlinsky S, Kugler S, Bar-Yosef O, Nissenkorn A, et al. Hereditary neuropathy with liability to pressure palsies (HNPP): intrafamilial phenotypic variability and early childhood refusal to walk as the presenting symptom. *Ital J Pediatr.* 2022;48(1):84.
7. Behse F, Buchthal F, Carlsen F, Knappeis GG. Hereditary neuropathy with liability to pressure palsies: electrophysiological and histopathological aspects. *Brain.* 1972;95:777–794.
8. Li J, Krajewski K, Lewis RA, Shy ME. Loss-of-function phenotype of hereditary neuropathy with liability to pressure palsies. *Muscle Nerve.* 2004;29(2):205–210.
9. Bertorini T, Narayanaswami P, Rashed H. Charcot-Marie-Tooth disease (hereditary motor sensory neuropathies) and hereditary sensory and autonomic neuropathies. *Neurologist.* 2004;10(6):327–337.
10. Martinez AC, Conde MC, Cajal SR, et al. Recurrent familial polyneuropathy with liability to pressure palsies: special regards to electrophysiological aspects of 25 members from 7 families. *Electromyogr Clin Neurophysiol.* 1977;17:101–124.
11. Stogbauer F, Young P, Kuhlenbaumer G, et al. Hereditary recurrent focal neuropathies: clinical and molecular features. *Neurology.* 2000;54:546–551.
12. Gouider R, LeGuern E, Gugenheim M, et al. Clinical, electrophysiologic and molecular correlations in 13 families with hereditary neuropathy with liability to pressure palsies and a chromosome 17p11.2 deletion. *Neuropathy.* 1995;45:2018–2023.
13. Chance PF, Lensch MW, Lipe H, et al. Hereditary neuralgic amyotrophy and hereditary neuropathy with liability to pressure palsies: two distinct genetic disorders. *Neurology.* 1994;44:2253–2257.
14. Stogbauer F, Young P, Kerschensteiner M, et al. Recurrent brachial plexus palsies as the only clinical expression of hereditary neuropathy with liability to pressure palsies associated with a de novo deletion of the peripheral myelin protein-22 gene. *Muscle Nerve.* 1998;21:1199–1201.

15. Andersson PB, Yuen E, Parko K, So YT. Electrodiagnostic features of hereditary neuropathy with liability to pressure palsies. *Neurology*. 2000;54(1):40–44.
16. Padua L, Coraci D, Lucchetta M, Paolasso I, et al. Different nerve ultrasound patterns in Charcot-Marie-Tooth types and hereditary neuropathy with liability to pressure palsies. *Muscle Nerve*. 2018;57(1):E18–E23.
17. Chrestian N. Hereditary neuropathy with liability to pressure palsies. *Gene Reviews*. 1998 (Last updated August 27, 2020).
18. Timmerman V, Nelis E, Van Hul W, et al. The peripheral myelin protein gene PMP-22 is contained within the Charcot-Marie-Tooth disease type 1A duplication. *Nat Genet*. 1992;1:171–175.
19. Snipes GJ, Suter U, Welcher AA, Shooter EM. Characterization of a novel peripheral nervous system myelin protein (PMP-22 SR13). *J Cell Biol*. 1992;117:225–238.
20. Welcher AA, Suter U, De Leon M, et al. A myelin protein is encoded by the homologue of a growth arrest-specific gene. *Proc Natl Acad Sci USA*. 1991;88:7195–7199.
21. Yoshikawa H, Nishimura T, Nakatsuji Y, et al. Elevated expression of messenger RNA for peripheral myelin protein 22 in biopsied peripheral nerves of patients with Charcot-Marie-Tooth disease type 1A. *Ann Neurol*. 1994;35:445–450.
22. Van de Wetering RA, Gabreels-Festen AA, Timmerman V, et al. Hereditary neuropathy with liability to pressure palsies with a small deletion interrupting the *PMP22* gene. *Neuromuscul Disord*. 2002;12(7–8):651–655.
23. Chapon F, Diraison P, Lechevalier B, et al. Hereditary neuropathy with liability to pressure palsies with a partial deletion of the region often duplicated in Charcot-Marie-Tooth disease, type 1A. *J Neurol Neurosurg Psychiatry*. 1996;61:535–536.
24. Bort S, Nelis E, Timmerman V, et al. Mutational analysis of the MPZ, PMP22 and Cx32 genes in patients of Spanish ancestry with Charcot-Marie-Tooth disease and hereditary neuropathy with liability to pressure palsies. *Hum Genet*. 1997;99: 746–754.
25. Nicholson GA, Valentijin LJ, Cherryson AK, et al. A frame shift mutation in the PMP22 gene in hereditary neuropathy with liability to pressure palsies. *Nat Genet*. 1994;6:263–266.
26. Young P, Wiebusch H, Stogbauer F, et al. A novel frameshift mutation in PMP22 accounts for hereditary neuropathy with liability to pressure palsies. *Neurology*. 1997;48:450–452.

65 CASE

An Elderly Woman With Foot Drop and Hand Weakness

A 76-year-old woman presented several days after a sudden onset of left foot drop that occurred immediately after a fall. She also complained of anorexia, weight loss, malaise, and numbness in both lower extremities for several weeks.

Past medical history was positive for coronary artery disease, carotid endarterectomy, aortic valve stenosis with valve replacement, hypertension, and hyperlipidemia. Medications included atenolol, hydrochlorothiazide, amlodipine, thyroid supplement, and aspirin.

She was referred for an EMG.

General physical examination was normal. On neurologic examination, strength was intact except for mild weakness in both hands and toe dorsiflexors on the right, and she could not dorsiflex the left foot and toes or evert the left foot. Reflexes were absent in the ankles, trace at the knees, and normal in the arms. She had absent vibration sense in the toes and ankles and decreased pinprick, temperature, and touch sensations in both lower extremities in a stocking distribution up to the calf. There was mildly decreased vibration sense and two-point discrimination in the fingers. The rest of the examination was normal.

WHAT IS THE DIFFERENTIAL DIAGNOSIS?

Clinically, this patient had a polyneuropathy with a superimposed left peroneal neuropathy. It was not completely clear if peroneal palsy was caused by stretch trauma from the fall or was spontaneous and caused the fall. The differential diagnosis included a diabetic polyneuropathy. Other causes of neuropathy were also considered, including a polyneuropathy from a microangiopathic vasculitis. She could also have had a polyneuropathy with an L5 radiculopathy, plexopathy, or a sciatic nerve lesion.

AN EMG TEST WAS PERFORMED

Motor Nerve Studies

Nerve and Site	Latency (ms)	Amplitude (mV)	Conduction Velocity (m/s)
Peroneal Nerve L.	**Normal ≤ 5.7**	**Normal ≥ 3**	**Normal ≥ 40**
Ankle	**NR**	**NR**	–
Fibular head	**NR**	**NR**	**NR**
Knee	**NR**	**NR**	**NR**

Motor Nerve Studies—cont'd

Nerve and Site	Latency (ms)	Amplitude (mV)	Conduction Velocity (m/s)
Peroneal Nerve L.[a]	**Normal ≤ 5.2**	**Normal ≥ 3**	**Normal ≥ 40**
Fibular head	3.3	**0.8**	–
Knee	6.0	**0.7**	**37**

[a]Recorded at the tibialis anterior muscle with needle electrode.

Motor Nerve Studies—cont'd

Nerve and Site	Latency (ms)	Amplitude (mV)	Conduction Velocity (m/s)
Tibial Nerve L.	**Normal ≤ 5.3**	**Normal ≥ 4**	**Normal ≥ 40**
Ankle	**NR**	**NR**	–
Pop. fossa	**NR**	**NR**	**NR**
Peroneal Nerve R.	**Normal ≤ 5.7**	**Normal ≥ 3**	**Normal ≥ 40**
Ankle	**6.6**	**0.3**	–
Fibular head	15.2	**0.2**	**31**
Knee	18.3	**0.2**	**32**
Nerve and Site	**Latency (ms)**	**Amplitude (mV)**	**Conduction Velocity (m/s)**
Peroneal Nerve R.[b]	**Normal ≤ 5.2**	**Normal ≥ 3**	**Normal ≥ 40**
Fibular head	3.1	7	–
Knee	5.3	6	45
Tibial Nerve R.	**Normal ≤ 5.3**	**Normal ≥ 4**	**Normal ≥ 40**
Ankle	4.6	**1.1**	–
Pop. fossa	14.4	**0.3**	**36**
Median Nerve R.	**Normal ≤ 4.2**	**Normal ≥ 6**	**Normal ≥ 50**
Wrist	4.2	**2**	–
Elbow	9.0	**1**	**44**
Ulnar Nerve R.	**Normal ≤ 3.6**	**Normal ≥ 8**	**Normal ≥ 50**
Wrist	3.2	**2**	–
Below elbow	6.7	**1**	**44**
Above elbow	9.1	**1**	50

[b]Recorded at tibialis anterior muscle.

Motor Nerve Studies—cont'd

Nerve and Site	Latency (ms)	Amplitude (mV)	Conduction Velocity (m/s)
Median Nerve L.	**Normal ≤ 4.2**	**Normal ≥ 6**	**Normal ≥ 50**
Wrist	4.0	16	–
Elbow	8.4	15	**45**

F-Wave and Tibial H-Reflex Studies

Nerve	Latency (ms)	Normal Latency ≤ (ms)
Peroneal nerve L.	**NR**	54
Tibial nerve L.	**NR**	54

F-Wave and Tibial H-Reflex Studies—cont'd

Nerve	Latency (ms)	Normal Latency ≤ (ms)
Peroneal nerve R.	**NR**	54
Tibial nerve R.	**NR**	54
Median nerve R.	28.3	30
Ulnar nerve R.	29.3	30
Median nerve L.	28.0	30
H-reflex L.	**NR**	34
H-reflex R.	**NR**	34

Sensory Nerve Studies

Superficial peroneal nerve R.—Absent
Sural nerve R.—Absent

EMG Data

Muscle	Insrt Activity	Fibs	Pos Waves	Fasc	Amp	Dur	Poly	Pattern
Biceps brachii R.	Norm	None	None	None	Norm	Norm	None	Full
Triceps R.	Norm	None	None	None	Norm	Norm	None	Full
Brachioradialis R.	Norm	None	None	None	Norm	Norm	None	Full
First dorsal interosseous R.	**Inc**	None	**1+**	None	**Lg**	**Inc**	None	**Red**
Abductor pollicis brevis R.	Norm	None	None	None	**Lg**	**Inc**	None	Full
Tibialis anterior R.	**Inc**	**2+**	**2+**	None	**Lg**	**Inc**	None	**Red**
Gastrocnemius R.	**Inc**	None	**2+**	None	**Lg**	**Inc**	None	**Red**
Vastus lateralis R.	Norm	None	None	None	Norm	Norm	None	Full
Rectus femoris R.	Norm	None	None	None	Norm	Norm	None	Full
Lumbar paraspinals L.	Norm	None	None	None	Norm	Norm	None	Full
Gluteus medius L.	Norm	None	None	None	Norm	Norm	None	Full
Tensor fasciae latae L.	Norm	None	None	None	Norm	Norm	None	Full
Biceps femoris (long head)	Norm	None	None	None	Norm	Norm	None	Full
Biceps femoris (short head)	Norm	None	None	None	Norm	Norm	None	Full
Vastus lateralis L.	Norm	None	None	None	Norm	Norm	None	Full
Tibialis anterior L.	**Inc**	**4+**	**4+**	None	**Lg**	**Inc**	None	**Red**
Peroneus longus L.	**Inc**	**4+**	**4+**	None	**Lg**	**Inc**	None	**Red**
Gastrocnemius L.	**Inc**	None	**1+**	None	**Lg**	**Inc**	None	**Red**

WHAT WERE THE EMG FINDINGS?

This test demonstrated an absent left tibial CMAP and peroneal CMAP when recording at the extensor digitorum brevis muscle and low-amplitude CMAP when recording at the tibialis anterior muscle. The nerve conduction velocity was mildly slow across the fibular head. The right peroneal and tibial nerves had low-amplitude CMAPs and decreased conduction velocities. The median and tibial nerves had decreased CMAP amplitudes and velocities.

F-responses were prolonged, except for the left peroneal and tibial nerves in which they were absent. SNAPs were absent in both sural and superficial peroneal nerves. The right median SNAP was normal, while the left had a prolonged latency and low amplitude.

Needle EMG showed denervation potentials in the left tibialis anterior and peroneus longus with reduced motor unit recruitment. There was also mild denervation on the right tibialis anterior and both gastrocnemius and first dorsal interosseous; other muscles were normal.

It was concluded that the patient had a predominantly axonal sensory and motor polyneuropathy with secondary demyelination affecting mainly the lower extremities with more severe involvement of the left peroneal nerve. The lack of denervation in the other L5, or paraspinal muscles argued against a radiculopathy. The normal hamstring muscles, particularly the short head of the biceps, were against a sciatic neuropathy.

THE FOLLOWING LABORATORY STUDIES WERE DONE

Electrolytes were normal except for a sodium of 126 mg/dL (normal, 135–155 mg/dL). Thyroid-stimulating hormone was elevated at 47.4 µV/mL (normal, 0.35–5.50 µV/mL) and glucose was 200 mg/dL. Lipid profile showed mild hyperlipidemia. Erythrocyte sedimentation rate (ESR) was 85 mm/h; fluorescent antinuclear antibody was negative.

CT scans of the chest and abdomen were normal.

Her symptoms improved with physical therapy and fluid restriction. Her thyroid supplement was adjusted. She was diagnosed with diabetic neuropathy, with hypothyroidism as a possible contributing factor, and a peroneal palsy.

FOLLOW-UP

She was referred for neurologic evaluation 2 months later because of acute onset of hand weakness in the right, more than the left.

General physical examination was unremarkable except for mottling bluish discoloration of fingers and feet. Strength was 2/5 in the right wrist and finger extensors, 3/5 in the left hand; hand flexion was 4/5, finger flexion was 4/5, and hand muscles were 4−/5. In addition, there was a left foot drop (Fig. 65-1). She had mild right foot dorsiflexion weakness. Motor examination was otherwise normal. Reflexes were 1 to 2+ in the left upper extremity, 0 in the right brachioradialis and biceps, and 1+ in the triceps. Knee and ankle reflexes were absent. She had absent vibration sense in feet, ankles, and fingers. Pinprick, touch, and temperature sensations were decreased to the mid-calf, left forearm, and right elbow. The rest of the examination was normal.

A SECOND EMG TEST WAS PERFORMED

Motor Nerve Studies

Nerve and Site	Latency (ms)	Amplitude (mV)	Conduction Velocity (m/s)
Peroneal Nerve L.	**Normal ≤ 5.7**	**Normal ≥ 3**	**Normal ≥ 40**
Ankle	**NR**	**NR**	–
Fibular head	**NR**	**NR**	**NR**
Peroneal Nerve L.[a]	**Normal ≤ 5.2**	**Normal ≥ 3**	**Normal ≥ 40**
Fibular head	13.1	**1**	–
Knee	16.5	**1**	**36**

[a]Recorded at tibialis anterior muscle.

Motor Nerve Studies—cont'd

Nerve and Site	Latency (ms)	Amplitude (mV)	Conduction Velocity (m/s)
Tibial Nerve L.	**Normal ≤ 5.3**	**Normal ≥ 4**	**Normal ≥ 40**
Ankle	5.3	**2**	–
Pop. fossa	14.9	**1**	**37**
Peroneal Nerve R.	**Normal ≤ 5.7**	**Normal ≥ 3**	**Normal ≥ 40**
Ankle	5.7	**1**	–
Fibular head	12.8	**1**	**36**

Motor Nerve Studies—cont'd

Nerve and Site	Latency (ms)	Amplitude (mV)	Conduction Velocity (m/s)
Median Nerve R.	**Normal ≤ 4.2**	**Normal ≥ 6**	**Normal ≥ 50**
Wrist	**6.3**	**0.1**	–
Elbow	13.0	**0.0**	**33**
Ulnar Nerve R.	**Normal ≤ 3.6**	**Normal ≥ 8**	**Normal ≥ 50**
Wrist	**8.1**	**0.0**	–
Below elbow	**NR**	**NR**	–
Radial Nerve R.	**NR**	**NR**	**NR**
Median Nerve L.	**Normal ≤ 4.2**	**Normal ≥ 6**	**Normal ≥ 50**
Wrist	4.2	**2.4**	–
Elbow	13.1	**0.1**	**23**
Ulnar Nerve L.	**Normal ≤ 3.6**	**Normal ≥ 8**	**Normal ≥ 50**
Wrist	**3.8**	**2.8**	–
Below elbow	8.8	**2.2**	**42**
Above elbow	12.9	**0.0**	**29**
Axilla	14.8	**0.0**	**47**
Radial Nerve L.	**NR**	**NR**	**NR**

F-Wave and Tibial H-Reflex Studies

Nerve	Latency (ms)	Normal Latency ≤ (ms)
Peroneal nerve R.	**NR**	54
Median nerve R.	**NR**	30
Ulnar nerve R.	**NR**	30
Median nerve L.	**NR**	30
Ulnar nerve L.	**NR**	30
H-reflex R.	**NR**	34

Sensory Nerve Studies

Nerve	Latency (ms)	Normal Latency ≤ (ms)	Amp (μV)	Normal Amp ≥ (μV)
Median nerve R.	**NR**	3.1	**NR**	20
Ulnar nerve R.	**NR**	3.1	**NR**	13
Radial nerve R.	**NR**	3.1	**NR**	30

EMG Data

Muscle	Insrt Activity	Fibs	Pos Waves	Fasc	Amp	Dur	Poly	Pattern
Deltoid L.	Norm	None	None	None	**Lg**	**Inc**	None	**Red**
Biceps brachii L.	Norm	None	None	None	Norm	Norm	None	**Red**
Extensor digitorum com. L.	Norm	None	None	None	**Lg**	**Inc**	None	Full
First dorsal interosseous L.	**Inc**	**3+**	**3+**	None	**Lg**	**Inc**	None	**Red**
Extensor carpi radialis L.	Norm	None	None	None	**Lg**	**Inc**	None	**Red**
Extensor digitorum com. L.	**Inc**	**2+**	**2+**	None	**Lg**	**Inc**	None	**Red**
Tibialis anterior L.	**Inc**	**2+**	**2+**	None	**Absent**	–	–	**Absent**
Gastrocnemius L.	**Inc**	**2+**	**2+**	None	**Lg**	**Inc**	None	**Red**

EMG Data—cont'd

Muscle	Insrt Activity	Fibs	Pos Waves	Fasc	Amp	Dur	Poly	Pattern
Deltoid R.	Norm	None	None	None	**Lg**	**Inc**	None	**Red**
Biceps brachii R.	Norm	None	None	None	**Lg**	**Inc**	None	**Red**
Extensor digitorum com. R.	**Inc**	**2+**	**2+**	None	**Lg**	**Inc**	None	**Red**
Flexor carpi radialis R.	**Inc**	**1+**	**1+**	None	**Lg**	**Inc**	None	**Red**
Flexor carpi ulnaris R.	**Inc**	**2+**	**2+**	None	**Lg**	**Inc**	None	**Red**
First dorsal interosseous R.	**Inc**	**2+**	**2+**	None	**Lg**	**Inc**	None	**Red**

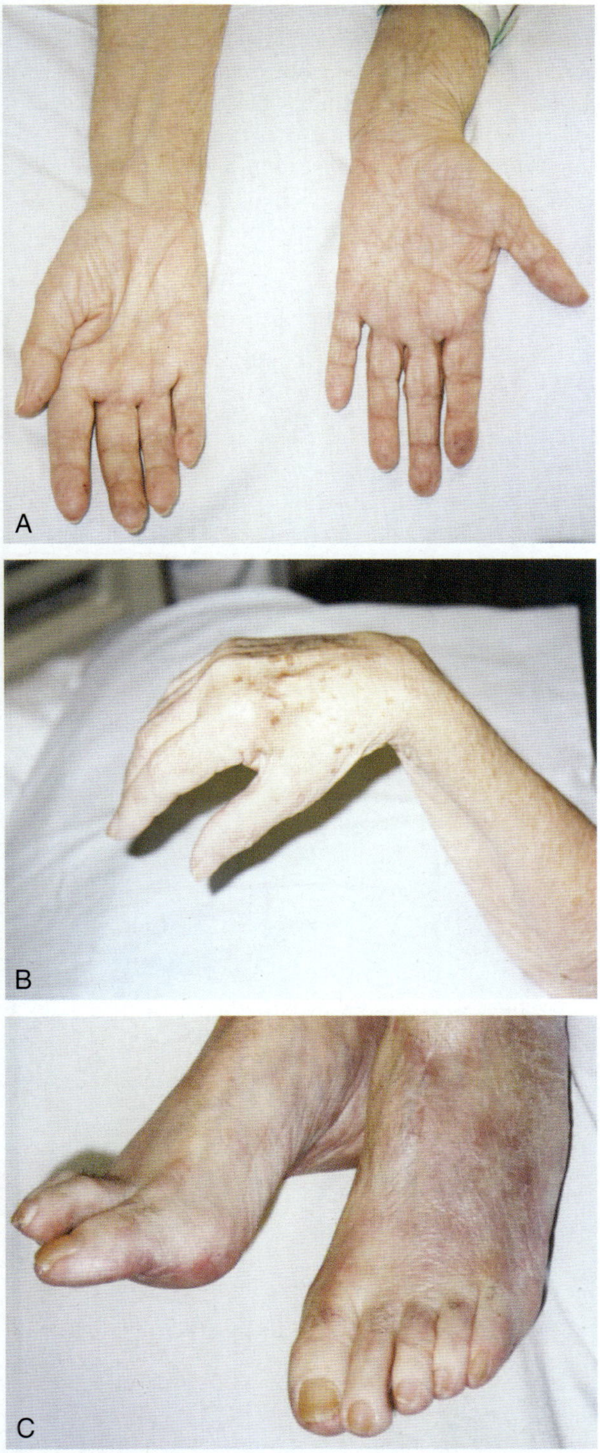

FIG. 65-1 A, Discoloration of the fingers and right thenar atrophy in this patient. **B**, Right wrist drop; notice atrophy of the first dorsal interosseous muscle. **C**, Left foot drop and also bluish mottling discoloration of the skin.

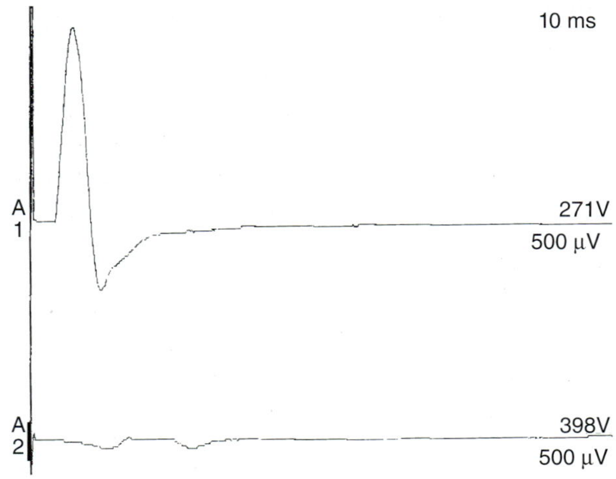

FIG. 65-2 Left median nerve CMAP obtained with wrist stimulation (*above*), and during elbow stimulation (*below*); notice conduction block (500 μV/10 ms).

WHAT WERE THE EMG FINDINGS?

This test showed interval worsening of the neuropathy with conduction blocks, most prominent in the left ulnar and median nerves (Fig. 65-2), and absent bilateral peroneal CMAPs. There was also diffuse denervation in both legs, as well as in the right median-, radial-, and ulnar-innervated muscles.

In summary, the test showed a severe asymmetric polyneuropathy with both axonal degeneration and demyelinating features with conduction blocks, consistent with mononeuritis multiplex.

Laboratory studies revealed normal chemistries, except for sodium 133 mg/dL and albumin 3 mg/dL. ESR was 105 mm/h (normal, <0–20 mm/h); FANA and HIV were negative. Circulating antineutrophil cytoplasmic antibodies (C-ANCA) IgG index titer was 0.20 (normal, <0.8). Anti-MPO perinuclear ANCA (P-ANCA) IgG titer was 4.6 (normal, <0.8). C3 and C4 complement were normal. Anti-SSA (RO) and SSB (LA) Sjögren antibodies were normal. Spinal fluid showed glucose of 96 mg/dL and protein of 31 mg/dL and had no cells.

The elevated ESR and P-ANCA with a normal C-ANCA supported the diagnosis of a vasculitis. Therefore sural nerve and quadriceps muscle biopsies were done.

WHAT DID THE NERVE AND MUSCLE BIOPSY SHOW?

The muscle biopsy showed neurogenic atrophy with atrophic angular fibers. The sural nerve biopsy showed a small- to mid-sized vasculitis with infiltration of the vessel wall having some fibrinoid necrosis (Fig. 65-3).

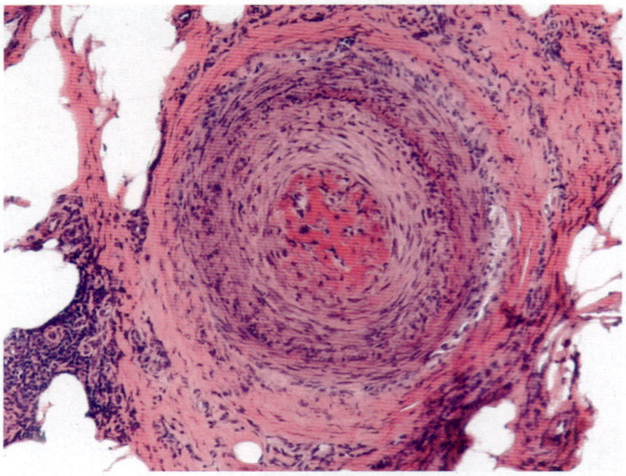

FIG. 65-3 Sural nerve biopsy showing a vessel with inflammatory infiltrates embedded in the vessel wall; there is also fibrinoid necrosis (H&E stain, ×200).

The patient was treated with prednisone 60 mg each day with improvement.

This therapy was used with some trepidation because of her diabetes, which was closely monitored. As her diabetes mellitus worsened and she developed significant cushingoid features, she was slowly switched to azathioprine with close monitoring of her ESR and ANCA titers.

SUMMARY

This patient presented initially with a polyneuropathy and a mononeuritis of the left peroneal nerve during a fall. Her sedimentation rate was elevated, and when a later workup revealed an elevated P-ANCA titer, a nerve biopsy showed vasculitis. She responded well to steroids and later to azathioprine.

For further discussion, important points, and references, see Case 66.

CASE 66

A Woman With Rheumatoid Arthritis Who Developed Numbness and Pain in the Feet

A 64-year-old woman with rheumatoid arthritis (RA) was being treated with oral prednisone, methotrexate 7.5 g weekly, and rofecoxib. She also received thyroid replacement, injections of Kineret (anakinra), a recombinant interleukin-1 receptor antagonist, and atenolol with hydrochlorothiazide for hypertension. She had a 4-month history of pain in the back of the thighs while sitting. This pain was so severe that she could not sit even for 10 minutes. An MRI of the thighs was normal.

Over the past 2 months, she developed tingling and numbness of the feet. She felt worse when she wore tight clothes or tennis shoes. She also had pain that shot down to the toes and numbness on the tips of her toes, mainly on the right side. The numbness had spread up to the middle right foot in the past month.

Past medical history included hysterectomy and chole cystectomy.

She did not smoke or drink. Family history was positive for RA in an aunt and two cousins. Her father died of amyotrophic lateral sclerosis.

Mentation and cranial nerves were unremarkable. There was no dryness of the mouth or conjunctiva. Some joint deformities were noticed. Strength and reflexes were normal, except for absent ankle jerks. There were no Babinski signs. Coordination and gait were normal. There were no Tinel's signs in the tibial nerves at the ankles.

Sensory examination revealed mildly decreased vibration sense over the great toes and thumbs. Pinprick sensation was decreased in an asymmetric fashion: on the right foot, it was decreased up to the ankle, and on the left just decreased at the tips of her toes. The rest of the examination was unremarkable.

WHAT IS THE MOST LIKELY DIAGNOSIS?

This patient with RA presented with burning feet. The possibility of tarsal tunnel syndrome needed to be considered. However, her sensory deficit included the dorsum of the feet and was up to the ankles, indicating a peripheral neuropathy that was asymmetric, suggesting a neuropathy from small vessel vasculitis associated with RA. This can also be seen in Sjögren syndrome, but she had no manifestation of this condition.

She also had hypothyroidism, which could cause a neuropathy, but was well maintained with thyroid supplement. In such cases other causes of a predominantly sensory neuropathy, such as diabetes, or B_{12} or other vitamin deficiencies, should also be considered. Secondary amyloidosis is rarely seen in patients with a known connective tissue disorder. She was not exposed to toxins or drugs and did not take an excessive amount of vitamins that could cause a neuropathy.

Her father had amyotrophic lateral sclerosis, but she had no symptoms or findings to suggest this disease, and her problem was typical of a neuropathy.

AN EMG TEST WAS PERFORMED

Motor Nerve Studies

Nerve and Site	Latency (ms)	Amplitude (mV)	Conduction Velocity (m/s)
Peroneal Nerve R.	**Normal ≤ 5.7**	**Normal ≥ 3**	**Normal ≥ 40**
Ankle	4.9	2	–
Fibular head	11.8	2	40
Knee	13.5	2	47
Tibial Nerve L.	**Normal ≤ 5.3**	**Normal ≥ 4**	**Normal ≥ 40**
Ankle	4.0	3	–
Pop. fossa	13.7	3	38
Ulnar Nerve R.	**Normal ≤ 3.6**	**Normal ≥ 8**	**Normal ≥ 50**
Wrist	2.8	11	–
Below elbow	6.0	10	56
Above elbow	12.0	10	60

F-Wave and Tibial H-Reflex Studies

Nerve	Latency (ms)	Normal Latency ≤ (ms)
Peroneal nerve R.	51.3	54
Tibial nerve L.	53.9	54
Ulnar nerve R.	29.7	30
H-reflex R.	NR	34
H-reflex L.	NR	34

Sensory Nerve Studies

Nerve	Onset Latency (ms)	Normal Onset Latency ≤ (ms)	Peak Latency (ms)	Normal Peak Latency ≤ (ms)	Amp (μV)	Normal Amp ≥ (μV)	Conduction Velocity (m/s)	Normal Conduction Velocity ≥ (m/s)
Sural nerve R.	3.5	3.5	3.9	4.0	9	11	40	40
Superficial peroneal nerve R.	3.2	3.5	3.7	4.0	5	8–10	44	40
Ulnar nerve R.	2.2	2.6	2.7	3.1	17	13	55	50

Sympathetic Skin Response

Hand R.—Normal
Foot R.—Absent

EMG Data

Muscle	Insrt Activity	Fibs	Pos Waves	Fasc	Amp	Dur	Poly	Pattern
Lumbar paraspinals R.	Norm	None	None	None	Norm	Norm	None	Full
Vastus lateralis R.	Norm	None	None	None	Norm	Norm	None	Full
Tibialis anterior R.	Norm	None	None	None	Norm	Norm	None	Full
Gastrocnemius R.	Inc	None	1+	None	Norm	Norm	None	Full
Extensor hallucis longus R.	Inc	None	None	None	Norm	Norm	None	Full
Lumbar paraspinals L.	Norm	None	None	None	Norm	Norm	None	Full
Gastrocnemius L.	Inc	None	1+	None	Norm	Norm	None	Full
First dorsal interosseus L.	Norm	None	None	None	Norm	Norm	None	Full

WHAT WERE THE EMG FINDINGS?

The motor nerve conduction velocity was borderline slow in the tibial nerve, and there was a low-amplitude peroneal CMAP. Sural and superficial peroneal nerve SNAPs were of low amplitude with normal latencies. The sympathetic skin response was absent in the foot and normal in the hand. There were absent H-reflexes. Needle tests showed some denervation potentials in distal muscles of both legs, particularly in the gastrocnemii.

These electrophysiologic findings were suggestive of a sensorimotor axonal neuropathy.

WHAT OTHER TESTS SHOULD BE DONE?

Complete metabolic panel, T4, thyroid-stimulating hormone, and immunoelectrophoresis were normal. DNA antibodies were elevated at 109 IU/mL (normal, <25 IU/mL) and C3 complement was low at 69 mg/dL (normal, 80–207 mg/dL). C4 complement was normal. Antinuclear ribonucleoprotein (anti-RNP) antibodies are negative. Serum creatine kinase was normal. Antinuclear antibodies were positive with a titer of 1:640. B_{12} and folate were normal. Serum immunofixation was normal. Erythrocyte sedimentation rate was 14 (normal, <30). Rheumatoid factor was 60 IU/mL (normal, <43 IU/mL).

An MRI of the spine was normal.

WHAT SHOULD BE DONE NEXT?

A muscle biopsy showed mild interstitial inflammation without necrosis and occasional atrophic angular fibers. A sural nerve biopsy showed axonal degeneration with demyelination and small vessel vasculitis (Fig. 66-1).

She was treated by increasing methotrexate to 15 mg weekly and adalimumab (Humira), a recombinant monoclonal antibody against tumor necrosis factor; Kineret was discontinued. Since this patient was seen, tumor necrosis factor antagonists have been reported to be associated with the development of autoimmune neuropathies. She, however, has been stable in the last three years.

SUMMARY

This woman with RA developed an asymmetric, predominantly sensory neuropathy in spite of being on immunosuppressant therapy. She was found to have a vasculitis and responded to an increased dose of methotrexate and adalimumab (Humira) injections.

DISCUSSION (CASES 65 AND 66)

Case 65 was an elderly woman who presented initially with a polyneuropathy and superimposed mononeuropathy of the

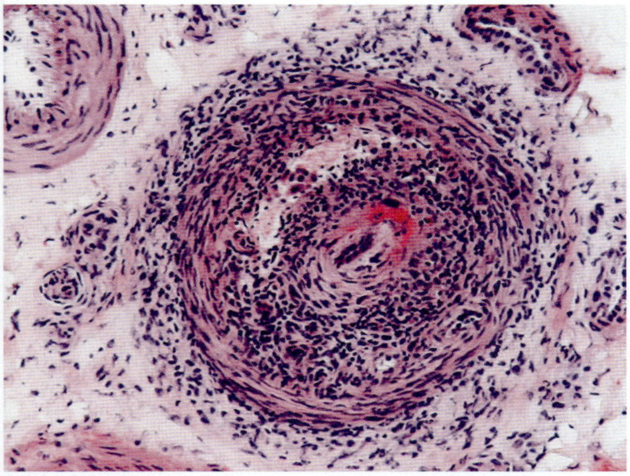

FIG. 66-1 Sural nerve biopsy showing vascular inflammation with invasion of the vessel wall. There is also a vessel occlusion with recanalization (H&E stain, ×200).

peroneal nerve. This was thought to be related to diabetes or trauma in spite of her elevated sedimentation rate. Later, she developed a mononeuritis multiplex. She had elevated perinuclear antineutrophil cytoplasmic antibodies (P-ANCAs) and a nerve biopsy showed vasculitis. The peroneal nerve is more frequently affected in vasculitis and likely was the initial manifestation in this case. Although vasculitis has been reported in focal diabetic neuropathies and in lumbosacral radiculoplexus neuropathy,[1] the presence of a diffuse mononeuritis multiplex and the positive ANCA titers were indicative of a systemic vasculitis.[2–7] She had no evidence of temporal arteritis[2] clinically, and only small- and medium-sized arteries were involved.

In periarteritis nodosa both P-ANCA and circulating antineutrophil cytoplasmic antibody (C-ANCA) titers are elevated. The P-ANCA elevation is, however, nonspecific and can be seen in other disorders.[8] There was no evidence of other systemic manifestations except for the skin changes; her hypertension was long-standing.

There were no signs or symptoms of other connective tissue disorders, such as Sjögren's disease, RA, or lupus. She had no lung manifestations to suggest Wegener granulomatosis, and in that disease, C-ANCA and not P-ANCA titers are elevated.[9]

It was concluded that she developed a vasculitic neuropathy[10,11] causing mononeuritis multiplex superimposed on a diabetic polyneuropathy. Conduction blocks were caused by the vasculitic neuropathy, likely from focal edema.[12,13]

Vasculitic neuropathy can occur in the setting of systemic necrotizing vasculitis, such as periarteritis nodosa with multiple manifestations (Fig. 66-2), and in Sjögren syndrome, Wegener granulomatosis, lupus, and RA. It can also occur in patients with giant cell arteritis.

In addition to peripheral nerves being involved in systemic vasculitis, a nonsystemic vasculitic neuropathy, or isolated peripheral nerve vasculitis, without other manifestations, is one of the most common causes of this type of neuropathy,[10] overall, after periarteritis nodosa and RA. It accounts for about 25% of cases.[2] The vasculitis affects both small and medium size arteries of the epineurium and perineurium and might represent a restrictive form of periarteritis nodosa with a more benign course.

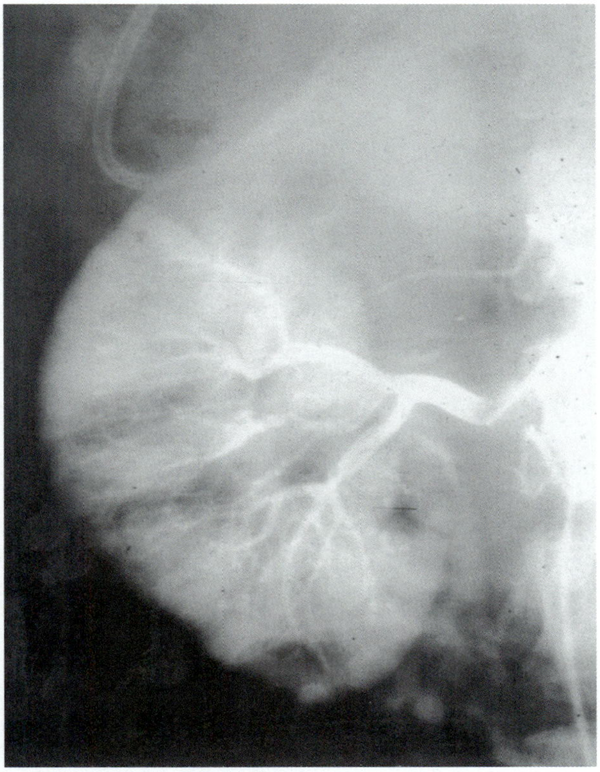

FIG. 66-2 Arteriogram of the kidney showing microaneurysm in a case with periarteritis nodosa.

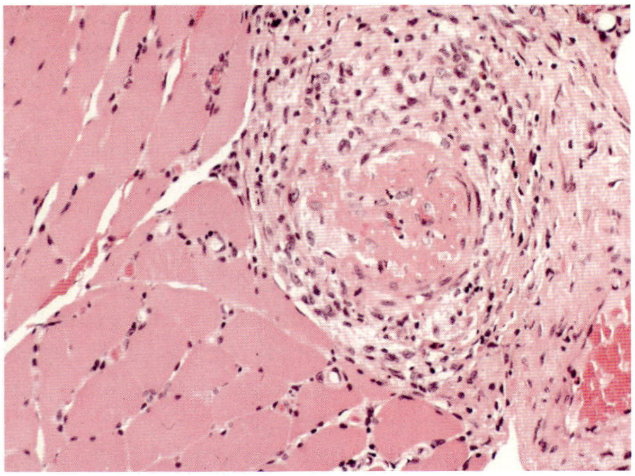

FIG. 66-3 Muscle biopsy of a case with periarteritis nodosa; notice vasculitis in the muscle with fibrinoid necrosis, not present in the sural nerve of this case (H&E stain, ×200).

In this case the vasculitis was proved with a peripheral nerve biopsy, but it is always wise to do a muscle biopsy together with a nerve biopsy, as vasculitis might be missed in nerves but present in muscles (Fig. 66-3).

The peripheral nerve manifestations of vasculitic neuropathy include pain, sensory loss, and weakness involving several individual nerves. It sometimes manifests diffusely as a polyneuropathy.[7,14] Patients present acutely or subacutely, and the disease could be steadily progressive. Some might give a history of exacerbation and remissions. EMG shows low-amplitude CMAPs and SNAPs and evidence of denervation.[7,14]

Pathologic studies show inflammatory cell infiltrates around and in the vessel wall; fibrinoid necrosis and hemorrhages can also be seen. Inflammatory cells are predominantly T cells and macrophages, with deposits of immunoglobulins and complement.[14] In chronic cases, there are deposits of hemosiderin with thrombosis and vascular recanalization. There is damage of both myelinated and unmyelinated axons with axonal degeneration. Focal myelinated fiber loss can also be seen.

Case 66 had RA,[15,16] and although she had an elevated FANA and low C4, there was no evidence of systemic lupus erythematosus. She developed a vasculitic neuropathy, in spite of being on immunosuppressive therapy for RA.

RA is an autoimmune disorder of unknown cause but might be related to an exaggerated immune response against some type of infectious agent. This produces activation of CD4 and CD8 cells in the joints with joint hypertrophy. There is also evidence that B cells produce polyclonal immunoglobulins that manifest as the rheumatoid factor.[15] This is elevated in 75% of cases and represents antibodies that react with the Fc portion of IgG. There is activation of cytokines and chemotactic proteins that produce joint destruction,[17,18] and the synovia plays a key pathogenic role in this process.[19] The clinical characteristics include malaise, fever, and joint pain and swelling. Patients might also develop rheumatoid nodes with splenomegaly and pericarditis (Felty syndrome).

Patients with RA could have multiple neurological manifestations.[20] In RA there could be pathologic evidence of vasculitis as initially described by Sokoloff.[21] Patients can also develop nerve entrapments, such as carpal tunnel syndrome, ulnar entrapments, and tarsal tunnel syndrome. They also might develop myelopathies due to subluxation of the atlas and cauda equina syndrome.[22]

A polyneuropathy occurs in about 25% of RA cases,[19–23] and about 10% have a vasculitic neuropathy.[24–27] This neuropathy is usually sensorimotor.[28] The peroneal nerve is more frequently affected, but other nerves could also be affected. Some patients might develop a mononeuritis multiplex.

Other neuropathies that can be seen with RA include chronic inflammatory demyelinating polyradiculoneuropathy (CIDP), an autonomic neuropathy, and Guillain–Barré syndrome.[29]

Patients with RA and other connective tissue disorders can also manifest the SICCA syndrome (*secondary* Sjögren's), or this syndrome can manifest alone (*primary* Sjögren's). The clinical characteristics include dry eyes (keratoconjunctivitis) and dry mouth (xerostomia) from inflammation in the salivary and lacrimal glands. Patients with Sjögren syndrome can develop a ganglioneuritis[30] and trigeminal neuralgia and could have other systemic manifestations.[15,17]

Tumor necrosis factor alpha antagonist could be associated with various autoimmune neruopathies.[31,32]

The treatment of vasculitic neuropathy consists of the use of steroids or immunosuppressants like cyclophosphamide, azathioprine, or methotrexate. Gamma globulin infusions are also of help.[14,33]

IMPORTANT POINTS

- The possibility of vasculitis should be considered in a patient presenting with mononeuropathy, mononeuritis multiplex, and even a peripheral polyneuropathy.
- An elevated sedimentation rate should be pursued aggressively in a patient with a neuropathy, as this could indicate a systemic cause such as vasculitis.
- P-ANCA antibodies are nonspecific and are elevated in vasculitis, while C-ANCA is elevated in Wegener granulomatosis. Both P-ANCA and C-ANCA elevations are seen in patients with polyarteritis nodosa.
- Focal slowing, conduction block, and temporal dispersion on EMG may be present in vasculitis.
- RA is an autoimmune disease characterized by arthralgia, joint deformities, malaise, fever, splenomegaly, and positive rheumatoid factor.
- RA can cause nerve entrapments, such as carpal tunnel syndrome, ulnar entrapment, or tarsal tunnel syndrome. It can also cause a symmetrical sensory neuropathy and a multifocal neuropathy from vasculitis. Other neuropathies reported in patients with RA include CIDP and Guillain–Barré syndrome. Those with Sjögren syndrome might also develop a ganglioneuritis and a trigeminal neuralgia.
- The mononeuritis multiplex in RA is caused by a small vessel vasculitis.
- Vasculitic neuropathy is treated with corticosteroids and immunosuppressant drugs.
- When using tumor necrosis factor antagonists to treat RA, it should be remembered that they could be associated with autoimmune neuropathies.[30]

This case was seen with Dr. Pushpa Narayanaswami.

REFERENCES

1. Dyck PJ, Norell JE, Dyck PJ. Microvasculitis and ischemia in diabetic lumbosacral radiculoplexus neuropathy. *Neurology*. 1999;53(9):2113–2121.
2. Collins M, Kissel JT, Mendell JR. Vasculitis of the peripheral nervous system. In: Antel J, Birnbaum G, Hartung P, eds. *Neuroimmunology*. Cambridge, MA: Blackwell Science; 1998: 316–339.
3. Lie JT. Systemic and isolated vasculitis: a rational approach to classification and pathologic diagnosis. *Pathol Annu*. 1989;24 (Part 1):25–114.
4. Moore PM, Fauci AS. Neurologic manifestations of systemic vasculitis: a retrospective study of the clinicopathologic features and responses to therapy in 25 patients. *Am J Med*. 1981;71: 517–524.
5. Dyck P, Conn DL, Okazaki H. Necrotizing angiopathy neuropathy: three-dimensional morphology of fiber degeneration related to sites of occluded vessels. *Mayo Clin Proc*. 1972;47:461–475.
6. Kissel JT, Slivka AP, Warmolts JR, Mendell JR. The clinical spectrum of necrotizing angiopathy of the peripheral nervous system. *Ann Neurol*. 1985;18:251–257.
7. Moore PM, Cupps TR. Neurological complications of vasculitis. *Ann Neurol*. 1983;14:155–167.

8. Zeek PM. Periarteritis nodosa: a clinical review. *Am J Clin Pathol.* 1952;22:777–790.
9. Hoffman GS, Kerr GS, Leavitt RY, et al. Wegener granulomatosis: an analysis of 158 patients. *Ann Intern Med.* 1992;116:488–498.
10. Kissel JT, Mendell JR. Vasculitic neuropathy. *Neurol Clin.* 1992;10: 761–781.
11. Harati Y, Niakan E. The clinical spectrum of inflammatory-angiopathic neuropathy. *J Neurol Neurosurg Psychiatry.* 1986;49: 1313–1316.
12. Ropert A, Metral S. Conduction block in neuropathies with necrotizing vasculitis. *Muscle Nerve.* 1990;13:102–105.
13. Jamieson PW, Giuliani MJ, Martinez AJ. Necrotizing angiopathy presenting with multifocal conduction blocks. *Neurology.* 1991;41: 442–444.
14. Kissell JT, Collins MP, Mendell JR. Vasculitic neuropathy. In: Mendell JR, Kissell JT, Cornblath DR, eds. *Diagnosis and Management of Peripheral Nerve Disorders.* In: Contemporary Neurology. Oxford: Oxford University Press; 2001:202–232.
15. Lipsky PE. Rheumatoid arthritis. In: Fauci AS, Braunwald E, Isselbacher KJ, eds. *Harrison's Principles of Internal Medicine.* 14th ed. New York, NY: McGraw-Hill; 1998:1880–1888.
16. Arnett FC, Edworthy SM, Bloch DA, et al. The American Rheumatism Association 1987 revised criteria for the classification of rheumatoid arthritis. *Arthritis Rheum.* 1988;31(3):315–324.
17. Collins MP, Kissel JT. Neuropathies with systemic vasculitis. In: Dyck PJ, Thomas PK, eds. *Peripheral Neuropathy.* Philadelphia, PA: Elsevier; 2005:2335–2404.
18. Cruickshank B. The arteritis of rheumatoid arthritis. *Ann Rheum Dis.* 1954;13:136–146.
19. Lee DM, Kiener HP, Agarwal SK, et al. Cadherin-11 in synovial lining formation and pathology in arthritis. *Science.* 2007;315(814): 1006–1010.
20. Piecyk ML, Schur PH. *Neurologic Manifestations of Rheumatoid Arthritis.* Waltham, MA: UpToDate; 2022.
21. Sokoloff L, Wilens SL, Bunim JJ. Arteritis of striated muscle in rheumatoid arthritis. *Am J Pathol.* 1951;27(1):157–173.
22. Gordon DA, Stein JL, Broder I. The extra-articular features of rheumatoid arthritis: a systemic analysis of 127 cases. *Am J Med.* 1973;54(4):445–452.
23. Good AE, Christopher RP, Koepke GH, et al. Peripheral neuropathy associated with rheumatoid arthritis: a clinical and electrodiagnostic study of 70 consecutive rheumatoid arthritis patients. *Ann Intern Med.* 1965;63:87–99.
24. Scott DG, Bacon PA, Tribe CR. Systemic rheumatoid vasculitis: a clinical and laboratory study of 50 cases. *Medicine.* 1981;60: 288–297.
25. Schmid FR, Cooper NS, Ziff M, McEwen C. Arteritis in rheumatoid arthritis. *Am J Med.* 1961;30:56–83.
26. Voskuyl AE, Zwinderman AH, Westedt ML, et al. Factors associated with the development of vasculitis in rheumatoid arthritis: results of a case-control study. *Ann Rheum Dis.* 1996;55:190–192.
27. Pallis CA, Scott JT. Peripheral neuropathy in rheumatoid arthritis. *Br Med J.* 1965;1:1141–1147.
28. Upreti S, Oudah M, Hauptman H, Minn H. Vasculitis neuropathy associated with rheumatoid arthritis, a case report. *J Community Hosp Intern Med Perspect.* 2019;9(5):430–432.
29. Mielke H, Daniel W, Deicher H, et al. A three-year prospective study of systemic manifestation in rheumatoid arthritis. *Clin Rheumatol.* 1987;7(2):26–34.
30. Kuntzer T, Antoine JC, Steck AJ. Clinical features and pathophysiological basis of sensory neuronopathies (ganglionopathies). *Muscle Nerve.* 2004;30(3):255–268.
31. Alshekhlee A, Basiri K, Miles JD, Ahmad SA, Katiji B. Chronic inflammatory demyelinating polyneuropathy associated with tumor necrosis factor-alpha antagonists. *Muscle Nerve.* 2010;41(5): 723–727.
32. Stubgen JP. Tumor necrosis factor-alpha antagonists and neuropathy. *Muscle Nerve.* 2008;37(3):281–292.
33. Gorson KC. Vasculitic neuropathy: an update. *Neurology.* 2007;13(1): 12–19.

67 CASE

A Woman With Granulomatous Lesions in the Lungs and a Peripheral Neuropathy

A 71-year-old woman presented initially to her internist with an acute episode of severe cough, mild fever, and weight loss. Chest x-ray and CT scan demonstrated bilateral granulomatous lesions (Fig. 67-1).

Laboratory studies showed a white blood cell count of 4000 cells/μL (normal, 3800–10,000 cells/μL). Hematocrit was 32.3% (normal, 35%–46%). Thyroid-stimulating hormone, B_{12}, glycosylated hemoglobin, and fasting blood sugar were normal. Anti-PR3 (antiproteinase 3; circulating antineutrophil cytoplasmic antibody [C-ANCA]) IgG titer was 0.97 EU/mL (normal, <6 EU/mL). The antimyeloperoxidase (anti-MPO; perinuclear ANCA [P-ANCA]) IgG was 0.01 EU/mL (normal, <6 EU/mL).

A lung biopsy showed a granulomatous lesion compatible with Wegener granulomatosis (Fig. 67-2).

She was started on oral cyclophosphamide 100 mg/day orally with the improvement of the cough and resolution of the lung lesions. The drug was discontinued after she developed severe leukopenia. She presented 6 months later with progressive numbness and tingling in the legs and hands.

Past medical history was positive for two C-sections, hemorrhoidectomy, cataract surgery, and hyperlipidemia for which she was taking simvastatin. She did not drink or smoke, and there was no family history of neurologic disorders.

Mentation and cranial nerve examinations were normal. Strength and reflexes were also normal, except for absent ankle jerks. She had decreased vibration sense in the toes, mildly decreased at the ankles, and normal at the knees, with decreased pinprick and pain sensations up to the midcalf. Hand sensation was normal. There were no Babinski signs. Coordination and gait were normal. There was no visceromegaly, and the rest of the examination was normal.

EMG AND QUANTITATIVE SENSORY TESTS WERE PERFORMED

Motor Nerve Studies

Nerve and Site	Latency (ms)	Amplitude (mV)	Conduction Velocity (m/s)
Peroneal Nerve R.	**Normal ≤ 5.7**	**Normal ≥ 3**	**Normal ≥ 40**
Ankle	**6.5**	7	–
Fibular head	14.3	6	40
Knee	16.3	6	**38**
Tibial Nerve L.	**Normal ≤ 5.3**	**Normal ≥ 4**	**Normal ≥ 40**
Ankle	4.4	13	–
Pop. fossa	15.7	7	**35**
Nerve and Site	**Latency (ms)**	**Amplitude (mV)**	**Conduction Velocity (m/s)**
Ulnar Nerve R.	**Normal ≤ 3.6**	**Normal ≥ 8**	**Normal ≥ 50**
Wrist	3.3	11	–
Below elbow	7.0	8	55
Above elbow	9.3	8	52
Axilla	11.4	8	61

F-Wave and Tibial H-Reflex Studies

Nerve	Latency (ms)	Normal Latency ≤ (ms)
Peroneal nerve R.	**58.0**	54
Tibial nerve L.	**66.9**	54
Ulnar nerve R.	27.4	30
H-reflex R.	**38.1**	34
H-reflex L.	**NR**	34

Sensory Nerve Studies

Nerve	Onset Latency (ms)	Normal Onset Latency ≤ (ms)	Peak Latency (ms)	Normal Peak Latency ≤ (ms)	Amp (μV)	Normal Amp ≥ (μV)	Conduction Velocity (m/s)	Normal Conduction Velocity ≥ (m/s)
Sural nerve R.	**3.7**	**3.5**	**4.2**	4.0	**5**	11	–	40
Superficial peroneal nerve R.	**NR**	3.5	**NR**	4.0	**NR**	10	**NR**	40
Ulnar nerve R.	2.3	2.6	2.8	3.1	23	13	52	50

Quantitative Sensory Testing

	Threshold JND	Normal/Abnormal
Vibration Detection Threshold		
Hand: 40%	13.5	Normal
Foot: 98%	**20.5**	**Abnormal**
Cold Detection Threshold		
Hand: 35%	6.75	Normal
Foot: 96%	**22.5**	**Abnormal**
Heat Pain Threshold		
Hand: 45%	16.5	Normal
Foot: 97%	**25.0**	**Abnormal**

JND, Just noticeable distortion.

EMG Data

Muscle	Insrt Activity	Fibs	Pos Waves	Fasc	Amp	Dur	Poly	Pattern
Vastus lateralis R.	Norm	None	None	None	Norm	Norm	None	Full
Tibialis anterior R.	Norm	None	None	None	**Lg**	**Inc**	None	**Red**
Gastrocnemius R.	Norm	None	None	None	Norm	Norm	None	Full
Extensor hallucis longus R.	Norm	None	None	None	Norm	Norm	None	**Red**
Tibialis anterior L.	Norm	None	None	None	**Lg**	**Inc**	None	**Red**
Gastrocnemius L.	Norm	None	None	None	Norm	Norm	None	**Red**

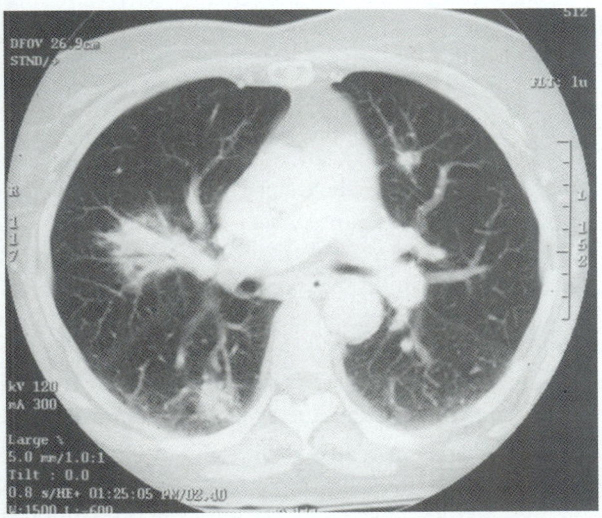

FIG. 67-1 Contrast CT scan of the chest showing the multiple lung nodes.

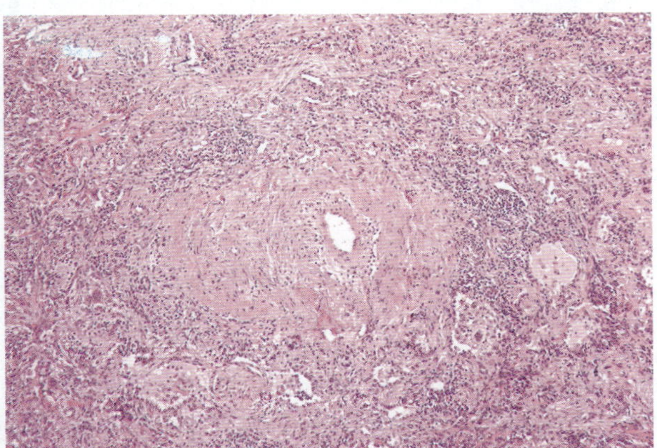

FIG. 67-2 Lung biopsy showing granulomatous material with lymphocytic accumulation (H&E stain, ×200).

WHAT WERE THE TEST FINDINGS?

The test revealed mildly decreased motor conduction velocity of the tibial nerve and of the peroneal nerve across the knee. Upper extremity motor conduction velocities, CMAP amplitudes and latencies, and SNAP amplitudes were normal. The sural SNAP was of low amplitude, and the superficial peroneal nerve SNAP was absent. Needle test showed large motor unit potentials and decreased motor unit recruitment in both distal legs. These findings indicate a mild, predominantly sensory peripheral neuropathy.

Quantitative sensory testing results indicated a distal deficit affecting both large myelinated and small unmyelinated fibers with increased cold, pain, and vibration detection thresholds.

WHAT TESTS SHOULD BE DONE NEXT?

There was a faint IgA kappa monoclonal protein on electrophoresis. Fluorescent antinuclear antibodies and anti-Hu antibody tests were negative. A 24-hour urine for Bence-Jones proteinuria was negative; sulfatide antibodies and MAG antibodies were not present.

Anti-PR3 (C-ANCA) was elevated at 47 EU/mL, and the anti-MPO (P-ANCA) was normal at 6 EU/mL; the erythrocyte sedimentation rate was 55 mm/h (normal, <30 mm/h).

A sural nerve biopsy showed a decreased number of myelinated fibers and some subperineural edema with small perivascular inflammatory infiltrates (Fig. 67-3).

WHAT IS THE MOST LIKELY DIAGNOSIS?

This patient with Wegener granulomatosis presented with a diffuse polyneuropathy. Her initial Wegener serology was negative when she presented with lung lesions, which improved

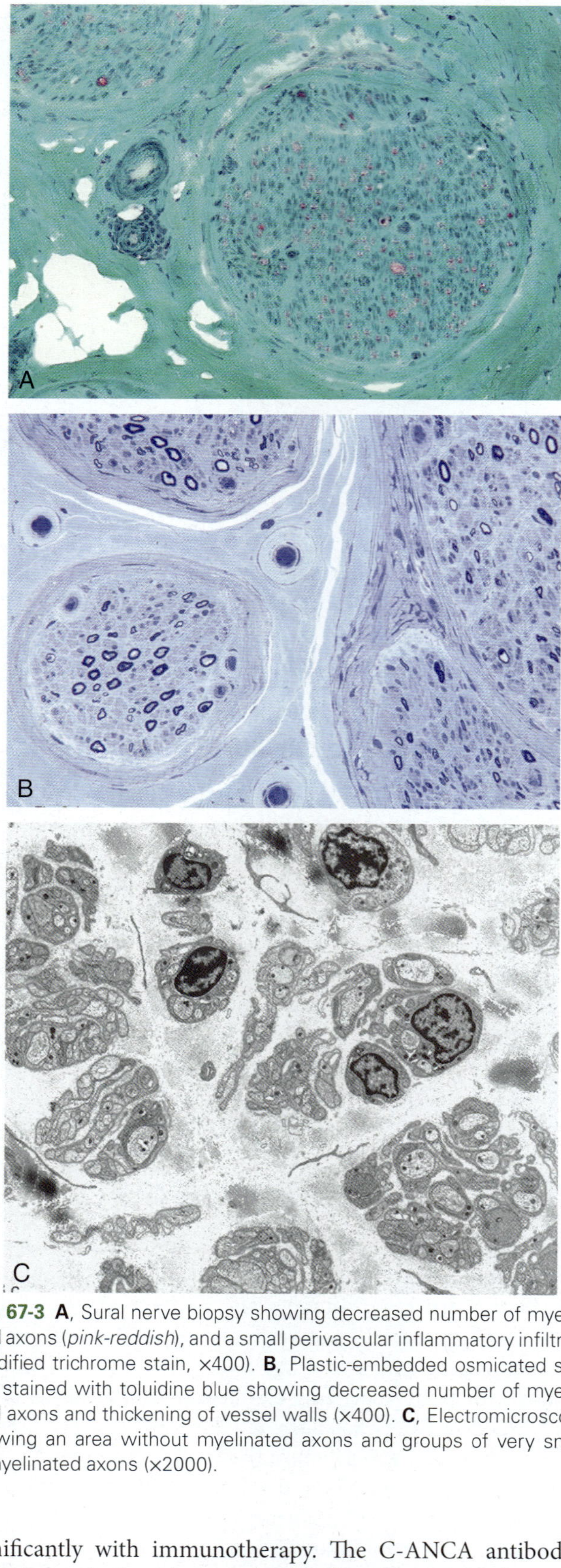

FIG. 67-3 **A**, Sural nerve biopsy showing decreased number of myelinated axons (*pink-reddish*), and a small perivascular inflammatory infiltrate (modified trichrome stain, ×400). **B**, Plastic-embedded osmicated section stained with toluidine blue showing decreased number of myelinated axons and thickening of vessel walls (×400). **C**, Electromicroscopy showing an area without myelinated axons and groups of very small unmyelinated axons (×2000).

significantly with immunotherapy. The C-ANCA antibodies were elevated when she presented with a polyneuropathy.

The differential diagnosis includes not only Wegener-associated polyneuropathy but also other common etiologies. Her blood sugar and B_{12} levels were normal, and she had no exposure to toxins. Workup for other causes was negative. As the initial protein electrophoresis suggested a monoclonal gammopathy, this was repeated and no abnormalities were detected. Immunoelectrophoresis was also normal. Her nerve biopsy showed no amyloid deposits but did show evidence of perivascular inflammatory infiltrates. This and her history of Wegener granulomatosis with positive serology suggest that her neuropathy was caused by that disease, and no clear histologic evidence of vasculitis was found in the nerve biopsy,[1] only perivascular infiltrates, but this did not rule out a vasculitis.[2]

The neuropathy involved the large myelinated and small sensory fibers.

She was treated with prednisone 40 mg/day with marked improvement; it was decided to hold cyclophosphamide due to leukopenia. She then developed cushingoid features, and prednisone was tapered off. Cyclophosphamide was started again with careful monitoring of her white blood cell count. She has remained stable for 3 years.

WHAT IS WEGENER GRANULOMATOSIS?

This is a form of systemic necrotizing vasculitis characterized by granulomatous lung lesions that can be associated with peripheral neuropathy in 15% of the cases.[3–7] This disorder is now called granuloma with polyangiitis (GAN). The other name is no longer used as Dr. Wegener was a Nazi physician who worked with a facility associated with unethical humane experimentation.[8] The disease is similar to Churg–Strauss syndrome which also presents with eosinophilia and asthma. Another vasculitis with positive ANCA serology is micro-angiopathic polyangiitis, characterized by purpura and rapidly progressive glomerulonephritis with lung involvement but without granulomatous formations. Some patients have an overlap of these conditions.

This vasculitis can manifest as mononeuritis or mononeuritis multiplex affecting most frequently the peroneal, posterior tibial, ulnar, radial, sensory, and sciatic nerves. It might also present as a polyneuropathy due to the simultaneous involvement of multiple nerves.[9] The neuropathy in this disorder is usually milder than in Churg–Strauss disease and microscopic polyangiitis.[10] Other primary vasculitic neuropathies also include periarteritis nodosa, giant cell arteritis, microscopic polyangiitis, and nonsystemic vasculitic neuropathies of the small vessels.

WHAT IS ANCA?

These are antibodies directed against cytoplasmic proteins of neutrophils and monocytes.

The name *antineutrophil cytoplasmic antibody* is based on the staining characteristic of ethanol-fixed neutrophils. This test could have a cytoplasmic pattern (C-ANCA), which is very specific for Wegener granulomatosis, and a perinuclear pattern (P-ANCA), which is seen in Churg–Strauss syndrome and microscopic polyangiitis. The target antigens for ANCA include PR3 of the alpha granules (C-ANCA) and a perinuclear staining that reacts with MPO (MPO-ANCA), which can

TABLE 67-1 **ANCA-Associated Disease**

Disease	Pattern	Antigen
Microscopic polyarteritis	C	MPO, PR3
Wegener granulomatosis	C	PR3, BPI
Henoch–Schönlein purpura	C	Unknown
Churg–Strauss syndrome	C, P	PR3, MPO, BPI
Kawasaki syndrome	C, P	PR3, MPO
Giant cell arteritis	P	MPO
Polyarteritis nodosa	C, P	PR3, MPO
Drug-induced vasculitis	P	MPO
Rapidly progressive glomerulonephritis	P, X	MPO, elastase, and h-lamp 2
Glomerular basement membrane disease	C, P	PR3, MPO
Rheumatoid arthritis (Felty syndrome)	X	Lactoferrin, cathepsin G
Rheumatoid arthritis (vasculitis)	P	MPO
Rheumatoid arthritis	X	Elastase, lactoferrin, and cathepsin G
Systemic lupus erythematosus	X	Elastase, lactoferrin, and cathepsin G
Autoimmune hepatitis, HIV, Crohn disease, and ulcerative colitis	X	Lysozyme, β-glucuronidase, cathepsin G, and lactoferrin

BPI, Bactericidal/permeability-increasing; *C*, circulating; *MPO*, myeloperoxidase; *P*, perinuclear; *PR3*, proteinase 3; *X*, atypical. Reprinted with permission from Nishino H, Rubino F, DeRemee RA, et al. Neurological involvement in Wegener's granulomatosis: an analysis of 324 consecutive patients at the Mayo Clinic. *Ann Neurol.* 1993;33:4–9.

be demonstrated by enzyme-linked immunosorbent analysis. A positive C-ANCA sera with PR3 antibodies is 80% sensitive and 97% specific for Wegener granulomatosis.[10,11] Both C-ANCA and P-ANCA antibodies might be present in periarteritis nodosa. An atypical staining (X-ANCA) has activation to different myeloid antigens, such as elastase, cathepsin G, and lysosomal and lactoferrin. P-ANCA and X-ANCA are not very specific and can also be seen in other autoimmune conditions[12] (Table 67-1).

WHAT IS THE PATHOGENESIS OF THE VASCULITIS IN WEGENER GRANULOMATOSIS?

In general, vasculitis might be secondary to infections such as Lyme disease, HIV, and hepatitis; they can also be drug-induced connective tissue disorders, sarcoidosis, cryoglobulinemia, and Behçet disease or have an autoimmune pathogenesis.

The vessel injury in autoimmune vasculitis is caused by various mechanisms, such as the formation of immune complexes that deposit in vessel walls,[13] or by antibodies directed to endothelial cell antigens[13] with activation of complement and the formation of membrane attack complexes, and generation of chemotactic factors resulting in adherence of leukocytes to endothelial cells. This causes the release of enzymes, toxic oxygen radicals, and cytokines that produce cell damage and promote the recruitment of inflammatory cells with perpetuation of the immune response.[9,14]

In cell-mediated vasculitis the effector cells are cytotoxic T lymphocytes directed against endothelial cells or toward exogenous antigens processed by these cells. ANCA might activate neutrophils to adhere to the endothelial cells causing their lysis.[15,16] In addition, endothelial cells express antigens to ANCA, such as PR3, which triggers the expression of adhesion molecules causing antibody-mediated cytotoxicity.[17]

WHAT IS THE TREATMENT FOR WEGENER GRANULOMATOSIS?

The treatment consists of the use of cyclophosphamide orally, 1–2 mg/kg daily or by intravenous infusions in severe cases and/or steroids, 1–2 mg/kg.[4] The disease may also respond to other immunotherapeutic drugs such as azathioprine. Rituximab and infliximab are very beneficial[18,19] and these can be used in combination with corticosteroids.[20]

SUMMARY

This patient has Wegener granulomatosis which manifested initially with lung granulomas. She responded to cyclophosphamide but presented later with a peripheral neuropathy and elevated TPR-3 C-ANCA when the drug was discontinued. The neuropathy responded to oral prednisone therapy, but this was discontinued when she developed severe cushingoid features. She then responded to a low-dose cyclophosphamide.

IMPORTANT POINTS

- Wegener granulomatosis is a form of vasculitis characterized by granulomas of the lungs, but can also affect kidneys and peripheral nerves.
- This and other types of vasculitis might present as a mononeuritis, a mononeuritis multiplex, or a polyneuropathy.
- In this condition the vessels are damaged from the activation of neutrophils by ANCA that degrade endothelial cells. ANCA might also target endothelial cell antigens such as PRs, causing the expression of adhesion molecules triggering an antibody-mediated cytotoxicity.
- The treatment of Wegener granulomatosis consists of immunosuppressant therapy such as cyclophosphamide, steroids, and rituximab.

REFERENCES

1. Prayson RA, Sedlock DJ. Clinicopathologic study of 43 patients with sural nerve vasculitis. *Hum Pathol.* 2003;34(5):484–490.
2. Vrancken AF, Notermans NC, Jansen GH, et al. Progressive idiopathic axonal neuropathy: a comparative clinical and histopathological study with vasculitic neuropathy. *J Neurol.* 2004;251(3):269–278.

3. Rao JK, Weinberger M, Oddone EZ, et al. The role of antineutrophil cytoplasmic antibody (c-ANCA) testing in the diagnosis of Wegener granulomatosis: a literature review and *meta*-analysis. *Ann Intern Med.* 1995;123:925–932.
4. Duna GF, Galperin C, Hoffman GS. Wegener's granulomatosis. *Rheum Dis Clin North Am.* 1995;21:949–986.
5. Nishino H, Rubino FA, Parisi JE. The spectrum of neurologic involvement in Wegener's granulomatosis. *Neurology.* 1993;43: 1334–1337.
6. Bajema I, Hagen E. Evolving concepts about the role of antineutrophil cytoplasm autoantibodies in systemic vasculitides. *Curr Opin Rheumatol.* 1999;11:34–40.
7. Nishino H, Rubino F, DeRemee RA, et al. Neurological involvement in Wegener's granulomatosis: an analysis of 324 consecutive patients at the Mayo Clinic. *Ann Neurol.* 1993;33:4–9.
8. Amato AA, Russell JA. Vasculitic neuropathies. *Neuromuscular Disorders.* New York, NY: McGraw Hill; 2016:371–383 (Chapter 15).
9. Kissel JT, Collins MP, Mendell JR. Vasculitis neuropathy Contemporary Neurology Series. In: Mendell JR, Kissel JT, Cornblath DR, eds. *Diagnosis and Management of Peripheral Nerve Disorders.* New York, NY: Oxford University Press; 2001: 202–232.
10. Cattaneo L, Chierici E, Pavone L, et al. Peripheral neuropathy in Wegener's granulomatosis, Churg–Strauss syndrome and microscopic polyangiitis. *Neurol Neurosurg Psychiatry.* 2007;78(10):1119–1123.
11. Ahmed AE, Aziz DC. Antineutrophil cytoplasmic autoantibodies. In: Peter JB, ed. *Use and Interpretation of Laboratory Tests in Neurology.* 4th ed. Santa Monica, CA: Specialty Laboratories; 1999:305–310.
12. Rowshani AT, Schot LJ, ten Berge IJ. c-ANCA as a serological pitfall. *Lancet.* 2004;364(9442):1313–1314.
13. Gauthier VJ, Mannik M. Immune complexes in the pathogenesis of vasculitis. In: LeRoy EC, ed. *Systemic Vasculitis: The Biological Basis.* New York, NY: Marcel Dekker; 1992:401–420.
14. Kekow J, Szmkowiak CH, Sticherling M, et al. Pro- and anti-inflammatory cytokines in primary systemic vasculitis. In: Gross WL, ed. *ANCA-Associated Vasculitis: Immunological and Clinical Aspects.* New York, NY: Plenum Press; 1993:341–344.
15. Ben-Baruch A, Michiel DF, Oppenheim JJ. Signals and receptors involved in recruitment of inflammatory cells. *J Biol Chem.* 1995; 270:11703–11706.
16. Chalk CH, Homburger HA, Dyck PJ. Anti-neutrophil cytoplasmic antibodies in vasculitis peripheral neuropathy. *Neurology.* 1993;43: 1826–1827.
17. Mayet WJ, Csernok E, Szymkowiak C, et al. Human endothelial cells express proteinase 3, the target antigen of anticytoplasmic antibodies in Wegener's granulomatosis. *Blood.* 1993;82: 1221–1229.
18. Holle JU, Dubrau C, Herlyn K, Heller M, et al. Rituximab for refractory granulomatosis with polyangiitis (Wegener's granulomatosis): comparison of efficacy in granulomatous versus vasculitic manifestations. *Ann Rheum Dis.* 2012;71(3): 327–333.
19. de Menthon M, Cohen P, Pagnoux C, Buchler M, et al. Infliximab or rituximab for refractory Wegener's granulomatosis: long-term follow up. A prospective randomised multicentre study on 17 patients. *Clin Exp Rheumatol.* 2011;29(1 suppl 64):S63–71.
20. Stone JH, Merkel PA, Spiera R, Seo P, Langford CA, et al. Rituximab versus cyclophosphamide for ANCA-associated vasculitis. *N Engl J Med.* 2010;363(3):221–232.

CASE 68

A Man With a Neuropathy, Weight Loss, and Lung Nodules

A 31-year-old black man was referred from another institution for evaluation of a neuropathy with a nerve biopsy suggestive of vasculitis. He had been healthy until 1 year before when he developed perioral dysesthesias followed by hand and leg weakness, with numbness in the legs and difficulty walking. He had a 60-lb weight loss.

The previous workup revealed a normal erythrocyte sedimentation rate and a spinal fluid protein of 60 mg/dL without cells. FANA was negative. A chest x-ray showed multiple pulmonary nodules.

Past medical history was unremarkable. His father had some type of lung disease, apparently chronic obstructive pulmonary disease, and was a non–insulin-dependent diabetic. The patient drank a six-pack of beer per month but did not smoke.

He appeared cachetic but had no visceromegaly or palpable nodes. Mentation and cranial nerves were normal except for decreased sensation in the right mental area and he had facial asymmetry from mild weakness of the right hemiface. There was weakness of the hand interossei muscles and bilateral foot drop with prominent weakness of the distal muscles in both legs. He had areflexia in the legs and arms, vibration sense was absent in the toes and ankles and decreased in the knees and toes, and there were decreased pinprick and touch sensations up to the midarm and up to the mid-calf. The ulnar nerves were thick.

Complete blood count and metabolic panel were normal. Antineutrophilic cytoplasmic antibody titers were normal. A spinal fluid test showed seven white blood cells, 97% lymphocytes, and three monocytes; cytology was negative for malignant cells, protein was 678 mg/dL. Acid-fast bacilli and fungus cultures were negative. Electrophoresis, human T-lymphotropic virus 1, and HIV tests were negative. Angiotensin-converting enzyme was elevated at 69 μg/L (normal, <52 μg/L).

WHAT IS THE DIFFERENTIAL DIAGNOSIS?

This patient had pulmonary nodules and a peripheral neuropathy. The differential diagnosis includes sarcoidosis, particularly as the angiotensin-converting enzyme was mildly elevated, but there was no evidence of a mediastinal mass. Another possibility is Wegener granulomatosis which presents with peripheral neuropathy and granulomatous lesions in the lungs. A malignant lymphoma and lymphoid granulomatosis could have a similar presentation. Tuberculosis does not cause a neuropathy; leprosy does not present with lung disease.

AN EMG TEST WAS PERFORMED

Motor Nerve Studies

Nerve and Site	Latency (ms)	Amplitude (mV)	Conduction Velocity (m/s)
Peroneal Nerve R.	**Normal ≤ 5.7**	**Normal ≥ 3**	**Normal ≥ 40**
Ankle	**NR**	**NR**	–
Fibular head	**NR**	**NR**	**NR**
Tibial Nerve L.	**Normal ≥ 5.3**	**Normal ≥ 4**	**Normal ≥ 50**
Ankle	**6.3**	**0.5**	–
Pop. fossa	**NR**	**NR**	**NR**

Nerve and Site	Latency (ms)	Amplitude (mV)	Conduction Velocity (m/s)
Median Nerve L.	**Normal ≤ 4.2**	**Normal ≥ 6**	**Normal ≥ 50**
Wrist	3.1	16	–
Elbow	8.4	12	58
Ulnar Nerve L.	**Normal ≤ 3.6**	**Normal ≥ 8**	**Normal ≥ 50**
Wrist	**4.2**	**3**	–
Below elbow	9.4	**3**	**44**
Above elbow	12.8	**3**	**35**

F-Wave Studies

Nerve	Latency (ms)	Normal Latency ≤ (ms)
Median nerve L.	27.6	30
Ulnar nerve L.	30	30

Sensory Nerve Studies

Nerve	Onset Latency (ms)	Normal Onset Latency ≤ (ms)	Peak Latency (ms)	Normal Peak Latency ≤ (ms)	Amp (μV)	Normal Amp ≥ (μV)	Conduction Velocity (m/s)	Normal Conduction Velocity ≥ (m/s)
Median nerve L.	2.4	2.6	2.9	3.1	17	20	54	50
Ulnar nerve L.	**NR**	2.6	**NR**	3.1	**NR**	13	**NR**	50
Sural nerve R.	**NR**	3.5	**NR**	4.0	**NR**	11	**NR**	40

EMG Data

Muscle	Insrt Activity	Fibs	Pos Waves	Fasc	Amp	Dur	Poly	Pattern
Biceps brachii L.	Norm	None	None	None	Norm	Norm	None	Full
Flexor carpi radialis L.	Norm	None	None	None	Norm	Norm	None	Full
Flexor carpi ulnaris L.	**Inc**	None	None	None	**Lg**	**Inc**	None	Full
Extensor digitorum com. L.	Norm	None	None	None	Norm	Norm	None	Full
First dorsal interosseus L.	**Inc**	None	**1+**	None	**Lg**	**Inc**	None	**Red**
Vastus lateralis L.	Norm	None	None	None	**Lg**	**Inc**	None	Full
Tibialis anterior L.	**Inc**	None	**1+**	None	**Lg**	**Inc**	None	**Red**
Gastrocnemius L.	**Inc**	None	**1+**	None	Norm	Norm	None	**Red**
Gastrocnemius R.	**Inc**	None	**1+**	None	Norm	Norm	None	**Red**

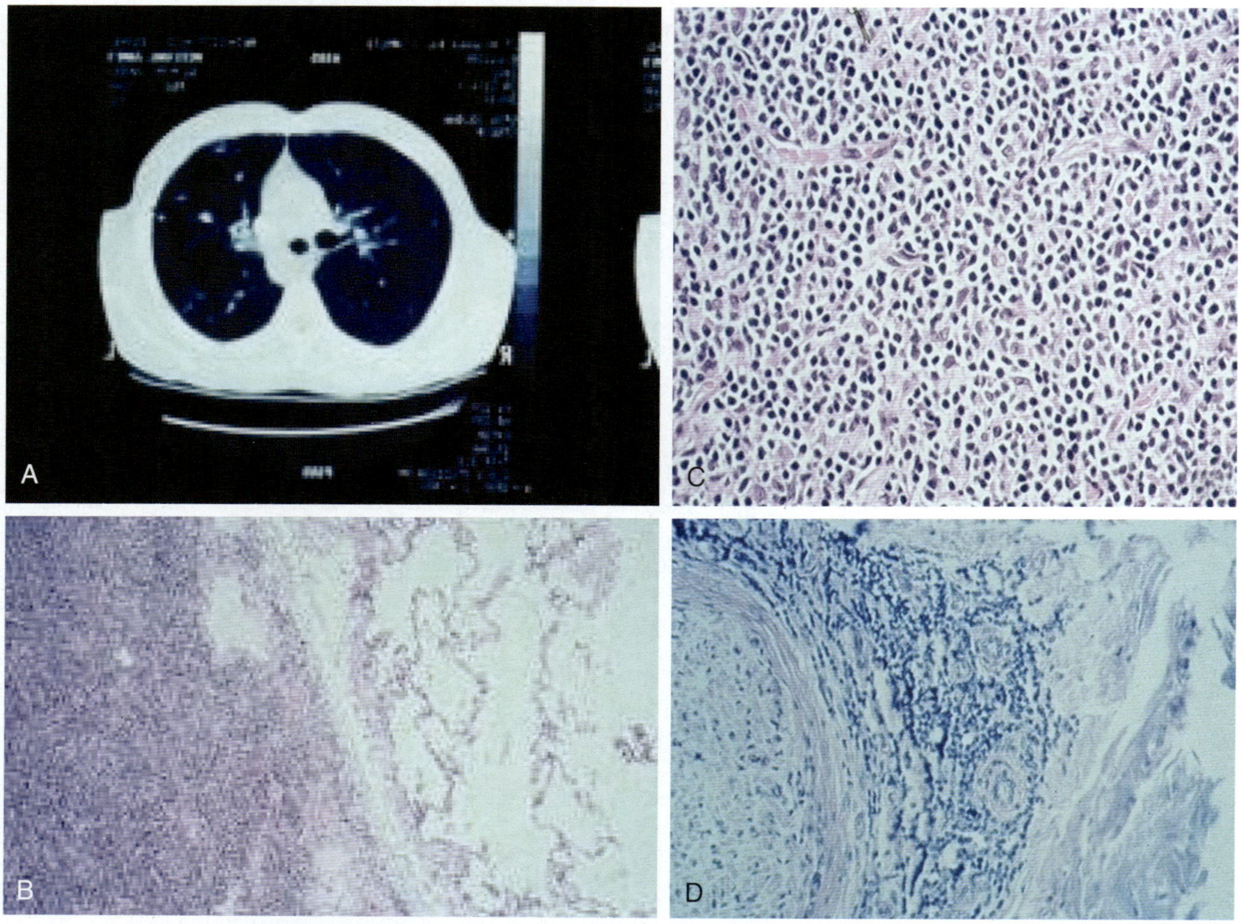

FIG. 68-1 **A**, Contrast CT scan of the chest showing multiple small nodes. **B**, Lung infiltrates consisting mostly of lymphocytes (H&E stain, ×100). **C**, Homogenous mononuclear cells in node (H&E stain, ×200). **D**, Perineural cellular infiltrate in sural nerve (toluidine blue stain, ×200).

WHAT WERE THE EMG FINDINGS?

The test showed peripheral neuropathy involving some nerves and sparing others. There were no recordable CMAPs from the tibial or peroneal nerve stimulation; there was slowing of the ulnar nerve conduction velocity with low-amplitude CMAP, but the median nerve was normal. The F-responses were normal. SNAPs were absent in the ulnar and sural nerves.

There was diffuse denervation and reduced motor unit recruitment in the legs.

It was concluded that he had a neuropathy with axonal degeneration, with features of a mononeuritis multiplex despite the apparent symmetrical clinical distribution of finding in the limbs.

A CT scan of the chest revealed multiple pulmonary nodules (Fig. 68-1A); lung biopsy showed granulomatous lymphocytic infiltrates with some hemorrhage (see Fig. 68-1B and C). The cells had irregular nuclei. There were both B and T lymphocytes, but mainly T cells. They appear malignant but a flow cytometry revealed no clear clonicity. Bone marrow biopsy showed similar findings.

WHAT SHOULD BE DONE NEXT?

The sural nerve biopsy was reviewed and showed evidence of axonal degeneration with lymphocytic infiltrations in the perineural area, some around vessels (see Fig. 68-1D). In some areas the endoneurium was also infiltrated.

The patient was treated with cyclophosphamide that produced remission. Eight months later, he became progressively worse and had multiple organ involvement with lymphocytic infiltrates. He did not respond to aggressive chemotherapy and died. No autopsy was performed.

DISCUSSION

This patient had multinodular infiltration of the lungs that appeared to be caused by T-cell non-Hodgkin lymphoma that was not well categorized.

He had a polyneuropathy, but some nerves were more affected than others, and the nerve biopsy showed pseudovasculitic infiltrates and also axonal degeneration. In some areas, the endoneurium was infiltrated by lymphoid cells.

Lymphomas can cause various neurological manifestations, including peripheral neuropathies from a metabolic or infectious process or by paraneoplastic mechanisms and tumor infiltration.[1] These include a sensorimotor polyneuropathy, Guillain–Barré syndrome (GBS), and a chronic inflammatory demyelinating polyneuropathy (CIDP), particularly in those with Hodgkin lymphoma.[1–6] Other manifestations include cranial neuropathies, as in this patient; they could also cause radiculopathies from infiltration of the dura and adjacent nerves. Lymphomas can also cause plexopathies, mononeuropathies, and mononeuritis multiplex.[7]

Non-Hodgkin lymphoma is the most common cause of a lymphomatous neuropathy. Hodgkin lymphoma, on the other hand, can also manifest with an autoimmune neuropathy, such as GBS or CIDP. Other manifestations of a lymphoma include vasculitis, cryoglobulinemia, motor neuron disorders, Isaacs syndrome, and stiff-person syndrome.[8–11]

The term *neurolymphomatosis* defines a malignant lymphomatous infiltration of nerves causing their focal or diffuse enlargement.[12–20] In this the cell types can be defined by flow cytometry and immunohistochemistry. The great majority are B cells; only about 10% represent T cells.

Other lymphomatous diseases that affect the nervous system include intravascular B-cell lymphoma or malignant angioendotheliomatosis in which the lymphoma is confined to the lumen of vessels, and this can cause strokes, but sometimes also mononeuropathies.[18] Lymphoid granulomatosis is an angiocentric nonneoplastic granulomatous disease associated with Epstein–Barr viral infection that could rarely manifest as a peripheral neuropathy.[21,22]

Detailed evaluation on patients with proper diagnostic techniques, particularly bone marrow and lymph node biopsy, are useful in determining, if possible, the exact type of lymphoma for treatment.[1] Therapy includes immunomodulation and immunotherapy.[23]

SUMMARY

This patient had multiple lung nodules and a neuropathy. In EMG some nerves were more affected than others with axonal degeneration. He had a lymphomatous infiltration of the lungs and peripheral nerves. He initially responded to chemotherapy, but later he developed multiorgan involvement.

IMPORTANT POINTS

- The differential diagnosis of patients with lung nodes and peripheral neuropathy includes sarcoidosis, infections, Wegener granulomatosis, lymphoid granulomatosis, and tumors, such as lymphoma.
- Neurolymphomatosis refers to invasion of peripheral nerves and/or central nervous system lymphoma.
- Lymphoma can manifest with polyneuropathy, mononeuropathies, plexopathies or radiculopathy, and, rarely, GBS, chronic inflammatory demyelinating polyradiculoneuropathy and other autoimmune disorders (such as cryoglobulinemia), vasculitis, stiff-person syndrome, and Isaacs syndrome.

REFERENCES

1. Kelly JJ, Karcher DS. Lymphoma and peripheral neuropathy: a clinical review. *Muscle Nerve.* 2005;31:301–313.
2. Baehring JM, Damek D, Martin EC, et al. Neurolymphomatosis. *Neuro-Oncology.* 2003;5:104–115.
3. Croft PB, Urich H, Wilkinson M. Peripheral neuropathy of sensorimotor type associated with malignant disease. *Brain.* 1967;90:31–66.
4. Hunt WE, Bouroncle BA, Meagher JN. Neurological complications of leukemia and lymphomas. *J Neurosurg.* 1959;16:135–151.
5. Germignani F, Melli G, Inglese C, Marbini A. Cryoglobulinemia is a frequent cause of peripheral neuropathy in undiagnosed referral patients. *J Peripher Nerv Syst.* 2002;7:59–64.
6. Creange A, Theodorou I, Sabourin JC, et al. Inflammatory neuromuscular disorders associated with chronic lymphoid leukemia: evidence for clonal B cells within muscle and nerve. *J Neurol Sci.* 1996;137:35–41.
7. Rahmani M, Birouk N, Amarti A, et al. T-cell lymphoma revealed by a mononeuritis multiplex: case report and review of literature. *Rev Neurol (Paris).* 2007;163(4):462–490.
8. Wada M, Kurita K, Tajima K, et al. A case of inflammatory demyelinating polyradiculoneuropathy associated with T-cell lymphoma. *Acta Neurol Scand.* 2003;107:62–66.
9. Walk D, Handelsman A, Beckmann E, et al. Mononeuropathy multiplex due to infiltration of lymphoma in hematologic remission. *Muscle Nerve.* 1998;21:823–826.
10. Ince PG, Shaw PJ, Fawcett PR, Bates D. Demyelinating neuropathy due to primary IgM kappa B cell lymphoma of peripheral nerve. *Neurology.* 1987;37:1231–1235.
11. Lahrmann H, Albrecht G, Drlicek M, et al. Acquired neuromyotonia and peripheral neuropathy in a patient with Hodgkin's disease. *Muscle Nerve.* 2001;24:834–838.
12. Borit A, Altrocchi PH. Recurrent polyneuropathy and neurolymphomatosis. *Arch Neurol.* 1971;24:40–49.
13. Diamond AL, Thomas FP. Clinical summaries. In: *Neurolymphomatosis.* San Diego, CA: Medlink; 2003. Available at http://www.medlink.com. Retrieved 14.04.04.

14. Trelles JO, Urquiaga C, Palomino L, Trelles L. Human peripheral neurolymphomatosis (reticuloendothelial polyradiculoneuritis). *J Neurol Sci*. 1976;28:187–202.
15. Diaz-Arrastia R, Younger DS, Hair L, et al. Neurolymphomatosis: a clinicopathologic syndrome re-emerges. *Neurology*. 1992;42: 1136–1141.
16. Gordon PH, Younger DS. Neurolymphomatosis. *Neurology*. 1996; 46:1191–1192.
17. Grisold W, Drlicek M, Jellinger K. Neurolymphomatosis. *Neurology*. 1992;43:1628–1629.
18. Vital C, Heraud A, Vital A, et al. Acute mononeuropathy with angiotropic lymphoma. *Acta Neuropathol (Berl)*. 1989;78:105–107.
19. Borit A, Altrocchi PH. Recurrent polyneuropathy and neurolymphomatosis. *Arch Neurol*. 1971;24:40–49.
20. Baehring JM, Damek D, Martin EC, et al. Neurolymphomatosis. *Neuro-Oncology*. 2003;5:104–115.
21. Bone RC, Vernon M, Sobonya RE, Rendon H. Lymphomatoid granulomatosis: report of a case and review of the literature. *Am J Med*. 1978;65:709–716.
22. Hogan PJ, Greenberg MK, McCarty GE. Neurologic complications of lymphomatoid granulomatosis. *Neurology*. 1981;31:619–620.
23. Melani C, Jaffe ES, Wilson WH. Pathobiology and treatment of lymphomatoid granulomatosis, a rare EBV-driven disorder. *Blood*. 2020;135(16):1344–1352.

A Woman With Difficulty Walking and Ataxia

A 67-year-old woman complained of weakness in both lower extremities for 3 months; she also had burning sensations in her feet and difficulty walking, with marked unsteadiness which caused her to fall and fracture her right ankle.

Previous studies that were reviewed included normal MRIs of the brain, neck, and lumbosacral spine. Cerebrospinal fluid abnormalities consisted of elevated glucose of 82 mg/dL (normal, 40–60 mg/dL) and protein of 126 mg/dL (normal, 20–40 mg/dL); there were no cells.

Past medical history was positive for hysterectomy, cholecystectomy, pulmonary fibrosis, and carcinoma of the right breast, treated only with mastectomy 10 years before.

Family and social history were noncontributory.

Neurologic examination revealed normal higher cortical functions and cranial nerves. There was mild weakness in the hands and intrinsic muscles of the feet. All deep tendon reflexes were absent. She had decreased vibration sense in the toes, ankles, knees, and fingers, decreased position sense in the toes, ankles, and fingers, and decreased two-point discrimination in fingers and toes. There were pain and touch sensory deficits to 5 cm above the ankles. Finger-to-nose and heel-to-shin testing were fairly well done but were very abnormal when performed with her eyes closed. Romberg's test was positive, and she had an ataxic gait. She had no Babinski signs.

WHAT IS THE DIFFERENTIAL DIAGNOSIS?

This patient presented with an unsteady gait and progressive sensory ataxia with significant proprioceptive deficits and minimal weakness, indicating an ataxic sensory neuropathy. The slow progression of symptoms is against the sensory ataxic variant of Guillain–Barré syndrome,[1,2] but the presentation is compatible with chronic sensory inflammatory demyelinating polyneuropathy.[3] A sensory neuropathy associated with Sjögren syndrome[4] is an important consideration, as in this condition there is an ataxic sensory neuronopathy caused by degeneration of the posterior root ganglia neurons with inflammation, but she had no symptoms of this disease. Table 69-1 lists the differential diagnosis of ganglionopathies.

Diabetic neuropathy can present with sensory ataxia and proprioceptive deficits, but this usually is seen in patients with a long-standing history of the disease, and this patient was not a diabetic.

She did not receive chemotherapy for her breast cancer nor did she take excessive pyridoxine, both of which can cause a sensory neuropathy.[5,6] That this patient had cancer could suggest autoimmune paraneoplastic neuronopathy,[7] which is usually associated with small cell carcinoma of the lung.

The possibility of combined degeneration of the spinal cord also had to be considered. The absence of Babinski signs or other evidence of spinal cord involvement, however, is against this diagnosis.[8] B_{12} deficiency, on the other hand, might rarely manifest only with a peripheral neuropathy. There were no pupillary abnormalities to suggest tabes dorsalis. The lack of sphincter problems and long tract signs is against a myelopathy, and she had a normal MRI of the neck.

AN EMG TEST WAS PERFORMED

Motor Nerve Studies

Nerve and Site	Latency (ms)	Amplitude (mV)	Conduction Velocity (m/s)
Peroneal Nerve R.	**Normal ≤ 5.7**	**Normal ≥ 3**	**Normal ≥ 40**
Ankle	4.2	4	–
Fibular head	12.0	4	44
Knee	14.0	4	50
Tibial Nerve L.	**Normal ≤ 5.3**	**Normal ≥ 4**	**Normal ≥ 40**
Ankle	5.0	9	–
Pop. fossa	14.9	7	41
Median Nerve R.	**Normal ≤ 4.2**	**Normal ≥ 6**	**Normal ≥ 50**
Wrist	3.8	8	–
Elbow	7.7	7	53
Nerve and Site	**Latency (ms)**	**Amplitude (mV)**	**Conduction Velocity (m/s)**
Ulnar Nerve R.	**Normal ≤ 3.6**	**Normal ≥ 8**	**Normal ≥ 50**
Wrist	2.8	13	–
Below elbow	6.6	11	53
Above elbow	8.8	10	55

F-Wave and Tibial H-Reflex Studies

Nerve	Latency (ms)	Normal Latency ≤ (ms)
Peroneal nerve R.	52.5	54
Tibial nerve L.	53.9	54
Median nerve R.	28.3	30
Ulnar nerve R.	28.6	30
H-reflex R.	**NR**	34
H-reflex L.	**NR**	34

Sensory Nerve Studies

Nerve	Onset Latency (ms)	Normal Onset Latency ≤ (ms)	Peak Latency (ms)	Normal Peak Latency ≤ (ms)	Amp (μV)	Normal Amp ≥ (μV)	Conduction Velocity (m/s)	Normal Conduction Velocity ≥ (m/s)
Sural nerve R.	**NR**	3.5	**NR**	4.0	**NR**	11	**NR**	40
Superficial peroneal nerve R.	**NR**	3.5	**NR**	4.0	**NR**	8–10	**NR**	40
Ulnar nerve R.	2.6	2.6	3.1	3.1	**2**	13	50	50
Median nerve R.	**2.8**	2.6	**3.3**	3.1	**4**	20	**46**	50

EMG Data

Muscle	Insrt Activity	Fibs	Pos Waves	Fasc	Amp	Dur	Poly	Pattern
Lumbar paraspinals R.	**Inc**	**1+**	**1+**	None	Norm	Norm	None	Full
Vastus lateralis R.	Norm	None	None	None	**Lg**	**Inc**	None	**Red**
Tibialis anterior R.	Norm	None	None	None	Norm	Norm	None	Full
Gastrocnemius R.	Norm	None	None	None	Norm	Norm	None	Full
Cervical paraspinals R.	Norm	None	None	None	Norm	Norm	None	Full
Deltoid R.	Norm	None	None	None	Norm	Norm	None	Full
Biceps brachii R.	Norm	None	None	None	Norm	Norm	None	Full
Brachioradialis R.	Norm	None	None	None	Norm	Norm	None	Full
First dorsal interosseus R.	Norm	None	None	None	**Lg**	**Inc**	None	**Red**
Lumbar paraspinals L.	**Inc**	**1+**	**1+**	None	Norm	Norm	None	Full
Vastus lateralis L.	Norm	None	None	None	**Lg**	**Inc**	None	**Red**

TABLE 69-1 Differential Diagnosis of Sensory Polyradiculopathy/Polyganglionopathy/Polygangl ioradiculoneuropathy

Sensory Polyradiculopathy/ Polyganglionopathy/ Polyganglioradiculoneuropathy	History	Physical Findings	Laboratory Abnormalities
MISP	Smoking history, weight loss, may have autonomic/CNS symptoms	Distal and proximal upper and lower limb symmetrical or asymmetrical hypesthesia, loss of deep tendon reflexes, normal strength, sensory ataxia, pseudoathetosis	Antineuronal nuclear antibodies, abnormal chest imaging; low-amplitude SNAPs; autonomic testing abnormalities
NISP, idiopathic	Hyperacute, acute, subacute, or chronic presentations	Distal and proximal upper and lower limb symmetrical or asymmetrical hypesthesia, loss of deep tendon reflexes, normal strength, sensory ataxia, pseudoathetosis	No distinctive features; low-amplitude SNAPs (must aggressively exclude serologic and imaging evidence of occult malignancy)
NISP, Sjögren-associated	Xerophthalmia, xerostomia	Distal and proximal upper and lower limb symmetrical or asymmetrical hypesthesia, loss of deep tendon reflexes, normal strength, sensory ataxia, pseudoathetosis	Elevated extractable nuclear antigen antibodies; positive Schirmer test; minor salivary gland inflammation; low-amplitude SNAPs
Toxic sensory polyganglionopathy Pyridoxin Cisplatin Paclitaxel Semisynthetic penicillins	Relevant exposure	Distal and proximal upper and lower limb symmetrical or asymmetrical hypoesthesia, loss of deep tendon reflexes, normal strength, sensory ataxia, pseudoathetosis	Normal CSF protein; low-amplitude SNAPs
Acute inflammatory demyelinating polyradiculoneuropathy (sensory variant)	Acute or subacute onset; ± antecedent febrile illness	Distal > proximal ascending findings, typically symmetrical	CSF albuminocytologic dissociation; nerve conductions suggesting demyelination; low-amplitude SNAPs
Chronic inflammatory demyelinating polyradiculoneuropathy (sensory variant)	Chronic progressive course	Distal > proximal deficits, typically symmetrical	CSF cytoalbuminologic dissociation; nerve conductions suggesting demyelination; low-amplitude SNAPs
IgM paraproteinemic neuropathy	Chronic progressive course	Distal > proximal deficits, typically symmetrical, sensory ataxia	IgM monoclonal paraproteinemia; low-amplitude SNAPs

CNS, Central nervous system; *CSF*, cerebrospinal fluid; *IgM*, immunoglobulin M; *MISP*, malignant inflammatory sensory polyganglionopathy; *NISP*, nonmalignant inflammatory sensory polyganglionopathy.

Reproduced with permission from Smith BE, Windebank A, Dyck PJ. Nonmalignant inflammatory sensory polyganglionopathy. In: Dyck PJ, Thomas P, eds. *Peripheral Neuropathy*. Vol. 2. 4th ed. Philadelphia, PA: Elsevier Saunders; 2005:2315.

WHAT WERE THE EMG FINDINGS?

The nerve conduction velocity and EMG test showed no SNAPs in the leg and SNAPs of low amplitude in the hand; H-reflexes were also absent. Motor nerve conduction velocities and CMAP amplitudes and latencies were normal. There were only minimal abnormalities on needle EMG with some large motor unit potentials in the first dorsal interosseous and vastus lateralis muscles, and only minimal paraspinal denervation, thus confirming the diagnosis of a predominantly sensory neuropathy/neuronopathy with only mild involvement of motor axons.

ARE OTHER TESTS NEEDED?

B_{12}, rapid plasma reagin (RPR), thyroid-stimulating hormone, liver functions, angiotensin-converting enzyme, serum lymphocyte-lymphoma panel, C3 and C4 complement, FANA, double-stranded DNA, sulfatide antibody and anti-Hu antibodies, myelin-associated glycoprotein antibodies, anti-SSA, SSB (Sjögren antibodies), HIV antibodies, cytomegalic virus titers, and serum immunoelectrophoresis were all normal.

Cerebrospinal fluid protein was 140 mg/dL and glucose 67 mg/dL; there were 10 lymphocytes with normal cytology. CT scan of the chest showed pulmonary fibrosis, and CT of the abdomen was normal.

Sural nerve biopsy showed scattered lymphocytes and macrophages in the endoneural area with axonal degeneration and decreased number of myelinated fibers (Fig. 69-1A). There was also some segmental demyelination seen on the teased nerve preparations (see Fig. 69-1B).

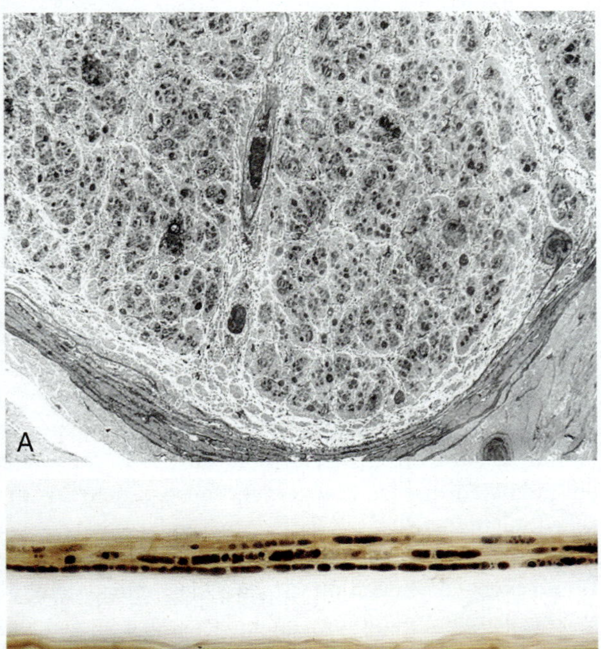

FIG. 69-1 A, Sural nerve showing decreased number of myelinated axons; there is apparent subperineural edema (osmicated, plastic-embedded and toluidine blue-stained sections, ×200). **B**, Teased nerve preparation showing segmental demyelination and axonal degeneration (×200).

The patient was started on IV IgG infusions monthly without significant improvement. Azathioprine 150 mg per day was added after 2 months; with this her symptoms showed mild improvement thereafter, and her gait stabilized.

Three months later she was admitted with marked worsening of truncal ataxia, pseudoathetosis, weakness, and severe proprioceptive deficit. Intravenous cyclophosphamide treatment did not produce any benefit.

Complete metabolic panel, C3, and C4 were normal. Repeat Hu antibody was inconclusive. FANA was normal.

She became progressively weaker in 1 week, became very ataxic and encephalopathic, and had a tonic/clonic seizure. An MRI showed an area of increased signal in the left temporal lobe (Fig. 69-2), and EEG demonstrated slowing with sharp waves in the left hemisphere. Cerebrospinal fluid test revealed 15 lymphocytes/mm^3; protein level was 70 mg/dL with oligoclonal bands, and there was an increased IgG index of 1.7 (normal, 0.3–0.7). Cytology and flow cytometry were negative. A CT scan of the chest showed pulmonary fibrosis and a left lower lung mass (Fig. 69-3). The patient became progressively more obtunded; her family opted for conservative management and she expired.

DISCUSSION

This woman developed a severe progressive sensory neuropathy and later limbic encephalopathy. This spectrum was indicative of a paraneoplastic disorder, despite previous normal CT of the chest and negative Hu antibodies. The left pulmonary infiltrate appeared very late in the disease course but may have been obscured by the pulmonary fibrosis.

Autopsy revealed a small cell carcinoma in the left lower lobe of the lung (Fig. 69-4) and limbic encephalitis (Fig. 69-5).

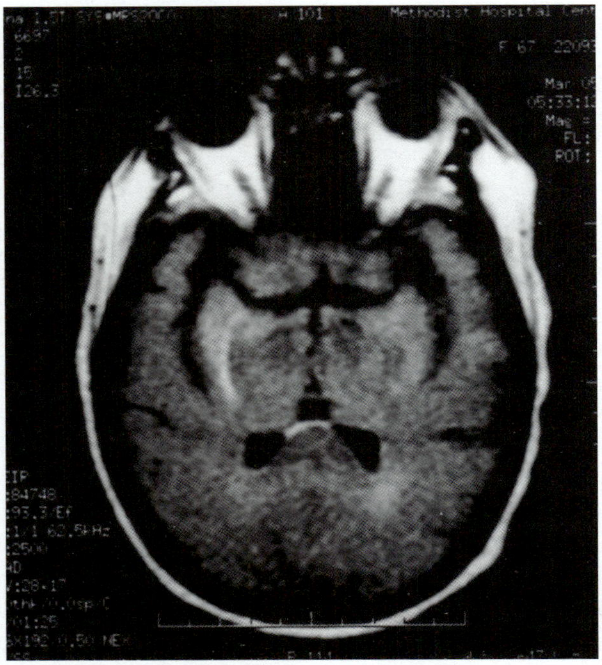

FIG. 69-2 MRI, T2-weighted image (axial view) showing increased signal in the left temporal lobe.

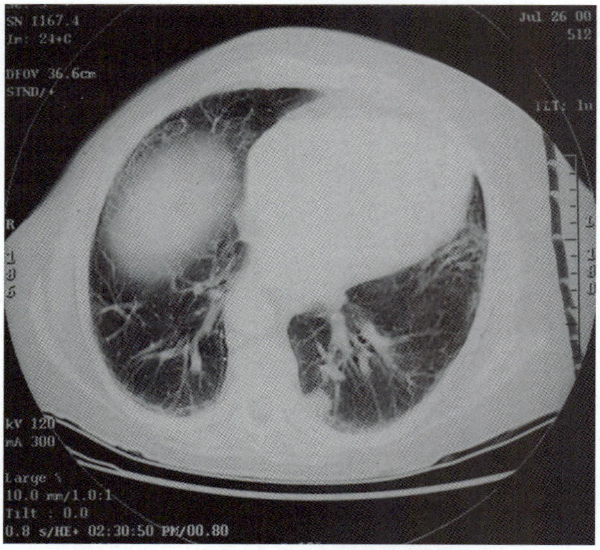

FIG. 69-3 CT scan of the chest showing the lung mass.

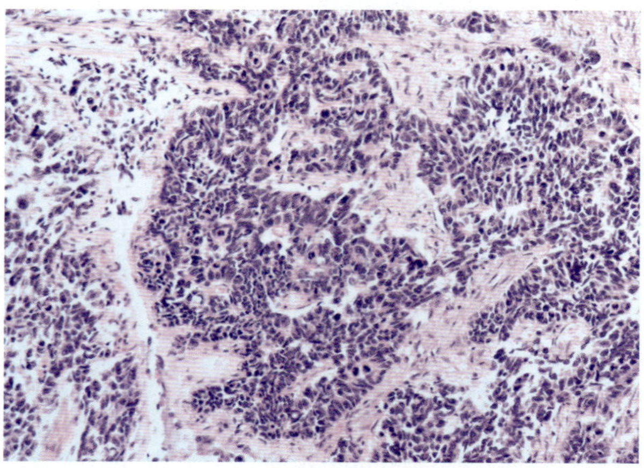

FIG. 69-4 Lung specimen showing the small cell cancer (H&E stain, ×200).

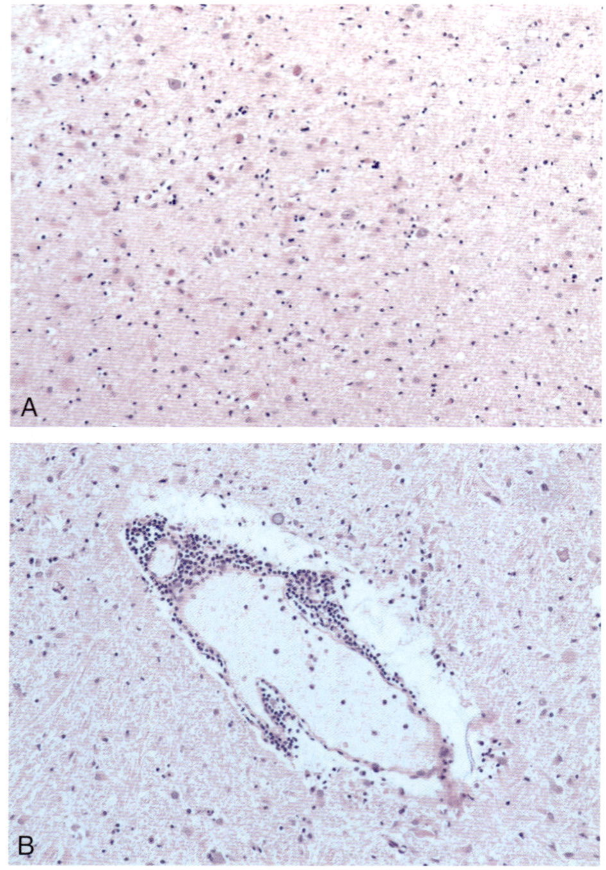

FIG. 69-5 **A**, Specimen of temporal lobe of the brain showing spongy vacuolated appearance with prominent astrocytes (H&E stain, ×200). **B**, Perivascular inflammatory infiltrates in the white matter of the temporal lobe (H&E stain, ×200).

She was diagnosed with paraneoplastic sensory neuropathy (PSN). This is a condition usually associated with small cell carcinoma and Hu antibodies, but it can also occur with lymphoma and tumors of the ovary and breast.[9] Patients might also have another paraneoplastic syndrome, such as limbic encephalopathy, which is usually characterized by personality changes, memory loss, hallucinations, and seizures.[9] Other paraneoplastic neurologic disorders are listed in Table 69-2 and their associated autoantibodies are listed in Table 69-3. (It should be clear that, although there is some syndromic association of neurologic disorders with particular antibodies or with specific tumors, some tumors are associated with several antibodies.)

PSN was first described in 1948 by Denny-Brown,[10] but the Hu–antibody association with the disease was not made until 1965.[11–14]

This is a subacute neuropathy characterized by numbness and painful paresthesias. Patients later develop gait ataxia, poor coordination, and, occasionally, dysautonomia. The neurologic examination reveals sensory loss of all modalities, predominantly vibration sense, gait ataxia, pseudoathetosis, and areflexia. Pupillary abnormalities may occur.[15]

The nerve conduction and EMG tests usually show decreased amplitude or absent SNAPs, while motor nerve conduction velocities are normal or minimally affected. The needle test is often normal.[16]

Pathologically, there are lymphocytic infiltrates in the dorsal root ganglia with gliosis, degeneration, and loss of sensory neurons, indicating that this is a primary neuronopathy. There could also be evidence of degeneration of the posterior roots and later of the posterior columns. It is considered a T cell–mediated disease that targets sensory neurons in the dorsal root ganglia.[17]

Sural nerve pathology might show diffuse perivascular infiltrates and axonal degeneration with loss of myelinated fibers.[18,19]

As the primary pathology in PSN is seen in the dorsal root ganglia, the condition is usually called a *paraneoplastic sensory neuronopathy* or *carcinomatous paraneoplastic sensory neuropathy*, but when the central nervous system is also involved, it is termed *paraneoplastic encephalomyelitis* and *subacute sensory neuronopathy* (PEM-SSN).[20–22] Patients frequently have nonspecific antinuclear antibodies[22]; these were termed anti-Hu in reference to the first patient studied.

TABLE 69-2 Paraneoplastic Neurologic Syndromes Associated With Immunologic Mechanisms

Central Nervous System
Paraneoplastic encephalomyelitis and focal encephalitis
  Limbic encephalitis
  Brainstem encephalitis
  Myelitis
  Multifocal: encephalomyelitis
Paraneoplastic cerebellar degeneration
Opsoclonus–myoclonus
Stiff-man syndrome
Paraneoplastic sensory neuropathy (dorsal root ganglia involvement)

Peripheral Nervous System
Paraneoplastic vasculitis of the nerve and muscle
Subacute peripheral neuropathies (Guillain–Barré, plexitis)
Peripheral neuropathy associated with malignant monoclonal gammopathies
Autonomic neuropathy[a]
Neuromyotonia[a]
Lambert–Eaton myasthenic syndrome[a]
Myasthenia gravis[a]
Dermatomyositis[a]
Acute necrotizing myopathy[a]

[a]Reviewed by Rudnicki and Dalmau.
Reprinted with permission from Bataller L, Dalmau J. Paraneoplastic neurologic syndromes: approaches to diagnosis and treatment. *Semin Neurol.* 2003;22:216.

TABLE 69-3 Antibodies Associated With Paraneoplastic Neurologic Syndrome

Antibody	Associated Cancer	Syndrome
Antibodies Associated With Paraneoplastic Neurologic Syndrome		
Anti-Hu	SCLC, other	Focal encephalitis, encephalomyelitis, cerebral degeneration, sensory neuropathy, autonomic dysfunction
Anti-Yo	Gynecological, breast	Cerebral degeneration
Anti-Ri	Breast, gynecological, SCLC	Cerebral ataxia, opsoclonus
Anti-Tr	Hodgkin lymphoma	Cerebellar degeneration
Anti-CV2 (for anti-CRMP5)	SCLC, other	Encephalomyelitis, cerebellar degeneration, peripheral neuropathy
Anti-Ma proteins	Germ-cell tumors	Limbic, brainstem encephalitis, cerebellar degeneration
Antiamphiphysin	Breast	Stiff-man syndrome, encephalomyelitis
Antibodies Associated With Neurologic Syndromes That Can Occur With or Without Cancer		
Anti-VGCC	SCLC	LEMS, cerebellar degeneration
Antiacetylcholine receptor	Thymoma	Myasthenia gravis
Anti-VGKC	Thymoma, others	Neuromyotonia, seizures, limbic encephalitis

LEMS, Lambert–Eaton myasthenic syndrome; *SCLC*, small cell lung cancer.
Reprinted with permission from Bataller L, Dalmau J. Paraneoplastic neurologic syndromes: approaches to diagnosis and treatment. *Semin Neurol.* 2003;22:216.

Later, anti-Hu antibodies were renamed *antineuronal nuclear antibody type 1* (ANNA1) or *anti-RI antibody*. Those that are associated with ataxia, and opsoclonic paraneoplastic syndromes are termed ANNA2 (or *anti-R2*).[22] There is also an ANNA3 antibody against Purkinje cells seen in patients with small cell carcinoma.

The anti-Hu antibody is a polyclonal complement-fixing IgG that reacts strongly with the nuclei and weakly with the cytoplasm of neurons. This antibody reacts to Hu antigens, which is a family of three RNA-binding proteins: HuD, HuC, and Hel-N1. These proteins are localized in neuronal nuclei, in cytoplasm, and also in carcinoma cells,[14,15] causing cross-reactivity. In a large series, lung cancer, usually of the small cell type, was detected in 88% of patients with anti-Hu antibodies.[23] It is recommended that antibody testing for disorders of the nervous system should include serum and spinal fluid to increase reliability.[24]

Cancer therapy and tumor radiation may improve PSN. Plasma exchange and chemotherapy drugs are usually of little benefit.[7]

It is important to recognize that the clinical presentation of this syndrome can precede the manifestations of cancer.

SUMMARY

This woman had a history of breast cancer and developed a progressive ataxic neuropathy. She had no evidence of Sjögren syndrome and was thought to have a paraneoplastic syndrome. Her evaluation for neoplasm was initially negative. Immunotherapy produced moderate improvement of her symptoms initially, but she then worsened and developed limbic encephalitis. A lung mass was found prior to her death, and on autopsy, this was demonstrated to be small cell carcinoma of the lung.

IMPORTANT POINTS

- Sensory ataxic neuronopathy can be idiopathic or associated with cancer or with Sjögren syndrome.
- The clinical characteristics are sensory ataxia, pseudoathetosis, mild weakness, and areflexia.
- Electrophysiologic studies show absent or low-amplitude SNAPs, but motor nerve conduction tests may be normal.
- Hu antibodies are seen in 90% of patients with PSN.
- Anti-Hu antibodies reflect the name of the initial patient and are also called neuronal nuclear antibodies type 1 (ANNA1).
- The presence of Hu antibodies is highly suggestive of a neoplasm.
- Pathologic findings in PSN include mononuclear inflammatory cells and nerve cell loss in the dorsal root ganglia; the sural nerve shows a decreased number of axons and axonal degeneration.

- Other paraneoplastic syndromes include limbic encephalitis or cerebellar degeneration, Eaton–Lambert syndrome, myasthenia gravis (thymoma) dermatomyositis, stiff-person syndrome, neuromyotonia, opsoclonus–myoclonus, encephalomyelitis, and other neuropathies (i.e., those with lymphoma or myeloproliferative disorders).
- Limbic encephalitis is characterized by personality changes, memory loss, confusion, and hallucinations and seizures; T2 hyperintensity of the temporal lobe may be noted on MRI.
- Aggressive immunotherapy and tumor removal may be of some benefit in PSN, but the disease usually progresses.

REFERENCES

1. Oh SJ, LaGanke C, Claussen GC. Sensory Guillain-Barré syndrome. *Neurology*. 2001;56:82–86.
2. Pan CL, Yuki N, Koga M, et al. Acute sensory ataxic neuropathy associated with monospecific anti-GD1b IgG antibody. *Neurology*. 2001;57:1316–1318.
3. Oh SJ, Joy JL, Kuruoglu R. Chronic sensory demyelinating neuropathy: chronic inflammatory demyelinating polyneuropathy presenting as a pure sensory neuropathy. *J Neurol Neurosurg Psychiatry*. 1992;55(8):677–680.
4. Griffin JW, Cornblath DR, Alexander E, et al. Ataxic sensory neuropathy and dorsal root ganglionitis associated with Sjögren's syndrome. *Ann Neurol*. 1990;27(3):304–315.
5. Quasthoff S, Hartung HP. Chemotherapy-induced peripheral neuropathy. *J Neurol*. 2002;249:9–17.
6. Schaumberg H, Kaplan J, Windebank A, et al. Sensory neuropathy from pyridoxine abuse: a new megavitamin syndrome. *N Engl J Med*. 1983;309:445–448.
7. Graus F, Keime-Guibert F, Rene R, et al. Anti-Hu-associated paraneoplastic encephalomyelitis: analysis of 200 patients. *Brain*. 2001;124:1138–1148.
8. McCombe PA, McLeod JG. The peripheral neuropathy of vitamin B12 deficiency. *J Neurol Sci*. 1984;66(1):117–126.
9. Bataller L, Dalmau J. Paraneoplastic neurologic syndromes: approaches to diagnosis and treatment. *Semin Neurol*. 2003;23(2): 215–224.
10. Denny-Brown D. Primary sensory neuropathy with muscular changes associated with carcinoma. *J Neurol Neurosurg Psychiatry*. 1948;11:73–87.
11. Wilkinson PC, Zeromski J. Immunofluorescent detection of antibodies against neurones in sensory carcinomatous neuropathy. *Brain*. 1965;88:529–583.
12. Graus F, Cordon-Cardo C, Posner JB. Neuronal antinuclear antibody in sensory neuronopathy from lung cancer. *Neurology*. 1985;35:538–543.
13. Horwich MS, Cho L, Porro RS, Posner JB. Subacute sensory neuropathy: a remote effect of carcinoma. *Ann Neurol*. 1977;2(1): 7–19.
14. Liu J, Dalmau J, Szabo A, et al. Paraneoplastic encephalomyelitis antigens bind to the AU-rich elements of mRNA. *Neurology*. 1995;3(Pt 1):544–550.
15. Elrington GM, Murray NM, Spiro SG, Newsom-Davis J. Neurological paraneoplastic syndromes in patients with small cell cancer: a prospective survey of 150 patients. *J Neurol Neurosurg Psychiatry*. 1991;54(9):764–767.
16. Kuntzer T, Antoine JC, Steck AJ. Clinical features and pathophysiological basis of sensory neuronopathies (ganglionopathies). *Muscle Nerve*. 2004;30(3):255–268.
17. Antoine JC, Camdessanché JP. Paraneoplastic disorders of the peripheral nervous system. *Presse Med*. 2013;42(6 Pt 2):e235–e244.
18. Antoine JC, Mosnier JF, Honnorat J, et al. Paraneoplastic demyelinating neuropathy, subacute sensory neuropathy, and anti-Hu antibodies: clinicopathological study of an autopsy case. *Muscle Nerve*. 1998;21(7):850–857.
19. Wanchitz J, Hainfellner JA, Kristoferitsch W, et al. Ganglionitis in paraneoplastic subacute sensory neuronopathy: a morphololologic study. *Neurology*. 1997;49(4):1156–1159.
20. Benyahia B, Liblau R, Merle-Beral H, et al. Cell-mediated autoimmunity in paraneoplastic neurological syndromes with Hu antibodies. *Ann Neurol*. 1999;45(2):162–167.
21. Dalmau J, Furneaux HM, Gralla RJ, et al. Detection of the anti-Hu antibody in the serum of patients with small cell cancer: a quantitative western blot analysis. *Ann Neurol*. 1990;27(5):544–552.
22. Jean WC, Dalmau J, Ho A, Posner JB. Analysis of the IgG subclass distribution and inflammatory infiltrates in patients with anti-Hu-associated paraneoplastic encephalomyelitis. *Neurology*. 1994; 44(1):140–147.
23. Lucchinetti CF, Kimmel DW, Lennon VA. Paraneoplastic and oncologic profiles of patients seropositive for type 1 antineuronal nuclear autoantibodies. *Neurology*. 1998;50(3):652–657.
24. Graus F, Vogrig A, Muniz-Castrillo S, Antoine Jean-Christophe G, et al. Updated diagnostic criteria for paraneoplastic neurologic syndrome. *Neurol Neuroimmunol Neuroinflamm*. 2021;8(4):e1014.

A Man With Progressive Neuropathy and Congestive Heart Failure

A 59-year-old man presented with a 3-year history of paresthesias in the legs, feet, and thighs and weakness in the legs, with difficulty going up stairs and getting up from a chair. He developed severe leg weakness and atrophy in the hands for approximately 6 months prior. He had an MRI of the lumbosacral spine that showed spinal stenosis.

The family history was positive. His father died of tuberculosis and a brother died at age 50 of congestive heart failure after a 6-year history that included peripheral neuropathy and carpal tunnel syndrome (CTS).

Past medical history was positive for a nonspecific lung nodule, for which he received isoniazide for 1 month until the results of the biopsy were reported negative for tuberculosis and otherwise nonspecific. He had hypertension and congestive heart failure from cardiomyopathy and had been previously operated on for a right carpal tunnel. He also had hiatal hernia, irritable bowel, chronic low back pain, and depression.

Physical examination revealed normal mentation and cranial nerves except for a dry tongue and mild decreased tearing in the eyes. Pupillary light responses were mildly sluggish. No cataracts or corneal opacities were detected. The fundi and extraocular movements were normal. Strength was normal in the neck and upper extremities, except 3+/5 in the hand muscles. Hip flexors were 4−/5, extensors 4/5; foot dorsiflexors were 3−/5, feet flexors 4/5. He had wasting in the hands and feet and was areflexic without pathologic reflexes. Sensory examination revealed a stocking/glove deficit to pain and temperature to the midforearm and midlegs with absent vibration sense in the toes and ankles. The rest of the examination was unremarkable.

This case was studied with Dr. Lance Wright.

WHAT IS THE DIFFERENTIAL DIAGNOSIS?

This patient presented with a progressive sensorimotor neuropathy with an apparent cardiomyopathy, autonomic dysfunction, and a history of CTS. There was no history of exposure to drugs, except for isoniazide, which can cause a neuropathy,[1] but he only took this medicine for 1 month, and his symptoms started years after its discontinuation. There was no exposure to alcohol or other toxins. He had a history of lumbar spinal stenosis, but this does not explain the upper extremity findings.

Diabetes is a primary consideration in a patient with this presentation, and patients with diabetic polyneuropathy have a predisposition to CTS.[2] It is also possible that the cardiac involvement was secondary to arteriosclerotic coronary disease related to diabetes, but he had no history of diabetes.

Another consideration would be neuropathy associated with monoclonal gammopathy with antibodies against myelin-associated glycoprotein, a sensorimotor neuropathy of older persons that shows predominantly distal demyelination (DADS).[3] This patient's neuropathy appeared to involve large and small nerve fibers.

Finally, the history of a lung mass could suggest the possibility of a paraneoplastic neuropathy[4] or Wegener granulomatosis.[5] Neither cancer nor inflammation was demonstrated by his biopsy.

The history of neuropathy in a brother with a similar presentation suggests a hereditary condition, such as Charcot–Marie–Tooth disease.[6] However, his problems appeared to have a late onset as opposed to that typically seen in these patients and would not explain the cardiomyopathy or his autonomic dysfunction, and prominent sensory findings are unusual in those.

The family history, cardiovascular manifestations, autonomic involvement, and CTS suggest familial amyloidosis, particularly the transthyretin (TTR) or Andrade type.[7]

AN EMG TEST WAS PERFORMED

Motor Nerve Studies

Nerve and Site	Latency (ms)	Amplitude (mV)	Conduction Velocity (m/s)
Median Nerve R.	**Normal ≤ 4.2**	**Normal ≥ 6**	**Normal ≥ 50**
Wrist	**6.0**	**0.5**	–
Elbow	12.8	**0.5**	**35**
Median Nerve L.	**Normal ≤ 4.2**	**Normal ≥ 6**	**Normal ≥ 50**
Wrist	**4.5**	**0.8**	–
Elbow	11.3	**0.8**	**36**
Ulnar Nerve R.	**Normal ≤ 3.6**	**Normal ≥ 8**	**Normal ≥ 50**
Wrist	3.4	**0.2**	–
Below elbow	8.6	**0.2**	**39**
Nerve and Site	**Latency (ms)**	**Amplitude (mV)**	**Conduction Velocity (m/s)**
Peroneal Nerve R.	**Normal ≤ 5.7**	**Normal ≥ 3**	**Normal ≥ 40**
Ankle	**NR**	**NR**	–
Fibular head	**NR**	**NR**	**NR**

Motor Nerve Studies—cont'd

Tibial Nerve R.	Normal ≤ 5.3	Normal ≥ 4	Normal ≥ 40
Ankle	5.0	**0.1**	–
Pop. fossa	15.0	**0.1**	40

F-Wave Responses

Nerve	Latency (ms)	Normal Latency ≤ (ms)
Median nerve R.	**NR**	30
Ulnar nerve R.	**32.8**	30
Peroneal nerve R.	**NR**	54
Tibial nerve R.	**NR**	54

Sensory Nerve Studies

Nerve	Latency (ms)	Normal Latency ≤ (ms)	Amp (μV)	Normal Amp ≥ (μV)
Sural nerve R.	**NR**	4.0	**NR**	11
Superficial peroneal nerve R.	**NR**	4.0	**NR**	10

Sensory Nerve Studies—cont'd

Nerve	Latency (ms)	Normal Latency ≤ (ms)	Amp (μV)	Normal Amp ≥ (μV)
Ulnar nerve R.	**NR**	3.1	**NR**	13
Median nerve R.	**NR**	3.1	**NR**	20
Median nerve L.	**NR**	3.1	**NR**	20

Autonomic Testing

	Normal Range	Patient's Values
Change in HR with deep respirations	>15 bpm	**8.1 bpm**
Valsalva ratio	>1.21	**1.0**
Sympathetic skin responses		
Upper limb	Present	**Absent**
Lower limb	Present	**Absent**
Sympathetic isometric exercise test: diastolic BP		
Base line	–	**68**
After 5 min	–	**76**
Difference (after 5 min base line)	>16	**8**

EMG Data

Muscle	Insrt Activity	Fibs	Pos Waves	Fasc	Amp	Dur	Poly	Pattern
Deltoid R.	**Inc**	**1+**	**1+**	None	**Lg**	**Inc**	None	Full
First dorsal interosseous R.	**Inc**	**2+**	**2+**	None	**Lg**	**Inc**	None	**Red**
Flexor carpi radialis R.	**Inc**	**2+**	**2+**	None	**Lg**	**Inc**	None	Full
Vastus lateralis R.	**Inc**	**1+**	**1+**	None	**Lg**	**Inc**	None	Full
Tibialis anterior R.	**Inc**	**2+**	**2+**	**Few**	**Lg**	**Inc**	None	**Red**
Gastrocnemius R.	**Inc**	**2+**	**2+**	None	**Lg**	**Inc**	None	**Red**

WHAT WERE THE EMG FINDINGS?

The nerve conduction tests showed low-amplitude CMAPs, indicating axonal degeneration, and also slowing of conduction velocities, which could suggest demyelination, but this was not out of proportion to the low-amplitude CMAPs. Distal motor latencies were prolonged only on the median nerve, indicating a median neuropathy at the wrist, likely CTS. The median F-response was absent, likely from axonal dropout, correlating with the low-amplitude CMAP. The ulnar F-response was mildly prolonged. The SNAPs were absent. On needle test there were denervation potentials, mainly in distal muscles, indicating axonal degeneration with large motor unit action potentials secondary to reinnervation.

In conclusion, these tests indicated a predominantly axonal sensory and motor neuropathy and bilateral CTS. The autonomic tests done indicated autonomic dysfunction.

Workup included complete blood counts, chemistry profile, glucose tolerance test, glycosylated hemoglobin, B_{12} level, fluorescent antinuclear antibody, erythrocyte sedimentation rate, thyroid function tests, and immunoelectrophoresis; all were normal.

Spinal fluid studies showed a protein of 65 mg/dL (normal, <45 mg/dL); the cerebrospinal fluid was otherwise normal.

WHAT SHOULD BE THE NEXT DIAGNOSTIC TEST?

A rectal, fat pad biopsy or a nerve biopsy could be useful in demonstrating deposits of amyloid and/or TTR using antibodies against this protein.[7] DNA testing for TTR mutations is a less invasive and useful test, but some TTR mutations might not be detected by commercially available methods.

A nerve biopsy was done and showed demyelination, axonal degeneration with the involvement of small unmyelinated fibers and deposits of amyloid, particularly in vessel walls, demonstrated by Crystal violet (Fig. 70A-1) and Congo red stains (Fig. 70A-2). The biopsy also showed birefringence on polarized light (Fig. 70A-3). The amyloid deposits also were seen on thick plastic sections and electromicroscopy (Figs. 70A-4 and 70A-5).

DNA testing by polymerase chain reaction amplification and automated sequencing detected one normal allele and one with an amino acid change of the TTR gene, diagnostic of TTR amyloidosis.

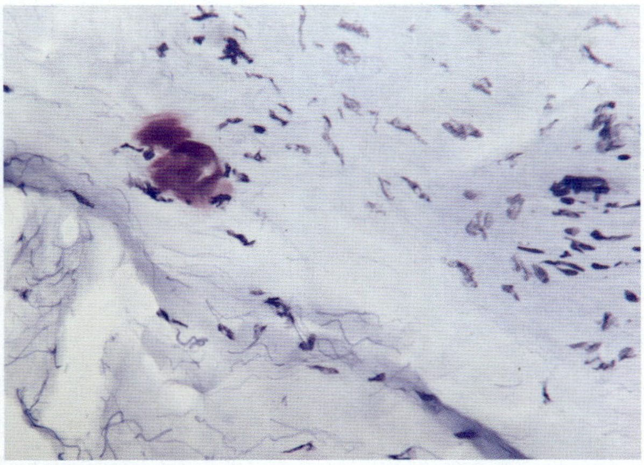

FIG. 70A-1 Sural nerve showing amyloid deposits demonstrated by Crystal violet stain (×400).

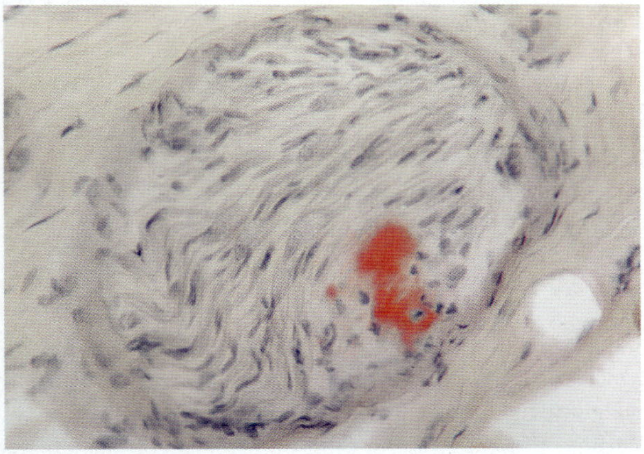

FIG. 70A-2 Congophilic reddish material seen on Congo red stain (×400).

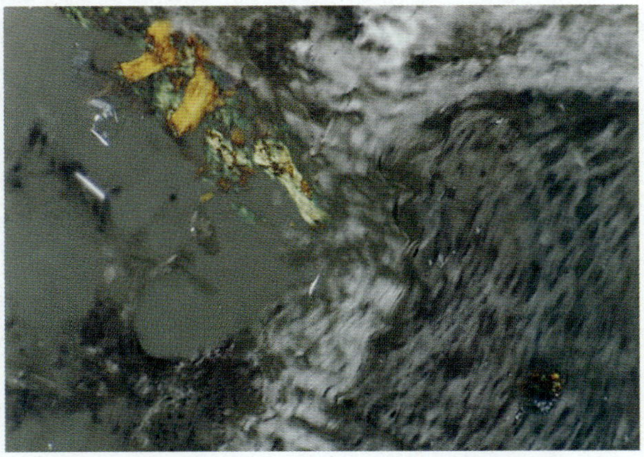

FIG. 70A-3 Amyloid deposits seen with polarized light giving the apple-green birefringence (×400).

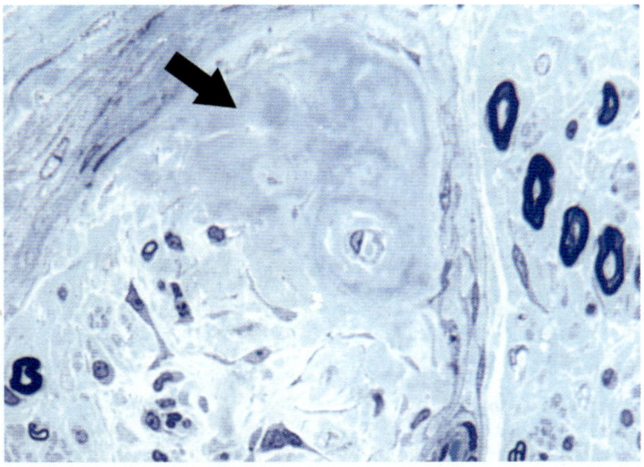

FIG. 70A-4 Amyloid deposits in the sural nerve (*arrow*), osmicated toluidine blue–stained section (×400).

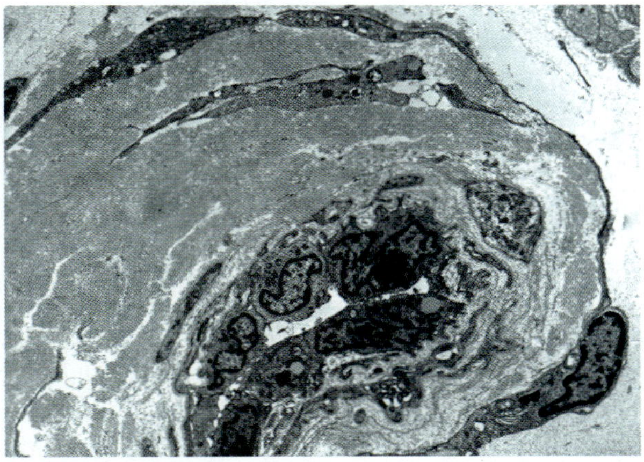

FIG. 70A-5 Amyloid in the vessel wall on electromicroscopy (×1000).

WHAT IS AMYLOIDOSIS?

Amyloidosis refers to a variety of conditions characterized by deposits of Congo red–positive materials in tissue; these are recognized by their apple-green birefringence under polarized light.

Amyloid deposits are β-pleated, nonbranching fibrillar proteins of about 7.5–10 nm in diameter. Their β-pleated structure consists of strands of polypeptides in a zigzag formation. They have the capacity to acquire more than one conformation and for this reason are called *chameleon* proteins.

Protein misfolding in amyloidosis develops in different ways; for example, a protein may have a propensity to have the abnormal conformation that becomes evident with aging, or when they are in higher concentrations, such as in β_2-microglobulin accumulation in uremics, or caused by the replacement of a single amino acid, as in the familial amyloidosis. Another mechanism is remodeling of protein precursors, as in the case of β amyloid precursor protein in Alzheimer disease. These mechanisms can act independently or in association. Other factors could also contribute to this propensity.[8]

The word "amyloid" was used initially to describe the normal "amylaceous" constituents of plants by Matthias Schleiden.[9] In 1854 Virchow[10] coined the term to describe the amyloid deposits in tissue, mistakenly thinking that the substance was a polysaccharide, based on its affinity for sulfuric acid and iodine.

Amyloid deposits occur in a variety of conditions, such as familial amyloidosis, cerebral amyloid angiopathy, Alzheimer disease, familial Creutzfeldt–Jakob disease, Gerstmann–Straussler–Scheinker disease, fatal familial insomnia, inclusion body myopathies, as well as Mediterranean fever and other familial diseases[8].

WHAT ARE THE DIFFERENT TYPES OF AMYLOIDOSIS AFFECTING PERIPHERAL NERVES?

Although there are many conditions caused by amyloid deposits in tissue, the amyloidoses affecting peripheral nerves are usually divided as follows:

1. *Primary systemic amyloidosis.* This is a nonfamilial disease associated with deposits of a light chain in tissues: these are usually lambda but also can be kappa light chains. The condition is also called *AL* for "amyloid light chains." Primary amyloidosis could be idiopathic, but some patients later develop multiple myeloma or lymphoproliferative disease.[11] Men are more affected than women and the abnormal monoclonal protein is detected in serum, urine, or both. The disease manifests nephrotic syndrome and renal failure. There could be deposits of amyloid in other tissues, including muscles, causing their pseudohypertrophy, and in nerves causing predominantly a painful sensory neuropathy. This is associated with CTS.
2. *Secondary systemic amyloidosis.* In this condition the deposits of amyloid are secondary to chronic infections and/or inflammatory diseases such as tuberculosis, leprosy, and rheumatoid arthritis. The abnormal protein is called *serum amyloid A*.[12] This type of amyloidosis has also been designated AA and is not associated with a significant neuropathy. A form of secondary amyloidosis also occurs in patients with renal failure having deposits of β_2 microglobulin in vessels and joints and manifesting CTS.[13] In some patients, particularly those with chronic infections, there might be diffuse tissue involvement with muscle weakness and polyneuropathy.[14] Eprosidate, a compound that inhibits the polymerization of amyloid fibrils and its deposits in tissues, slows the progression of renal disease in secondary amyloidosis and could theoretically be applied to other forms of amyloidosis.[15]
3. *Familial amyloidosis* represents a group of inherited disorders with various presentations associated by deposits of amyloid proteins in tissues. They are caused by genetic defects of autosomal-dominant inheritance. Those affecting the peripheral nerve system include the following:
   a. *TTR amyloidosis.* This disease, which was the diagnosis in this case, is caused by deposits of TTR (also known as prealbumin), a plasma protein that transports thyroxine and retinol. This form of amyloidosis was initially described by Andrade in Portuguese families[14] and is called *familial amyloid polyneuropathy* (FAP) or familial amyloidosis I. A group of patients in Indiana families of Swiss extraction were initially reported by Rukavina (called *FAP II*).[16]

This disorder has a variable phenotype associated with various mutations of chromosome 18.[17] The clinical manifestations include sensorimotor neuropathy, autonomic dysfunction, vitreous opacities, and cardiomyopathy with cardiac failure and a neuropathy (Table 70-1). CTS is common.

The disease is diagnosed by rectal, fat pad, or sural nerve biopsy with Congo red and immunofluorescence using antibodies against TTR and by DNA analysis. In some cases of TTR amyloidosis the clinical features could be confused with chronic inflammatory demyelinating polyneuropathy; the nerve biopsy also could be misleading. DNA analysis should be performed, particularly in patients with length-dependent polyneuropathy with significant autonomic dysfunction and cardiac involvement.[18,19] TTR amyloidosis can be treated with liver transplantation, which halts the progression.[20] Plasma exchange and immunoabsorption do not produce a significant benefit. We now have a number of treatments available, particularly for TTR amyloidosis. Patisiran is a small RNA interference drug given intravenously. The FDA just approved the use of vutrisiran for subcutaneous use. Diflunisal is an antiinflammatory drug that binds the thyroxine binding sites of the TTR tetramers stabilizing the protein and preventing amyloid deposits, and this is a promising therapy.[21] Inotersen is an antisense oligonucleotide which inhibits hepatic production of TTR and is used in TTR neuropathy.[21] Dezamizumab is a monoclonal antibody that targets serum amyloid peak component (SAP), a glycoprotein present in TTR. Tafamidis is a small molecule that binds to the thyroxine binding site of TTR producing kinetic stabilization, and tauroursodeoxycholic acid and doxycycline, which disrupt TTR fibers, are possible new therapies not yet approved for this use.[22]

   b. *Apolipoprotein A-I amyloidosis.* This form is classified as the Iowa type and was initially reported by Van Allen. Also called *FAP III*,[23] it is caused by deposits of apolipoprotein A-I. This rare disorder usually manifests at a later age but might present earlier. It is characterized by a sensory neuropathy with some variable motor involvement, accompanied by hearing loss, peptic ulcers, endocrinopathy,

TABLE 70A-1 Features Associated With Polyneuropathy That Suggest TTR-Related FAP

Family history consistent with autosomal-dominant inheritance, early age of onset, although it may present later
Small-fiber polyneuropathy, or sensory-motor neuropathy, with carpal tunnel syndrome
Autonomic failure (orthostatic hypotension, alternating constipation/diarrhea, gastric distention, impotence, urinary hesitancy, dry skin, sicca syndrome, blurred vision)
Other organ system involvement
Vitreous deposits
Cardiac (arrhythmia or cardiomyopathy)
Kidney (usually glomerular involvement causing proteinuria and, rarely, azotemia)
GI tract (dyspepsia, anorexia, nausea, constipation, or malabsorption)
Spleen (splenomegaly, usually not associated with leukopenia or anemia)
Liver (hepatomegaly, rarely of clinical importance)
Leptomeninges (headache, ataxia, seizures, dementia, fluctuating level of consciousness, focal signs, and subarachnoid bleeding from vascular amyloid deposition)

Reproduced with permission from Nardin R, Lachmann H. Familial amyloid polyneuropathy: presentation, diagnosis and treatment. *J Clin Neuromuscul Dis.* 2001;2(4):221–226.

and renal failure. The disease is caused by a gene defect in chromosome 11.[24] No treatment is available.

c. *Gelsolin amyloidosis.* This form corresponds to the group of patients in Finnish families described by Meretoja; it is called *FAP IV*.[25] It is autosomal dominant and presents later in life with the involvement of cranial nerves, particularly trigeminal and facial nerves with corneal lattice dystrophy. The peripheral neuropathy is very mild. Patients have decreased turgor of the skin, particularly in the face. The life span is usually not affected. FAP IV is caused by a mutation in chromosome 9.[26] No treatment is available.

d. *Primary cardiac amyloidosis* is an aggressive and life-threatening nonhereditary disorder caused by ATTRwt (amyloid TTR wild-type). Tafamidis appears to be beneficial in this disorder.[22]

For further discussion, important points and references see Case 70B.

SUMMARY

This patient had a sensorimotor neuropathy with autonomic dysfunction and a history of CTS and congestive heart failure. The diagnosis of familial amyloidosis was made by demonstrating deposits of amyloid in the sural nerve and a mutation of the TTR gene in chromosome 18.

70B CASE

A Woman With a Demyelinating and Axonal Neuropathy

A 50-year-old female was referred for a progressive neuropathy, possible CIDP which did not respond to IVIG treatment. She started having symptoms 2 years prior to presentation with burning pain in the feet and leg weakness with numbness. The pain was present day and night. She had no real tingling. She received gabapentin with some improvement of the pain, but the numbness persisted. The patient was adopted.

Past medical history is only remarkable for hypothyroidism treated with radiation, and she is on thyroid supplementation.

On exam, vital signs and mentation were normal. Cranial nerve examination was unremarkable, except for poorly reactive pupils to light and accommodation. There was distal weakness in the upper and lower extremities at 4–4.5/5 in the legs. She had weakness in the upper extremities. There was minimal interossei weakness. Reflexes were normal in the arms and absent in the legs. She had diminished vibration and pinprick sensations in both legs. There was diminished pain and temperature up to the mid-calf bilaterally. There was decreased position sense in the toes. She had minimal high arches, but there was no atrophy of the feet muscles. No prominent atrophy was seen in the legs.

WHAT IS THE DIFFERENTIAL DIAGNOSIS?

This patient has a progressive neuropathy, and she was initially diagnosed with CIDP, but the prominent small-fiber sensory deficit is unusual for this disorder.

Other possibilities to consider include a hereditary neuropathy such as Charcot–Marie–Tooth disease, but because she was adopted, there was no family medical history.

The pupillary abnormalities indicate an autonomic nervous system dysfunction; although such dysfunction occurs in CIDP, it is rare. Other possibilities include TTR amyloidosis which is a neuropathy with demyelinating and axonal features and has prominent dysautonomic symptoms.

WHAT TESTS WILL BE DONE?

Thyroid antibodies, T4, T3, methylmalonic acid, glucose tolerance test, homocysteine, and immunoelectrophoresis were all unremarkable.

EMG

This EMG showed a mixed neuropathy showing axonal and demyelinating features with distal denervation. There was also absent sympathetic skin response.

OTHER TESTS

A lumbar puncture was not done.

A nerve and muscle biopsy were done, and it showed evidence of amyloid deposits with some demyelination and axonal degeneration. The muscle biopsy showed neurogenic atrophy and amyloid deposits (Fig. 70B-1).

DNA testing for *TTR* gene revealed a pathogenic variant of PGLU-T-4GLY (E74G) heterogenous.

WHAT IS THE DIAGNOSIS?

This patient was diagnosed as having familial TTR amyloidosis. The patient was worked up for cardiomyopathy, and there were minor changes in the left ventricle on cardiac MRI. She is currently receiving diflunisal, inotersen, and tafamidis as well as doxycycline and is stable.

SUMMARY

A 50-year-old female presented with a demyelinating and axonal neuropathy with dysautonomia. She failed IVIG therapy and was diagnosed having TTR amyloidosis and is currently on medication and is stable.

DISCUSSION FOR CASES 70A AND 70B

These two patients have amyloid TTR polyneuropathy. The difference between the two cases is that when the first case was seen the only treatment available was a liver transplant which the patient declined. Since then, the second case who had a prominent neuropathy with demyelinating and axonal features with dysautonomia is currently being treated with medications for amyloidosis and is doing well.

Familial TTR amyloidosis affects the small myelinated and unmyelinated fibers presenting with pain, paresthesias, and autonomic symptoms. Patients may have disassociated sensory abnormalities initially with the progression of neuropathy; large sensory and motor fibers are involved. Careful observation of autonomic disturbance is important in the evaluation of patients with a neuropathy. Patients may also develop gait abnormalities and falls. The examination may show weakness, but the sensory findings are predominant and usually in a length-dependent pattern. Patients may also present with an entrapment neuropathy. A common misdiagnosis is CIDP,[19] although the presentation in CIDP affects primarily large fibers. Pain occurs more

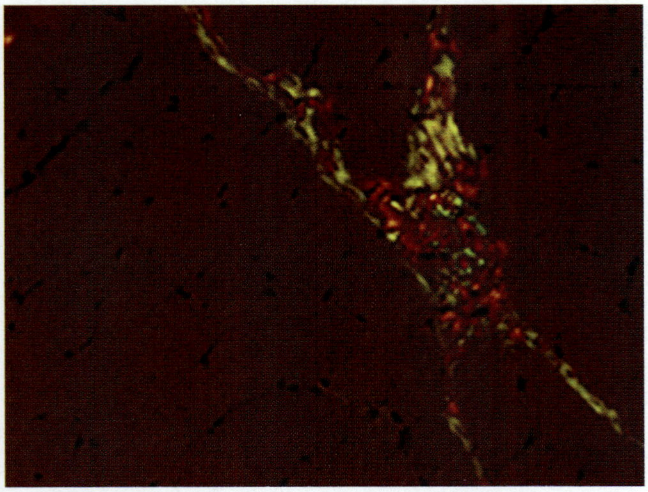

FIG. 70B-1 Congo red stain showing birefringent amyloid deposits in nerve (×200).

frequently in amyloid neuropathy, and autonomic dysfunction is seen in about one-third of CIDP cases, but up to 75% of amyloid neuropathies. The most common focal neuropathy is bilateral median neuropathy at the wrist and it may also affect peripheral nerves in the lumbosacral plexus forming tumor-like deposits.

Screening for nonneurological systemic features of amyloidosis is important, but those symptoms are nonspecific and would include findings related to complication of cardiac disorders and hypertension.

Early diagnosis is crucial in familial TTR amyloidosis. This is caused by 30 different mutations of the *TTR* gene. The incidence of this varies across the globe, with 8.7 per million per year in Portugal and only 0.3 cases in the United States. The symptoms can be neurological, cardiac, and/or mixed.

There are several newer treatments that are useful particularly in TTR amyloidosis including patisiran and vutrisiran, antiinflammatory drugs, a small RNA interfering molecule, and antisense oligonucleotides. Liver transplant can be used in severe cases that do not respond to therapy.

IMPORTANT POINTS

- Amyloidoses are conditions associated with amyloid deposits in tissue, demonstrated with Congo red–positive material by birefringence; these are formed by aggregates of β-pleated fibrillar proteins of 7.5–10 nm in diameter.
- The histological diagnosis of amyloidosis is made using rectal, fat pad, or sural nerve biopsy.
- TTR familial amyloidosis is caused by deposits of TTR in tissues, due to a defect in chromosome 18q. The disease has variable presentations with sensorimotor neuropathy, carpal tunnel syndrome, autonomic dysfunction, vitreous opacities, cardiomyopathy, and renal failure.
- Nerve biopsy and particularly DNA testing for amyloidosis should be done in atypical CIDP patients particularly with prominent small-fiber and autonomic dysfunction.
- Therapy for TTR amyloidosis now includes several new drugs that are beneficial. These also include antiinflammatory drugs, small interferon RNA molecules, and antisense oligonucleotides to prevent the formation of amyloid.

REFERENCES

1. Jones WA, Jones GP. Peripheral neuropathy due to isoniazid; report of two cases. *Lancet*. 1953;1(22):1073–1074.
2. Vinik AI. Diabetic neuropathy: pathogenesis and therapy. *Am J Med*. 1999;107(2B):17S–26S.
3. Ellie E, Vital A, Steck A, et al. Neuropathy associated with “benign” anti-myelin-associated glycoprotein IgM gammopathy: clinical, immunological, neurophysiological pathological findings and response to treatment in 33 cases. *J Neurol*. 1996; 243(1):34–43.
4. Croft PB, Urich H, Wilkinson M. Peripheral neuropathy of sensorimotor type associated with malignant disease. *Brain*. 1967;90(1):31–66.
5. Duna GF, Galperin C, Hoffman GS. Wegener’s granulomatosis. *Rheum Dis Clin North Am*. 1995;21(4):949–986.
6. Harding AE, Thomas PK. The clinical features of hereditary motor and sensory neuropathy types I and II. *Brain*. 1980;103(2): 259–280.
7. Nardin R, Lachmann H. Familial amyloid polyneuropathy: presentation, diagnosis and treatment. *J Clin Neuromuscul Dis*. 2001;4:221–226.
8. Merlini G, Bellotti V. Molecular mechanisms of amyloidosis. *N Engl J Med*. 2003;349(6):583–596.
9. Kyle RA, Kelly JJ, Dyck PJ. Amyloidosis and neuropathy. In: Dyck PJ, Thomas PK, eds. *Peripheral Neuropathy*. 4th ed. Philadelphia, PA: Elsevier-Saunders; 2005:2427–2451.
10. Virchow R. Uber einem Gehim und Rfichekenmark des Menschen aufgefundene Substanz mit der chemischen Reaction der cellulose virchows. *Arch Pathol Anat*. 1854;7:135–138.
11. Kyle RA, Gertz MA. Systemic amyloidosis. *Crit Rev Oncol Hematol*. 1990;10(1):49–87.
12. Benson MD, Kleiner E. Synthesis and secretion of serum protein A (SAA) by hepatocytes in mice treated with Casein. *J Immunol*. 1980;124:495–499.
13. Drueke TB. Beta$_2$-microglobulin and amyloidosis: a review. *Nephrol Dial Transplant*. 2000;15(Suppl 1):17–24.
14. Andrade C. A peculiar form of peripheral neuropathy: familial atypical generalized amyloidosis with special involvement of peripheral nerves. *Brain*. 1952;75:408–427.
15. Dember LM, Hawkins PN, Hazenberg BP, et al. Eprodisate for the treatment of renal disease in AA amyloidosis. *N Engl J Med*. 2007;356(23):2349–2360.
16. Rukavina JC, Block WD, Jackson CE, et al. Primary systemic amyloidosis: a review and an experimental, genetic and clinical study of 29 cases with particular emphasis on the familial form, 1956. *Medicine*. 1993;72:45–63.
17. Connors LH, Richardson AM, Theberge R, Costello CE. Tabulation of transthyretin (TTR) variants of 1/1/2000. *Amyloid*. 2000;7:54–69.
18. Planté-Bordeneuve V, Ferreira A, Lalu T, et al. Diagnostic pitfalls in sporadic transthyretin familial amyloid polyneuropathy (TPR-FAP). *Neurology*. 2007;69(7):693–698.
19. Pinto MV, Dyck PJ, Liewluck T. Neuromuscular amyloidosis: unmasking the master of disguise. *Muscle Nerve*. 2021;64:23–36.

20. Suhr QB, Frimman S, Ericzon BG. Early liver transplantation improves familial amyloidotic polyneuropathy patients' survival. *Amyloid*. 2005;12:233–238.
21. Tojo K, Sekijima Y, Kelly JW, Ikeda S. Diflunisal stabilizes familial amyloid polyneuropathy-associated transthyretin variant tetramers in serum against disassociation required for amyloidogenesis. *Neurosci Res*. 2006;56(4):441–449.
22. Muller ML, Butler J, Heidecker B. Emerging therapies in transthyretin amyloidosis – a new wave of hope after years of stagnancy? *Eur J Heart Fail*. 2020;22(1):39–53.
23. Karathanasis SK, Zannis VI, Breslow JL. Isolation and characterization of the human apolipoprotein A-I gene. *Proc Natl Acad Sci USA*. 1983;80:6147–6151.
24. Meretoja J. Familial systemic paramyloidosis with lattice dystrophy of the cornea, progressive cranial neuropathy, skin changes and various internal symptoms: a previously unrecognized heritable syndrome. *Ann Clin Res*. 1969;1:314–324.
25. Benson MD, Kinkaid JC. The molecular biology and clinical features of amyloid neuropathy. *Muscle Nerve*. 2007;36:411–423.
26. Kwiatkowski DJ, Westbrook CA, Bruns GA, Morton CC. Localization of gelsolin proximal to ABL on chromosome 9. *Am J Hum Genet*. 1988;42:565–572.

An Elderly Woman With a Progressive Neuropathy

A 75-year-old woman with congestive heart failure and coronary artery disease was evaluated for progressive numbness and weakness in the feet and legs for the past 3 months. She had been on lanoxin, furosemide, and amiodarone. Past medical and family histories were unremarkable, and she did not smoke or drink. Gait was normal; the rest of the neurologic examination was unremarkable.

Examination revealed normal mentation and gross cognitive function. Cranial nerves were normal. There was 4–4+/5 weakness in all extremities; the iliopsoas and glutei were 3–4−/5 bilaterally; quadriceps, adductors, and hamstrings were 5−/5; foot dorsiflexors 4/5; evertors 4/5; flexors 5−/5. There was decreased pinprick in a stocking distribution up to the midarm and midcalf. She was areflexic, and her toes were downgoing.

WHAT IS THE DIFFERENTIAL DIAGNOSIS?

This woman presented with progressive motor and sensory neuropathy. There was no history of diabetes or renal disease, but she had congestive heart failure and a negative family history.

Other conditions such as connective tissue disorder, an autoimmune polyneuropathy, a toxic neuropathy, or a neuropathy associated with carcinoma needed to be considered. The congestive heart failure could also suggest amyloidosis.

The patient was on amiodarone which could cause a peripheral neuropathy.

WHAT SHOULD BE DONE?

A complete metabolic panel was normal except for mildly elevated sugar of 182 mg/dL (normal, <110 mg/dL). Erythrocyte sedimentation rate was 52 mm/h (normal, <30 mm/h) and when repeated was 39 mm/h. Fluorescent antinuclear antibody was positive 1:80. C3 and C4 complement and extractable nuclear antibody titers were normal.

AN EMG TEST WAS PERFORMED

Motor Nerve Studies

Nerve and Site	Latency (ms)	Amplitude (mV)	Conduction Velocity (m/s)
Peroneal Nerve L.	**Normal ≤ 5.7**	**Normal ≥ 4**	**Normal ≥ 40**
Ankle	4.6	**2**	–
Fibular head	10.9	**2**	**37**
Knee	12.4	**2**	**39**

Motor Nerve Studies—cont'd

Nerve and Site	Latency (ms)	Amplitude (mV)	Conduction Velocity (m/s)
Tibial Nerve L.	**Normal ≤ 5.3**	**Normal ≥ 4**	**Normal ≥ 40**
Ankle	4.4	**3**	–
Pop. fossa	12.6	**2**	**37**
Median Nerve L.	**Normal ≤ 3.6**	**Normal ≥ 8**	**Normal ≥ 50**
Wrist	2.7	**7**	–
Elbow	6.3	**7**	**49**

F-Wave and Tibial H-Reflex Studies

Nerve	Latency (ms)	Normal Latency ≤ (ms)
Peroneal nerve L.	51.5	54
Tibial nerve L.	52.8	54
Median nerve L.	28.9	30
H-reflex L.	**NR**	34
H-reflex R.	**NR**	34

Sensory Nerve Studies

Nerve	Peak Latency (ms)	Normal Peak Latency ≤ (ms)	Amp (μV)	Normal Amp ≥ (μV)
Sural nerve L.	**NR**	4.0	**NR**	11
Superficial peroneal nerve L.	**NR**	4.0	**NR**	8–10
Median nerve L.	**NR**	3.1	**NR**	13

EMG Data

Muscle	Insrt Activity	Fibs	Pos Waves	Fasc	Amp	Dur	Poly	Pattern
Vastus lateralis L.	Norm	None	None	None	Norm	Norm	None	Full
Tibialis anterior L.	Norm	None	None	None	**Lg**	**Inc**	None	**Red**
Peroneus longus L.	**Inc**	None	None	None	Norm	Norm	None	Full
Gastrocnemius L.	**Inc**	None	**1+**	None	**Lg**	**Inc**	None	**Red**
Vastus lateralis R.	Norm	None	None	None	**Lg**	**Inc**	None	**Red**
Tibialis anterior R.	**Inc**	None	None	None	**Lg**	**Inc**	None	**Red**
Gastrocnemius R.	**Inc**	None	**1+**	None	Norm	Norm	None	Full
First dorsal interosseous L.	Norm	None	None	None	**Lg**	**Inc**	None	**Red**
Flexor carpi ulnaris L.	Norm	None	None	None	Norm	Norm	None	Full

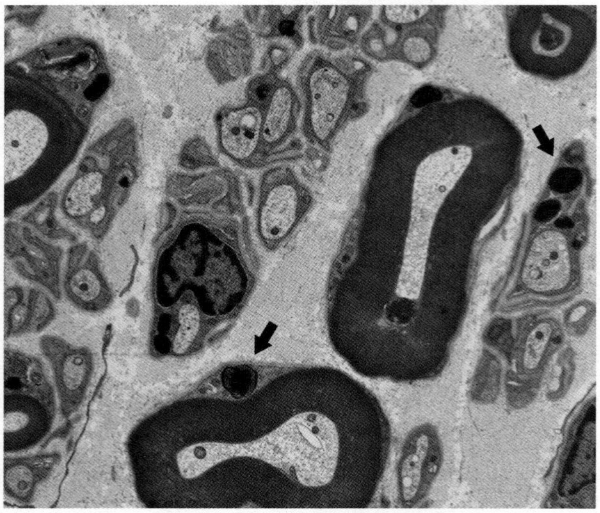

FIG. 71-1 Electromicroscopy on sural nerve biopsy showing osmiophilic inclusions in cytoplasm of Schwann cells (*arrows*) (×10,000).

WHAT WERE THE EMG FINDINGS?

These electrophysiologic studies revealed mild slowing of nerve conduction velocities with low-amplitude median and peroneal CMAPs; all tested SNAPs were absent.

There was mild denervation in the distal legs.

It was concluded that this patient had a mild demyelinating and axonal polyneuropathy.

A nerve biopsy showed some axonal degeneration, segmental demyelination, and osmiophilic inclusions in the endoneural area (Fig. 71-1).

The patient was diagnosed having an amiodarone-induced neuropathy, and the drug was discontinued. She was treated with physical therapy and slowly improved.

TABLE 71.1 Drug-induced Neuropathies: Anatomical Site of Disease

Axonopathy	Axonopathy—cont'd
Almitrine	Nitrous oxide
Amiodarone	Phenytoin
Amitriptyline	Sulfapyridine
Bortezomib	Sulfasalazine
Carbamide	Statins?
Chloramphenicol	Seramin
Chloroquine	Taxanes
Cisplatin	Thalidomide
(predominantly	Vancomycin
dorsal root ganglia)	Vinca alkaloids
Clioquinol	**Anterior Horn Cell**
Colchicine	Dapsone
Cyanate	**Dorsal Root Ganglion**
Disopyramide	Pyridoxine
Disulfiram	Cisplatin
Epothilones	Etoposide
Ethambutol	**Schwann Cell, myelin**
Ethionamide	Allopurinol ?
Hydralazine	Amiodarone
Gold	AZA C
Glutethimide	Check point inhibitors
Isoniazid	Indomethacin
Lithium	Perhexiline
Methaqualone	Suramin
Metronidazole	Tumor necrosis factor alpha
Misonidazole	antagonists
Nitrofurantoin	ARAZ
Oxaliplatin	Zimeldine
Perhexiline	Gentamicin
	Streptokinase
	Eosinophilia-myalgia syndrome

Modified with permission from Brown WF, Bolton CF, Aminoff MJ (eds): Drug-Related Neuropathies from Neuromuscular Function and Disease, vol 2. Philadelphia, WB Saunders, 2002, p. 1128.

DISCUSSION

This elderly woman presented with a polyneuropathy that was thought to be caused by amiodarone, and she improved after discontinuing this drug. Other medications that could cause a neuropathy are summarized in Table 71-1.[1]

Amiodarone is an iodinated benzoforan derivative used in the treatment of cardiac arrhythmias. The drug can cause several systemic side effects, such as thyroid disease, skin rash, pulmonary fibrosis, and corneal disease.[2,3] It could also cause neurologic problems, which occur in about 54% of the cases. Most frequently, this consists of tremors, ataxia, and, rarely, optic neuropathy.[4,5] Amiodarone also can cause a peripheral neuropathy,[5–9] myopathy,[10] or neuromyopathy.[11–13]

Amiodarone neuropathy could be predominantly demyelinating, axonal, or both. EMGs could show signs of denervation as well, but also small, polyphasic motor unit action potentials. Some patients could have elevated serum creatine kinase.

The muscle biopsy shows atrophy[12,13] or some vacuolization with lipidlike inclusions[11–13]; a necrotizing myopathy has also been reported.[9]

Nerve biopsies demonstrate loss of myelinated axons with degeneration[6,10] and demyelination.[13] The characteristic finding is the presence of electron-dense inclusions in the Schwann cells, endoneural cells, and interstitial cells.[7,11] These osmophilic inclusions can also be caused by other amphiphilic drugs and are likely of lysosomal origin.[14] The demyelination is believed to be produced by Schwann cell dysfunction with secondary axonal degeneration.[13] The long half-life of the drug is likely predisposed to its tissue accumulation.[11,15]

The treatment of the neurologic manifestations of amiodarone toxicity includes discontinuation of the drug and physical therapy.

SUMMARY

This elderly woman presented with a severe peripheral neuropathy. Her nerve biopsy showed an accumulation of osmiophilic occlusions in several areas of the nerve. This was thought to be caused by amiodarone toxicity. She improved upon withdrawal of the drug.

IMPORTANT POINTS

- The neurologic manifestations of amiodarone toxicity include tremor, ataxia, a neuropathy, and a myopathy.
- Amiodarone neuropathy can be axonal, demyelinating, or both.
- The characteristic finding of a nerve biopsy of amiodarone neuropathy is the presence of osmiophilic bodies within the Schwann cells and other areas of the peripheral nerve.
- The treatment consists of discontinuation of the drug and management of contributing factors.

This case was evaluated with Dr. Thomas Arnold.

REFERENCES

1. Luciano CA, Caraballo-Cartagena S. Treatment and management of infectious, granulomatous, and toxic neuromuscular disorders. In: Bertorini TE, ed. *Neuromuscular Disorders: Treatment and Management*. Amsterdam, Netherlands: Elsevier; 2022:345–379.
2. Hilleman D, Miller MA, Parker R, et al. Optimal management of amiodarone therapy: efficacy and side effects. *Pharmacotherapy*. 1998;18:138S–145S.
3. Dovie JM, Gurwood AS. Acute onset of halos and glare: bilateral corneal epithelial edema with cystic eruptions: atypical presentation of amiodarone keratopathy. *Optometry*. 2006;77(2):76–81.
4. Charness ME, Morady F, Scheinman MM. Frequent neurologic toxicity associated with amiodarone therapy. *Neurology*. 1986;34:669–671.
5. Azzam I, Tov N, Elias N, Naschitz JE. Amiodarone toxicity presenting as pulmonary mass and peripheral neuropathy: the continuing diagnostic challenge. *Postgrad Med J*. 2006;82(963):73–75.
6. Martinez-Arizala A, Sobol SM, McCarty GE, et al. Amiodarone neuropathy. *Neurology*. 1983;33:643–645.
7. Pellissier JF, Pouget J, Cros D, et al. Peripheral neuropathy induced by amiodarone chlorohydrate: a clinicopathological study. *J Neurol Sci*. 1984;63:251–266.
8. Lemaire JF, Autret A, Biziere K, et al. Amiodarone neuropathy: further arguments for human drug-induced neurolipidosis. *Eur Neurol*. 1982;21:65–68.
9. Fraser AG, McQueen IN, Watt AH, et al. Peripheral neuropathy during long-term high dose amiodarone therapy. *J Neurol Neurosurg Psychiatry*. 1985;48:576–578.
10. Clouston PD, Donnelly PE. Acute necrotizing myopathy associated with amiodarone therapy. *Aust N Z J Med*. 1989;19:483–485.
11. Miere C, Kauer B, Muller U, et al. Neuromyopathy during chronic amiodarone treatment: a case report. *J Neurol*. 1979;220:231–239.
12. Roth RF, Itabashi H, Louie J, et al. Amiodarone toxicity: myopathy and neuropathy. *Am Heart J*. 1990;119:1223–1225.
13. Pulipaka U, Lacomis D, Omalu B. Amiodarone-induced neuromyopathy: three cases and a review of the literature. *J Clin Neuromuscul Dis*. 2002;3:97–105.
14. Lullmann H, Lullmann-Rauch R, Wasserman O. Lipidosis induced by amphiphilic cationic drugs. *CRC Crit Rev Toxicol*. 1975;4:185–218.
15. Adams PC, Holt DW, Storey GC, et al. Amiodarone and its desethyl metabolite: tissue distribution and morphologic changes. *Circulation*. 1985;72:1064–1075.

72A CASE

A Young Woman With Difficulty Swallowing

A 20-year-old woman presented for evaluation of progressive dysphagia for approximately 2 years, worsening during the last 4 months. She had lost 70 lb. For these reasons, she had chest x-rays and various endoscopic procedures and was later referred for neurologic evaluation.

Past medical history was significant for a nonspecific arthritis at the age of 10 that lasted for 2 years.

Neurologic examination revealed normal mentation. Extraocular movements were normal, and she had only minimal ptosis on the left. She had a horizontal smile (Fig. 72A-1) and bilateral facial weakness, her speech had a nasal quality, and her palate did not move. Her tongue was not atrophic but was weak. Other cranial nerves were normal. Neck flexors and extensors were 5−/5, and she had 4/5 weakness of the proximal muscles of the arms with mild fatigue. There was no muscle wasting or scapular winging. Reflexes were brisk but normal and symmetrical. Sensory examination and coordination were normal. No fasciculations were detected in the tongue or limbs. There were no Babinski signs. Gait and the rest of the examination were unremarkable.

WHAT IS THE DIFFERENTIAL DIAGNOSIS?

This patient had weakness and difficulty swallowing; progressive spinal muscular atrophy is unlikely due to the recent onset of symptoms, the hyperreflexia, and the lack of fasciculations. Other motor neuron diseases are also unlikely, particularly because of her age. The differential diagnosis should include myasthenia gravis or a myopathy, such as polymyositis. Oculopharyngeal and facioscapulohumeral muscular dystrophy are unlikely because of the lack of family history, the recent onset of symptoms, and the lack of facial weakness, or the characteristic muscle atrophy in the latter. The lack of systemic manifestations and normal eye movements is against a mitochondrial myopathy.

WHAT TESTS SHOULD BE DONE?

Serum creatine kinase and thyroid-stimulating hormone tests were normal. An edrophonium test demonstrated mild improvement of speech and horizontal smile. Complete blood count and metabolic profile were normal, as were FANA and a CT scan of the chest. Acetylcholine receptor antibodies were not elevated. Her insurance company refused to pay for muscle-specific protein kinase antibody measurements.

AN EMG TEST WAS PERFORMED

Motor Nerve Study

Nerve and Site	Latency (ms)	Amplitude (mV)	Conduction Velocity (m/s)
Ulnar Nerve R.	**Normal ≤ 3.6**	**Normal ≥ 8**	**Normal ≥ 50**
Wrist	3.6	8	–
Below elbow	7.9	8	56
Above elbow	10.9	8	60

F-Wave Study

Nerve	Latency (ms)	Normal Latency ≤ (ms)
Ulnar nerve R.	29.1	30

Repetitive Stimulation of Ulnar Nerve R.

Potential Number	Amp (mV)	Amp Decrement (%)	Area Decrement (%)
Before Exercise			
1	6.30	0	0
2	5.11	**19**	**20**
3	4.21	**33**	**32**
4	3.98	**37**	**36**
5	3.96	**37**	**36**
Posttetanic			
1	5.47	0	0
2	4.98	9	**12**
3	4.82	**12**	**12**
4	4.76	**13**	**14**
5	4.77	**13**	**15**
1 min Postexercise			
1	5.51	0	0
2	4.16	**25**	**26**
3	3.47	**37**	**37**
4	3.29	**40**	**41**
5	3.28	**40**	**41**
2 min Postexercise			
1	6.25	0	0
2	5.15	**18**	**25**
3	4.25	**34**	**33**
4	3.99	**37**	**38**
5	3.95	**37**	**39**

EMG Data

Muscle	Insrt Activity	Fibs	Pos Waves	Fasc	Amp	Dur	Poly	Pattern
Deltoid R.	Norm	None	None	None	**Variable**	Norm	None	Full
Biceps brachii R.	Norm	None	None	None	**Variable**	Norm	None	Full
Extensor digitorum com. R.	Norm	None	None	None	Norm	Norm	None	Full
First dorsal interosseous R.	Norm	None	None	None	Norm	Norm	None	Full

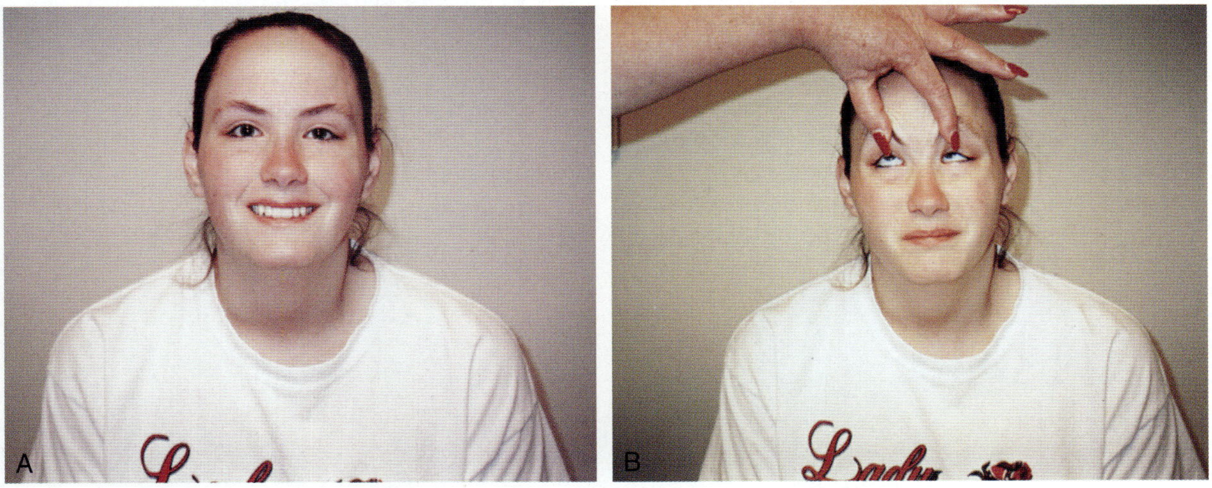

FIG. 72A-1 **A**, Patient showing horizontal smile. There is only slight ptosis of the left eye; notice prominent orbicularis oculi weakness (**B**).

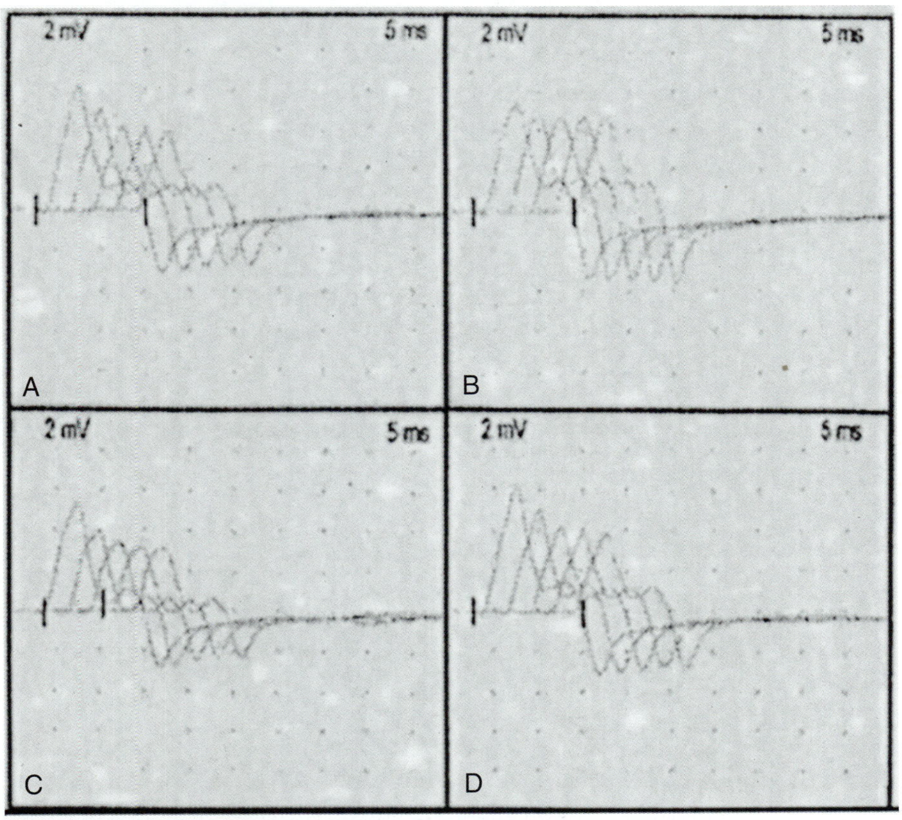

FIG. 72A-2 **A**, Repetitive stimulation test of the ulnar nerve, at 3 Hz recording at the ADM muscle; notice the significant CMAP area decrement. **B**, The decrement diminished after 15 s of tetanic contraction. There was no significant posttetanic facilitation; notice increased decrements after 1 (**C**) and 2 (**D**) min of the tetanic contraction.

WHAT WERE THE EMG FINDINGS?

This test showed normal ulnar motor nerve conduction velocity and distal latency with borderline low CMAP amplitude, and a normal ulnar SNAP.

Needle test showed unstable motor unit potentials in the deltoid and biceps muscles; some were small and polyphasic. Otherwise, the test was normal. There were no denervation potentials.

The repetitive stimulation test showed a significant area decrement of the CMAP in the abductor digiti minimi muscle stimulating the ulnar nerve at 3 Hz up to 26%. There was no significant posttetanic facilitation, but there was a reduced decrement level after a 15-second tetanic contraction, and there was a postactivation exhaustion (Fig. 72A-2). The test was diagnostic of myasthenia gravis.

She was placed on pyridostigmine 60 mg four times a day and prednisone with increasing dosage to 60 mg each day; she also underwent plasmapheresis and later a trans-sternal thymectomy. Prednisone was slowly tapered, and she continued to do well.

SUMMARY

This young woman had difficulty swallowing, which initially was thought to be caused by gastrointestinal problems for which she had numerous tests. Her examination showed a mild horizontal smile and facial and tongue weakness without ptosis or extraocular movement involvement.

She had positive edrophonium and repetitive stimulation tests characteristic of myasthenia gravis but had no elevation of acetylcholine receptor antibodies. She improved after immunotherapy and thymectomy.

For further discussion, important points and references see Case 72B.

A Young Woman With Intermittent Weakness and a Positive Family History of Similar Problems

A 22-year-old woman presented with a 3-month history of weakness, some instability of gait, and difficulty swallowing. The symptoms fluctuated somewhat during the day.

Past medical history was negative. She was on birth control pills. Family history was positive for her mother having myasthenia gravis (MG).

General physical examination and mentation were normal. Cranial nerve examination revealed mild ptosis on the left without clear evidence of fatigue. There was no diplopia or ophthalmoplegia, but there was mild orbicularis oculi and oris weakness. She had proximal weakness of about 4+/5 in the neck and shoulder muscles and 4/5 in the hips. Reflexes, sensation, and coordination were normal. There were no Babinski signs. The examination was otherwise unremarkable.

WHAT IS THE DIFFERENTIAL DIAGNOSIS?

The differential diagnosis of this patient with limb and facial weakness includes facioscapulohumeral dystrophy,[1] because of the family history, as her mother presented with similar weakness, but for that diagnosis, one has to assume that the mother's diagnosis of MG was incorrect. Furthermore, this patient did not have prominent muscle atrophy, and there was no history of progression; ptosis is not common in that disorder. Another hereditary disease of similar presentation is oculopharyngeal dystrophy, but this usually presents at an older age, and she did not have the typical astronomers' sign or prominent ptosis, and her symptoms fluctuated during the day. An acquired endocrine or autoimmune myopathy should be considered, but they usually do not present with facial weakness, nor does periodic paralysis, which presents with episodic rather than a fluctuating weakness as in this case. Hyperthyroidism could present with weakness and ophthalmoplegia, but the symptoms usually do not fluctuate.[2]

Patients with sarcoidosis might have proximal weakness from myositis and develop bilateral seventh and sixth nerve palsies, but these do not fluctuate.[3] Mitochondrial myopathies might present with ophthalmoplegia and ptosis, but in those patients the symptoms are usually slowly progressive.

The apparent autosomal-dominant inheritance could also suggest slow channel syndrome, but in that disease weakness is more prominent in the finger extensors.[4]

Autoimmune MG is not hereditary, but there are reports of the disease occurring in families,[5–8] and thus MG should be considered in the differential diagnosis because of the recently acquired weakness and asymmetric ptosis.

AN EMG TEST WAS PERFORMED

Motor Nerve Studies

Nerve and Site	Latency (ms)	Amplitude (mV)	Conduction Velocity (m/s)
Median Nerve R.	**Normal ≤4.2**	**Normal ≥ 6**	**Normal ≥ 50**
Wrist	4.1	16	–
Elbow	8.4	16	59

Nerve and Site	Latency (ms)	Amplitude (mV)	Conduction Velocity (m/s)
Ulnar Nerve R.	**Normal ≤ 3.6**	**Normal ≥ 8**	**Normal ≥ 50**
Wrist	2.9	11	–
Below elbow	6.3	10	63

F-Wave Studies

Nerve	Latency (ms)	Normal Latency ≤ (ms)
Median nerve R.	27.4	30
Ulnar nerve R.	27.6	30

Sensory Nerve Studies

Nerve	Onset Latency (ms)	Normal Onset Latency ≤ (ms)	Peak Latency (ms)	Normal Peak Latency ≤ (ms)	Amp (μV)	Normal Amp ≥ (μV)	Conduction Velocity (m/s)	Normal Conduction Velocity ≥ (m/s)
Median nerve R.	2.6	2.6	3.1	3.1	38	20	50	50
Ulnar nerve R.	1.9	2.6	2.4	3.1	20	13	63	50

Repetitive Stimulation of Ulnar Nerve R.

Potential Number	Amp (mV)	Amp Decrement (%)	Area Decrement (%)
Before Exercise			
1	8.19	0	0
2	7.68	6	7
3	7.09	**13**	**15**
4	6.82	**17**	**20**
5	6.80	**17**	**20**
Posttetanic			
1	8.22	0	0
2	8.17	1	0
3	8.11	1	2
4	8.11	1	1
5	8.15	1	0
1 min Postexercise			
1	8.35	0	0
2	7.92	5	3
3	7.39	**11**	**12**
4	7.18	**14**	**15**
5	7.25	**13**	**15**

Repetitive Stimulation of Ulnar Nerve R.—cont'd

Potential Number	Amp (mV)	Amp Decrement (%)	Area Decrement (%)
2 min Postexercise			
1	8.63	0	0
2	8.26	4	7
3	7.61	**12**	**17**
4	7.34	**15**	**22**
5	7.29	**16**	**22**
3 min Postexercise			
1	8.63	0	0
2	8.09	6	4
3	7.40	**14**	**15**
4	7.27	**16**	**18**
5	7.30	**15**	**18**

EMG Data

Muscle	Insrt Activity	Fibs	Pos Waves	Fasc	Amp	Dur	Poly	Pattern
Extensor digitorum com. R.	Norm	None	None	None	**Variable**	Norm	None	Full
Deltoid R.	Norm	None	None	None	**Variable**	Norm	**Few**	Full

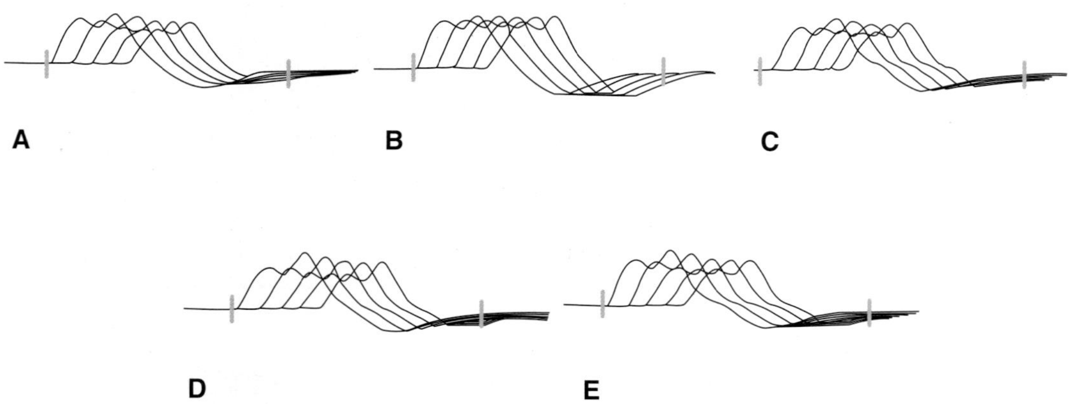

FIG. 72B-1 **A**, Ulnar nerve repetitive stimulation recording at the ADM muscle at 2–3 Hz; notice CMAP amplitude area decrement. **B**, Posttetanic facilitation and disappearance of the decrement. The decrement was then again present at 1 **(C)**, 2 **(D)**, and 3 **(E)** min after tetanic contraction (2 ms/5 mV).

WHAT WERE THE EMG FINDINGS?

This test showed normal nerve conduction velocities and normal amplitudes and latencies of the CMAPs and SNAPs. She had the characteristic decrement of the CMAP area upon repetitive stimulation of the ulnar nerve at 3 Hz with posttetanic facilitation and postactivation exhaustion, diagnostic of MG (Fig. 72B-1). There was no evidence of repetitive after-discharges on the CMAP as seen in congenital slow channel syndrome. There were also some polyphasic motor units and motor unit variability in the deltoid muscle, as occur in disorders of neuromuscular transmission.

WHAT SHOULD YOU DO NEXT?

Complete metabolic panel, complete blood count, and thyroid-stimulating hormone test were normal for this patient. Her fluorescent antinuclear antibody (FANA) was positive at 1:40 with a homogenous pattern.

An edrophonium test produced mild improvement of limb weakness. This test and the EMG findings were diagnostic of MG. Acetylcholine (ACh) receptor antibody levels were elevated at 85 nmol/L (normal, <0.02 nmol/L). Her mother's records were reviewed and showed that she had typical autoimmune myasthenia with elevated antibody titers.

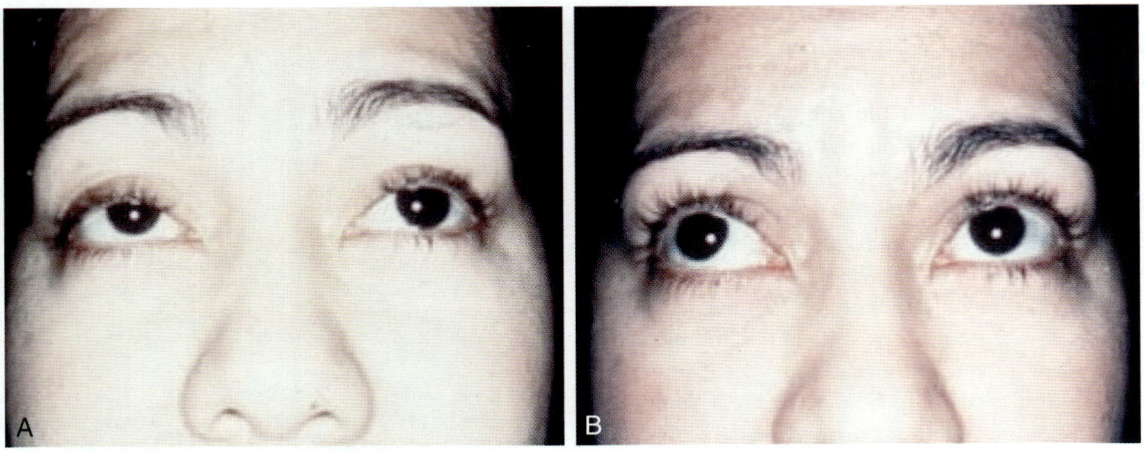

FIG. 72B-2 **A**, Notice limitation of upward gaze and right ptosis on the patient. **B**, Improvement after edrophonium.

The patient was treated with pyridostigmine with improvement.

CT scan of the chest showed mild enlargement of the thymus gland. This was removed by endoscopic suprasternal thymectomy elsewhere at her request and showed thymus hyperplasia.

She did very well after her thymectomy and was maintained on only pyridostigmine 60 mg four times a day.

FOLLOW-UP

Two years later, she presented with increasing droopiness of her eyelids and difficulty swallowing. An edrophonium test again produced improvement (Fig. 72B-2).

A repeated CT scan of the chest showed no residual thymus.

She was treated with azathioprine 100 mg daily with marked improvement. She declined an exploratory thoracotomy for the removal of possible residual thymus tissue not seen on CT scan.

SUMMARY

This 22-year-old woman with MG improved after endoscopic thymectomy but had a recurrence of the disease afterward. She responded to azathioprine therapy.

The patient's mother had MG. Although MG is an acquired autoimmune disease, there is a genetic predisposition, and there are reports of inherited cases.

DISCUSSION (CASES 72A AND 72B)

Cases 72A and 72B had MG, which was documented by positive edrophonium test and decremental responses on repetitive stimulation tests. *Case 72B* also had elevated ACh receptor antibodies.

This woman is of particular interest because her mother had MG and because the recurrence of symptoms after a partial thymectomy raised the possibility that there could have been residual thymus. This is known to occur after endoscopic surgery, which is the reason most recommend a complete thymectomy.

Case 72A emphasizes that even though extraocular and eyelid muscles are more frequently affected in MG, these are not involved in all patients.[9,10] This patient also had tongue weakness but did not have the characteristic forked tongue seen in MG. This and pharyngeal muscle weakness likely caused the difficulty swallowing. This case also emphasizes the difficulties in applying the old Osserman classification of MG,[11] as she had neither ocular nor clinical evidence of generalized muscle weakness and that classification does not include a category linked to only facial and bulbar weakness. She, however, appeared to correspond to type 3B of Myasthenia Gravis Association of America classification, which is more complete and useful.[12] She tested negative for ACh receptor antibodies, and her insurance company did not allow her to be tested for muscle-specific tyrosine kinase (MuSK) antibodies, which raised concerns regarding the possible indication for a thymectomy, as this appears not to be beneficial in patients who are MuSK antibody positive,[13] and thymic hyperplasia is not seen in MuSK positive patients.[14] Nevertheless, this case was recommended for a thymectomy.

MG is an acquired autoimmune postsynaptic disorder of neuromuscular transmission, in which antibodies block and cause a complement-mediated destruction of ACh receptors, resulting in weakness and fatigability. Close to 90% of the patients have measurable ACh receptor antibodies,[15] and 37%–70% of patients that are ACh antibody negative have antibodies against MuSK.[13,14] MuSK mediates agrin-induced clustering of ACh receptors during synapse formation. Thus, this antibody likely affects the formation of ACh receptors. There are other antibodies that can be present in MG but are not frequently used in diagnosis. These include LRP4 and agrin striated muscle antibodies in those with thymoma and titin and ryanodine antibodies that can be seen in older myasthenics without thymoma.

The incidence of MG is 6–11 per million population.[16] Hereditary susceptibility to developing the disease depends on ACh epitope presentation to major histocompatibility complex proteins with a higher incidence of human leukocyte antigens (HLAs) A1, B8, and Dr3 in young White women.[17] There also appear to be other genes that increase the susceptibility. There are isolated reports of MG occurring in the same family with autosomal-dominant[6–8] or recessive patterns.[5]

The electrophysiologic diagnosis of MG is based on repetitive stimulation tests following the Association of Neuromuscular and Electrodiagnostic Medicine practice parameters,[18] and for this, ulnar nerve stimulation is chosen first because it is less painful. However, only about 40% of patients with generalized myasthenia show decrements in the abductor digiti minimi. The yield increases with stimulating nerves to proximal muscles such as the spinal accessory which raises the sensitivity to 90%.[19] Facial stimulation also increases the diagnostic yield but is less tolerable. Single-fiber EMG is a very sensitive diagnostic test that is positive in up to 99% of cases.[20] The sensitivity is high even in ocular myasthenia and has been reported to reach 100% in severe ocular myasthenia.[21] Microelectrode studies in MG show normal miniature end plate potentials (EPPs) frequency, but they could be decreased in amplitude. The EPP quantal content could be normal or decreased, but their amplitude decreases during repetitive nerve stimulation. In normal people during repetitive stimulation, the EPPs decrease in amplitude but remain above the threshold to generate muscle action potential; this is called *safety factor*. In MG there is a decreased safety factor, and as the EPPs become smaller, they might not generate muscle action potentials.[22] The consequence of this is smaller CMAPs during the clinical repetitive stimulation test.

MG was initially described by Willis in 1672 in patients who developed weakness and difficulty speaking during the day.[17] In 1895 Jolly described the disease as "myasthenia gravis pseudoparalytica"[23] and found a decreased muscle tetanic tension that worsened upon repetitive nerve stimulation and improved with rest. He also suggested that pyridostigmine could be beneficial. In 1941 Harvey and Masland[24] reported the decremental response of the CMAP on repetitive nerve stimulation, and Lindsley[25] demonstrated the variability of the motor unit action potentials on routine EMG, while more recently Stålberg and colleagues described the characteristic single-fiber EMG abnormalities of increased neuromuscular jitter and blocking.[26]

The history of MG is filled with other extraordinary clinical observations that led to the current knowledge of its autoimmune etiology and to its treatment.[27] Walker in 1934[28] suggested that anticholinesterase drugs could be beneficial. An autoimmune etiology was proposed by Simpson,[29] based on the association of MG with other autoimmune disorders, the fluctuation of weakness, and the development of myasthenic symptoms in children born of myasthenic mothers.

Patrick and Lindstrom reproduced myasthenic weakness in rabbits immunized with electric eel ACh receptors,[30] and later the disease was reproduced in several other animal species (Fig. 72B-3). Lindstrom and coworkers reported that patients with MG have ACh receptor antibodies.[31] The ultrastructural localization of IgG and complement at the neuromuscular junction in experimental and human myasthenics was demonstrated by Engel and collaborators.[32,33]

In 1939 Blalock reported the benefit of thymectomy in a patient with thymoma[34] and later summarized his experience in 20 cases that underwent thymectomy.[35]

About 15% of patients with MG have a thymoma, while 65% have thymus hyperplasia.[36] Thymectomy has generally been recommended, particularly in the treatment of younger individuals.[37,38] A complete thymectomy is recommended,[37] because an endoscopic thymectomy might miss an ectopic thymus[38] and might not remove the gland completely.

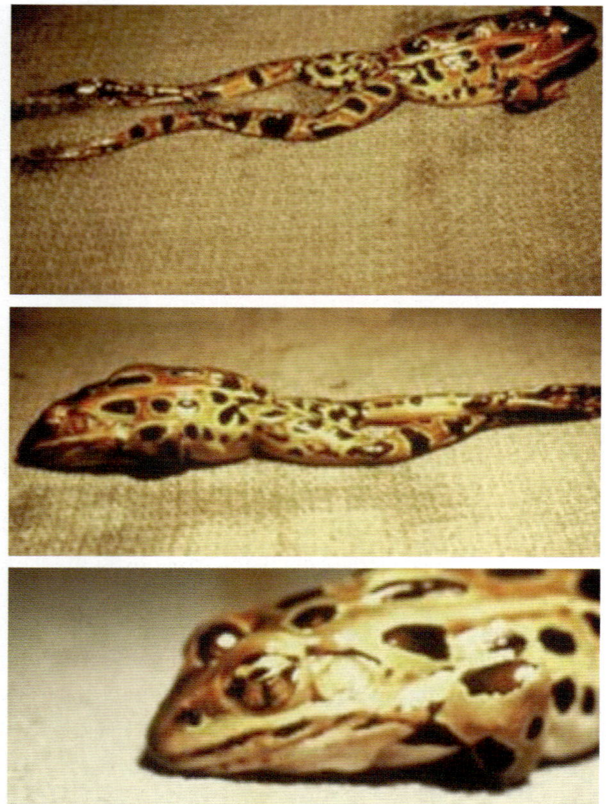

FIG. 72B-3 Myasthenic frog immunized with ACh receptors; notice the dropped head (*center, bottom*) following prostigmin injection (*top*). Courtesy Dr. D. Feinreider and Dr. D. Grob.

The role of the thymus in MG is likely related to the presence of myoid cells in the gland, as these cells have ACh receptors.[39] They do not have HLA type II molecules and thus cannot present antigens to T cells, but they are associated with interdigitation reticulum cells, which are HLA II antigen–presenting cells.[17] The hyperplastic thymus is enriched with ACh receptor–specific T cells[40] and has an increased number of B cells.[41] Also, myasthenic patients have reductions of antibody titers and activated T cells[41] after thymectomy, which are associated with clinical improvement.

The medical treatment of MG includes the use of anticholinesterase drugs,[17] corticosteroids, and immunosuppressants, such as azathioprine, cyclophosphamide, or cyclosporine.[15] Mycophenolate mofetil has recently been proven to be beneficial with less toxic side effects.[42] Plasma exchange[43] and immunoglobulin infusions[44] and rituximab[45] are helpful. (Table 72B-1 summarizes the workup and treatment of patients with MG.) Patients should avoid many drugs that could impair neuromuscular transmission and precipitate weakness (Table 72B-2). D-Penicillamine can actually cause autoimmune MG.[46]

The treatment of MG has progressed significantly and recently eculizumab, a monoclonal antibody that binds C5 and blocks degeneration, has been beneficial in ACh receptor–positive

TABLE 72B-1 Workup and Treatment of Myasthenia Gravis

Ice pack test edrophonium test when available, or the neostigmine test
Acetylcholine receptor antibodies and, if negative, MuSK antibodies
Repetitive stimulation, if negative single-fiber EMG
Routine EMG for motor unit variability and to rule out other disorders
CT scan of the chest, B_{12}, CBC, CMP, T4, TSH, and FANA
Initiate anticholinesterase drugs
Add steroids slowly depending on the severity
If disabling ocular myasthenia, plan thymectomy
Plasmapheresis or IgG infusions 2 weeks prior to thymectomy in generalized myasthenia
Thymectomy
Taper steroids
Taper anticholinesterase drugs: if worsening, add steroids; if there are side effects or no response, add an immunosuppressant (mycophenolate or azathioprine), taper steroids if significant side effects
Consider eculizumab, zilucoplan, ravulizumab, efgartigimod

myasthenia.[47] This is given biweekly. Zilucoplan is a synthetic peptide that inhibits C5 and is given subcutaneously and is also beneficial.[48] Ravulizumab is a compound similar to eculizumab and has been engineered to last longer and is given every 2 months.[49] The monoclonal antibody efgartigimod is an FcRN receptor antagonist and is proven beneficial in MG by promoting the degradation of antibodies. This drug is given every week, 10 mg/kg, and could be repeated when symptoms recur.[50] Rituximab can also help in refractory cases.

TABLE 72B-2 Drugs That Adversely Affect Myasthenia Gravis (MG)

Type of Adverse Effect	Name of Drug or Toxin
Unmask or exacerbate MG	Adrenocorticosteroids and ACTH (temporarily)
	Thyroid preparations
	Neuromuscular blocking agents (including Botox)
	Anesthetic agents (including alcohol)
	Magnesium salts, epsom salts
	Antiarrhythmics: quinidine, procainamide, phenytoin, gabapentin, verapamil, and intravenous lidocaine or procaine
	Antibiotics
	Aminoglycosides: systemic gentamicin, tobramycin, neomycin, paromomycin, amikacin, kanamycin, and streptomycin
	Polypeptides: polymyxin B, colistin, and colistimethate
	Tetracyclines: chlortetracycline, oxytetracycline, demeclocycline, methacycline, doxycycline, and minocycline
	Miscellaneous: clindamycin, lincomycin, ciprofloxacin, high-dose ampicillin, and intravenous erythromycin
May induce MG by precipitating an autoimmune reaction	D-Penicillamine, trimethadione, chloroquine, α-interferon, interleukin-2, wasp stings, and coral snake bite
Implicated in isolated instances of MG exacerbation[a]	Cimetidine, citrate, chloroquine, cocaine, diazepam, lithium carbonate, quinine, β-blockers including timolol maleate eyedrops, trihexyphenidyl hydrochloride, radiocontrast media (ophthalmic acid, meglumine diatrizoate), gemfibrozil (Lopid), and hydroxymethylglutaryl-coenzyme A reductase inhibitors ("statins")

[a]Not every MG patient is expected to react adversely to these medications.

Modified and reproduced with permission from Keesey JC. Clinical evaluation and management of myasthenia gravis. *Muscle Nerve.* 2004;29(4):495.

IMPORTANT POINTS (FOR CASES 72A AND 72B)

- MG is an autoimmune disease with some genetic predisposition.
- The characteristic clinical findings of MG include ptosis, diplopia, facial weakness, dysphagia, and proximal muscle weakness which fluctuates. Patients have normal reflexes on sensory examination. Some might not have abnormalities of extraocular movements or ptosis.
- The diagnosis of MG is based on a positive edrophonium test, if available, or a pyridostigmine test; ice pack test is also useful, and abnormal repetitive stimulation tests, and elevation of ACh receptor antibodies. An edrophonium test, or pyridostigmine test, should always be done in patients with dysphagia, if there are no other obvious causes.
- Antibody-negative myasthenics could have MuSK antibodies. The workup of MG also includes repetitive stimulation tests, a CT or MRI of the chest (to rule out a thymoma), thyroid studies, and FANA.
- Determination of variability of motor units on routine EMG is helpful in the diagnosis. Single-fiber EMG is a highly sensitive test, particularly in facial muscles.
- MG can be associated with other autoimmune disorders such as lupus, pernicious anemia, and thyroid disease.
- The treatment of MG consists of the use of anticholinesterase drugs, corticosteroids, and immunosuppressants as well as complement inhibitors and FcRn antagonists. Plasma exchange and immunoglobulin therapy are beneficial.
- Thymectomy is beneficial in AChR-positive and likely AChR-negative MG.

REFERENCES

1. Bertorini TE. Clinical evaluation and clinical laboratory tests. In: Bertorini TE, ed. *Clinical Evaluation and Diagnostic Tests for Neuromuscular Disorders*. Boston, MA: Butterworth-Heinemann; 2002:15–98.
2. Jacobson DM. Dysthyroid orbitopathy. *Semin Neurol*. 2000;20(1):43–54.
3. Stern BJ, Krumholz A, Johns C, et al. Sarcoidosis and its neurological manifestations. *Arch Neurol*. 1985;42(9):909–917.
4. Engel AG, Lambert EH, Mulder DM, et al. A newly recognized congential myasthenic syndrome attributed to a prolonged open time of the acetylcholine-induced ion channel. *Ann Neurol*. 1982;11(6):553–569.

5. Bergoffen J, Zmijewski CM, Fischbeck KH. Familial autoimmune myasthenia gravis. *Neurology*. 1994;4:551–554.
6. Li F, Szobor A, Croxen R, et al. Dominantly inherited myasthenia gravis as a separate genetic entity without involvement of definite candidate gene loci. *Int J Mol Med*. 2001;7:289–294.
7. Marrie RA, Sahlas DJ, Bray GM. Familial autoimmune myasthenia gravis: four patients involving three generations. *Can J Neurol Sci*. 2000;27:307–310.
8. Szobor A. Familial myasthenia gravis: nine patients in two generations. *Acta Med Hung*. 1991;48(3–4):145–149.
9. Chia LG. Facial weakness without ocular weakness in myasthenia gravis. *Muscle Nerve*. 1988;11(2):185–186.
10. Grob D, Brunner NG, Namba T. The natural course of myasthenia gravis and effect of therapeutic measures. *Ann NY Acad Sci*. 1981;377:652–669.
11. Osserman KE. *Myasthenia Gravis*. New York, NY: Grune & Stratton; 1958:77–80.
12. Jaretzki A III, Barohn RJ, Ernstoff RM, et al. Myasthenia gravis: recommendations for clinical research standards. Task Force of the Medical Scientific Advisory Board of the Myasthenia Gravis Foundation of America. *Neurology*. 2000;55(1):16–23.
13. Sanders DB, El-Salem K, Massey JM, et al. Clinical aspects of MuSK antibody positive seronegative MG. *Neurology*. 2003; 60(12):1978–1980.
14. Lauriola L, Ranelletti F, Maggiano N, et al. Thymus changes in anti-MuSK–positive and –negative myasthenia gravis. *Neurology*. 2005;64:536–538.
15. Seybold ME. Treatment of myasthenia gravis. In: Engel AG, ed. *Myasthenia Gravis and Myasthenic Disorders*. New York, NY: Oxford University Press; 1999:167–201.
16. Robertson NP, Deans J, Compston DA. Myasthenia gravis: a population based epidemiological study in Cambridgeshire, England. *J Neurol Neurosurg Psychiatry*. 1998;65(4):492–496.
17. Engel AG, Hohfield R. Acquired autoimmune myasthenia gravis. In: Engel AG, Franzini-Armstrong C, eds. *Myology*. 3rd ed. New York, NY: McGraw Hill; 2004:1775–1790.
18. AAEM Quality Assurance Committee Practice parameter for repetitive nerve stimulation and single fiber EMG evaluation of adults with suspected myasthenia gravis or Lambert-Eaton myasthenic syndrome: summary statement. *Muscle Nerve*. 2001;24(9):1236–1238.
19. Keesey JC. AAEM minimonograph 33: electrodiagnostic approach to defect of neuromuscular transmission. *Muscle Nerve*. 1989;12(8):613–626.
20. Minggioli MN, Sanders DB. Myasthenia gravis: diagnosis. In: Pascuzzi RM, ed. *Seminars of Neurology in Myasthenia Gravis*. New York, NY: Thieme; 2004:31–39.
21. Katzberg HD, Hans D, Bril V. A comparison of electrodiagnostic tests in ocular myasthenia gravis. *J Clin Neuromuscul Dis*. 2005; 6:109–113.
22. Maselli RA. Role of in vitro intracellular microelectrode studies in the diagnosis of neuromuscular disorders. In: Bertorini TE, ed. *Clinical Evaluation and Diagnostic Tests for Neuromuscular Disorders*. Boston, MA: Butterworth-Heinemann; 2002:295–329.
23. Jolly F. Uber myasthenia gravis pseudoparalytica. *Berl Klin Wychenshf*. 3218951–7.
24. Harvey AM, Masland RL. The electromyogram in myasthenia gravis. *Bull John Hopkins Hosp*. 1941;69:1–13.
25. Lindsley DB. Myographic and electromyographic studies of myasthenia gravis. *Brain*. 1935;58:470–482.
26. Stålberg EJ, Trontelj JV, Schwartz MS. Single-muscle-fiber recording of the jitter phenomenon in patients with myasthenia gravis and in members of their families. *Ann NY Acad Sci*. 1976; 274:189–202.
27. Keesey JC. "Crisis" in myasthenia gravis: an historical perspective. *Muscle Nerve*. 2002;26(1):1–3.
28. Walker MB. Treatment of myasthenia gravis with physostigmine. *Lancet*. 1934;1:1200–1201.
29. Simpson JA. Myasthenia gravis, a new hypothesis. *Scott Med J*. 1960;5:419–436.
30. Patrick J, Lindstrom J. Autoimmune response to acetylcholine receptor. *Science*. 1973;180(88):871–872.
31. Lindstrom JM, Seybold ME, Lennon VA, et al. Antibody to acetylcholine receptor in myasthenia gravis: prevalence, clinical correlates, and diagnostic value. *Neurology*. 1976;26(11): 1054–1059.
32. Engel AG, Fumagalli G. Mechanisms of acetylcholine loss from the neuromuscular junction. In: Everest D, Whelan J, eds. *Receptors, Antibodies and Disease, CIBA Foundation Symposium 90*. London, England: Pitman Medical; 1982:197–224.
33. Engel AG, Arahata K. The membrane attack complex of complement at the endplate in myasthenia gravis. *Ann NY Acad Sci*. 1987;505:326–332.
34. Blalock A, Mason MF, Morgan HJ, Riven S. Myasthenia gravis and tumors of the thymic region: report of a case in which the tumor was removed. *Ann Surg*. 1939;110:544–561.
35. Blalock A. Thymectomy in the treatment of myasthenia gravis: report of 20 cases. *J Thorac Surg*. 1944;13:316–339.
36. Viets HR, Schwab RS. Thymectomy for myasthenia gravis. In: Viets HR, ed. *Records of Experience of Massachusetts General Hospital*. Springfield, IL: Charles Thomas Publishers; 1960: 597–607.
37. Molnar J, Szobor A. Myasthenia gravis: effect of thymectomy in 425 patients: a 15-year experience. *Eur J Cardiothorac Surg*. 1990;4(1):8–14.
38. Wolfe GI, Kaminski HJ, Abn IB, et al. Randomized trial of thymectomy in myasthenia gravis. *N Engl J Med*. 2016;375(6): 511–522.
39. Schluep M, Willcox N, Vincent A, et al. Acetylcholine receptors in human thymic myoid cells in situ: an immunohistological study. *Ann Neurol*. 1987;22(2):212–222.
40. Melms A, Schalke BC, Kirchner T, et al. Thymus in myasthenia gravis: isolation of T-lymphocytic lines specific for the nicotinic acetylcholine receptor from thymuses of myasthenic patients. *J Clin Invest*. 1988;81(3):902–908.
41. Durelli L, Massazza U, Poccardi G, et al. Increased thymocyte differentiation in myasthenia gravis: a dual-color immuno-fluorescence phenotypic analysis. *Ann Neurol*. 1990;27(2): 174–180.
42. Ciafaloni E, Massey JM, Tucker-Lipscomb B, Sanders DB. Mycophenolate mofetil for myasthenia gravis: an open-label pilot study. *Neurology*. 2001;56(1):97–99.
43. [No authors listed]. Assessment of plasmapheresis. Report of the therapeutics and technology assessment subcommittee of the American Academy of Neurology. *Neurology*. 1996;47:840–843.
44. Zinmon L, Ng E, Bril V. IV immunoglobulin in patients with myasthenia gravis: a randomized controlled trial. *Neurology*. 2007;68:837–841.
45. Tandan R, Hehir MK 2nd, Waheed W, Howard DB. Rituximab treatment of myasthenia gravis: a systemic review. *Muscle Nerve*. 2017;56(2):185–196.
46. Fawcett PR, McLachlan SM, Nicholson LV, et al. D-Penicillamine-associated myasthenia gravis: immunological and electrophysiological studies. *Muscle Nerve*. 1982;5(4):328–334.

47. Muppidi S, Utsugisawa K, Benatar M, Murai H, et al. Long-term safety and efficacy of eculizumab in generalized myasthenia gravis. *Muscle Nerve*. 2019;60(1):14–24.
48. Howard JF, Nowak RJ, Wolfe GI, Freimer ML, et al. Clinical effects of the self-administered subcutaneous complement inhibitor Zilucoplan in patients with myasthenia gravis: results of a phase 2 randomized, double-blind, placebo-controlled, multicenter clinical trial. *JAMA Neurol*. 2020;77(5):582–592.
49. Vu T, Melsel A, Mantegazza R, Annane D, et al. Terminal complement inhibitor ravulizumab in generalized myasthenia gravis. *N Engl J Med*. 2022;1(5). https://doi.org/10.1056/EVIDoa2100066.
50. Howard JF, Bril V, Burns TM, et al. Randomized phase 2 study of FcRn antagonist efgartigimod in generalized myasthenia gravis. *Neurology*. 2019;92(23):e2661–e2673. https://doi.org/10.1212/WNL.00000000000007600.

73 CASE

A Weak Woman With a Weak Baby

A 30-year-old G2POA1 African American female developed diplopia and fatigue during the late second trimester of pregnancy. A year earlier, she had experienced similar symptoms briefly, but they improved spontaneously. She had one previous pregnancy resulting in a spontaneous abortion at about 10 weeks. During the second pregnancy, her weakness worsened and she underwent a Cesarean section at 34 weeks gestation after polyhydramnios was discovered. The baby had Apgar scores of 3 at 1 minute and 6 at 5 minutes. He was floppy and areflexic and had to be intubated. Blood chemistries including serum creatine kinase were normal.

The mother remained weak after delivery and initial neurology consultation documented mild dysarthria and decreased neck flexion. She had positive edrophonium testing and characteristic decrement was demonstrated on repetitive stimulation on both the facial and the peroneal motor studies. She was started on pyridostigmine but subsequently decompensated and was admitted to the hospital. On examination she had bifacial weakness, ophthalmoplegia, nasal speech, and 4/5 strength in the proximal extremities with 4+/5 strength distally. She demonstrated labored respirations and had a forced vital capacity of 0.95 L. By that time, AChR antibody testing had returned negative.

WHAT TO DO NEXT?

Muscle-specific kinase (MuSK) antibody titers were drawn and found to be present on radioimmunoassay immunoprecipitation performed by Athena Diagnostics. She was treated initially with intravenous immunoglobulin (IVIG) with little improvement, but she responded well to subsequent plasmapheresis.

Although he did not have electrophysiological testing, the baby received 5 mg/kg of pyridostigmine on days 10–14 when the mother's workup appeared consistent with myasthenia gravis. He initially showed little improvement and underwent exchanged transfusion on day 11. He was then switched to intravenous neostigmine on days 15–39 with minimal response. IVIG was initiated on day 23 and given for 4 days. He improved during the course of IVIG with increased spontaneous respirations and movements. On day 40, he was weaned off neostigmine and was extubated on day 44. At 9 weeks, he appeared normal. At 2 years of age, he had normal development and neurological examination was unremarkable.

The mother was treated with steroids and later azathioprine which she did not tolerate and mycophenolate, but she required intermittent IgG infusions. She later was treated with rituximab and she responded very well and is very stable.

SUMMARY

A young woman with MuSK antibody-positive myasthenia delivered a child with transient weakness. She responded to plasmapheresis and the baby responded to IVIG. The baby has been asymptomatic for 6 years and the mother is being treated with immunotherapy. This case is an example of the difficulties in myasthenia during pregnancy. This case also demonstrates that MuSK antibody myasthenia can manifest in the baby as a transient myasthenia.

DISCUSSION

The patient had a MuSK antibody-positive myasthenia and her baby had transient weakness likely secondary to the antibodies crossing the placenta.[1] New-onset myasthenia may occur in pregnancy; 41% of myasthenic patients have an exacerbation during pregnancy and 28% have an exacerbation in postpartum.[2–4] Patients with MuSK myasthenia and their baby should be observed carefully as they develop weakness.[5] Fortunately for the baby this weakness is transitory.

About 10% of patients with myasthenia are acetylcholine receptor antibody-negative and among them about 40% have antibodies against MuSK, a disorder that manifests with somewhat different phenotypes.[6–10] These patients also do not seem to respond to thymectomy and anticholinesterase drugs.[11] In myasthenia, there could be transitory weakness in the baby and this can occur before delivery and may result in polyhydramnios.[3] There is an association of severity with an increased ratio of fetal to maternal antibody titers.[9] These have not been demonstrated in MuSK myasthenia.

Anti-MuSK myasthenia can be difficult to recognize because patients manifest with bulbar signs which can be confused with signs of a motor neuron disease. Patients respond to plasma exchange and IVIG, but the response to anticholinesterase drugs is not very good. It appears that rituximab is the best treatment for MuSK-positive myasthenia.[12,13]

IMPORTANT POINTS

- MuSK antibody myasthenia gravis antibodies can be transmitted to the newborn causing transitory weakness similar to acetylcholine receptor-positive myasthenia.
- Patients' babies should be treated symptomatically and if necessary using immunotherapy, but weakness is transitory.
- MuSK antibody-positive myasthenia responds well to rituximab.

- MuSK antibody-positive myasthenia might present with prominent bulbar signs.
- The response to anticholinesterase drugs and thymectomy is not good in MuSK-positive myasthenia.

This case was reported in O'Carroll P, Bertorini TE, Jacob G, Mitchell CW, Graff J. Transient neonatal myasthenia gravis in a baby born to a mother with new-onset anti-MuSK-mediated myasthenia gravis. J Clin Neuromuscul Dis. 2009;11(2):69–71.

REFERENCES

1. Hoff J, Dalveit A, Gilhus N. Myasthenia gravis: consequences for pregnancy, delivery and the newborn. *Neurology*. 2003;61: 1362–1366.
2. Plauche W. Myasthenia gravis in mothers and their newborns. *Clin Obstet Gynecol*. 1991;34:82–99.
3. Verspyck E, Nandelbrot L, Dommergues M, et al. Myasthenia gravis with polyhydramnios in the fetus of an asymptomatic mother. *Prenat Diagn*. 1993;13:539–542.
4. Oskout M, Jacobson L, Chung W, et al. Fetal acetylcholine receptor inactivation syndrome and maternal myasthenia gravis. *Neurology*. 2008;72:2010–2012.
5. Niks E, Verrips A, Semmekrot B, et al. A transient neonatal myasthenia syndrome with anti MuSK antibodies. *Neurology*. 2008;70:1215–1216.
6. Sanders DB, El-Salem K, Massey J, et al. Clinical aspects of MuSK antibody positive seronegative MG. *Neurology*. 2003;60:1978–1980.
7. Zhou L, McConville J, Chaundhry V, et al. Clinical comparison of muscle-specific tyrosine kinase (MuSK) antibody positive and negative myasthenic patients. *Muscle Nerve*. 2004;30:55–60.
8. Shigemoto K. Myasthenia gravis induced by autoantibodies against MuSK. *Acta Myol*. 2007;26:185–191.
9. Farrugia ME, Melms A, Vincent A. Myasthenia gravis with MuSK antibodies. *Pract Neurol*. 2005;5:356–359.
10. Meriggioli MN, Sanders DB. Myasthenia gravis diagnosis. *Semin Neurol*. 2004;24:31–39.
11. Hatanaka Y, Hemmi S, Morgan MB, et al. Nonresponsiveness to anticholinesterase agents in patients with MuSK antibody positive MG. *Neurology*. 2005;65:1508–1509.
12. Diaz-Manera J, Martínez-Hernández E, Querol L, Klooser R, et al. Long-lasting treatment effect of rituximab in MuSK myasthenia. *Neurology*. 2012;78(3):189–193.
13. Hehir MK, Hobson-Webb LD, Benatar M, Barnett C, et al. Rituximab as treatment for anti-MuSK myasthenia gravis: multicenter blinded prospective review. *Neurology*. 2017;89(10): 1069–1077.

74 CASE

A Woman With Muscle Weakness and Areflexia

A 52-year-old woman presented with a history of weakness and fatigue in the legs with difficulty going upstairs and downstairs for over 1 year. She also had burning paresthesias in the thighs and was treated with amitriptyline 50 mg every night for depression and fibromyalgia. She had a loss of appetite and had had a 20-lb weight loss.

Previous neurologic workup included an EMG that showed brief polyphasic motor unit potentials and increased insertional activity in proximal muscles; her serum creatine kinase was normal; a muscle biopsy showed type II muscle fiber atrophy; and a nerve biopsy was unremarkable. A CT scan of the chest showed benign hilar adenopathy. Other previous tests included a fluorescent antinuclear antibody titer of 1:160 homogenous pattern, normal thyroid function tests, acetylcholine receptor antibodies, protein electrophoresis, 24-hour heavy metals, porphyrins, extractable nuclear Ag, and C3 and C4.

She was treated with 30 mg of prednisone daily without benefit and was referred to us.

Past medical history included a hysterectomy and oophorectomy in the remote past. She smoked one pack of cigarettes a day and did not drink. She worked as a secretary. Family history was positive for a daughter with cystic fibrosis.

Neurologic examination revealed normal mentation and cranial nerves. The pupils, disks, extraocular movements, face, palate movement, and tongue strength were normal, but her tongue was dry. Strength examination showed mild proximal weakness without fatigue. She was areflexic. Vibration sense was diminished in the toes, but pinprick sensation was normal. Coordination was also normal. There was no evidence of muscle atrophy or fasciculations.

WHAT IS THE DIFFERENTIAL DIAGNOSIS?

This patient presented with progressive muscle weakness mainly in the legs with paresthesias. For this, spinal stenosis is a consideration, although she did not have back pain. Another possibility would be an inflammatory myopathy such as polymyositis and inclusion body myositis, but she had normal serum creatine kinase, and both were ruled out by her muscle biopsy. Endocrine myopathies, such as from hypothyroidism or hyperparathyroidism, might manifest with predominant lower extremity weakness, and their muscle biopsies might show type II muscle fiber atrophy, as in this patient.

She had some clinical suggestion of a neuropathy, as she had paresthesias and was areflexic, but her previous nerve conduction test and EMG were against that diagnosis. The lack of fasciculations, the small motor units reported on the EMG, and the muscle biopsy findings are against a motor neuron disease.

Another possibility is a disorder of neuromuscular transmission, particularly because of her history of fatigue and lack of significant muscle atrophy. The lack of diplopia or ptosis and the areflexia are against myasthenia gravis, but not Eaton–Lambert syndrome. She also had a dry mouth as in that disorder, but this could have been caused by the amitriptyline.

AN EMG TEST WAS PERFORMED

Motor Nerve Studies

Nerve and Site	Latency (ms)	Amplitude (mV)	Conduction Velocity (m/s)
Peroneal Nerve L.	**Normal ≤ 4.2**	**Normal ≥ 6**	**Normal ≥ 50**
Ankle	3.9	**2**	–
Fibular head	10.6	**2**	42
Nerve and Site	**Latency (ms)**	**Amplitude (mV)**	**Conduction Velocity (m/s)**
Ulnar Nerve L.	**Normal ≤ 3.6**	**Normal ≥ 8**	**Normal ≥ 50**
Wrist	3.0	**2.5**	–
Below elbow	7.7	**2.5**	50

F-Wave Studies

Nerve	Latency (ms)	Normal Latency ≤ (ms)
Peroneal nerve L.	53.8	54
Ulnar nerve L.	26.7	30

Sensory Nerve Studies

Nerve	Onset Latency (ms)	Normal Onset Latency ≤ (ms)	Peak Latency (ms)	Normal Peak Latency ≤ (ms)	Amp (μV)	Normal Amp ≥ (μV)	Conduction Velocity (m/s)	Normal Conduction Velocity ≥ (m/s)
Sural nerve L.	3.3	3.5	3.8	4.0	14	11	42	40
Ulnar nerve L.	2.1	2.6	2.4	3.1	15	13	57	50

EMG Data

Muscle	Insrt Activity	Fibs	Pos Waves	Fasc	Amp	Dur	Poly	Pattern
Cervical paraspinals L.	Norm	None	None	None	Norm	Norm	Norm	Full
Deltoid L.	Norm	None	None	None	**Variable**[a]	Norm	Norm	**Red**
Biceps brachii L.	Norm	None	None	None	Norm	Norm	Norm	Full
Gluteus medius L.	Norm	None	None	None	Norm	Norm	Norm	Full
Vastus lateralis L.	Norm	None	None	None	**Variable**[a]	Norm	Norm	**Red**
Tibialis anterior L.	Norm	None	None	None	Norm	Norm	Norm	Full
Peroneus longus L.	Norm	None	None	None	Norm	Norm	Norm	Full
Abductor hallucis L.	Norm	None	None	None	Norm	Norm	Norm	**Red**
Tibialis anterior R.	Norm	None	None	None	Norm	Norm	Norm	Full
Peroneus longus R.	Norm	None	None	None	Norm	Norm	Norm	Full
Gastrocnemius R.	Norm	None	None	None	Norm	Norm	Norm	Full

[a]Low amplitude.

Repetitive Stimulation of Ulnar Nerve R.

Potential Number	Amp (mV)	Amp Decrement (%)	Area Decrement (%)
Before Exercise			
1	2.50	–	–
2	2.17	**12**	**12**
3	1.94	**21**	**22**
4	1.80	**26**	**31**
5	1.46	**38**	**38**
6	1.46	**38**	**40**
7	1.20	**40**	**44**
Posttetanic			
1	4.54	–	–
2	4.29	6	7
3	3.98	**12**	**15**
4	3.79	**17**	**20**
5	3.69	**19**	**23**
6	3.47	**24**	**26**
7	3.39	**25**	**28**
8	3.33	**27**	**28**

Repetitive Stimulation of Ulnar Nerve R.—cont'd

Potential Number	Amp (mV)	Amp Decrement (%)	Area Decrement (%)
1 min Postexercise			
1	3.17	–	–
2	2.86	10	16
3	2.35	**26**	**28**
4	2.33	**26**	**26**
5	2.06	**35**	**33**
6	2.00	**37**	**39**
7	1.92	**39**	**39**
8	1.86	**41**	**40**
2 min Postexercise			
1	2.70	–	–
2	2.37	**12**	**12**
3	2.14	**21**	**22**
4	2.00	**26**	**31**
5	1.66	**38**	**38**
6	1.67	**38**	**40**
7	1.61	**40**	**44**

Repetitive Stimulation of Accessory Nerve R.

	Amp (mV)	Area (mV/ms)
Before exercise	2.9	**12.2**
Posttetanic	**4.9**	**19.7**

WHAT WERE THE EMG FINDINGS?

This test showed normal sural SNAP and normal motor nerve conduction velocities and latencies. The CMAPs, however, were of low amplitude.

She also had scattered small motor unit action potentials with amplitude variability in the deltoid and quadriceps muscles. There were no denervation potentials.

Repetitive stimulation test in the ulnar nerve showed a low initial CMAP amplitude and a decrement of the CMAP amplitude and area at low-frequency stimulation and a prominent posttetanic facilitation of over 100% (Fig. 74-1).

The CMAP of the trapezius muscle showed a markedly increased area after a tetanic contraction using a single stimulation of the accessory nerve (Fig. 74-2).

She was diagnosed with Eaton–Lambert syndrome.

A repeat chest CT scan showed a perihilar mass, diagnosed as small cell lung carcinoma on needle biopsy. She was treated with radiation and chemotherapy with some improvement; 3,4-diaminopyridine 10 mg four times a day was added with an improvement of her weakness and fatigue.

The patient later developed diffuse metastasis from her tumor and died.

SUMMARY

This woman, who smoked, presented with muscle weakness and areflexia. Electrophysiologic studies demonstrated a low-amplitude CMAP, which increased markedly after a tetanic contraction.

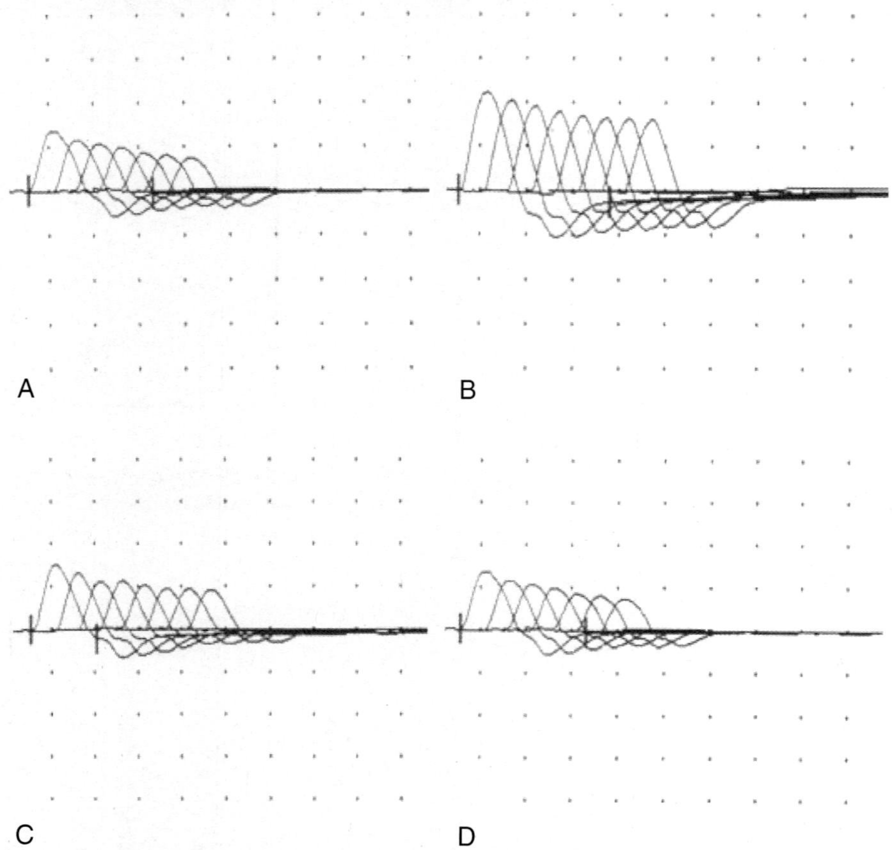

FIG. 74-1 Repetitive stimulation of the ulnar nerve at 3 Hz. Notice the low-amplitude CMAP with decrement (**A**) and significant posttetanic facilitation after 10 s of tetanic contractions (**B**); but there is still a decrement even after facilitation. There are lower-amplitude responses with decrements at 1 (**C**) and 2 (**D**) min after tetanic contractions (2 ms/2 mV).

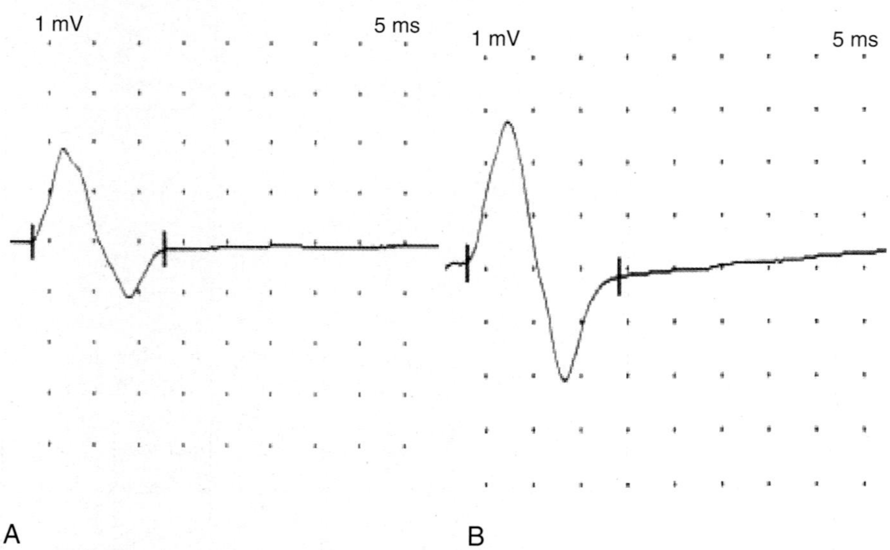

FIG. 74-2 Trapezius muscle CMAP during stimulation of the accessory nerve; one single stimulus before (**A**) and after (**B**) tetanic contraction.

She was later found to have small cell carcinoma of the lung and improved with therapy of the tumor and 3,4-diaminopyridine.

For further discussion, important points, and references, see Case 75.

CASE 75

An Elderly Woman With Proximal Weakness

A 76-year-old woman presented with a 6-month history of progressive weakness in the arms and legs.

Past medical history was positive for hypertension, hypothyroidism, and a left mastectomy for localized cancer 10 years previously. She was on sertraline HCl, diltiazem HCl, and thyroid replacement.

Family history was noncontributory. She did not smoke or drink.

She complained of a crawling sensation in her leg muscles periodically and noticed that her fingernails were not growing. She also was losing weight.

Previous EMG done elsewhere revealed a "mild demyelinating neuropathy."

Mentation and cranial nerve examination were unremarkable. The pupils were equal and reactive, and the disks were flat. The tongue was not atrophic, dry, or weak. She had mild weakness in the proximal muscles with some fatigue, although at times this had a "giveaway" characteristic. There was no improvement after repetitive motion. She had difficulty rising up from a chair, could not sit up from a supine position, and was not able to walk on her tiptoes or squat. Reflexes were trace in the upper extremities and knees, and absent in the ankles. These did not change with repetitive testing. There were no Babinski signs. She had decreased vibration sense in the toes, but pinprick was normal. No atrophy or fasciculations were noted. Coordination was normal.

WHAT IS THE DIFFERENTIAL DIAGNOSIS?

This patient had a history of proximal muscle weakness and had evidence of a mild peripheral neuropathy clinically and by her previous EMG. An acquired demyelinating neuropathy such as chronic inflammatory demyelinating polyneuropathy is a consideration. Her proximal weakness could also be secondary to hypothyroidism or hyperparathyroidism. Other possibilities include polymyositis, and, particularly because of her age, inclusion body myositis, but the distribution of weakness is against the latter. The lack of fasciculations is against progressive spinal muscular atrophy. This and hyporeflexia are against amyotrophic lateral sclerosis. Another possibility would be a disorder of neuromuscular transmission. She had no ptosis or bulbar muscular weakness, and the decreased reflexes are against myasthenia gravis but could suggest Lambert–Eaton syndrome. She, however, had no history of fatigue or improvement after a short period of muscle activity, nor did she have dry mouth or abnormal pupils to suggest this syndrome.

Complete blood count, serum creatine kinase and metabolic panel, T4, thyroid-stimulating hormone, B_{12}/folate, and acetylcholine receptor antibodies were normal. Antinuclear antibody titer was greater than 1:320; C-reactive protein and complements were normal.

AN EMG TEST WAS PERFORMED

Motor Nerve Studies

Nerve and Site	Latency (ms)	Amplitude (mV)	Conduction Velocity (m/s)
Ulnar Nerve R.	**Normal ≤ 3.6**	**Normal ≥ 8**	**Normal ≥ 50**
Wrist	3.5	**2.3**	–
Below elbow	10.7	**2.4**	**37**
Peroneal Nerve R.	**Normal ≤ 5.7**	**Normal ≥ 3**	**Normal ≥ 40**
Ankle	5.5	**2**	–
Fibular head	12.6	**1**	40
Tibial Nerve L.	**Normal ≤ 5.3**	**Normal ≥ 4**	**Normal ≥ 40**
Ankle	3.7	4	–
Pop. fossa	12.8	4	42

F-Wave and H-Reflex Studies

Nerve	Latency (ms)	Normal Latency ≤ (ms)
Peroneal nerve R.	**54.3**	54
Tibial nerve L.	**55.2**	54
Ulnar nerve R.	30.0	30
H-reflex R.	**NR**	34
H-reflex L.	**NR**	34

Sensory Nerve Studies

Nerve	Onset Latency (ms)	Normal Onset Latency ≤ (ms)	Peak Latency (ms)	Normal Peak Latency ≤ (ms)	Amp (μV)	Normal Amp ≥ (μV)	Conduction Velocity (m/s)	Normal Conduction Velocity ≥ (m/s)
Sural nerve R.	3.5	3.5	4.0	4.0	**6**	11	40	40
Ulnar nerve R.	2.5	2.6	3.0	3.1	**12**	13	50	50

EMG Data

Muscle	Insrt Activity	Fibs	Pos Waves	Fasc	Amp	Dur	Poly	Pattern
Deltoid R.	Norm	None	None	None	Norm	Norm	None	Full
Biceps brachii R.	Norm	None	None	None	**Variable**	Norm	None	**Red**
Flexor carpi ulnaris R.	Norm	None	None	None	Norm	Norm	None	Full
First dorsal interosseous R.	Norm	None	None	None	**Variable**	Norm	None	Full
Vastus lateralis R.	Norm	None	None	None	Norm	Norm	None	Full
Tibialis anterior R.	Norm	None	None	None	Norm	Norm	None	Full
Gastrocnemius R.	Norm	None	None	None	Norm	Norm	None	Full
Tibialis anterior L.	Norm	None	None	None	Norm	Norm	None	Full
Gastrocnemius L.	Norm	None	None	None	Norm	Norm	None	Full

Repetitive Stimulation of Ulnar Nerve R.

Potential Number	Amp (mV)	Amp Decrement (%)	Area Decrement (%)
Before Exercise			
1	2.30	0	0
2	1.93	**12**	**15**
3	1.77	**18**	**21**
4	1.71	**20**	**22**
5	1.65	**11**	**18**
Posttetanic			
1	5.95	0	0
2	5.73	2	1
3	5.69	3	4
4	5.38	6	7
5	5.13	9	8

Repetitive Stimulation of Ulnar Nerve R.—cont'd

Potential Number	Amp (mV)	Amp Decrement (%)	Area Decrement (%)
1 min Postexercise			
1	3.80	0	0
2	3.85	1	1
3	3.86	2	1
4	3.84	1	3
5	3.89	2	3
2 min Postexercise			
1	3.42	0	0
2	3.15	8	9
3	2.90	**15**	**13**
4	2.84	**17**	**18**
5	2.83	**17**	**18**

WHAT WERE THE EMG FINDINGS?

This electrophysiologic test showed mildly decreased SNAPs amplitudes and absent H-reflexes, indicating a neuropathy. All of the CMAPs had decreased amplitudes. There was no significant slowing, temporal dispersion, conduction blocks, or prolonged distal latencies and F-responses to suggest chronic inflammatory demyelinating polyradiculoneuropathy. Lack of denervation or fasciculations on the needle test was against a motor neuron disease. There were no low-amplitude polyphasic motor unit potentials to suggest myositis; there was some evidence of motor unit action potential variability and characteristic of a neuromuscular transmission defect.

WHAT SHOULD ONE DO NEXT?

A repetitive stimulation test of the ulnar nerve showed low-amplitude CMAP with decremental response, at low stimulation rates and marked posttetanic facilitation of over 300%, characteristic of a presynaptic transmission defect such as Lambert–Eaton myasthenic syndrome (LEMS) (Fig. 75-1) in addition to a mild neuropathy.

Calcium channel binding antibodies N-type titer was 77 pmol/L (normal, <20 pmol/L); calcium channel binding antibody P/Q-type was 1402 pmol/L (normal, <20 pmol/L), and striated muscle antibodies were normal.

The patient had a workup for malignancy which revealed an enlarged uterus. On biopsy, this was diagnostic of an endometrial carcinoma, which was removed.

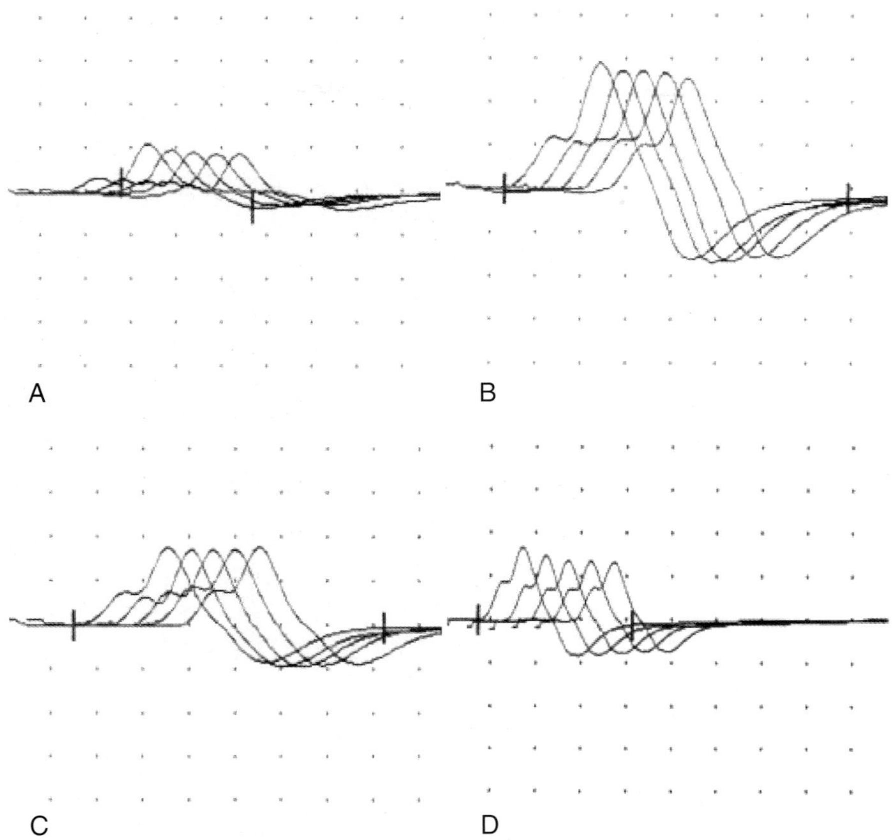

FIG. 75-1 Repetitive stimulation of the ulnar nerve recording at the ADM muscle at 3 Hz; notice low-amplitude CMAP with a decrement (**A**), posttetanic fasciculation (**B**), and return to low-amplitude CMAP with a decrement of 1 (**C**) and 2 (**D**) min after the tetanic contraction (2 mV/5 ms).

She was treated with monthly immunoglobulin infusion and 3,4-diaminopyridine and has remained mildly symptomatic for the last 4 years.

SUMMARY

This elderly woman with a history of an autoimmune thyroiditis, cancer of the breast, and also was found to have endometrial carcinoma of the uterus presented with muscle weakness and diminished reflexes. On EMG, she had low-amplitude CMAPs with marked posttetanic facilitation and had antibodies against the voltage-gated calcium channel (VGCC). Her LEMS could have been related to thyroiditis or the carcinoma.

DISCUSSION (CASES 74 AND 75)

Cases 74 and *75* had LEMS; *Case 74* also had predominantly leg weakness and cancer of the lung.

Case 75 had a remote cancer of the breast and a history of thyroiditis. She was also found to have endometrial cancer, presented mainly with proximal weakness, and had elevated titers of VGCCs typical of LEMS. She had no significant autonomic symptoms or findings. She had stable weakness rather than fatigue or improvement of weakness after physical activities, and her EMG showed some motor unit variability. She also had a mild sensory neuropathy. Her breast cancer was remote, but either the thyroiditis or the uterine cancer could be related to the syndrome. She also had an elevated FANA but no evidence of lupus. This case emphasizes that in patients with low-amplitude CMAP during nerve conduction test, the CMAP should also be measured after tetanic contraction, or, more importantly, the patient should undergo a complete repetitive stimulation test, particularly if the low-amplitude CMAP is not associated with signs of denervation on EMG.

LEMS was initially reported by Lambert, Eaton, and Rooke in 1956.[1] Eaton and Lambert later reviewed the disease in detail in 1957.[2] Prior to this, Anderson and colleagues reported a patient who apparently had myasthenia and cancer of the lung as the antigenic stimulus.[3]

Approximately 60% of patients with LEMS have small cell lung cancer; other malignancies include other carcinomas, such as breast and prostate, and lymphoproliferative disorders. Some patients do not have a malignancy but could have other autoimmune conditions such as vitiligo, pernicious anemia, psoriasis, Addison disease, and thyroiditis. Generally, older patients have the association with carcinoma more often.[4] These two cases emphasize the need for aggressive workup for cancer in patients with LEMS.

In this disease, there is a defective release of acetylcholine from the presynaptic terminal of the neuromuscular junctions and autonomic neurons,[5,6] causing weakness and autonomic dysfunction such as dry mouth and pupillary abnormalities. The IgG antigens in LEMS are known to block the VGCCs, particularly the P/Q-type. Some patients, particularly those with cancer, have antibodies against the N-type VGCCs.[6]

The clinical characteristics include predominantly proximal limb (mainly leg) weakness and fatigability with a temporary increase in strength after voluntary exercise, and depressed or absent reflexes which temporarily increase during repetitive tapping. There is a relatively poor response to anticholinesterase drugs.[4] Other symptoms include slurred speech and dysphagia. Examination could show some droopy eyelids, a weak voice, and pupillary abnormalities. Autonomic dysfunctions occur in 80% of patients.[4] These could include constipation, poor bladder control, and impaired sweating.

Electrophysiologic abnormalities of LEMS were described in the initial report by Lambert et al.[1] and Eaton and Lambert,[2] who demonstrated low-amplitude muscle responses on nerve stimulation, with marked facilitation at fast stimulation rates of 40 Hz.[2] Microelectrode studies revealed normal amplitude but low-frequency miniature endplate potentials (EPPs). There was a greatly reduced and variable amplitude of the EPPs.[7,8] The quantal content of the EPP was reduced, and this increased with the addition of calcium to the preparation and during fast stimulation rates.[8] Later, it was also found that IgG from LEMS patients reduced the quantal content of the EPPs in mice.[9]

Freeze-fracture electromicroscopy studies demonstrated a reduced density of the active zones, particularly of the nerve terminals of the neuromuscular junction; these appeared clustered instead of having their normal appearance in parallel rows.[10] The active zone particles represent VGCCs; the clustering is caused by the antibodies associated with the disease.[10–12] It is of interest that small cell lung carcinoma, which is an ectodermal tumor, has a high concentration of VGCCs. In these cancer cells, the calcium currents are inhibited by LEMS IgG,[13,14] indicating disimmune pathogenesis in which the P/Q VGCC channel is the target antigen. In addition, LEMS patients could have antibodies against synaptotagmin, a calcium-binding protein that plays a role in synaptic vesicle docking and forms a complex with the N-type VGCC.[15,16]

Routine electrodiagnostic findings are characteristic during the repetitive stimulation test.[17–20] This shows low-amplitude CMAPs with decremental responses at low stimulation rates and a pronounced posttetanic facilitation, in which the CMAPs increase to over 100% after a tetanic muscle contraction, and also during fast stimulations. Recently, Oh and collaborators suggested a 60% increment is sufficient for diagnosis.[21] These results are different from those in myasthenia, in which the amplitude of the initial CMAP is normal and there is a decrement at slow stimulation rates and an increased decrement 1–2 minutes after a tetanic contraction. The posttetanic facilitation is of a much smaller degree in myasthenia than in LEMS. During stimulated single-fiber EMG in LEMS, there is increased jitter at low frequencies that disappears during fast-frequency stimulation.[22]

The treatment includes the use of the potassium channel blocker 3,4-diaminopyridine at a dosage of 20–80 mg four times a day. 3,4-Diaminopyridine and 3,4-diaminopyridine phosphate are both beneficial.[23] This increases acetylcholine release and improves muscle strength and autonomic disturbances without serious side effects,[24–27] although seizures can occur with higher doses. Guanidine has been used in the past, but this can cause hepatotoxicity, cardiac arrhythmias, and dermatitis.[28,29] Anticholinesterase drugs produce mild or no improvement, but could add to the effects of 3,4-diaminopyridine.[24] Some use anticholinesterase drugs with 3,4-diaminopyridine or low doses of guanidine.[25] Long-term prednisone therapy has been helpful in individual cases.[30] Plasma exchange[31–34] and intravenous gamma globulin produce clinical improvement[33] with a significant drop in the antibodies.[34] Removal of the tumor can improve symptoms.[35]

IMPORTANT POINTS

- LEMS manifests with proximal leg weakness (more than arm weakness), autonomic dysfunction, areflexia, and normal sensory examination.
- LEMS should be a consideration in patients with low-amplitude CMAPs out of proportion with SNAP amplitudes, particularly if there is a lack of denervation on EMG. In those, the CMAPs should be measured before and after a tetanic contraction, and, in particular, a repetitive stimulation test should be performed.
- LEMS is a presynaptic disorder caused by antibodies against the VGCCs of neuromuscular junctions and autonomic neurons. The disease is associated with cancers, as well as with autoimmune conditions.
- The electrodiagnostic findings in LEMS during a repetitive stimulation test consist of low-amplitude CMAP with a decrement at slow stimulation rates. There is a marked increment during fast stimulation or after a tetanic contraction.
- Needle electromyography shows the variability of motor units without denervation. Stimulated single-fiber EMG shows increased jitter at low-frequency stimulation. This improves at faster rates of stimulation.
- In vitro studies in LEMS show reduced acetylcholine quantal content. The EPP amplitudes and quantal release increase at fast-frequency nerve stimulation. The electrophysiologic abnormalities are caused by antibodies against the P/Q VGCCs.
- LEMS patients should be worked up carefully for a neoplasm.
- The treatment of LEMS includes immunosuppressant therapy and removal of the tumor. 3,4-Diaminopyridine and 3,4-diaminopyridine phosphate produce symptomatic improvement, and weakness improves with removal of the tumor. Anticholinesterase drugs produce only mild benefit; the addition of anticholinesterase drugs is helpful.

REFERENCES

1. Lambert EH, Eaton LM, Rooke ED. Defect of neuromuscular conduction associated with malignant neoplasms. *Am J Physiol.* 1956;187:612–613.
2. Eaton LM, Lambert EH. Electromyography and electrical stimulation of nerves in diseases of the motor unit: observations on myasthenic syndrome associated with malignant tumors. *JAMA*. 1957;163:1117–1124.
3. Anderson HJ, Churchill-Davidson HC, Richardson AT. Bronchial neoplasm with myasthenia: prolonged apnea after administration of succinylcholine. *Lancet*. 1953;2:1291–1293.
4. O'Neill JH, Murray NM, Newsom-Davis J. The Lambert-Eaton myasthenic syndrome: a review of 50 cases. *Brain*. 1988;111: 577–596.
5. Waterman SA, Lang B, Newsom-Davis J. Effect of Lambert-Eaton myasthenic syndrome antibodies on autonomic neurons in the mouse. *Ann Neurol.* 1997;42:147–156.
6. Lennon VA, Kryzer TJ, Griesmann GE, et al. Calcium-channel antibodies in the Lambert-Eaton syndrome and other paraneoplastic syndromes. *N Engl J Med.* 1995;332(22):1467–1474.
7. Elmqvist D, Lambert EH. Detailed analysis of neuromuscular transmission in a patient with the myasthenic syndrome sometimes associated with bronchogenic carcinoma. *Mayo Clin Proc*. 1968;43:689–713.
8. Lambert EH, Elmqvist D. Quantal components of end-plate potentials in the myasthenic syndrome. *Ann NY Acad Sci.* 1971;183:183–199.
9. Lang B, Newsom-Davis J, Peers C, et al. The effect of myasthenic syndrome antibody on presynaptic calcium channels in the mouse. *J Physiol.* 1987;390:257–270.
10. Fukunaga H, Engel A, Osame M, Lambert EH. Paucity and disorganization of presynaptic membrane active zones in the Lambert-Eaton myasthenic syndrome. *Muscle Nerve*. 1982;5: 686–697.
11. Fukunaga H, Engel AG, Lang B, et al. Passive transfer of Lambert-Eaton myasthenic syndrome with IgG from man to mouse depletes the presynaptic membrane active zones. *Proc Natl Acad Sci USA*. 1983;80:7636–7640.
12. Nagel A, Engel AG, Lang B, et al. Lambert-Eaton myasthenic syndrome IgG depletes presynaptic membrane active zone particles by antigenic modulation. *Ann Neurol.* 1988;24:552–558.
13. Roberts A, Perera S, Lang B, et al. Paraneoplastic myasthenic syndrome IgG inhibits 45Ca2+ flux in a human small cell carcinoma line. *Nature*. 1985;317(6039):737–739.
14. Newsom-Davis J. The Lambert-Eaton myasthenic syndrome. In: Engel A, Franzini-Armstrong C, eds. *Myology*. New York, NY: McGraw Hill; 2004:1791–1799.
15. Takamori M, Hamada T, Komai K, et al. Synaptotagmin can cause an immune-mediated model of Lambert-Eaton myasthenic syndrome in rats. *Ann Neurol.* 1994;35:74–80.
16. Takamori M, Iwasa K, Komai K. Antigenic sites of the voltage-gated calcium channel in Lambert-Eaton myasthenic syndrome. *Ann NY Acad Sci.* 1998;841:625–635.
17. Henriksson KG, Nilsson O, Rosen I, Schiller HH. Clinical, neurophysiological and morphological findings in Eaton-Lambert syndrome. *Acta Neurol Scand.* 1977;56:117–140.
18. Jablecki C. Lambert-Eaton myasthenic syndrome. *Muscle Nerve.* 1984;7:250–257.
19. Maselli RA. Electrodiagnosis of disorders of neuromuscular transmission. *Ann NY Acad Sci.* 1998;841:696–711.
20. Keesey JC. AAEM minimonograph 33: electrodiagnostic approach to defects of neuromuscular transmission. *Muscle Nerve.* 1989;12:613–626.
21. Oh SJ, Kurokawa K, Claussen GC, Ryan HF Jr. Electrophysiological diagnostic criteria of Lambert-Eaton myasthenic syndrome. *Muscle Nerve.* 2005;32(4):515–520.
22. Schwartz MS, Stalberg E. Myasthenic syndrome studied with single fiber electromyography. *Arch Neurol.* 1975;32:815–817.
23. Oh SJ. Amifampridine for the treatment of Lambert-Eaton myasthenic syndrome. *Expert Rev Clin Immunol.* 2019;15(10): 991–1007.
24. Lundh H, Nilsson O, Rosen I. Treatment of Lambert-Eaton syndrome: 3,4-diaminopyridine and pyridostigmine. *Neurology.* 1984;34:1324–1330.
25. Oh SJ. Treatment and management of disorders of neuromuscular junction Chapter 19. In: Bertorini TE, ed. *Neuromuscular Disorders: Treatment and Management*. Amsterdam, Netherlands: Elsevier; 2022. 2nd ed.
26. McEvoy KM, Windebank AJ, Daube JR, Low PA. 3,4-Diaminopyridine in the treatment of Lambert-Eaton myasthenic syndrome. *N Engl J Med.* 1989;321:1567–1571.
27. Sanders DB. 3,4-Diaminopyridine (DAP) in the treatment of Lambert-Eaton myasthenic syndrome (LEMS). *Ann NY Acad Sci.* 1998;841:811–816.
28. Oh SJ, Kim KW. Guanidine hydrochloride in the Eaton-Lambert syndrome: electrophysiologic improvement. *Neurology.* 1973;23:1084–1090.
29. Cherington M. Guanidine and germine in Eaton-Lambert syndrome. *Neurology*. 1976;26:944–946.
30. Streib EW, Rothner DA. Eaton-Lambert myasthenic syndrome: long-term treatment of three patients with prednisone. *Ann Neurol.* 1981;10:448–453.
31. Dau PC, Denys EH. Plasmapheresis and immunosuppressive drug therapy in the Eaton-Lambert syndrome. *Ann Neurol.* 1982;11: 570–575.
32. Newsom-Davis J, Murray NM. Plasma exchange and immunosuppressive drug treatment in the Lambert-Eaton myasthenic syndrome. *Neurology*. 1984;34:480–485.
33. Bird SJ. Clinical and electrophysiologic improvement in Lambert-Eaton syndrome with intravenous immunoglobulin therapy. *Neurology*. 1992;42:1422–1423.
34. Bain PG, Motomura M, Newsom-Davis J, et al. Effects of intravenous immunoglobulin on muscle weakness and calcium-channel autoantibodies in the Lambert-Eaton myasthenic syndrome. *Neurology*. 1996;47:678–683.
35. Sanders DB. Lambert-Eaton myasthenic syndrome: diagnosis and treatment. *Ann NY Acad Sci.* 2003;998:500–508.

76 CASE

An Elderly Woman With Ptosis, Areflexia, and Weakness

A 55-year-old nonsmoker African American woman presented with a 2-week history of severe bilateral arm and leg weakness, along with a 4-month history of ptosis and double vision (Fig. 76-1). These symptoms were aggravated by activity. She also had constipation and dry mouth.

On examination, she showed severe bilateral ptosis and ophthalmoplegia (Fig. 76-1). Pupils were equal and reactive to light. The patient showed generalized weakness, more proximal than distal, along with areflexia that did not improve on repetitive tapping. Sensory exam was unremarkable and an edrophonium test was positive.

WHAT IS THE DIFFERENTIAL DIAGNOSIS?

This patient has many features that are suggestive of myasthenia gravis (MG),[1,2] including ptosis and ophthalmoplegia with recent onset, and the positive response to the edrophonium. The dry mouth and constipation are somewhat unusual, but she could also have Sjögren syndrome. Botulism may present like this, but this patient did not have pupillary involvement.

Another possibility is that this patient has Lambert–Eaton myasthenic syndrome (LEMS), but prominent ptosis is unusual in this condition.[3,4]

WHAT DO YOU DO NEXT?

Lab analysis showed negative AChR, MuSK, and VGCC antibodies. CT of the chest showed no evidence of neoplasm or thymus enlargement.

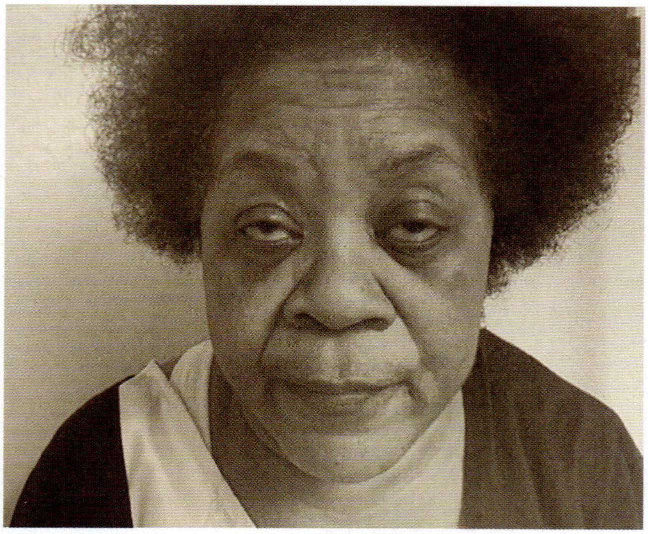

FIG. 76-1 Showing patient having bilateral ptosis.

The patient underwent repetitive stimulation test and nerve conduction studies showing: left ulnar amplitude—4.30 mV pre and 9.10 mV on tetanic contraction, right median amplitude—6.90 mV pre and 11.00 mV on tetanic contraction. Initial decremental response of 67.3% was observed in the right abductor digiti-quinti muscle at 3 Hz stimulation. Immediately after 15 seconds of tetanic contraction, there was a 106% incremental response (Fig. 76-2). Nerve conduction studies were normal showing no evidence of peripheral neuropathy, and needle EMG showed no denervation and scattered small polyphasic motor unit action potentials with mild variability.

WHAT TO DO NEXT?

Antibodies against VGCC and antibodies against LRP4 agrin were also negative.

WHAT IS THE MOST LIKELY DIAGNOSIS?

This patient has features of MG of which a small percentage of cases are antibody-negative.[1] The significant posttetanic facilitation and somewhat small CMAP are features of Lambert-Eaton myasthenic syndrome (LEMS) in which the facilitation is usually over 60%,[5] so it appears that she had features of a presynaptic disorder such as Lambert-Eaton and MG. This has also been called MG–Lambert-Eaton overlap syndrome (MLOS).[6] It is interesting that this patient did not show antibodies characteristic of either of these disorders.

WHAT TO DO NEXT?

This patient was treated with pyridostigmine 60 mg four times a day, IVIG, and later tapering doses of steroids. The IVIG was later discontinued. She was switched to azathioprine as a steroid-sparing agent.

DISCUSSION

A 55-year-old female who developed ophthalmoplegia and ptosis had generalized weakness with areflexia. She had characteristic findings of myasthenia, because of severe ophthalmoplegia with ptosis, a positive response to edrophonium testing, and the decremental response on repetitive stimulation testing. She also has features of LEMS, because of profound weakness, constipation, dry mouth, and areflexia, and a significant, over 60%, incremental response on posttetanic contraction.[5]

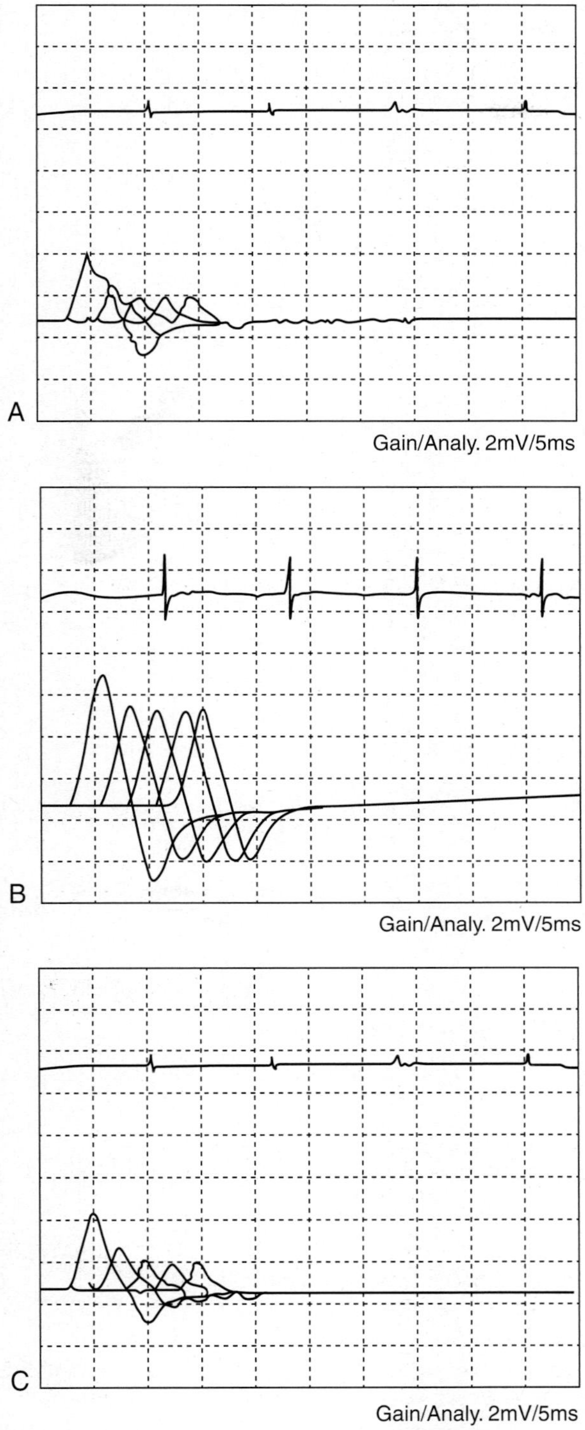

FIG. 76-2 Repetitive stimulation test of the right ulnar nerve recording at the adductor digiti-quinti muscle. **A**, Baseline 3 Hz stimulation; **B**, repetitive stimulation after 15 s of tetanic contraction; and **C**, 2 min after tetanic contraction (2 mV/5 ms).

She tested negative for acetylcholine-receptive MuSK and VGCC antibodies. Furthermore, antibodies against agrin and LRP4[7,8] were also negative, so she is a patient without antibodies associated with MG or LEMS. The patient was treated aggressively with immunotherapy and remained asymptomatic. Up to date, there are only two patients with MLOS with MG, Lambert–Eaton overlap syndrome, who have been tested for all three antibodies, one patient has positive MuSK and VGCC, and one patient tested negative for all three. This case will be the second case in which tests were negative for all three antibodies, and the first patient with MLOS also tested negative for LRP4 and agrin.[7,8]

It is unclear why the antibodies tested were negative; it could be that the antibody test used was not sensitive enough, or perhaps there are additional antibodies that affect neuromuscular transmission which were not studied at this time. Recently, antibodies against Cortactin and Dok 7 subgroup have been reported. These are postsynaptic proteins involving AChR clustering along with LRP4 and agrin.[9] Antibodies against these components should be added to the list of those studies in patients with double-negative MG. Additional antibodies against clustering AChR have also been reported in 38.1% of patients who were double-seronegative.[10]

IMPORTANT POINTS

- There are rare cases with features of MG and Lambert-Eaton syndrome, thus MG/ Lambert-Eaton overlap syndrome (MLOS) that have no detectable antibodies.
- Posttetanic facilitation of more than 60% is characteristic of MLOS.
- Patients with MLOS respond well to immunotherapy.
- The presence of prominent increased posttetanic facilitation and decremental response is characteristic of MLOS.

This case was reported in Maturana MA, Bertorini TE, Mei L, et al. J Clin Neuromuscul Dis. 2019;21(2):103–106.

REFERENCES

1. Engel AG, Hohlfield R. Acquired autoimmune myasthenia gravis. In: Engel AG, Franzini-Armstrong C, eds. *Myology*. 3rd ed. New York, NY: McGraw Hill; 2004:1775–1790.
2. Sanders DB, El-Salem K, Massey JM, et al. Clinical aspects of MuSK positive and negative myasthenia gravis. *Neurology*. 2005; 64:536–538.
3. Ciafloni E, Massey JM. Repetitive stimulation tests Chapter 9. In: Bertorini T, ed. *Neuromuscular Disorders*. Boston, MA: Butterworth-Heinemann; 2009:290–291.
4. Merino-Ramirez MA, Bolton CF. Review of the diagnostic challenges of Lambert-Eaton syndrome revealed through three case reports. *Can J Neurol Sci*. 2016;43:1–13.
5. Oh SJ, Kurokawa K, Claussen GC, et al. Electrophysiological diagnostic criteria of Lambert-Eaton myasthenic syndrome. *Muscle Nerve*. 2005;32:515–520.
6. Oh SJ. Myasthenia gravis Lambert-Eaton overlap syndrome. *Muscle Nerve*. 2016;53:20–26.
7. Zhang B, Shen C, Bealmear B, et al. Autoantibodies to agrin in myasthenia gravis patients. *PLoS One*. 2014;9:e91816.

8. Zhang B, Tzartos JS, Bealimezi M, et al. Autoantibodies to lipoprotein-related protein 4 in patients with double-seronegative myasthenia gravis. *Arch Neurol.* 2012;69:445–451.
9. Cortés-Vicente E, Gallardo E, Martínez MA, et al. Clinical characteristics of patients with double-seronegative myasthenia gravis and antibodies to cortactin. *JAMA Neurol.* 2016;73:1099–1104.
10. Rodriguez Cruz PM, Al-Hajjar M, Huda S, et al. Clinical features and diagnostic usefulness of antibodies for clustered acetylcholine receptors in the diagnosis of seronegative myasthenia gravis. *JAMA Neurol.* 2015;72:642–649.

CASE 77

A Young Woman With Distal Upper Extremity Weakness

A 22-year-old woman presented with an 8-year history of progressive muscle weakness and fatigue, particularly in the hand muscles after physical activities; this became severe over the past year. Her estranged father had an ill-defined muscle weakness during his youth that improved with time.

Serum creatine kinase (CK), antinuclear antibodies, thyroid studies, and blood chemistries were normal.

Examination revealed normal cranial nerves without evidence of ptosis, ophthalmoplegia, or eyelid fatigue. There was mild proximal muscle and finger extensor weakness with fatigue on repetitive testing. Reflexes were symmetric 1–2+, and plantar reflexes were flexor. There was no evidence of myotonia or fasciculations. Sensory examination and coordination were normal and symmetrical.

WHAT IS THE DIFFERENTIAL DIAGNOSIS?

Multiple disorders can cause hand weakness. This is accompanied by pain or sensory deficits in cervical spinal canal disease, such as spondylosis, intramedullary tumors, and syringomyelia. *Multifocal motor neuropathy* frequently starts in the upper extremities but is often associated with fasciculations; the patient also has a characteristic EMG and conduction block in motor nerve conduction tests.

Distal autoimmune myasthenia gravis is a likely possibility in this patient. Although myasthenia gravis usually presents with ptosis and extraocular and proximal muscle weakness, some patients could manifest with distal weakness.[1] They have the characteristic decremental response on a repetitive nerve stimulation test, and usually have elevated acetylcholine antibody titers or muscle-specific protein kinase (MuSK) antibodies.

Slow-channel myasthenic syndrome (SCMS) is a hereditary, postsynaptic disease of neuromuscular transmission that manifests in weakness of the finger extensors with mild extraocular muscle weakness and ptosis. An afterresponse or afterdischarge is seen after the initial compound muscle action potential during routine motor nerve conduction studies and during the repetitive stimulation test, and there is also a decrement of the CMAP amplitude during this test. Acetylcholine receptor and MuSK antibodies are negative. Edrophonium test may show mild improvement. These patients usually have DNA mutations of the acetylcholine receptor subunit gene.[2–4]

SCMS can present in adolescence or later in life, whereas most other congenital or hereditary myasthenic syndromes usually start in infancy (Table 77-1). (Table 77-2 lists the differential diagnosis of the congenital myasthenic syndromes.) SCMS has an autosomal-dominant inheritance, but there is not always a positive family history. A hereditary condition was possible in this patient due to her father's transient childhood weakness, and thus SCMS should be included in the differential diagnosis.

Distal muscular dystrophy, particularly the Welander type, is an autosomal-dominant disease that is slowly progressive and not fluctuating. Patients do not have a positive edrophonium test or a decremental response on repetitive stimulation testing. The serum CK is mildly elevated, and muscle biopsy shows characteristic dystrophic changes and rimmed vacuoles.[5–9]

Myotonic dystrophy can manifest with ptosis and distal extremity weakness; patients also have facial or neck flexor weakness with myotonia demonstrated clinically or by EMG.[10]

Adult onset debranching enzyme deficiency is an autosomal-recessive glycogen storage disease that manifests with distal weakness, but patients usually also have an elevated serum CK and characteristic muscle biopsy showing glycogen accumulation.[11]

Sporadic inclusion body myositis starts in mid-life or later. Patients have predominantly distal lower extremity and upper extremity weakness with prominent quadriceps weakness, elevated serum CK, and a characteristic muscle biopsy demonstrating rimmed vacuoles and inclusion bodies.[12] *Familial inclusion body myopathy* also shows distal muscle weakness presenting in younger persons but is predominantly in the lower extremities, sparing the quadriceps muscles.[13]

Myofibrillar myopathies are in a heterogeneous group that manifests with distal upper extremity weakness or cardiomyopathy. The serum CK is mildly elevated, and muscle biopsies show characteristic hyaline cytoplasmic inclusions with desmin accumulation.[14–17]

Nephrotic calcinosis is an autosomal-recessive lysosomal storage myopathy that produces distal hand weakness and renal failure. The biopsy shows a vacuolar myopathy.[18]

Oculopharyngodistal myopathy is characterized by oculopharyngeal and distal upper extremity and lower extremity weakness.[19]

TABLE 77-1 Classification of Congenital Myasthenic Syndromes

Presynaptic Conditions
Congenital caused by choline acetyltransferase (ChAT) deficiency (also referred to as congenital myasthenic syndrome associated with episodic apnea)
Congenital myasthenia with paucity of synaptic vesicles
Congenital myasthenia with quantal release deficiency
Episodic ataxia with myasthenic weakness
Postsynaptic Conditions
Synthetic defect, AChendplate deficiency
Slow-channel congenital myasthenic syndrome
Fast-channel congenital myasthenic syndrome
Receptor deficiency due to mutations in acetylcholine receptor genes
Receptor deficiency due to mutations in rapsyn
MuSK deficiency
DOK7 (limb-girdle weakness)
Plectin deficiency
DOK deficiency
Glycosylation deficiency (limb-girdle weakness)

MuSK, Muscle-specific protein kinase.
Reprinted from Oh S. Treatment and management of disorders of neuromuscular junction. In: Bertorni TE, ed. *Neuromuscular Disorders: Treatment and Management*. Amsterdam, Netherlands: Elsevier; 2022:477. Chapter 19.

TABLE 77-2 Differential Diagnosis of Congenital Myasthenic Syndromes

Neonatal Period, Infancy, Childhood
Spinal muscular atrophy
Congenital myopathies (central core disease, nemaline myopathy, myotubular myopathy)
Congenital muscular dystrophies
Infantile myotonic dystrophy
Mitochondrial myopathy
Brainstem anomaly
Möbius syndrome
Infantile botulism
Seropositive and seronegative autoimmune myasthenia gravis[a]
Older Patients
Motor neuron disease
Radial nerve palsy[b]
Peripheral neuropathy[b]
Limb-girdle or facioscapulohumeral muscular dystrophy
Mitochondrial myopathy
Chronic fatigue syndrome
Seropositive and seronegative autoimmune myasthenia gravis

[a]Not reported in the first year of life.
[b]This diagnosis has been made in some cases of the slow-channel congenital myasthenic syndromes.
Reprinted with permission from Engel A. Congenital myasthenic syndromes. In: Katirji B, Kaminski H, Preston D, et al., eds. *Neuromuscular Disorders in Clinical Practice*. Boston, MA: Butterworth-Heimemann; 2002:955.

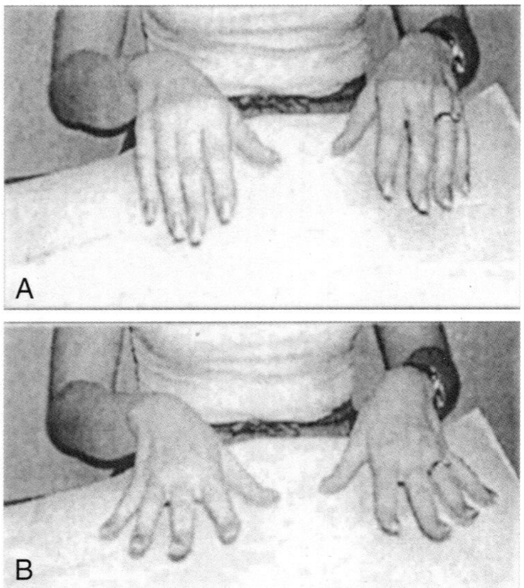

FIG. 77-1 **A**, Notice the patient's weakness of the finger extensors. **B**, The patient's weakness improved with edrophonium.

BASED ON THESE POSSIBILITIES, WHAT TESTS SHOULD BE DONE?

The patient's acetylcholine receptor antibodies were normal. MuSK antibodies were not tested. FANA, thyroid function tests, and serum chemistry profile were normal.

Edrophonium test produced mild improvement of the finger extensor weakness (Fig. 77-1).

AN EMG TEST WAS PERFORMED

Motor Nerve Studies

Nerve and Site	Latency (ms)	Amplitude (mV)	Conduction Velocity (m/s)
Median Nerve L.	**Normal ≤ 4.2**	**Normal ≥ 6**	**Normal ≥ 50**
Wrist	3.3	10	–
Elbow	7.1	9	57
Ulnar Nerve L.	**Normal ≤ 3.6**	**Normal ≥ 8**	**Normal ≥ 50**
Wrist	3.2	**6**	–
Below elbow	6.4	**6**	58

F-Wave Studies

Nerve	Latency (ms)	Normal Latency ≤ (ms)
Median nerve L.	27.3	30
Ulnar nerve L.	27.8	30

Sensory Nerve Studies

Nerve	Onset Latency (ms)	Normal Onset Latency ≤ (ms)	Peak Latency (ms)	Normal Peak Latency ≤ (ms)	Amp (μV)	Normal Amp ≥ (μV)	Conduction Velocity (m/s)	Normal Conduction Velocity ≥ (m/s)
Median nerve L.	2.2	2.6	2.7	3.1	38	20	59	50
Ulnar nerve L.	2.2	2.6	2.7	3.1	29	13	55	50

Repetitive Stimulation of Ulnar Nerve L.

Potential Number	Amp (mV)	Amp Decrement (%)	Area Decrement (%)
Before Exercise			
1	6.24	0	0
2	6.19	4	3
3	6.17	6	9
4	6.17	6	9
5	6.17	6	9
Posttetanic			
1	6.05	0	0
2	6.02	1	0
3	5.65	2	4
4	5.65	2	6
5	5.67	2	7
1 min Postexercise			
1	6.36	0	0
2	5.99	5	2
3	5.70	9	5
4	5.70	9	7
5	5.69	9	7
2 min Postexercise			
1	6.60	0	0
2	6.24	4	2
3	6.09	6	3
4	6.02	5	5
5	6.01	5	5

Repetitive Stimulation of Accessory Nerve L.

Potential Number	Amp (mV)	Amp Decrement (%)	Area Decrement (%)
Before Exercise			
1	15.96	0	0
2	15.65	4	0
3	15.51	6	5
4	14.45	7	7
5	15.39	8	9
Posttetanic			
1	15.55	0	0
2	15.41	6	2
3	15.39	6	4
4	15.33	7	6
5	15.31	7	6

Repetitive Stimulation of Accessory Nerve L.—cont'd

Potential Number	Amp (mV)	Amp Decrement (%)	Area Decrement (%)
1 min Postexercise			
1	15.36	0	0
2	14.99	5	4
3	14.73	9	7
4	14.71	9	9
5	14.70	9	9
2 min Postexercise			
1	15.55	0	0
2	15.18	5	3
3	15.17	5	5
4	14.91	9	8
5	14.89	9	8

Repetitive Stimulation of Facial Nerve L.

Potential Number	Amp (mV)	Amp Decrement (%)	Area Decrement (%)
Before Exercise			
1	15.45	0	0
2	15.06	6	5
3	14.83	**10**	**10**
4	14.76	**11**	**12**
5	14.76	**11**	**12**
Posttetanic			
1	15.50	0	0
2	15.50	0	0
3	15.44	5	6
4	15.44	5	7
5	15.42	5	7
1 min Postexercise			
1	15.44	0	0
2	15.05	6	7
3	14.85	**11**	**11**
4	14.83	**11**	**15**
5	14.83	**11**	**15**
2 min Postexercise			
1	15.33	0	0
2	14.94	6	7
3	14.71	**10**	9
4	14.69	**11**	**11**
5	14.69	**11**	**11**

EMG Data

Muscle	Insrt Activity	Fibs	Pos Waves	Fasc	Amp	Dur	Poly	Pattern
Cervical paraspinals L.	Norm	None	None	None	Norm	Norm	None	Full
Deltoid L.	Norm	None	None	None	**Variable**	**Brief**	**Few**	Full
Biceps brachii L.	Norm	None	None	None	**Variable**	**Brief**	**Few**	Full
Triceps L.	Norm	None	None	None	Norm	Norm	None	Full
Extensor digitorum com. L.	Norm	None	None	None	**Variable**	Norm	None	Full
Flexor carpi radialis L.	Norm	None	None	None	Norm	Norm	None	Full
Flexor carpi ulnaris L.	Norm	None	None	None	Norm	Norm	None	Full
First dorsal interosseous L.	Norm	None	None	None	Norm	Norm	None	Full

What Were the EMG Findings?

This test showed normal nerve conduction results, except for mildly decreased CMAP amplitude upon ulnar nerve stimulation, with a mild decremental response of the CMAP area (12%) and 15% 1 minute after tetanic contraction, and amplitude upon repetitive stimulation of the facial nerve at 3 Hz, but not after stimulating other nerves. There were small polyphasic motor unit action potentials in proximal arm muscles.

The normal CK, the decremental response with the repetitive stimulation tests, and mild improvement with edrophonium were all against a diagnosis of primary myopathy. Her EMG not only showed small motor units as can be seen in myopathies and disorders of neuromuscular transmission, but there was also motor unit variability, as seen in the latter. The lack of myotonia was against myotonic dystrophy.

The patient was diagnosed with probable distal autoimmune myasthenia gravis that was antibody negative. The absence of repetitive response of the initial CMAP was against the diagnosis of SCMS. A chest CT scan was normal.

She was treated with pyridostigmine up to 90 mg four times a day with mild improvement. Later corticosteroids were added but without benefit.

A SECOND EMG TEST WAS PERFORMED

Motor Nerve Studies

Nerve and Site	Latency (ms)	Amplitude (mV)	Conduction Velocity (m/s)
Median Nerve L.	**Normal ≤ 4.2**	**Normal ≥ 6**	**Normal ≥ 50**
Wrist	3.4	9	–
Elbow	8.0	9	54

Nerve and Site	Latency (ms)	Amplitude (mV)	Conduction Velocity (m/s)
Ulnar Nerve L.	**Normal ≤ 3.6**	**Normal ≥ 8**	**Normal ≥ 50**
Wrist	3.4	8	–
Below elbow	6.4	8	56

F-Wave Studies

Nerve	Latency (ms)	Normal Latency ≤ (ms)
Median nerve L.	27.2	30
Ulnar nerve L.	26.6	30

Repetitive Stimulation of Ulnar Nerve L.

Potential Number	Amp (mV)	Amp Decrement (%)	Area Decrement (%)
Before Exercise			
1	7.39	0	0
2	7.35	1	**10**
3	7.29	1	**14**
4	7.10	3	**14**
5	7.10	3	**13**
Posttetanic			
1	8.01	0	0
2	7.99	1	**10**
3	7.98	1	**11**
4	7.98	1	**10**
5	7.92	2	**10**

Repetitive Stimulation of Ulnar Nerve L.—cont'd

Potential Number	Amp (mV)	Amp Decrement (%)	Area Decrement (%)
1 min Postexercise			
1	6.45	0	0
2	6.06	6	**15**
3	5.83	**10**	**20**
4	5.76	**11**	**22**
5	5.76	**11**	**22**
2 min Postexercise			
1	6.97	0	0
2	6.49	7	**15**
3	6.18	**12**	**19**
4	6.23	**12**	**19**
5	6.19	**12**	**18**

Repetitive Stimulation of Accessory Nerve L.

Potential Number	Amp (mV)	Amp Decrement (%)	Area Decrement (%)
Before Exercise			
1	17.18	0	0
2	17.00	1	3
3	16.67	2	4
4	16.65	2	**11**
5	16.60	2	**12**
Posttetanic			
1	16.62	0	0
2	16.58	4	1
3	16.51	5	4
4	16.35	5	5
5	15.78	5	5
1 min Postexercise			
1	16.84	0	0
2	16.54	5	0
3	16.48	5	8
4	16.47	5	**10**
5	15.70	7	**11**

Repetitive Stimulation of Accessory Nerve L.—cont'd

Potential Number	Amp (mV)	Amp Decrement (%)	Area Decrement (%)
2 min Postexercise			
1	16.77	0	0
2	16.57	4	6
3	16.41	3	7
4	16.28	2	**12**
5	16.00	5	**12**
3 min Postexercise			
1	17.07	0	0
2	16.84	9	0
3	16.62	6	9
4	16.47	7	**11**
5	15.52	**10**	**11**

EMG Data

Muscle	Insrt Activity	Fibs	Pos Waves	Fasc	Amp	Dur	Poly	Pattern
Deltoid L.	Norm	None	None	None	**Variable**	**Brief**	**Few**	Full
First dorsal interosseous L.	Norm	None	None	None	**Variable**	Norm	None	Full
Vastus lateralis L.	Norm	None	None	None	**Variable**	Norm	None	Full

What did the second EMG test show?

This EMG also showed normal nerve conduction tests and a decremental response of the CMAP during repetitive stimulation of the ulnar (Fig. 77-2) and spinal accessory nerves, characteristic of a neuromuscular transmission disorder. There were small polyphasic motor unit action potentials with a variation of amplitude.

The patient's treatment for myasthenia gravis was continued. Neither plasma exchange nor IgG was beneficial, and she had increased weakness and developed mild ptosis.

WHAT SHOULD BE DONE NEXT?

She underwent a third repetitive nerve stimulation test at 3 Hz recording in the trapezius, the abductor pollicis brevis (APB), extensor digitorum brevis, abductor digiti minimi, and anconeus muscle, stimulating their respective motor nerves (Fig. 77-3).

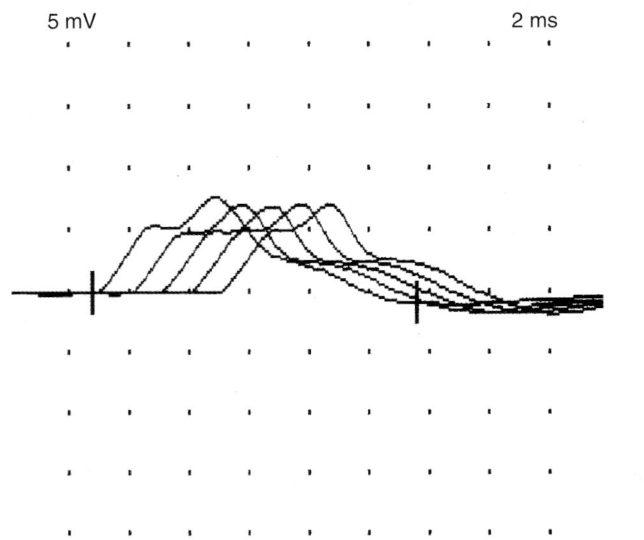

FIG. 77-2 Decrement response of the CMAP during repetitive stimulation of the ulnar nerve while recording at the ADM muscle at 3 Hz. *ADM*, Abductor digiti minimi.

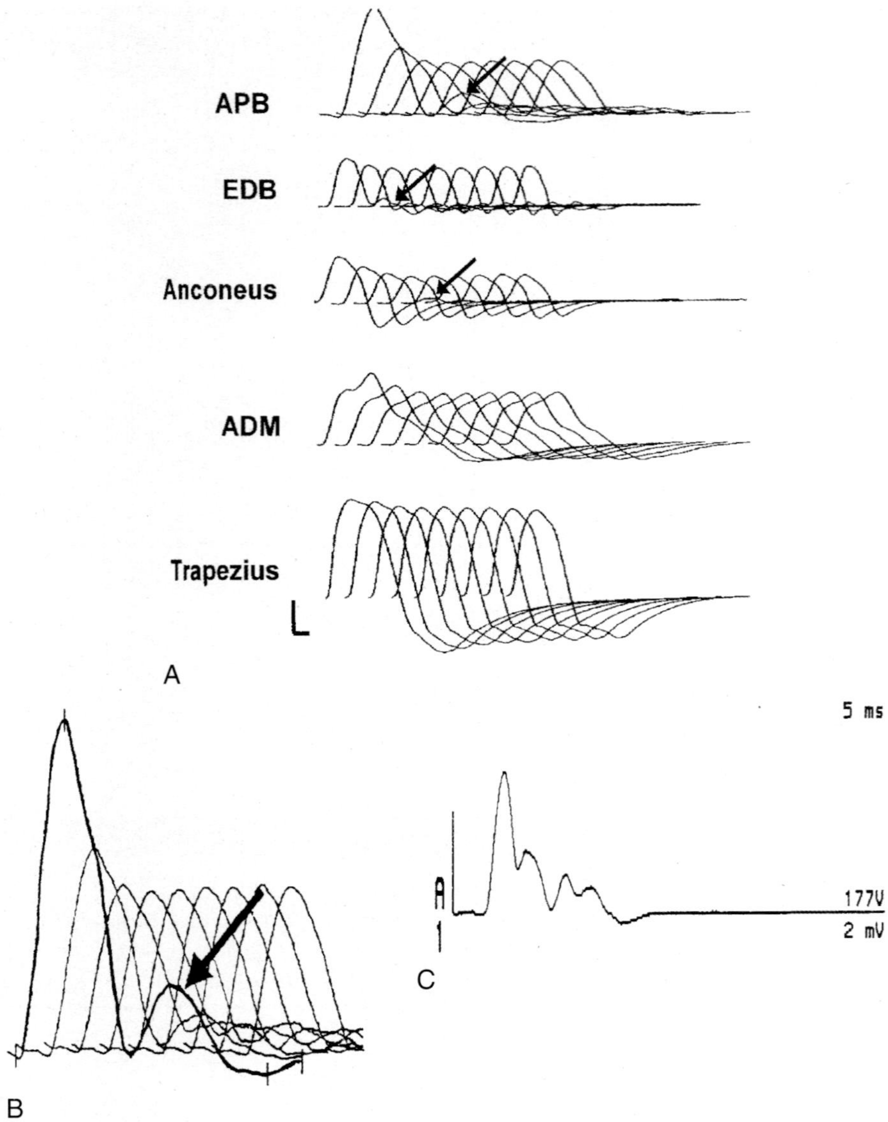

FIG. 77-3 A, Repetitive stimulation test at 3 Hz (5 mV/2 ms). Notice an afterdischarge when stimulating the median nerve and recording at the APB muscle (*arrow*). A second repetitive response is seen in the extensor digitorum brevis muscle stimulating the peroneal nerve (*arrow*) and a very small afterdischarge in the anconeus muscle when stimulating the radial nerve (*arrow*). There is no evidence of an afterdischarge in the ADM muscle when stimulating the ulnar nerve or in the trapezius muscle when stimulating the spinal accessory nerve. **B**, CMAP of the APB muscle when stimulating the median nerve at 3 Hz; notice the afterdischarge (*arrow*) (2 mV/2 ms). **C**, several afterdischarges are seen in the extensor digitorum communis muscle when stimulating the radial nerve (2 mV/5 ms). *ADM*, Abductor digiti minimi; *APB*, abductor pollicis brevis.

A THIRD EMG TEST WAS PERFORMED

Motor Nerve Studies

Nerve and Site	Latency (ms)	Amplitude (mV)	Conduction Velocity (m/s)
Ulnar Nerve L.	Normal ≤ 3.6	Normal ≥ 8	Normal ≥ 50
Wrist	3.2	8	–
Elbow	7.9	8	58

Repetitive Stimulation

Potential Number	Amp (mV)	Amp Decrement (%)	Area Decrement (%)
Median Nerve L.			
1	9.32	0	0
2	6.53	**30**	**25**
3	5.41	**42**	**34**
4	4.76	**49**	**41**
5	4.48	**52**	**48**

Repetitive Stimulation

Potential Number	Amp (mV)	Amp Decrement (%)	Area Decrement (%)
Peroneal Nerve L.			
1	8.05	0	0
2	6.82	**15**	**11**
3	6.82	**15**	**15**
4	6.44	**20**	**18**
5	6.44	**20**	**20**
Ulnar Nerve L.			
1	6.70	0	
2	5.70	**15**	**12**
3	5.30	**21**	**18**
4	5.03	**25**	**23**
5	4.76	**29**	**29**

Repetitive Stimulation—cont'd

Potential Number	Amp (mV)	Amp Decrement (%)	Area Decrement (%)
Radial Nerve L.			
1	12.18	0	0
2	9.99	**18**	**21**
3	8.29	**32**	**28**
4	7.19	**41**	**40**
5	6.70	**45**	**44**
Accessory Nerve L.			
1	9.21	0	0
2	8.20	**11**	**10**
3	8.20	**11**	**13**
4	8.02	**13**	**13**
5	7.83	**15**	**15**

What did the third EMG test show?

This test showed a significant decremental response of the CMAPs. There was no clear second afterdischarge during the ulnar or the spinal accessory nerve stimulations. However, a second hidden response and a marked decrement were obtained by stimulating the median nerve when recording at the APB muscle and when stimulating the radial nerve and recording at the anconeus muscle (see Fig. 77-3A and B). A single stimulus of the radial nerve while recording at the extensor digitorum communis muscle revealed multiple responses of the CMAP (see Fig. 77-3C).

Because of this, molecular genetic analysis was done at the Mayo Clinic for slow-channel syndrome. This demonstrated a mutation in which serine was substituted for glycine at codon 153 of the alpha subunit of the acetylcholine receptor gene.

The patient was treated with quinidine sulfate 200 mg four times a day, producing significant improvement.

DISCUSSION

This patient presented with distal upper extremity weakness and later developed ptosis. She was initially diagnosed as having antibody-negative distal myasthenia gravis due to her positive edrophonium test and the decremental response on repetitive stimulation test, and because she had no clear positive family history. Although her father's history of childhood weakness that improved later was suspicious of a hereditary disease, his exact diagnosis was never made. She did not have afterdischarges of the CMAP on the initial repetitive nerve stimulation to suggest she had SCMS.

She did not show significant improvement with anticholinesterase drugs or corticosteroids.

During reevaluation there were second wave or repetitive afterdischarges after the initial CMAP when stimulating the median and radial nerves; this was characteristic of SCMS. The diagnosis was confirmed by molecular diagnostic tests.

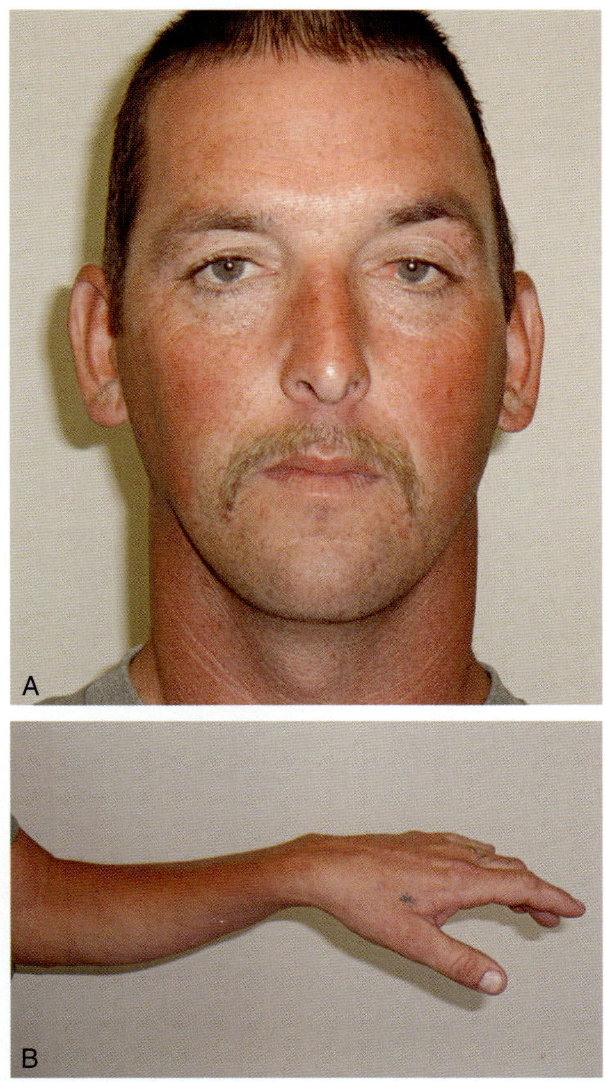

FIG. 77-4 Another patient with SCMS. **A**, Notice mild ptosis. **B**, There is also limitation of wrist extension and particularly finger extension. *SCMS*, Slow-channel myasthenic syndrome.

This case emphasizes that SCMS should be considered in patients with finger extensor weakness. The initial CMAP should be studied for the characteristic CMAP afterdischarges during single-nerve stimulation and during repetitive stimulation testing, and, if the syndrome is suspected, nonconventional nerves, such as radial and median nerves, should be studied to demonstrate these discharges, particularly in weak muscles. The CMAP afterdischarges are characteristic of slow-channel syndrome but can also be seen in congenital endplate cholinesterase deficiency, anticholinesterase overmedication, and organophosphate poisoning. When the diagnosis of SCMS is considered, molecular diagnostic tests should be done.

The SCMS was initially described by Engel and coworkers in 1982[2] as an autosomal-dominant disease characterized by weakness of the finger extensors (Fig. 77-4) and also extraocular muscles with mild ptosis and scapular and cervical muscle weakness. Generalized weakness and even respiratory failure can also occur. The weakness may improve for months or even years without an apparent cause. We recently saw a 20-year-old man who presented previously with undiagnosed weakness as a child and did well without treatment and even played football in school. He came with respiratory failure and weakness. He had characteristic EMG findings and had the DNA mutation and responded well to 60 mg of fluoxetine a day.

Muscle biopsy shows type I muscle fiber predominance with variations in fiber size and internalized nuclei; there are also tubular aggregates. Abnormal accumulation of calcium is seen at the endplates with normal cholinesterase staining. On electromicroscopy, there is disruption of the junctional folds with pinocytotic vesicles and abnormal membranous network. In severe cases, there is degeneration of the junctional folds.[4]

The syndrome is caused by mutations of the genes of the acetylcholine receptor subunit. Over 20 mutations have been reported.[4,20–22] These genetic defects produce an increased affinity of acetylcholine to its receptor with an increased prolonged opening of the receptor channel, and an excessive entrance of cations, causing a prolonged depolarization of the endplate and a prolongation of the decay phase of the miniature endplate potentials (Fig. 77-5), miniature endplate currents, and endplate potentials. The excessive calcium ingress causes a deleterious effect of muscle proteins with degeneration of the junctional folds.[4] The afterdischarge that occurs after the main CMAP is the electrodiagnostic consequence of these abnormalities,[4] and a decrement is observed during repetitive nerve stimulation. As in this case, the second response can be hidden or partially buried within the CMAP or not obvious in some muscles.

Anticholinesterase drugs are usually of no benefit or provide only mild temporary improvement in this disease. Quinidine, a blocker of the sodium channel that is also an acetylcholine receptor blocker[23] contraindicated in autoimmune myasthenia, produces clinical improvement.[24] Another acetylcholine receptor blocker, the antidepressant fluoxetine, is also helpful at high doses[25] and can produce long-term beneficial effects.[26,27]

SUMMARY

This patient presented with distal upper extremity weakness, developed mild ptosis, and had some improvement with anticholinesterase drugs but not with immunosuppressants. She had

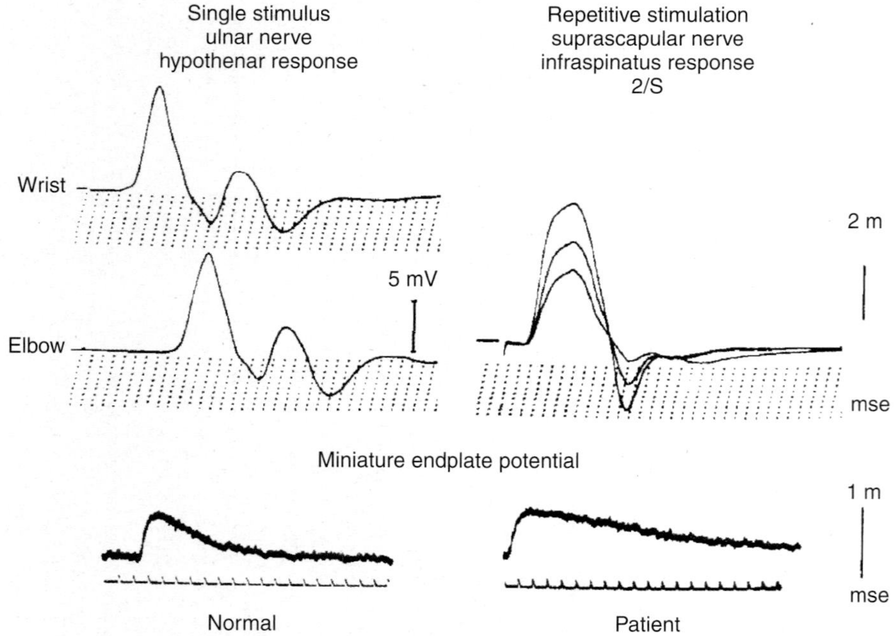

FIG. 77-5 Stimulus-linked CMAP in hypothenar muscles (*upper left*); decremental response of the infraspinatus muscle CMAP during 2 Hz stimulation of suprascapular nerve (*upper right*); duration of decay time of the miniature endplate potential is longer in patient (*lower right*) than in normal control (*lower left*). Reproduced with permission from Engel AG, Lambert EH, Mulder DM, et al. A newly recognized congenital myasthenic syndrome attributed to a prolonged open time of the acetylcholine-induced ion channel. *Ann Neurol.* 1982;11:553–569.

nondetectable receptor antibodies. She was initially assumed to have seronegative distal autoimmune myasthenia but was later proved to have congenital SCMS.

This case is particularly interesting because the characteristic afterdischarges were not obvious during initial routine nerve stimulation tests but were demonstrated when less frequently used nerves were studied.

She responded to quinidine, a drug contraindicated in autoimmune myasthenia gravis.

IMPORTANT POINTS

- Distal upper extremity weakness could be caused by a variety of neuromuscular disorders. Among them is congenital SCMS.
- The syndrome is caused by mutations of the acetylcholine receptor subunits which cause an increased affinity of acetylcholine to its receptor and prolonged opening of the receptor-producing prolonged endplate and miniature endplate potentials. The prolonged depolarization is manifested during nerve stimulations, showing a decrement of the CMAP during repetitive stimulation with afterdischarges of the CMAP.
- The afterdischarges can also be seen in congenital cholinesterase deficiency, anticholinesterase overmedication, and organophosphate poisoning.
- The afterdischarges of congenital SCMS could be missed on routine nerve stimulation. One should stimulate other, less frequently used nerves when the condition is suspected.
- DNA testing for acetylcholine receptor channel mutations is used to confirm the diagnosis of congenital SCMS.
- Treatment with cholinesterase drugs is of little benefit in the SCMS, and steroids produce no improvement. Quinidine, which is contraindicated in autoimmune myasthenia gravis, is helpful in these patients. Fluoxetine is also beneficial.

This case was reported as Bedlack RS, Bertorini TE, Sanders DB. Hidden afterdischarges in slow channel congenital myasthenic syndrome. J Clin Neuromuscul Dis. 2000;1:186–189.

REFERENCES

1. Nations SP, Wolfe GI, Amato AA, et al. Distal myasthenia gravis. *Neurology*. 1999;52:632–634.
2. Engel AG, Lambert EH, Mulder DM, et al. A newly recognized congenital myasthenic syndrome attributed to a prolonged open time of the acetylcholine-induced ion channel. *Ann Neurol*. 1982; 11:553–569.
3. Engel AG, Ohno K, Sine SM. Congenital myasthenic syndromes: recent advances. *Arch Neurol*. 1999;56:163–167.
4. Engel AG, Ohno K, Sine SM. Myasthenic syndromes. In: Engel A, Franzini-Armstrong C, eds. *Myology*. 2nd ed. New York, NY: McGraw-Hill; 2004:1801–1844.
5. Barohn RJ, Amato AA. Distal myopathies. *Semin Neurol*. 1999;19: 45–58.
6. Welander L. Myopathia distalis tarda hereditaria: 249 examined cases in 72 pedigrees. *Acta Med Scand*. 1951;141(265):1–124.
7. Griggs RC, Markesbery WR. Distal myopathies. In: Engel A, Franzini-Armstrong C, eds. *Myology*. 2nd ed. New York, NY: McGraw-Hill; 1994:1246–1257.
8. Lindberg C, Borg K, Edstrom L, et al. Inclusion body myositis and Welander distal myopathy: a clinical, neurophysiological and morphological comparison. *J Neurol Sci*. 1991;103:76–81.
9. Borg K, Ahlberg G, Borg J, Edstrom L. Welander's distal myopathy: clinical, neurophysiological and muscle biopsy observations in young and middle-aged adults with early symptoms. *J Neurol Neurosurg Psychiatry*. 1991;54:494–498.
10. Moxley RT III. The myotonias: their diagnosis and treatment. *Comp Ther*. 1996;22:8–21.
11. DiMauro S, Hartwig GB, Hays A, et al. Debrancher deficiency: neuromuscular disorder in 5 adults. *Ann Neurol*. 1979;5: 422–436.
12. Bertorini TE. Histopathology of the inflammatory myopathies. In: Dalakas MC, ed. *Polymyositis and Dermatomyositis*. Boston, MA: Butterworth-Heinemann; 1987:157–194.
13. Eisenberg I, Grabov-Nardini G, Hochner H, et al. Mutations spectrum of GNE in hereditary inclusion body myopathy sparing the quadriceps. *Hum Mutat*. 2003;21(1):99.
14. Goebel HH. Desmin-related neuromuscular disorders. *Muscle Nerve*. 1995;18:1306–1320.
15. Horowitz SH, Schmalbruch H. Autosomal dominant distal myopathy with desmin storage: a clinicopathologic and electrophysiologic study of a large kinship. *Muscle Nerve*. 1994;17:151–160.
16. Amato AA, Kagan-Hallet K, Jackson CE, et al. The wide-spectrum of myofibrillar myopathy suggests a multifactorial etiology and pathogenesis. *Neurology*. 1998;51:1646–1655.
17. Selcen D, Engel AG. Mutations in myotilin cause myofibrillar myopathy. *Neurology*. 2004;62(8):1363–1371.
18. Charnas LR, Luciano CA, Dalakas M, et al. Distal vacuolar myopathy in nephropathic cystinosis. *Ann Neurol*. 1994;35: 181–188.
19. Amato AA, Jackson CE, Ridings L, Barohn RJ. Childhood-onset oculopharyngodistal myopathy with chronic intestinal pseudo-obstruction. *Muscle Nerve*. 1995;18:842–847.
20. Sine SM, Ohno K, Bouzat C, et al. Mutation of the acetylcholine receptor alpha subunit causes a slow-channel myasthenic syndrome by enhancing agonist-binding affinity. *Neuron*. 1995;15:229–239.
21. Ohno K, Hutchinson DO, Milone M, et al. Congenital myasthenic syndrome caused by prolonged acetylcholine receptor channel openings due to a mutation in the M2 domain of the epsilon subunit. *Proc Natl Acad Sci USA*. 1995;92:758–762.
22. Engel AG, Ohno K, Milone M, et al. New mutations in the acetylcholine receptor subunit genes reveal heterogeneity in the slow-channel congenital myasthenic syndrome. *Hum Mol Genet*. 1996;5:1217–1227.
23. Fukudome T, Ohno K, Brengman JM, Engel AG. Quinidine normalizes the open duration of slow-channel mutants of the acetylcholine receptor. *Neuroreport*. 1998;9:1907–1911.
24. Harper CM, Engel AG. Quinidine sulfate therapy for the slow-channel congenital myasthenic syndrome. *Ann Neurol*. 1998;43:480–484.
25. Harper CM, Fukudome T, Engel AG. Treatment of slow channel congenital myasthenic syndrome with fluoxetine. *Neurology*. 2003;60:1710–1713.
26. Colomer J, Muller JS, Vernet A, et al. Long-term improvement of slow-channel congenital myasthenic syndrome with fluoxetine. *Neuromuscular Disord*. 2006;16:329–333.
27. Engel AG Congenital myasthenic syndromes. In: Rosenberg's Molecular and Genetic Basis of Neurological and Psychiatric Disease. Vol. 2. Amsterdam: Elsevier; 2020:539–558.

78 CASE

A Young Man With Episodic Weakness

An 18-year-old man was evaluated for intermittent muscle weakness that occurred mainly in the mornings after eating pizza the previous night. This started about 6 months earlier. A recent attack prompted him to make an emergency room visit, where he had a potassium level of 3.0 mEq/L (normal, 3.5–5.0 mEq/L) and was treated with an oral potassium supplement.

Past medical history was unremarkable. His father had complained of similar problems with weakness following rest after exercise and heavy meals. There was no other family history. He was a college student who did not drink alcohol or smoke.

Examination revealed normal mentation and cranial nerves. Muscle strength was normal. Reflexes were normal and symmetrical, and there were no Babinski signs. Sensation and coordination were normal. There was no clinical myotonia. The neurological examination was otherwise normal.

WHAT IS THE DIFFERENTIAL DIAGNOSIS?

This patient presented with intermittent weakness. Myasthenia gravis is a consideration, but the weakness did not include cranial nerves and was episodic and related to heavy meals, and it did not fluctuate during the day as in that disease; the patient was otherwise completely normal between attacks.

A mitochondrial myopathy is also a possibility, as those patients can present with intermittent weakness and fatigue; however, this occurs mainly during exercise, and they also usually have other manifestations. In other metabolic myopathies there are exercise-induced muscle pains.

The history was rather suggestive of a periodic paralysis. The clinical presentation, symptoms in his father, and his low serum potassium during an attack are characteristic of

TABLE 78-1 Characteristics and Treatment of Hypokalemic Periodic Paralysis (HypoPP)

	Periodic Paralysis With Cardiac Arrhythmia	Calcium Channel Periodic Paralysis	Sodium Channel Periodic Paralysis	Potassium Channel Periodic Paralysis	Periodic Paralysis With Thyroid Disease
Clinical Features	Andersen Syndrome With Normo-, Hypo-, or Hyperkalemic Periodic Paralysis	HypoPP 1	HypoPP 2	HypoPP	Hypokalemic Thyrotoxic Periodic Paralysis
Inheritance	Dominant	Dominant	Dominant	Dominant	Sporadic; occasionally dominant
Gene defect	Chromosome 17; affects Kir2.1 potassium channel	Chromosome 2; affects skeletal muscle calcium channel	Chromosome 17; affects skeletal muscle sodium channel	Chromosome 11; affects MiRP2 subunit of potassium channel	Unknown
Age of onset; myopathy infrequent	First or second decade typical; also short stature; dysmorphic features; prolonged QT interval on ECG; ventricular arrhythmias	First to third decade; moderate common late; vacuoles frequently seen on biopsy	First to third decade; not yet determined	Second to third decade; not yet determined	Third decade (males 20:1)
Myotonia; provocative stimuli	No Rest after exercise, oral glucose	No High-carbohydrate meals, rest after exercise, cold; emotional stress/ excitement	No High-carbohydrate meals, rest after exercise, cold; emotional stress/ excitement	No Usually by strenuous exercise followed by rest; less consistent provocation after high carbohydrate intake	No High-carbohydrate meals, rest after exercise, acetazolamide
Therapy for symptoms	Mild exercise, glucose, high sodium intake, acetazolamide	Acetazolamide, dichlorphenamide, potassium, spironolactone	Potassium, spironolactone	Acetazolamide	Propranolol, restoration of euthyroid state, oral potassium, spironolactone

ECG, Electrocardiography.

Reprinted with permission from Moxley R. Channelopathies affecting skeletal muscle: myotonic disorders including myotonic dystrophy and periodic paralysis. In: Jones HR, DeVivi DC, Darras BT, eds. *Neuromuscular Disorders of Infancy, Childhood, and Adolescence: A Clinician's Approach*. Boston, MA: Butterworth-Heinemann; 2003:787.

TABLE 78-2 Characteristics and Treatment of Hyperkalemic Periodic Paralysis

	Sodium Channel Myotonia with Periodic Paralysis			Sodium Channel Periodic Paralysis without Myotonia
Inheritance	Dominant	Dominant	Dominant	Dominant
Gene defect	Chromosome 17; affects skeletal muscle sodium channel	Chromosome 17; affects skeletal muscle sodium channel	Chromosome 17; affects skeletal muscle sodium channel	Chromosome 17; affects skeletal muscle sodium channel
Age of onset	First decade	First decade	First decade	First decade
Myopathy	Very rare	Rare	Infrequent	Infrequent
Myotonia	Especially paradoxical myotonia of the eyelids and grip	Especially paradoxical myotonia of the eyelids and grip	Especially paradoxical myotonia of the eyelids	No
Provocative stimuli	Cold exposure followed by exercise leads to focal paralysis; occasionally exercise provokes stiffness	Oral potassium load, rest after exercise mainly in morning (hyperkalemic weakness), cold exposure followed by exercise (focal paralysis)	Rest after exercise, cold, and oral potassium	Rest after exercise, cold, and oral potassium
Therapy for symptoms	Mexiletine, mild exercise, keep patient warm	Mild exercise, thiazides, mexiletine, and tocainide	Thiazides, acetazolamide, dichlorphenamide, and sodium restrictions	Thiazides, acetazolamide, dichlorphenamide, and sodium restrictions

Reprinted with permission from Moxley R. Channelopathies affecting skeletal muscle: myotonic disorders including myotonic dystrophy and periodic paralysis. In: Jones HR, DeVivo DC, Darras BT, eds. *Neuromuscular Disorders of Infancy, Childhood, and Adolescence: A Clinician's Approach*. Boston, MA: Butterworth-Heinemann; 2003:788.

hypokalemic periodic paralysis (HypoPP). Tables 78-1 and 78-2 describe the various periodic paralyses.

AN EMG TEST WAS PERFORMED

Motor Nerve Studies

Nerve and Site	Latency (ms)	Amplitude Latency (mV)	Conduction Velocity (m/s)
Peroneal Nerve R.	**Normal ≤ 5.7**	**Normal ≥ 3**	**Normal ≥ 40**
Ankle	5.0	6	–
Fibular head	12.6	6	42
Ulnar Nerve R.	**Normal ≤ 3.6**	**Normal ≥ 8**	**Normal ≥ 50**
Wrist	3.6	13	–
Below elbow	7.5	13	62

F-Wave Studies

	Latency (ms)	Normal Latency ≤ (ms)
Peroneal nerve R.	48.6	54
Ulnar nerve R.	28.2	30

WHAT WERE THE EMG FINDINGS?

This test was normal. Serum creatine kinase (CK) and a complete metabolic panel were also normal.

Sequencing of the calcium channel gene showed a point mutation in the calcium channel gene with a change of guanine for adenine in base 242 (Fig. 78-1).

He was treated with spironolactone 25 mg/day, and his potassium increased; thereafter he did reasonably well maintaining normal electrolyte levels.

DISCUSSION

This patient had HypoPP, an autosomal-dominant disease with decreased penetrance in women. It is characterized by weakness after exercise and heavy meals, particularly those with high carbohydrates, and also by stress, infections, pregnancy, and menstruation. Local anesthetics and antiinflammatory drugs might also trigger an attack.[1] Breathing is usually not affected but can be when attacks are severe. Patients might also have muscle pains after a severe paralysis from muscle necrosis.

Some patients with HypoPP may have more frequent attacks later in life and can develop a persistent myopathy[2,3]; in some, these may disappear in late adulthood. EMG studies are usually

Sensory Nerve Studies

Nerve	Onset Latency (ms)	Normal Onset Latency ≤ (ms)	Peak Latency (ms)	Normal Peak Latency ≤ (ms)	Amp (μV)	Normal Amp ≥ (μV)	Conduction Velocity (m/s)	Normal Conduction Velocity ≥ (m/s)
Sural nerve R.	3.2	3.5	3.7	4.0	18	11	44	40
Ulnar nerve R.	2.1	2.6	2.6	3.1	20	13	57	50

EMG Data

	Insrt Activity	Fibs	Pos Waves	Fasc	Amp	Dur	Poly	Pattern
Deltoid R.	Norm	None	None	None	Norm	Norm	None	Full
Biceps brachii R.	Norm	None	None	None	Norm	Norm	None	Full
Triceps R.	Norm	None	None	None	Norm	Norm	None	Full
First dorsal interosseous R.	Norm	None	None	None	Norm	Norm	None	Full
Iliopsoas R.	Norm	None	None	None	Norm	Norm	None	Full
Tensor fasciae latae R.	Norm	None	None	None	Norm	Norm	None	Full
Vastus lateralis R.	Norm	None	None	None	Norm	Norm	None	Full
Gastrocnemius R.	Norm	None	None	None	Norm	Norm	None	Full

normal between attacks, but during a paralytic episode there is decreased insertional activity, and the motor units appear small. Nerve stimulation may produce low-amplitude CMAPs, whereas the SNAPs are normal (Fig. 78-2). To confirm the diagnosis, long electrophysiological exercise testing is recommended.[2] The long exercise test is used in the diagnosis of periodic paralysis. In this test there is late CMAP amplitude decrease in periodic paralysis. (Table 78.3)

Serum potassium levels are low during attacks, and this can cause EKG changes. Serum CK is usually normal, but might rise after paralysis, from hypokalemia-induced muscle fiber necrosis.

When the diagnosis is in doubt, provocative tests can be done with the use of oral or intravenous administration of glucose and/or insulin and epinephrine.[4] These tests should be done with careful observation and EKG monitoring, as they may precipitate a severe weakness and cause cardiac arrhythmias.

Muscle biopsy could be normal but may show characteristic vacuolated fibers (Fig. 78-3); the vacuoles are components of the T-tubular system and sarcoplasmic reticulum. There could also be T-tubular aggregates, but these are more common in hyperkalemic periodic paralysis (Fig. 78-4).

HypoPP is caused by two types of genetic mutations. *HypoPP 1* is associated with abnormalities in the gene of the alpha subunit of the voltage-gated L-type calcium channel or *CaCNA1AS* in chromosome 1q31–032.[5] This channel is the dihydropteridine calcium receptor.[6] *HypoPP 2*, on the other hand, is caused by mutations of the *SCN4A* sodium channel gene in chromosome 17q.[7,8] The CaCNA1AS mutations are more common.

Attacks are associated with sustained membrane depolarization caused by hypokalemia from an increased insulin release. In HypoPP 1 there is a reduction of the calcium currents, lowering the voltage threshold for inactivation and slowing the rate of channel activation.[8] In HypoPP 2 sodium channel inactivation is enhanced, causing reduced current amplitudes and hyperpolarizing shifts.[9] The Andersen–Tawil syndrome is a rare autosomal-dominant disorder that presents with episodic paralysis which could be either hyper- or hypokalemic accompanied by cardiac arrythmia, short stature, and skeletal anomalies. The disease is caused by the mutation in the gene in chromosome 17q23 that expresses the inward rectifying potassium channel.[2]

The treatment of HypoPP includes avoidance of heavy meals, particularly those high in carbohydrates. The paralytic attacks are treated with 2–10 g of potassium chloride orally. Intravenous replacement should be used *only* in severe cases and, in the ICU or ER, under close observation with cardiac monitoring.[1] Measurements to prevent attacks include low- sodium/low- carbohydrate diets with avoidance of excessive exercise and alcohol. The medications of choice for prevention in HypoPP 1 are acetazolamide or dichlorphenamide[10,11]; both are carbonic anhydrase inhibitors.[11] The symptoms of some patients might worsen with

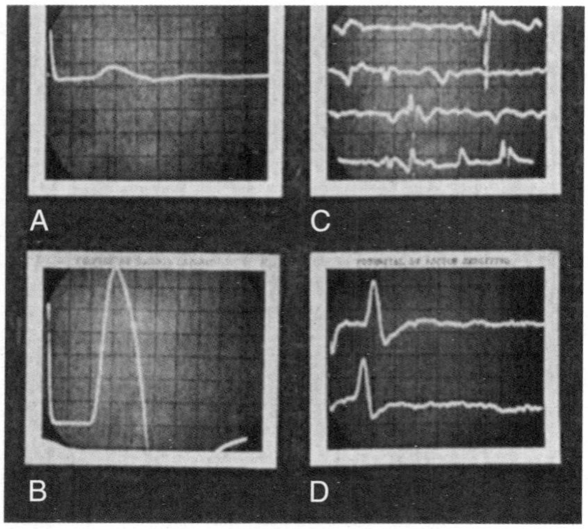

FIG. 78-2 **A**, Low-amplitude CMAP of the ulnar nerve recording in the abductor digiti minimi muscle during an attack of HypoPP. **B**, Normal CMAP after the attack (2 mV/2 ms). **C**, Low-amplitude motor unit potentials during an attack (100 mV/10 ms). **D**, Normal SNAPs of the ulnar nerve during and after an attack (20 µV/2 ms). *HypoPP*, Hypokalemic periodic paralysis. Courtesy Dr. Julio Cesar Alfaro, Lima, Peru.

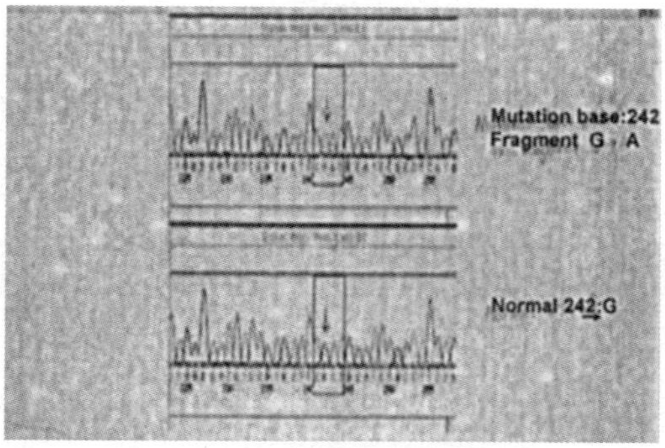

FIG. 78-1 Sequencing of the calcium channel gene in the receptor, exon 11 showing a change of G for A in base 242.

TABLE 78-3 Exercise Tests in Channelopathies

Short Exercise Test (Fournier, E., Viala K, Gervais, H. et al. Cold extends electromyography distinction between ion channel mutation causing myotonia. Annals of Neurology, 60, 356-365. 2006. Streib, E. W. AANEM Minimonograph # 27: Differential diagnosis of myotonic syndromes. Muscle and Nerve, 10, 603-615)

1. The hand to be tested is rested for 10 minutes before resting.
2. The hand is immobilized, and CMAPs are recorded over the ADM with surface electrodes and supramaximal stimulation of the ulnar nerve at the wrist.
3. Baseline CMAP is recorded every 60 seconds for 2 minutes.
4. The ADM is maximally contracted by forceful abduction of the 5th digit against resistant for 10 seconds.
5. The CMAP is recorded again immediately after exercise and every 10 seconds until no change in amplitude is observed. The test may be repeated three times with 60 seconds of rest between trials.
6. The percentage change in amplitude is calculated as follows:
   Increase = 100 x (greatest amplitude after exercise -amplitude before exercise) / amplitude before exercise.
   Decrease = 100 x (greatest amplitude after exercise -smallest amplitude after exercise) / greatest amplitude after exercise.
   The normal limit for amplitude increase is less than 10%.

Long Exercise Test (Kuntzer, T., Flocard F., Vial C., et al. Exercise test in muscle channelopathies and other muscle disorders. Muscle and Nerve, 23, 1089-1094. 2000. McManis, P.G., Lambert E. H., & Daube J.R. The exercise test in periodic paralysis. Muscle and Nerve 9, 794-710. 1986**)**

1. The hand to be tested is rested for 10 minutes before testing.
2. The hand is immobilized and CMAPs are recorded over the ADM with surface electrodes and supramaximal stimulation of the ulnar nerve at the wrist.
3. Baseline CMAP is recorded every 60 seconds for 2 minutes.
4. The ADM is maximally contracted by forceful abduction of the fifth digit against resistance for 5 minutes with 3 to 5 second rest periods every 30 seconds.
5. The CMAP is recorded very minute post exercise for 50 minutes or until no change in amplitude is noted for 5 minutes.
6. The percentage change in CMAP amplitude is calculated as for the short exercise test.

Normal limit for amplitude increase is less than 30% and for amplitude decrease is less than 41%.

ADM, Abductor digiti minimi. CMAP, compound muscle action potential.

Note
During the short exercise test: The CMAP transiently decreases in myotonia congenita; it first increases and later decreases in paramyotonia congenita. It increases in hyperkalemic periodic paralysis, and it is unchanged in hypokalemic periodic paralysis. During the long exercise test: The CMAP does not change in myotonia congenita, decreases in paramyotonia congenita, and decreases late in hypokalemic paralysis. It increases early then decreases in hyperkalemic paralysis.

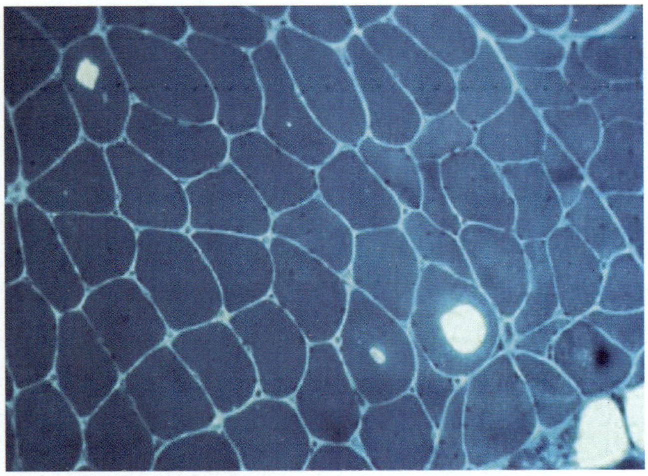

FIG. 78-3 Vacuolated fibers in a patient with HypoPP (modified trichrome stain, ×200). *HypoPP*, Hypokalemic periodic paralysis.

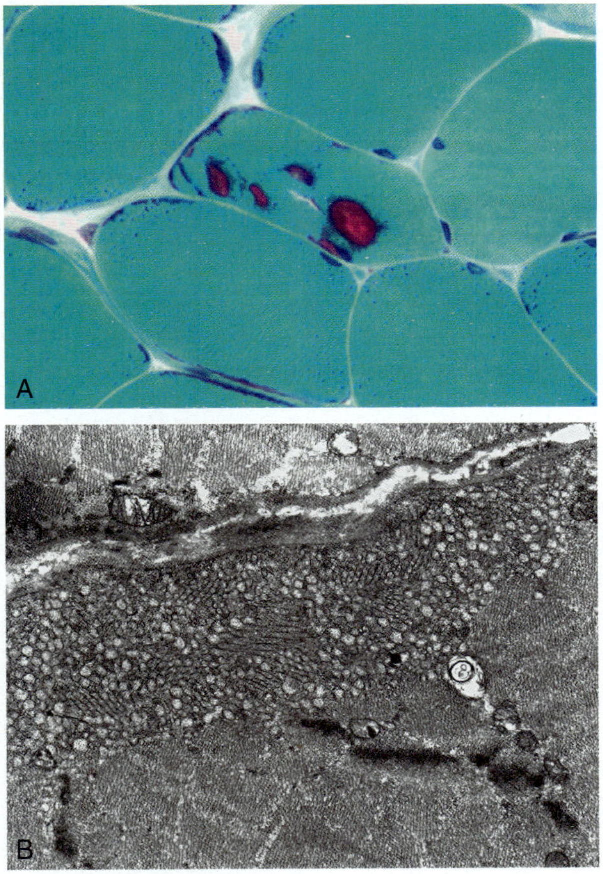

FIG. 78-4 A, Muscle biopsy of a patient with hyperkalemic periodic paralysis tubular aggregates (modified trichrome stain, ×400). **B**, Tubular aggregates seen in electromicroscopy on the same patient (×30,000).

acetazolamide, and thus they should be observed carefully during the initiation of therapy. Some also need low doses of potassium supplements, but, as this could trigger attacks of HypoPP 2, those patients are better treated with potassium-sparing diuretics, such as triamterene and spironolactone.[10] Lithium can be used but has a low therapeutic range and should be restricted to patients who do not respond to other therapies.[12] The treatment of the Andersen–Tawil syndrome should be aimed at cardiac protection using antiarrhythmics[11] and patients should be evaluated to see if the attacks are hyper- or hypokalemic.[13–15]

SUMMARY

This patient has HypoPP, an autosomal-dominant disease caused by a mutation in the calcium channel, or HypoPP 1.

He was treated with a potassium-sparing diuretic and low-dose potassium supplements and did reasonably well.

IMPORTANT POINTS

- HypoPP is caused by mutations of the calcium channel causing a change of function; the disease is characterized by attacks of hypokalemia-associated weakness. Some patients have mutation in the sodium channel (HypoPP 2).
- Weakness is precipitated by heavy meals or alcohol.
- Serum CK is usually normal but could be elevated after an attack; this is caused by hypokalemia-induced muscle necrosis.
- Muscle biopsy could show a vacuolar myopathy.
- EMG might show reduced excitability of muscles with decreased insertional activity during attacks; also, the CMAPs could be of low amplitude, while the SNAPs are normal.
- The treatment consists of using carbonic anhydrase inhibitors and potassium-sparing diuretics like spironolactone, particularly in periodic paralysis 2.

REFERENCES

1. Lehmann-Horn F, Rudel R, Jurkat-Rott K. Altered excitability of the cell membrane: nondystrophic myotonia and periodic paralysis. In: Engel AG, Franzini-Armstrong C, eds. *Myology*. Vol. 2. New York, NY: McGraw-Hill; 2004:1257–1300.
2. Boegle AK, Narayanaswami P. Treatment and management of disorders of neuromuscular hyperexcitability and periodic paralysis Chapter 18. In: Bertorini TE, ed. *Neuromuscular Disorders: Treatment and Management*. Amsterdam, Netherlands: Elsevier; 2022:pages 414–445. 2nd ed.
3. Stevens JR. Familial periodic paralysis, myotonia, progressive amyotrophy, and pes cavus in members of a single family. *AMA Arch Neurol Psychiatry*. 1954;72:726–741.
4. Bertorini TE. Clinical evaluation and clinical laboratory tests. In: Bertorini TE, ed. *Clinical Evaluation and Diagnostic Tests for Neuromuscular Disorders*. Boston, MA: Butterworth-Heinemann; 2002:15–98.
5. Jurkat-Rott K, Lehmann-Horn F, Elbaz A, et al. A calcium channel mutation causing hypokalemic periodic paralysis. *Hum Mol Genet*. 1994;3:1415–1419.
6. Fontaine B, Vale-Santos J, Jurkat-Rott K, et al. Mapping of the hypokalemic periodic paralysis (HypoPP) locus to chromosome 1q31–32 in three European families. *Nat Genet*. 1994;6:267–272.
7. Bulman DE, Scoggan KA, van Oene MG, et al. A novel sodium channel mutation in a family with hypokalemic periodic paralysis. *Neurology*. 1999;53:1932–1936.
8. Sternberg D, Maisonobe T, Jurkat-Rott K, et al. Hypokalemic periodic paralysis type 2 caused by mutations at codon 672 in the muscle sodium channel gene SCN4A. *Brain*. 2001;124:1091–1099.
9. Lapie P, Goudet C, Nargeot J, et al. Electrophysiological properties of the hypokalemic periodic paralysis mutation (R528H) of the skeletal muscle alpha 1s subunit as expressed in mouse L cells. *FEBS Lett*. 1996;382(3):244–248.
10. Morrill JA, Cannon SC. Effects of mutations causing hypokalemic periodic paralysis on the skeletal muscle L-type Ca 2+ channel expressed in *Xenopus laevis* oocytes. *J Physiol*. 1999;520:321–336.
11. Sansone VA, Burge J, McDermott MP, Smith PC, et al. Randomized, placebo-controlled trials of dichlorphenamide in periodic paralysis. *Neurology*. 2016;86(15):1408–1416.
12. Tawil R, McDermott MP, Brown R Jr, et al. Randomized trials of dichlorphenamide in the periodic paralyses. Working Group on Periodic Paralysis. *Ann Neurol*. 2000;47:46–53.
13. LoVecchio F, Jacobson S. Approach to generalized weakness and peripheral neuromuscular disease. *Emerg Med Clin North Am*. 1997;15:605–623.
14. Sansone V, Tawil R. Management and treatment of Andersen-Tawil syndrome (ATS). *Neurotherapeutics*. 2007;4(2):233–237.
15. Confavreux C, Garassus P, Vighetto A, Aimard G. Familial hypokalemic periodic paralysis: prevention of paralytic attacks with lithium gluconate. *J Neurol Neurosurg Psychiatry*. 1991;54:87–88.

CASE 79

An African American Man With Hyperthyroidism and Acute Paralysis

A 68-year-old African American man developed weakness in the legs that got progressively worse during the 2 days prior to the point that he became unable to walk. He fell at home, could not get up on his own, and was brought to the emergency room (ER). In the ER he was found to be severely weak and had a serum potassium level of 2.1 mEq/dL (normal, 3.5–5.1 mEq/dL); troponin level was increased, but cardiac workup was negative. The patient was loaded with IV potassium chloride under cardiac monitoring.

Past medical history included hyperthyroidism for which he was on methimazole 50 mg in the morning and 20 mg at night and atenolol with triamterene/hydrochlorothiazide for hypertension. He had a previous coronary angioplasty.

Family history was negative. The patient did not use drugs but used to smoke up until 1 year before. He did not drink alcohol.

Review of systems revealed no chest pains, shortness of breath, difficulty swallowing, or diplopia.

Examination the following day showed normal mentation and cranial nerves. There was minimal weakness of the proximal muscles of the legs, at about 5−/5. Gait was normal. Reflexes were trace in the legs and 1+ in the arms. Sensation to pinprick, touch, and vibration were normal. Coordination was normal. There was no myotonia.

The patient was observed and discharged home on potassium supplements of 20 mEq a day orally.

DISCUSSION

This patient had thyrotoxic periodic paralysis, but in this case it was clearly secondary to hyperthyroidism. Secondary periodic paralysis could have many causes,[1] and is similar to hypokalemic paralysis. This condition is more often described in the Japanese population, and 75% of cases occur in those of Asian extraction, but it has been reported in other populations,[2–4] including African Americans.[5]

The attacks are characterized by weakness with hyporeflexia, and thyrotoxicosis might appear simultaneously with the paralytic attacks in more than 80% of patients.[6] The thyrotoxic signs could be mild.

Typically, attacks are characterized by proximal weakness that occurs after exercise or heavy meals. The hypokalemia is caused by insulin-induced entrance of potassium into muscle fibers. At the end of the attack, potassium is released from the muscle and might cause rebound hyperkalemia.[7]

The relationship between periodic paralysis and the thyroid disorder is not clear, and the genetic defect in these patients is unknown.

Muscle biopsy shows nonspecific changes, but there could be vacuolization as in HypoPP. The EMG reveals myopathic motor units during attacks.

Acetazolamide is not efficient in preventing attacks and could even precipitate them, whereas propranolol is beneficial.[8,9] Treatment of thyrotoxicosis is most important; low-carbohydrate and low-sodium diets and potassium supplements can sometimes help.

SUMMARY

This patient with hyperthyroidism had an attack of weakness with hypokalemia; he was diagnosed with thyrotoxic paralysis.

IMPORTANT POINTS

- Symptoms of thyrotoxic periodic paralysis are similar to those of HypoPP.
- Hypokalemic periodic paralysis and thyrotoxic periodic paralysis can present in any race.
- Management of an acute attack of paralysis in those with thyroid disease is similar to that used for those without thyroid disease.
- Attacks of muscle weakness in HypoPP are associated with the slow membrane depolarization, which is caused by insulin release lowering serum potassium levels.

REFERENCES

1. Stapleton LJ. Hypokalaemia periodic paralysis. *Scott Med J*. 2018; 63(1):28–31.
2. Ober KP. Thyrotoxic periodic paralysis in the United States: report of 7 cases and review of the literature. *Medicine (Baltimore)*. 1992; 71:109–120.
3. Reisin RC, Martinez O, Moran M, et al. Thyrotoxic periodic paralysis in Caucasians: report of 8 cases. *Neurologia*. 2000;15: 222–225.
4. Pichon B, Lidove O, Delbot T, et al. Thyrotoxic periodic paralysis in Caucasian patients: a diagnostic challenge. *Eur J Intern Med*. 2005;16(5):372–374.
5. Kilpatrick RE, Seiler-Smith S, Levine SN. Thyrotoxic hypokalemic periodic paralysis: report of four cases in black American males. *Thyroid*. 1994;4:441–445.

6. Engel AG. Thyroid function and periodic paralysis. *Am J Med.* 1961;30:327–333.
7. Manoukian MA, Foote JA, Crapo LM. Clinical and metabolic features of thyrotoxic periodic paralysis in 24 episodes. *Arch Intern Med.* 1999;159:601–606.
8. Birkhahn RH, Gaeta TJ, Melniker L. Thyrotoxic periodic paralysis and intravenous propranolol in the emergency setting. *J Emerg Med.* 2000;18:199–202.
9. Tran HA. Thyrotoxic periodic paralysis. *Mayo Clin Proc.* 2005; 80(7):960–961.

A Boy With Large Muscles, Leg Pain, and Elevated Serum Creatine Kinase

A 7-year-old White boy was referred because of an elevated serum creatine kinase (CK). For 6 months he had experienced swelling of the right thumb and later of the first metacarpal phalangeal and interphalangeal joints of both hands. The diagnosis of juvenile rheumatoid arthritis (JRA) was tentatively made, and he was treated with nonsteroidal antiinflammatory drugs with marked improvement. His parents also noted "large muscles" since his early childhood, and his pediatrician found elevated serum enzymes with an alanine transaminase of 237 IU/L (normal, <45 IU/L) and aspartate transaminase of 187 U/L (normal, <36 IU/L). L-Lactate dehydrogenase was 1941 IU/L (normal, 110–220 IU/L) and CK of 8724 IU/L (normal, <200 IU/L).

He was born to a 39-year-old gravida III, para II mother at term and from an uncomplicated pregnancy. Labor lasted 4 hours, and because of breech presentation, he was delivered by C-section. Birth weight was 6 lb, 7 oz. He cried immediately. There were no prenatal complications. He sat at 4 months, crawled at 9 months, pulled to standing at 10 months, and walked at 1 year of age. Speech development was thought to be normal. He was repeating the first grade but was doing fairly well in school. The mother reported that he often complained of his legs hurting. This was more severe over the past 2-month period, particularly after exercise. He had no significant weakness and kept up with other children.

Family history was negative. He had no siblings.

Past medical history was remarkable for hernia surgery at 2 years of age; otherwise, there had been no other hospitalizations or injuries. The review of systems was in all other aspects negative.

Physical examination showed an alert, cooperative young boy. Height was normal at 115.8 cm. There were no birthmarks. Cranial nerves were normal. Muscle strength testing showed no evidence of distal or proximal weakness. However, he had rather large calves, and the triceps, quadriceps, gastrocnemius, and abdominal wall muscles appeared hypertrophic (Fig. 80-1), although the consistency of the muscle appeared normal. The heel cords were not tight. Finger-to-nose, heel-to-shin, and rapid alternating movements were well performed. He showed no Gowers maneuver when rising from the floor. Gait and stance were normal. There was no muscle tenderness or myotonia. The examination was otherwise unremarkable.

WHAT IS THE DIFFERENTIAL DIAGNOSIS?

This patient presented initially with joint pains and was diagnosed with JRA; he also had muscle hypertrophy. The differential diagnosis of muscle hypertrophy includes myotonias, such as myotonia congenita and Schwartz–Jampel syndrome, but he had neither clinical myotonia nor dysmorphic features. Hypothyroidism could cause muscle hypertrophy and elevated CK, but there were no clinical features of this disease. Another consideration was Becker dystrophy, but the lack of weakness is somewhat against this diagnosis. Other dystrophies, such as limb-girdle muscular dystrophy (LGMD) and centronuclear myopathy, are considerations, as they could also cause muscle hypertrophy but mainly of the calf muscles. They all are associated with muscle weakness, but LGMD 2I, caused by mutations of the fukutin-related protein gene, is important in the differential diagnosis, because these patients manifest with not only muscle hypertrophy and weakness but also a cardiomyopathy similar to Becker dystrophy.

Metabolic myopathies should also be considered because of the exercise-induced muscle pains, but these do not cause muscle hypertrophy.[1] He also had arthritis, which improved with nonsteroidal antiinflammatories; thus an associated myositis, causing muscle pain and swelling, should be included in the differential diagnosis, but the lack of weakness is also against this diagnosis.

Patients with spinal muscular atrophy rarely have large muscles, particularly in the calf, but the lack of weakness and the markedly elevated serum CK are against that diagnosis.[1] Stiff-person syndrome and Isaacs syndrome cause muscle stiffness and large muscles, but these are unusual in children. Furthermore, the affected muscles are prominent mainly in the trunk, and these disorders do not cause such a high CK.

WHAT SHOULD BE DONE NEXT?

Complete metabolic panel was normal, except for elevated alanine transaminase and aspartate transaminase. Thyroid-stimulating hormone, FANA, rheumatoid factor, and erythrocyte sedimentation rate were normal. Serum CK was high at 8300 IU/L (normal, <200 IU/L).

Motor Nerve Responses

Nerve and Site	Latency (ms)	Amplitude (mV)	Conduction Velocity (m/s)
Median Nerve R.	**Normal ≤ 4.2**	**Normal ≥ 6**	**Normal ≥ 50**
Wrist	3.6	10	–
Elbow	6.6	10	60

F-Wave Study

Nerve	Latency (ms)	Normal Latency ≤ (ms)
Median nerve R.	26.8	30

Sensory Nerve Study

Nerve	Onset Latency (ms)	Normal Onset Latency ≤ (ms)	Peak Latency (ms)	Normal Peak Latency ≤ (ms)	Amp (μV)	Normal Amp ≥ (μV)	Conduction Velocity (m/s)	Normal Conduction Velocity ≥ (m/s)
Median nerve R.	2.3	2.6	2.8	3.1	36	20	57	50

EMG Data

Muscle	Insrt Activity	Fibs	Pos Waves	Fasc	Amp	Dur	Poly	Pattern
Deltoid R.	Norm[a]	None	None	None	**Dec**	**Brief**	**Many**	Full[b]
Biceps brachii R.	Norm[a]	None	None	None	**Dec**	**Brief**	**Many**	Full[b]
First dorsal interosseous R.	Norm[a]	None	None	None	Norm	Norm	**Few**	Full

[a]No myotonic discharges seen on EMG examination.
[b]Rapid recruitment of motor unit action potentials.

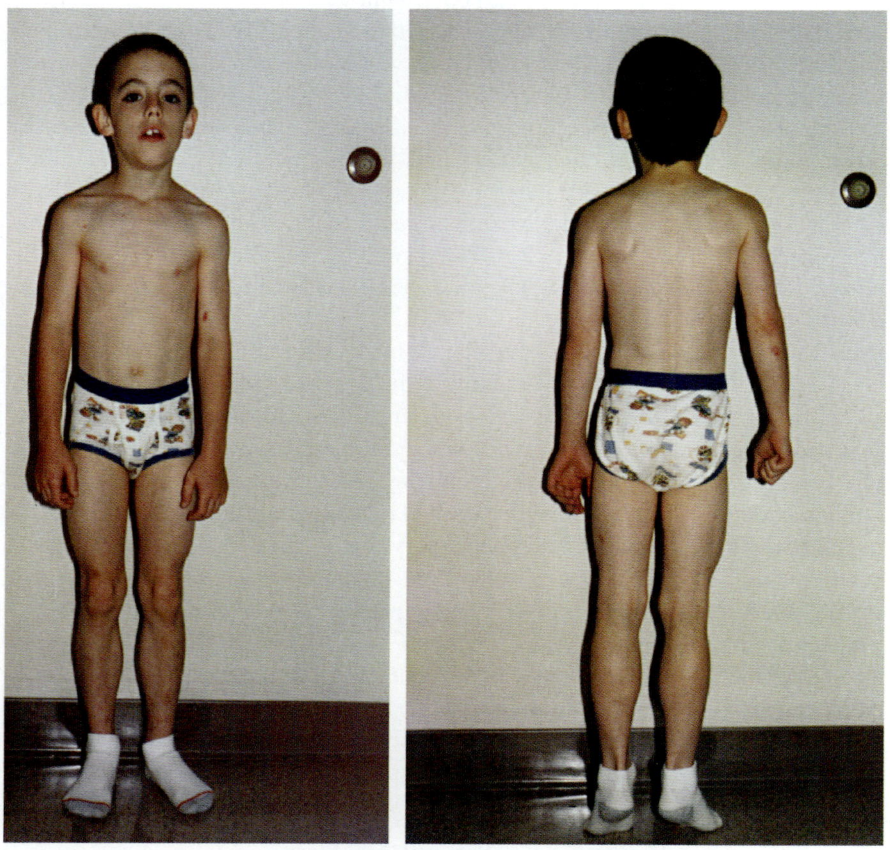

FIG. 80-1 Patient showing muscle hypertrophy.

AN EMG TEST WAS PERFORMED

What Were the EMG Findings?

The nerve conduction tests were normal. The needle test showed an absence of spontaneous activity, but many brief polyphasic motor unit potentials were seen during voluntary contractions. These findings were against the myotonias, other diseases of muscle irritability, or spinal muscular atrophy and indicate a primary myopathy.

WHAT SHOULD BE DONE NEXT?

The next test done was DNA testing in lymphocytes using PCR multiplex for dystrophinopathy; it showed no evidence of

DNA mutations. On follow-up, the patient's arthritic symptoms disappeared.

WHAT SHOULD BE THE NEXT DIAGNOSTIC TEST?

A quadriceps muscle biopsy showed variation of fiber size, increased connective tissue, and frequent regenerating fibers with no evidence of necrosis. There was a patchy decreased staining for dystrophin (Fig. 80-2) and (see Fig. 1.11 in Chapter 1) suggesting a dystrophinopathy like Becker dystrophy. This was confirmed by the Western blot test that showed dystrophin of normal size (about 400 kDa) but reduced in quantity to 20% of normal, confirming the diagnosis of a dystrophinopathy, such as Becker dystrophy.

WHAT ARE DYSTROPHINOPATHIES?

Dystrophinopathies are conditions caused by either the absence (Duchenne muscular dystrophy [DMD])[2] (Fig. 80-3) or a deficiency (Becker muscular dystrophy [BMD]) of dystrophin (Fig. 80-4); these are allelic disorders.[3] BMD is usually of later onset and has a more benign course. It can sometimes manifest in adulthood as a quadriceps myopathy, a cardiomyopathy, or even only with muscle cramps and elevated CK, depending on the degree of dystrophin deficiency and the structure of the protein.[3,4] (Fig.80-5 is a diagram of the steps in the evaluation of a patient with possible dystrophinopathy.) The incidence of BMD is between 1/14,000 and 1/31,000 live male births,[5] compared with the incidence of DMD, which is about 1/3500.

The initial description of the characteristics of childhood muscular dystrophy is attributed to Duchenne from his reports in 1861[6]; however, there were earlier reports by Bell in 1830,[7,8] and in 1836 Conte and Gioja[9] emphasized muscle hypertrophy in children. In 1851 Meryon[10] made the first clinical and pathologic correlation. Becker in 1953 described a more benign condition, also of an X-linked inheritance, but of later onset (BMD).[11] The initial case described by Bell might also have had BMD, as the patient's condition started at the age of 10 years and was reported at age 18.

There are several animals with dystrophinopathy, such as the mdx mouse, the golden retriever, Rottweiler and Japanese Spitz dogs, and the dystrophic cat[12] (Table 80-1). Muscle hypertrophy is particularly prominent in the latter; asphyxiation

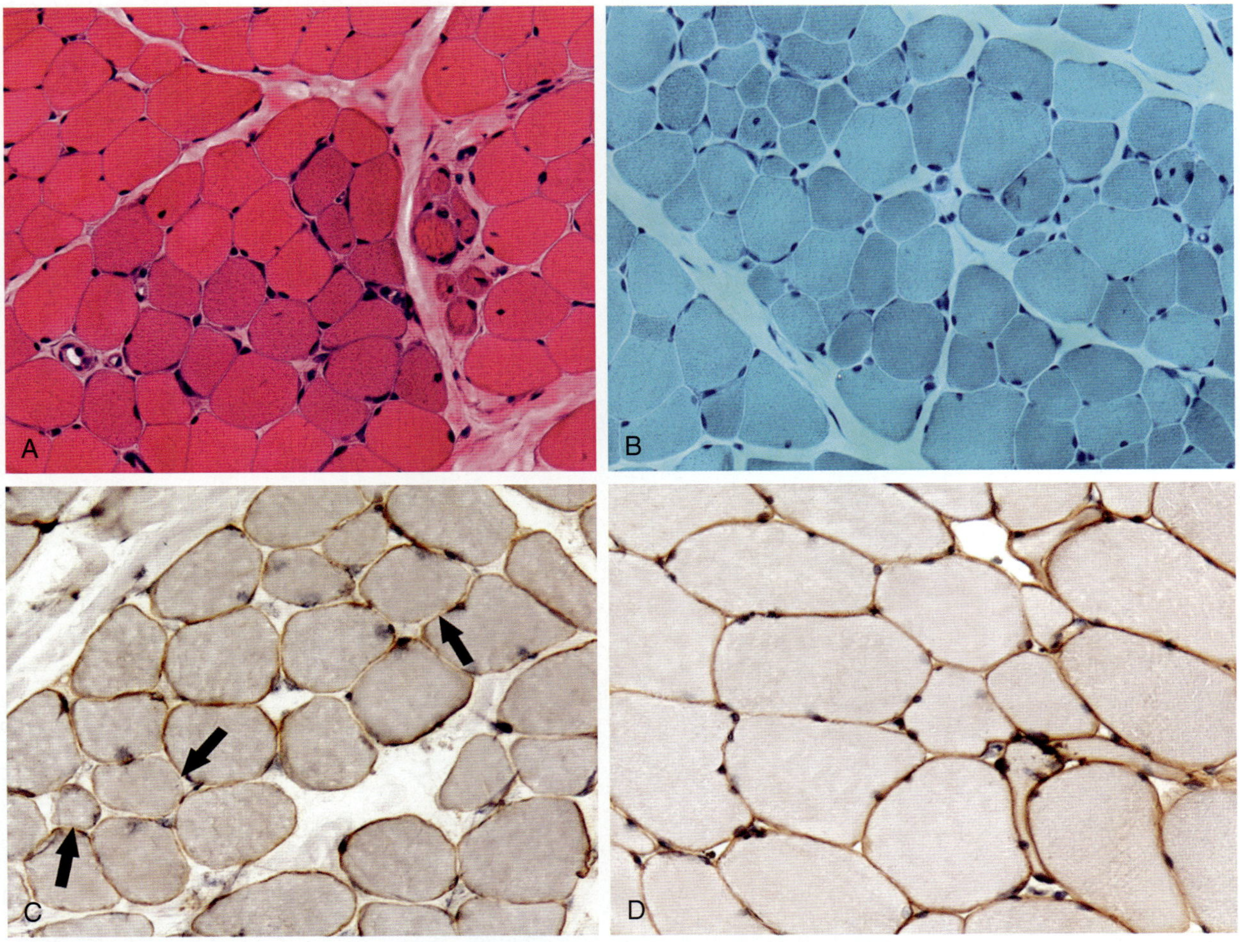

FIG. 80-2 **A**, Muscle biopsy showing variation of muscle fiber size, internalized nuclei, and mildly increased endomysial connective tissue (H&E stain, ×200). **B**, Scattered regenerating fibers (trichrome stain, ×200). **C**, Immunohistology staining for dystrophin showing patchy fibers with decreased stain (*arrows*); compare with a control (**D**) (immunoperoxidase stain, ×400).

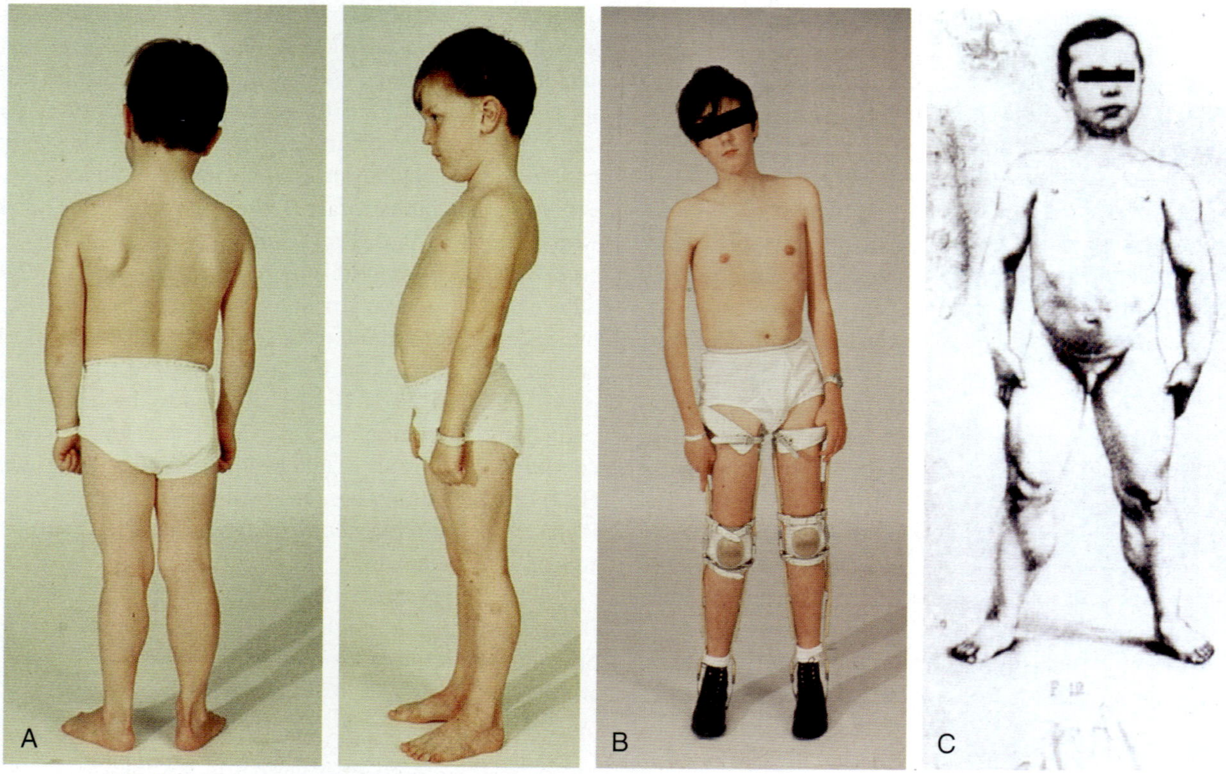

FIG. 80-3 **A**, A patient with typical Duchenne dystrophy; notice prominent lordosis and winging of the scapulae and mild calf muscle enlargement. **B**, Older Duchenne's patient showing muscle atrophy and wearing long leg braces. **C**, Initial case reported by Duchenne.

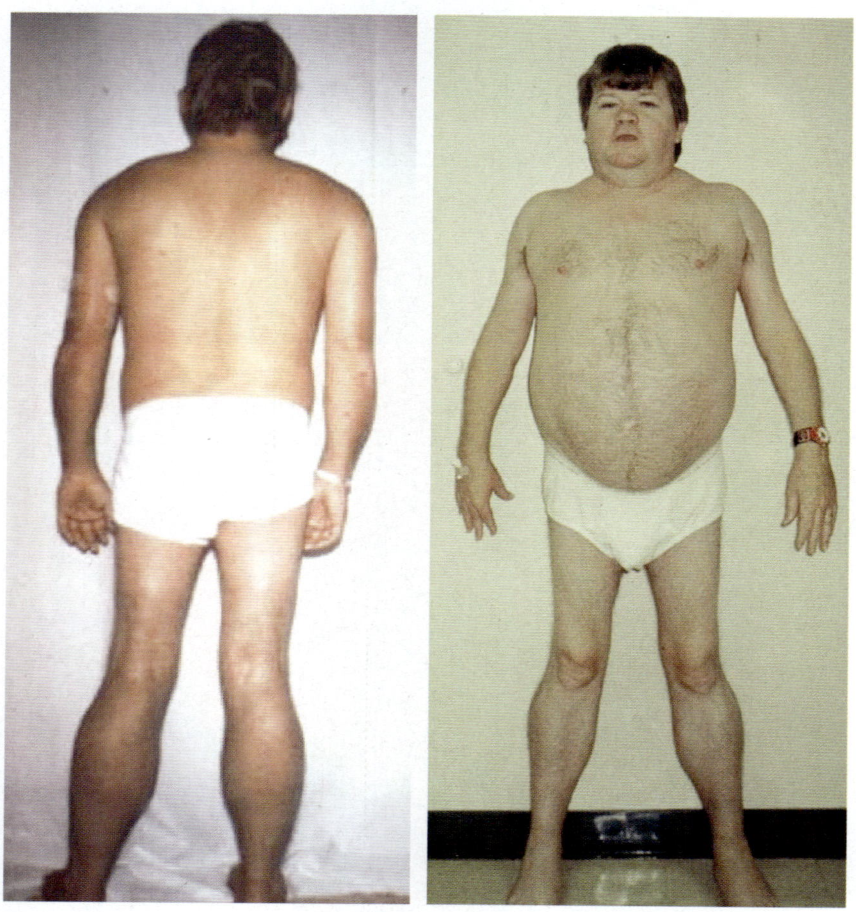

FIG. 80-4 Classic Becker dystrophy patient; notice lordosis and calf hypertrophy.

from tongue hypertrophy may occur (Fig. 80-6). The exact cause of muscle hypertrophy is not clear but could be secondary to necrosis, edema, or true muscle fiber hypertrophy.

Human dystrophinopathies are caused by mutations of the *dystrophin* gene in the X chromosome at Xp21. This is a large gene with 79 exons and 8 tissue-specific promoters that spread over 3 million base pairs of DNA. The gene expresses dystrophin, which is a 427-kDa protein that has four domains: an amino terminus, a rodlike domain, a cysteine-rich domain, and a C-terminus (Table 80-2). The protein is similar to spectrin and has an important role as a transmembrane protein. It is present in the heart, striate muscle, smooth muscle, and brain.[2]

Dystrophin binds to actin, the dystroglycans, and the sarcoglycans, forming the dystrophin–glycoprotein complex, and deficiencies of some of these proteins cause several forms of limb-girdle dystrophy.[13]

The mutations causing BMD occur most often in the rod domain,[3,4] resulting in a deficiency, but not the absence, of the protein. These mutations are usually in nonstop codons, thus are "in-frame" mutations that could be deletions, duplications, or point mutations of important amino acids. The frame-shift rule, however, has exceptions, as frame-shift mutations of exons 3–7 can also produce a less severe phenotype. Different

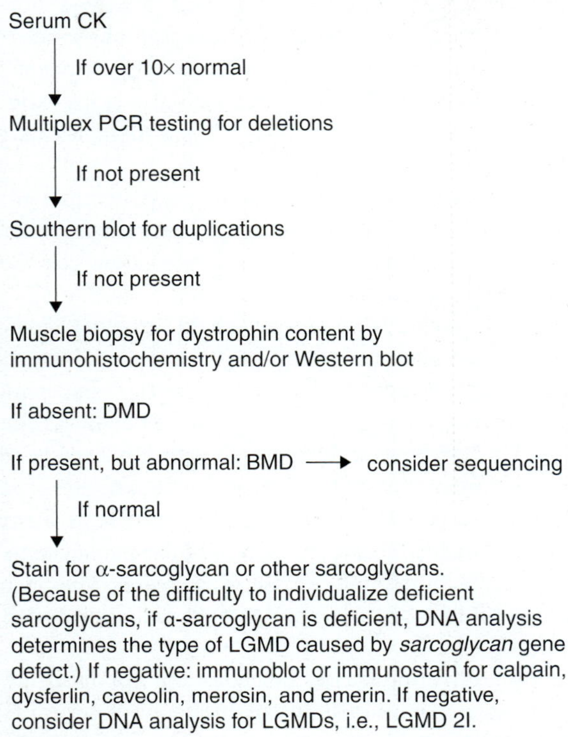

FIG. 80-5 Diagram of steps taken in the evaluation of a child with a possible dystrophinopathy.

TABLE 80-1 Dystrophinopathies

Classical Duchenne muscular dystrophy
Outliers (intermediate)
Classical Becker muscular dystrophy, mild, moderate
Dystrophinopathy (Becker's type) in Turner and Klinefelter syndromes
Quadriceps myopathy
Cardiomyopathy with and without mild weakness
Muscle cramps with high creatine kinase
Asymptomatic serum creatine kinase elevation
Manifesting female carriers
Dystrophic dogs (golden retriever, rottweiler, Japanese spitz)
Dystrophic cat
Mdx mouse

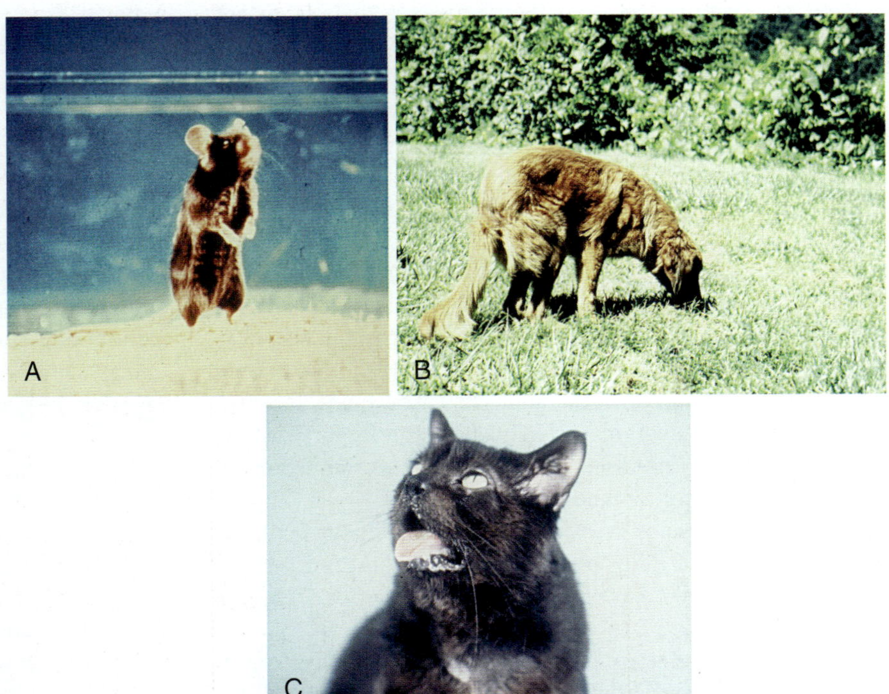

FIG. 80-6 **A**, Dystrophic mouse. **B**, Dystrophic dog. **C**, Dystrophic cat; notice tongue hypertrophy. Courtesy Dr. E. Hoffman, Washington, D.C.

TABLE 80-2 Characteristics of Dystrophin

Rodlike component of the membrane cytoskeleton of myofibers similar to spectrin
3685 amino acids, 427 kDa
Binds to actin, dystroglycans, and sarcoglycans (the dystrophin–glycoprotein complex), providing structural integrity to muscle membrane and linking the cytoskeleton with the extracellular matrix
Four domains: an amino terminus, a rod domain, a cysteine-rich domain, and a C-terminus
Normally present in skeletal muscle, heart, smooth muscle, and brain
Absent in Duchenne muscular dystrophy and present but abnormal in Becker muscular dystrophy

phenotypes have been associated with various mutations.[14] Missense mutations of the N-terminus are usually associated with BMD. Deletion of the proximal portion of the N-terminus is associated with more severe BMD than those in the most distal portions. Deletions in exon 45–48 are associated with cardiomyopathy and mild BMD.[15] Mutations that enhance or induce exon skipping or splicing are associated with milder phenotypes.[16]

The diagnosis of a dystrophinopathy could be made noninvasively by multiplex PCR amplification or Southern blot analysis, but, as in this case, these tests do not detect point mutations. For this reason, Western blot studies and histologic staining for dystrophin are still very valuable. Gene sequencing could also be considered in suspected cases.

Multiplex PCR amplification and Southern blot analysis detect partial gene deletions in about 55%–65% of DMD/BMD cases and duplications in 5%. These deletions and duplications occur in areas of the gene that are called "hot spots." Of the other remaining 30%–35%, some are small (1 or 2 exons) duplications or deletions that are missed by Southern blot analysis, or are point mutations.[17,18] Detection of point mutations requires the use of gene sequencing, which is difficult and time-consuming due to size and complexity of the gene and also because the mutations are scattered.

Recently, automated simplified methods have been used for the detection of mutations.[15,17–20] Sequencing is now commercially available but is expensive.

There is currently no cure for BMD. Steroids have been found to delay the progression of Duchenne dystrophy,[21,22] and, although it has not been proved, this drug might also help BMD. Dantrolene has been used in DMD to ameliorate muscle pains which sometimes occur after increased physical activity.[23] Proper cardiac workup and management is important, and transplant is sometimes used in patients with severe cardiomyopathy, particularly if weakness is mild.[24]

Tendon stretching is used to prevent or ameliorate contractures.[25] In Duchenne dystrophy myoblast implants produce dystrophic expression but have not been proven to produce clinical benefit.

New therapies that are promising in Duchenne dystrophy include gene therapy using adeno-associated viral vectors and a *microdystrophin* gene that restores dystrophin in animals.[26] Stem cell therapy has produced the expression of dystrophin in the mdx mouse.[27] Ataluen is a protein that could restore the normal expression of dystrophin by bypassing the nonsense mutations,[28] and antisense oligonucleotides can restore the reading frame with long-term production of dystrophin in animals.[29–31]

Antisense oligonucleotide binds selected sequences of RNA and regulates the expression of genes that are complementary and the "sense strand" that regulates protein synthesis is restored.[32] Several exon-skipping antisense oligonucleotides have been used. Eteplirsen skips exon 51 and is beneficial.[33] Although Golodirsen skips 53, vitolarsen also skips exon 53.[34] Calcinersen is used to skip exon 45.[33] These therapies are given weekly.[34]

The upregulation of utrophin, another sarcolemmal protein, is under trial. Therapies include drugs that reduce inflammation, regulate calcium, and reduce fibrosis. Stem cell therapy and gene modification have also been used.[35]

Blockade of myostatin, a muscle-specific growth factor/cytokine that induces muscle wasting, has been reported to produce functional improvement in dystrophic muscle.[36] Experimental studies in murine dystrophy demonstrated a beneficial effect of HCT 1026, a derivative of flurbiprofen with nitric oxide release and antiinflammatory activity.[37] Also, the angiotensin II receptor-blocker losartan, which might help the cardiac performance in advanced Duchenne cases, was found to be beneficial in dystrophic muscle function.[38] Albuterol increases muscle mass, producing mild functional improvement, as demonstrated in a short clinical trial.[39]

Genetic testing and carrier detection are important in dystrophinopathies. These include measurement of serum CK as screening, as well as Southern blot or PCR multiplex evaluation for duplications or deletions similar to those in the affected persons. Linkage analysis and muscle biopsy are also useful, and in pregnant women amniocentesis, chorionic villus DNA testing, or fetal muscle biopsy can also be used.

SUMMARY

This child presented with muscle hypertrophy and had an elevated serum CK. Electromyography showed small polyphasic motor unit action potentials, and DNA testing for dystrophinopathy mutations in lymphocytes was negative. A muscle biopsy showed decreased dystrophin staining and a decreased amount of dystrophin of normal size on Western blot.

IMPORTANT POINTS

- Muscle hypertrophy in children can be seen in the myotonias, hypothyroidism, Isaacs syndrome, Schwartz–Jampel syndrome, some cases of spinal muscular atrophy, and limb-girdle dystrophies, dystrophinopathies, and other myopathies.
- Dystrophin is a large molecule of 427 kDa, the deficiency of which is caused by several mutations of the *dystrophin* gene, presenting with variable phenotypes such as Becker and Duchenne dystrophies.
- Becker dystrophy is an X-linked recessive disorder usually caused by in-frame mutations of the *dystrophin* gene,

resulting in a deficiency of dystrophin or a dystrophin molecule of abnormal structure.

- Becker dystrophy usually manifests by muscle weakness, elevated CK, and cardiomyopathy with hypertrophy of the calf and other muscles. These can sometimes be severe. Some cases might manifest only with muscle cramps without weakness or high serum CK or with an isolated cardiomyopathy.
- Some mutations correlate with the phenotype.
- DNA testing with PCR multiplex or Southern blot is used in the diagnosis of dystrophinopathies by demonstrating deletions or duplications. These are not found when the disease is caused by point mutations; in those, the diagnosis is made by muscle biopsy using Western blot and dystrophin staining, or sequencing.
- The treatment of Becker dystrophy is conservative; steroids and dantrolene may be helpful. Cardiac transplant has been done in patients with mild weakness but severe cardiomyopathy.
- Duchenne dystrophy can be treated with gene therapy and antisense oligonucleotides.

This case was studied with Dr. Masanori Igarashi.

REFERENCES

1. Bertorini TE. Clinical evaluation and clinical laboratory tests. In: Bertorini TE, ed. *Clinical Evaluation and Diagnostic Tests for Neuromuscular Disorders*. Boston, MA: Butterworth-Heinemann; 2002:15–98.
2. Hoffman EP, Brown RH Jr, Kunkel LM. Dystrophin: the protein product of the Duchenne muscular dystrophy locus. *Cell*. 1987;51: 919–928.
3. Monaco AP, Bertelson CJ, Liechti-Gallati S, et al. An explanation for the phenotype differences between patients bearing partial deletions of the DMD locus. *Genomics*. 1988;2:90–95.
4. Koenig M, Beggs AH, Moyer M, et al. The molecular basis for Duchenne vs Becker muscular dystrophy: correlation of severity with type of deletion. *Am J Hum Genet*. 1989;45(4):498–506.
5. Bushby KM, Thambyayah M, Gardner-Medwin D. Prevalence and incidence of Becker's muscular dystrophy. *Lancet*. 1991;337(8748): 1022–1024.
6. Duchenne de Boulogne GBA. *De l' electrisation localisée et de son application a la pathologie et a la therapeutique*. 3rd ed. Paris: JB Balliere et Fils; 1872.
7. Bell CH. *The Nervous System of the Human Body*. London, England: Longman Rees Orme Borman and Green; 1830.
8. Tyler KL. Origins and early descriptions of "Duchenne muscular dystrophy". *Muscle Nerve*. 2003;28:402–422.
9. Conte G, Gioja L. Scrofola del sistema muscolare. *Annali Clinici dell Ospedale Degli Incurabili di Napoli*. 1836;2:66–79.
10. Meryon E. Granular and fatty degeneration of the voluntary muscles. *Med Clin Trans*. 1852;35:73–84.
11. Becker PE. *Dystrophia Muscularum Progressiva*. Stuttgart, Germany: Thieme Verlag; 1953.
12. Shelton GD, Engvall E. Canine and feline models of human inherited muscle diseases. *Neuromuscul Disord*. 2005;15:127–138.
13. Matsumura K, Campbell KP. Deficiency of dystrophin-associated proteins: a common mechanism leading to muscle cell necrosis in severe childhood muscular dystrophies. *Neuromuscul Disord*. 1993;3:109–118.
14. Muntoni F, Torelli S, Ferlin A. Dystrophin and mutations: one gene, several proteins, multiple phenotypes. *Lancet Neurol*. 2003; 2(12):731–740.
15. Aartsma-Rus A, VanDeutekom JCT, Fokkema IF, Van Ommen Gert-Jan B, et al. Entries in the Leiden Duchenne muscular dystrophy mutation database: an overview of mutation types and paradoxical cases that confirm the reading-frame rule. *Muscle Nerve*. 2006;34(2):135–144.
16. Novakovic I, Bojic D, Todorovic S, Apostolski S, et al. Proximal dystrophin gene deletions and protein alterations in Becker muscular dystrophy. *Ann NY Acad Sci*. 2005;1048:406–410.
17. Bennett RR, den Dunnen J, O'Brien KF, et al. Detection of mutations in the dystrophin gene via automated DHPLC screening and direct sequencing. *BMC Genet*. 2001;2(1):17–28.
18. Hofstra RM, Mulder IM, Vossen R, et al. DGGE-based whole-gene mutation scanning of the dystrophin gene in Duchenne and Becker muscular dystrophy patients. *Hum Mutat*. 2004;23:57–66.
19. Flanigan KM, von Niederhausern A, Dunn DM, et al. Rapid direct sequence analysis of the dystrophin gene. *Am J Hum Genet*. 2003;72:931–939.
20. Dent KM, Dunn DM, von Niederhausern AC, et al. Somatic mosaicism in a DMD carrier detected by use of direct sequence (SCAIP) analysis. *Neurology*. 2005;64(Suppl 1):A81.
21. Mendell JR, Moxley RT, Griggs RC, et al. Randomized, double-blind six-month trial of prednisone in Duchenne's muscular dystrophy. *N Engl J Med*. 1989;320(24):1592–1597.
22. Bonifati MG, Ruzza G, Bonometto P, et al. A multicenter, double-blind, randomized trial of deflazacort vs prednisone in Duchenne muscular dystrophy. *Muscle Nerve*. 2000;23(9):1344–1347.
23. Bertorini TE, Palmieri GM, Griffin J, et al. Effect of dantrolene in Duchenne muscular dystrophy. *Muscle Nerve*. 1991;14:503–507.
24. Donofrio PD, Challa VR, Hackshaw BT. Myocardial pathology in a patient with Becker's muscular dystrophy undergoing cardiac transplantation. *Neurology*. 1987;37(Suppl 1):197.
25. Bertorini TE. Muscular dystrophies. In: Pourmand R, ed. *Neuromuscular Diseases: Expert Clinicians' Views*. Boston, MA: Butterworth-Heinemann; 2001:227–299.
26. Chamberlain JR, Chamberlain JS. Progress toward gene therapy for Duchenne muscular dystrophy. *Mol Ther*. 2017;25(5): 1125–1131.
27. Gussoni E, Soneoka Y, Strickland CD, et al. Dystrophin expression in the mdx mouse restored by stem cell transplantation. *Nature*. 1999;401(6751):390–394.
28. McDonald CM, Campbell C, Torricelli RE, Finkel RS, et al. Ataluren in patients with nonsense mutation Duchenne muscular dystrophy (ACT DMD): a multicentre, randomised double-blind, placebo-controlled, phase 3 trial. *Lancet*. 2017;390(10101): 1489–1498.
29. Lu DL, Rabinowitz A, Chen YC, et al. Systemic delivery of antisense oligoribonucleotide restores dystrophin expression in body-wide skeletal muscle. *Proc Natl Acad Sci USA*. 2005;102: 198–203.
30. Gebski BL, Errington SJ, Johnsen RD, et al. Terminal antisense oligonucleotide modifications can enhance induced exon skipping. *Neuromuscul Disord*. 2005;15:622–629.
31. Van Deutekom JC, Janson AA, Ginjaar IB, et al. Local dystrophin restoration with antisense oligonucleotide PRO051. *N Eng J Med*. 2007;357:2677–2688.
32. Goyal N, Narayanswami P. Making sense of antisense oligonucleotides: a narrative review. *Muscle Nerve*. 2018;57(3): 356–370.

33. Mendell JR, Goemans N, Lowes LP, Alfano LN, et al. Longitudinal effect of eteplirsen vs historical control on ambulation in Duchenne muscular dystrophy. *Ann Neurol.* 2016;79(2):257–271.
34. Roshmi RR, Yokota T. Viltolarsen for the treatment of Duchenne muscular dystrophy. *Drugs Today (Barc.).* 2019;55(10):627–639.
35. Tesi Rocha C, Escolar DM. Treatment and management of muscular dystrophies Chapter 20. In: Bertorini TE, ed. *Neuromuscular Disorders: Treatment and Management.* Amsterdam, Netherlands: Elsevier; 2022:492–527. 2nd ed.
36. Bogdanovich S, Krag TO, Barton ER, et al. Functional improvement of dystrophic muscle by myostatin blockade. *Nature.* 2002;420(6914):418–421.
37. Brunelli S, Sciorati C, Antona GD, et al. Nitric oxide release combined with nonsteroidal anti-inflammatory activity prevents muscular dystrophy pathology and enhances stem cell therapy. *Proc Natl Acad Sci USA.* 2007;104:264–269.
38. Cohn RD, van Erp C, Habashi JP, et al. Angiotensin II type 1 receptor blockade attenuates TGF-B induced failure of muscle regeneration in multiple myopathic states. *Nat Med.* 2007;13: 204–210.
39. Skura CI, Fowler EG, Wetzel GT, et al. Albuterol increases lean body mass in ambulatory boys with Duchenne or Becker muscular dystrophy. *Neurology.* 2008;70:137–143.

CASE 81

A Woman With Proximal Muscle Weakness, Calf Hypertrophy, Heel Contractures, and Elevated Serum Creatine Kinase

A 23-year-old obese White woman was referred because of weakness in the legs, an EMG that showed a "myopathy," and a very elevated serum creatine kinase (CK) level. She had normal thyroid-stimulating hormone and FANA and a normal spinal MRI.

She stated that she had walked on her toes since age 10 and was seen by an orthopedic surgeon who placed her in braces for years. She later noticed difficulty going upstairs, bending, and squatting and had a tendency to fall; she had no numbness. There was no family history of neurologic disorders.

Neurologic examination revealed normal mentation and cranial nerves. She had mild hypertrophy of the calf muscles, contractures of the ankles, and difficulty walking on her heels and rising from a chair (Fig. 81-1). Manual muscle testing revealed 4/5 neck flexor weakness and 5−/5 in shoulder extension and abduction; biceps and triceps were 5/5; hip flexors, abduction, and extensors were 4/5; thigh muscles were 5−/5; and foot dorsiflexion was 4−/5; foot flexion, inversion, and eversion, and other muscle groups were normal. Reflexes and sensory examination were normal.

WHAT IS THE DIFFERENTIAL DIAGNOSIS?

This patient had a long-standing history of muscle weakness since childhood with contractures of the heel cords and large calves. The differential diagnosis includes spinal muscular atrophy, although the previous report of a "myopathic" EMG and the elevated CK suggests that she had a primary myopathy. Her long-standing history made inflammatory myopathy unlikely. There was no history of hypotonia or early-childhood-onset weakness to suggest a congenital myopathy, although nemaline or rod myopathy, myotubular myopathy, and central core disease could have their initial manifestation in late childhood or even adulthood. The rather high CK, however, makes most of these myopathies unlikely. Metabolic myopathies, such as acid maltase deficiency and mitochondrial disorder, cannot be ruled out. However, they usually do not have calf hypertrophy, and there was no evidence of extraocular muscle impairment, decreased hearing, or other systemic manifestations to suggest the latter. Endocrine myopathies, particularly hypothyroidism, manifest with an elevated CK, but the patient's thyroid-stimulating hormone was normal.

Other possibilities include limb-girdle muscular dystrophy or the manifest carrier state of a dystrophinopathy, in spite of the negative family history.

AN EMG TEST WAS PERFORMED

Motor Nerve Studies

Nerve and Site	Latency (ms)	Amplitude (mV)	Conduction Velocity (m/s)
Median Nerve R.	**Normal ≤ 4.2**	**Normal ≥ 6**	**Normal ≥ 50**
Wrist	3.9	14	–
Elbow	7.8	13	55
Ulnar Nerve R.	**Normal ≤ 3.6**	**Normal ≥ 8**	**Normal ≥ 50**
Wrist	2.8	16	–
Below elbow	6.0	15	66
Nerve and Site	**Latency (ms)**	**Amplitude (mV)**	**Conduction Velocity (m/s)**
Peroneal Nerve R.	**Normal ≤ 5.7**	**Normal ≥ 3**	**Normal ≥ 40**
Ankle	4.5	4	–
Fibular head	9.9	4	51
Knee	11.7	4	52

F-Wave and Tibial H-Reflex Studies

Nerve	Latency (ms)	Normal Latency ≤ (ms)
Median nerve R.	25.8	30
Ulnar nerve R.	25.7	30
Peroneal nerve R.	43.7	54
H-reflex R.	32.0	34
H-reflex L.	32.2	34

Sensory Nerve Studies

Nerve	Onset Latency (ms)	Normal Onset Latency ≤ (ms)	Peak Latency (ms)	Normal Peak Latency ≤ (ms)	Amp (μV)	Normal Amp ≥ (μV)	Conduction Velocity (m/s)	Normal Conduction Velocity ≥ (m/s)
Median nerve R.	2.4	2.6	2.9	3.1	53	20	54	50
Ulnar nerve R.	2.2	2.6	2.7	3.1	20	13	55	50
Sural nerve R.	3.1	3.5	3.6	4.0	18	11	45	40

EMG Data

Muscle	Insrt Activity	Fibs	Pos Waves	Fasc	Amp	Dur	Poly	Pattern
Deltoid R.	Norm	None	None	None	**Dec**	**Brief**	**Many**	Full[a]
Biceps brachii R.	Norm	None	None	None	**Dec**	**Brief**	**Many**	Full[a]
Triceps R.	Norm	None	None	None	**Dec**	**Brief**	**Few**	Full[a]
First dorsal interosseous R.	Norm	None	None	None	Norm	Norm	None	Full
Iliopsoas R.	Norm	None	None	None	**Dec**	**Brief**	**Few**	Full
Tensor fasciae latae R.	Norm	None	None	None	**Dec**	**Brief**	**Few**	Full
Tibialis anterior R.	Norm	None	None	None	Norm	Norm	None	Full

[a]Rapid recruitment of motor unit action potentials.

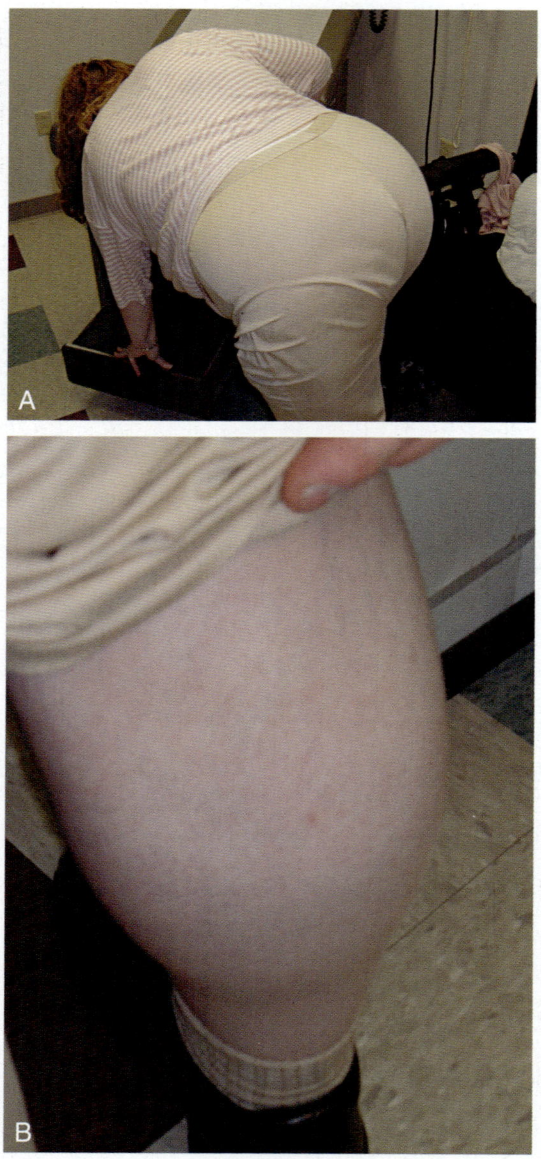

FIG. 81-1 A, Patient, trying to get off a chair, has to push with her arms over her thighs. **B**, Marked hypertrophy of the calf.

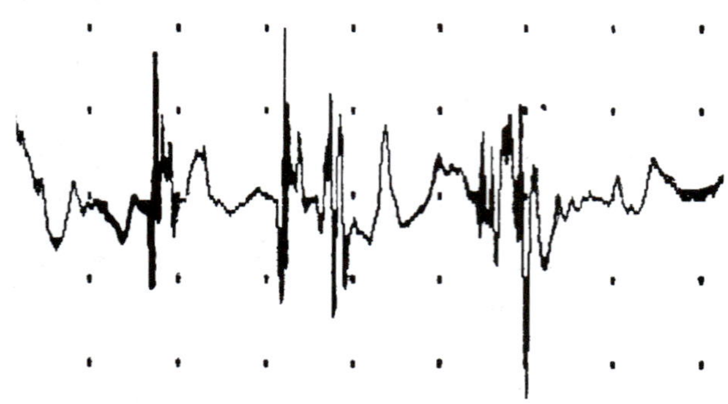

FIG. 81-2 Small polyphasic motor unit action potential in the deltoid muscle (100 μV/10 ms).

What Were the EMG Findings?

The test showed normal nerve conduction studies. Frequent small polyphasic motor unit potentials were seen on the needle test (Fig. 81-2). There were no fibrillations or myotonic potentials, making the possibility of inflammatory myopathy or acid maltase deficiency less likely. This also ruled out a spinal muscular atrophy.

WHAT OTHER TESTS SHOULD BE DONE?

A muscle biopsy showed variations in fiber size with some atrophic and hypertrophic fibers, increased number of internalized nuclei, and mild proliferation of connective tissue. She had patchy fibers with decreased dystrophin staining (Fig. 81-3), and Western blot analysis revealed dystrophin deficiency.

We concluded that she had a dystrophinopathy, and thus, she is a manifest carrier. Later DNA testing was done and showed a deletion of exon 45–62.

The patient later developed severe cardiomyopathy.

DISCUSSION

This woman presented with a long-standing history of muscle weakness without a previous family history. She also had ankle

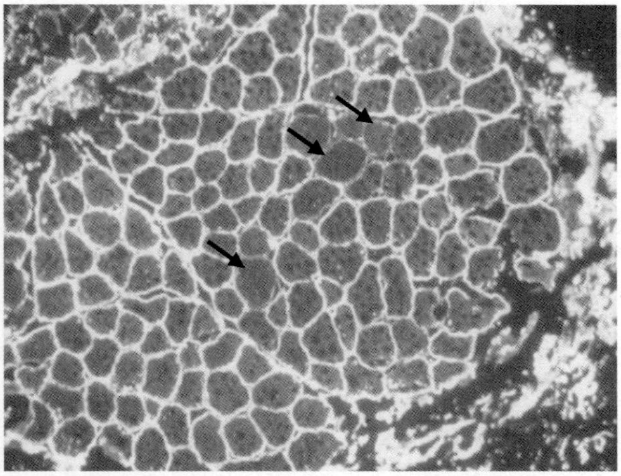

FIG. 81-3 Immunohistochemistry of muscle biopsy for dystrophin showing scattered dystrophin-negative fibers (*arrows*) (×200).

contractures, calf hypertrophy, and elevated CK, and she was demonstrated to have dystrophin deficiency. The patient's clinical presentation is characteristic of a manifest carrier of muscular dystrophy.

Whereas most women carriers of a dystrophin mutation are entirely asymptomatic, some may present with significant weakness as in this case. Still others may only have an elevated CK, depending on the amount of dystrophin present.[1–6] Some cases have muscle pain and fatigue.[7]

In one study, signs of myopathy were present in 22% of cases and cardiomyopathy in 7%.[5,8] This could be serious.[9]

Hausmanowa-Petrusewicz and associates demonstrated dystrophin deficiency in isolated females who had a previous diagnosis of limb-girdle dystrophy and elevated CK and emphasized the need for a definite diagnosis either by DNA testing or by muscle biopsy for proper genetic counseling.[10] Rarely, the only manifestation of the disease could be a cardiomyopathy.[11]

Mora and colleagues[12] found no correlation between the clinical phenotypes and elevations of CK with the degree of dystrophin deficiencies, while Hoffman et al. noted a clear correlation between the clinical severity and the dystrophin deficiency.[13]

A female carrier could become symptomatic because of skewed inactivation of the mutated X chromosome; this could be caused by translocation between an X and an autosome or from a chromosomal abnormality such as in Turner syndrome.[14]

During the early stages of development, females have two X chromosomes; one becomes inactivated in each cell, leaving only one active X chromosome.[14] In carriers of the mutation, each muscle fiber segment is controlled by one nucleus, either the mutated or the wild-type, as only one of them can be active.[15] For carriers to manifest a dystrophinopathy, there could be a skewed inactivation of the normal X chromosome and thus a larger number of the mutant nuclei, particularly in groups producing many dystrophin-negative fibers and muscle weakness *(manifest carriers)*. However, if the wild-type mutant nuclei are intimately mixed, dystrophin presents in adjacent muscle fiber segments,[16,17] causing no significant deficiency or weakness *(nonmanifest carriers)*. Histologically, in carriers there is variable presence of dystrophin in fibers of different muscles.[18,19]

There is currently no cure for these patients, but steroids appear to be beneficial.[20]

This case emphasizes the need for proper diagnosis and for genetic counseling in an isolated woman presenting with possible limb-girdle myopathy.

SUMMARY

This young adult woman had slowly progressive weakness, elevated CK, and an abnormal EMG with small polyphasic motor unit action potentials. She was found to have a deficiency of dystrophin histologically and had a reduced amount of the protein determined by Western blot.

Proper diagnosis in patients with this presentation is important for adequate management and counseling.

IMPORTANT POINTS

- The diagnosis of a manifest carrier of Duchenne/Becker muscular dystrophy needs to be considered in women with weakness and/or an elevated serum CK, even without a family history, for proper management and counseling.
- About 20% of manifest carriers might have weakness and an asymptomatic cardiomyopathy. Some might have a severe cardiomyopathy.
- The Duchenne phenotype occurs in patients who have chromosomal translocations or other chromosome abnormalities, such as Turner syndrome.
- Weakness occurs in a woman from a skewed inactivation of the normal X chromosome.
- The muscle biopsy of manifest carriers shows myopathic features and decreased or nonuniform staining of dystrophin in muscle fibers.

REFERENCES

1. Moser H, Emery AE. The manifesting carrier in Duchenne muscular dystrophy. *Clin Genet*. 1974;5(4):271–284.
2. Hoffman EP, Arahata K, Minetti C, et al. Dystrophinopathy in isolated cases of myopathy in females. *Neurology*. 1991;42(5):967–975.
3. Engel A, Olawa E. Dystrophinopathies. In: Engel AG, Franzini-Armstrong C, eds. *Myology*. 2nd ed. New York, NY: McGraw-Hill; 2004:961–1025.
4. Grain L, Cortini-Borja M, Fofar C, et al. Cardiac abnormalities and skeletal muscle weakness in carriers of Duchenne and Becker muscular dystrophies and controls. *Neuromuscul Disord*. 2001;1:186–191.
5. Ishizaki M, Kobayashi M, Adachi K, Matsumura T, Kimura E. Female dystrophinopathy: review of current literature. *Neuromuscul Disord*. 2018;28(7):572–581.
6. Zhong J, Xie Y, Bhandari V, Chen G, et al. Clinical and genetic characteristics of female dystrophinopathy carriers. *Mol Med Rep*. 2019;19(4):3035–3044.
7. Drivsholm P, Werlauff U. Pain and fatigue in manifesting carriers of Duchenne and Becker muscular dystrophy. *Neuromuscul Disord*. 2016;26(2):S123.

8. Hoogerwaard EM, Bakker E, Ippel PF, et al. Signs and symptoms of Duchenne muscular dystrophy and Becker muscular dystrophy among carriers in The Netherlands: a cohort study. *Lancet.* 1999;353:2116–2119.
9. Lim KRQ, Sheri N, Nguyen Q, Yokota T. Cardiac involvement in dystrophin-deficient females: current understanding and implications for the treatment of dystrophinopathies. *Genes (Basel).* 2020;11(7):765.
10. Hausmanowa-Petrusewicz I, Fidzianska A, Niebroj-Dobosz I, et al. Dystrophinopathies in females. *Folia Neuropathol.* 2000; 38(1):7–12.
11. Mirabella M, Servidei S, Manfredi G, et al. Cardiomyopathy may be the only clinical manifestation in female carriers of Duchenne muscular dystrophy. *Neurology.* 1993;43:2342–2345.
12. Mora M, Morandi L, Piccinelli A, et al. Dystrophin abnormalities in Duchenne and Becker dystrophy carriers: correlation with cytoskeletal proteins and myosins. *J Neurol.* 1993;240(8):455–461.
13. Hoffman EP, Arahata K, Minetti C, Bonilla E, Rowland LP. Dystrophinopathy in isolated cases of myopathy in females. *Neurology.* 1992;42(5):967–975.
14. Avner P, Heard E. X-chromosome inactivation: counting, choice and initiation. *Nat Rev Genet.* 2001;2:59–67.
15. Anderson LVB. Dystrophinopathies. In: Karpati G, ed. *Structural and Molecular Basis of Skeletal Muscle Diseases.* Basel, Switzerland: International Society of Neuropath Press; 2002:6–23.
16. Kong J, Anderson JE. Dynamic restoration of dystrophin to dystrophin-deficient myotubes. *Muscle Nerve.* 2001;24:77–88.
17. Doriguzzi C, Palmucci L, Mongini T, et al. Variable histological expression of dystrophinopathy in two females. *Acta Neuropathol (Berl).* 1999;97:657–660.
18. Vainzof M, Pavanello RC, Pavanello I, et al. Dystrophin immunofluorescence pattern in manifesting and asymptomatic carriers of Duchenne's and Becker muscular dystrophies of different ages. *Neuromuscul Disord.* 1991;1:177–183.
19. Muntoni F, Mateddu A, Marrosu MG, et al. Variable dystrophin expression in different muscles of a Duchenne muscular dystrophy carrier. *Clin Genet.* 1992;42:35–38.
20. Dubrovsky A, Pirra LN, Lautre A, et al. Deflazacort treatment in DMD symptomatic carriers. *Neurology.* 2005;A174(Suppl 1):64.

A Young Man With Distal Leg Wasting and Normal Sensation

An 18-year-old Black man presented with a 5-year history of limping and difficulty walking and going upstairs. He denied pain, numbness, cramps, fasciculations, or difficulties swallowing. His family and social histories were negative.

On examination he had normal mentation and cranial nerves. He had thin muscles, particularly in the distal legs with marked atrophy of the posterior compartment, but his feet muscles appeared normal, as did his upper extremities (Fig. 82-1). Muscle strength testing revealed that his neck flexors, shoulder adductors, and elbow flexors and extensors were 4/5; wrist extensors and flexors were 4−/5. Interossei muscles were 5/5. Hip extension and flexion were 4−/5, knee extension and knee flexion were 3+/5, and feet flexors were 3/5; feet dorsiflexion was 4/5, eversion and inversion were 5/5. Feet muscles were normal. Reflexes were normal, except for trace ankle jerks. Sensation and coordination were normal. No fasciculations or myotonia was detected. The examination was otherwise normal.

WHAT IS THE MOST LIKELY DIAGNOSIS?

The distal more than proximal weakness suggests a neuropathy, but he had normal sensation and relatively preserved reflexes. A hereditary motor sensory neuropathy such as Charcot–Marie–Tooth disease does manifest with distal leg weakness and atrophy and minimal sensory abnormalities initially; however, reflexes are diminished in those, particularly in the demyelinating type, and patients usually have weakness and atrophy of the feet muscles with high arches and hammertoes. Other predominantly motor neuropathies, such as those caused by porphyria and lead intoxication, are considerations, but the chronicity of symptoms and distribution of findings are against those. Patients with distal spinal muscular atrophy could have a similar presentation but usually are areflexic and have fasciculations. His presentation was rather suggestive of distal myopathy, particularly because of the atrophic legs with normal feet, sensation, and reflexes.

WHAT SHOULD BE DONE NEXT?

Serum creatine kinase (CK) level was 28,867 IU/L (normal, <210 IU/L); aspartate transaminase 270 IU/L (normal, 0–43 IU/L); alanine transaminase 228 IU/L (normal, 0–45 IU/L); L-lactate dehydrogenase 917 IU/L (normal, 100–270 IU/L); FANA, T4, and thyroid-stimulating hormone were normal.

AN EMG TEST WAS PERFORMED

Motor Nerve Studies

Nerve and Site	Latency (ms)	Amplitude (mV)	Conduction Velocity (m/s)
Peroneal Nerve R.	**Normal ≤ 5.7**	**Normal ≥ 3**	**Normal ≥ 40**
Ankle	5.4	13	–
Fibular head	12.0	12	46
Knee	14.2	12	46
Tibial Nerve L.	**Normal ≤ 5.3**	**Normal ≥ 4**	**Normal ≥ 40**
Ankle	4.3	22	–
Pop. fossa	15.9	18	42

Nerve and Site	Latency (ms)	Amplitude (mV)	Conduction Velocity (m/s)
Ulnar Nerve R.	**Normal ≤ 3.6**	**Normal ≥ 8**	**Normal ≥ 50**
Wrist	3.2	9	–
Below elbow	7.4	9	58
Above elbow	9.3	9	60
Median Nerve R.	**Normal ≤ 4.2**	**Normal ≥ 6**	**Normal ≥ 50**
Wrist	2.6	6	–
Elbow	8.1	6	50

Nerve and Site	Latency (ms)	Amplitude (mV)	Conduction Velocity (m/s)
Median Nerve L.	**Normal ≤ 4.2**	**Normal ≥ 6**	**Normal ≥ 50**
Wrist	3.0	6	–
Elbow	8.0	6	53

F-Wave and Tibial H-Reflex Studies

Nerve	Latency (ms)	Normal Latency ≤ (ms)
Peroneal nerve R.	50.1	54
Tibial nerve L.	52.7	54
Ulnar nerve R.	28.2	30
Median nerve R.	29.2	30
H-reflex R.	**NR**	34
H-reflex L.	**NR**	34

Sensory Nerve Studies

Nerve	Onset Latency (ms)	Normal Onset Latency ≤ (ms)	Peak Latency (ms)	Normal Peak Latency ≤ (ms)	Amp (μV)	Normal Amp ≥ (μV)	Conduction Velocity (m/s)	Normal Conduction Velocity ≥ (m/s)
Sural nerve R.	3.5	3.5	4.0	4.0	39	11	40	40
Ulnar nerve R.	2.6	2.6	3.1	3.1	24	13	50	50
Median nerve R.	2.6	2.6	3.1	3.1	24	20	50	50
Median nerve L.	2.5	2.6	3.0	3.1	28	20	52	50

EMG Data

Muscle	Insrt Activity	Fibs	Pos Waves	Fasc	Amp	Dur	Poly	Pattern
Vastus lateralis R.	**Inc**	**2+**	**2+**	None	**Red**	**Brief**	**Many**	Full[a]
Tibialis anterior R.	Norm	None	None	None	**Red**	**Brief**	**Many**	Full[a]
Tibialis anterior L.	**Inc**	**2+**	**2+**	None	**Red**	**Brief**	**Few**	Full[a]
Gastrocnemius L.	**Inc**	**2+**	**2+**	None	**Red**	**Brief**	**Few**	Full
Biceps brachii R.	Norm	None	None	None	**Red**	**Brief**	**Many**	Full[a]
First dorsal interosseous R.	Norm	None	None	None	**Red**	**Brief**	**Few**	Full

[a]Rapid recruitment of motor unit action potentials.

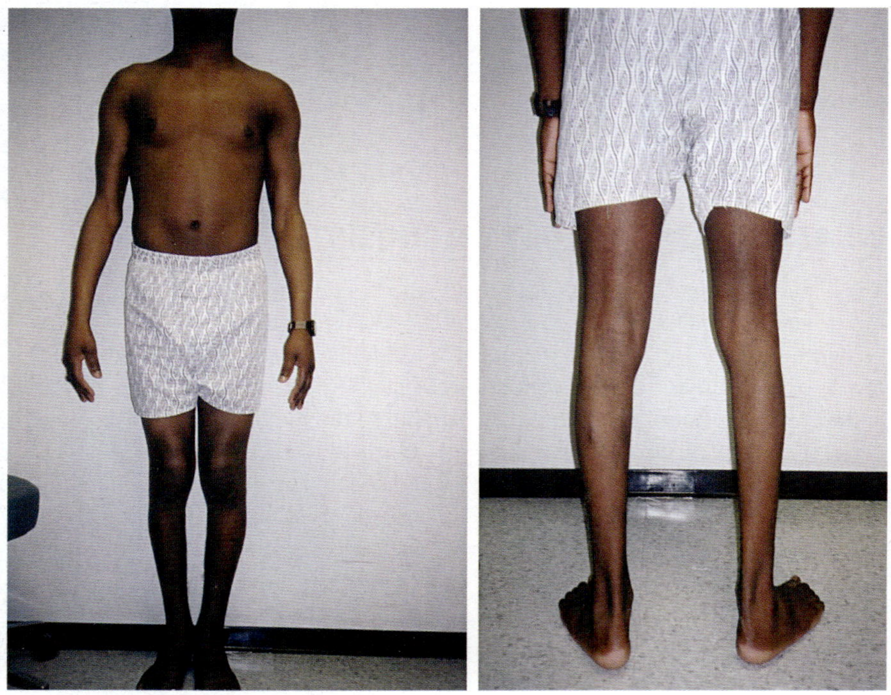

FIG. 82-1 Patient showing prominent calf muscle atrophy.

WHAT WERE THE EMG FINDINGS?

The nerve conduction tests were normal, except for the absence of H-reflexes, which was assumed to be caused by the severe atrophy of the calf muscles. The needle test showed fibrillation potentials without fasciculations and small polyphasic motor unit potentials of rapid recruitment in several muscles. The lack of large motor units with decreased recruitment and fasciculations was against a diagnosis of a motor neuron disease. The normal nerve conduction tests were against a peripheral neuropathy. This combination of findings on EMG is not only seen in inflammatory myopathies but also occurs in other myopathies, particularly when there is significant muscle necrosis, which was supported by his elevated serum CK. All of these findings indicated that this patient had a distal myopathy.

In patients with distal myopathies one should consider several disorders, such as inclusion body myositis, unlikely in this case due to the patient's age, but there is also a familial distal myopathy with inclusion bodies seen in younger persons, as discussed later. Myotonic dystrophy and oculopharyngeal distal dystrophy are also unlikely because of the lack of facial weakness, ptosis, or myotonia clinically or by EMG. Emery–Dreifuss muscular dystrophy could present with distal weakness, but such patients have prominent muscle contractures. Centronuclear myopathy, as well as debrancher enzyme deficiency, can also manifest distal weakness, but this is particularly present in the hands. The differential diagnosis also includes distal muscular dystrophies.[1,2]

WHAT SHOULD BE DONE NEXT?

The patient underwent a biceps muscle biopsy which showed prominent muscle fiber necrosis with mild inflammation; dysferlin deficiency was demonstrated by Western blot and immunohistology (Fig. 82-2). No DNA testing was done.

DISCUSSION

This patient was diagnosed as having a distal muscular dystrophy. This is a group of hereditary disorders characterized by prominent distal weakness and wasting, resembling neuropathies. They are caused by different genetic defects, age of onset, and clinical presentations, as summarized in Table 82-1. These include the following:

Miyoshi myopathy, or *posterior compartment distal muscular dystrophy* of autosomal-recessive inheritance, is a disease that manifests between ages 15 and 30 years and begins in the calves, as did this patient's. Later, these patients develop proximal weakness.[3] Reflexes are normal except for the ankle reflexes that are decreased or absent; there is a markedly elevated serum CK, and the EMG is myopathic. The histologic findings include muscle necrosis, fibrosis, and interstitial inflammatory infiltrates, as seen in this case. Miyoshi myopathy is linked to chromosome 2p13[4]; the gene expresses the protein dysferlin. There are other genes associated with this phenotype listed in Table 82-1.

Nonaka distal myopathy of the anterior compartment has an autosomal-recessive inheritance, with weakness beginning in the late second or third decade, particularly in the anterior compartment of the legs, ankle dorsiflexors, and toe extensors. Patients may present with a foot drop and develop proximal weakness later. Serum CK is usually elevated up to five times normal, and the EMG shows myopathic features.[5]

The muscle biopsy characteristically shows rimmed vacuoles with granular, basophilic material and nuclear or cytoplasmic 15–18 nm filaments as seen on electron microscopy (EM). The histochemical features are identical to the quadriceps-sparing vacuolar myopathy or familial-inclusion body myopathy

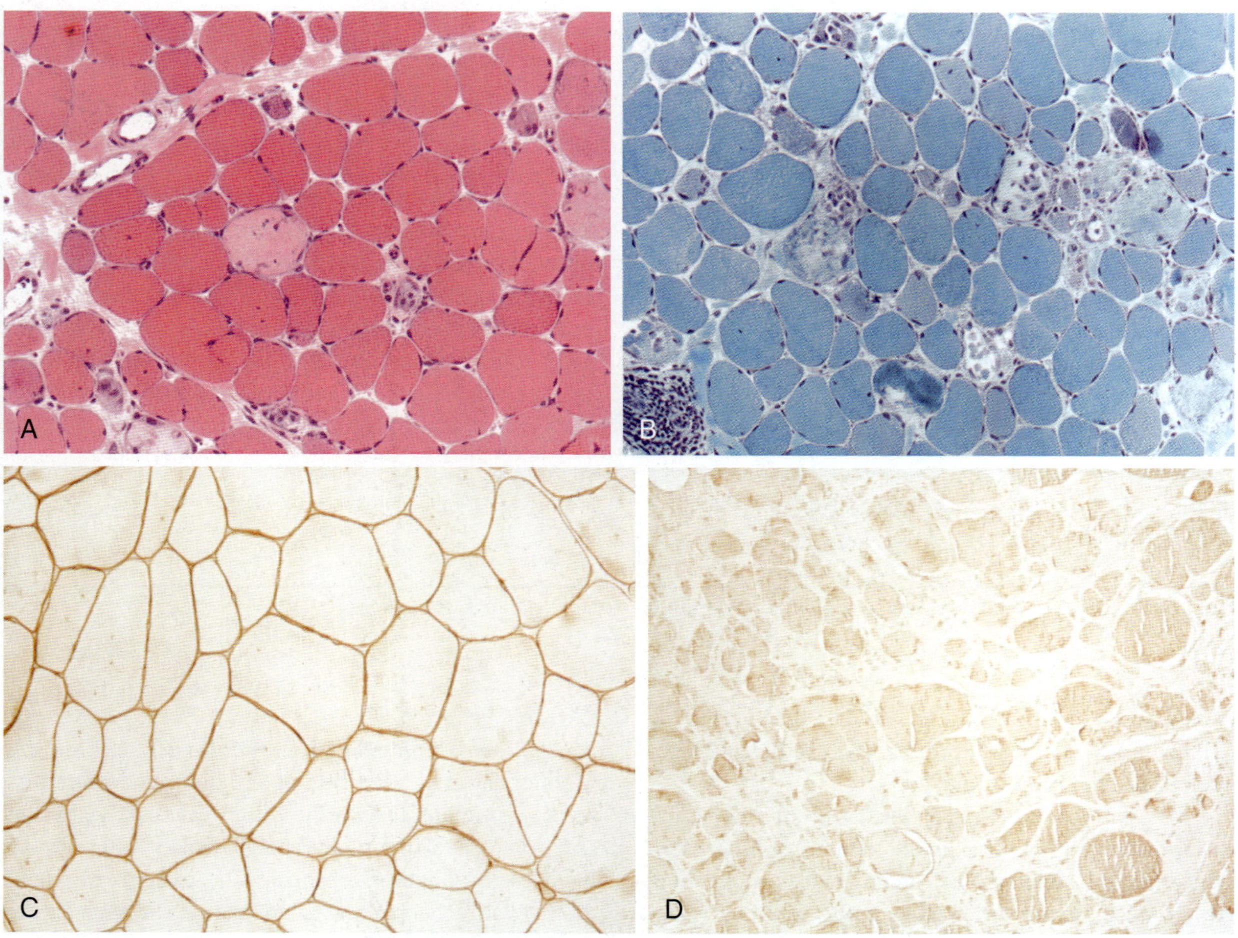

FIG. 82-2 **A** and **B**, Muscle biopsy showing necrotic fibers and mild inflammation (H&E and trichrome stains, ×100). **C**, Immunoperoxidase stain for dysferlin. **D**, Notice the absent dysferlin staining in the patient; compare with part (**C**), normal dysferlin staining of control (×200).

TABLE 82-1 Distal Muscular Dystrophies

Type and Eponym	Gene Localization	Gene Product	Initial Weakness	Serum CK Level	Biopsy
Autosomal-Dominant					
Late adult onset, predominantly in hands (Welander)	2p13	*TIA1* gene	Hands: finger/wrist extensors	Normal or slightly increased	Myopathic: vacuoles in most cases
Late adult onset, predominantly in legs (Markesbery–Griggs)	10q22. 3–23.2	Titin	Legs: anterior compartment	Normal or slightly increased	Vacuolar myopathy, sarcolemmal disruption, and accumulation of myofibrillar
Udd	2q31		Same as above	Same as above	
Autosomal-Recessive					
Early adult onset, anterior compartment in legs (Nonaka type, quadriceps-sparing myopathy), some sporadic	9p1-q1	SNF (UDP-N-acetyl)-2-epimerase/ N-acetylmannosamine kinase	Legs: anterior compartment	Increased, usually <5× normal	Vacuolar myopathy
Early adult onset, posterior compartment	2p12.13 Chromosome 10	Dysferlin (allelic to LGMD 2B)	Legs: posterior compartment	Increased, 10–150× normal	Myopathic, necrosis, no vacuoles: dysferlin deficiency
Miyoshi 1	11p14	Unknown	Asymmetric	Variable onset	
Miyoshi 2		Anoctamin 5	Asymmetric	Variable onset	Dystrophic changes
Miyoshi 3		ANO53			Dystrophic changes
Early adult onset (Laing)	14q11	Myosin heavy chain 7	Legs: anterior compartment, neck flexors	Slightly increased, <3× normal	Moderate myopathic changes; no vacuoles
Distal myopathy with vocal cord and pharyngeal weakness (onset in fourth to sixth decades)	5q31	Matrin 3	Legs: anterior compartment; finger extensors may first be involved	Normal to moderately increased	Vacuolar myopathy
Myofibrillar myopathy (onset in childhood to fifth decade)	2q35 11q21–23 5q22	Desmin, αβ-crystallin, filamin *ZASP*	Hands or legs, some with scapuloperoneal syndrome	Moderately increased, <5× normal	Myopathic, usually with vacuoles; subsarcolemmal granules or cytoplasmic bodies: accumulation of desmin, and other myofibrillar proteins
Autosomal-dominant or sporadic	7q-32.1 1p36	Myotilin Selenopathy			
Autosomal-recessive X-linked	10q22.3				
Others					
Some caveolinopathies	3p25	Caveolin	Variable presentation	Elevated	Dystrophic changes, caveolin deficiency
Nebulin gene mutations	2q	Nebulin	Young adults, tibial and facial weakness	Normal	Some small nemaline rods
HIBM with Paget disease and frontotemporal dementia	9p13–p12	Valosin-containing protein	Juvenile onset	CK normal or mildly elevated	Vacuolar myopathy
HIBM 3 (AD)	17p13.1	Myosin heavy chains	Variable presentation Juvenile onset Variable presentation	CK normal or mildly elevated	Vacuolar myopathy

CK, Creatine kinase; *HIBM*, Hereditary inclusion body myopathy; *LGMD*, limb-girdle muscular dystrophy.

(Fig. 82-3), and likely the disorders are allelic.[6] Nonaka myopathy has been linked to chromosome 9p1-q1.[7]

Laing autosomal-dominant distal myopathy of early adult onset was reported in 1995.[8] It is an autosomal-dominant disease characterized by weakness in the anterior compartment of the legs and neck flexors, followed by finger extensor weakness. Serum CK is mildly elevated, and muscle biopsy shows nonspecific myopathic changes. This disease is linked to chromosome 14q11.

Autosomal-dominant late adult-onset distal myopathy. Markesbery et al.[9] and Udd et al.[10] described a late-onset autosomal-dominant myopathy with weakness beginning in the anterior compartment of the legs, usually after age 40; it also involves the finger extensors. Some patients might have cardiomyopathy. Serum CK is normal or slightly elevated. EMG is "myopathic" and muscle biopsy shows prominent vacuoles. The disease was thought to be linked to chromosome 2q31[11] and caused by a defect in the gene-expressing protein titin. A recent

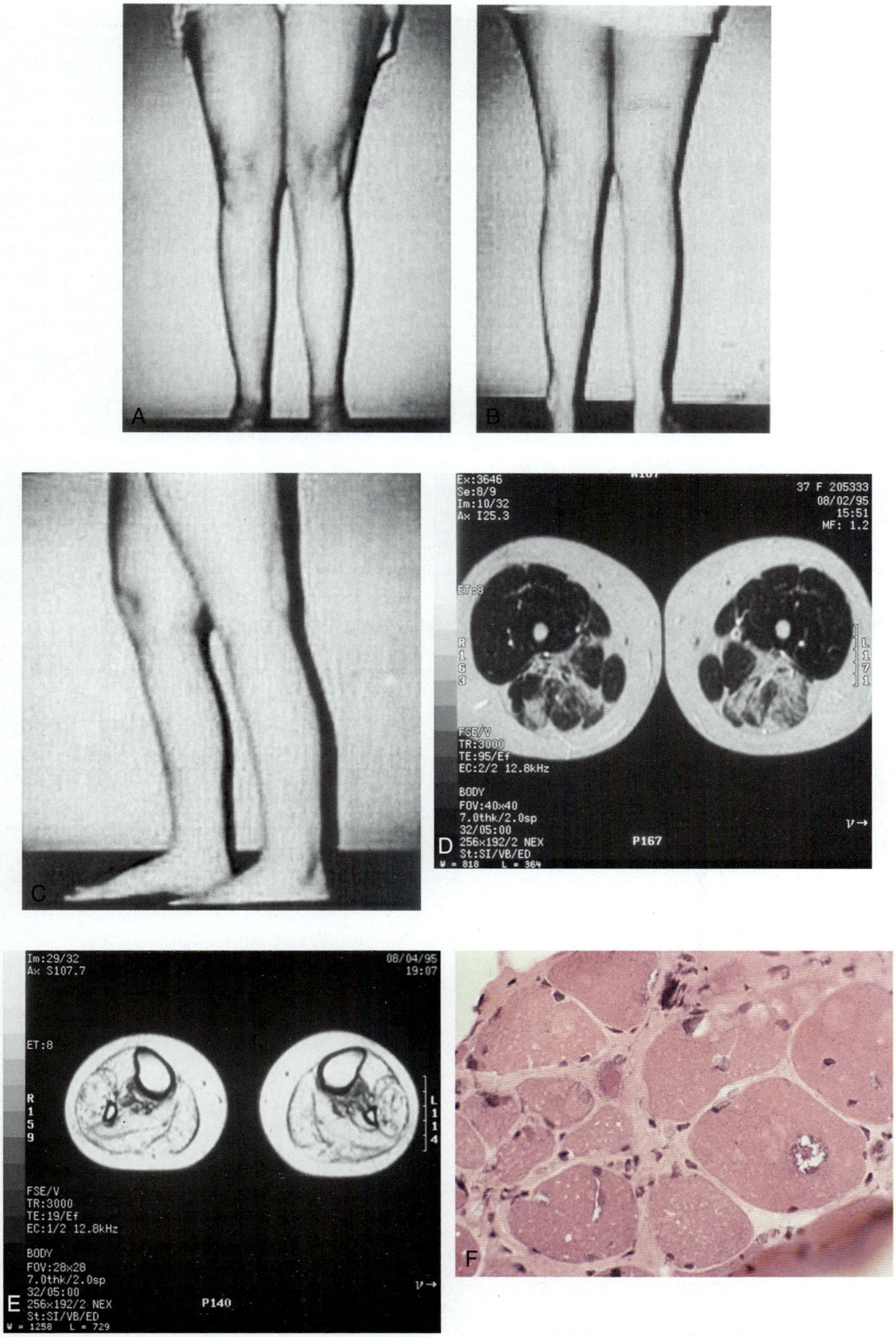

FIG. 82-3 **A–C**, Patient with quadriceps-sparing distal muscular atrophy; notice distal leg atrophy. **D**, MRI, T1-weighted image of the thighs of this patient, normal quadriceps, and atrophic hamstrings. **E**, MRI of the legs, T1-weighted image; notice atrophy and fat replacement of anterior and posterior compartments of the legs. **F**, Muscle biopsy of the patient with quadriceps-sparing myopathy showing rimmed vacuoles, fiber atrophy, and proliferation of connective tissue (H&E stain, ×400).

report, however, documented a mutation of the Z-band alternatively spliced PDZ-motif–containing protein.[12]

Welander distal myopathy appears in adulthood and was initially reported in Scandinavian families, having autosomal-dominant inheritance with weakness of neck flexors and the upper extremities[13] (Fig. 82-4). Serum CK is usually mildly elevated, EMG shows myopathic features, and muscle biopsy shows rimmed vacuoles. Welander myopathy is linked to chromosome 2p13,[14] as are Miyoshi myopathy and limb-girdle dystrophy 2B. In Welander myopathy, however, there is no dysferlin deficiency.

Distal myopathy with vocal cord paralysis and pharyngeal weakness usually begins in the anterior compartment of the legs and later develops in the finger extensors. Muscle biopsy reveals myopathy with rimmed vacuoles. Molecular genetics has been linked to chromosome 5q31.[15]

Other distal myopathies include *myofibrillary myopathies*, which may present with distal weakness, although the presentation is heterogenous. In some cases weakness begins in the hands and in others in the distal lower extremities. A scapuloperoneal distribution and cardiomyopathy have been reported. The diseases have been linked to mutations of the desmin gene in chromosome 2q31,[16] the αβ-crystallin gene in chromosome 11q21/23,[17] and the myotilin gene.[18] Patients with limb-girdle dystrophy caused by caveolin deficiency could also present with distal weakness.[19] Recently, an autosomal-dominant distal myopathy affecting the posterior legs and anterior upper limbs was reported; the disease was not linked to any genetic defect associated with other distal dystrophies.[20]

The patient in this case had Miyoshi myopathy, a disease that manifests with predominant weakness and atrophy of the gastrocnemius/soleus muscles.[21-23] Frequently, however, patients later develop upper extremity and proximal leg weakness and become wheelchair-bound. Some patients present with asymptomatic hyperkalemia, proximal/distal weakness, or limb-girdle muscular dystrophy (LGMD) 1B.[24]

The genetic defect in this myopathy is located in chromosome 2p13 in the gene that expresses dysferlin,[25,26] a muscle transmembrane protein. Absence of dysferlin is demonstrated by Western blot and immunohistology. As discussed, the muscle biopsy shows dystrophic changes and prominent necrosis early; inflammatory reactions can also be seen. Dysferlin belongs to the ferlin family of proteins which may have a role in myogenesis and repair[27] and have interaction with caveolin-3 for signaling.[28] Dysferlin-deficient mice are susceptible to autoimmune disease,[29] and a similar mechanism could underline the inflammation seen in the muscles of patients with this disease.

There is currently no treatment for Miyoshi myopathy other than palliative care, bracing, and proper genetic counseling.

Miyoshi myopathy is allelic to LGMD 2B that is also associated with dysferlin deficiency but manifests with proximal muscle weakness,[23] suggesting that the phenotypic variation is caused by modifier genes. A late-onset distal muscular dystrophy affecting the posterior compartment, not caused by dysferlin deficiency, was recently described by Katz and colleagues. (Fig. 82-5 shows a patient with limb-girdle dystrophy).[30] There is no cure for this condition. Deflazacort did not help.[31] There is a single case with a response to prednisone, alternating daily with a low dose.[32] Obviously, no conclusion could be made from a single case. Experimental antisense therapy appears very promising.[33]

IMPORTANT POINTS

- Distal muscle weakness usually indicates a neuropathy but can be seen in some spinal muscular atrophies and myopathies.
- Myopathies with distal presentation include distal muscular dystrophies, inclusion body myositis, debrancher enzyme deficiency, myofibrillary myopathy, myotonic dystrophy, and rare cases of myotubular myopathy.
- There are various genetic defects and clinical presentations of distal dystrophies.
- Miyoshi myopathy affects the posterior compartment of the legs with preservation of feet muscles which are usually affected in neuropathies, and this is a clue in the diagnosis.

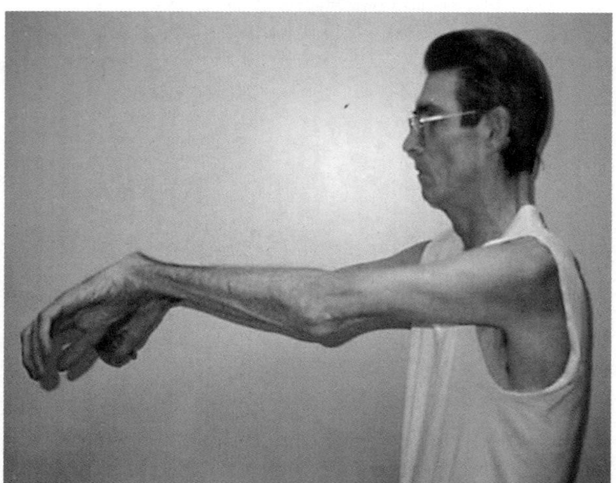

FIG. 82-4 Patient with Welander-type distal muscular dystrophy; notice distal atrophy and wrist drop.

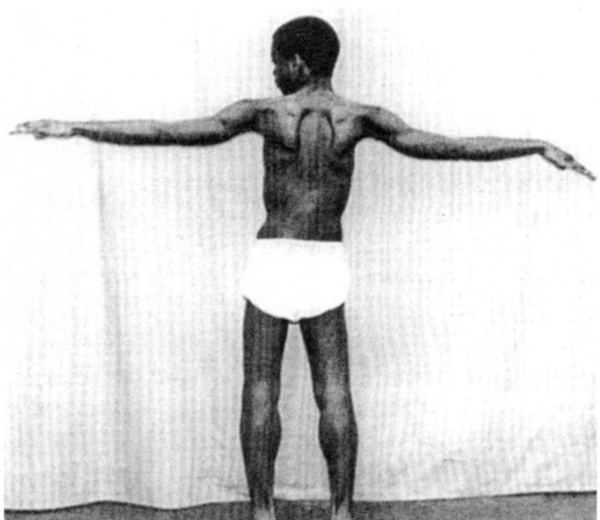

FIG. 82-5 Patient with limb-girdle muscular dystrophy with prominent proximal muscle wasting (compare with Fig. 82-1).

- Miyoshi myopathy is caused by a defect in chromosome 2p13 which causes a deficiency of dysferlin. The disease is allelic to LGMD 2B.
- There is currently no cure for Miyoshi myopathy.

REFERENCES

1. Penisson-Besnier I. Distal myopathies. *Rev Neurol (Paris)*. 2004; 160(2):211–216.
2. Saperstein DS, Amato AA, Barohn RJ. Clinical and genetic aspects of distal myopathies. *Muscle Nerve*. 2001;24(11):1440–1450.
3. Miyoshi K, Kawai H, Iwasa M, et al. Autosomal recessive distal muscular dystrophy: seventeen cases in eight families including an autopsy case. *Brain*. 1986;109:31–54.
4. Takahashi T, Aoki M, Tateyama M, et al. Dysferlin mutations in Japanese Miyoshi myopathy: relationship to phenotype. *Neurology*. 2003;60(11):1799–1804.
5. Nonaka I, Sunohara N, Ishiura S, Satoyoshi E. Familial distal myopathy with rimmed vacuole and lamellar (myeloid) body formation. *J Neurol Sci*. 1981;51(1):141–155.
6. Nishino I, Noguchi S, Murayama K, et al. Distal myopathy with rimmed vacuoles is allelic to hereditary inclusion body myopathy. *Neurology*. 2002;59(11):1689–1693.
7. Ikeuchi T, Asaka T, Saito M, et al. Gene locus for autosomal recessive distal myopathy with rimmed vacuoles maps to chromosome 9. *Ann Neurol*. 1997;42(4):432–437.
8. Laing NG, Laing BA, Meredith C, et al. Autosomal dominant distal myopathy: linkage to chromosome 14. *Am J Hum Genet*. 1995;56(2):422–427.
9. Markesbery WR, Griggs RC, Leach RP, Lapham LW. Late onset hereditary distal myopathy. *Neurology*. 1974;24(2): 127–134.
10. Udd B, Kaarianen H, Somer H. Muscular dystrophy with separate clinical phenotypes in a large family. *Muscle Nerve*. 1991;14(11):1050–1058.
11. Udd B, Haravouri H, Griggs R. Tibial muscular dystrophy (TMD) late onset distal myopathy (LODM, Markesbery and Griggs): an update. *Muscle Nerve*. 1998;21(Suppl 7):S656.
12. Griggs R, Vihola A, Hackman P, et al. Zaspopathy in a large classic late-onset distal myopathy family. *Brain*. 2007;130: 1485–1496.
13. Welander L. Myopathia distalis tarda hereditaria: 249 examined cases in 72 pedigrees. *Acta Med Scand Suppl*. 1951;265:S1–S124.
14. Ahlberg G, von Tell D, Borg K, et al. Genetic linkage of Welander distal myopathy to chromosome 2p13. *Ann Neurol*. 1999;46(3):399–404.
15. Feit H, Silbergleit A, Schneider LB, et al. Vocal cord and pharyngeal weakness with autosomal dominant distal myopathy: clinical description and gene localization to 5q31. *Am J Hum Genet*. 1998;63(6):1732–1742.
16. Dalakas MC, Park KY, Semino-Mora C, et al. Desmin myopathy, a skeletal myopathy with cardiomyopathy caused by mutations in the desmin gene. *N Engl J Med*. 2000;342(11):770–780.
17. Vicart P, Caron A, Guicheney P, et al. A missense mutation in the alpha B-crystallin chaperone gene causes desmin-related myopathy. *Nat Genet*. 1998;20(1):92–95.
18. Selcen D, Engel AG. Mutations in myotilin cause myofibrillar myopathy. *Neurology*. 2004;62(8):1363–1371.
19. Woodman SE, Sotgia F, Galbiati F, et al. Caveolinopathies: mutations in caveolin-3 cause four distinct autosomal dominant muscle diseases. *Neurology*. 2004;62(4):538–543.
20. Williams DR, Reardon K, Roberts L, et al. A new dominant distal myopathy affecting posterior leg and anterior upper extremity muscles. *Neurology*. 2005;64:1245–1254.
21. Yildiz H, Emre U, Coskun O, et al. Distal muscular dystrophy of the Miyoshi type. *Clin Neuropathol*. 2003;22(4):204–208.
22. Khadilkar SV, Singh RK, Kulkarni K, Chitale AL. A study of clinical and laboratory features of 14 Indian patients with dysferlinopathy. *J Clin Neuromuscul Dis*. 2004;6:1–8.
23. Mahjneh I, Passos-Bueno MR, Zatz M, et al. The phenotype of chromosome 2p-linked limb-girdle muscular dystrophy. *Neuromuscul Disord*. 1996;6:483–490.
24. Nguyen K, Bassez G, Krahn M, et al. Phenotype study in 40 patients with dysferlin gene mutations high frequency of atypical phenotypes. *Arch Neurol*. 2007;64(8):1176–1182.
25. Bejaoui K, Hirabayashi K, Hentati F, et al. Linkage of Miyoshi myopathy (distal autosomal recessive muscular dystrophy) locus to chromosome 2p12–14. *Neurology*. 1995;45:768–772.
26. Bushby KM. Dysferlin and muscular dystrophy. *Acta Neurol Belg*. 2000;100(3):142–145.
27. Bansal D, Miyake K, Vogel SS, et al. Defective membrane repair in dysferlin-deficient muscular dystrophy. *Nature*. 2003;423 (6936):168–172.
28. Matsuda C, Hayashi YK, Ogawa M, et al. The sarcolemmal proteins dysferlin and caveolin-3 interact in skeletal muscle. *Hum Mol Genet*. 2001;10:1761–1766.
29. Matsubara S, Kitaguchi T, Kawata A, et al. Experimental allergic myositis in SJL/J mouse: reappraisal of immune reaction based on changes after single immunization. *J Neuroimmunol*. 2001;119(2):223–230.
30. Katz JS, Rando TA, Barohn RJ, et al. Late-onset distal muscular dystrophy affecting the posterior calves. *Muscle Nerve*. 2003; 28(4):443–448.
31. Walter MC, Reilich P, Thiele S, Schessl J, et al. Treatment of dysferlinopathy with deflazacort: a double-blind, placebo-controlled clinical trial. *Orphanet J Rare Dis*. 2013;8:26. Online.
32. Takahashi K.. Effects of prednisone on a patient with dysferlinopathy assessed by maximal voluntary isometric contraction: alternate-day low-dose administration for a 17-year period. *Case Rep Neurol*. 2019;11:10–16.
33. Lee JJA, Maruyama R, Duddy W, Sakurai H, et al. Identification of novel antisense-mediated exon skipping targets in DYSF for therapeutic treatment of dysferlinopathy. *Mol Ther Nucleic Acids*. 2018;13:596–604.

83 CASE

A Boy With Proximal Weakness and Cardiomyopathy

A 14-year-old Caucasian boy presented for the evaluation of muscle weakness. He was born full-term to a 27-year-old multipara. The pregnancy was complicated by spotting during the first trimester as well as an episode of abdominal pain accompanied by nausea and vomiting at four months of gestation. The mother recalls active fetal movement. Labor was uncomplicated and the child was delivered vaginally. Birth weight was 9 lb 9 oz. Although early motor milestones were not recalled well, the mother stated that the patient was walking by 14 months of age. Toe-walking was noted early on. Although he played several sports as a child, he did not have the same endurance as other children. By the age of 11, he could not run at all. He became ill at the age of 13 with vomiting, jaundice, and multiple organ failure. Evaluation revealed a dilated cardiomyopathy. This was presumed to be viral in etiology, and he subsequently received a cardiac transplant elsewhere. After the transplant, he was noted to have difficulty climbing stairs as well as arising from the floor without using his arms. He did complain of occasional myalgias in the lower extremities. He denied muscle stiffness.

His medical history was significant only for a history of mild intermittent asthma. He rarely used an inhaler. Medications included tacrolimus, mycophenolate mofetil, citalopram, and montelukast. The immunosuppressives were to prevent rejection of his recent transplant. Family history was notable for parkinsonism in his mother aged 41. There are two siblings, a brother and a sister who are both normal. A maternal uncle, aged 33, is also normal.

On examination the patient was alert and cooperative. Mental status exam was appropriate for age. Cranial nerves II–XII were intact with the exception of a mildly enlarged tongue. Motor examination was notable for markedly enlarged calves. No atrophy was noted. Manual motor testing showed proximal weakness. Neck flexion was 4+. Deltoids, biceps, and triceps were 4/5, while wrist extension and grip were 5/5. Hip abduction was 3/5 and hip flexion was 4/5. Knee flexion was 5/5, while knee extension was 4/5. Foot dorsiflexion was 4/5. Foot plantar flexion was 5/5. The patient arose from the floor with a modified Gower maneuver. Reflexes were 1+ throughout and toes were downgoing to plantar stimulation. Sensation was intact to light touch, vibration, and pinprick. No dysmetria on finger-to-nose or heel-to-shin was noted. His gait was waddling with moderate toe-walking.

Initial laboratory studies from his referring physician were notable for an elevated creatine kinase (CK) of 13,103 units/L (normal, <200 units/L).

WHAT IS THE DIFFERENTIAL DIAGNOSIS FOR AN ADOLESCENT WITH PROXIMAL MUSCLE WEAKNESS AND CARDIOMYOPATHY?

The patient's proximal muscle weakness with retained reflexes, normal sensory exam, elevated CK, and possible cardiac involvement point strongly toward a myopathy. Possibilities include the following:

- Dystrophinopathies
  - Duchenne muscular dystrophy (DMD)
- Becker muscular dystrophy (BMD)
- Limb-girdle muscular dystrophy (LGMD)
- X-linked Emery–Dreifuss dystrophy
- Myotonic dystrophy type 2/proximal myotonic myopathy (PROMM)
- Disorders of carbohydrate metabolism
  - Acid maltase deficiency/glycogenosis type II
  - Debrancher deficiency/glycogenosis type III
  - Branching enzyme deficiency/glycogenosis type IV
- Carnitine deficiency
- Mitochondrial myopathy
- Inflammatory myopathies
- Hypothyroid myopathy

DMD is an X-linked disorder caused by mutations in the enormous gene *DMD* on Xp21 which codes for the sarcolemmal protein *dystrophin*. Most cases of DMD are caused by large deletions or duplications within this gene. The disease is characterized by normal gross motor milestones until the age of 2–3 years when parents may note that the affected child does not run or jump. Calf hypertrophy is common. While periods of stabilization may be noted, the disease is relentlessly progressive: the ability to walk is lost around 10–13 years of age.[1] Dilated cardiomyopathy is common and, given the availability of effective respiratory support, is now the most common cause of death. The posterobasal and lateral aspects of the left ventricle are predominantly affected. In contrast, the right ventricle is relatively preserved. Conduction abnormalities are uncommon until the cardiomyopathy is advanced.[2]

BMD is also caused by mutations within the gene for *dystrophin*. While the mutations in DMD typically result in a nonfunctioning or absent protein, those in BMD result in a protein that is present in reduced amounts or reduced function. This partial loss of *dystrophin* correlates with a milder phenotype.[3]

Symptoms of skeletal muscle weakness usually occur between 5 and 15 years of age and the ability to walk is maintained into adulthood. A range of disabilities exists, however, with some patients ambulating beyond the fifth decade. Death occurs from respiratory failure or cardiomyopathy.[4] The pattern of cardiac involvement is similar to DMD.[2] Cardiomyopathy may even be the presenting feature of BMD4. Some patients may only have cardiomyopathy with an elevated CK yet no muscle weakness. These patients can benefit tremendously from cardiac transplantation. Female carriers of DMD/BMD are also increasingly recognized as having dilated cardiomyopathy despite normal muscle strength or only mild weakness.[2] CK levels in DMD/BMD are usually elevated >10 times the upper limit of normal, especially within the first 3 years of illness. Levels may then decline as atrophy dominates. Of note, the degree of CK elevation does not distinguish between the major dystrophinopathies.[4]

LGMD is a clinically and genetically heterogeneous syndrome characterized by proximal weakness that has a variable age of onset and is often less severe than DMD, although some forms can mimic DMD/BMD. Calf hypertrophy is, as a whole, seen less commonly than in the dystrophinopathies. Both autosomal-dominant (AD) and autosomal-recessive (AR) patterns of inheritance have been described; however, the majority of cases are autosomal-recessive. Cardiomyopathy is a feature of some forms of LGMD, especially LGMD1B, 2I, and the sarcoglycanopathies (LGMD2C–F).

CK levels in the LGMDs vary from normal or mildly elevated to markedly abnormal as in the dystrophinopathies.

X-linked Emery–Dreifuss muscular dystrophy is a disorder due to mutation of the gene coding for the nuclear envelope protein *emerin*. An autosomal-dominant variant is also recognized and is listed under the LGMDs as LGMD1B. This may present with weakness in a limb-girdle or scapuloperoneal pattern. They also have early contractures at the elbow and ankle which are often more problematic than weakness. In addition, they are prone to cardiac conduction abnormalities and rarely dilated cardiomyopathy.[2] The CK is often elevated, up to around 10 times the upper limit of normal, although levels decline with age.

Myotonic dystrophy type 2/PROMM is less common than myotonic dystrophy type 1. It is notable for proximal rather than distal weakness and less muscle atrophy. Other manifestations such as endocrinopathy, balding, and cataracts are present but probably less common than in myotonic dystrophy type 1. Cardiac conduction abnormalities and cardiomyopathy may occur but are often late features and are thought to be less prominent than in myotonic dystrophy 1. The CK is usually elevated but not often more than five times the upper limit of normal.[5]

Disorders of carbohydrate metabolism, or glycogenoses often cause exercise intolerance, cramps, and myoglobinuria with or without affecting other organ systems such as the liver or heart. Some of these disorders, however, can cause fixed weakness. It should be noted that the cardiomyopathy associated with the glycogenoses is usually hypertrophic rather than a primary dilated cardiomyopathy. *Acid maltase deficiency (glycogenosis type II)* may present as a juvenile form with limb-girdle weakness and calf hypertrophy. A distinguishing feature of this disorder as well as some of the other glycogenoses is the presence of myotonia on electromyography (EMG). In contrast to the infantile form, cardiomyopathy is uncommon.[6] *Debrancher deficiency (glycogenosis type III)* can also present in a juvenile age group with fixed weakness and cardiomyopathy; however, the weakness is usually distal rather than proximal. Also, additional features such as exercise intolerance or myoglobinuria can occur.[6,7]

Brancher deficiency (glycogenosis type IV) may also present in childhood with myopathy and cardiomyopathy.[6,7] CK levels in the glycogenosis are often elevated to variable degree.

Carnitine deficiency, whether primary or secondary to systemic illness, has been reported to cause a myopathy as well as a hypertrophic cardiomyopathy. In systemic primary carnitine deficiency, presentation usually occurs before the age of 10.

Associated features include hepatomegaly, encephalopathy, and hyperammonemia (Reye syndrome–like illness). Serum carnitine levels are low as are muscle carnitine levels in the systemic primary form.[6] Carnitine deficiency causes moderate elevation of the CK.

Mitochondrial myopathies are characterized by proximal weakness and findings of ragged red fibers and/or COX-negative fibers on muscle biopsy. Several clinical syndromes exist, although genotype–phenotype correlations are poor. In addition to the proximal weakness the presence of sensorineural deafness, myoclonic epilepsy, heart block, ophthalmoplegia, or stroke-like episodes should raise the suspicion of a mitochondrial process. Plasma and CSF lactate may be elevated.[1,6] The CK may be normal or moderately elevated in mitochondrial myopathy.

Inflammatory myopathies are uncommon in the pediatric group. Polymyositis is believed to be particularly rare. Among the inflammatory myopathies, *dermatomyositis* is probably the most frequent.[8]

Hypothyroid myopathy may present with proximal weakness, myalgias, and muscle hypertrophy as well as cardiomyopathy in severe cases. Additional features suggesting the diagnosis include myoedema and constitutional symptoms. The CK level is often elevated.[9]

WHICH OF THESE DISORDERS IS MORE LIKELY TO AFFECT THE PATIENT?

Although one cannot be certain just from the history that the cardiac disease is related to the patient's muscle weakness, it is assumed that this is the case. While a number of the above conditions could account for our patient's findings, the most likely diagnosis is BMD. The next most plausible diagnosis would be an LGMD with a BMD-like phenotype. X-linked Emery–Dreifuss is less likely since the patient had only mild contractures at the ankle after significant weakness developed. Additionally, presentation with a primary dilated cardiomyopathy would be unusual for X-linked Emery–Dreifuss. Myotonic dystrophy type 2/PROMM appears unlikely, as there was neither clinical myotonia nor any systemic manifestation of the disease. Although hypertrophic cardiomyopathy may progress to a dilated cardiomyopathy, the severity and early appearance of systolic failure in this patient make carnitine deficiency and the glycogenoses less likely. Also, with the exception of acid maltase deficiency, a myopathy of the severity seen in this case is uncommon in the disorders of carbohydrate metabolism.

A mitochondrial myopathy is a consideration, although this is less common than BMD or LGMD. Additionally, no mitochondrial "red flags" as discussed above were noted in our patient. The low incidence of inflammatory myopathies in this age group along with the absence of dermatologic abnormalities in this case makes dermatomyositis and systemic sclerosis/overlap syndrome unlikely. Hypothyroidism in males of this age group is uncommon, and no additional findings support this diagnosis.

WHAT DIAGNOSTIC TESTING WOULD BE HELPFUL IN ESTABLISHING THE DIAGNOSIS?

Definitive diagnosis of DMD/BMD can often be accomplished noninvasively with the use of multiplex PCR or Southern blotting analysis of the *DMD* gene.

Approximately 30%–35% of cases will have false-negative results with this test. These patients have point mutations, small insertions/deletions, or splicing errors. Sequencing of the gene may be useful for these cases; this was not available at the time of the initial evaluation.

When genetic testing fails to identify a mutation, muscle biopsy is recommended. Immunostaining for *dystrophin* is then performed. Staining is nearly or completely absent in DMD, while it is often reduced or patchy in BMD. Unfortunately, immunostaining in BMD can occasionally be normal. Western blotting in these instances often shows a dystrophin molecule with an abnormal molecular weight, confirming the diagnosis. Muscle biopsy may also be diagnostic for the glycogenoses, mitochondrial myopathy, dermatomyositis, and certain forms of LGMD.

In the glycogenoses causing fixed weakness the muscle shows vacuoles containing periodic acid–Shiff positive material.[7] Mitochondrial myopathies often have ragged red fibers and/or COX-negative fibers. In childhood dermatomyositis, perifascicular atrophy is the most specific histologic feature. Histochemical studies are routinely available for only a few LGMDs such as LGMD2A, 2B, and 2C–F.

EMG is unnecessary for diagnosing DMD/BMD except in the rare instances where one needs to rule out spinal muscular atrophy. EMG can be helpful, however, in finding subclinical myotonia in PROMM or the glycogenoses.

Additional laboratory testing such as TSH and carnitine levels could be done. Serum or CSF lactate/pyruvate is also prudent when a mitochondrial disorder is suspected. Serologic tests such as ANA, ENA, and other autoantibodies may be done if the suspicion for dermatomyositis/overlap syndrome is high.

Finally, genetic testing is available for a number of the other myopathies listed above including PROMM.

RESULTS OF INITIAL DIAGNOSTIC TESTING

Genetic testing for DMD/BMD by multiplex PCR was negative. An EMG was not performed. The patient underwent biopsy of the deltoid muscle (see Fig. 83-1). On H&E and trichrome stains, there is fiber size variability with small round fibers. There were necrotic fibers and an increase in connective tissue. There was no inflammation seen. Notably, dystrophin staining by immunoperoxidase was entirely normal. Western blotting for dystrophin was not performed in this case. Staining for α-sarcoglycan was diminished in a patchy distribution. Staining for the remaining sarcoglycans was normal. Dysferlin staining (for LGMD2B) was also unremarkable.

What Is the Differential Diagnosis Now?

At this point, an LGMD is the most likely diagnosis. To date, 9 AD forms (LGMD1A–L) and 26 AR forms (LGMD2) have been described. This information is according to the classification of LGMD proposed by the European Neuromuscular Center of Classification in 2018, and this modifies the previous classification of 1995 which included disorders such as dystrophinopathies, and Pompe disease, for example (see Table 83-1). Gene products for most of these are known. While some LGMDs are due to mutations in structural proteins related to the dystrophin–glycoprotein complex, others alter nonstructural proteins and may have unique pathogenic mechanisms.

Although it may be difficult to clinically distinguish the various LGMDs, some novel differences exist. Some of the forms have only been described in a few families in certain countries.[10] Additionally, the frequency and prominence of cardiomyopathy vary. This occurs in LGMD1B, LGMD1C2–F, or LGMDR1 to 6 using the new classification and LGMD21.[11]

LGMD1B is a rare disorder, described in only four unrelated families at present. Its singularly unique feature is the presence of a marked dysarthria. No cases outside of Brazil have been reported.[10]

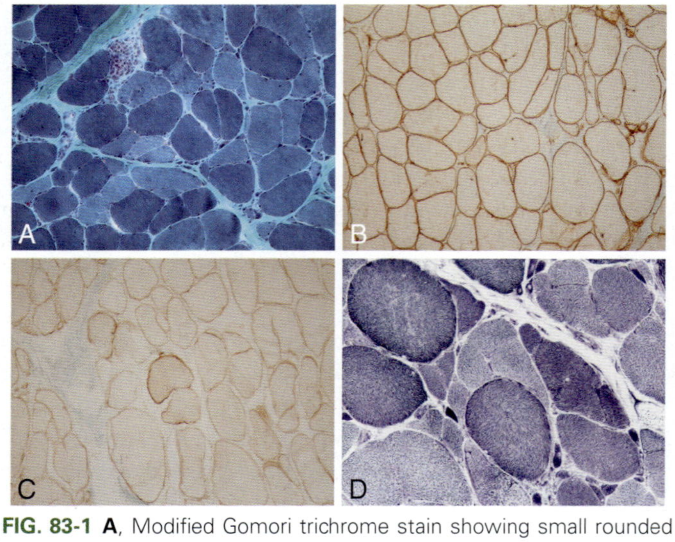

FIG. 83-1 A, Modified Gomori trichrome stain showing small rounded fibers, phagocytosis of a necrotic fiber and increased connective tissue (magnification ×200). **B**, Immunostain for dystrophin showing a normal pattern (magnification ×200). **C**, Immunostain for α-sarcoglycan showing patchy, slightly diminished staining (magnification ×200). **D**, NADH-TR stain showing atrophy of both fiber types (magnification ×200).

TABLE 83-1 Pathophysiological Classifications of Muscular Dystrophies

Disease		Locus	Gene	
Limb-girdle muscular dystrophy (LGMD) caused by sarcolemma or cytosolic protein defects				
X-linked				
Beckers, Duchenne's muscular dystrophy		XP21	Dystrophin	X-linked
Autosomal Dominant				
LGMD-1A (myofibrillar myopathy)	X	5q31	Myotilin	AD
LGFMD-1B (Emery-Dreyfuss muscular dystrophy	X	1q21	Lamin AVC	AD
LGMD-1C (rippling muscle disease)	X	3p25	Caveolin	AD
LGMD-1D (DNAJ86-related LGMD)	D1	7q36	DNAJB6	AD
LGMD-1E (myofibrillar myopathy)	X	6q23	Desmin	AD
LGMD-1F (TNPO3-related LGMD)	D2	7q32	Transportin-3	AD
LGMD-1G (HNRNPDL-related LGMD)	D3		HNRDL	AD
LGMD-1H	X	3p23-25	unknown-not confirmed	AD
LGMD-1L (calpain-3-related LGMD)	D4	15q15.1	Calpain-3	AD
LGMD-5	D5	COL6A1	collagen type 6 alpha 1 chain	AD
Autosomal Recessive				
LGMD-2A (calpain-3r elated LGMD)	R1	15q15.1	Calpain-3	AR
LGMD-2B (dysferlin-related LGMD)	R2	2p13.1	Dysferlin	AR
LGMD-2C (γ-sarcoglycan-related LGMD)	R5	13q12	Gamm-sarcoglycan	AR
LGMD-2D (α-sarcoglycan-related LGMD)	R3	17q21	Alpha-sarcoglycan	AR
LGMD-2E (β-sarcoglycan-relaed LGMD)	R4	4q12	Beta-sarcogycan	AR
LGMD-2F (δ-sarcoglycan-related LGMD)	R6	5q33	Delta-sarcoglycan	AR
LGMD-2G (-telethonin-related LGMD)	R7	17q11.2	Telethonin (TCAP)	AR
LGMD-2H (TRIM 32-related LGMD)	R8	9q31-q33	Tripartite motif-containing	AR
			32 (TRIM32)	AR
LGMD-I (-FKRP-related LGMD)	R9	13q13.3	Fukutin-related protein	AR
			(FKRP)	AR
LGMD 2J (-titan-related LGMD)	R10	2q31	Titin	AR/AD
LGMD-2K (-POMT1-related LGMD)	R11	9q34.1	Protein-O-mannosyl-	AR
			transfererase (POMT1)	AR
LGMD-2L (-anoctamin 5-related LGMD)	R12	11p14.3	ANO5	AR
LGMD-2M (-fukutin-related LGMD)	R13	9q31	Fukutin-related protein	AR
LGMD-2N (-fukutin-related LGMD)	R14	14q24	POMT2	AR
LGMD-2O (POMGNT1-rleated LGMD)	R15	1p32	POMGnT1	AR
LGMD-2P (α-dystroglycan-related LGMD)	R16	3p21	DAG1	AR
LGMD-2Q (plectin-related LGMD)	R17	8q24	Plectin 1f	AR
LGMD-2R (myofibrillar myopathy)	X	2q35	Desmin	AR
LGMD 2S (TRAPPC11-related LGMD)	R18	4q35	TRAPPC11	AR
LGMD-2T (GMPPB-related LGMD)	R19	3p21	GMPPB	AR
LGMD-2U (ISPD-related LGMD)	R20	7p21	ISPD	AR
LGMD-2V (Pompe disease)	X	17q25	GAA	AR
LGMD-2W (PINCH-2-related myopathy)	X	2q14	LIMS2	AR
LGMD-2X (BVES-related myopathy)	X	6p21	BVES	AR
LGMD-2Y (TOR1AiP1-related myopathy)	X	3q13.33	POGLUT1	AR
LGMD2Z	R21	6q21	POPDC1	AR
AR 22	R22	COL6A1	collagen 6 subunit	AR
AR 23	R23	LAMA2	Laminin 2 subunit alpha 2	AR
AR 24	R24	POMP6GT	protein O linked	
			Manose N acetyl glucosaminyl Transferase 2 (beta 1,4-)	AR

From Tesi-Rocha C, Escolar D. Treatment and management of muscular dystrophy. In: Bertorini TE, ed. *The Treatment and Management of Neuromuscular Disorders*. 2nd ed. Amsterdam, Netherlands: Elsevier; 2022. Table 20.1, Chapter 20; Straub BA, Murphy A, Udd V, LGMD working group. 229 ENMC international workshop on limb girdle muscular dystrophies nomenclature and refined classification. *Neuromuscular Disorders*. 2018;28(8):702–710; Bushby KM, Diagnostic Criteria for the limb-girdle muscular dystrophy report of the ENMC consortium of the limb girdle dystrophies. *Neuromuscular Disorders*. 1995;5(1):71–79.

Note: Those that with an X indicate that the disorder is not included in the classification of 2018.

LGMDB is caused by mutations within the *LMNA* gene. This is a single gene that can produce two gene products—*lamin A* or *lamin C*—via alternative splicing.

These proteins are ubiquitously expressed structural members of the nuclear envelope. Mutations within *LMNA* give rise to a surprising variety of conditions including CMT2B 1, Hutchinson–Gilford progeria syndrome, and LGMD1 B/autosomal Emery–Dreifuss muscular dystrophy. Patients with LGMD1B have a phenotype that is very similar to X-linked Emery–Dreifuss. This form of LGMD is also associated with prominent cardiomyopathy as well as conduction abnormalities and a high incidence of sudden death.[4]

LGMD1C is an uncommon condition caused by mutations in the gene coding for *caveolin-3*, a major structural component of skeletal muscle caveolae. Caveolae are 50–100 nm invaginations of the sarcolemma that are posited to have roles in cell signaling.[12] In addition to limb-girdle weakness, these patients may rarely have symptoms of rippling muscle disease.[12] This syndrome is characterized by subjective muscle cramping, pain or stiffness in addition to two phenomena: myoedema and muscle "rippling." Myoedema is a mounding of the muscle belly in response to percussion. The "rippling" of muscles refers to an electrically silent, slow-moving wave across the muscle that is precipitated by stretch. Dilated cardiomyopathy has not been reported with this disorder.[2]

LGMD1 D and *LGMD2 E–H* have been linked to separate chromosomes. There is, as yet, no distinguishing feature to these forms.

LGMD2A is thought to be a relatively common form of LGMD. The causative mutation is in the gene coding for *calpain-3*. Alterations of this calcium-dependent protease may result in apoptosis through its interaction with the NF-KB pathway. Alternatively, it may compromise remodeling of the cytoskeleton during myoblast fusion and repair.[2] Patients with LGMD2B may have prominent atrophy of the posterior leg compartment and/or hip adductor weakness out-of-proportion to surrounding muscles. Although a single case report of cardiac arrest as the presenting feature has been reported,[13,14] cardiac involvement is felt to be uncommon.

LGMD2B is caused by mutations in the *DYSF* gene encoding the protein *dysferlin*. Patients with mutations in this gene may present with a typical LGMD phenotype, a distal myopathy with prominent atrophy of the posterior leg compartment (Myoshi myopathy), or some combination of proximal and distal weakness.[4] Cardiomyopathy has not been reported.

LGMD2C–F are collectively referred to as sarcoglycanopathies as they result from mutations in the genes encoding for γ-, α-, β- and δ-sarcoglycans respectively. Sarcoglycans form an important component of the dystrophin–glycoprotein complex. The clinical phenotype is relatively severe and resembles DMD/BMD. Associated cardiac involvement is common in the p and 8 mutations, but rare in the others.[2]

LGMD2I or LGMDR9 is a form of LGMD caused by mutations in the *FKRP* gene coding for the *fukutin-related protein* (FKRP). Mutations in this gene cause a spectrum of findings from a severe congenital muscular dystrophy (MDClC) to the LGMD to asymptomatic carriers. *FKRP* is a putative glycosyltransferase. Evidence for its role in glycosylation derives from its structural similarity to other Golgi-resident glycosyltransferases. Additionally, immunostaining for sarcoglycans and α-dystroglycan is reduced, and the molecular weight of these proteins is lower than normal.[14] The clinical phenotype varies from a severe DMD-like disease to a mild, slowly progressive LGMD syndrome. Calf hypertrophy is common. Dilated cardiomyopathy and respiratory failure are not uncommon. In a recent series, 6/13 patients had evidence of cardiac dysfunction including one who died from heart failure and one other patient who was awaiting heart transplantation.[15]

Isolated cardiomyopathy without clinical muscle weakness has also been reported.[16]

WHAT IS THE NEXT STEP IN DIAGNOSING THIS PATIENT?

Although it was not done in this case, Western blotting for dystrophin would be quite reasonable to completely exclude BMD. The next logical step would be to perform genetic testing for LGMDs. Nowadays, next-generation sequencing will be most useful in screening, but this was not available when this patient was seen. Analysis of the *FKRP* gene disclosed two mutations. One allele had a 4 base-pair insertion at codon 165–166 resulting in a frameshift. The other allele had a cytosine to adenine substitution at nucleotide 826, resulting in an amino acid change of leucine to isoleucine at codon 276. This second mutation is very common in LGMD2I. It has been suggested that practically all patients with LGMD2I will be detected by evaluation of codon 276. Patients who are homozygous for this mutation are often less severely affected than those who are compound heterozygotes like our patient.

LGMD2I is increasingly recognized as a cause for a DMD/BMD phenotype with negative *DMD* gene testing and *dystrophin* immunostaining. The prominent cardiomyopathy, as described above, only strengthens the similarity. In a study of 102 sporadic male cases with clinical findings suggestive of DMD/BMD but no large deletion/duplication of *DMD*, 3 patients with mutations of *FKRP* were discovered.[17]

There is no specific finding on muscle biopsy in LGMD2I patients. Reduced immunostaining for α-dystroglycan and α-sarcoglycan can be seen as mentioned previously. One should be careful not to erroneously label these patients with LGMD2D based on this alone. In LGMD2D, immunostaining for any or all of the sarcoglycans will be reduced or absent.

It was concluded that this patient had LGMD 2DI caused by FKRP mutation, a disorder of muscle glycosylation.

What Is the Treatment for This Patient?

Currently, there is no specific treatment for LGMD2I or for any of the other LGMDs. The defect in glycosylation of elements in the dystrophin–glycoprotein complex that is responsible for LGMD2I has received some attention from researchers. It has been shown that enhancement of glycosylation of proteins by upregulating other enzymes can have a beneficial effect in animal models of muscular dystrophy, even when the primary defect is not in a glycosyltransferase.[18,19]

While corticosteroids have been shown to be of benefit to patients with DMD, there are no trials of this class of medications for patients with LGMDs. Creatine monohydrate has been investigated in DMD/BMD as well as some LGMDs such as the sarcoglycanopathies. There have not, to our knowledge, been any trials including patients with LGMD2I. The benefit in the studied groups is modest with no demonstrated functional improvement; however, side effects are also minimal.[20] Therefore some patients may elect to take creatine. Doses of 0.1 mg/kg/day are reasonable.

Given the frequency with which cardiomyopathy develops in LGMD2I, special attention should be given to monitoring this complication. Although no evidence base or consensus exists for LGMD2I, we can refer to a published expert consensus for DMD/BMD.[21] It is reasonable that a cardiologist evaluates all patients at the time of diagnosis, regardless of age. Cardiology visits should occur at least every 2 years until the age of 10 when they should become yearly. The ECG and Holter monitoring are useful in periodic monitoring of those with suspected arrhythmias. Echocardiography is frequently used, but in patients who are wheelchair-bound with significant scoliosis and resultant poor acoustic windows, MUGA should be considered. Once cardiomyopathy develops, medical treatment with ACE inhibitors or angiotensin-receptor blockers (sartans), blockers, digoxin, and a reduction in dietary sodium may be helpful as in any other patient. ACE inhibitors may also play a role in the prevention of cardiomyopathy as shown by a recent clinical trial that tested perindopril in boys with DMD.[22]

In those with left ventricular dysfunction and arrhythmias, an implantable cardioverter/defibrillator is recommended. Finally, cardiac transplantation can be done with a significant prolongation of life.[11]

In addition to cardiac surveillance, routine respiratory care is also recommended.

A consensus statement is available for DMD, and we can extrapolate their conclusions.[23] Monitoring of respiratory function should be done at each visit. Once a patient is using a wheelchair or has an FVC <80% predicted, they should be followed by a pulmonologist twice yearly. Additionally, the pneumonia vaccine should be administered as well as yearly influenza vaccines. Surgical intervention for scoliosis may be considered when it develops. Physical therapy and bracing as needed are also therapies that should be offered to these patients.

Because LGMD2I is a disorder of glycosylation, ribitol or a pentose alcohol formed by reduction of ribose partially restores the function of mannosylation of α-dystroglycan. In an animal model of muscular dystrophy, increasing levels of ribitol phosphate in skeletal and cardiac muscle lead to a reduction of pathology[24] and this can improve muscle function.[25] Ribitol has been beneficial in a phase 2 trial in the human form of this muscular dystrophy.[26]

IMPORTANT POINTS

- LGMDs may resemble DMD/BMD.
- Cardiomyopathy is common in inherited diseases of muscle and is a prominent component of LGMD1B, and LGMD2I, and the sarcoglycanopathies as well as DMD/BMD and X-linked Emery–Dreifuss dystrophy.
- LGMD2I is caused by mutations in FKRP, a putative glycosyltransferase.
- LGMD2I should be considered in all patients with a DMD/BMD phenotype with negative genetic testing and biopsy for these disorders.
- Treatment of LGMD2I is similar to DMD/BMD with the exception that the use of corticosteroids has not been evaluated in LGMD2I.
- Ribitol is a promising new therapy to improve glycosylation and function in this type of muscular dystrophy.

This case was reported by Mitchell CW, Bertorini TE, Shadle M. A boy with proximal muscle weakness and cardiomyopathy. J Clin Neuromuscul Dis. 2006;8(2):83–91.

REFERENCES

1. Bradley D, Fenichel J, Daroff R. *Neurology in Clinical Practice.* Boston, MA: Elsevier; 2004:2463–2510. 4th ed.
2. Muntoni F. Cardiomyopathy in muscular dystrophies. *Curr Opin Neural.* 2003;16:577–583.
3. Melanci P, Fanin M, Danieli GA, et al. Myocardial involvement is very frequent among patients affected with subclinical Becker's muscular dystrophy. *Circulation.* 1996;94:3168–3175.
4. Darras B. Muscular dystrophies. *Continuum.* 2006;12:33–75.
5. Day JW, Ricker K, Jacobsen J, et al. Myotonic dystrophy type 2: molecular, diagnostic and clinical spectrum. *Neurology.* 2003;60:657–664.
6. Walsh R. Metabolic myopathies. *Continuum.* 2006;12:76–120.
7. Tsujino S, Nonaka I, DiMauro S. Glycogen storage myopathies. *Neurol Clin.* 2000;18:125–150.
8. Dalakas M, Hohlfeld R. Polymyositis and dermatomyositis. *Lancet.* 2003;362:971–982.
9. Aminoff M. *Neurology and General Medicine.* 3rd ed. Cambridge, MA: Academic Press; 2001:317–339.
10. Laval SH, Bushby KMD. Limb-girdle muscular dystrophies – from genetics to molecular pathology. *Neuropathol Appl Neurobiol.* 2004; 30:91–105.
11. Spurney CF, Schramm JE. Cardiac complications of neuromuscular disorders. Chapter 3. In: Bertorini TE, ed. *Neuromuscular Disorders: Treatment and Management.* 2nd ed. Amsterdam, Netherlands: Elsevier; 2022:52–78.
12. Fee DB, So YT, Barraza C, et al. Phenotypic variability associated with Arg26Gln mutation in caveolin3. *Muscle Nerve.* 2004;30:375–378.
13. Dirik E, Aydin A, Kurul S, et al. Limb girdle muscular dystrophy type 2A presenting with cardiac arrest. *Pediatr Neurol.* 2001;24: 235–237.
14. Brown S, Torelli S, Brockington M, et al. Abnormalities in a-Dystroglycan expression in MDClC and LGMD2I muscular dystrophies. *Am J Pathol.* 2004;164:727–737.
15. Boito C, Melacini P, Vianello A, et al. Clinical and molecular characterization of patients with limb girdle muscular dystrophy type 2I. *Arch Neurol.* 2005;62:1894–1899.
16. Muller T, Krasnianski M, Witthaut R, et al. Dilated cardiomyopathy may be an early sign of the C826A fukutin-related protein mutation. *Neuromuscul Disord.* 2005;15:372–376.

17. Schwartz M, Hertz JM, Sveen ML, et al. LGMD2I presenting with a characteristic Duchenne or Becker muscular dystrophy phenotype. *Neurology*. 2005;64:1635–1637.
18. Barresi R, Michele D, Kanagawa M, et al. LARGE can functionally bypass alpha-dystroglycan glycosylation defects in distinct congenital muscular dystrophies. *Nat Med*. 2004;117:953–964.
19. Nguyen HH, Jayasinha V, Xia B, et al. Overexpression of the cytotoxic T cell GalNAc transferase in skeletal muscle inhibits muscular dystrophy in mdx mice. *Proc Natl Acad Sci USA*. 2002;99:5616–5621.
20. Tamopolsky M, Martin J. Creatine monohydrate enhances strength and body composition in Duchenne muscular dystrophy. *Neurology*. 2004;62:1771–1777.
21. Section on Cardiology and Cardiac Surgery Cardiovascular health supervision for individuals affected by Duchenne or Becker muscular dystrophy. *Pediatrics*. 2005;116:1569–1573.
22. Duboc D, Meune C, Lerebours G, et al. Effect of perindopril on the onset and progression of left ventricular dysfunction in Duchenne muscular dystrophy. *JACC*. 2005;45:855–857.
23. Finder JD. Respiratory complications in neuromuscular disorders Chapter 2. In: Bertorini TE, ed. *Neuromuscular Disorders: Treatment and Management*. 2nd ed. Amsterdam, Netherlands: Elsevier; 2022:40–51.
24. Cataldi MP, Lu P, Beaeser A, Lu. QL. Ribitol restores functionally of glycosylated α-dystroglycan and improves muscle function in dystrophin FKRP mutant mice. *Nat. Commun*. 2018;9(1):3448. https://doi.org/10.1038/s41467-018-05990-z.
25. Kanagawa M. Dystroglycanopathy: from elucidation of molecular and pathological mechanisms to development of treatment methods. *Int J Mol. Sci*. 2021;22(23):13162. https://doi.org/10.3390/ijms22231313162.
26. Harper A, Langsley R, Rodriquez H, et al. Open label phase 2 study of RVP-418 in patients with limb girdle dystrophy, type 2I. In: *Presented at the annual clinical and scientific conference*. MDA, Nashville, TN; 2022.

A Woman With Droopy Eyelids and Difficulty Swallowing

A 71-year-old woman presented with a 5-year history of progressive difficulty swallowing, mild hoarseness, and droopy eyelids. She had an esophageal dilatation procedure with some improvement in swallowing 3 years before presentation. She had some difficulty handling saliva and noticed a nasal twang in her voice but had no limb muscle weakness.

The family history was positive for a brother, her mother, maternal grandmother, and several cousins with difficulty swallowing. Past medical history was unremarkable.

On examination, she had normal mentation and cranial nerves. Extraocular movements were intact. She had ptosis with contraction of the forehead when looking straight ahead, demonstrating Hutchinson or "astronomer's" sign (Fig. 84-1). There was minimal weakness of the orbicularis oculi and of the neck flexors; limb muscle strength was normal. Reflexes were 1+ throughout without pathologic reflexes. Gait, sensory examination, and coordination were unremarkable.

Chemistry profile was normal, serum creatine kinase (CK) was 300 U/L (normal, <200 U/L) and serum lactate was normal.

WHAT IS THE DIFFERENTIAL DIAGNOSIS?

The differential diagnosis of this patient with difficulty swallowing and droopy eyelids includes mitochondrial myopathies which in adults could manifest as progressive external ophthalmoplegia[1] with ptosis and dysphagia but could have a more prominent proximal weakness. These can be sporadic or recessive and, rarely, are autosomal-dominant. Serum CK and lactate are frequently elevated, and muscle biopsy demonstrates the characteristic ragged red fibers.

Myasthenia gravis[2] should always be considered in patients with ptosis. That diagnosis, in this case, was unlikely because the symptoms did not fluctuate, and there was a positive family history. If myasthenia gravis is suspected, patients should be worked up for this disease, including a repetitive stimulation test; this test also helps to diagnose Lambert–Eaton myasthenic syndrome, which could present with mild ptosis and some dysphagia, but generalized weakness, fatigue, and areflexia are more typical.

Patients with inclusion body myositis[3] might have difficulty swallowing, but they have no ptosis and have distal weakness and prominent weakness in the quadriceps muscles. Patients with familial-inclusion body myopathy experience significant limb weakness, excluding the quadriceps, and have no dysphagia or ptosis,[4] except for familiar groups that also manifest with ophthalmoplegia.

Individuals with myotonic dystrophy[5] might have ptosis and later develop difficulty swallowing, but usually have typical facial features, distal weakness, and myotonia. There is also an autosomal-recessive oculopharyngeal-distal muscular dystrophy.

Other diseases that manifest with dysphagia, but without ptosis, include amyotrophic lateral sclerosis, bulbospinal neuromuscular atrophy (Kennedy disease), and polymyositis.

The most likely diagnosis in this patient is oculopharyngeal muscular dystrophy (OPMD).[6]

AN EMG TEST WAS PERFORMED

Motor Nerve Studies

Nerve and Site	Latency (ms)	Amplitude (mV)	Conduction Velocity (m/s)
Ulnar Nerve R.	Normal ≤ 3.6	Normal ≥ 8	Normal ≥ 50
Wrist	3.5	15	–
Below elbow	7.6	15	52
Above elbow	9.7	15	60

Repetitive Stimulation Study

Facial Nerve R.	Normal

Sensory Nerve Study

Nerve	Onset Latency (ms)	Normal Onset Latency ≤ (ms)	Peak Latency (ms)	Normal Peak Latency ≤ (ms)	Amp (μV)	Normal Amp ≥ (μV)	Conduction Velocity (m/s)	Normal Conduction Velocity ≥ (m/s)
Ulnar nerve L.	2.2	2.6	2.8	3.1	15	13	54	50

EMG Data

Muscle	Insrt Activity	Fibs	Pos Waves	Fasc	Amp	Dur	Poly	Pattern
Deltoid R.	Norm	None	None	None	**Dec**[a]	**Brief**	**Many**	Full[b]
Biceps brachii R.	Norm	None	None	None	**Dec**[a]	**Brief**	**Many**	Full[b]
Triceps R.	Norm	None	None	None	**Dec**[a]	**Brief**	**Few**	Full
Flexor carpi ulnaris R.	Norm	None	None	None	Norm	Norm	None	Full
Flexor carpi radialis R.	Norm	None	None	None	Norm	Norm	None	Full
Extensor digitorum com. R.	Norm	None	None	None	Norm	Norm	None	Full
First dorsal interosseous R.	Norm	None	None	None	Norm	Norm	None	Full

[a]No variability of motor unit action potentials was noticed.
[b]Rapid recruitment of motor action potentials.

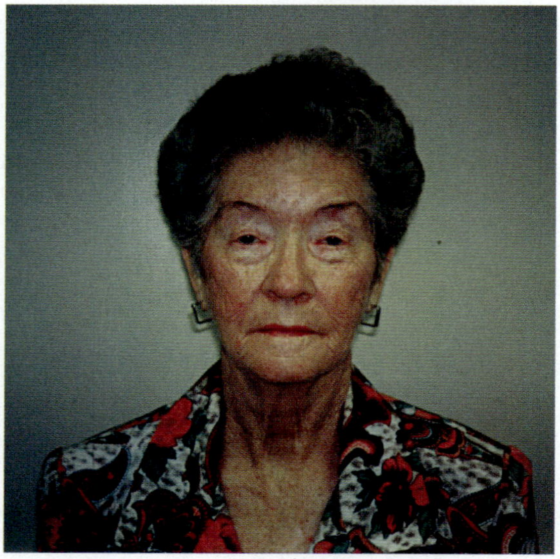

FIG. 84-1 Patient showing ptosis and the astronomer's sign, with contraction of forehead muscles.

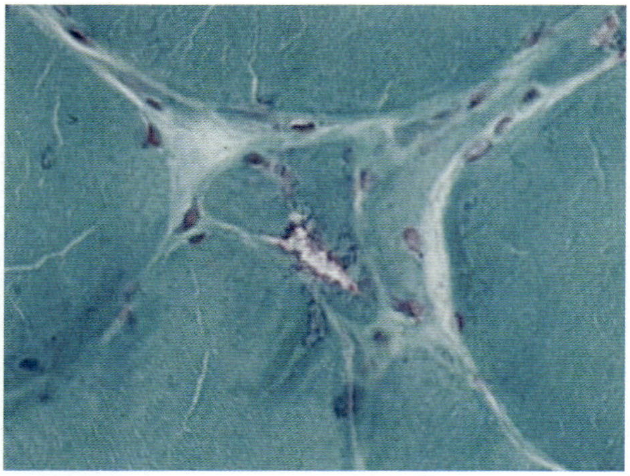

FIG. 84-2 Deltoid muscle biopsy showing a rimmed vacuole in an atrophic fiber (modified trichrome stain, ×400).

WHAT WERE THE EMG FINDINGS?

Motor and sensory nerve conduction velocities and CMAP amplitude and latencies were normal. Needle electromyography showed scattered small polyphasic motor unit action potentials with full interference patterns in the deltoid, biceps, and triceps muscles. No denervation potentials were seen. A repetitive stimulation test on the facial nerve was normal. These findings indicated that she had a myopathy.

An edrophonium test was not done, and acetylcholine receptor antibodies were not measured because of the positive family history, elevated serum CK, and normal repetitive stimulation results.

A left deltoid muscle biopsy showed a variation in muscle fiber size, an increased number of internalized nuclei, and small fibers with rimmed vacuoles characteristic of OPMD (Fig. 84-2). The patient later had DNA testing using PCR technology when this became available, and this showed six GCG repeats in 1 allele and 10 in the other (normal, <6) in the poly A-binding protein nuclear 1 (*PABP 1*) gene in chromosome 14q.

WHAT IS THE MEANING OF HUTCHINSON'S, OR ASTRONOMER'S POSTURE?

The astronomer's posture is a tendency for the patient to contract the forehead muscles to assist in raising the eyelids. This is classically demonstrated in the patient's photograph in Fig. 84-1.

DISCUSSION

This patient was diagnosed with OPMD, a condition reported initially by Taylor in 1915.[7] Later, in 1962, Victor et al.[8] described the disease in detail and used the current descriptive name. Patients usually present in late adulthood and characteristically have difficulty swallowing and ptosis, although some patients may develop proximal weakness, mainly in the upper extremities.

Serum CK is mildly elevated; the EMG could demonstrate small polyphasic motor units, and muscle biopsy shows characteristic rimmed vacuoles and atrophic muscle fibers.

The vacuoles (see Fig. 77-2) contain myeloid bodies and filaments of 15–18 mm in diameter. There are also characteristic 8.5 nm diameter filaments in the myonuclei.[8] The specimen could sometimes be normal, if unaffected muscles are biopsied.

OPMD has an autosomal-dominant inheritance, although, rarely, there are autosomal-recessive cases. The autosomal-dominant form has been reported in many countries, with the most frequent clusters occurring in the French-Canadian population, and apparently in individuals of Mexican origin in the American southwest. The highest disease frequency is found among the Bukhara Jews settled in Israel. OPMD is caused by short GCG repeat expansions in the *PABP 1*, previously abbreviated as *PABP 2*,[9,10] producing an accumulation of cellular aggregates. Patients who are homozygous are more severely affected. Two percent of the normal population has CGC7 exon expansion and patients who are heterozygous to the CGC mutations are more severely affected.[8–13]

The mutation causes the lengthening of a predicted N-terminus of the polyalanine domain. PABP 1 is an abundant nuclear protein involved in the polyadenylation of messenger RNAs[11]; it has been postulated that in OPMD there is a polyalanine toxic gain of function.[12–14] The protein in the intracellular inclusions is tagged with ubiquitin without being degraded. This suggests that the mutated *PABP 1* acquires new pathogenic characteristics and causes fibrillary accumulations by polymerization of misfolded polyalanine,[15] forming B-sheets which are resistant to nuclear proteasomal degradation, thereby interfering with cellular functions.

There is no cure for OPMD. There are currently very promising experimental studies with the use of adenovirus vectors, increasing the wild-type PABPN, and also the use of monoclonal antibodies that inhibit myostatin as well as improving mitochondrial function. Also because the mutated PABN1 may be toxic, pharmacological methods to decrease aggregates are very promising. The most important newer therapy is the use of autologous myoblast transplants from nonaffected to affected muscles.[16] Eyelid surgery[17] and cricopharyngeal myotomy are helpful[18]; gastrostomy can also be used.

SUMMARY

This woman presented with ptosis and difficulty swallowing. Her disease was autosomal-dominant, and her muscle biopsy, characteristic of OPMD, was found to have the *PABP 1* gene in chromosome 14q.

IMPORTANT POINTS

- Myasthenia gravis should always be considered in a patient presenting with dysphagia, ptosis, and ophthalmoplegia, as this is a treatable disease and can be diagnosed with proper tests.
- Other conditions with this presentation include oculopharyngeal dystrophy, mitochondrial myopathy, and myotonic dystrophy. Dysphagia, without ptosis or ophthalmoplegia, can also be seen in motor neuron diseases and polymyositis.
- The astronomer's sign refers to the characteristic of patients with OPMD to contract the frontalis muscles to elevate the eyelids.
- Muscle biopsies of OPMD show fiber atrophy and rimmed vacuoles with myeloid bodies and characteristic nuclear filaments.
- OPMD is usually of autosomal-dominant inheritance; however, there are autosomal-recessive cases. The dominant form is seen most frequently in French Canadians, but it is also prevalent in the Bukhara Jews living in Israel. The disease is caused by short GCG repeat expansions in chromosome 14q of the *PABP 1* gene. The repeat expansion stretches the first exon of the *PABP 1* gene.
- Patients with OPMD can be treated with eyelid surgery and cricopharyngeal myotomy.

REFERENCES

1. Holt IJ, Harding AE, Cooper JM, et al. Mitochondrial myopathies: clinical and biochemical features of 30 patients with major deletions of muscle mitochondrial DNA. *Ann Neurol.* 1989;26(6):699–708.
2. Drachman DB. Myasthenia gravis. *N Engl J Med.* 1994;330: 1797–1810.
3. Bertorini TE. Inflammatory myopathies (polymyositis, dermatomyositis, inclusion body myositis). *Comp Ther.* 1998;24:494–502.
4. Argov Z. Hereditary inclusion body myopathies. In: Engel A, Franzini-Armstrong C, eds. *Myology.* 3rd ed. New York, NY: McGraw-Hill; 2004:1211–1320.
5. Bertorini TE. Muscular dystrophies. In: Pourmand R, ed. *Neuromuscular Diseases: Expert Clinicians' Views.* Boston, MA: Butterworth-Heinemann; 2001:227–296.
6. Brais B, Rouleau GA, Bouchard JP. Oculopharyngeal muscular dystrophy. *Semin Neurol.* 1999;19(1):59–66.
7. Taylor EW. Progressive vagus-glossopharyngeal paralysis with ptosis: a contribution to the group of family diseases. *J Nerv Ment Dis.* 1915;42:129–139.
8. Victor M, Hayes R, Adams RD. Oculopharyngeal muscular dystrophy: a familial disease of late life characterized by dysphagia and progressive ptosis of the eyelids. *N Engl J Med.* 1962;20: 1267–1272.
9. Fan X, Rouleau GA. Progress in understanding the pathogenesis of oculopharyngeal muscular dystrophy. *Can J Neurol Sci.* 2003; 30(1):8–14.
10. Robinson DO, Hammans SR, Read SP, Sillibourne J. Oculopharyngeal muscular dystrophy (OPMD): analysis of the PABPN1 gene expansion sequence in 86 patients reveals 13 different expansion types and further evidence for unequal recombination as the mutational mechanism. *Hum Genet.* 2005;116(4):267–271.
11. Wahle E, Ruegsegger U. 3′-End processing of pre-mRNA in eukaryotes. *FEMS Microbiol Rev.* 1999;23(3):277–295.
12. Zoghbi HY, Orr HT. Glutamine repeats and neurodegeneration. *Ann Rev Neurosci.* 2000;23:217–247.
13. Brais B. PABPN1, dysfunction in oculopharyngeal muscular dystrophy. In: Karpati G, ed. *Structural and Molecular Basis of Skeletal Muscle Disorders.* Basel, Switzerland: ISN Neuropath Press; 2002:115–118.
14. Brais B. Oculopharyngeal muscular dystrophy: a late-onset polyalanine disease. *Cytogenet Genome Res.* 2003;100(1–4): 252–260.
15. Scheuermann T, Schulz B, Blume A, et al. Trinucleotide expansions leading to an extended poly-L-alanine segment in the poly (A) binding protein PABPN1 cause fibril formation. *Protein Sci.* 2003; 12:2685–2692.
16. Kang DH, Koo SHE, Ahn DS, et al. Correction of blepharoptosis in oculopharyngeal muscular dystrophy. *Ann Plast Surg.* 2002; 49(4):419–423.
17. St Guily JL, Perie S, Willig TN, et al. Swallowing disorders in muscular diseases: functional assessment and indications of cricopharyngeal myotomy. *Ear Nose Throat J.* 1994;73(1):34–40.
18. Yamashita S. Recent progress in oculopharyngeal muscular dystrophy. *J Clin Med.* 2021;10(7):1375. https://doi.org/10.3390/jcm10071375.

85 CASE

A Man With Facial and Shoulder Muscle Weakness

A 22-year-old man with a strong family history of muscular dystrophy (his father and one brother) complained of difficulty raising his arms. He denied weakness in the legs.

On examination, there was a mildly asymmetric smile and weak orbicularis oculi and oris muscles. Cranial nerves were otherwise normal. There was bilateral atrophy and weakness of the spinati, pectoralis, biceps, and trapezius muscles (Fig. 85-1). The deltoids were not atrophic and were strong when the shoulder was fixed by the examiners; there was prominent winging of the scapulae, as well as weakness of the biceps and triceps muscles. Distal upper extremity and lower extremity strength were normal. Reflexes were normal and symmetrical; coordination was intact; sensation was also normal to all modalities. No fasciculations were seen. There were no Babinski signs, and the rest of the neurologic examination was unremarkable.

WHAT IS THE DIFFERENTIAL DIAGNOSIS?

Spinal muscular atrophy is a consideration, but in these patients there is limb weakness and areflexia, and facial weakness is seen only rarely. Myasthenia gravis and myasthenic syndromes can affect facial muscles, but these are fluctuating rather than progressive, and patients usually do not have muscle atrophy. Polymyositis is another consideration, but this disease is not hereditary and only rarely affects the facial muscles. Mitochondrial myopathies can have limb and facial muscle weakness but also ophthalmoplegia, and the inheritance is not autosomal-dominant. Scapuloperoneal syndromes affect the scapulae and distal leg muscles, sparing the face.

The most likely diagnosis is facioscapulohumeral muscular dystrophy (FSHD), based on the positive family history of apparent autosomal-dominant inheritance, with facial as well as scapular and arm weakness and prominent winging of the scapulae.

AN EMG TEST WAS PERFORMED

Motor Nerve Studies

Nerve and Site	Latency (ms)	Amplitude (mV)	Conduction Velocity (m/s)
Median Nerve R.	**Normal ≤ 4.2**	**Normal ≥ 6**	**Normal ≥ 50**
Wrist	3.5	16	–
Elbow	7.3	16	57
Ulnar Nerve R.	**Normal ≤ 3.6**	**Normal ≥ 8**	**Normal ≥ 50**
Wrist	3.0	10	–
Below elbow	7.4	10	54
Above elbow	9.4	10	60

Nerve and Site	Latency (ms)	Amplitude (mV)	Conduction Velocity (m/s)
Peroneal Nerve R.	**Normal ≤ 5.7**	**Normal ≥ 3**	**Normal ≥ 40**
Ankle	3.9	8	–
Fibular head	10.6	8	44
Knee	12.8	8	45

F-Wave Studies

Nerve	Latency (ms)	Normal Latency ≤ (ms)
Median nerve R.	26.4	30
Ulnar nerve R.	26.7	30
Peroneal nerve R.	48.9	54

Sensory Nerve Studies

Nerve	Onset Latency (ms)	Normal Onset Latency ≤ (ms)	Peak Latency (ms)	Normal Peak Latency ≤ (ms)	Amp (μV)	Normal Amp ≥ (μV)	Conduction Velocity (m/s)	Normal Conduction Velocity ≥ (m/s)
Median nerve R.	2.4	2.6	2.9	3.1	35	20	54	50
Ulnar nerve R.	2.2	2.6	2.7	3.1	18	13	55	50
Superficial peroneal nerve R.	3.1	3.5	3.6	4.0	16	8–10	45	40

EMG Data

Muscle	Insrt Activity	Fibs	Pos Waves	Fasc	Amp	Dur	Poly	Pattern
Trapezius R.	Norm	None	None	None	**Dec**	**Brief**	**Many**	Full
Infraspinatus R.	Norm	None	None	None	Norm	Norm	None	Full
Deltoid R.	Norm	None	None	None	Norm	Norm	None	Full
Biceps brachii R.	Norm	None	None	None	**Dec**	**Brief**	**Many**	Full
Triceps R.	Norm	None	None	None	Norm	Norm	None	Full
First dorsal interosseous R.	Norm	None	None	None	Norm	Norm	None	Full
Trapezius L.	Norm	None	None	None	**Dec**	**Brief**	**Many**	Full
Biceps brachii L.	Norm	None	None	None	**Dec**	**Brief**	**Many**	Full
Vastus lateralis R.	Norm	None	None	None	Norm	Norm	None	Full

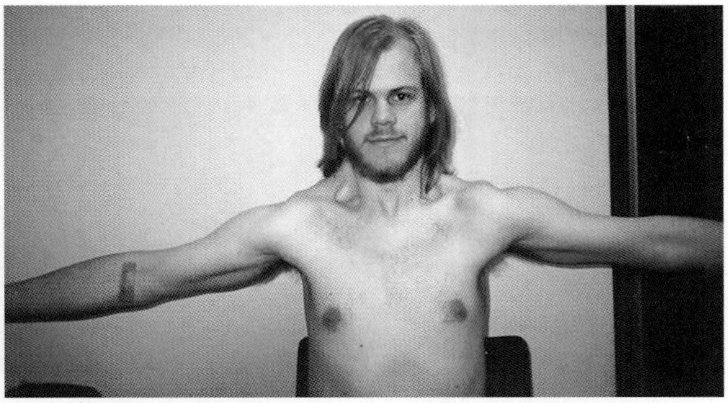

FIG. 85-1 Patient showing a mildly asymmetric smile and a trapezius "hump," as this muscle is atrophic and its apparent prominence is the elevated scapulae.

WHAT WERE THE EMG FINDINGS?

This study showed normal motor and sensory conduction tests. Needle studies showed no spontaneous activity but brief polyphasic motor unit action potentials, particularly in the trapezius and biceps muscles, suggesting a primary myopathy.

Serum creatine kinase was mildly elevated at 280 IU/L (normal, <200 IU/L). A muscle biopsy was not done.

WHAT SHOULD BE DONE NEXT?

Whole blood DNA testing was done by EcoRI and EcoRL-BInI using endonuclease digestion and Southern blot analysis; this showed one normal FSHD allele of over 48 kb and one abnormal allele of 23 kb (normal, >42 kb; borderline, 38–41 kb; FSHD, 12–37 kb), diagnostic for FSHD 1A.

DISCUSSION

This patient had FSHD 1A that defines the group of patients with FSHD with a known genetic defect. This case emphasizes that with the advances in molecular genetics, invasive tests such as biopsies, and even an EMG, might not be necessary, if the proper tests are ordered according to the clinical presentation.

FSHD is an autosomal-dominant muscular dystrophy with an incidence of 1/8,000–22,000, initially described by Duchenne,[1,2] but the disease is also called *Landouzy–Dejerine* form of muscular dystrophy after the detailed report by these authors.[3]

Later papers documented the autosomal-dominant inheritance,[4] and in a large study Tyler and Stephens reported a large pedigree that confirmed this form of inheritance and demonstrated the variable presentation in members of the same family.[5]

Characteristically, patients with FSHD manifest facial weakness prominently in the orbicularis oris and oculi (Fig. 85-2) and could have an asymmetric smile. There is prominent muscle weakness, usually asymmetric, with atrophy of the sternocleidomastoid, scapular fixator, and pectoralis muscles. There is usually winging of the scapulae that can become more evident during forward movements and during dressing and undressing.[6]

Weakness of scapular fixators causes the bone position to be more upward and forward, producing the "trapezius hump" (Figs. 85-3 and 85-4), giving the false appearance of a prominent upper trapezius muscle when observed from the front, when in fact this muscle is atrophic and the prominence is caused by the raised scapulae.

The deltoids are usually not affected or are only mildly weak, and patients may acquire a "Popeye" appearance because of biceps atrophy (see Fig. 85-4), while having fairly normal forearm muscles, except for the commonly atrophic brachioradialis. Weakness is frequently asymmetric and slowly progressive, although the progression can be stepwise.

The disease manifests in young adults, but the onset varies from ages 7 to 27 years[6,7]; earlier presentations are also seen. Patients might note a decreased athletic ability initially, and it has been suggested that increased muscle activity might trigger a decline in strength.[6]

Weakness of the lower extremities appears later, starting with the foot dorsiflexors. Sensory examination and reflexes are usually normal early, except that the biceps reflex might be depressed.

In some cases, there are retinal vasculopathy and hearing loss, and, rarely, patients develop difficulty swallowing.

Although FSHD is autosomal-dominant, some cases lack a positive family history. There is a suggestion of anticipation, but some children from affected parents might not be as weak, whereas mildly affected persons might have severely affected children. Early-onset cases may also manifest mental retardation.

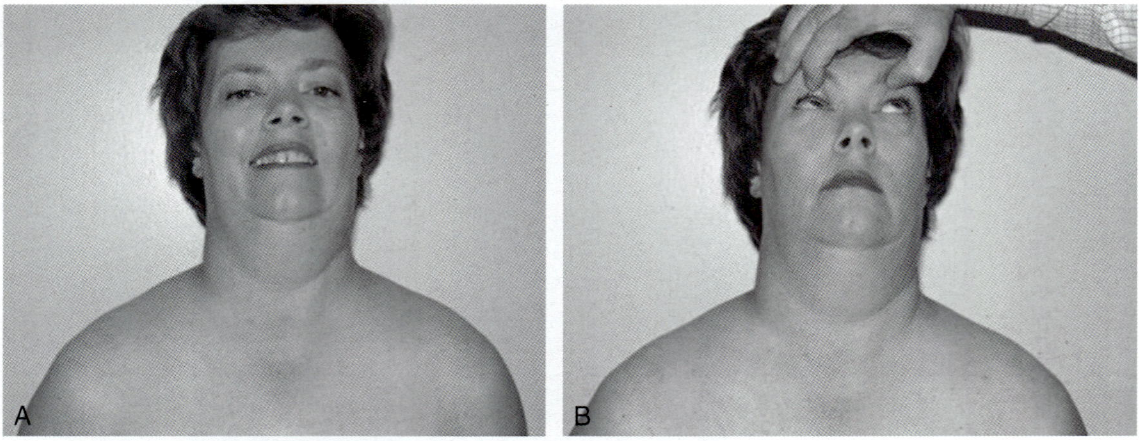

FIG. 85-2 **A**, A patient with FSHD showing a horizontal, asymmetric smile. **B**, The same patient showing weakness of the orbicularis oculi. *FSHD*, Facioscapulohumeral muscular dystrophy.

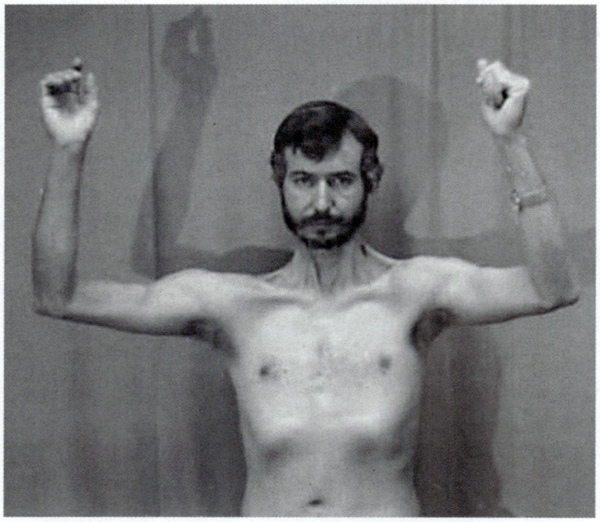

FIG. 85-3 A patient with FSHD showing atrophic trapezius, pectoralis, and biceps muscles; the deltoids appear normal. *FSHD*, Facioscapulohumeral muscular dystrophy.

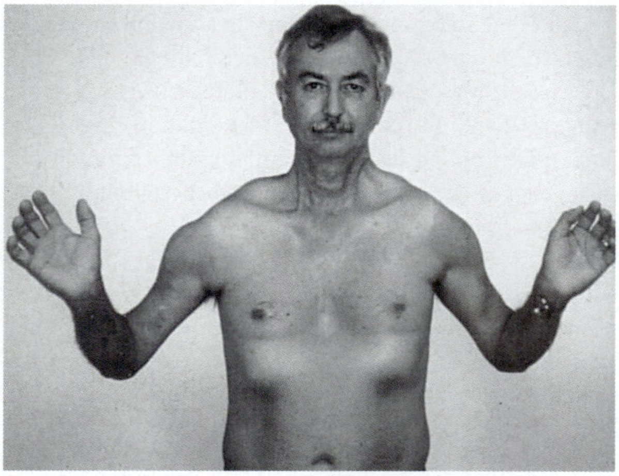

FIG. 85-4 A patient with FSHD showing a trapezius "hump" and atrophic arm muscles. *FSHD*, Facioscapulohumeral muscular dystrophy.

Serum creatine kinase is mildly or moderately high, and the EMG shows small polyphasic motor units in affected muscles. Muscle biopsy might show dystrophic changes and lobulated fibers (Fig. 85-5), and in some cases when the clinically

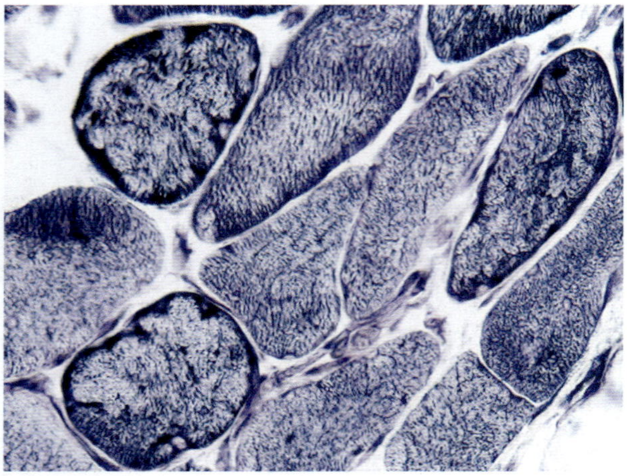

FIG. 85-5 A biceps muscle biopsy from a patient with FSHD showing lobulated fibers (NADH-TR, ×200). *FSHD*, Facioscapulohumeral muscular dystrophy.

unaffected muscle is biopsied, the findings are normal or nonspecific. Focal inflammation is not uncommon.

FSHD 1 was mapped in 1991 to the 4q telomere,[8] and the locus is at 4q35.[9] As discussed, some families are not linked to this locus.[10]

FSHD 1 is caused by a polymorphism of the EcoRI fragment in chromosome 4q35 that consists of multiple copies of a 3.3 kb tandem repeat (D4Z4 repeat). A smaller than normal number of repeats results in the disease.[11] The normal allele has 42–300 kb. In FSHD, they are usually smaller than 35 kb (FSHD 1A).

FSHD1 is the most common form of the disease in which there is decompaction of the D4Z4 resulting in contraction of the repeats increasing the expression of the distal homeobox protein (DUX4) which is toxic to muscle causing oxidative stress and apoptosis.[12]

In FSHD2, the less common form, there is a mutation of the epigenetic modifiers *SMCHD1* and *DNMD3B* genes which does involve chromatin metalation and also results in increasing the expression of DUX4 causing myotoxicity.[13]

The diagnosis of the FSHD is made with Southern blot analysis, but there could be some problems with this test, as the probes used in the analysis also hybridize to a segment in chromosome 10q,[14] complicating the interpretation, and this genome region that evolved independently from the 4q35 region has no disease association.[15] The use of restriction endonucleases obviates the problem; they cleave the 10q fragment leaving the 4q35 fairly intact.[11]

The treatment of FSHD is conservative. Fixation of the scapulae with straps, or using surgical wiring of the scapulae to the rib cage, might improve function (Fig. 85-6). Pain might be treated with nonsteroidal antiinflammatory drugs. Gentle exercise could be helpful and aerobic training appears to improve performance.[16,17] There are several therapeutic approaches to either diminish the increase of DUX4 or modify the effects. This includes the use of β2 agonists that appear beneficial, but albuterol showed only minor benefit.[14] A more potent inhibitor of DUX4 is clenbuterol that is promising but the benefits have not yet been confirmed. Myostatin inhibitors seem to increase muscle mass, but there is no clear evidence of increased muscle performance.

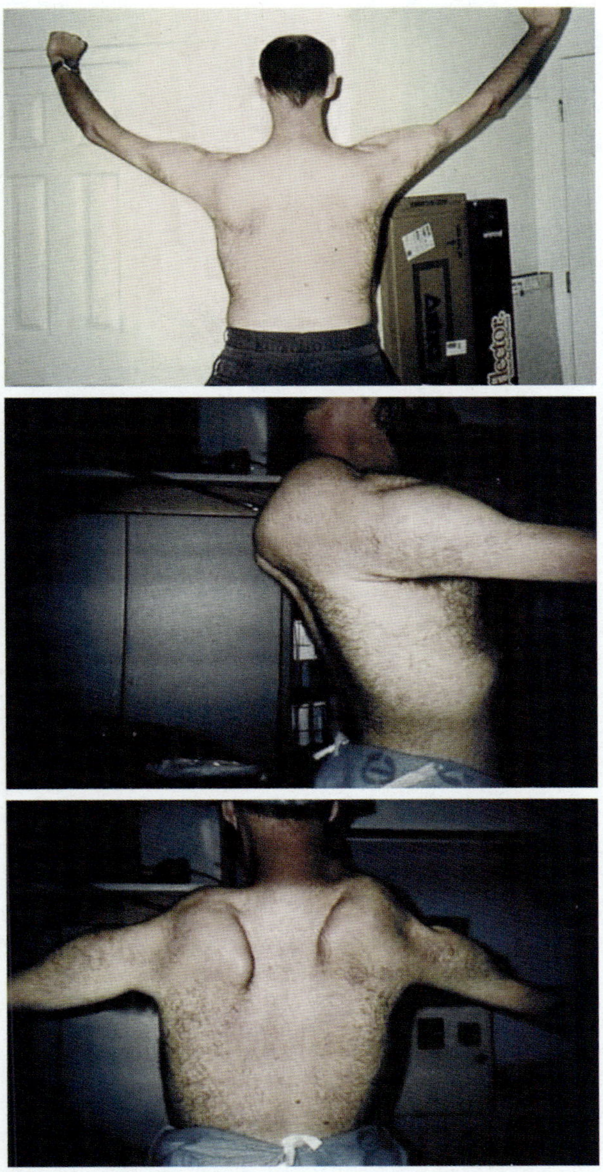

FIG. 85-6 A patient with FSHD after scapular fixation (*top*) recovering the ability to raise his arms. Compare the patient prior to surgery, when he was unable to raise his arms, lateral (*middle*) and posterior (*bottom*) views. *FSHD*, Facioscapulohumeral muscular dystrophy.

Aminoacyl-tRNA synthetases are enzymes that participate in the production of proteins and some like physiocrines have antiinflammatory effects and have been used in small trials.[13]

Creatine supplementation appears beneficial but has not been proven in clinical trials. Testosterone-recombinant human growth factor appears promising. Losmapimod AP38MAPK inhibitor appears to inhibit DUX4 and is undergoing trials. Antisense oligonucleotides inhibit DUX4 expression by interfering with mRNA slicing and processing or targeting mRNA degradation, and they have promising effects in animals. Finally, CRISP modification also has been found to be of beneficial effect in animal models.[12]

SUMMARY

This patient had a familial disorder characterized by facial and scapular weakness and was diagnosed to have FSHD. He had a genetic abnormality characteristic of the disease.

IMPORTANT POINTS

- FSHD is an autosomal-dominant progressive disease characterized by scapular and facial weakness. The disease is associated with a mutation of 4q35 in most cases (FSHD 1A). FSHD2 is caused by mutation of the *SMCHD1* and *DNMT3B;* both cause expression of DUX4 which is toxic to cells.
- The differential diagnosis of FSHD includes inflammatory myopathies, spinal muscular atrophy, scapuloperoneal syndrome, and mitochondrial myopathy.
- The best way to make the diagnosis of FSHD is DNA analysis in suspected cases, obviating the need for a muscle biopsy.
- There is no cure for this disease. Treatment includes straps or fixation of scapulae with surgery.
- Beta 2 agonist and creatine supplementation could be helpful. Losmapimod is a compound that appears promising. Myostatin inhibitors produce some benefit by increasing muscle mass but not performance. Physiocrines are currently being tested. Antisense oligonucleotides and the use of CRISP genetic therapies are very promising.

REFERENCES

1. Duchenne G. Recherches sur la paralysie musculaire pseudo-hypertrophique, ou paralysie myosclerosique. *Arch Gen Med.* 1868;11:5–25.
2. Duchenne G. *Album de photographies pathologiques.* Paris, France: JB Bailliere; 1862.
3. Landouzy L, Dejerine J. De la myopathie atrophique progressive. *Revue de Medicine Francaise.* 1885;5:81–117. 253–366.
4. Pearson K. Two new pedigrees of muscular dystrophy. *Ann Eugen.* 1933;5:179–191.
5. Tyler FH, Stephens FE. Studies in disorders of muscle, II: clinical manifestations and inheritance of facioscapulohumeral dystrophy in a large family. *Ann Intern Med.* 1950;32:640–660.
6. Flanigan K. Facioscapulohumeral muscular dystrophy in scapuloperoneal disorders. In: Engel AG, Franzini-Armstrong C, eds. *Myology*. 3rd ed. New York, NY: McGraw-Hill; 2004:1123–1133.
7. Walton JN, Nattrass FJ. On the classification, natural history and treatment of the myopathies. *Brain.* 1954;77:169–231.

8. Wijmenga C, Padberg GW, Moerer P, et al. Mapping of facioscapulohumeral muscular dystrophy gene to chromosome 4q35-qter by multipoint linkage analysis and in situ hybridization. *Genomics.* 1991;9:570–575.
9. Wijmenga C, Hewitt JE, Sandkuijl LA, et al. Chromosome 4q DNA rearrangements associated with facioscapulohumeral muscular dystrophy. *Nat Genet.* 1992;2:26–30.
10. Gilbert JR, Stajich JM, Wall S, et al. Evidence for heterogeneity in facioscapulohumeral muscular dystrophy (FSHD). *Am J Hum Genet.* 1993;53:401–408.
11. Fisher J, Upadhyaya M. Molecular genetics of facioscapulohumeral muscular dystrophy (FSHD). *Neuromuscul Disord.* 1997;7:55–62.
12. Lim KRQ, Yokota T. Genetic approaches for the treatment of facioscapulohumeral muscular dystrophy. *Front Pharmacol.* 2021;12:642858.
13. Cohen J, DeSimone A, Lek M, Lek A. Therapeutic approaches in facioscapulohumeral muscular dystrophy. *Trends Mol Med.* 2021;27(2):123–137.
14. Wilson C, Bellen HJ, Gehring WJ. Position effects on eukaryotic gene expression. *Annu Rev Cell Dev Biol.* 1990;6:679–714.
15. Winokur ST, Chen YW, Masny PS, et al. Expression profiling of FSHD muscle supports a defect in specific stages of myogenic differentiation. *Hum Mol Genet.* 2003;12:2895–2907.
16. Olsen DB, Orngreen MC, Vissing J. Aerobic training improves exercise performance in facioscapulohumeral muscular dystrophy. *Neurology.* 2005;64:1064–1066.
17. Tawil R, Van Der Maarel SM. Facioscapulohumeral muscular dystrophy. *Muscle Nerve.* 2006;34:1–15.

A Boy Born Floppy With Severe Weakness and, Later, Contractures

This patient was initially evaluated elsewhere when he presented as a "floppy baby." He was born at term of a 26-year-old primigravida; he was a 9-lb product of a 41-week gestation; the pregnancy was complicated by pyelonephritis. Respirations were normal at birth, but he was noted to be hypotonic and to have a weak cry. He was found to have torticollis at the age of 2 months. His scalp was mildly asymmetric; he was able to sit up at 5 months but could not pull himself up independently or raise his head against gravity at 2 years. He had never been able to walk.

MRI showed an increased signal on the T2-weighted image white matter. EKG and EEG were normal.

Family history was positive for porphyria in a cousin, a maternal grandfather, and a great-grandfather, and a first cousin of the mother had Charcot–Marie–Tooth disease.

AN EMG TEST WAS PERFORMED

Motor Nerve Studies

Nerve and Site	Latency (ms)	Amplitude (mV)	Conduction Velocity (m/s)
Ulnar Nerve R.	**Normal ≤ 3.5**	**Normal ≥ 5.6**	**Normal ≥ 49**
Wrist	2.0	6	–
Above elbow	3.6	6	51
Peroneal Nerve R.	**Normal ≤ 5.7**	**Normal ≥ 2.2**	**Normal ≥ 41**
Ankle	3.2	3	–
Knee	6.4	2.6	47

F-Wave Studies

Nerve	Latency (ms)	Normal Latency ≤ (ms)
Ulnar nerve R.	25.1	31
Peroneal nerve R.	42.0	52

EMG Data

Muscle	Insrt Activity	Fibs	Pos Waves	Fasc	Amp	Dur	Poly	Pattern
Vastus lateralis R.	Norm	None	None	None	**Low**	**Brief**	**Many**	Full
Tibialis anterior R.	Norm	None	None	None	**Low**	Norm	None	Full
Deltoid R.	Norm	None	None	None	**Low**	**Brief**	**Many**	Full
Biceps brachii R.	Norm	None	None	None	Norm	**Brief**	**Many**	Full
First dorsal interosseous R.	Norm	None	None	None	Norm	Norm	None	Full

WHAT WERE THE EMG FINDINGS?

Nerve conduction tests were normal. EMG demonstrated "myopathic changes" with many polyphasic motor unit action potentials. Serum creatine kinase (CK) was 1225 IU/L (normal, <200 IU/L). Left quadriceps biopsy showed "marked variation of fiber size, internalized nuclei, hypertrophic fibers, and no ragged red fibers." Histochemistry was reported as normal. He was diagnosed as having a congenital muscular dystrophy.

At the age of 2½ years his general physical examination and intellectual function appeared normal. He had contractures of the left elbow at about 20 degrees and had a limited range of motion of the ankles. The joints were normal. He was alert and responded properly to questions. Cranial nerves were normal except for mild bilateral facial weakness. There was diffuse hypotonia with wasting in the elbows. Reflexes were absent throughout. Pain perception appeared normal.

At the age of 14 years he had evidence of severe weakness with contractures and developed respiratory failure requiring tracheostomy (Fig. 86-1). He also developed staring spells and had generalized tonic/clonic seizures. EEG showed frontal sharp waves on the right side.

WHAT IS THE DIFFERENTIAL DIAGNOSIS?

This patient presented as a floppy baby. The differential diagnosis of this includes spinal muscular atrophy, but the lack of fasciculations and denervation on the EMG is against this disease. The lack of significant facial weakness and ptosis are against congenital myasthenic syndrome. The differential diagnosis should include central core, disease, nemaline myopathy, and myotubular myopathy that are unlikely because of the rather high serum CK, but this can be seen in congenital muscular dystrophy and congenital myotonic dystrophy. Acid maltase deficiency was a consideration, as this patient presented with only weakness and hypotonia, unlike the infantile form of Pompe disease, which also manifests with visceromegaly. The lack of myotonia on EMG is against this diagnosis. There was no evidence of a neuropathy.

Some mitochondrial myopathies could have similar MRI findings, but the reported absence of ragged red fibers in the biopsy is against this diagnosis.

A quadriceps muscle biopsy showed dystrophic changes with proliferation of endomysial connective tissue and fat with lack of merosin staining (Fig. 86-2).

The MRI was reviewed and this showed diffuse white matter changes on T2-weighted images (Fig. 86-3). The MRI and biopsy findings are diagnostic of merosin-deficiency congenital muscular dystrophy. (Figs. 86-4 to 86-9 show patients and biopsy findings of various other congenital myopathies.)

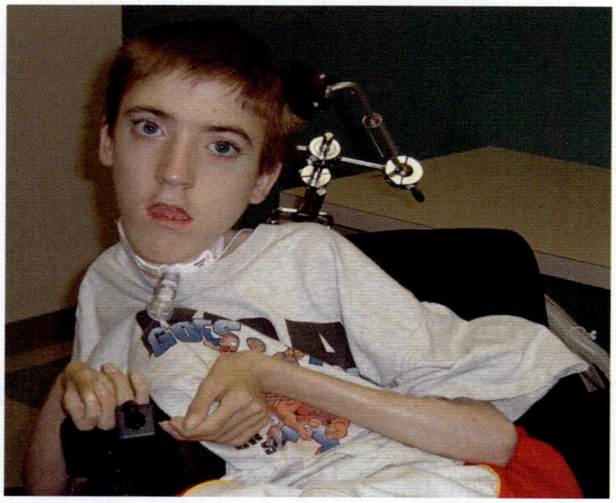

FIG. 86-1 The patient at age 14 with a tracheostomy and prominent contractures.

DISCUSSION

This patient was evaluated in early childhood for severe weakness and hypotonia and later at the age of 14 years when he presented with seizures. He was diagnosed as having congenital muscular dystrophy (CMD) with merosin deficiency.

Several forms of CMD have been reported since the initial description by Batten in 1903[1] (Table 86-1). Some of these might present with severe mental retardation. The most common form of CMD is caused by a deficiency of laminin α-2, or merosin (CMD 1A), as in this patient. This occurs in up to 50% of the cases.[2,3] It has an incidence of 1:30,000. The clinical characteristics of CMD 1A are relatively uniform in those with severe disease, caused by complete absence of the protein. They manifest early, even during pregnancy, with diminished fetal movement and may require respiratory support at birth.[4] Patients could have facial muscle weakness, but the extraocular muscles are not affected. The weakness in limb muscles is more proximal than distal. There is muscle atrophy and joint contractures but no muscle hypertrophy. A partial merosin deficiency might cause hypotonia and delayed motor milestones,[5,6] but many patients can remain ambulatory and even appear normal in adulthood or have a very mild limb-girdle syndrome.[7,8]

Serum CK usually is markedly elevated, unlike most other congenital myopathies (listed in Table 86-2).

Thirty percent of the cases develop seizures.[4] The degree of white matter changes is variable, and some patients have a low IQ. There is usually increased protein in the cerebrospinal fluid.

The characteristic white matter findings on brain MRI could be explained in part by the fact that laminin α-2 also expresses in the basal lamina of the brain blood vessels, including the capillaries that form the blood–brain barrier. There are, however, no apparent structural abnormalities in the nerve tissue,[9,10] and the exact etiology of central nervous system involvement is unclear.

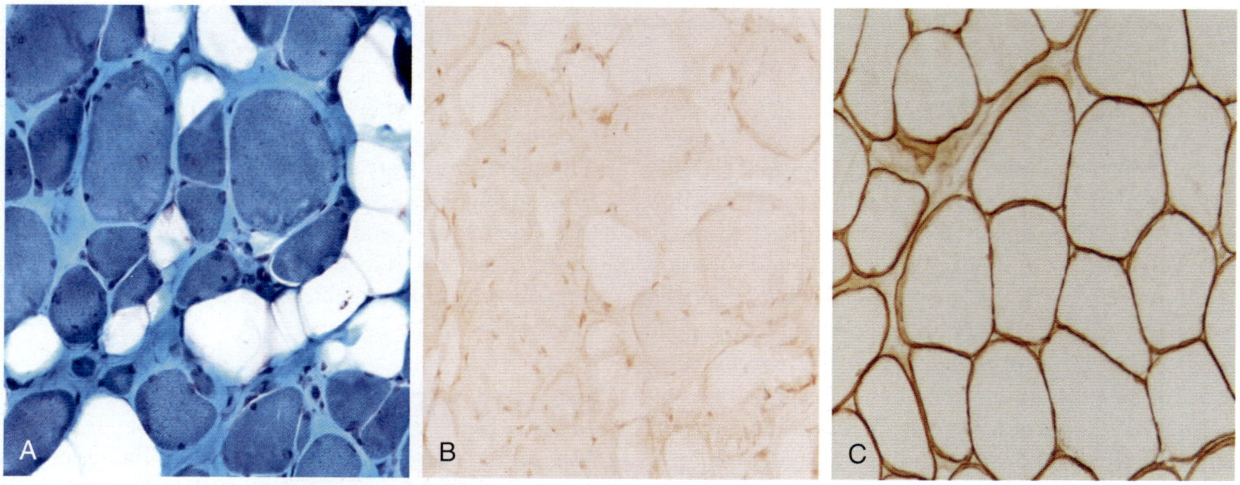

FIG. 86-2 **A**, Muscle biopsy showing dystrophic changes (modified trichrome, ×200). **B**, Absent merosin staining compared with normal control (**C**) (immunoperoxidase, ×200).

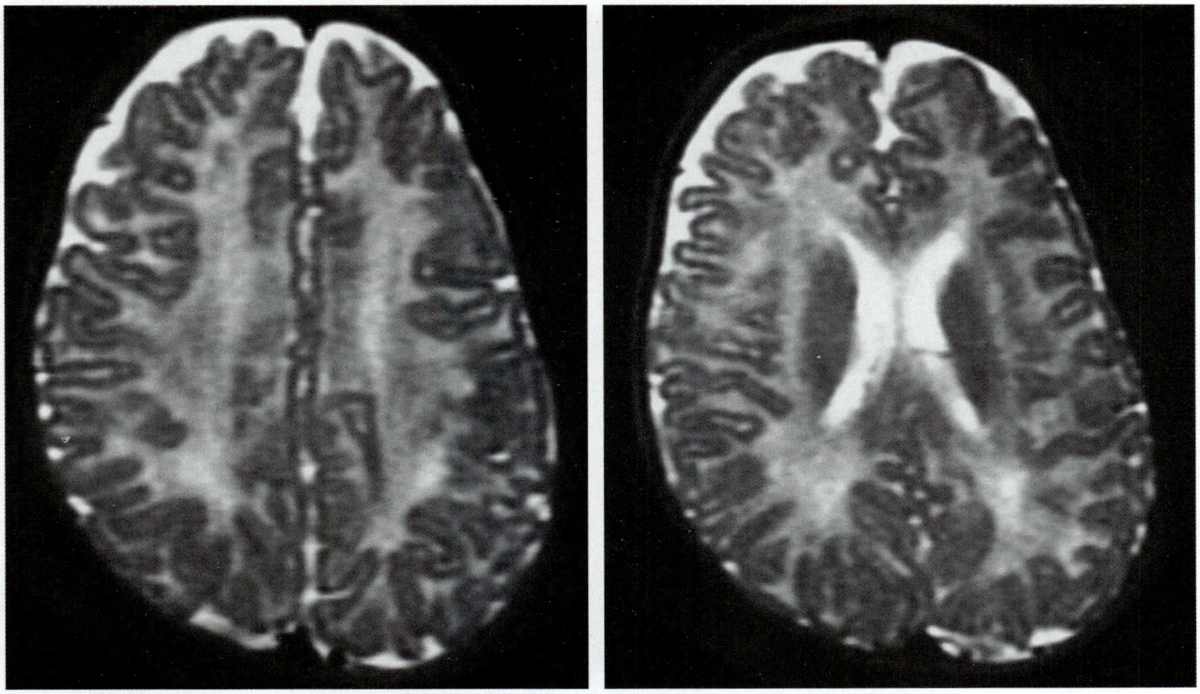

FIG. 86-3 MRI of the head of the patient at age 2; notice increased white matter signal in the T2-weighted images.

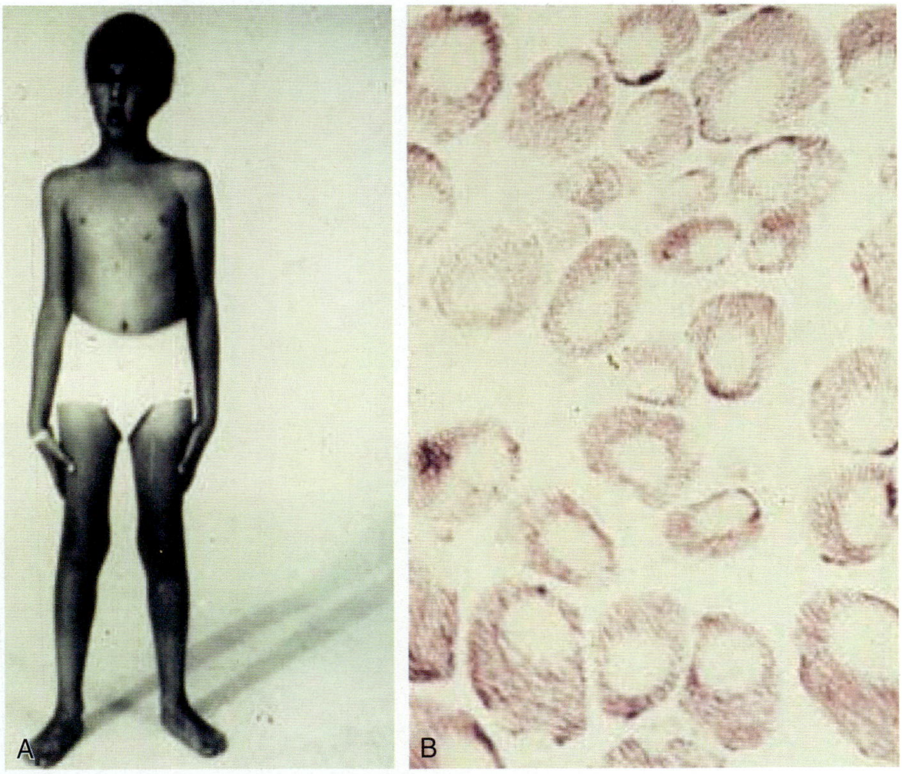

FIG. 86-4 A, A boy with central core disease. B, Muscle biopsy showing the cores with lack of oxidative stain (NADH-TR, ×200).

Merosin is also expressed in the endoneurium surrounding myelinated fibers and Schwann cells, causing demyelination which could result in nerve conduction slowing.[11] The protein also expresses in the heart, but cardiomyopathy does not occur. The skin in CMD 1A also reveals a deficiency of the protein between the junction of dermis and epidermis,[12] but this is not associated with clinical changes.

The muscle pathology in laminin deficiency demonstrates dystrophic changes with complete or partial absence of the protein, as in this case.

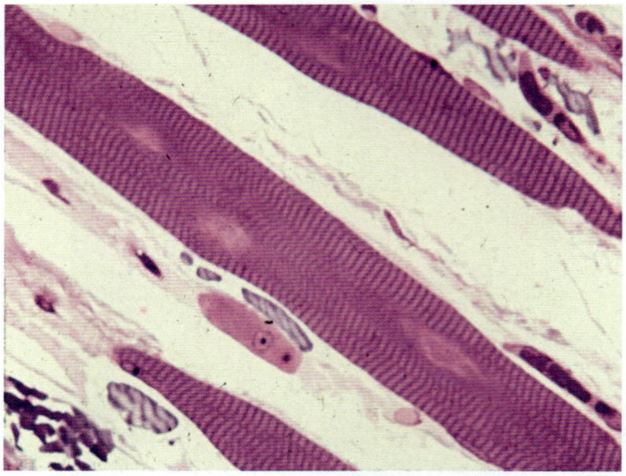

FIG. 86-5 Mini-core disease biopsy showing multiple small cores and proliferation of connective tissue (toluidine blue–stained, plastic-embedded section, ×400).

CMD 1A is caused by mutations of the *LAMA-2* gene in chromosome 6q2.[5,13] Merosin deficiency, however, has also been reported in cases not linked to this defect.

The laminins are important glycoprotein components of the basal lamina of most tissues, connecting the membrane with the extracellular matrix. They are secreted by the cells to the extracellular matrix where it forms polymers that bind a number of other macromolecules.[14] Merosin is important in the survival of myotubes, which could explain the muscle abnormalities of affected children.[15]

The treatment of CMD 1A includes physical therapy with stretching to alleviate contractures; anticonvulsant therapy could be necessary. There is currently no cure. There are many experimental therapies in animal models with the disease, and this includes the use of metformin and medications to reduce oxidative stress. Other therapies being considered include using the CRISPS method and stem-cell therapy.[16]

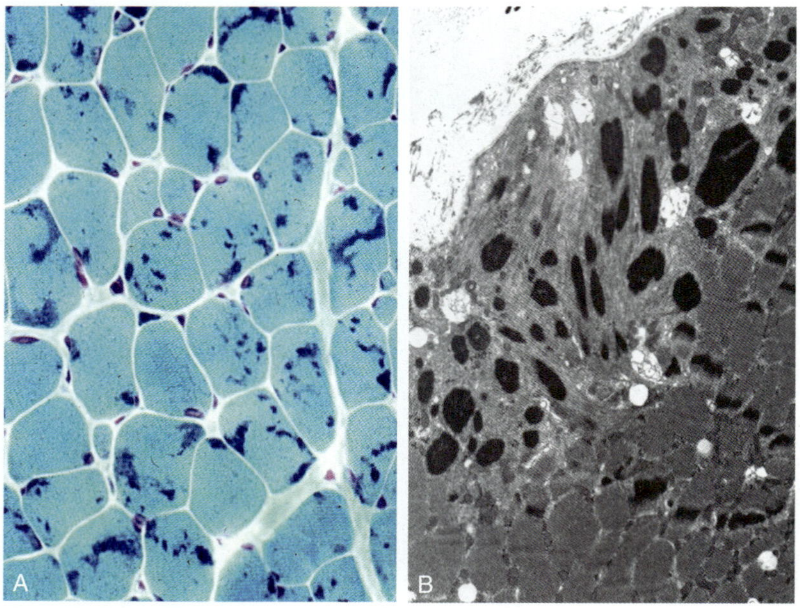

FIG. 86-6 Nemaline rod myopathy; notice the red nemaline rods on trichrome stain (×200) (**A**) and on electromicroscopy (×3000) (**B**).

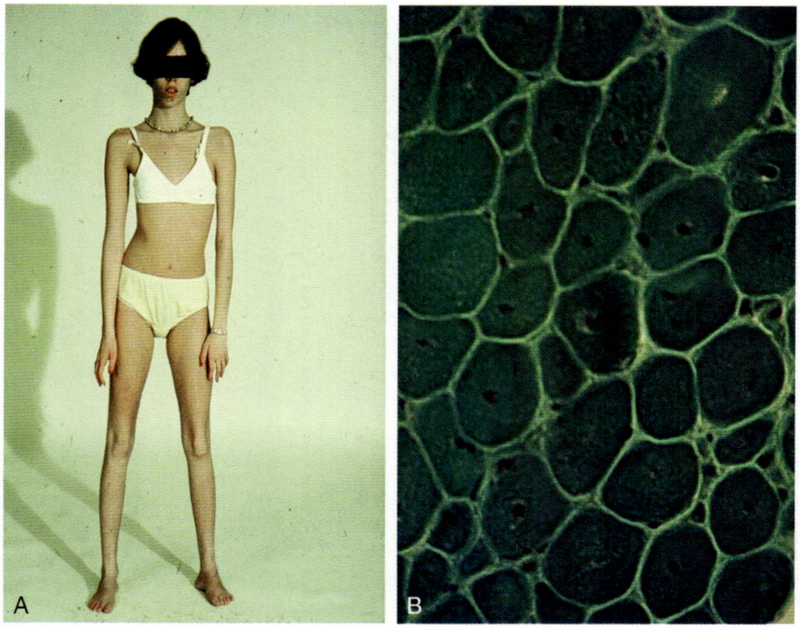

FIG. 86-7 **A**, A patient with myotubular myopathy; notice muscle atrophy and lordosis. (She also had ptosis.) **B**, Modified trichrome stain showing many fibers with centrally located nuclei; there is also fiber atrophy and proliferation of connective tissue (×200).

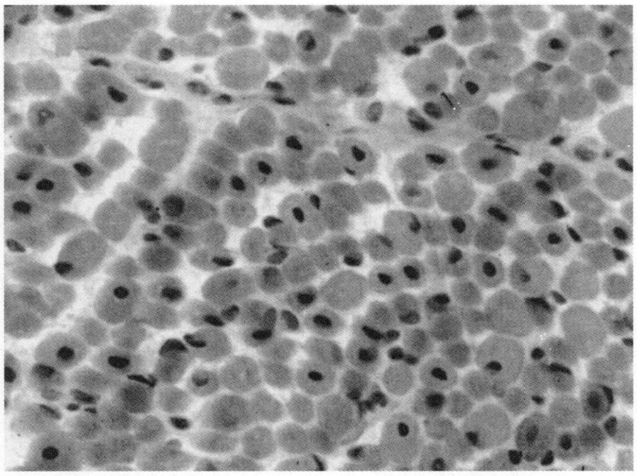

FIG. 86-8 Muscle biopsy of severe infantile myotubular myopathy showing many atrophic fibers and centrally located internalized nuclei (modified trichrome stain, ×200).

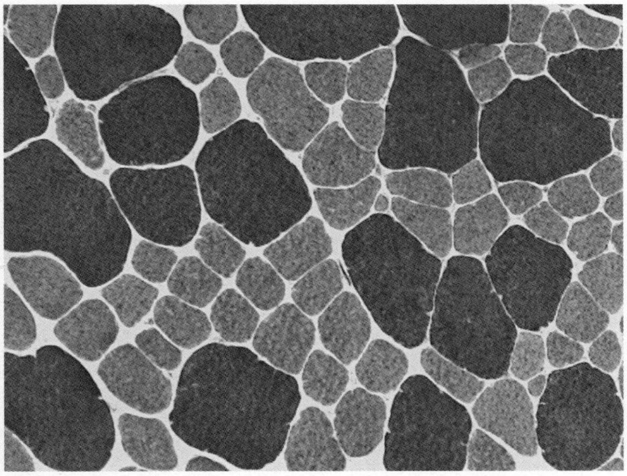

FIG. 86-9 Biopsy of a case with congenital fiber-type disproportion (ATPase stain, pH 9.4, ×200).

TABLE 86-1 Congenital Muscular Dystrophies (CMDs)

Anatomic Site/Disease	Gene
Extracellular Space	
Ullrich CMD/Bethlem myopathy[a]	Collagen VI subunits
Laminin α2 deficiency	Laminin α2 (merosin)
Transmembrane Attached to Laminin α2	
α-Dystroglycan, abnormal glycosylation	
Fukuyama CMD	Fukutin
Muscle–eye–brain disease	*POMGNT1*
Walker–Warburg syndrome	*POMT1*
CMD 1C/LGMD 2I	Fukutin-related protein
CMD 1D (1 patient)	*LARGE*
Other transmembrane	
Integrin α7 (4 patients)	*ITA7*
Within Myofiber	
CMD with early rigid spine	Selenoprotein-N
Unknown	
CMD 1B (2 families)	Unknown
Others	–

[a]Bethlem myopathy is not usually classified as a CMD, although it results in mutations of the same genes as Ullrich disease; the two share some clinical and pathological features.
Reprinted with permission from Walsh RS, Greenberg SA. Molecular diagnosis of neuromuscular disease: genetic testing in neuromuscular disease. *Muscle Nerve.* 2005;31:418–430.

TABLE 86-2 The Genetics of Congenital Myopathies

Gene	Subtype	Inheritance Pattern	Protein	Primary Subcellular Involvement	Possible Pathogenesis
ACTA 1	• NM	AD, AR	Actin, alpha skeletal muscle	Thin filament involvement	Abnormal thin filament structure
	• Cap disease (NM variant)	AD			
	• Zebra body myopathy (NM variant)	AD			
	• Congenital fiber-type disproportion	AD			
TPM3	• NM (NM variant)	AD, AR	Tropomyosin 3		
	• Cap disease (NM variant)	AD			
	• Congenital fiber-type disproportion	AD			
TPM2	• NM	AD	Tropomyosin 2 (beta)		
	• Cap disease (NM variant)	AD			
TNNTI	• NM	AR	Troponin T type 1 (skeletal, slow)		
NEB	• NM	AR	Nebulin		Thin filament remodeling ± stability
	• Core–rod myopathy				
LMOD3	• NM	AR	Leiomodin 3		
KBTBD13	• NM	AD	Kelch repeat and BTB (POZ) domain–containing protein 13		
CFL2	• NM	AR	Cofilin 2 (muscle)		

(Continued)

TABLE 86-2 The Genetics of Congenital Myopathies—cont'd

Gene	Subtype	Inheritance Pattern	Protein	Primary Subcellular Involvement	Possible Pathogenesis
KLHL40	• NM	AR	Kelch-like family member 40		
KLHL41	• NM	AR	Kelch-like family member 41		
MYO18B	• NM	AR	Myosin 18B	Unknown	Unknown
RYR1	• Central core myopathy • Multiminicore myopathy • Core–rod myopathy • NM • Congenital fiber-type disproportion • Centronuclear myopathy • Congenital neuromuscular disease with uniform type 1 fiber	AD, AR AR AD, AR AR AR AR AD	Ryanodine receptor I	Triad involvement	Abnormal EC coupling
CACNASI	• Congenital fiber-type disproportion	AR	DHPR		
STAC3	• Native American myopathy	AR	SH3 and cysteine-rich domain–containing protein 3		
ORA11	• Tubular aggregate myopathy	AD	Transmembrane protein 142A		Abnormal SOCE
ST1M1	• Tubular aggregate myopathy	AD	Stromal interaction molecule 1		
SEPN1	• Multiminicore myopathy • Congenital fiber-type disproportion	AR AR	Selenoprotein N1		Oxidative defects
CCDC78	• Centronuclear myopathy	AD	Coiled-coil domain–containing protein 78		Abnormal EC coupling?
BIN 1	• Centronuclear myopathy	AR, AD	Amphiphysin		Membrane remodeling ± stability.
DNM2	• Centronuclear myopathy	AD	Dynamin 2		
MTM1	• Myotubular myopathy	XR	Myotubularin 1		
MTMR14[a]	• Centronuclear myopathy		Myotubularin-related protein 14		
SPEG	• Centronuclear myopathy with dilated cardiomyopathy	AR	SPEG complex locus		
PTPLA (=*HCDA1*)	• Congenital myopathy related to PTPLA	AR	Protein tyrosine phosphatase-like (3-hydroxyacyl-CoA dehydratase)		
TTN	• Centronuclear myopathy • Congenital myopathy with fatal cardiomyopathy	ARAR	Titin		
MYH7	• Myosin storage myopathy • Myosin storage myopathy with cardiomyopathy • Congenital fiber-type disproportion	AD AR AD	Myosin, heavy-chain 7, cardiac muscle		Abnormal ATPase and actin-binding properties Structural abnormalities
MYH2	• Myosin IIa myopathy	AD, AR	Myosin, heavy-chain 2, skeletal muscle	Heavy-chain NJ	Abnormal ATPase and actin-binding properties
CNTN1	• Compton–North congenital myopathy	AR	Contactin-1		Structural abnormalities Aberrant NJ adhesion?
MEGF10	• Early-onset myopathy, areflexia respiratory distress, and dysphagia • Minicores	AR AR	Multiple EGF-like domains 10	Satellite cells	Abnormal regulation of satellite cells
ZAK	• Congenital fiber-type disproportion	AR	Sterile alpha motif and leucine zipper containing kinase AZK	Unknown	MAPK signaling pathway

[a]Until now MTMR14 has been proven to produce a myopathy only in animal models.

AD, Autosomal-dominant; *AR*, autosomal-recessive; *AZK*, Sterile alpha motif and leucine zipper containing kinase; *BTB*, Broad-Complex, Tramtrack, and Bric a brac; *DHPR*, dihydropyridine receptor; *EC*, excitation–contraction; *EGF*, epidermal growth factor; *MAPK*, mitogen-activated protein kinase; *NJ*, neuromuscular junction; *NM*, nemaline myopathy; *POZ*, Pox virus and Zinc finger; *SOCE*, store-operated calcium entry; *XR*, X-linked recessive.

Geschwind DH, Paulson HL, Klein C, eds. Neurogenetics, Part II. In: *Handbook of Clinical Neurology*. Vol. 148 (3rd series). Amsterdam, Netherlands: Elsevier. https://doi.org/10.1016/B978-0-444-64076-5.00036-3.

Adapted from Kaplan JC, Hamroun D. The 2016 version of the gene table of monogenic neuromuscular disorders (nuclear genome). *Neuromuscul Dis*. 2015;25:991–1020.

SUMMARY

This child had CMD with characteristic MRI changes and muscle biopsy showing dystrophic changes and merosin deficiency.

IMPORTANT POINTS

- Congenital muscular dystrophies manifest as floppy babies.
- The differential diagnosis includes primary cerebral disorders, spinal muscular atrophy, disorders of the neuromuscular junction, congenital neuropathies and myopathies, and metabolic myopathies, such as acid maltase deficiency.
- CMD 1A is caused by a deficiency of laminin α-2, or merosin, and has variable phenotypes, depending on the degree of protein deficiency.
- Brain MRI showing diffusely increased white matter signals on a T2-weighted image is characteristic of CMD 1A. Muscle biopsies show absent or decreased merosin in immunohistochemistry and Western blot.
- CMD 1A is caused by a defect of chromosome 6q2.
- The laminins are important components of the basal lamina of most tissue.
- There is no cure for merosin deficiency.

REFERENCES

1. Batten FE. Three cases of myopathy, infantile type. *Brain*. 1903;26:147–148.
2. Dubowitz V, Fardeau M. *Workshop Report: Proceedings of the 27th ENMC Sponsored Workshop on Congenital Muscular Dystrophy*, 22–24 April 1994, The Netherlands. *Neuromuscul Disord*. 1995;3:253–258.
3. Dubowitz V. *41st ENMC International Workshop on Congenital Muscular Dystrophy*, March 8–10, 1996, Naarden, The Netherlands. *Neuromuscul Disord*. 1996;6:295–306.
4. Jones KJ, Morgan G, Johnston H, et al. The expanding phenotype of laminin alpha 2 chain (merosin) abnormalities: case series and review. *J Med Genet*. 2001;38:649–657.
5. Pegoraro E, Marks H, Garcia C, et al. Laminin alpha 2 muscular dystrophy: genotype/phenotype studies of 22 patients. *Neurology*. 1998;51(1):101–110.
6. Mora M, Moroni I, Uziel G, et al. Mild clinical phenotype in a 12-year-old boy with partial merosin deficiency and central and peripheral nervous system abnormalities. *Neuromuscul Disord*. 1996;6:377–381.
7. Herrmann R, Straub V, Meyer K, et al. Congenital muscular dystrophy with laminin alpha 2 chain deficiency: identification of a new intermediate phenotype and correlation of clinical findings to muscle immunohistochemistry. *Eur J Pediatr*. 1996;155:968–976.
8. Bushby K, Anderson LV, Pollitt C, et al. Abnormal merosin in adults: a new form of late onset muscular dystrophy not linked to chromosome 6q2. *Brain*. 1998;121:581–588.
9. Jucker M, Tian M, Norton DD, et al. Laminin alpha 2 is a component of brain capillary basement membrane: reduced expression in dystrophic dy mice. *Neuroscience*. 1996;71(4):1153–1161.
10. Villanova M, Malandrini A, Sabatelli P, et al. Localization of laminin alpha 2 chain in normal human central nervous system: an immunofluorescence and ultrastructural study. *Acta Neuropathol (Berl)*. 1997;94:567–571.
11. Shorer Z, Philpot J, Muntoni F, et al. Demyelinating peripheral neuropathy in merosin-deficient congenital muscular dystrophy. *J Child Neurol*. 1995;10:472–475.
12. Sewry CA, D'Alessandro M, Wilson LA, et al. Expression of laminin chains in skin in merosin-deficient congenital muscular dystrophy. *Neuropediatrics*. 1997;28(4):217–222.
13. Helbling-Leclerc A, Zhang X, Topaloglu H, et al. Mutations in the laminin alpha 2-chain gene (LAMA2) cause merosin-deficient congenital muscular dystrophy. *Nat Genet*. 1995;11:216–218.
14. Colognato H, Yurchenco PD. Form and function: the laminin family of heterotrimers. *Dev Dyn*. 2000;218(2):213–234.
15. Vachon PH, Loechel F, Xu H, et al. Merosin and laminin in myogenesis: specific requirement for merosin in myotube stability and survival. *J Cell Biol*. 1996;134(6):1483–1497.
16. Smeets HJM, Verbrugge B, Springuel P, et al. *MDC1A Workshop Group. Merosin Deficient Congenital Muscular Dystrophy Type 1A: An International Workshop on the Road to Therapy*, November 15–17, 2019. Maastricht, The Netherlands. *Neuromuscul Disord*. 2021;31(7):673–680.

87 CASE

A Woman With Long-standing Weakness and Foot Deformities

A 43-year-old woman had had progressive leg weakness for 6 years, but she stated that she had been mildly weak since childhood when she had several falls. She had always walked on her tiptoes and was diagnosed as having "tight heel cords." She was told then that she might have some form of muscular dystrophy.

The patient was the product of a normal delivery; she was not floppy, sat at 8 months, spoke at 10 months, and started walking at the age of 2 years. Her mother and maternal grandfather had similar problems. Past medical history included polycystic kidney disease.

Examination revealed normal mentation and cranial nerves. There was no muscle atrophy. She had difficulty arising from a chair (Fig. 87-1A). Manual muscle testing revealed strength in neck flexors 4+/5 and shoulder abduction of 4+/5; biceps, triceps, and forearm muscles were 5/5 hip flexors, extensors, and thigh muscles were 4/5; and foot dorsiflexors were 4−/5. Reflexes were normal in the arms and only trace at the knees and ankles. Sensation to touch, vibration, and pinprick were normal. Coordination was normal. There were no Babinski signs or fasciculations. She had contractures of the Achilles tendons and small feet with mildly high arches (see Fig. 87-1B). The examination was otherwise unremarkable.

WHAT IS THE DIFFERENTIAL DIAGNOSIS?

This woman had weakness and high arches mainly in the legs and depressed reflexes suggesting a hereditary neuropathy; however, there was no other clinical suggestion of a neuropathy, and the weakness was more proximal. She could also have had spinal muscular atrophy, but the lack of fasciculations and normal reflexes was against that diagnosis. The lack of fluctuation and cranial nerve involvement was against a disorder of neuromuscular transmission.

She appeared to have a myopathy, and those considered in the differential diagnosis were congenital myopathies of slow progression, such as central core disease (CCD) and some cases with congenital-fiber-type disproportion. Most other congenital myopathies are more progressive and severe, although cases of rod or nemaline myopathy may start later (adult-onset rod myopathy).[1] A limb-girdle muscular dystrophy or a manifest carrier state of a dystrophinopathy are also considerations; an endocrine myopathy and polymyositis seem very unlikely as the weakness was long-lasting and she had a positive family history. Other possibilities include acid maltase and carnitine deficiencies, but the apparent pattern in inheritance is not autosomal-recessive as in those disorders. A mitochondrial myopathy and proximal myotonic myopathy (PROMM) are also considerations. The lack of myotonia is against the latter diagnosis, but this may not be clinically obvious at times.

The family history, which suggests an autosomal-dominant inheritance, narrows the differential diagnosis to either CCD or limb-girdle dystrophy type I (LGMD 1) and, less likely, PROMM.

WHAT TESTS SHOULD BE DONE?

Complete metabolic panel and thyroid-stimulating hormone were normal. Serum creatine kinase was mildly elevated up to 260 IU/L (normal, <200 IU/L).

AN EMG TEST WAS PERFORMED

Motor Nerve Studies

Nerve and Site	Latency (ms)	Amplitude (mV)	Conduction Velocity (m/s)
Peroneal Nerve R.	Normal ≤ 5.7	Normal ≥ 3	Normal ≥ 40
Ankle	4.5	4	–
Fibular head	10.4	3	46
Knee	11.8	3	58

F-Wave and Tibial H-Reflex Studies

Nerve	Latency (ms)	Normal Latency ≤ (ms)
Peroneal nerve R.	44.0	54
H-reflex R.	28.6	34

Sensory Nerve Study

Nerve	Onset Latency (ms)	Normal Onset Latency ≤ (ms)	Peak Latency (ms)	Normal Peak Latency ≤ (ms)	Amp (μV)	Normal Amp ≥ (μV)	Conduction Velocity (m/s)	Normal Conduction Velocity ≥ (m/s)
Sural nerve R.	3.0	3.5	3.5	4.0	17	11	47	40

EMG Data

Muscle	Insrt Activity	Fibs	Pos Waves	Fasc	Amp	Dur	Poly	Pattern
Lumbar paraspinals R.	Norm	None	None	None	Norm	Norm	None	Full
Deltoid R.	Norm	None	None	None	**Dec**	**Brief**	**Many**	Full[a]
Iliopsoas R.	Norm	None	None	None	**Dec**	**Brief**	**Many**	Full
Tensor fasciae latae R.	Norm	None	None	None	**Dec**	**Brief**	**Few**	Full[a]
Vastus lateralis R.	Norm	None	None	None	**Dec**	**Brief**	**Few**	Full[a]
Tibialis anterior R.	Norm	None	None	None	**Dec**	**Brief**	**Few**	Full
Gastrocnemius R.	Norm	None	None	None	Norm	Norm	None	Full

[a]Rapid recruitment of motor unit action potentials.

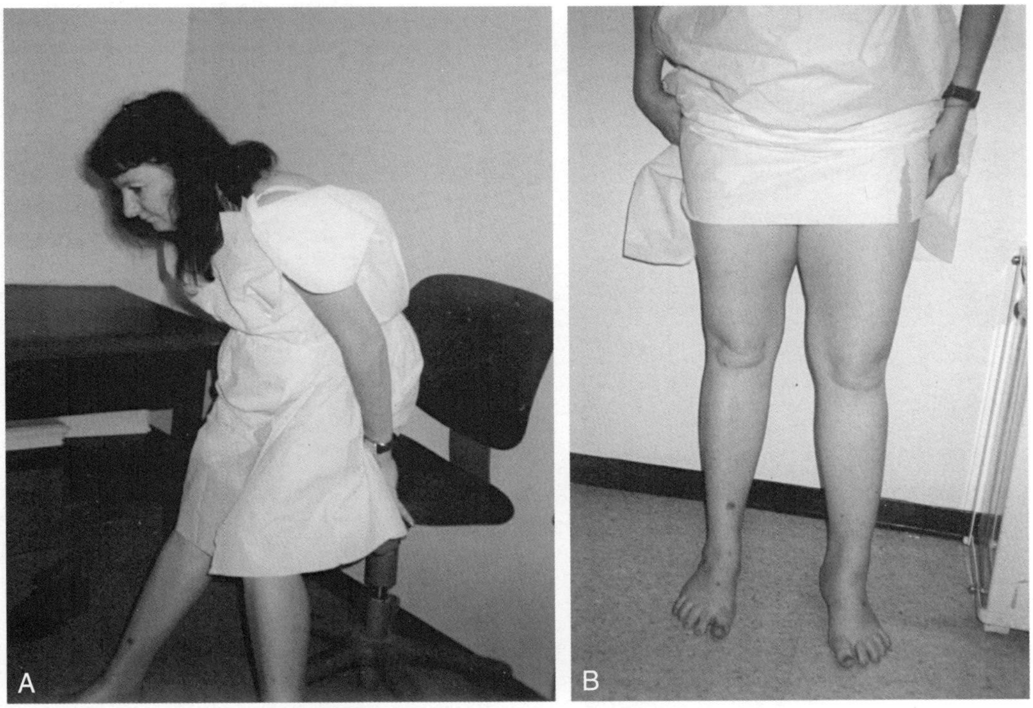

FIG. 87-1 **A**, Patient showing difficulty in rising up from a chair; note that she has to use her hands to stand up. **B**, The patient showing a lack of muscle atrophy and mild foot deformities.

WHAT WERE THE EMG FINDINGS?

Nerve conduction tests were normal. The needle test showed many short-duration polyphasic motor unit potentials with increased recruitment for the level of effort, highly suggestive of a myopathy. No denervation potentials were detected at rest. This test thus ruled out peripheral neuropathy and spinal muscular atrophy. The lack of fibrillations is against, but cannot rule out, an inflammatory myopathy, and the lack of electrical myotonia is against PROMM and adult-onset acid maltase deficiency.

WHAT SHOULD BE DONE NEXT?

A muscle biopsy showed small type I muscle fibers with type I fiber predominance; many fibers had centrally located cores (Fig. 87-2). The diagnosis of CCD was made.

WHAT ARE CENTRAL CORES?

Central cores are large areas of muscle fibers devoid of oxidative enzyme activity. The cores run along the long axis of the muscle fiber across various sarcomeres, often measuring up to 300 µm. They could be located centrally or peripherally and can be single or multiple.[2] They might all have small rims of increased oxidative staining but these are different in appearance and less intense than targets seen in denervating diseases. Both the cores and their rims contain increased amounts of desmin, vimentin, developmental myosin heavy chains, and tubulin.[3] The ryanodine receptor (RYR1) protein might be identified within the cores.[4] Cores and nemaline bodies can appear, but only rarely, intermixed in the same biopsy in patients with CCD.[2] On electromicroscopy the cores either consist of areas within the myofibers that have the same structure of the sarcomeres with variation in orientation to the other myofibrils (structured

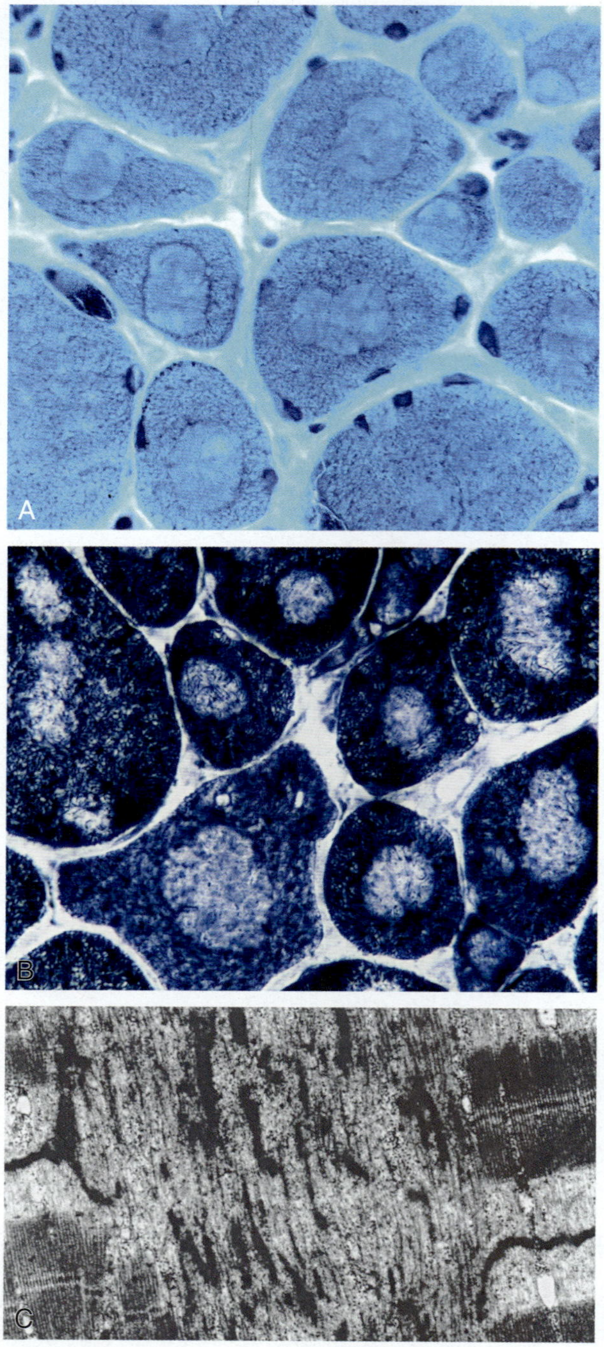

FIG. 87-2 **A**, The patient's muscle biopsy showing central cores on trichrome stain, also showing proliferation of connective tissue and fiber atrophy (×400). **B**, NADH-TR showing cores lacking oxidative staining (×400). **C**, Electromicroscopy showing an unstructured core (×12,000).

cores) or are disorganized, and the structure of the sarcomeres is not preserved (unstructured cores).[2]

Type I fiber predominance is common in CCD and other congenital myopathies, and this is not caused by reinnervation, as occurs in fiber-type grouping[5] (see Case 86 and Table 86-2).

DISCUSSION

This woman had CCD, the first reported congenital myopathy identified by Shy and Magee in 1956.[6] The disease manifests as floppy infant syndrome with generalized hypotonia and trunk and limb weakness. Motor milestones might be delayed, but the progression is very slow. Although patients might end up in a wheelchair, some have a much more benign course.[6–8] Characteristically, CCD manifests with more proximal than distal weakness and hypotonia, and reflexes are normal or mildly decreased. Patients might also have hip dislocation, flat feet, or other skeletal anomalies, including high arches[7] and scoliosis.[9]

CCD is an autosomal-dominant disorder caused by mutations in chromosome 19q12–13.2 on the ryanodine (RyR1) Ca^{2+} receptor gene region.[10,11] All mutations causing the disease are missense mutations, and the majority affect the N terminal or the rod domains of the protein.[11,12] Only a few mutations affect the C terminal. Autosomal-recessive cases are rare and more severe.[13]

The ryanodine receptor protein is one of the calcium-release channels. Malignant hyperthermia (MH) syndrome is also caused by mutations of this gene and thus is allelic to CCD, and patients with CCD are susceptible to developing MH.[14–16] This is a condition in which susceptible individuals develop severe attacks of fever, contractures, and rhabdomyolysis when exposed to certain anesthetics, such as halothane. Not all MH cases have CCD, and an MH-like syndrome can occur in other myopathies, such as muscular dystrophy, myotonic dystrophy, and some metabolic myopathies.[16,17]

The treatment of CCD remains conservative. Genetic counseling is appropriate and should stress the predisposition of MH to patients and their relatives. The caffeine contracture test in muscle biopsies can be used in screening a subject's risk.[17] MH is prevented by avoidance of known trigger anesthetics; attacks are treated with intravenous dantrolene and correction of the metabolic derangements caused by the attack.[18,19]

SUMMARY

This woman had proximal muscle weakness with some skeletal anomalies which started in childhood and had delayed developmental motor milestones.

Her EMG was "myopathic," and she had a muscle biopsy characteristic of CCD, a congenital myopathy of relatively benign prognosis caused by mutation of the ryanodine receptor gene in chromosome 19q.

IMPORTANT POINTS

- Some congenital myopathies might have a benign course, and patients might not seek medical attention until later in life.
- The differential diagnosis of adult patients with slowly progressive proximal muscle weakness includes LGMD, polymyositis, CCD, adult-onset nemaline myopathy, acid maltase deficiency, carnitine deficiency, endocrine myopathies (e.g., hyperparathyroidism), PROMM, manifest carriers of Duchenne dystrophy, mitochondrial myopathy, and spinal muscular atrophy.
- Small polyphasic motor unit potentials are highly suggestive of a myopathy. The lack of increased insertional activity, fibrillations, and myotonia is against the diagnosis of polymyositis but does not rule out the disease. This is also against

acid maltase deficiency, PROMM, and adult-onset nemaline myopathy.

- CCD is an autosomal-dominant disease caused by mutations in chromosome 19q, and the disease is allelic to MH syndrome; patients with CCD are predisposed to this syndrome.
- Cores are areas of muscle fibers characterized by lack of oxidative staining. On electromicroscopy these either show disruption of the sarcomere (unstructured cores) or preserve the normal structure but have a different orientation from the rest of the myofibrils (structured cores).
- There is no cure for CCD, but genetic counseling and physical therapy are important.

REFERENCES

1. Chahin N, Selcen D, Engel AG. Sporadic late onset nemaline myopathy. *Neurology*. 2005;65:1158–1164.
2. Golbel HH. Central core disease. In: Kaptai G, ed. *Structural and Molecular Basis of Skeletal Muscle Diseases*. Basel, Switzerland: ISN Neuropathy Press; 2002:65–67.
3. Vita G, Migliorato A, Baradello A, et al. Expression of cytoskeleton proteins in central core disease. *J Neurol Sci*. 1994;124:71–76.
4. Scacheri PC, Hoffman EP, Fratkin JD, et al. A novel ryanodine receptor gene mutation causing both cores and rods in congenital myopathy. *Neurology*. 2000;55:1689–1696.
5. Bertorini TE, Stålberg E, Juson CP, Engel WK. Single-fiber electromyography in neuromuscular disorders: correlation of muscle histochemistry, single-fiber electromyography, and clinical findings. *Muscle Nerve*. 1994;17:345–353.
6. Shy GM, Magee KR. A new congenital non-progressive myopathy. *Brain*. 1956;79:610–621.
7. Shuaib A, Paasuke RT, Brownell KW. Central core disease: clinical features in 13 patients. *Medicine (Baltimore)*. 1987;66:389–396.
8. Manzur AY, Sewry CA, Ziprin J, et al. A severe clinical and pathological variant of central core disease with possible autosomal recessive inheritance. *Neuromuscul Disord*. 1998;8:467–473.
9. Mertz KD, Jost B, Glatzel M, Min K. Progressive scoliosis in central core disease. *Eur Spine J*. 2005;14:900–905.
10. Lynch PJ, Tong J, Lehane M, et al. A mutation in the transmembrane/luminal domain of the ryanodine receptor is associated with abnormal Ca2+ release channel function and severe central core disease. *Proc Natl Acad Sci USA*. 1999;96: 4164–4169.
11. Haan EA, Freemantle CJ, McCure JA, et al. Assignment of the gene for central core disease to chromosome 19. *Hum Genet*. 1990;86:187–190.
12. Kausch K, Lehmann-Horn F, Janka M, et al. Evidence for linkage of the central core disease locus to the proximal long arm of human chromosome 19. *Genomics*. 1991;10(3):765–769.
13. Castro D, Henriquez A. Treatment and management of spinal muscular atrophy and congenital myopathies Chapter 13. In: Bertorini TE, ed. *Neuromuscular Disorders: Treatment and Management*. Amsterdam, Netherlands: Elsevier; 2022:261–277. 2nd ed.
14. McCarthy T, Quane KA, Lynch PJ. Ryanodine receptor mutations in malignant hyperthermia and central core disease. *Hum Mutat*. 2000;15(5):410–417.
15. Jurkat-Rott K, McCarthy T, Lehmann-Horn F. Genetics and pathogenesis of malignant hyperthermia. *Muscle Nerve*. 2000; 23(1):4–17.
16. Brandt A, Schleithoff L, Jurkat-Rott K, et al. Screening of the ryanodine receptor gene in 105 malignant hyperthermia families: novel mutations and concordance with the in vitro contracture test. *Hum Mol Genet*. 1999;8(11):2055–2062.
17. Bertorini TE. Myoglobinuria, malignant hyperthermia, neuroleptic malignant syndrome and serotonin syndrome. *Neurol Clin*. 1997;15:649–671.
18. Bertorini TE. Malignant hyperthermia. In: Katirji B, Kaminski HJ, Preston DC, eds. *Neuromuscular Disorders in Clinical Practice*. Boston, MA: Butterworth-Heinemann; 2002:1021–1027.
19. Bertorini TE, Finder JD, Bassam BA. Perioperative management of patients with neuromuscular disorders. In: Bertorini TE, ed. *Neuromuscular Disorders: Treatment and Management*. Amsterdam, Netherlands: 2nd ed.

88 CASE

A floppy baby who later developed malignant hyperthermia

The patient was a 4600-g product of a 37-week gestation complicated by spotting, cramping, and viral infection. Medications during pregnancy included medroxyprogesterone acetate, penicillin G potassium, and phenobarbital sodium. Immediately after birth, the newborn was noticed to have paucity of movement and a weak cry, and he was treated for pneumonia with antibiotics.

At 3 weeks of age, he was profoundly weak. Minimal retractions of the chest and pectus excavatum were noted. Heart and lungs were normal. Generalized hypotonic included severe weakness in all four extremities, with retraction and adduction of the upper extremities and minimal movement of the shoulders. Proximal muscles were weaker than distal. Sensory examination was intact to pinprick. Deep tendon reflexes could not be elicited.

Laboratory studies included normal serum creatine kinase and normal nerve conduction velocities. On electromyogram there was an increased number of polyphasic potentials of short duration. A muscle biopsy specimen at 7 months of age was studied with a complete battery of histochemical stains and by electron microscopy. There was evidence of atrophy of both fiber types, but mainly of type I fibers; many fibers of primary type I had small areas devoid of oxidative enzyme activity (Fig. 88-1), and there was no evidence of necrosis or phagocytosis. Electron microscopy showed that there were no mitochondria in the core areas and that the myofibers were disorganized.

At 9 months of age the patient would lie in a pithed frog position. By 18 months he could not sit independently but needed to prop himself on his arms. He attempted to crawl but could not support his body weight. He was fitted with a parapodium for standing. At 18 months of age there was evidence of a mild thoracic scoliosis, and a grade 1/6 systolic murmur was heard at the left sternal border. He had frequent respiratory tract infections, and at 28 months of age he developed congestive heart failure.

He was admitted for cardiac catheterization one month later and was premedicated with meperidine hydrochloride (Demerol), 20 mg intramuscularly and hydroxyzine hydrochloride (Vistaril), 10 mg intravenously (IV). Because he was irritable, he received ketamine hydrochloride 10 mg IV as well. Six milliliters of 1% lidocaine hydrochloride with epinephrine was used for local infiltration. Cardiac cath revealed an atrial septal defect with a large left–right shunt and mitral regurgitation. The child was transferred to the recovery room where he was lethargic, clammy, and pale with an axillary temperature of 37.3°C. One hour later, his rectal temperature was 40.9°C and his heart rate was 210 beats per minute.

He was treated with dantrolene sodium and cooling and was intubated. During the next 12 hours his condition gradually deteriorated. He was in shock with unmeasurable blood pressure despite maximum support including dopamine hydrochloride, epinephrine, sodium nitroprusside drip, sodium bicarbonate, calcium chloride, methylprednisolone sodium succinate (Solu-Medrol), glucose, and insulin. He remained hypotensive and 26 hours after cardiac cath had a cardiac arrest with no response to any form of resuscitation.

Pertinent autopsy findings were a patent foramen ovale, a fenestrated valve, dilated atrium, and a markedly hypertrophic right ventricle with some focal wall thickening and minimal fibrosis. Skeletal muscle specimen showed endomysial fibrosis with internal nuclei and many necrotic atrophic basophilic fibers. Although this specimen was not studied by histochemistry or by electron microscopy, the paraffin-embedded sections showed segmental areas of rarefaction that appear to be the multicores seen on histochemical preparation. The spinal cord appeared normal with the normal number of neurons in the anterior horns. Cultures from the heart and lung were negative.

DISCUSSION

This patient was a floppy infant with histologic findings characteristic of multicore disease.[1] Children previously described as having multicore disease presented with generalized hypotonia, diffuse weakness, decreased muscle bulk, and delayed motor development.[1–10] Two patients had lordosis[5,8] and one had a high arched palate.[10] Most patients were not suspected of having muscle disease until 8 or 9 months of age when they were delayed in their ability to sit independently or to crawl. All ultimately became ambulatory but had great difficulty sitting up from supine and rising from a chair without handrails.[1–11]

This case was noted to be extremely weak and hypotonic immediately after birth. Initially, a clinical diagnosis of Werdnig–Hoffmann disease was made. No DNA testing was available at that time. Muscle biopsy findings at 7 months of age were diagnostic for multicore disease. In contrast to other reported patients with multicore disease, this patient remained very weak. He was severely limited in motor skills, needing adaptive equipment to feed himself and external support for independent sitting, and a parapodium was prescribed to allow him to stand. At age 2 1/2 years, prior to developing congestive heart failure, there was no significant improvement in muscle strength to suggest that he was near the point of being able to walk.[12,13]

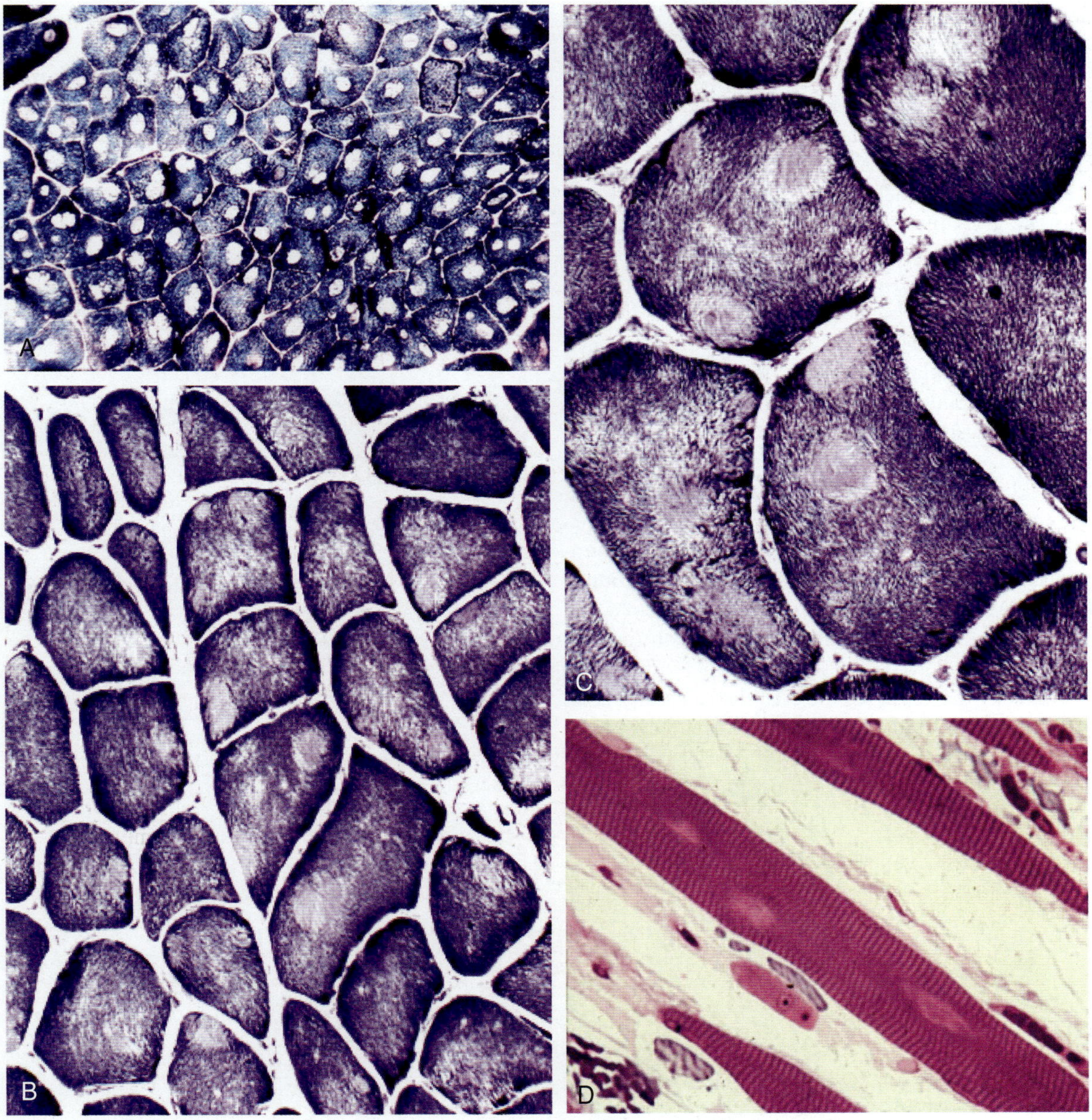

FIG. 88-1 **A**, NADH-TR shows many muscle fibers with small cores (×100). **B**, Fibers with many cores (×200). **C**, NADH-TR showing several cores in individual muscle fibers (×400). **D**, Mini-core disease biopsy showing multiple small cores and proliferation of connective tissue (toluidine blue–stained, plastic-embedded section, ×400).

One other reported patient with multicore disease had cardiac involvement and an atrial septal defect. Her course was much different, and at age 11 years, she had only limitations in bike riding and stair climbing.[1] This case was asymptomatic from his cardiac disease from birth to 18 months of age, with a normal respiratory rate, heart rate, and without hepatosplenomegaly. He did have several upper respiratory tract infections between 18 and 28 months, which may have been related to his cardiac disease or his weak respiratory musculature. At 28 months, he developed congestive heart failure that was controlled with medication. In fact, he was asymptomatic of heart failure at the time of admission for cardiac catheterization.

Central core and multicore disease have some striking similarities in their pathologic lesions,[8] and this could suggest related pathogenetic mechanisms resulting in these two diseases. Central core disease and multicore disease have been associated with malignant hyperthermia syndrome (MHS) during anesthesia.[14–17] Multiple mini-core myopathies have variable phenotypes that are present in childhood or adolescence. The most typical presentation includes weakness, respiratory involvement, and spinal deformities. Those disorders are caused by mutations of the *RYR1* gene of the ryanodine receptor affecting EC coupling.

The patient developed a high, unexplained fever, acidosis, and tachycardia after receiving lidocaine and ketamine agents previously associated with malignant hyperthermia.[18,19] Hyperthermia could have been precipitated by medication or the stress of cardiac catheterization.[18,20] He did not have muscle rigidity, elevated creatine kinase levels, or myoglobinuria as would have been expected for malignant hyperthermia.

However, nonrigid forms of the syndrome have been described.[21] Laboratory tests cannot identify all patients with his condition.[22] Although the cause of death could have been an allergic reaction to the contrast media,[23] or from sepsis, the clinical and autopsy findings do not support those diagnoses and the cause of death is more likely related to anesthesia.

MHS is a condition characterized by severe muscle rigidity, fever, cardiac arrythmia, and rhabdomyolysis. It occurs particularly with exposure to general anesthesia such as halothane and the paralyzing muscle relaxants. Other manifestations include acidosis, hypermetabolism, fever, hyperkalemia, cardiac arrythmia, and initial hyperkalemia and initial hypercalcemia due to intracellular calcium accumulation. The incidence of MHS is 1 in 1500 children and 1 in 50,00 adults.[24] It is an usual autosomal disorder more frequently associated with the RYR1 mutation.[25] It has also been reported in patients with the dihydropyridine voltage-gated calcium channel,[26] and these voltage channels are involved in muscle calcium release. Attacks of MH are caused by the excessive release of calcium by the sarcoplasmic reticulum (SR) under certain conditions. The mutations of MH cells appear to lower the threshold for calcium release by the SR altering the excitation–contraction coupling.

During the attacks, the increased intracellular calcium causes muscle contractures that lead to increased oxygen consumption, glycogenolysis, and depletion of high-energy phosphate compounds with an elevation of body temperature. There is also limitation of calcium reuptake by the SR for muscle relaxation increasing muscle contractures with further increased intramuscular calcium accumulation (Fig. 88-2). This results in leakage of phosphate and potassium into the bloodstream that can cause cardiac arrythmias. Serum uric acid and lactic acid, creatine kinase, and myoglobin are increased and can cause renal failure[16,27] (Table 88-1). It should be mentioned that although

TABLE 88-1 Clinical Events and Laboratory Findings During Malignant Hyperthermia

Clinical Events
Unexplained, sudden increase in end-tidal CO_2
Unexplained tachycardia, tachypnea, labile blood pressure, or arrhythmias
Masseter muscle rigidity or generalized muscle rigidity
Unanticipated respiratory or metabolic acidosis
Increasing patient temperature
Cola-colored urine (myoglobinuria)
Mottled, cyanotic, hot skin; sweating; decreased SpO_2
Laboratory Findings
Arterial blood gases; $PaCO_2 \geq 60$ mm Hg, base excess more negative than −8 mEq/L, pH <7.25
Potassium ion >6 mEq/L
Creatine kinase >10,000 IU/L after anesthetic without succinylcholine
Serum myoglobin >170 µg/L

Modified from Karlet MC. Malignant hyperthermia: considerations for ambulatory surgery. *J Perianesth Nurs.* 1998;13:306, with permission.

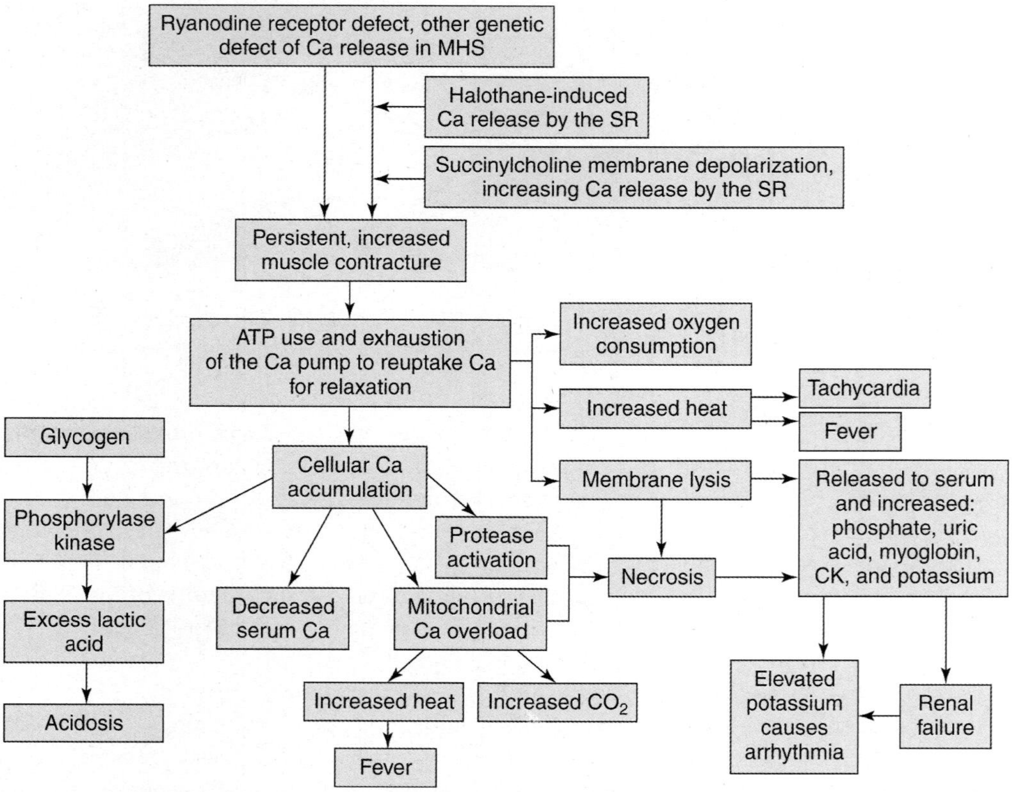

FIG. 88-2 Possible mechanisms of clinical and laboratory abnormalities in malignant hyperthermia syndrome. *ATP,* Adenosine 5′-triphosphate; *Ca,* calcium; *CK,* creatine kinase; *CO_2,* carbon dioxide; *MHS,* malignant hyperthermia syndrome; *SR,* sarcoplasmic reticulum. Modified from Bertorini TE. Myoglobinuria, malignant hyperthermia, neuroleptic malignant syndrome and serotonin syndrome. *Neurol Clin.* 1997;15:658.

TABLE 88-2 Individuals at Risk for Malignant Hyperthermia or Malignant Hyperthermia-Like Syndrome

Family history of malignant hyperthermia
King–Denborough syndrome
Evans myopathy
Central core disease
Multicore diseases
Muscular dystrophy (dystrophinopathy, myotonic dystrophy)
Periodic paralysis
Myotonia congenita
Carnitine palmitoyltransferase deficiency
Phosphorylase deficiency; possibly other glycogen storage myopathies
Brody disease
Idiopathic hyperCkemia

halothane and paralyzing skeletal muscle relaxants are the drugs more often implicated in triggering this disorder, several other medications have been reported to cause MHS.

The diagnosis of MHS is based on the clinical presentation and should be suspected early in those who developed masseter contractures and then generalized muscle rigidity with a rapid rise in body temperature, tachycardia, acidosis, and hypermetabolism, and this etiology should suspect MH in patients who have early excessive masseter contractions. Recognition of individuals and risks for surgery is important, and patients and physicians should consider these risks, particularly those patients with a strong family history of MHS or myopathies such as mini-core or central core disorders of being predisposing of the disease (Table 88-2) and consider the performance of muscle contracture test, but this test is not universally available.

Treatment and management of malignant hyperthermia consist in correction of fluid and electrolyte imbalance, reduction in temperature, and specifically the use of dantrolene, a muscle relaxant that decreases calcium release by the SR and inhibits muscle contractions (Table 88-3). Perioperative dantrolene is recommended in patients who are at risk of receiving anesthetics that can trigger an attack. Operating rooms and emergency departments should be instructed and prepared to treat disease complications (Table 88-3).

TABLE 88-3 Recommended Steps in Managing Patients With Suspected Malignant Hyperthermia

Discontinue the anesthetic and deliver 100% oxygen.
Administer dantrolene IV, 2–3 mg/kg every 5 min for a total of 10 mg/kg.
Get help; consult the malignant hyperthermia hotline for guidance. http://www.mhous.org, United States and Canada: 1-800-644-9737, other countries: 209-417-3722.
Administer sodium bicarbonate and ice in IV saline infusion, avoiding Ringer lactate.
Cover the stomach, bladder, and rectum with iced saline and use cooling blankets while closely monitoring body temperature.
Treat arrhythmias by reducing hyperkalemia with antiarrhythmic drugs but not calcium channel blockers.
Monitor end-tidal CO_2 and blood gases; increase end-tidal CO_2.
Treat hyperkalemia with hyperventilation, bicarbonate, glucose, and insulin; in life-threatening cases, use calcium chloride.
Ensure urine output is greater than 2 mL/kg/h by hydration, or by use of mannitol, furosemide, or both diuretics.
Treat unexpected cardiac arrests in children by treating hyperkalemia first.
Monitor blood gases, potassium, and calcium and check for the presence of myoglobulin in urine in the recovery room or ICU for a minimum of 24 h. Monitor coagulation parameters; correct if necessary.
Administer dantrolene IV 1 mg/kg every 6 h for 24–48 h or up to 10 mg/kg/day followed by oral dantrolene for another day.
Observe patient in the ICU for at least 36 h.
Refer the patient and family to a malignant hyperthermia testing center; provide genetic counseling
Obtain information from the following: http://www.mhaus.org. http://www.mhreg.org. http://www.emhg.org.

ICU, Intensive care unit.
Modified from Malignant Hyperthermia Association of the United States (MHAUS). *Emergency Therapy for Malignant Hyperthermia.* New York, NY: Malignant Hyperthermia Association of the United States; 1995. Updated in 2018.

SUMMARY

A floppy child was diagnosed as having mini-core disease. After cardiac catheterization, for which he received meperidine hydrochloride (Demerol), he developed malignant hyperthermia and died in spite of aggressive treatment.

IMPORTANT POINTS

- Mini-core disease and central core disease are causes of floppy infant syndrome. Both conditions are caused by mutations of the *RYR1* gene.
- Malignant hyperthermia can be seen in patients with mini-core and central core disease and other myopathies.
- Special precaution should be taken during surgery to prevent malignant hyperthermia and the patient should be medicated with sodium dantrolene, which should be available in all operating rooms.

This case was reported in Koch B, Bertorini T, Eng G, Boehm R. Severe multicore disease associated with reaction to anesthesia. Arch Neurol. 1985;42:1204–1206.

REFERENCES

1. Engel AG, Gomez MR, Groover RV. Multicore disease: a recently recognized congenital myopathy with multifocal degeneration of muscle fibers. *Mayo Clin Proc.* 1971;48:666–681.
2. Mykoyama M, Matouka Y, Kato H, et al. Multicore disease. *Rinsho Shinkeigaku.* 1973;13:221–227.
3. Tanimura R, Suzuki H, Yokota J, et al. Multicore myopathy: a case of congenital nonprogressive myopathy with 'multicore' changes of muscle fibers. *Rinsho Shinkeigaku.* 1974;14:613–622.
4. Currie S, Noronha M, Harriman D. Minicore disease. In: Bradley WG, ed. *III. International Congress on Muscle Disease.* In:

International Congress Series No. 334. Amsterdam, Netherlands: Excerpta Medica; 1974:12.
5. Heffner R, Cohen M, Duffner P, et al. Multicore disease in twins. *J Neurol Neurosurg Psychiatry*. 1976;39:602–608.
6. DeLumley L, Vallat JM, Catanzano G. Etude clinique et ultrastructure d'un cas myopathic congenital a foyers multiples. *Ann Pediatr*. 1978;23:333–336.
7. Taratuto AL, Sfaello ZM, Rezzojico C, et al. Multicore disease: report of a case with lack of fibre type differentiation. *Neuropediatria*. 1978;9:285–297.
8. Dubowitz V. Muscle disorders in childhood. In: *The Congenital Myopathies*. Vol. 16: Muscle Disorders in Children. Philadelphia, PA: WB Saunders Co.; 1978:73–77.
9. Ricoy JR, Cabelle A, Golzueta G. Myopathy with multiple minicores: report of two siblings. *J Neurol Sci*. 1980;48:81–92.
10. Issacs H, Badenhorst M. Multicore disease. *S Afr Med J*. 1980;57:543–546.
11. Bonnette H, Roelofs R, Olson WH. Multicore disease: report of a case with onset in middle age. *Neurology*. 1974;24:1039–1044.
12. Brooks MH, Engle WR. The histographic analysis of human muscle biopsies with regard to fiber types, I: adult male and female. *Neurology*. 1969;19:221–233.
13. Brooks MH, Engle WK. The histographic analysis of human muscle biopsies with regard to fiber types, IV: children's biopsies. *Neurology*. 1969;19:591–605.
14. Eng GD, Epstein BS, Engel WK, et al. Malignant hyperthermia and central core disease in a child with dislocating hips. *Arch Neurol*. 1978;35:189–197.
15. Denbrough MA, Dennett X. Anderson RMcD: central core disease and malignant hyperpyrexia. *Br Med J*. 1973;1:272–273.
16. Quane KA, Healy JM, Keating KE, et al. Mutations n the ryanodine receptor gene in central core disease and malignant hyperthermia. *Nat Genet*. 1993;5(1):51–55.
17. Frank JP, Harati Y, Butler IJ. Central core disease and malignant hyperthermia syndrome. *Ann Neurol*. 1980;7:11–17.
18. Stehling LC. Anesthesia update 86. *Orthop Rev*. 1980:9–33.
19. Roervic S, Stovner J. Ketamine induced acidosis, fever and creatine kinase rise. *Lancet*. 1974;2:1384.
20. Wingard DW. Malignant hyperthermia: a human stress syndrome. *Lancet*. 1974;2:1450–1451.
21. Britt BA, Kalow W. Malignant hyperthermia: a statistical review. *Can Anesth Soc J*. 1970;17:293–315.
22. Roland LP. Malignant hyperpyrexia: a reply. *Muscle Nerve*. 1980;3:443–444.
23. Lalli AF. Contrast media reactions: data analysis and hypothesis. *Radiology*. 1980;134:1–12.
24. Bertorini T. Malignant hyperthermia. In: Kaminski HJ, ed. *Neuromuscular Disorders in Clinical Practice*. Boston, MA: Butterworth-Heinemann; 2002:1021–2017.
25. Quane KA, Healy JM, Keating KE, et al. Mutations in the ryanodine receptor gene in central core disease and malignant hyperthermia. *Nat Genet*. 1993;5:51–55.
26. Kim JH, Jarvik GP, Browning BL, et al. Exome sequencing reveals novel rare variants in the ryanodine receptor and calcium channel genes in malignant hyperthermia families. *Anesthesiology*. 2013;119(5):1054–1065.
27. Bertorini TE. *Perioperative Management of Neuromuscular Case Studies*. Philadelphia, PA: Butterworth-Heinemann; 2008:352–356.

A Woman With Droopy Eyelids and Ophthalmoplegia

A 40-year-old Black woman presented with progressive droopy eyelids and blurred vision for the past 15 years. Her symptoms improved somewhat periodically, but during the past year, she developed intermittent diplopia, and her symptoms were worse in the afternoons.

She denied difficulty swallowing or breathing, limb weakness, or headaches. Previous workup included a normal MRI of the head.

Past medical history included a motor vehicle accident 5 years prior to this evaluation. The accident caused her to have glass fragments in her eyes and blurred vision. Four weeks later, her vision cleared; however, the patient stated that her eyelid droopiness had never been normal since then. She had a history of hypertension.

Family history was negative for neurologic disorders.

Examination revealed ptosis and ophthalmoplegia to all movements, worse on lateral gaze. The ptosis increased somewhat with sustained upward gaze and partially worsened in either eye with the examiner holding the opposite eyelid (Fig. 89-1). Pupils were equal and reactive without evidence of retinopathy. There was mild weakness of the orbicularis oculi. Facial muscles were strong, and other cranial nerves were normal, although neck flexors were mildly weak. She had no weakness of her extremity muscles, either distally or proximally, and there was no muscle fatigue during repetitive contractions. Reflexes, sensation, and coordination were normal. The examination was otherwise unremarkable.

T4 and thyroid-stimulating hormone were normal, erythrocyte sedimentation rate was 35 mm/h (normal, 0–30 mm/h), and acetylcholine receptor antibody titer was normal or less than 0.8 nmol/L. Complete blood count and a comprehensive metabolic profile were normal. Serum lactate was 10 mg/dL (normal, 9–18 mg/dL), and serum creatine kinase (CK) was 97 IU/L (normal, <200 IU/L).

WHAT IS THE DIFFERENTIAL DIAGNOSIS?

In this patient with bilateral ophthalmoplegia and ptosis having normal pupils and without long tract signs, a central nervous system disorder seemed unlikely.

Myasthenia gravis should be considered because of the fluctuation of symptoms, fatigue, and the enhancement of ptosis of either eye while the examiner held the opposite eyelid. A patient like this should be worked up for that disease with edrophonium and repetitive stimulation tests. If the latter is negative, single-fiber electromyography (SFEMG) should be done, and acetylcholine receptor antibodies should be measured.[1] If this test is negative, muscle-specific protein kinase (MuSK) antibody levels should be ordered.

The long-standing symptoms and the symmetry of the ophthalmoplegia, however, are somewhat against myasthenia gravis.

Progressive external ophthalmoplegia (PEO) also occurs in mitochondrial myopathy as the manifestation of a more severe disorder, such as Kearns–Sayre syndrome.[2,3] The ophthalmoplegia could also be isolated, or patients might have mild proximal limb weakness. Another possibility is oculopharyngeal dystrophy, but this patient did not have a family history or difficulty swallowing to support this diagnosis.[4] Slow channel congenital myasthenic syndrome was a consideration,[5,6] but she did not have the finger extensor weakness characteristic of this disease; and in this, ptosis and ophthalmoplegia are not prominent. Thyroid eye disease could manifest with ophthalmoplegia and ptosis but is usually accompanied by exophthalmos. This condition could resemble myasthenia gravis or can be associated with myasthenia.[7]

WHAT SHOULD BE THE WORKUP?

The serum lactate and thyroid function tests in this patient were normal. Acetylcholine receptor antibodies were also normal. An edrophonium test was negative. MuSK antibody test was not available then.

The normal thyroid tests ruled out thyroid disease, and normal serum lactate and CK are somewhat against, but do not rule out, a mitochondrial myopathy. The edrophonium test is a sensitive test for myasthenia; however, it could be negative in some patients. Acetylcholine receptor antibodies could also be negative, particularly when weakness is limited to the eye muscles.[1]

AN EMG TEST WAS PERFORMED

Motor Nerve Studies

Nerve and Site	Latency (ms)	Amplitude (mV)	Conduction Velocity (m/s)
Median Nerve L.	Normal ≤ 4.2	Normal ≥ 6	Normal ≥ 50
Wrist	3.7	26	–
Elbow	7.3	25	60

F-Wave Studies

Nerve	Latency (ms)	Normal Latency ≤ (ms)
Median nerve L.	25.5	30

Repetitive Stimulation of Accessory Nerve L.

Potential Number	Amp (mV)	Amp Decrement (%)	Area Decrement (%)
Before Exercise			
1	5.28	0	0
2	5.11	3	2
3	5.06	3	1
4	5.05	4	3
5	4.90	8	4
Posttetanic			
1	5.58	0	0
2	5.51	1	5
3	5.26	6	10
4	5.26	7	10
5	5.26	7	10
1 min Postexercise			
1	5.70	0	0
2	5.52	3	8
3	5.48	4	10
4	5.48	5	10
5	5.48	6	10
2 min Postexercise			
1	5.65	0	0
2	5.59	1	3
3	5.47	3	1
4	5.32	6	10
5	5.29	6	10
3 min Postexercise			
1	5.76	0	0
2	5.56	3	0
3	5.44	6	2
4	5.45	5	1
5	5.45	5	2

Repetitive Stimulation of Facial Nerve L. —cont'd

Potential Number	Amp (mV)	Amp Decrement (%)	Area Decrement (%)
Before Exercise			
1	2.64	0	0
2	2.69	2	3
3	2.59	2	0
4	2.47	6	4
Posttetanic			
1	2.75	0	0
2	2.73	1	1
3	2.66	3	3
4	2.64	4	4
1 min Postexercise			
1	3.27	0	0
2	3.40	4	1
3	3.24	1	1
4	3.19	2	3
2 min Postexercise			
1	3.32	0	0
2	3.36	1	1
3	3.36	1	1
4	3.30	1	0
3 min Postexercise			
1	3.10	0	0
2	3.07	5	3
3	3.01	4	1
4	2.96	2	2

EMG Data

Muscle	Insrt Activity	Fibs	Pos Waves	Fasc	Amp	Dur	Poly	Pattern
Deltoid L.	Norm	None	None	None	Norm	**Brief**	**Few**	Full
Biceps brachii L.	Norm	None	None	None	Norm	**Brief**	**Few**	Full
First dorsal interosseous L.	Norm	None	None	None	Norm	Norm	None	Full
Tensor fasciae latae L.	Norm	None	None	None	Norm	Norm	None	Full
Vastus lateralis L.	Norm	None	None	None	Norm	Norm	None	Full

Single-Fiber EMG

	Jitter Values	
	Patient	Normal Controls
Extensor Digitorum Communis R.		
Mean MCD	27	36
Maximal MCD	44	52
Frontalis R.		
Mean MCD	28	30
Maximal MCD[a]	**47**	45

[a]Three pairs above normal limits.
MCD, Mean consecutive differences.

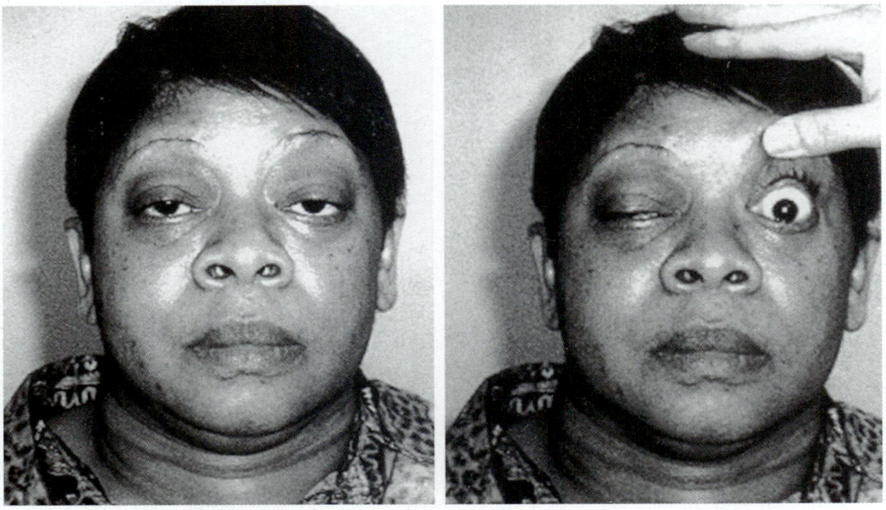

FIG. 89-1 Patient with ptosis; notice enhancement of right ptosis when the examiner holds the left eyelid.

WHAT WERE THE EMG FINDINGS?

The nerve conduction tests were normal. Small scattered polyphasic motor unit potentials were seen on EMG which are compatible with myasthenia as well as myopathy. There was no motor unit variability to suggest myasthenia. Repetitive stimulation test in the facial muscles was normal. When recording the trapezius muscle stimulating the spinal accessory nerve at 3 Hz, there was a 10% decrement 1 minute after exercise. This is in the upper limits of normal and was reproducible.

SFEMG of the extensor digitorum communis muscle was normal. The maximal mean of consecutive differences (MCD) in the frontalis muscle was 47 μs (normal, <45 μs), and three pairs had an abnormal jitter with MCDs above the normal limits, but the mean MCD was normal, 28 μs (normal, <30 μs). There were no blocks.

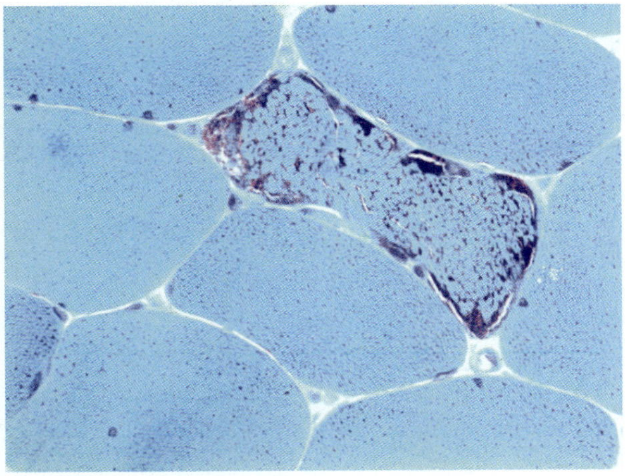

FIG. 89-2 Ragged red fibers on the modified trichrome stain (×400).

WHAT DOES THIS TEST MEAN?

These test results are suggestive, but not diagnostic, of a neuromuscular transmission defect such as myasthenia gravis; however, increased jitter values have also been reported in other disorders, including mitochondrial myopathy.[8]

The lack of an afterdischarge in the CMAP is against slow channel congenital myasthenic syndrome and acetylcholinesterase deficiency.

WHAT SHOULD BE DONE NEXT?

The patient received a trial of pyridostigmine and, later, steroids for 3 months, and neither helped. For that reason, she underwent a deltoid muscle biopsy that was characteristic of mitochondrial myopathy (Figs. 89-2 and 89-3). A mitochondrial DNA deletion test using Southern blot analysis in muscle showed a single mitochondrial DNA deletion, consistent with the diagnosis of PEO.[9,10]

WHAT IS PROGRESSIVE EXTERNAL OPHTHALMOPLEGIA?

PEO is a disorder that manifests by ophthalmoplegia and ptosis, and patients may have a mild proximal weakness. This is a mitochondrial disease that is classified with the group of *mitochondrial encephalomyopathies*.

PEO could start in childhood, adolescence (Fig. 89-4), or later in life (Fig. 89-5). As demonstrated in this case, patients may lack other manifestations or can have mild proximal muscle weakness, or they might have a more severe disorder with short stature, ophthalmoplegia, ptosis, atypical retinitis pigmentosa, ataxia, deafness, cardiomyopathy, and high protein in the spinal fluid (Kearns–Sayre syndrome). These conditions are caused by deletions of mitochondrial DNA.

As in this case, most mitochondrial diseases are caused by deletions of mitochondrial DNA, although some myopathies causing defects of the mitochondrial respiratory chains are caused by nuclear DNA deletions.

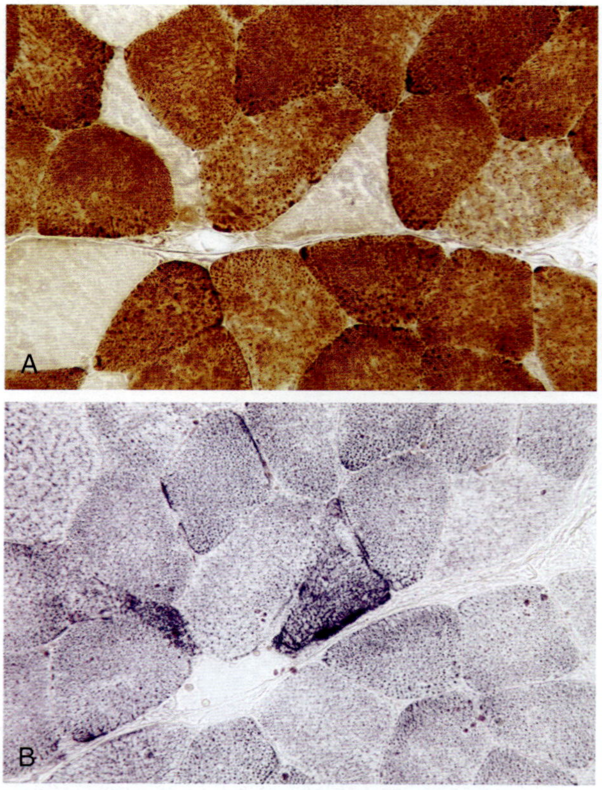

FIG. 89-3 A, Muscle biopsy showing decreased staining for cytochrome oxidase. **B**, The same fiber showing increased activity on the SDH stain (×200). *SDH*, Succinic dehydrogenase.

Mitochondrial DNA deletions are maternally inherited,[11] but PEO is frequently sporadic, because the mutations occur during oogenesis or early embryogenesis with very rare exceptions. There is no paternal inheritance in mitochondrial disorders because the sperm do not contain mitochondria.[12] The oocytes of normal women contain about 150,000 mitochondrial DNA,[12] and only a few of them have deletions. As the embryo only receives maternal mitochondrial DNA, only some of the mutant DNA might enter the blastocyte. In the case of PEO, there are more mutant mitochondrial DNA, and these are increased and might segregate only in muscle or occur in three layers of the blastocyte and manifest as a multisystem disorder such as Kearns–Sayre syndrome. The functional abnormalities in the mitochondrial encephalomyopathies are caused by impaired adenosine triphosphate production, and the manifestations are more severe in tissues that are more dependent on oxidative metabolisms, such as muscle and brain.[12]

An important concept of mitochondrial disorders is heteroplasmy, which indicates that only a few of the mitochondrial DNA in each cell have pathologic mutations, and the number of mutated mitochondrial genes in each cell determines the expression of the disease. The symptoms appear because mitotic segregation during cell division varies and because the threshold to cause the disease is surpassed. In normals, all mitochondrial DNA are identical; this is called *homoplasmy*. The majority of patients with PEO have large single mitochondrial DNA deletions similar to those in Kearns–Sayre syndrome, a severe childhood disorder;

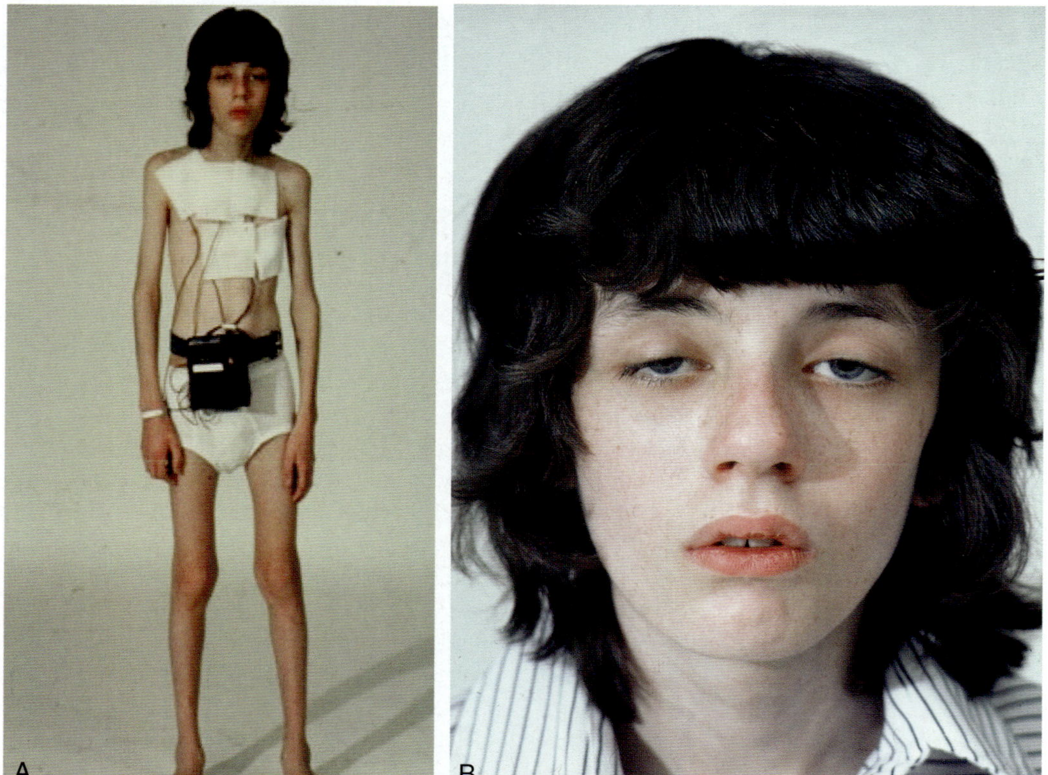

FIG. 89-4 A, Patient with Kearns–Sayre syndrome; notice proximal muscle atrophy (she is wearing a cardiac monitor). **B**, Prominent ptosis in the same patient.

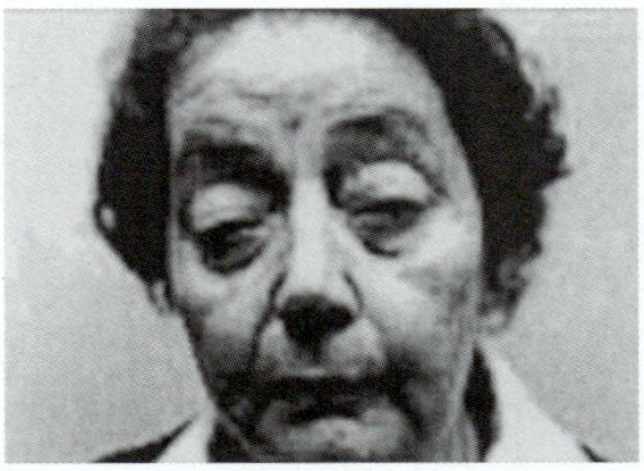

FIG. 89-5 Older woman with ophthalmoplegia and ptosis; she had a late-onset mitochondrial myopathy.

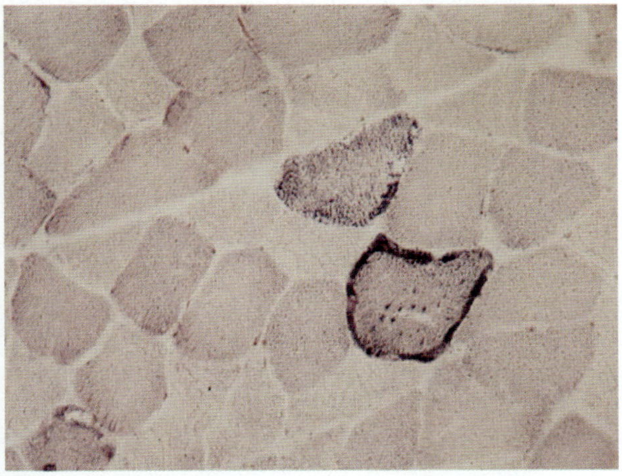

FIG. 89-6 A muscle fiber with increased SDH staining ("ragged blue" fiber, ×400). *SDH*, Succinic dehydrogenase.

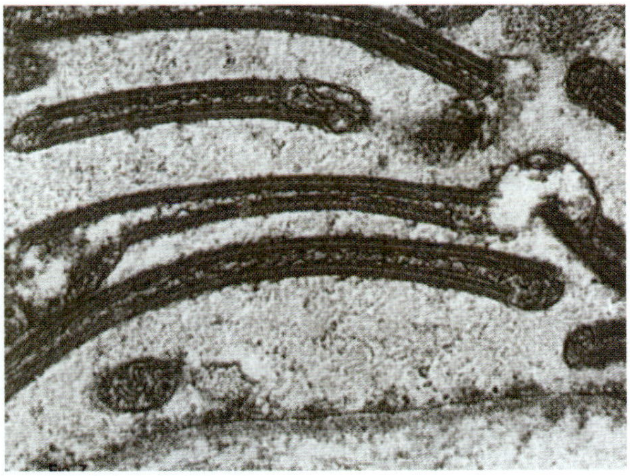

FIG. 89-7 Mitochondrial paracrystalline inclusions in mitochondrial myopathy (×12,000).

patients also have retinopathy, deafness, and heart block.[13–15] Autosomal-recessive PEO is most commonly associated with mutations of the nuclear genes such as the polymerase gamma (*POLG*) gene or *TWINKLE* gene and the ribonucleotide reductase small subunit of p53 (RRM2B).

Characteristic biopsy findings are the presence of ragged red fibers, seen in the trichrome stain; they lack cytochrome oxidase activity and stain dark with oxidative stains, particularly the succinic dehydrogenase stain (Fig. 89-6), and EM shows numerous abnormal mitochondria with paracrystalline inclusions (Fig. 89-7).

There is no cure for PEO; eyelid crutches might help, and these were recommended but were not helpful. She then underwent eyelid surgery with marked benefit as she was able to see more clearly. There are several therapeutic trials for mitochondrial disorders such as the use of elamipretide (see also Case 90).[14–16]

WHAT IS THE EXPLANATION FOR THE ENHANCEMENT OF PTOSIS UPON HOLDING THE OPPOSITE EYELID?

Since Hering first observed, "the two eyes are so related to one another that one cannot be moved independently from the other; rather the musculature of both eyes react simultaneously to one and the same impulse of will,"[17,18] similar observations of this simultaneous innervation have been documented in the levator palpebrae muscles.[11,19–24] Primate studies have demonstrated that innervation to the levator palpebrae superioris is supplied by an unpaired subnucleus of the oculomotor nuclear complex, which lies ventral to the Edinger–Westphal nucleus in the rostral midbrain.[25] Eyelid opening is accomplished through the contraction of the levator palpebrae muscles, with lesser contributions made by the frontalis and Mueller's muscles.[26] Ptosis may be observed in various disorders involving the oculomotor complex, causing weakness of the levator muscles. In unilateral ptosis there is often retraction of the contralateral eyelid. If the ptotic eyelid is closed or lifted, then the contralateral eyelid develops ptosis, or this increases. The phenomenon has been described as *enhanced ptosis*.[27] In accordance with Hering's law the weakness in the lesser-involved eyelid is masked, as an increased drive in central innervation is needed to elevate the weakened contralateral eyelid. Thus, by lifting or closing the ptotic eyelid, weakness in the contralateral eyelid is revealed. Disease processes that do not involve the neuromuscular junction are less likely to demonstrate enhanced ptosis, and most studies have demonstrated the clinical sign in myasthenic patients.[11,18,21] Several authors propose the concept of eye dominance as an explanation for the variability of this sign, such as when ptosis involving the dominant eye is severe enough to create visual impairment; then innervation is increased to compensate for levator weakness.[27–29] Nonetheless, when present, enhanced ptosis is a valuable bedside test in patients with myasthenia gravis,[29] but as discussed, could occur in other disorders.

Initially, this patient was thought to have myasthenia gravis, because of the fluctuating symptoms, the enhanced ptosis, and borderline abnormal decrement on repetitive stimulation testing, and also the increased jitter on SFEMG; however, it should be noted that increased jitter occurs not only in disorders of the neuromuscular junction but also in other conditions, and, as discussed, has been reported in patients with mitochondrial myopathies.[8] The negative edrophonium test, absence of acetylcholine antibodies, and poor response to immunosuppression trial were clues prompting further investigation, which ultimately resulted in mitochondrial DNA testing, leading to the correct diagnosis.

IMPORTANT POINTS

- Enhancement of ptosis upon passively holding the contralateral eyelid can be seen not only in central nervous system disorders and in myasthenia gravis but also in mitochondrial myopathies.
- Some patients with myasthenia might not have elevated acetylcholine receptor antibodies, and patients with mitochondrial myopathy might have normal serum lactate and CK.
- Increased jitter on SFEMG can be seen in mitochondrial myopathies.
- PEO is a disorder caused by mitochondrial DNA deletions, manifesting as isolated extraocular muscle weakness or with more generalized symptoms, such as the Kearns–Sayre syndrome characterized by short stature, weakness, cardiomyopathy, endocrinopathy, atypical retinitis pigmentosa, deafness, and high protein in spinal fluid.
- Management for external ophthalmoplegia is conservative, but eyelid surgery might be helpful.

This case was presented by Owens W, Gupta D, Bertorini T. 50th Annual Meeting of the American Association of Electrodiagnostic Medicine. San Francisco, CA; 2003.

REFERENCES

1. Keesey JC. Clinical evaluation and management of myasthenia gravis. *Muscle Nerve.* 2004;29(4):484–505.
2. Moraes CT, DiMauro S, Zeviani M, et al. Mitochondrial DNA deletions in progressive external ophthalmoplegia and Kearns-Sayre syndrome. *N Engl J Med.* 1989;320:1293–1299.
3. Petty RK, Harding AE, Morgan-Hughes JA. The clinical features of mitochondrial myopathy. *Brain.* 1986;109:915–938.
4. Bertorini TE, Igarashi M. Muscular dystrophies. In: Pourmand R, ed. *Neuromuscular Diseases: Expert Clinicians' Views.* Boston, MA: Butterworth-Heinemann; 2001:227–294.
5. Engel AG, Lambert EH, Mulder DM, et al. A newly recognized congenital myasthenic syndrome attributed to a prolonged open time of the acetylcholine-induced ion channel. *Ann Neurol.* 1982; 11:553–569.
6. Engel A, Franzini-Armstrong C. *Myology.* 3rd ed. New York, NY: McGraw-Hill; 2004:1801–1844.
7. Amato AA. Endocrine myopathies and toxic myopathies. In: Brown WF, Bolton CH, Aminoff M, eds. *Neuromuscular Function and Disease.* Philadelphia, PA: WB Saunders; 2002:1339–1428.
8. Krendel DA, Sanders DB, Massey JM. Single fiber electromyography in chronic progressive external ophthalmoplegia. *Muscle Nerve.* 1987;10:299–302.
9. Moraes CT, Ciacci F, Silvestri G, et al. Atypical clinical presentations associated with the MELAS mutation at position 3243 of human mitochondrial DNA. *Neuromuscul Disord.* 1993;3:43–50.
10. Nonaka I. Mitochondrial diseases. *Curr Opin Neurol Neurosurg.* 1992;5:622–632.
11. Walsh FB, Hoyt WF. *Clinical Neuro-Ophthalmology.* 5th ed. Baltimore, MD: Williams & Wilkins; 1998:1555.
12. DiMauro S, Schon EA. Mitochondrial respiratory-chain diseases. *N Engl J Med.* 2003;348:2656–2668.
13. Tinker RJ, Lim AZ, Stefanetti RJ, McFarland R. Current and emerging clinical treatment in mitochondrial disease. *Mol Diagn Ther.* 2021;25(2):181–206.
14. DiMauro S, Schon EA, Carelli V, Hirano M. The clinical maze of mitochondrial neurology. *Nat Rev Neurol.* 2013;9(8):429–444.
15. Milone M, Wong L-J. Diagnosis of mitochondrial myopathies. *Mol Genet Metab.* 2013;110(1–2):35–41.
16. O'Ferrell E. *Mitochondrial Myopathies: Treatment.* Waltham, MA: UpToDate; 2022.
17. Hering E. *The Theory of Binocular Vision.* New York, NY: Plenum Press; 1977.
18. Hering E. *Die Lehre v Binokularne Sehen.* Leipzig, Germany: Engleman; 1868.
19. Gupta JS, Jain IS, Kumar K. Lid retraction secondary to contralateral ptosis. *Br J Ophthalmol.* 1964;48:626–627.
20. Jain JS. Lid retraction in the non-paretic eye in acquired ophthalmoplegia. *Br J Ophthalmol.* 1963;47:757–759.
21. Lewallen WM Jr. Lid retraction syndrome due to secondary deviation. *Am J Ophthalmol.* 1958;45:565–567.
22. Gay AJ, Salmon ML, Windsor CE. Hering's law, the levators and their relationship in disease states. *Arch Ophthalmol.* 1967; 77:157–160.
23. Schechter RJ. Ptosis with contralateral lid retraction due to excessive innervation of the levator palpebrae superiorus. *Ann Ophthalmol.* 1978;10(10):1324–1328.
24. Lepore FE. Unilateral ptosis and Hering's law. *Neurology.* 1988;38(2):319–322.
25. Warwick R. Representation of the extraocular muscles in the oculomotor nuclei of the monkey. *J Comp Neurol.* 1953;98:449–503.
26. Brazis PW, Masdeu JC, Biller J. Localization in Clinical Neurology. Philadelphia, PA: Lippincott Williams & Wilkins; 2001:213–216. 4th ed.
27. Gorelick PB, Rosenberg M, Pagano RJ. Enhanced ptosis in myasthenia gravis. *Arch Neurol.* 1981;38:531.
28. Meyer DR, Wobig JL. Detection of contralateral eyelid retraction associated with blepharoptosis. *Ophthalmology.* 1992;99:366–375.
29. Barton JJ, Fouladvand M. Ocular aspects of myasthenia gravis. *Semin Neurol.* 2000;20:7–20.

CASE 90

A Man With Weakness and Swelling in the Neck

A 47-year-old man presented with a 15-year history of progressive proximal muscle weakness in the arms and legs. He also noted thinning of muscle and voluminous swelling of the back of the neck which was progressively worsening. He had some difficulty drinking liquids and a 10-year history of hearing loss.

Family history revealed that his parents had no such symptoms, but two sisters and one brother of a total of nine siblings are similarly affected. Another brother had only muscle weakness and exercise intolerance. The patient had two healthy children.

Laboratory studies including a comprehensive metabolic panel, complete blood count, and thyroid-stimulating hormone were all normal, except a serum creatine kinase test that was mildly elevated at 300 IU/L (normal, <200 IU/L). Serum cortisol and lactate levels were normal.

An EMG done prior to the referral showed normal nerve conduction velocities and small polyphasic motor unit potentials.

A muscle biopsy, done previously and studied with paraffin sections, showed nonspecific findings. A specimen was fixed in glutaraldehyde and was sent to us. The patient refused a second biopsy. Examination revealed mild facial weakness, bilateral sensory neural hearing loss, and thinning of proximal limb muscles, particularly in the arms and thighs. Muscle strength testing revealed neck flexors to be 5−/5; shoulder muscles and pectoralis, 4/5; biceps and triceps, 4+/5; wrist extensors and flexors, 5−/5; hip flexors and extensors, 4/5; quadriceps and iliopsoas, 4+/5; and hamstrings, 5−/5. Distal leg, forearm, and hand muscles were normal, as were reflexes and sensation. He had a prominent posterior neck mass that had the consistency of fat (Fig. 90-1). The examination was otherwise normal.

WHAT IS THE DIFFERENTIAL DIAGNOSIS?

This patient and his family have muscle weakness and prominent fat accumulation in the neck. He also has hearing loss. The condition appeared to be hereditary.

The EMG findings were against spinal muscular atrophy. He could have a limb-girdle dystrophy, but the lack of symptoms in either of his parents and the lack of definite trapezius muscle wasting and scapular winging are against a diagnosis of facioscapulohumeral dystrophy. A metabolic myopathy is a possibility; however, the lack of myotonia on the EMG is against acid maltase deficiency.

The patient's hearing loss and large lipoma of the neck in family members suggest a multisystem disorder such as mitochondrial myopathy which can manifest with variable phenotypes.[1]

AN EMG TEST WAS PERFORMED

Motor Nerve Studies

Nerve and Site	Latency (ms)	Amplitude (mV)	Conduction Velocity (m/s)
Peroneal Nerve R.	**Normal ≤ 5.7**	**Normal ≥ 3**	**Normal ≥ 40**
Ankle	5.2	9	–
Fibular head	12.7	9	41
Nerve and Site	**Latency (ms)**	**Amplitude (mV)**	**Conduction Velocity (m/s)**
Ulnar Nerve R.	**Normal ≤ 3.6**	**Normal ≥ 8**	**Normal ≥ 50**
Wrist	3.6	15	–
Below elbow	8.0	15	56

F-Wave Studies

Nerve	Latency (ms)	Normal Latency ≤ (ms)
Peroneal nerve R.	51.2	54
Ulnar nerve R.	26.6	30

Sensory Nerve Studies

Nerve	Onset Latency (ms)	Normal Onset Latency ≤ (ms)	Peak Latency (ms)	Normal Peak Latency ≤ (ms)	Amp (μV)	Normal Amp ≥ (μV)	Conduction Velocity (m/s)	Normal Conduction Velocity ≥ (m/s)
Sural nerve R.	3.2	3.5	3.7	4.0	16	11	44	40
Ulnar nerve R.	2.4	2.6	2.9	3.1	21	13	50	50

EMG Data

Muscle	Insrt Activity	Fibs	Pos Waves	Fasc	Amp	Dur	Poly	Pattern
Infraspinatus R.	Norm	None	None	None	**Dec**	**Brief**	**Many**	Full
Deltoid R.	Norm	None	None	None	**Dec**	**Brief**	**Many**	Full
Biceps brachii R.	Norm	None	None	None	**Dec**	**Brief**	**Few**	Full
Triceps R.	Norm	None	None	None	Norm	Norm	None	Full
First dorsal interosseous R.	Norm	None	None	None	Norm	Norm	None	Full
Tensor fasciae latae R.	Norm	None	None	None	Norm	Norm	None	Full
Tibialis anterior R.	Norm	None	None	None	Norm	Norm	None	Full

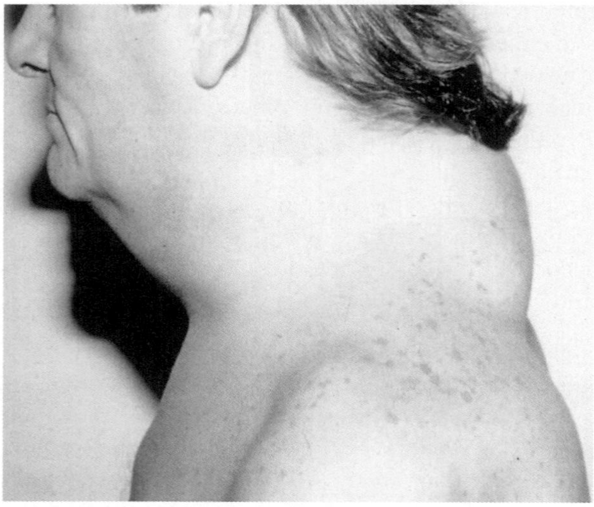

FIG. 90-1 Lateral view of the patient showing the prominent mass in the posterior neck.

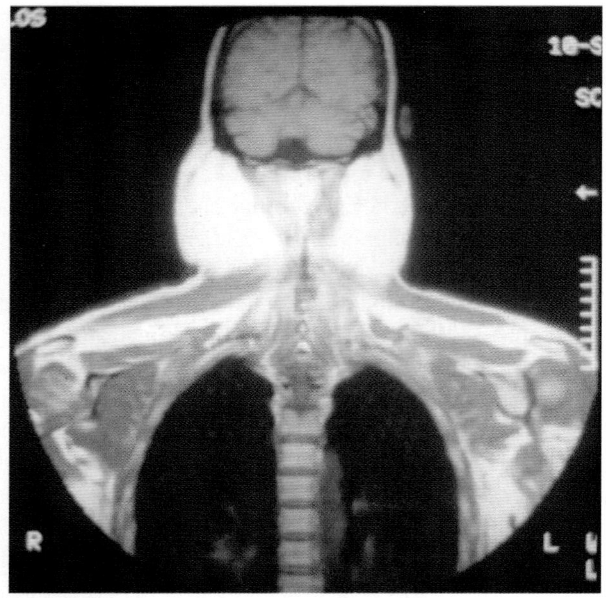

FIG. 90-2 T1-weighted MRI image (coronal view); notice the fat accumulation in the neck.

WHAT WERE THE EMG FINDINGS?

This EMG showed small polyphasic motor units compatible with a myopathy. An MRI of the neck showed atrophy of the paraspinal muscles in the neck with a prominent subcutaneous fatty mass (Fig. 90-2).

The muscle biopsy was studied with a trichrome stain and demonstrated scattered ragged red fibers. The EM showed abnormal mitochondrial paracrystalline inclusions (Fig. 90-3). DNA analysis in lymphocytes in Dr. S. DiMauro's laboratory showed a G8363 mitochondrial tRNA mutation.

DISCUSSION

This patient and his siblings appear to have a mitochondrial myopathy characterized by weakness and a large lipoma in the neck. These lipomas are a prominent feature in multiple symmetric lipomatosis (MSL), a disorder first described by Brodie in 1846[2] and later by Launois and Bensaude in 1898[3] and Madelung in 1888.[4] This condition has been reported as occurring mainly in Mediterranean countries.[5,6] Many of those patients were alcoholics and had a polyneuropathy.[5–8] Frequently, however, there is no history of excessive alcohol intake, and there are several reported familial cases of MSL with a neuropathy, associated with a mitochondrial dysfunction and mitochondrial DNA mutations.[9–11] It is that likely that the conditions described by Brodie, Launois and Bensaude, and Madelung are not caused by alcoholism, but excessive alcohol intake could be an aggravating factor. Schoffer and Grant recently reported an alcoholic man who had lipomas and a peripheral neuropathy and who later developed proximal weakness, which they found to be associated with a mitochondrial disorder and a myoclonic epilepsy with ragged red fibers (MERRF) DNA mutation.[12] As discussed, mitochondrial gene mutations have also been found in patients with MSL. The majority of these are sporadic but could also be familial. In one study 16% had MERRF mutations, and 12% had multiple small or single large deletions.[11]

Patients with MSL have large lipomas in the neck or other areas, and in some, this could be the only manifestation of the MERRF mutation.[13,14] Those with lipomas like this patient are also classified as type I, while type II have lipomas in other areas also and on the abdomen.[15]

It is of particular interest that fat accumulation occurs frequently in areas of normal brown fat in animals, and the fat of the lipomas of MSL has features of brown fat with abundant mitochondria on electromicroscopy.[16]

Brown fat is used for thermogenesis in mammals, and its mitochondria have an uncoupling protein that bypasses

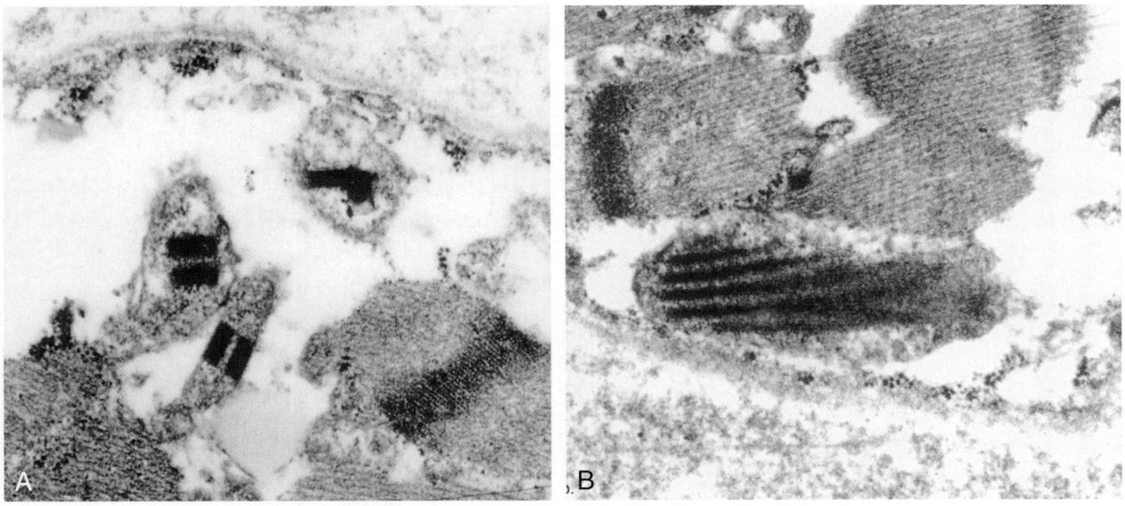

FIG. 90-3 Mitochondrial inclusions on electromicroscopy, ×10,000 (**A**) and ×30,000 (**B**).

adenosine triphosphate production; thus the energy generated by fatty acid oxidation is expressed as heat.[17] Brown fat has a high rate of lipolysis, and it is likely that a mitochondrial dysfunction impairs lipolysis, causing fat accumulation in MSL. Excessive alcohol intake could have a predisposing effect for this fat accumulation because alcohol impairs fatty acid β-oxidation and utilization. Lipomas and mitochondrial myopathies have also been associated with antiretroviral therapy.[18] Randomized crossover and dose–escalation trials with elamipretide in adults are beneficial in mitochondrial myopathy.[19,20]

SUMMARY

This man and members of his family had muscle weakness with massive fat accumulation in the neck. He had a mitochondrial DNA mutation in tRNA.

IMPORTANT POINTS

- MSL, or Launois–Bensaude or Madelung syndrome, in many patients likely represents a mitochondrial defect causing lipid accumulation in the neck and trunk, with a myopathy or neuropathy.
- A mitochondrial disorder could affect lipolysis of brown fat, which is normally used for thermogenesis in mammals. This could be the origin of the lipoma in the neck and trunk, where brown fat accumulates in mammals.
- MSL could be familial and also associated with excessive alcohol intake.
- Disorder of mitochondrial function could manifest as myopathies with exercise intolerance and with multiple system dysfunction, such as hearing loss, lipomas, seizures, cardiomyopathy, encephalopathy, optic atrophy, retinopathy, and neuropathy.

This case was studied with Dr. Juan Altamirano, Lima, Peru.

REFERENCES

1. DiMauro S, Gurgel-Giannetti J. The expanding phenotype of mitochondrial myopathy. *Curr Opin Neurol.* 2005;18(5):538–542.
2. Brodie BC. *Lectures Illustrative of Various Subjects in Pathology and Surgery*. London, England: Longman; 1846:275–276.
3. Launois PE, Bensaude R. De L'adenolipomatose symetrique *Bull Mem Soc Med Hosp Paris.* 11898298–318.
4. Madelung OW. Uber den fetthals (diffuses lipom des Halses). *Arch Klin Chir.* 1888;37:106–130.
5. Enzi G. Multiple symmetric lipomatosis: an updated clinical report. *Medicine.* 1984;63:56–64.
6. Enzi G, Angelini C, Negrin P, et al. Sensory, motor, and autonomic neuropathy in patients with multiple symmetric lipomatosis. *Medicine (Baltimore).* 1985;64:388–393.
7. Ruzicka T, Vieluf D, Landthaler M, Braun-Falco O. Benign symmetric lipomatosis Launois-Bensuade: report of ten cases and review of the literature. *J Am Acad Dermatol.* 1987;17:663–674.
8. Pollock M, Nicholson GI, Nukada H, et al. Neuropathy in multiple symmetric lipomatosis: Madelung's disease. *Brain.* 1988;111:1157–1171.
9. Silvestri G, Ciafaloni E, Santorelli FM, et al. Clinical features associated with the A → G transition at nucleotide 8344 of mtDNA ("MERRF mutation"). *Neurology.* 1993;43:1200–1206.
10. Gamez J, Playan A, Andreu AL, et al. Familial multiple symmetric lipomatosis associated with the A8344G mutation of mitochondrial DNA. *Neurology.* 1998;51(1):258–260.
11. Austin SA, Vriesendorp FJ, Thandroyen FT, et al. Expanding the phenotype of the 8344 transfer RNAlysine mitochondrial DNA mutation. *Neurology.* 1998;51(5):1447–1450.
12. Schoffer K, Grant I. Multiple lipomas, alcoholism, and neuropathy: Madelung's disease or MERRF? *Muscle Nerve.* 2006;33:142–146.
13. Chong P, Vucic S, Hedley-Whyte T, et al. Multiple symmetric lipomatosis (Madelung's disease) caused by the MERRF (A8344G) mutation. *J Clin Neuromuscul W Dis.* 2003;5:1–7.
14. Holme E, Larsson NG, Oldorfs A, et al. Multiple symmetric lipomas with high levels of mtDNA with the tRNA (Lys) A → G (8344) mutation as the only manifestation of disease in a carrier of the myoclonus epilepsy and ragged-red fibers (MERRF) syndrome. *Am J Hum Genet.* 1993;52:551–556.

15. Maximiano LF, Gaspar MT, Nakahira ES. Madelung disease (multiple symmetric lipomatosis). *Autops Case Rep*. 2018;8(3):e2018030.
16. Zancanaro C, Sbarbati A, Morroni M, et al. Multiple symmetric lipomatosis: ultrastructural investigation of the tissue and preadipocytes in primary culture. *Lab Invest*. 1990;63:253–258.
17. Nechad M. Structure and development of brown adipose tissue. In: Trayhurn P, Nicholls DG, eds. *Brown Adipose Tissue*. Baltimore, MD: Edward Arnold; 1986:1–30.
18. Guzman, N, Vijayan V. HIV-associated lipodystrophy. In: *StatPearls [Internet]*. Last updated May 8, 2022.
19. Karaa A, Haas R, Goldstein A, Vockley J, et al. Randomized dose-escalation trial of elamipretide in adults with primary mitochondrial myopathy. *Neurology*. 2018;90(14):e1212–e1221. https://doi.org/10.1212/WNL.0000000000005255. Epub Mar 2, 2018.
20. Karaa A, Haas R, Goldstein A, Vockley J, et al. A randomized crossover trial of elamipretide in adults with primary mitochondrial myopathy. *J Cachexia Sarcopenia Muscle*. 2020;11(4):909–918.

A Woman With Muscle Pains and Dark Urine

An 18-year-old woman presented with acute renal failure. She had been at a church youth function at which the activities required running. She subsequently suffered exhaustion and muscle cramps. Later that night the cramping became severe, and her urine became dark, which she thought was from blood, and she was taken to the hospital. She denied similar episodes in the past but did recall a long history of exercise intolerance with severe cramping. Exercise also caused shortness of breath, and she had been diagnosed with asthma as a child. She had not engaged in much physical activity since then.

Current medications included phenergan and an unnamed over-the-counter decongestant. Social history was negative for tobacco or drug use. She lived with her parents, and her family history was negative for neurologic diseases.

Physical examination revealed an obese girl whose general examination was unremarkable. Higher cortical function and cranial nerve testing were normal. Motor examination showed profound weakness of 2/5 throughout. She complained of severe pain with passive movements of the extremities. Sensory examination was normal. Reflexes were 1+ in the arms and knees, 2+ in the ankles; they were symmetrical.

WHAT IS THE DIFFERENTIAL DIAGNOSIS?

This patient presented with a severe paralyzing illness and diffuse muscle pains. The pigmenturia is against a disorder of neuromuscular transmission. Neuropathies, such as Guillain–Barré syndrome, can present with pain, severe weakness, and areflexia, but this patient had normal reflexes. Another possibility is porphyria, which presents in a similar manner to Guillain–Barré syndrome but with pigmenturia. The muscle pain with exercise intolerance and normal reflexes are rather atypical for neuropathy and most likely represent primary myopathy.

The symptoms are indicative of rhabdomyolysis, and the history of exercise intolerance is suggestive of a metabolic myopathy, such as in the glycogenosis, including phosphorylase kinase, myophosphorylase, phosphoglycerate mutase, phosphofructokinase, lactate dehydrogenase, and β-enolase deficiencies.[1] Typically, these patients report a history of difficulty with high-intensity exercise such as running. Diseases of fatty acid transport, such as carnitine palmitoyltransferase deficiency, can also present with exercise intolerance but usually only during prolonged exercise or fasting.[2] Sustained exercise intolerance and the ability to perform only brief bursts of exercise are symptoms that help to differentiate this disorder from disorders of glucose metabolism.

Mitochondrial disorders should be considered, as they may present with rhabdomyolysis.[3,4] The possibility of an inflammatory myopathy seems unlikely given the patient's long history of exercise intolerance without previous overt muscle weakness, although rhabdomyolysis may be the initial presentation of an inflammatory myopathy.[5–8] Drug ingestion (including alcohol), thyroid disease, and uremia and electrolyte imbalances[1] are also conditions to consider.

WHAT DIAGNOSTIC TESTING SHOULD BE PERFORMED NEXT?

Her serum creatine kinase (CK) level was elevated at 40,893 IU/L (normal, <200 IU/L); aspartate transaminase was 455 IU/L (normal, 0–40 IU/L); alanine transaminase, 306 IU/L (normal, 30–65 IU/L); creatinine, 9.4 mg/dL (normal, <1.5 mg/dL); and blood urea nitrogen, 102 μg/dL (normal, <20 μg/dL). She therefore required hemodialysis, and this gradually normalized. Testing for thyroid-stimulating hormone, antinuclear antibodies, human immunodeficiency virus, and hepatitis A, B, and C were all negative. Her urinalysis showed dark urine (Fig. 91-1) that was positive for "blood," but had only eight RBCs. However, a test for myoglobin in the urine was positive.

An exercise test was not performed.

WHAT IS RHABDOMYOLYSIS?

She was diagnosed as having *rhabdomyolysis*, a term that means destruction of skeletal muscle, and this is caused by a variety of mechanisms, such as trauma, toxins, infections, or metabolic derangements[9] (Table 91-1).

Rhabdomyolysis leads to leakage of muscle contents including the oxygen-binding protein myoglobin, and thus the terms *myoglobinuria* and *rhabdomyolysis* are used interchangeably.

Rhabdomyolysis was apparently recorded first in the Bible in the Book of Numbers, wherein it states that the Israelites became ill after eating quail which had probably fed on hemlock seeds.[2]

AN EMG TEST WAS PERFORMED

Motor Nerve Studies

Nerve and Site	Latency (ms)	Amplitude (mV)	Conduction Velocity (m/s)
Peroneal Nerve L.	Normal ≤ 5.7	Normal ≥ 3	Normal ≥ 40
Ankle	5.7	10	–
Fibular head	14.2	10	41

Motor Nerve Studies—cont'd

Nerve and Site	Latency (ms)	Amplitude (mV)	Conduction Velocity (m/s)
Tibial Nerve R.	**Normal ≤ 5.3**	**Normal ≥ 4**	**Normal ≥ 40**
Ankle	5.3	22	–
Pop. fossa	15.0	22	42
Median Nerve R.	**Normal ≤ 4.2**	**Normal ≥ 6**	**Normal ≥ 50**
Wrist	3.2	16	–
Elbow	7.2	15	53
Ulnar Nerve R.	**Normal ≤ 3.6**	**Normal ≥ 8**	**Normal ≥ 50**
Wrist	3.0	12	–
Below elbow	6.7	12	59

F-Wave and Tibial H-Reflex Studies

Nerve	Latency (ms)	Normal Latency ≤ (ms)
Peroneal nerve L.	50.0	54
Tibial nerve R.	51.6	54
Median nerve R.	27.8	30
Ulnar nerve R.	28.8	30
H-reflex L.	31.6	34
H-reflex R.	32.0	34

Sensory Nerve Studies

Nerve	Onset Latency (ms)	Normal Onset Latency ≤ (ms)	Peak Latency (ms)	Normal Peak Latency ≤ (ms)	Amp (μV)	Normal Amp ≥ (μV)	Conduction Velocity (m/s)	Normal Conduction Velocity ≥ (m/s)
Sural nerve L.	3.1	3.5	3.6	4.0	22	13	45	40
Median nerve R.	2.2	2.6	2.7	3.1	40	20	59	50
Ulnar nerve R.	2.0	2.6	2.5	3.1	25	13	60	50

EMG Data

Muscle	Insrt Activity	Fibs	Pos Waves	Fasc	Amp	Dur	Poly	Pattern
Deltoid R.	Norm	None	None	None	Norm	**Brief**	**Few**	Norm
Flexor carpi ulnaris R.	Norm	None	None	None	Norm	**Brief**	**Few**	Norm
Rectus femoris R.	**Inc**	**2+**	**2+**	None	Norm	Norm	None	Norm
Tibialis anterior R.	Norm	None	None	None	Norm	Norm	None	Norm

WHAT WERE THE EMG FINDINGS?

Nerve conduction studies were normal. On the needle test there were small polyphasic motor unit potentials with normal recruitment. Denervation potentials were seen only in the quadriceps muscle, compatible with a necrotizing myopathy.

A muscle biopsy showed abundant necrotic fibers and absence of phosphorylase staining and glycogen accumulation (Fig. 91-2). Nowadays, genetic testing can be done with blood in suspected cases.

DISCUSSION

This patient had myophosphorylase deficiency, a disease reported initially by McArdle in 1951.[10] He described this metabolic myopathy in a patient who presented with exercise intolerance and cramps. The defect blocks the formation of adenosine triphosphate from glycogen as a source of energy, as this is not converted to glucose 1-phosphate, particularly during early stages of exercise that utilize anaerobic metabolism. Although characteristically the symptoms in this disease are brought on by exercise, there are some case reports of a severe childhood presentation with respiratory failure and even sudden infant death syndrome.[11]

The phenotype of classic McArdle disease varies, and some patients may be more severely affected. This could be related to a genetic polymorphism,[12] and other factors may play a role in the clinical manifestations. Patients usually complain of muscle cramps and pigmenturia during or after exercise. They also usually have a "second wind" of tolerance to exercise after a brief period of rest. The neurologic examination is usually normal. The baseline serum CK is typically elevated.

Electrophysiologic examination at the time of an attack is characterized by normal motor and sensory nerve conduction tests. The needle EMG may be normal or may show fibrillation potentials and polyphasic motor units with increased recruitment. Myotonia or complex repetitive discharges, particularly in the paraspinal muscles, have been reported.[13]

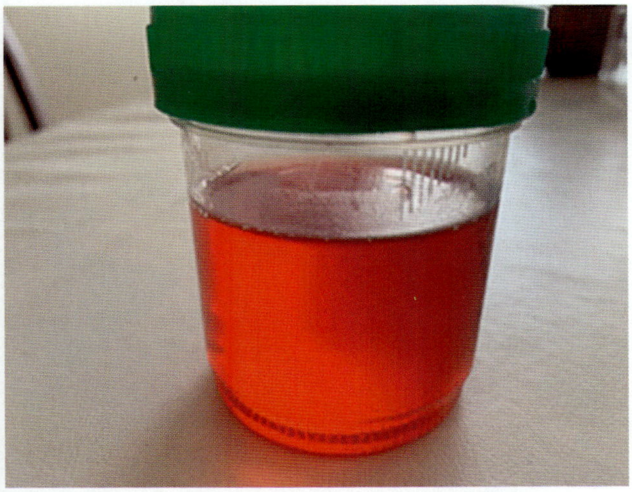

FIG. 91-1 Notice the dark urine of the patient with myoglobinuria.

The pathognomonic electromyographic finding is an absence of electrical muscle activity on needle examination during a muscle cramp (silent cramp).

The ischemic exercise test, which demonstrates a lack of rise of serum lactate with a normal rise of ammonia levels, is used for screening. This test could produce tissue ischemia. A nonischemic[14] and a modified semiischemic exercise are being used to diagnose glycogen storage diseases providing reproducible results.[15]

A lack of increase in serum lactate and pyruvate during this test is also seen in other glycogen storage diseases, such as *phosphofructokinase* and *phosphoglycerate mutase* deficiencies. In *phosphorylase B kinase* deficiency the rise is blunted, and in lactate *dehydrogenase deficiency* there is a lack of increase in lactate but a pyruvate level rise. (Fig. 91-3 shows the different glycogen storage diseases.) In all these conditions ammonia levels rise normally, whereas in *myoadenylate deaminase deficiency*, there is a normal increase of lactate, but not of ammonia, during the exercise test.[1]

Because the test does not distinguish between the various glycogen storage disorders, a muscle biopsy remains the gold standard for their differentiation, particularly using enzyme histochemical and biochemical analysis. DNA testing is increasingly being used in diagnosis.

McArdle disease has an autosomal-recessive inheritance caused by mutations in chromosome 11q13 in the *GGAV* gene. There is molecular heterogenicity, and various mutations have been reported. The most common are mutations at R50x (previously known as R49x), and in those the diagnosis can be made by molecular analysis of blood cells.[16,17]

Patients with this disorder should avoid excessive exercise, and they should be properly hydrated when performing physical activity. A high-carbohydrate, low-fat diet could be helpful; creatine 60 mg/kg daily has been found to improve exercise tolerance.[18] The ACE inhibitor ramipril appears beneficial.[19] This has been used as more phenotypes are associated with mutations that increase ACE activities. Sucrose ingestion before exercises improves exercise tolerance.[20]

TABLE 91-1 Causes of Myoglobinuria

Metabolic exhaustion
Excessive exercise in healthy persons
Seizures, delirium, tetanus, and strychnine
Heat stroke
Cold exposure
Metabolic myopathies, particularly during exercise: carnitine palmityl transferase deficiency, very-long-chain acyl–CoA deficiency, myoadenylate deaminase deficiency, mitochondrial disease, and glycogen storage diseases (phosphorylase, phosphofructokinase, phosphorylase kinase, phosphoglycerate mutase, phosphoglycerate kinase, and lactate dehydrogenase deficiencies)
Malignant hyperthermia
Neuroleptic malignant syndrome, serotonin syndrome
Diabetic acidosis
Ischemic (coma, arterial occlusion)
Trauma (crush syndrome)
High-voltage shock
Myopathies, nonmetabolic
Dystrophinopathies
Infectious myositis (influenza virus, HIV, toxic shock, bacterial infections, e.g., clostridium, legionnaires' disease)
Autoimmune myositis (dermatomyositis, polymyositis)
Toxins, abuse substances
Alcohol
Lysergic acid diethylamide
Cocaine
Plasmoid
Methadone
Heroin
Phencyclidine
Amphetamines
Envenomations (e.g., wasps, spiders, and snakes)
Cicuta
Haff disease
Medications
Cholesterol-lowering drugs
Hypokalemia-causing drugs (e.g., diuretics, amphotericin B), licorice
Azidothymidine
Salicylate overdose
Azathioprine
Theophylline
Lithium
Epsilon aminocaproic acid
Fluid, electrolyte imbalance
Hypokalemia
Hypernatremia
Hyponatremia
Hypophosphatemia
Hyperosmolar states
Water intoxication

CoA, Coenzyme A; *HIV*, human immunodeficiency virus.
Modified from Bertorini TE. Myoglobinuria, malignant hyperthermia, neuroleptic malignant syndrome and serotonin syndrome. *Neurol Clin.* 1997;15(3):649–671.

Some cases may also develop perioperative myoglobinuria. To prevent this, patients should be properly hydrated during this time.[21]

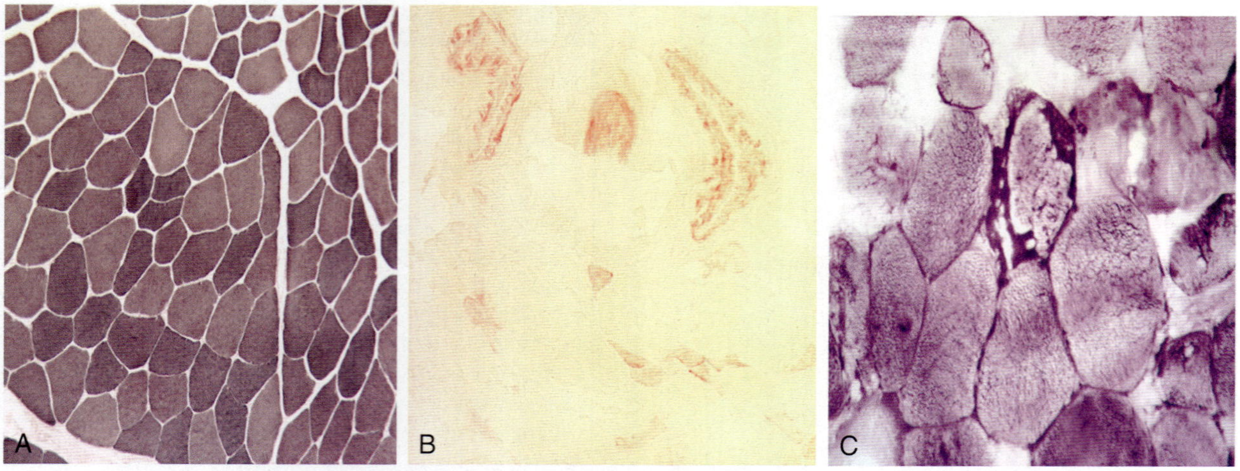

FIG. 91-2 **A**, Control muscle biopsy (phosphorylase stain, ×100). **B**, Note lack of staining for phosphorylase in muscle fiber in the patient, but its presence in the vessel wall (phosphorylase stain, ×200). **C**, Muscle biopsy showing glycogen accumulation in the periodic acid–Schiff stain (×200).

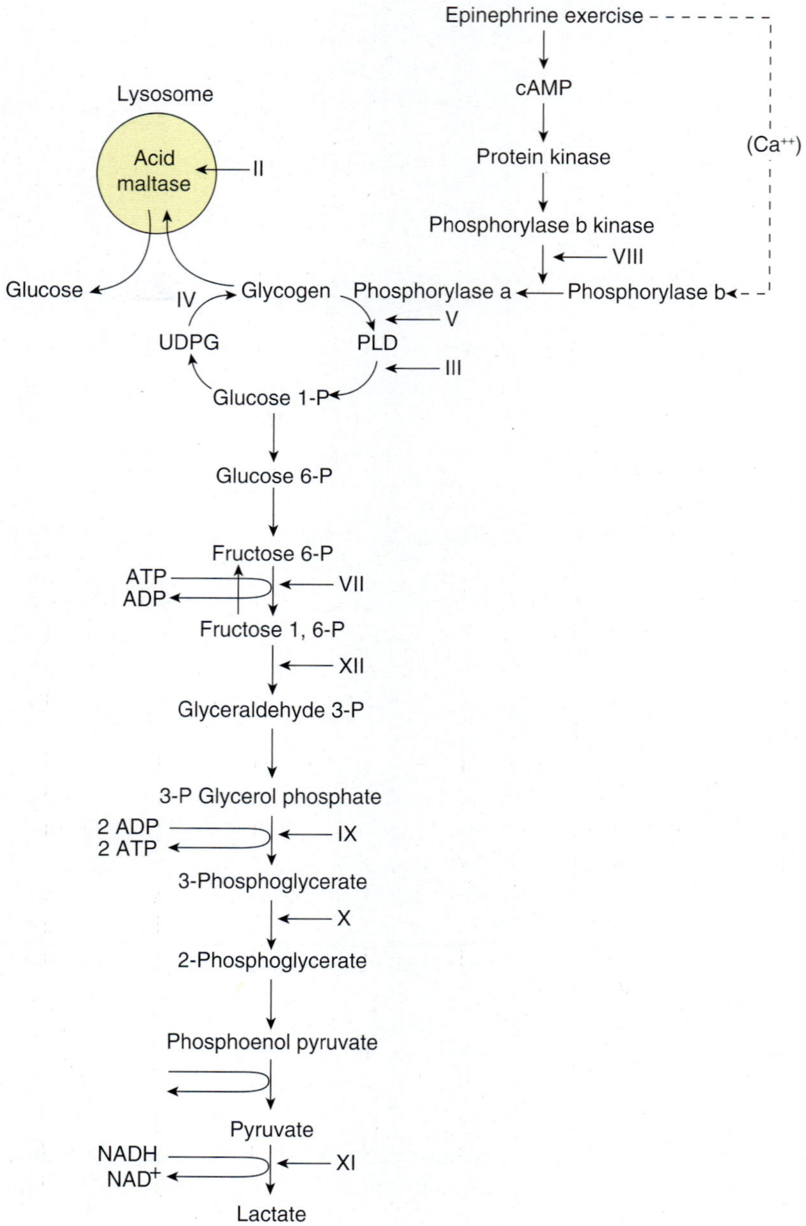

FIG. 91-3 General scheme of muscle metabolism. On the left, outside the mitochondrion, is a representation of glycogen metabolism and glycolysis. Roman numerals in this area of the diagram (II–XII) indicate enzymes whose deficiencies are associated with muscle glycogenosis (II, acid maltase; III, debrancher; IV, brancher; V, myophosphorylase; VII, phosphofructokinase; VIII, phosphorylase B kinase; IX, phosphoglycerate kinase; X, phosphoglycerate mutase; XI, lactate dehydrogenase; XII, aldolase). Modified from DiMauro S, Shanske S, Naini A, Krishna S. Biochemical evaluation of metabolic myopathies. In: Bertorini TE, ed. *Clinical Evaluation and Diagnostic Tests for Neuromuscular Disorders.* Boston, MA: Butterworth-Heinemann; 2002:535–564.

TABLE 91-2 Pathogenesis and Management of Systemic Complications of Rhabdomyolysis

Complication	Pathogenesis	Management
Acute tubular necrosis	Toxic effect of urinary myoglobulin	Intravascular volume expansion (normal saline, mannitol) to maintain urine output > 200–300 mL/h
	Hypotension (renal ischemia)	Hemodialysis or continuous hemofiltration if diuresis cannot be established
	Myoglobin and urate crystal formation at low urine pH	Urinary alkalinization (sodium bicarbonate) with close monitoring of urine and plasma pH
	Protease release from injured muscle	Minimize nephrotoxic agents
	? Free radical formation catalyzed by ferrihemate	? Dantrolene
	Lipid peroxidation	? Antioxidants, iron chelators, 21-aminosteroids (unproven)
	? Release of renal vasoconstrictor substances (cytokines, prostaglandins, and endothelin) by myoglobin, scavenging of nitric oxide	? Dopamine (unproven)
Hyperkalemia	Muscle breakdown, ARF	Calcium gluconate (severe), diuresis, hemodialysis if refractory
Hypocalcemia	Binding by damaged muscle hyperphosphatemia; decreased renal 1,25 (OH)-D formation	Await spontaneous correction
Hypercalcemia (late)	Release of calcium from muscle binding sites, impaired renal excretion	Promote diuresis
Hyperphosphatemia, tissue calcification	Release of organic and inorganic phosphates, excess solubility product for calcium phosphate	Promote diuresis
Hypovolemia, hypoalbuminemia, and anemia	Massive intramuscular capillary destruction with leakage of intravascular contents	Intravascular volume expansion, transfusion
DIC	Release of tissue thromboplastins, microthrombus formation	? Heparin, fresh frozen plasma
Compression palsies	Immobility, crush injury, and compartment syndrome	Early fasciotomy for compartment syndrome

ARF, Acute renal failure; *DIC*, disseminated intravascular coagulation. ? = Unproven
Reprinted with permission from Warren JD, Blumbergs PC, Thompson PD. Rhabdomyolysis: a review. *Muscle Nerve.* 2002;25(3):335.

The management of an acute myoglobinuric attack includes proper hydration and monitoring of urinary output. Alkalinization with sodium bicarbonate is used to prevent myoglobin deposits in the kidneys. Hyperkalemia, caused by muscle breakdown, should be monitored carefully and treated with diuresis, and when severe, with calcium gluconate. Hypocalcemia, caused by calcium accumulation in muscle fibers, is treated conventionally and only if symptomatic. Hypercalcemia might occur in late stages; hyperphosphatemia can also occur, and this is prevented and treated with proper diuresis. Hemodialysis might be necessary (Table 91-2).

SUMMARY

This patient developed weakness and had an elevated serum CK and pigmenturia. Likely the positive "blood in urine" indicated myoglobin from rhabdomyolysis.

She had a history of exercise intolerance and was diagnosed as having McArdle disease, or myophosphorylase deficiency.

IMPORTANT POINTS

- The presence of "blood" in the urine could indicate myoglobulin, particularly when microscopic examination shows rare or no RBCs.
- Myoglobinuria is caused by massive muscle necrosis or rhabdomyolysis.
- Exercise intolerance, myoglobinuria, and lack of increase in serum lactate during exercise are characteristic of McArdle disease. It is diagnosed by lack of phosphorylase in muscle biopsy, using histochemistry and biochemical analysis.
- McArdle disease is caused by a genetic defect in chromosome 11. Testing could be done so biopsy may not be necessary.
- Myoglobinuria is treated with proper hydration, diuresis, and urine alkalinization.

REFERENCES

1. Bertorini TE. Clinical evaluation and clinical diagnostic tests. In: Bertorini TE, ed. *Clinical Evaluation and Diagnostic Tests for Neuromuscular Disorders*. Boston, MA: Butterworth-Heinemann; 2002:15–97.

2. Bertorini TE. Myoglobinuria, malignant hyperthermia, neuroleptic malignant syndrome and serotonin syndrome. *Neurol Clin*. 1997; 15(3):649–671.
3. Kwon JH, Kim JS. Rhabdomyolysis in a patient with MELAS syndrome. *Eur Neurol*. 2003;50:123–124.
4. Melberg A, Holme E, Oldfors A, Lundberg PO. Rhabdomyolysis in autosomal dominant progressive external ophthalmoplegia. *Neurology*. 1998;50:299–300.
5. Tabarki B, Thabet F, Selmi H, et al. Acute rhabdomyolysis disclosing polymyositis in children. *Arch Pediatr*. 2001;8:51–54.
6. Thakur V, DeSalvo J, McGrath H Jr, et al. Case report: polymyositis-induced myoglobinuric acute renal failure. *Am J Med Sci*. 1996;312(2):85–87.
7. Rose MR, Kissel JT, Bickley LS, Griggs RC. Sustained myoglobinuria: the presenting manifestation of dermatomyositis. *Neurology*. 1996;47:119–123.
8. Lewington AJ, D'Souza R, Carr S, et al. Polymyositis: a cause of acute renal failure. *Nephrol Dial Transplant*. 1996;11:699–701.
9. Warren JD, Blumbergs PC, Thompson PD. Rhabdomyolysis: a review. *Muscle Nerve*. 2002;25(3):332–347.
10. McArdle B. Myopathy due to a defect in muscle glycogen breakdown. *Clin Sci*. 1951;10:13–33.
11. El-Schahawi M, Bruno C, Tsujino S, et al. Sudden infant death syndrome (SIDS) in a family with myophosphorylase deficiency. *Neuromuscul Disord*. 1997;7(2):81–83.
12. Martinuzzi A, Sartori E, Fanin M, et al. Phenotype modulators in myophosphorylase deficiency. *Ann Neurol*. 2003;53:497–502.
13. Pourmand R, Sanders DB, Corwin HM. Late-onset McArdle's disease with unusual electromyographic findings. *Arch Neurol*. 1983;40(6):374–377.
14. Hogrel JY, Laforet P, Ben Yaou R, et al. A non-ischemic forearm exercise test for the screening of patients with exercise intolerance. *Neurology*. 2001;56(12):1733–1738.
15. Bruno C, Bado M, Minetti C, Cordone G. Forearm semi-ischemic exercise test in pediatric patients. *J Child Neurol*. 1998;13(6): 288–290.
16. Tsujino S, Shanske S, DiMauro S. Molecular genetic heterogeneity of myophosphorylase deficiency (McArdle's disease). *N Engl J Med*. 1993;329(4):241–245.
17. el-Schahawi M, Tsujino S, Shanske S, DiMauro S. Diagnosis of McArdle's disease by molecular genetic analysis of blood. *Neurology*. 1996;47(2):579–580.
18. Vorgerd M, Grehl T, Jager M, Muller K, et al. Creatine therapy in myophosphorylase deficiency (McArdle disease): a placebo-controlled crossover trial. *Arch Neurol*. 2000;57(7):956–963.
19. Martinuzzi A, Liava A, Trevisi, Frare M, et al. Randomized, placebo-controlled, double-blind pilot trial of ramipril in McArdle's disease. *Muscle Nerve*. 2008;37(3):350–357.
20. Andersen ST, Haller RG, Vissing J. Effect of oral sucrose shortly before exercise on work capacity in McArdle disease. *Arch Neurol*. 2008;65(60):786–789.
21. Bollig G, Mohr S, Ræder J. McArdle's disease and anaesthesia: case reports. Review of potential problems and association with malignant hyperthermia. *Acta Anaesthesiol Scand*. 2005;49(8): 1077–1083.

A Woman With Progressive Proximal Muscle Weakness

A 36-year-old Black woman presented with progressive muscle weakness of 8 months; she had had increasing difficulty climbing stairs and rising from a chair and later raising her arms above her head. She was treated with prednisone (100 mg/day for 3 months) and later azathioprine (150 mg/day) without improvement and was referred to us after she developed difficulty breathing.

She denied muscle cramps, myotonia, fasciculations, sensory difficulties, or pigmenturia. A sister died at age 39 after a 5-year course of progressive weakness that had been diagnosed and treated as polymyositis. A maternal aunt had had similar problems, stopped walking in her 20s, and died after several years without being evaluated.

Cardiovascular and respiratory examinations were unremarkable except for labored respiration that caused some difficulty with speech. There was no visceromegaly. Neurologic examination showed a waddling gait. There was generalized hypotonia and mild atrophy of proximal muscles. Neck flexor and extensor muscles were 4/5; deltoids, 3/5; and trapezius, 3+ to 4/5. Distal muscles of the arms and hands were 5/5. Iliopsoas strength was 2/5; quadriceps, 3/5; adductors, 2/5; glutei, 3−/5; hamstrings, 4/5; foot dorsiflexors, flexors, invertors, and evertors were 5/5. Reflexes were absent throughout except 2+ at the ankles. Sensation and coordination were normal. No fasciculations were seen. There was no grip or percussion myotonia. Cranial nerves were normal. There was no evidence of tongue atrophy or hypertrophy. (Fig. 92-1 shows the patient after the disease progressed and she needed a cuirass respirator.)

WHAT IS THE DIFFERENTIAL DIAGNOSIS?

This woman presented with progressive weakness that was assumed to be from polymyositis but did not respond to treatment. The positive family history of a sister and probably an aunt having the same problem suggested an inherited disorder. This presentation could suggest adult-onset familial spinal muscular atrophy; the absence of most reflexes is compatible with this disorder, but the lack of fasciculations is against. The lack of cranial nerve involvement, the atrophy, and the progressive nature of the disease are against a disorder of neuromuscular transmission.

A mitochondrial disorder should be considered, but the lack of extraocular involvement and systemic manifestations are against this. Proximal myotonic myopathy should also be considered, but in that disease, the inheritance is autosomal-dominant and she had no clinical myotonia. Assuming that the sister's and aunt's conditions were unrelated, other possibilities should include an endocrine myopathy[1] and polymyositis,[2] a condition rarely seen in families. For this, it would have to be assumed that the disease was refractory to treatment.

A limb-girdle muscular dystrophy and a metabolic myopathy, such as acid maltase deficiency (AMD), also are considerations.

WHAT TESTS SHOULD BE DONE?

Routine laboratory studies (including liver function tests and serum electrolytes) and thyroid-stimulating hormone test were normal. Serum creatine kinase level was 650 IU/L (normal, <200 IU/L), and erythrocyte sedimentation rate was 55 mm/h (normal, <30 mm/h).

AN EMG TEST WAS PERFORMED

Motor Nerve Studies

Nerve and Site	Latency (ms)	Amplitude (mV)	Conduction Velocity (m/s)
Peroneal Nerve R.	**Normal ≤ 5.7**	**Normal ≥ 3**	**Normal ≥ 40**
Ankle	5.1	8	–
Fibular head	11.4	8	46
Knee	13.2	8	44
Ulnar Nerve R.	**Normal ≤ 3.6**	**Normal ≥ 8**	**Normal ≥ 50**
Wrist	3.3	10	–
Below elbow	6.7	9	60
Above elbow	8.5	9	67

F-Wave Studies

Nerve	Latency (ms)	Normal Latency ≤ (ms)
Peroneal nerve R.	51.2	54
Ulnar nerve R.	26.4	30

Sensory Nerve Studies

Nerve	Onset Latency (ms)	Normal Onset Latency ≤ (ms)	Peak Latency (ms)	Normal Peak Latency ≤ (ms)	Amp (μV)	Normal Amp ≥ (μV)	Conduction Velocity (m/s)	Normal Conduction Velocity ≥ (m/s)
Sural nerve R.	3.3	3.5	3.8	4.0	15	11	42	40
Ulnar nerve R.	2.2	2.6	2.7	3.1	22	13	54	50

EMG Data

Muscle	Insrt Activity	Fibs	Pos Waves	Fasc	Amp	Dur	Poly	Pattern
Deltoid R.[a]	**Myot**	**3+**	**3+**	None	**Dec**	**Brief**	**Many**	Full[a]
Biceps brachii R.	**Inc**	**3+**	**3+**	None	**Dec**	**Brief**	**Many**	Full[a]
Triceps R.	**Inc**	**3+**	**3+**	None	**Dec**	**Brief**	**Few**	Full
Brachioradialis R.	**CRD**	**1+**	**1+**	None	**Dec**	**Brief**	**Few**	Full
First dorsal interosseus R.	**Inc**	**1+**	**1+**	None	**Dec**	**Brief**	**Few**	Full[a]
Tensor fasciae latae R.	**CRD**	None	None	None	**Dec**	**Brief**	**Few**	Full[a]
Vastus lateralis R.	**Myot**	**2+**	**2+**	None	**Dec**	**Brief**	**Few**	Full
Tibialis anterior R.	**Inc**	**2+**	**2+**	None	**Dec**	**Brief**	**Few**	Full

[a]Rapid recruitment of motor unit action potentials.

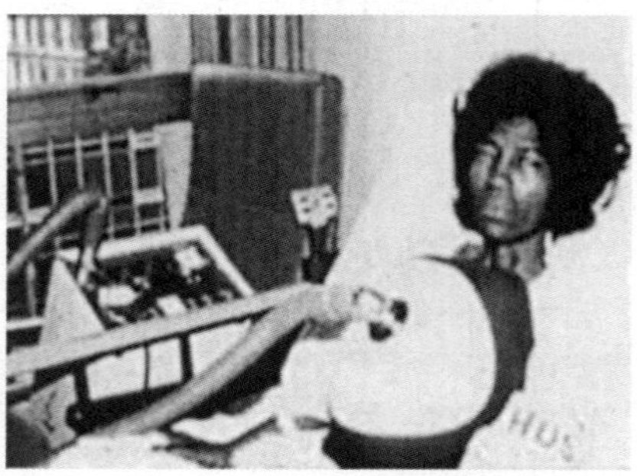

FIG. 92-1 Patient using a negative pressure chest cuirass ventilator for assistance in breathing.

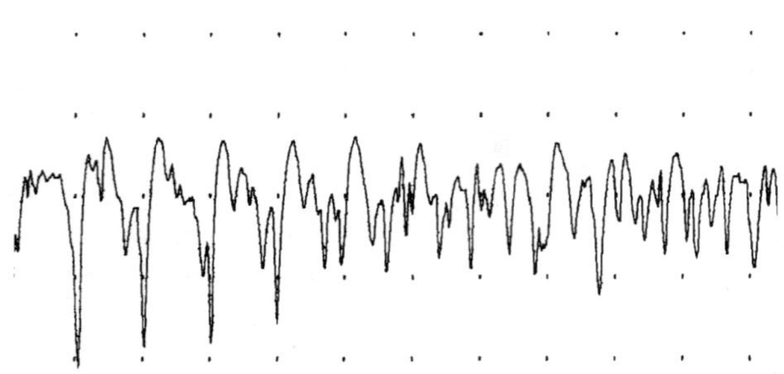

FIG. 92-2 EMG of the deltoid muscle showing myotonia (100 μV/10 ms).

WHAT WERE THE EMG FINDINGS?

This EMG showed normal nerve conduction studies. Needle electromyography showed frequent myotonic discharges (Fig. 92-2). Abundant small polyphasic motor units and fibrillation potentials were seen particularly in the proximal muscles.

Causes of proximal weakness and elevated creatine kinase without clinical myotonia, but with electromyographic myotonia and small polyphasic motor unit action potentials, include AMD, myositis, toxic myopathies, and cytoplasmic body myopathy.[3]

A left deltoid muscle biopsy revealed frequent internalized nuclei with variation in fiber size and scattered necrotic fibers. Many vacuoles were noted within muscle fibers; these stained positively with periodic acid–Schiff and acid phosphatase (Fig. 92-3A–C). There was a predominance of type I muscle fibers, many of which showed pale centers (NADH-TR stain). Electron microscopy revealed membrane-bound glycogen, as well as some free glycogen accumulation (see Fig. 92-3D). There was also myofibril disorganization.

The diagnosis of AMD was confirmed by biochemical analysis (acid maltase, 4.5% of normal; neutral maltase, 84% of normal).

She was treated with respiratory assistance and respiratory treatment and had a fulfilling life for over 20 years.

DISCUSSION

This patient had adult-onset AMD; acid maltase is an acid α-1,4- and α-1,6-glycosidase. This is a disease that manifests with progressive weakness and is one of the glycogen storage disorders that manifest in this form. Others include debrancher and brancher enzyme deficiencies, and aldolase A deficiency.[4] The clinical presentation, electrical myotonia, and the characteristic vacuolated muscle fibers with increased lysomal activity are typical of AMD, which is confirmed by biochemical analysis.

AMD might present in the neonatal period with hepatosplenomegaly, hypotonia and weakness, glossomegaly, and cardiomyopathy with premature death (Pompe disease) (Fig. 92-4). Late infantile and childhood forms of the disease

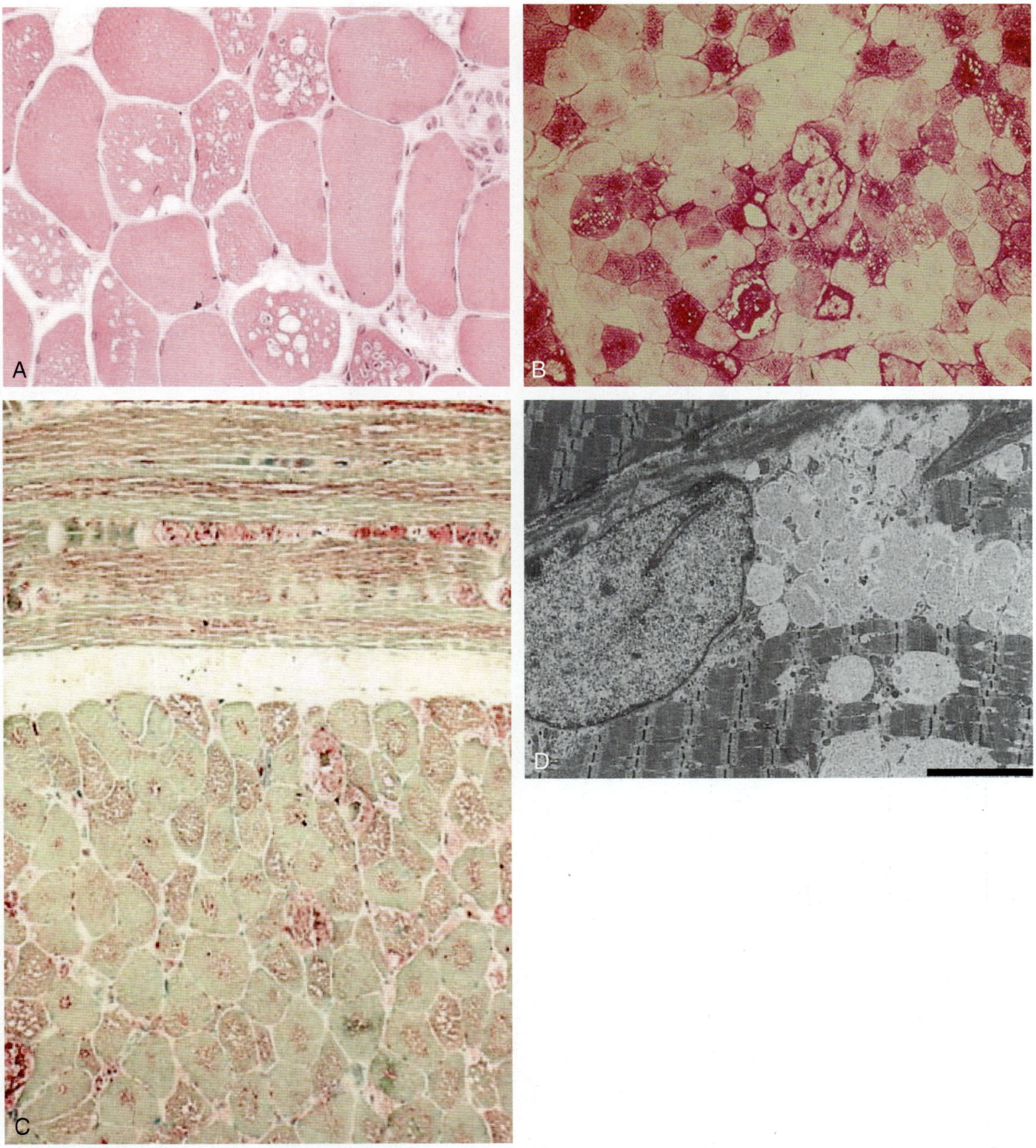

FIG. 92-3 **A**, Muscle biopsy showing multiple vacuoles in muscle fibers (H&E stain, ×400). **B**, Granular accumulation of glycogen on the PAS stain (×200). **C**, Increased acid phosphatase activity (from increased lysosomal activation) staining red; longitudinal (*top*), transverse section (*bottom*) (×200). **D**, Electromicroscopy showing multiple large lysosomes next to a myofiber nucleus (×3000).

also start early in life with weakness but without visceromegaly (Figs. 92-5 and 92-6).

Adult-onset AMD is characterized by a progressive myopathy resembling limb-girdle muscular dystrophy (Fig. 92-7), and as in this case, it could be confused with polymyositis. Patients could have significant respiratory involvement and manifest initially with respiratory insufficiency.[5–12] Prominent thigh adductor weakness and hypotonia are other characteristic clinical findings. Tongue hypertrophy can be seen (Fig. 92-8). The EMG could show fibrillation potentials, myotonia, and complex repetitive discharges with small motor unit action potentials.

The muscle biopsy shows fiber degeneration with vacuoles having glycogen accumulation and proliferation of lysosomes, which are likely pathogenic from their space-occupying effect and focal cell damage from "bursting of the lysomes." The diagnosis can also be made noninvasively by measuring the enzyme activity in lymphocytes.[13,14] This test or DNA analysis in dry blood should be done in suspected cases, particularly because electromyographic myotonia or histologic glycogen accumulation might not be seen in some adult cases.

AMD is caused by a defect in chromosome 17q21–23.[15] Deletions and nonsense mutations are associated with the

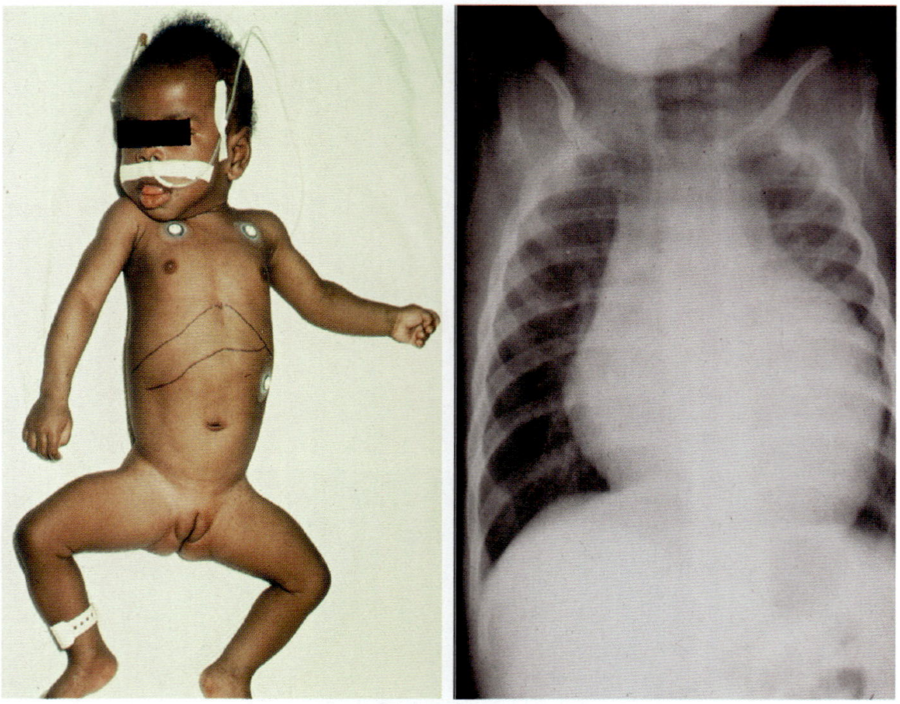

FIG. 92-4 A patient with Pompe disease showing glossomegaly, hypotonia, and hepatomegaly; chest x-ray shows cardiomegaly.

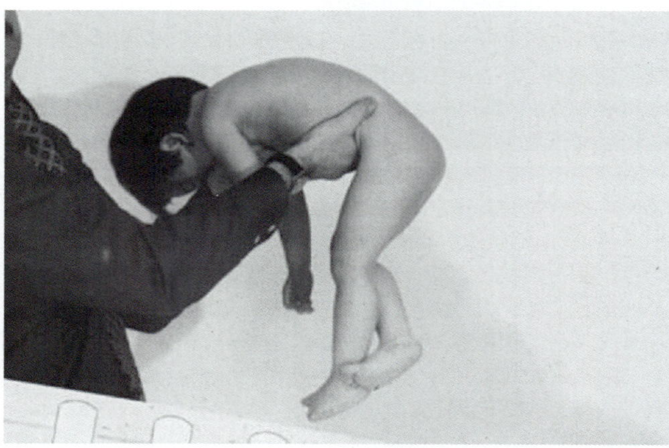

FIG. 92-5 A child with late infantile AMD (he had no visceromegaly), brother of the patient in Fig. 84-6. *AMD*, Acid maltase deficiency.

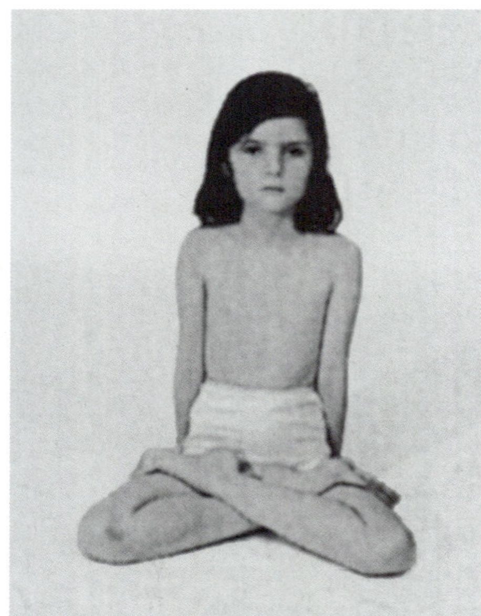

FIG. 92-6 A patient with childhood AMD showing hyperextensibility of the joints. *AMD*, Acid maltase deficiency.

infantile form, whereas "leaky" mutations, such as the common IVS1–13T > G splice-site mutation, are associated with the adult form.[14]

The lack of severe and systemic involvement of the adult and childhood forms might be explained by the small but crucial amount of residual acid maltase present in tissues in those cases.

There is no specific therapy for AMD at this time, but promising results have been obtained in vitro and in vivo using recombinant adenovirus encoding α-1,4-glucosidase.[16] Other viral therapies administered in muscles and liver are promising. Enzyme replacement (ERT) could be beneficial, and intravenous injections of the recombinant human enzyme corrected the enzyme defect in animals[17] and in Pompe disease in humans.[18,19] Patients might develop influenza-like reactions or may develop neutralizing antibodies that reduce efficacy. There are guidelines that recommend to discontinue therapy.[20] The combination of ERT and beta 2 agonist enhance efficacy. The use of enzyme therapy in combination with a chaperone improves stability[21] Because of the development of antibodies, sometimes the therapeutic effect is diminished and for this, concerns have been reported about when to start and stop enzyme replacement.[22] Gene therapy is promising. Respiratory care and assistance as well as gentle exercises are important in the management of these patients.

SUMMARY

This woman had progressive muscle weakness and respiratory insufficiency. Her sister died after having been diagnosed and

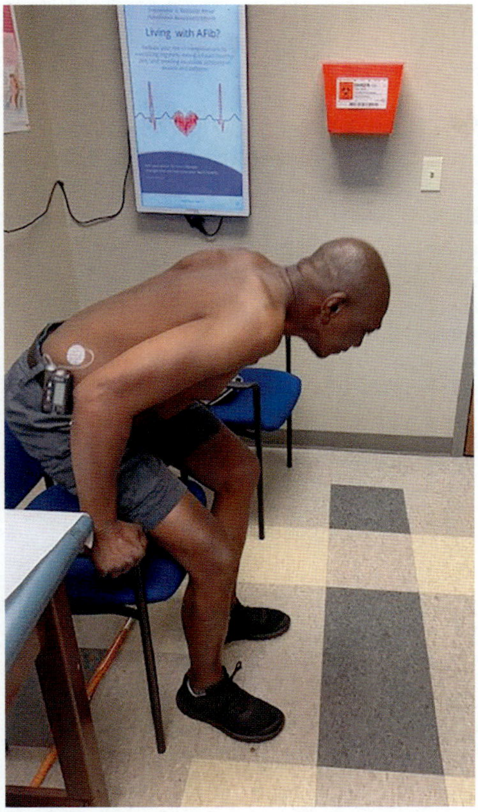

FIG. 92-7 An adult patient with AMD with difficulty arising from a chair. *AMD*, Acid maltase deficiency.

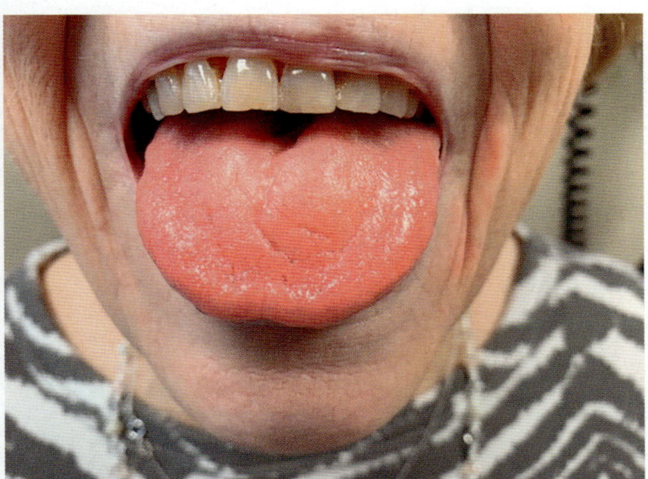

FIG. 92-8 A large tongue in a patient with AMD. *AMD*, Acid maltase deficiency.

treated for polymyositis, but her autopsy revealed evidence of vacuolated fibers. The patient was diagnosed as having AMD.

IMPORTANT POINTS

- Adult-onset acid maltase or α-1,4-glycosidase deficiency is a glycogen storage disease characterized by proximal muscle weakness and prominent respiratory insufficiency that can manifest in children and adults. There is also an infantile form that presents with multisystem involvement (Pompe disease).
- Patients with AMD have myotonia on EMG without clinical myotonia.
- A myopathic EMG with electrical myotonia, but without clinical myotonia can also be seen in polymyositis, hypothyroidism, drug-induced myopathy, and some cytoplasmic body myopathies.
- The genetic defect of AMD is in the long arm of chromosome 17.
- There is currently no cure for AMD although enzyme replacement is beneficial, and gene therapy appears promising.
- Proper respiratory care is important because patients can have a long survival with respiratory assistance.

This case was reported by Moufarrej N, Bertorini TE. Respiratory insufficiency in adult-type acid maltase deficiency. J South Med Assoc. 1993;86(5):560–567.

REFERENCES

1. Bertorini TE. Clinical evaluation and clinical laboratory tests. In: Bertorini TE, ed. *Clinical Evaluation and Diagnostic Tests for Neuromuscular Disorders*. Boston, MA: Butterworth-Heinemann; 2002:15–97.
2. Bertorini TE. Inflammatory myopathies (polymyositis, dermatomyositis, inclusion body myositis). *Compr Ther*. 1998;24(10): 494–502.
3. Kimura J. Routine needle electromyography. In: Bertorini TE, ed. *Clinical Evaluation and Diagnostic Tests for Neuromuscular Disorders*. Boston, MA: Butterworth-Heinemann; 2002:331–364.
4. DiMauro S, Shanske S, Naini A, Krishna S. Biochemical evaluation of metabolic myopathies. In: Bertorini TE, ed. *Clinical Evaluation and Diagnostic Tests for Neuromuscular Disorders*. Boston, MA: Butterworth-Heinemann; 2002:535–564.
5. Kuenen RW, Lambregts PC, Op de Coul AA, et al. Respiratory failure as initial symptom of acid maltase deficiency. *J Neurol Neurosurg Psychiatry*. 1984;47:549–552.
6. Smith J, Zellweger H, Afifi AK. Muscular form of glycogenosis type II (Pompe). *Neurology*. 1967;17:537–549.
7. Swaiman KF, Kennedy WR, Sauls HS. Late infantile acid maltase deficiency. *Arch Neurol*. 1968;18:642–648.
8. Bordiuk JM, Legato MJ, Lovelace RE, et al. Pompe's disease: electromyographic, electron microscopic, and cardiovascular aspects. *Arch Neurol*. 1970;23:113–119.
9. Schlenska GK, Heene R, Spalke G, et al. The symptomatology, morphology and biochemistry of glycogenosis type II (Pompe) in the adult. *J Neurol*. 1976;212:237–252.
10. Karpati G, Carpenter S, Eisen A, et al. The adult form of acid maltase (alpha-1,4 glucosidase) deficiency. *Ann Neurol*. 1977;1: 276–280.
11. Swash M, Schwartz MS, Apps MC. Adult onset acid maltase deficiency: distribution and progression of clinical and pathological abnormality in a family. *J Neurol Sci*. 1985;68(1):61–74.
12. Raben N, Nichols RC, Boerkoel C, Plotz P. Genetic defects in patients with glycogenosis type II (acid maltase deficiency). *Muscle Nerve*. 1995;3(Suppl):S70–S74.

13. Mehler M, DiMauro S. Residual acid maltase activity in late-onset acid maltase deficiency. *Neurology*. 1977;27:178–184.
14. Engel A, Hirschhorn R, Huie ML. Acid maltase deficiency. In: Engel AG, Franzini-Armstrong C, eds. *Myology*. 3rd ed. New York, NY: McGraw-Hill; 2004:1559–1586.
15. Kroos MA, Van der Kraan M, Van Diggelen OP, et al. Two extremes of the clinical spectrum of glycogen storage disease type II in one family: a matter of genotype. *Hum Mutat*. 1997;9:17–22.
16. Yang HW, Kikuchi T, Hagiwara T, et al. Recombinant human acid alpha glucosidase corrects acid alpha-glucosidase-deficient human fibroblasts, quail fibroblasts, and quail myoblasts. *Pediatr Res*. 1998;43:374–380.
17. Bijvoet AGA, van de Kamp EH, Kroos MA, et al. Generalized glycogen storage and cardiomegaly in a knockout mouse model of Pompe disease. *Hum Mol Genet*. 1998;7:53–62.
18. van der Beek NA, Hagemans ML, van der Ploeg AT, et al. Pompe disease (glycogen storage disease type II): clinical features and enzyme replacement therapy. *Acta Neurol Belg*. 2006;106(2):82–86.
19. Kishnani PS, Corzo D, Nicolino M, et al. Recombinant human acid alpha-glucosidase: major clinical benefits in infantile-onset Pompe disease. *Neurology*. 2007;68(2):99–109.
20. Pauly DF, Johns DC, Matelis LA, et al. Complete correction of acid alpha-glucosidase deficiency in Pompe disease fibroblasts in vitro, and lysosomally targeted expression in neonatal rat cardiac and skeletal muscle. *Gene Ther*. 1998;5:473–480.
21. Meena NK, Raben N. Pompe disease: new developments in an old lysosomal storage disorder. *Biomolecules*. 2020;10(9):1339.
22. van der Ploeg AT, Kruijshaar ME, Toscano A, Laforet P, et al. European consensus for starting and stopping enzyme replacement therapy in adult patients with Pompe disease: a 10-year experience. *Eur J Neurol*. 2017;24(6):768-e31. First published May 06, 2017. https://doi.org/10.1111/ene.13285.

A Sedentary Man With Acute Respiratory Failure and Myoglobinuria

A 51-year-old man came with a 4-day history of general malaise, cough, fever, and muscle aches. He had no previous similar episodes.

The patient's parents were first-degree cousins. He required resuscitation at birth, but other details of the perinatal history were not available. He always had impaired vision and mild bilateral spasticity that was thought to be related to trauma or anoxia at birth. His lifestyle was always sedentary, and he was deferred from military service. He worked as a salesman. Essential hypertension was discovered at age 46 and treated with hydrochlorothiazide and spironolactone (each 25 mg/day). During a routine medical evaluation, his serum creatine kinase (CK) was high at 1200 IU/L (normal, <200 IU/L) without an obvious cause. He had occasional chest pain that was not related to exercise or fasting and did not coincide with rises in serum CK.

There was no family history of neuromuscular disease.

Vital signs were normal except for a temperature of 38°C. His vital capacity was 380 mL. He developed respiratory distress and an endotracheal tube was inserted. He then received respiratory assistance for 11 days.

Visual acuity was limited to counting fingers. His optic disks were atrophic and of small diameter with a paucity of vessels. There was weakness of the left lateral rectus and bilateral nystagmus on horizontal gaze. Muscle tests showed mild proximal weakness and spasticity with hyperreflexia in the legs, but there were no Babinski signs. The rest of the examination was unremarkable.

The following laboratory data on admission were normal: complete blood cell and differential count, sedimentation rate, blood urea nitrogen (BUN), calcium, bilirubin, alkaline phosphatase, cholesterol, uric acid, protein electrophoresis, and thyroid function studies. Serum creatinine was 1 mg/dL; sodium, 127 mEq/L; potassium, 2.9 mEq/L; chloride, 96 mEq/dL; and CO_2, 28 mEq/L.

Serum CK was 36,000 IU/L (normal, 60–210 IU/L); alanine transaminase, 942 IU/L (normal, 9–42 IU/L); lactate dehydrogenase, 912 IU/L (normal, 50–200 IU/L); and aldolase, 92 IU/L (normal, 0–6 IU/L). His urine was dark brown with a specific gravity of 1.018, pH 6, 0–5 red cells per high-power field, and a few white cells. The protein reaction was 3+, and tests for glucose, ketones, and bilirubin were negative. Radial immunodiffusion was positive for myoglobin. Acute and convalescent complement fixation titers for coxsackie, influenza, and parainfluenza viruses were normal. Blood and sputum cultures were negative. Electrocardiogram was normal. Chest radiograms were normal except for a mild left ventricular hypertrophy. A CT scan of the head showed mild cerebral atrophy.

Despite proper therapy for myoglobinuria, on the 10th day of his hospital stay his BUN had increased to 100 µg/dL and creatinine to 6.5 µg/dL, but his urinary output continued to be more than 1200 mg/day, indicating high-output renal failure. This was treated by hemodialysis. He improved slowly and was removed from the ventilator; his respiratory function and his renal function gradually returned to normal.

AN EMG TEST WAS PERFORMED

Motor Nerve Studies

Nerve and Site	Latency (ms)	Amplitude (mV)	Conduction Velocity (m/s)
Peroneal Nerve R.	**Normal ≤ 5.7**	**Normal ≥ 3**	**Normal ≥ 40**
Ankle	5.2	3	–
Fibular head	12.0	3	40
Knee	14.0	3	45
Ulnar Nerve R.	**Normal ≤ 3.6**	**Normal ≥ 8**	**Normal ≥ 50**
Wrist	3.6	9	–
Below elbow	7.3	8	55
Above elbow	9.4	8	57

F-Wave and Tibial H-Reflex Studies

Nerve	Latency (ms)	Normal Latency ≤ (ms)
Peroneal nerve R.	52.6	54
Ulnar nerve R.	28.5	30
H-reflex R.	34.0	34
H-reflex L.	33.6	34

Sensory Nerve Studies

Nerve	Onset Latency (ms)	Normal Onset Latency ≤ (ms)	Peak Latency (ms)	Normal Peak Latency ≤ (ms)	Amp (μV)	Normal Amp ≥ (μV)	Conduction Velocity (m/s)	Normal Conduction Velocity ≥ (m/s)
Sural nerve R.	3.4	3.5	3.9	4.0	12	11	41	40
Ulnar nerve R.	2.2	2.6	2.7	3.1	15	13	55	50

EMG Data

Muscle	Insrt Activity	Fibs	Pos Waves	Fasc	Amp	Dur	Poly	Pattern
Pectoralis major R.	**CRD**	None	None	None	Norm	Norm	**Many**	Full
Deltoid R.	Norm	None	None	None	Norm	Norm	None	Full
Biceps brachii R.	Norm	None	None	None	Norm	Norm	None	Full
First dorsal interosseous R.	Norm	None	None	None	Norm	Norm	None	Full
Iliopsoas R.	Norm	None	None	None	Norm	Norm	None	Full
Vastus lateralis R.	Norm	None	None	None	Norm	Norm	None	Full
Gastrocnemius R.	Norm	None	None	None	Norm	Norm	None	Full

CRD = complex repetitive discharges

WHAT WERE THE EMG FINDINGS?

This test showed normal motor nerve conduction velocities and normal CMAP and SNAP amplitudes and latencies. Needle electromyography showed complex repetitive discharges only in the pectoralis muscle. Motor unit action potentials appeared normal, except for the presence of frequent polyphasic motor units in the pectoralis muscle, although cooperation was less than optimal. The test was not diagnostic.

WHAT IS THE DIFFERENTIAL DIAGNOSIS?

This patient, whose congenital blindness and spasticity were of unknown cause, developed respiratory failure and myoglobinuria. The initial differential diagnosis included a viral myositis. He did not drink alcohol and was not on statins or other drugs that could cause myoglobinuria. The myoglobinuria was not related to exercise, so the possibility of a glycogen storage disease seemed unlikely. Other causes, such as trauma, seizures, or toxins, were not evident. Metabolic disorders, such as mitochondrial myopathy, carnitine palmitoyl transferase (CPT) deficiency, and autoimmune, or infectious myositis, had to be considered in the differential diagnosis.[1]

WHAT OTHER TESTS ARE INDICATED?

An ischemic exercise test showed a normal raise in serum lactate, pyruvate, and ammonia.

A right vastus lateralis muscle biopsy showed occasional necrotic muscle fibers (Fig. 93-1). Many fibers, particularly type I, had numerous small vacuoles. These were positive for neutral fat in Oil Red O staining and confirmed to be fat accumulation by electromicroscopy. The biopsy showed no ragged red fibers, and periodic acid–Schiff, phosphorylase, cytochrome oxidase, deaminase, and phosphofructokinase stains were normal.

WHAT SHOULD BE DONE NEXT?

Biochemical analysis showed muscle carnitine levels of 28.5 mol/mg/ncp (normal, 11.6–26.4 mol/mg/ncp). Glycogen and glycogen enzyme content were normal.

CPT level was 7.70 pmol (normal, 43.8–100.7 pmol). This assay did not separate CPT I from CPT II.

It was concluded that this patient has CPT deficiency or DiMauro disease.

Six months later, he had an episode of right lower lobe pneumonitis accompanied by fever, malaise, and generalized weakness. Sputum cultures for bacteria and fungi were negative; complement fixation titers for influenza, parainfluenza, ECHO, coxsackie and adenoviruses, respiratory syncytial virus titers, cytomegalic inclusion virus, and lymphochoriomeningitis were all normal and did not increase during convalescence. Titers for *Mycoplasma pneumoniae* rose from 1:16 to 1:64. During this episode, serum CK was 4000 U/L, but there was no evidence of myoglobinuria. He recuperated from this uneventfully.

DISCUSSION

This patient was admitted initially with acute respiratory failure and myoglobinuria and was found to have muscle CPT deficiency. This disease, first described by DiMauro and DiMauro in 1973, is the most common disorder of lipid metabolism of muscle and the most common hereditary cause of myoglobinuria.[1]

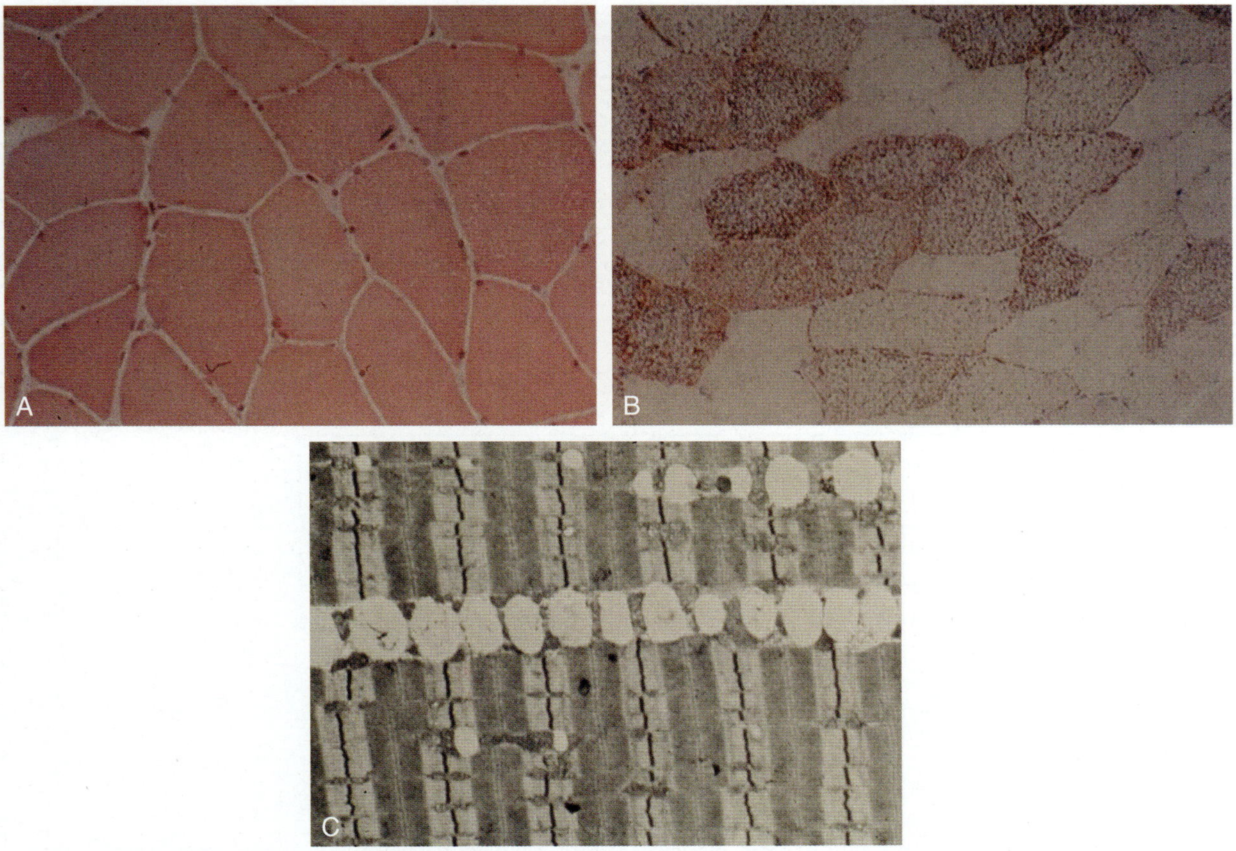

FIG. 93-1 **A**, Essentially normal right pectoralis muscle biopsy, except for very small vacuoles (H&E stain, ×400). **B**, Oil Red O stain showing increased neutral fat in muscle fibers (×200). **C**, Lipid accumulation seen on electromicroscopy (×7000).

Other possible causes[2] were considered and excluded. The patient was not alcoholic and had not been exposed to toxins. Muscle phosphorylase and phosphofructokinase deficiencies and other glycogen storage diseases were excluded by the normal rise in serum lactate after ischemic work, normal content of glycogen in muscle, and direct assay of muscle enzymes. Serum potassium was 2.9 mEq/L on admission, and hypokalemia could cause rhabdomyolysis, but values were higher than usually reported for patients with hypokalemia-induced myoglobinuria.[3,4] His potassium level was normal during his second episode of weakness and elevated serum CK.

Viral myositis, particularly from influenza virus infections, can cause myoglobinuria.[5,6] In this patient the muscle necrosis seemed to be precipitated by a viral infection, but antibody titers for influenza and other viruses were not abnormal. We could not rule out that other organisms or viruses, for which titers were not obtained, could have been responsible for the respiratory infection. Later, *Mycoplasma* pneumonitis was associated with an elevation of serum CK.

Viral and bacterial infections inhibit ketogenesis in experimental animals.[7] Similar inhibition of ketogenesis in a patient with already impaired fatty acid incorporation in the mitochondria and production of ketones from CPT deficiency could deprive muscles of this important source of energy during a stressful situation, leading to myoglobinuria, which likely occurred in this case.

An unusual and unexplained feature of this case was that his first attack of rhabdomyolysis occurred at age 51, much later than in classic cases of CPT deficiency.[1,8–15] His sedentary lifestyle, caused by blindness, could have delayed the attacks. These may also have occurred earlier without being recognized. This possibility seems unlikely, however, because he could not recall any episode of severe muscle aches, weakness, or respiratory distress during physical activity or previous respiratory infections.

Respiratory paralysis accompanied by generalized muscle weakness has been described in other patients with CPT deficiency.[9,10,13] This could have been caused by increased metabolic demands of respiratory muscles during his respiratory infection. The CPT system is composed of two acyl transferases: CPT I, located in the inner side of the outer mitochondrial membrane, and CPT II, located in the inner side of the inner mitochondrial membrane (Fig. 93-2).

These enzymes facilitate the transfer of fatty acids across the mitochondrial membrane as a source of energy. CPT I deficiency is not associated with neuromuscular disease. CPT II deficiency can manifest in three phenotypes: *type 1* is the characteristic myopathic juvenile form associated with myoglobinuria; *type 2*

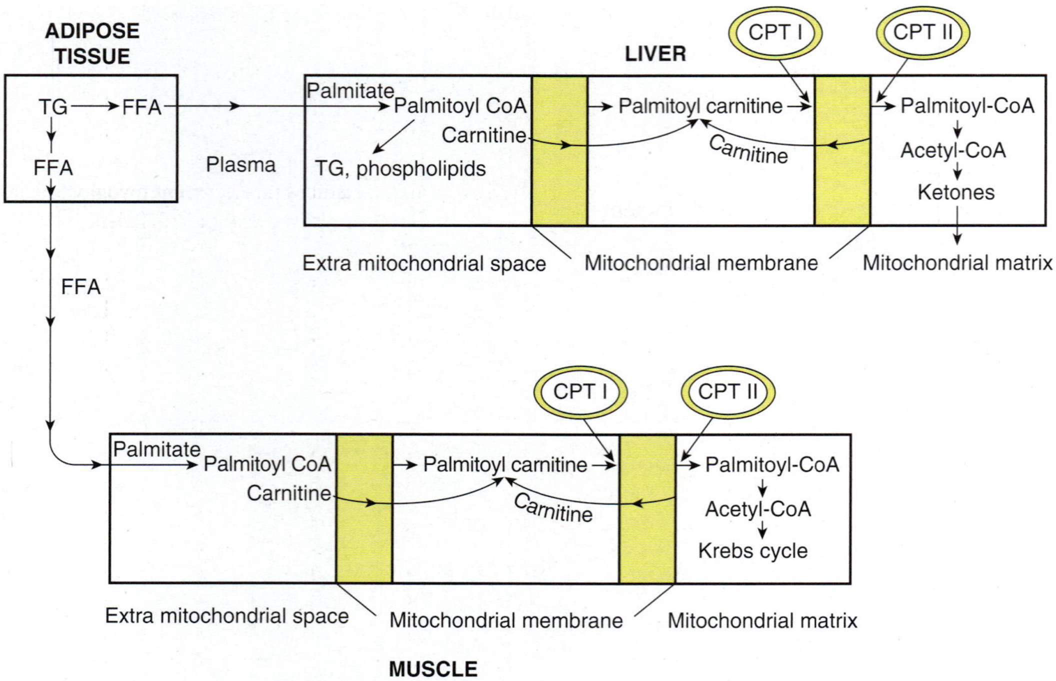

FIG. 93-2 Diagram of the incorporation of fatty acids into the mitochondria in muscle and liver. *CPT*, Carnitine palmitoyl transferase; *FFA*, free fatty acids; *TG*, triglycerides.

is a severe life-threatening infantile form with hepatic, muscular, and cardiac involvement; *type 3* is a fatal neonatal-onset disease with developmental abnormalities.[16]

Myopathic CPT II deficiency, as in this patient, is characterized by exercise-induced pain and muscle tightness, but usually without cramps. Muscle pain was the most frequent complaint in a recent review, in which 21% of the cases had no history of myoglobinuria.[17]

Rhabdomyolysis in DiMauro disease occurs during prolonged exercise when fatty acids are used as a primary source of energy, not during short bursts of exercise as occurs in the glycogen storage disorders; CPT-deficient patients do not have a second-wind phenomenon.

The attacks of myoglobinuria in CPT II deficiency could also occur in other situations, such as febrile illness, cold temperatures, and stress. There are also cases reported associated with malignant hyperthermia or triggered by medications.[16,18,19] The disease occurs more frequently in men, suggesting that hormonal factors and/or gender-related differences, including exercise activity, might play a role.[16]

The genetic defect is located in chromosome 1p32,[20] and most mutations are private, but a prevalent mutation (Ser113Leu)[21] occurs in about 50% of mutant alleles of patients. Testing for mutations in blood cells is an efficient and noninvasive method for arriving at this diagnosis.[22]

DiMauro disease (CPT II, type 1) is usually relatively benign, but there are exceptions,[16] and a neonatal myopathy with weakness has been reported.[23]

There is no cure for this condition. Oral glucose does not appear to be helpful, but intravenous glucose increases exercise tolerance.[24] A low-fat carbohydrate-rich diet that contains polysaccharides can be beneficial[25] with frequent and regularly scheduled meals, with intravenous glucose during attacks can be beneficial. Oral triheptanoin appears beneficial: bezafibrate increased palmitoylcarnitine oxidation in muscle mitochondria but it was found not to be beneficial in a controlled study.[26] Similarly, we have used medium-chain triglycerides (MCT) during febrile episodes, as these do not require CPT enzymes to incorporate in the mitochondria as a form of fuel.

SUMMARY

This sedentary patient manifested an attack of myoglobinuria after a viral infection. He was found to have CPT deficiency, or DiMauro disease, the most common metabolic myopathy causing myoglobinuria. The attacks of this disease can occur during prolonged exercise or fasting and could also be caused by infections or exposure to cold, stress, or surgery.

IMPORTANT POINTS

- Myoglobinuria is caused by massive muscle necrosis (rhabdomyolysis).
- Treatment of myoglobinuria includes hydration and alkalinization to prevent renal failure.
- Metabolic myopathies should be considered in patients with myoglobinuria of unclear causes before assuming they are "idiopathic."
- The CPT system is necessary for the incorporation of fatty acids in the mitochondria as a source of fuel, particularly during prolonged exercise or fasting or febrile episodes, when these are mobilized.

- CPT II deficiency is the most common familial metabolic cause of myoglobinuria and usually presents in young individuals.
- Muscle biopsy in CPT deficiency could be histologically normal or show evidence of lipid accumulation. Biochemical analysis is usually necessary to establish the diagnosis, but lymphocyte DNA testing is a nontraumatic and efficient way to diagnose suspected individuals.
- The disease is caused by a defect in chromosome 1p32.
- There is no cure for CPT deficiency, but intravenous glucose, high-carbohydrate diets with polysaccharides or MCT oil could be beneficial to prevent attacks of myoglobinuria.

This case was reported in Bertorini T, Yeh Y, Trevisan C, et al. Carnitine palmitoyl transferase deficiency: myoglobinuria and respiratory failure. Neurology. 1980;30(3):263–271.

REFERENCES

1. DiMauro S, DiMauro PM. Muscle carnitine palmitoyl transferase deficiency and myoglobinuria. *Science*. 1973;182:929–931.
2. Bertorini TE. Myoglobinuria, malignant hyperthermia, neuroleptic malignant syndrome, serotonin syndrome. In: Pourmand R, ed. *Acquired Neuromuscular Diseases*. Philadelphia, PA: WB Saunders; 1997:649–671.
3. Gross EG, Dexter JD, Roth RG. Hypokalemic myopathy with myoglobinuria associated with licorice ingestion. *N Engl J Med*. 1966;274:602–606.
4. Jensen OB, Mosdal C, Reske-Nielsen E. Hypokalemic myopathy during treatment with diuretics. *Acta Neurol Scand*. 1977;55: 465–482.
5. Mejlszenkier JD, Safran AP, Healy JJ, et al. The myositis of influenza. *Arch Neurol*. 1973;29:441–443.
6. Minow RA, Gorbach S, Johnson BL, et al. Myoglobinuria associated with influenza A infection. *Ann Intern Med*. 1974;80:359–361.
7. Neufeld HA, Kaminski MV Jr, Wannemacher RW Jr. Effect of inflammatory and noninflammatory stress on ketone bodies and free fatty acids in rats. *Am J Clin Nutr*. 1977;30:1357–1358.
8. Bank WJ, DiMauro S, Bonilla E, et al. A disorder of muscle lipid metabolism and myoglobinuria: absence of carnitine palmitoyl transferase. *N Engl J Med*. 1975;292:443–449.
9. Carroll JE, Brooke MH, DeVivo DC, et al. Biochemical and physiological consequences of carnitine palmitoyl transferase deficiency. *Muscle Nerve*. 1978;1:103–110.
10. Reza MJ, Kar NC, Pearson C, et al. Recurrent myoglobinuria due to carnitine palmityl transferase deficiency. *Ann Intern Med*. 1978;88:610–615.
11. DiDonato S, Cornelio F, Pacini L, et al. Muscle carnitine palmitoyl transferase deficiency: a case with enzyme deficiency in cultured fibroblasts. *Ann Neurol*. 1978;4:465–467.
12. Hostetler KY, Hoppel CL, Romine JS, et al. Partial deficiency of muscle carnitine palmitoyl transferase with normal ketone production. *N Engl J Med*. 1978;298:553–557.
13. Patten BM, Wood JM, Harati Y, et al. Familial recurrent rhabdomyolysis due to carnitine palmitoyl transferase deficiency. *Am J Med*. 1979;67:167–171.
14. Herman J, Nadler HL. Recurrent myoglobinuria and muscle carnitine palmitoyl transferase deficiency. *J Pediatr*. 1977;91: 247–250.
15. Layzer RB, Havel RJ, Becker N, et al. Muscle carnitine palmitoyl transferase deficiency: a case with diabetes and keturia (Abstr). *Neurology (Minneap)*. 1977;27:379–380.
16. DiDonato S, Taroni F. Disorders of lipid metabolism. In: Engel A, Franzini-Armstrong C, eds. Myology. Vol 2. 3rd ed. New York, NY: McGraw-Hill; 2004:1587–1621.
17. Deschauer M, Wieser T, Zierz S. Muscle carnitine palmitoyltransferase II deficiency: clinical and molecular genetic features and diagnostic aspects. *Arch Neurol*. 2005;62:37–41.
18. Katsuya H, Misumi M, Ohtani Y, Miike T. Postanesthetic acute renal failure due to carnitine palmitoyl transferase deficiency. *Anesthesiology*. 1988;68:945–948.
19. Vladutiu GD, Hogan K, Saponara I, et al. Carnitine palmitoyl transferase deficiency in malignant hyperthermia. *Muscle Nerve*. 1993;16:485–491.
20. Gellera C, Verderio E, Floridia G, et al. Assignment of the human carnitine palmitoyl transferase II gene (CPT1) to chromosome 1p32. *Genomics*. 1994;24:195–197.
21. Taroni F, Verderio E, Dworzak F, et al. Identification of a common mutation in the carnitine palmitoyl transferase II gene in familial recurrent myoglobinuria patients. *Nat Genet*. 1993;4:314–320.
22. DiMauro S, Shanske S, Naini A, Krishna S. Biochemical evaluation of metabolic myopathies. In: Bertorini TE, ed. *Clinical Evaluation and Diagnostic Tests for Neuromuscular Disorders*. Boston, MA: Butterworth-Heinemann; 2002:535–564.
23. Land JM, Mistry S, Squier M, et al. Neonatal carnitine palmitoyl transferase-2 deficiency: a case presenting with myopathy. *Neuromuscul Disord*. 1995;5:129–137.
24. Orngreen MC, Olsen DB, Vissing J. Exercise tolerance in carnitine palmitoyl transferase II deficiency with IV and oral glucose. *Neurology*. 2002;59:1046–1051.
25. Orngreen MC, Ejstrup R, Vissing J. Effect of diet on exercise tolerance in carnitine palmitoyl transferase II deficiency. *Neurology*. 2003;61(4):559–561.
26. Vorgard M, Deschauer M. Treatment and management of hereditary metabolic myopathies Chapter 23. In: Bertorini TE, ed. *Neuromuscular Disorders: Treatment and Management*. 2nd ed. Amsterdam, Netherlands: Elsevier; 2022:572–594.

94 CASE

An Elderly Man With New Onset Weakness

A 70-year-old male with hypertension, hyperlipidemia with a past medical history of chronic migraine, chronic lower back pain and coronary artery disease, and S/P triple bypass was referred for progressive proximal extremity weakness over the past 6 months. The weakness started with both lower extremities and later involved the upper extremities and neck, not associated with myalgia.

The patient was on atorvastatin, which was stopped, but the weakness did not improve. He denied dysarthria, dyspnea, dysphagia, worsening lower back pain, numbness, cramps, and fasciculations.

On physical examination he was noted to have normal cognition on screening. Cranial nerve examination revealed left cranial nerve VI palsy (secondary to prior ischemic cranial nerve VI); otherwise, cranial nerve exam was unremarkable. On motor exam there was moderate weakness appreciated in the deltoids, hip flexors, quadriceps, and hamstrings. Deep tendon reflexes were 2+ and symmetrical bilaterally. Sensory examination revealed minimal decreased vibration sensation in the toes. Coordination was intact. The patient had difficulty walking with an unsteady gait.

Serum CK was 2612 IU/L (normal, <200 IU/L), aspartate aminotransferase (AST) was 54 IU/L, and ALT 85 IU/L, and the rest of the lab tests were within normal limits including normal thyroid stimulating hormone (TSH), T3, T4, HIV, and ANA. Myositis panel was negative, which included anti-5-nucleotidase, cytosolic IA (NT5C1A), anticysolic 5-nucleotidase 1A (CN1A) antibody, anti-3-hydroxy-3-methylglutaryl-coenzyme A reductase (HMGCR) antibody. HIV was negative.

AN EMG TEST WAS PERFORMED

Motor Nerve Conduction

Nerve and Site	Latency (ms)	Amplitude (mV)	Segment	Latency Difference (ms)	Conduction Velocity
Peroneal nerve L.					
Ankle	4.8	10.1	Extensor digitorum brevis–ankle	4.8	
Fibula (head)	10.8	9.6	Ankle–fibula (head)	6.0	50 m/s
Popliteal fossa	12.5	9.9	Fibula (head)–popliteal fossa	1.7	53 m/s
Tibial nerve L.					
Ankle	5.1	9.6	Abductor–hallucis–ankle	5.1	m/s
Popliteal fossa	14.0	5.9	Ankle–popliteal fossa	8.9	51 m/s
Tibial nerve R.					
Ankle	5.0	13.4	Abductor–hallucis–ankle	5.0	m/s
Popliteal fossa	14.4	4.6	Ankle–popliteal fossa	9.4	44 m/s
Peroneal nerve R.					
Ankle	5.1	6.6	Extensor digitorum brevis–ankle	5.1	m/s
Fibula (head)	11.0	6.0	Ankle–fibula (head)	5.9	51 m/s
Popliteal fossa	12.4	6.0	Fibula (head)–popliteal fossa	1.4	64 m/s

F-Wave Studies

Nerve	M-Latency	F-Latency
Peroneal nerve L.	12.5	46.9
Tibial nerve L.	14.0	49.5
Tibial nerve R.	5.0	51.7
Peroneal nerve R.	13.1	51.5

Sensory Nerve Conduction

Nerve and Site	Onset Latency (ms)	Peak Latency (ms)	Amplitude (μV)	Segment	Latency Difference (ms)	Conduction Velocity
Sural nerve L.						
Lower leg	2.8	3.6	26	Ankle–lower leg	2.8	m/s
Superficial peroneal nerve L.						
Ankle	2.5	3.2	16	Dorsum of foot–ankle	2.5	m/s
Superficial peroneal nerve R.						
Ankle	2.4	3.4	19	Dorsum of foot–ankle	2.4	m/s
Sural nerve R.						
Lower leg	2.7	3.4	17	Ankle–lower leg	2.7	m/s

WHAT IS THE DIFFERENTIAL DIAGNOSIS?

The patient initially started having weakness of proximal muscles which has been progressing and required walking aides to ambulate. CK levels were elevated.

The differential diagnosis to consider includes statin-induced necrotizing autoimmune myopathy. Statins are commonly used for patients with hyperlipidemia and secondary prevention for established patients with atherosclerotic cardiovascular disease. This patient has been taken off the statin in the past without the improvement of symptoms and has tested negative for hydroxy-methyl-glutaryl-coenzyme A, reductase (HGCR) antibodies, making this diagnosis unlikely.

Inclusion body myositis (IBM) is a progressive disease of skeletal muscles, which is present at this age, affecting the quads, finger flexors, and ankles dorsiflexor.[1,2] Electromyography (EMG) shows fibrillation potentials and positive sharp waves with occasional large motor units. The CK levels typically are less than 5× of the upper limit of normal. The muscle biopsy of the involved muscle demonstrates an inflammatory process and rimmed vacuoles, which may not always be seen as process, is patchy and ragged red fibers. Occasionally autoantibody to antinucleotidase cytosolic 1A can be positive.[3,4] IBM is unlikely in our patient as the distribution of weakness is not typical.

Pompe disease is a lysosomal storage disease that results from a lysosomal acid alpha-glucosidase deficiency. The infantile form typically presents in the first several months of life with muscular hypotonia and cardiomyopathy. The juvenile and adult form presentation ranges from asymptomatic to severe progressive myopathy. Early diaphragm involvement is common.[5] Respiratory failure is typically the cause of death. This affects pure motor weakness. The adult form of Pompe disease is possible in our patient due to progressive weakness with myopathic features on EMG. Serum CK levels typically are not as high as in this patient.

Myotonic dystrophy type 2 (MD2) is an autosomal-dominant disorder caused by unstable tetranucleotide (CCTG) repeat expansion in the first intron at the cellular nucleic acid–binding protein (*CNBP*) gene. Typically, this disease is characterized by progressive weakness, myotonia, and early-onset cataracts. The weakness is usually progressive and more proximal (neck flexors, hip flexors, and hip extensors) and prominent muscle pain with typically described as aching or stiffness. In these patients EMG studies reveal the characteristic waxing and waning myotonic discharges which occasionally present without clinical myotonia. This patient had progressive weakness, but no myotonia, or muscle pains or ocular pathology. The lack of a family history, is somewhat against this diagnosis. The serum CK, however, is never this high in myotonic dystrophy.

Adult-onset limb-girdle muscular dystrophy (LGMD). This is a group of inherited diseases that affect proximal muscles. Although hereditary, there are cases without a family history. Patients have progressive weakness and muscle atrophy affecting shoulder and/or pelvic girdle. Some of these patients have cardiac involvement. Creatine kinase levels are modestly elevated. Muscle biopsy should be considered if genetic testing is unavailable or uninformative, this typically shows dystrophic changes with degeneration and regeneration of the muscle fibers, fiber-splitting, internal nuclei, fibrosis, moth-eaten, and whorled fibers. This patient does not have any family history of weakness, but sporadic mutations are reported. Patients typically present at a younger age, however, age is variable, and late-onset LGMD have been reported such as in this case by Dr. Shofer diagnosed with LGMD 2 at the age of 54.[6]

Becker muscular dystrophy could be considered as some cases are late onset caused by a mutation of the dystrophin gene.

Mitochondrial myopathies. As mitochondria is involved in fat and carbohydrate oxidation in individuals, this affects the mitochondria usually present with symptoms during periods of high metabolic demand like fasting, long exercise, and superimposed illness. Patients with a mitochondrial myopathy could have hypoacusis, ptosis, ophthalmoparesis, seizures, lipoma (head/neck), cardiomyopathy, peripheral neuropathy. However, some patients with mitochondrial myopathies present with only weakness.

Polymyositis. This idiopathic inflammatory myopathy presents with symmetrical proximal muscle weakness and there is evidence of muscle inflammation on biopsy which is required for this diagnosis which will show cellular infiltration within the fascicle with inflammatory cells invading individual muscle fibers.

Hypothyroid myopathy. Patients typically present with myalgias, muscle cramps, fatigue, and muscle weakness that is exacerbated with exertion.[7] Hypothyroid myopathy affects proximal muscles such as shoulder and pelvic girdle muscles. Myoedema can be seen in these patients. CK is frequently elevated. This diagnosis is unlikely as thyroid stimulator hormone, and thyroxine levels were within normal limits.

Muscle carnitine deficiency is a very rare disorder. Carnitine is the intermediate compound responsible for transferring long-chain fatty acids across the mitochondrial membrane. While primary carnitine deficiency is caused by mutation in sodium-dependent carnitine transporter gene organic cation/carnitine transporter 2 (OCTN) or also known as solute carrier family 22 member 5 (*SLCC22A5*) gene, which is located on chromosome 5q33.1. This entity typically presents with slowly progressive proximal weakness, fatigue, and exercise-related pains. The EMG typically appears myopathic with one case series describing myotonic discharges.[8] Muscle biopsy may show accumulated lipid droplets in muscle fibers. The serum carnitine levels (both free and total) are required for diagnosis. The cause of the secondary disease was not apparent in this patient.

Amyloid myopathy. Amyloid myopathy is a manifestation of primary systemic amyloidosis. Patients will typically present with a combination of cardiomyopathy, peripheral neuropathy, and nephrotic syndrome. Proximal weakness that is progressive along with macroglossia and muscle pseudohypertrophy may be present in setting of elevated serum CK levels. Congo red staining of muscle will show amyloid accumulation. This patient's muscle section did not show evidence of amyloid accumulation.

WHAT TO DO NEXT?

Nerve conduction studies were normal and on EMG testing showed positive sharp waves, fibrillations, high-frequency discharges, and waning myotonic discharges at rest. These findings could suggest disorders of muscle irritability including adult-onset Pompe disease, inflammatory myopathy (polymyositis, IBM, necrotizing myositis), and rarely late-onset muscular dystrophy, MD2, as well as other rare muscle diseases. MD2 could manifest with proximal weakness with these EMG findings without clinical myotonia.

WHAT TO DO NEXT?

Muscle biopsy of the left deltoid was done and on H&E stain noted to have many vacuolization. Oil Red O stain noted to have a marked increase in all fat content. Scattered lymphocytes were noted especially around necrotic fibers on anti-CD45

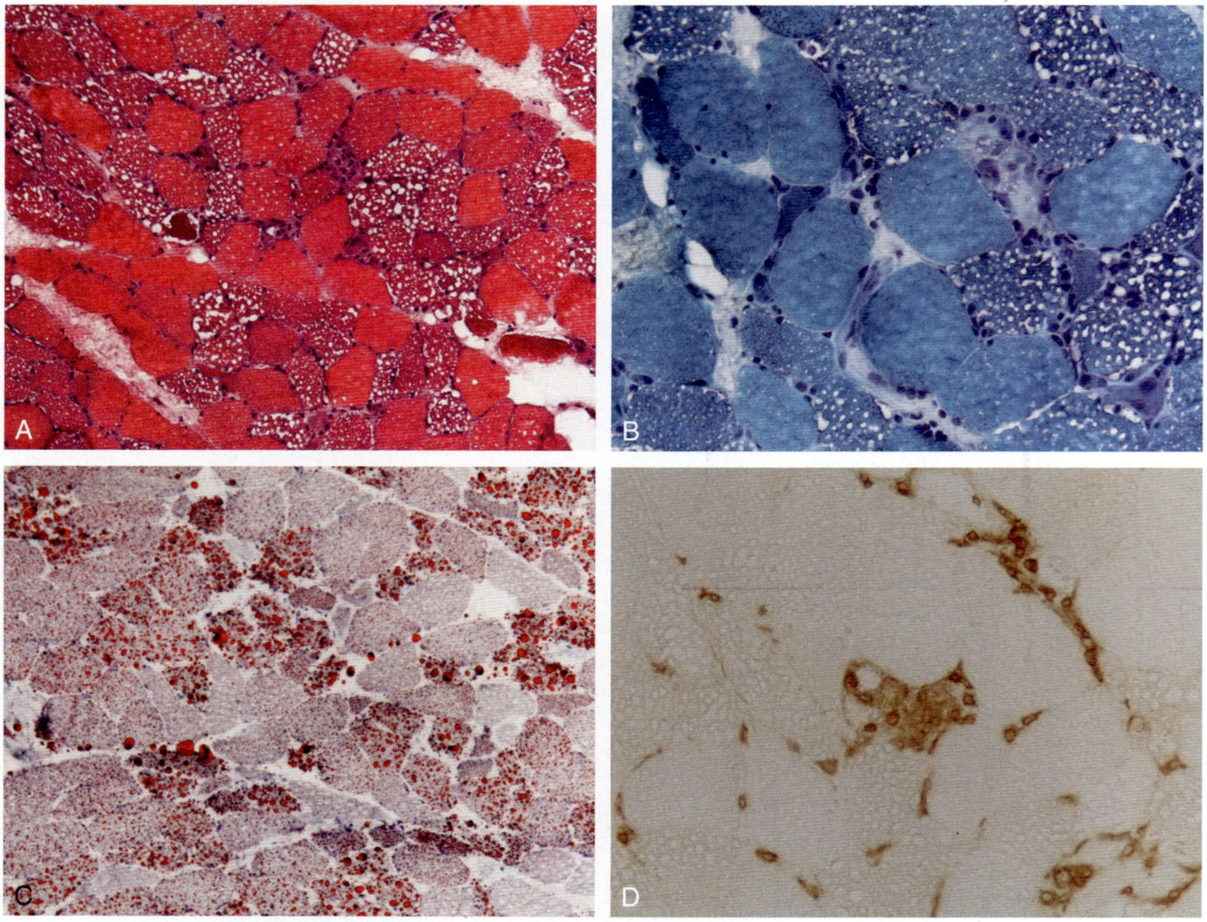

FIG. 94-1 A, H&E stain showing many small vacuoles (×100). **B**, Trichome stain also showing the small vacuoles (×200). **C**, Oil Red O stain shows that the vacuoles have lipid content (×100). **D**, CD45 stain shows scattered lymphocytic accumulation (×100).

staining (Fig. 94-1) and anti-MH1C staining showing mild patchy upregulation.

Biochemistry revealed the total skeletal muscle carnitine levels significantly reduced to 23% of normal, and free carnitine levels significantly reduced to 20% of normal.

DISCUSSION

This elderly patient presented with progressive proximal weakness and hyperCKemia. Statin-induced myopathy was not likely as the patient did not improve with the withdrawal of a statin and HMGCR antibodies were negative. IBM is less likely as the pattern of weakness was not typical for this disease and the anti-5-nucleotidase, cytosolic 1A antibody testing was negative and did not have typical features of IBM on muscle biopsy. No skin lesions were noted on skin inspections making dermatomyositis unlikely. The CK level was too low to suggest adult-onset Pompe disease. The deltoid biopsy showed significant lipid accumulation with inflammation and necrosis. The total muscle carnitine levels and serum-free carnitine levels were found to be significantly reduced. The inflammation on the muscle biopsy was likely secondary. He resumed prednisone 30 mg daily with mild improvement. The patient was tried on carnitine 1 g b.i.d. with CO Q10 400 mg b.i.d. and showed marked improvement.

There was no history of conditions to suggest a secondary cause of carnitine deficiency. No signs of malabsorption were noted (such as anemia, GI symptoms, changes, fatigue, and skin change/lesion). Carnitine is a vital transporter in fatty acid oxidation. Oxidation of long-chain fatty acids and very long–chain fatty acids requires carnitine palmitoyltransferase system, while short- and medium-chain fatty acids can bypass the carnitine palmitoyltransferase and enter the mitochondria directly for beat oxidation.

Primary systemic carnitine deficiency is an autosomal-recessive disorder, caused by mutation in solute carrier family 22 member 5 (*SLCC22A5*) gene that encodes carnitine transporter organic cation/carnitine transfer 2 (OCTN2).

Clinical manifestations of primary systemic carnitine deficiency can vary widely and mainly occurs in the younger population,[9] but can also be seen in older persons.[10] There is a report of carnitine deficiency presenting with rhabdomyolysis in an older person.[11]

In this case, DNA testing was denied by the patient's insurance provider.

SUMMARY

This elderly patient presented progressive weakness without sensory involvement. He had an elevated CK, the EMG showed myotonic discharges, and the biopsy showed lipid vacuoles. He had a significant reduction in carnitine levels, and he responded to carnitine supplementation.

IMPORTANT POINTS

- Weakness and elevated CK in elderly patients with hyperlipidemia could suggest a statin-induced myopathy, particularly caused by HMGCR antibody–related myositis, signal recognition particle antibodies, polymyositis, IBM, limb-girdle dystrophy, toxic myopathies, adult-onset Pompe disease, and MD2, although in this, CK is not that high.
- Myotonic discharges on EMG without clinical myotonia and can be seen in myotonic dystrophies, myotonia congenita, polymyositis, rarely limb-girdle dystrophy, adult-onset Pompe disease, hypothyroid myopathy, several myopathies, and carnitine deficiency.
- Carnitine deficiency is a rare cause of the recent onset of the disease, and the response to carnitine supplementation is very good.
- Carnitine deficiency can be primary or secondary to other conditions such as liver disease and could be primary without any other clinical manifestations of this disorder.
- Patients who are carnitine-deficient respond to carnitine supplementation.

This case was reported in Mirman I, Bertorini T. Case study of an elderly patient with new onset weakness. Clin Neuromuscul Dis. 2022;23(3):148–152.

REFERENCES

1. Phillips BA, Cala LA, Thickbroom GW et al. Patterns of muscle involvement in inclusion body myositis: clinical and magnetic resonance imaging study. *Muscle Nerve*. 2001;24(11):1526–1534.
2. Badrising UA, Maat-Scheieman MLC, van Houwelingen JC et al. Inclusion body myositis. Clinical features and clinical course of the disease in 64 patients. *J Neurol*. 2005;252(12): 1448–1454. https://doi.org/10.1007/s00415-005-0884-y.
3. Kang JH. Rechallenging statin therapy in veterans in statin-induced myopathy post vitamin D replenishment. *J Pharm Pract*. 2017;30(5):521–527.
4. Pluk H, van Hoeve BJA, van Dooren SHJ et al. Autoantibodies to cytosolic 5 nucleotidase 1A in inclusion body myositis. *Ann Neurol*. 2013;73(3):397–407.
5. Nabatame S, Taniike M, Sakai N et al. Sleep disordered breathing in childhood-onset acid maltase deficiency. *Brain Dev*. 2009;31(3):234.
6. Schofer MD, Patzer T, Quante M. Atypical manifestation of late onset limb girdle muscular dystrophy presenting with recurrent falling and shoulder dysfunction: a case report. *Cases J*. 2008;1:402.
7. Bassan BA, Bertorini TE. Neuromuscular manifestations of acquired metabolic endocrine and nutritional disorders (Chapter 21). In: Bertorini TE, ed. *Neuromuscular Disorders: Treatment and Management*. 2nd ed. Amsterdam, Netherlands: Elsevier; 2022:528–553.
8. Snyder TM, Little BW, Roman-Campos G, et al. Successful treatment of familial idiopathic lipid storage myopathy with L carnitine and modified lipid diet. *Neurology*. 1982:32.
9. Magoulas PL, El-Hattab AW. Systemic primary carnitine deficiency: an overview of clinical manifestations, diagnosis, and management. *Orphanet J Rare Dis*. 2012;7:68.
10. Martin JJ, Vercruyssen A, de Barsy T, Ceutrick C. Muscle carnitine deficiency in old age. Case report and therapeutic results. *Clin Neurol Neurosurg*. 1985;87(4):275–281.
11. Echaniz-Laquna A, Biancalana V, Gaignard P, et al. Primary carnitine deficiency in a 57 year old patient with recurrent exertional rhabdomyolysis. *BMJ Case Rep*. 2018. https://doi.org/10.1136/bcr-2018-224272.

95 CASE

A Uremic Man With Proximal Muscle Weakness

A 57-year-old right-handed White man with renal failure from glomerulonephritis had been on dialysis for 3 years and was evaluated for weakness and stiffness of his arms and legs which began 1 year before. He could not extend his right arm without experiencing pain in the biceps. There was also severe stiffness in both knees.

Neurologic examination revealed normal mentation and cranial nerves. Motor testing demonstrated that his neck flexors and extensors were normal. He had 4−/5 weakness of the proximal muscles in the arms and legs, distal legs were 3−/5, wrist extensors were 4/5, and flexors were 4+/5. Weakness was 3/5 in both hands with interossei wasting, and he had flexor contractures of the upper and lower extremities (Fig. 95-1). Reflexes were absent throughout. There were no Babinski signs. Sensory examination showed decreased vibration in the toes and decreased pinprick up to the mid-legs. Coordination was normal. The rest of the examination was unremarkable.

WHAT SHOULD BE DONE NEXT?

A comprehensive metabolic panel was normal except for blood urea nitrogen of 68 mg/dL (normal, <20 mg/dL); creatinine, 8 mg/dL (normal, <1.5 mg/dL); alkaline phosphatase, 132 IU/dL (normal, <12 IU/dL). Serum creatine kinase was 226 IU/L (normal, <200 IU/L); hematocrit was 34% (normal, 26%–50%), and hemoglobin, 11 g/dL (normal, 12–16 g/dL). Calcium was 9.9 mg/dL (normal, 8.6–10.3 mg/dL), and phosphorus, 5.2 mg/dL (normal, 2.5–5 mg/dL).

AN EMG TEST WAS PERFORMED

Motor Nerve Studies

Nerve and Site	Latency (ms)	Amplitude (mV)	Conduction Velocity (m/s)
Peroneal Nerve R.	**Normal ≤ 5.7**	**Normal ≥ 3**	**Normal ≥ 40**
Ankle	**NR**	**NR**	–
Fibular head	**NR**	**NR**	**NR**
Knee	**NR**	**NR**	**NR**
Peroneal Nerve R. (Tibialis Anterior Recording-Needle)			
Fibular head	6.6	**1**	–
Knee	9.5	**1**	**34**

Motor Nerve Studies—cont'd

Nerve and Site	Latency (ms)	Amplitude (mV)	Conduction Velocity (m/s)
Tibial Nerve L.	**Normal ≤ 5.3**	**Normal ≥ 4**	**Normal ≥ 40**
Ankle	**NR**	**NR**	–
Pop. fossa	**NR**	**NR**	**NR**
Median Nerve R.	**Normal ≤ 4.2**	**Normal ≥ 6**	**Normal ≥ 50**
Wrist	3.8	6	–
Elbow	8.8	6	**40**
Ulnar Nerve R.	**Normal ≤ 3.7**	**Normal ≥ 8**	**Normal ≥ 50**
Wrist	3.4	**6**	–
Below elbow	6.8	**6**	**36**
Above elbow	9.8	**6**	**25**
Median Nerve L.	**Normal ≤ 4.2**	**Normal ≥ 6**	**Normal ≥ 50**
Wrist	**5.2**	**5**	–
Elbow	10.6	**5**	**43**

F-Wave and Tibial H-Reflex Studies

Nerve	Latency (ms)	Normal Latency ≤ (ms)
Peroneal nerve R.	**NR**	54
Tibial nerve L.	**NR**	54
Median nerve R.	30	30
Ulnar nerve R.	30	30
Median nerve L.	30	30
H-reflex R.	**NR**	34
H-reflex L.	**NR**	34

Sensory Nerve Studies

Nerve	Onset Latency (ms)	Normal Onset Latency ≤ (ms)	Peak Latency (ms)	Normal Peak Latency ≤ (ms)	Amp (μV)	Normal Amp ≥ (μV)	Conduction Velocity (m/s)	Normal Conduction Velocity ≥ (m/s)
Sural nerve R.	**NR**	**3.5**	**NR**	4.0	**NR**	11	**NR**	40
Median nerve R.	**NR**	**2.6**	**NR**	3.1	**NR**	20	**NR**	50
Ulnar nerve R.	2.4	2.6	2.9	3.1	**5**	13	50	50
Median nerve L.	**NR**	**2.6**	**NR**	3.1	**NR**	20	**NR**	50

EMG Data

Muscle	Insrt Activity	Fibs	Pos Waves	Fasc	Amp	Dur	Poly	Pattern
Iliopsoas R.	Norm	None	None	None	**Dec**	**Brief**[a]	**Many**	Full
Vastus lateralis R.	**Inc**	None	None	None	**Dec**	**Brief**[a]	**Many**	Full
Tibialis anterior R.	**Inc**	**3+**	**3+**	None	**Lg**	**Inc**	**Few**	**Red**
Gastrocnemius R.	**Inc**	**3+**	**3+**	None	**Lg**	**Inc**	None	**Red**
Deltoid R.	**Inc**	None	None	None	**Dec**	**Brief**[a]	**Few**	Full
Biceps brachii R.	**Inc**	None	None	None	**Dec**	**Brief**[a]	**Few**	Full
Triceps R.	**Inc**	None	**1+**	None	**Dec**	**Brief**	**Few**	Full
Flexor carpi ulnaris R.	Norm	None	None	None	Norm	Norm	None	Full
First dorsal interosseous R.	**Inc**	**2+**	**2+**	None	**Lg**	**Inc**	None	**Red**

[a]No amplitude variability.

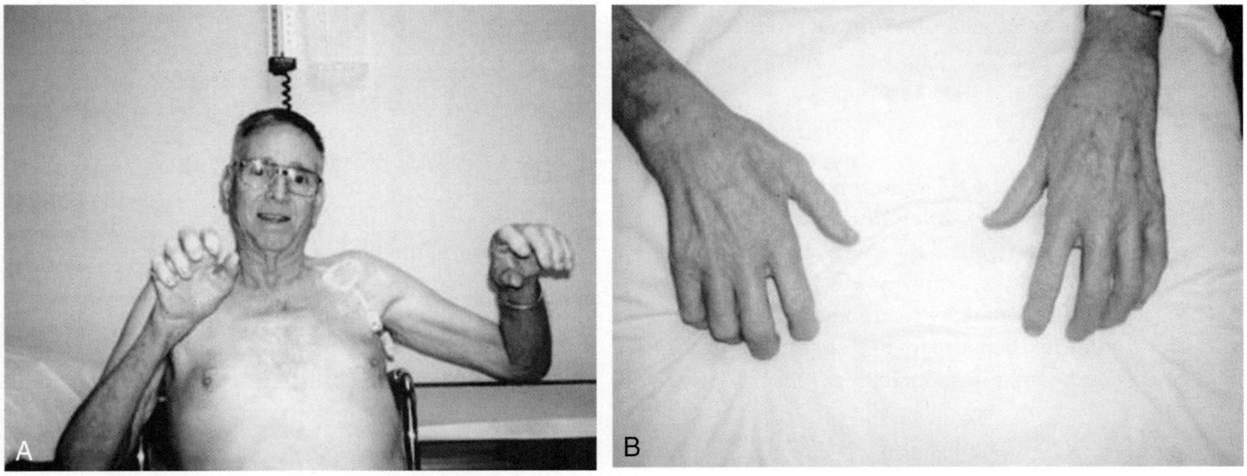

FIG. 95-1 A, Patient showing marked proximal muscle weakness with contractures. **B**, Interossei muscle atrophy with interphalangeal joint contractures.

WHAT WERE THE EMG FINDINGS?

Nerve conduction studies showed slow conduction velocities of the median and ulnar nerves with low amplitude CMAPs and prolonged distal latencies.

There were no elicitable CMAPs in the legs when recording in the feet, and there was slow motor nerve conduction velocity of the peroneal nerve when recording the tibialis anterior muscle with a needle electrode. Tibial H-reflexes and sural and median SNAPs were absent. The ulnar SNAP was of low amplitude. F-responses had normal latency in the arms but were absent in the legs.

The needle test showed denervation potentials in the distal muscles in the upper and lower extremities with large motor unit action potentials of decreased recruitment in the distal muscles, indicating axonal degeneration with reinnervation. There were frequent small polyphasic motor unit potentials with normal recruitment in the proximal muscles, particularly in the legs.

It was concluded that the patient had a motor and sensory polyneuropathy, predominantly axonal with demyelination that was thought to be secondary. There was also a suggestion of a myopathy, because of the presence of many brief motor unit potentials without amplitude variability in the proximal muscles.

WHAT IS THE DIFFERENTIAL DIAGNOSIS?

This patient had a peripheral neuropathy, likely from uremia; however, other contributing causes needed to be considered, particularly diabetes, vitamin deficiencies, and vasculitis, as well as secondary amyloidosis.

He also appeared to have a myopathy, although the scattered brief motor units seen in the proximal muscles on EMG could be secondary to disuse. The lack of proximal muscle denervation suggested that this was not caused by an inflammatory myopathy, and the normal recruitment of these motor units indicated that they were not caused by the neuropathy. The fairly recent onset of proximal weakness was against muscular dystrophy or an inherited metabolic myopathy. Uremics are predisposed to a number of causes of proximal weakness, such as hyperparathyroidism with vitamin D deficiency, carnitine deficiency, and hypophosphatemia, as well as β_2-microglobulin–associated amyloidosis (Table 95-1). These were all considerations, and a muscle biopsy was recommended.

A muscle biopsy of the right biceps demonstrated neurogenic atrophy and type II muscle fiber atrophy. In some areas there was β_2-microglobulin accumulation in the vessels; there appeared to be some perifascicular fiber atrophy and degeneration in the area of the fascicles located closest to the affected vessels (Fig. 95-2). A fat pad biopsy showed an accumulation of β_2-microglobulin in the vessels.

Two tests of serum β_2-microglobulin showed levels of 20,543 and 30,995 µg (normal, 2400 µg); parathyroid hormones were 90.9 and 95.5 pg/mL (normal, 11–64 pg/mL).

Thyroid function tests and serum protein electrophoresis were normal.

He was managed medically with a phosphate-binding agent and vitamin D supplementation. Microfiltration hemodialysis was instituted for optimal removal of the β_2-microglobulin–associated amyloid. This resulted in physical improvement to the point that he regained his ability to ambulate, although the contractures remained. He died a year later of complications of renal failure and congestive heart failure.

DISCUSSION

This patient had renal failure with a neuropathy but also appears to have had a myopathy, likely secondary to β_2-microglobulin accumulation and secondary hyperparathyroidism. Although distal weakness is seen in uremics from uremic neuropathy, proximal muscle weakness also occurs, and there is no clear association between the degree of weakness and azotemia.[1,2] About 20% of patients undergoing hemodialysis have elevated serum creatine kinase and its isoenzymes[2] that could have many causes. The most common is secondary hyperparathyroidism.[3,4] It is likely that parathyroid hormone impairs energy production, transfer, and utilization in skeletal muscles.[4] The myopathy might be associated with impaired oxidation of long-chain fatty acids. This is caused by a reduction of carnitine palmitoyl transferase, a key enzyme for the transport of long-chain fatty acids into the mitochondrial matrix.[5] Another possible cause of uremic myopathy is carnitine deficiency,[6–9] which also

TABLE 95-1 Causes of Uremia-Associated Myopathy

Secondary hyperparathyroidism
Aluminum intoxication
Iron overload
β_2-microglobulin–associated amyloidosis
Vitamin D deficiency
Chronic phosphate depletion
Hypokalemia
Hyperkalemia
Hypercalcemia
Carnitine deficiency
Azotemic vasculopathy (necrotizing myopathy)
Disuse atrophy (mainly type II muscle fiber)
Associated vasculitides
Connective tissue disease
Myopathy in dialysis-associated systemic fibrosis
Idiopathic

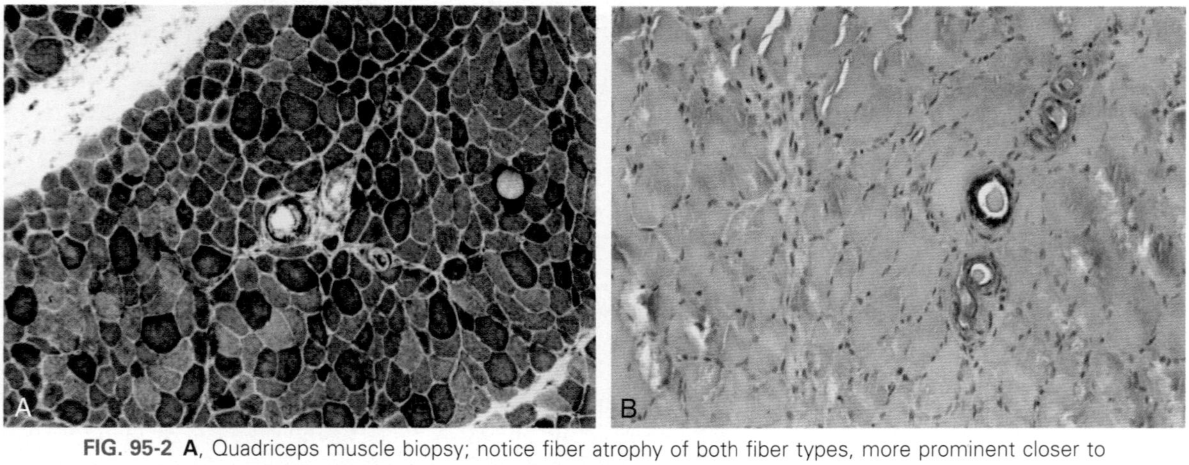

FIG. 95-2 A, Quadriceps muscle biopsy; notice fiber atrophy of both fiber types, more prominent closer to the perifascicular and perivascular areas (NADH-TR stain, ×200). **B**, Paraffin-fixed muscle, immunoperoxidase stained for β_2-microglobulin; notice accumulation of β_2-microglobulin in the vessel wall (×200).

impairs the utilization of these fatty acids. Iron accumulation, caused by excessive iron supplementation or from repeated transfusions, particularly in predisposed patients, can also cause weakness. The water used for dialysis was the cause of aluminum intoxication in the past, and although it is no longer a problem, the use of aluminum-containing binders for hyperphosphatemia could also cause aluminum intoxication. Metal accumulations improve with the use of the chelating agent desferroxamine.[10] β_2-microglobulin amyloidosis, which is a common cause of carpal tunnel syndrome in uremics,[11] has also been associated with deposits of this protein in vessels accompanied by atrophy of muscle fibers[12] and oxidiative stress, plays an important role.[13] This cause of uremic myopathy improves with dialysis ultrafiltration and, ideally, renal transplantation.

Vitamin D deficiency, hypophosphatemia, and electrolyte imbalance can also cause proximal weakness,[14–16] and uremics might develop weakness from connective tissue disorders. Dialysis-associated systemic fibrosis is a condition in which there are skin changes, joint contractions with weakness, and myofiber degeneration.[17,18]

This patient received vitamin D and ultrafiltration with a reduction of β_2-microglobulins to 1000 µg, associated with moderate improvement. However, he did not undergo renal transplantation and eventually died of congestive heart failure.

SUMMARY

This uremic man had a peripheral neuropathy and developed proximal weakness and joint contractures. He had hyperparathyroidism and elevated β_2-microglobulin in serum and had deposits of this protein in vessels associated with muscle atrophy. He improved with vitamin D supplementation and dialysis with ultrafiltration.

IMPORTANT POINTS

- The most common neuromuscular complication of uremia is neuropathy, but uremics can also present with a myopathy.
- Uremic myopathy has multiple causes which include, among others, hyperparathyroidism, malnutrition, carnitine deficiency, metal accumulation, and β_2-microglobulin deposits in muscle.
- β_2-microglobulin is a form of amyloid that deposits in vessels and soft tissue and is a common cause of carpal tunnel syndrome in uremics and an uncommon cause of myopathy.
- The treatment of β_2-microglobulin accumulation consists of the use of microfiltration hemodialysis and, preferentially, kidney transplantation.

REFERENCES

1. Ravid M, Robson M. Proximal myopathy caused by intragenic phosphate depletion. *JAMA*. 1976;236(12):1380–1381.
2. Quintanilla AP, Sahgal V. Uremic myopathy. *Int J Artif Organs*. 1984;7(5):239–242.
3. Baczynski R, Massry SG, Magott M, et al. Effect of parathyroid hormone on energy metabolism of skeletal muscle. *Kidney Int*. 1985;28(5):722–727.
4. Smogorzewski M, Piskorska G, Borum PR, Massry SG. Chronic renal failure, parathyroid hormone and fatty acids oxidation in skeletal muscle. *Kidney Int*. 1988;33(2):555–560.
5. Lennon DL, Shrago E, Madden M, et al. Carnitine status, plasma lipid profiles, and exercise capacity of dialysis patients: effects of a submaximal exercise program. *Metabolism*. 1986; 35(8):728–735.
6. Wanner C, Forstner-Wanner S, Rossle C, et al. Carnitine metabolism in patients with chronic renal failure: effect of L-carnitine supplementation. *Kidney Int*. 1987;22(Suppl):S132–S135.
7. Bohmer T, Bergrem H, Eiklid K. Carnitine deficiency induced during intermittent haemodialysis for renal failure. *Lancet*. 1978;1(8056):126–128.
8. Wanner C, Horl WH. Potential role of carnitine in patients with renal insufficiency. *Klin Wochenschr 1*. 1986;64(13):579–586.
9. Wanner C, Wieland H, Wackerle B, et al. Ketogenic and antiketogenic effects of L-carnitine in haemodialysis patients. *Kidney Int*. 1989;27(Suppl):S264–S268.
10. Pierides AM. Dialysis dementia, osteomalacic fractures and myopathy: a syndrome due to chronic aluminum intoxication. *Int J Artif Organs*. 1978;1(5):206–208.
11. Vaziri ND, Barnes J, Khosrow M, et al. Compression neuropathy subsequent to renal transplantation. *Urology*. 1976;7(2):145–147.
12. Hauglustaine D, Waer M, Michielsen P, et al. Haemodialysis membranes, serum beta 2-microglobulin, and dialysis amyloidosis. *Lancet*. 1986;1(8491):1211–1212.
13. Kaltasatou A, Sakkas GK, Poulianiti KP. Uremic myopathy: is oxidative stress implicated in muscle dysfunction in uremia? *Front Physiol*. 2015;6:102. https://doi.org/10.3389/fphys.2015.00102.
14. Wanic-Kossowska M, Grzegorzewska A, Plotast H, Bombicki K. Does calcitriol therapy improve muscle function in uremic patients? *Perit Dial Int*. 1996;16(Suppl 1):S305–S308.
15. Zumrutdal A, Bakinen O, Ucan H, et al. Relationship between uremic myopathy and false-positive cardiac troponin *T*-test. *Nephron*. 2000;86(4):522–523.
16. Al-Hayk EA, Bertorini TE. Neuromuscular complications in uremics: a review. *Neurologist*. 2007;13:131–137.
17. Levine JM, Taylor RA, Elman LB, et al. Involvement of skeletal muscle in dialysis-associated systemic fibrosis (nephrogenic fibrosing dermopathy). *Muscle Nerve*. 2004;30(5):569–577.
18. Shamam YM, de Jesus O. Nephrogenic Systemic Fibrosis. In: *StatPearls [Internet]*. Last updated 12:2023.

96 CASE

A Woman With Weakness, Elevated Cholesterol, and Serum Creatine Kinase Levels

A 64-year-old woman was referred because of a 5-year history of difficulty getting up from a chair, going up and down stairs, and muscle tightness with pain particularly in the thighs after exercising. Workup revealed an elevated serum creatine kinase (CK).

She had been on atorvastatin calcium for hyperlipidemia, and her problems were thought to be related to the drug. The drug was discontinued, but she remained symptomatic.

Previous workup revealed a normal EMG, and a myelogram that showed a mild lumbar stenosis.

The patient was hypertensive on diltiazem and on clopidogrel. She had no difficulty swallowing or breathing, and her review of systems was negative. She did not smoke or drink alcohol. Family history was negative.

Examination showed normal mentation and cranial nerves without facial, tongue, or palatal weakness. She had difficulty rising from a chair and sitting from a supine position, but gait was normal; there was iliopsoas and glutei weakness of 4−/5. Other muscle groups were normal. There was no atrophy or fasciculations. Reflexes were normal without slow relaxation. There was no myoedema during muscle percussion. There were no Babinski signs. Sensory examination to position, vibration, pain, and temperature was normal. Coordination was also normal. No myotonia was detected.

Blood work, including erythrocyte sedimentation rate, was normal except for serum CK of 1484 IU/L (normal, <200 IU/L); aspartate transaminase was 95 IU/L (normal, 0–40 IU/L), and alanine transaminase was 88 IU/L (normal, 30–65 IU/L).

AN EMG TEST WAS PERFORMED

Motor Nerve Studies

Nerve and Site	Latency (ms)	Amplitude (mV)	Conduction Velocity (m/s)
Peroneal Nerve R.	**Normal ≤ 5.7**	**Normal ≥ 3**	**Normal ≥ 40**
Ankle	5.7	5	–
Fibular head	12.4	4	40
Knee	14.2	4	42
Tibial Nerve L.	**Normal ≤ 5.3**	**Normal ≥ 4**	**Normal ≥ 40**
Ankle	4.4	10	–
Pop. fossa	12.7	8	46

Nerve and Site	Latency (ms)	Amplitude (mV)	Conduction Velocity (m/s)
Ulnar Nerve R.	**Normal ≤ 3.6**	**Normal ≥ 8**	**Normal ≥ 50**
Wrist	3.4	11	–
Below elbow	6.8	11	54

F-Wave and Tibial H-Reflex Studies

Nerve	Latency (ms)	Normal Latency ≤ (ms)
Peroneal nerve R.	50.4	54
Tibial nerve L.	53.3	54
Ulnar nerve R.	28.8	30
H-reflex R.	33.3	34
H-reflex L.	33.3	34

Sensory Nerve Studies

Nerve	Onset Latency (ms)	Normal Onset Latency ≤ (ms)	Peak Latency (ms)	Normal Peak Latency ≤ (ms)	Amp (μV)	Normal Amp ≥ (μV)	Conduction Velocity (m/s)	Normal Conduction Velocity ≥ (m/s)
Sural nerve R.	3.5	3.5	4.0	4.0	11	11	40	40
Ulnar nerve R.	2.3	2.6	2.8	3.1	15	13	52	50

EMG Data

Muscle	Insrt Activity	Fibs	Pos Waves	Fasc	Amp	Dur	Poly	Pattern
Deltoid R.	Norm	None	None	None	Norm	Norm	None	Full
Biceps brachii R.	Norm	None	None	None	Norm	Norm	**Few**	Full
Vastus lateralis R.	Norm	None	None	None	**Lg**	**Inc**	None	Full

EMG Data—cont'd

Muscle	Insrt Activity	Fibs	Pos Waves	Fasc	Amp	Dur	Poly	Pattern
Tibialis anterior R.	Norm	None	None	None	**Lg**	**Inc**	None	Full
Gastrocnemius R.	**Inc**	None	**1+**	None	Norm	Norm	None	Full
Tibialis anterior L.	Norm	None	None	None	**Lg**	**Inc**	None	Full
Gastrocnemius L.	**Inc**	None	None	None	Norm	Norm	None	Full

WHAT WERE THE EMG FINDINGS?

This electrophysiologic test showed normal motor and sensory conduction velocities, amplitudes, and latencies. There were scattered, rare, and large motor unit action potentials in the legs with mild denervation only in the gastrocnemius muscle. These findings were nonspecific, and it was thought that they could have been caused by her spinal disease.

WHAT IS THE DIFFERENTIAL DIAGNOSIS?

The differential diagnosis in this patient includes polymyalgia rheumatica because of the muscle pains, but weakness, elevated serum CK, and normal erythrocyte sedimentation rate were against this possibility. The normal reflexes and lack of fasciculations were against a motor neuron disorder. These and an elevated CK were also against Eaton–Lambert myasthenic syndrome.

She could have polymyositis causing pain and weakness. Other myopathies such as inclusion body myositis, a late-onset limb-girdle dystrophy, and acid maltase deficiency should be in the differential diagnosis, although they usually do not manifest with pain.

A myopathy caused by her statin medication[1] was a possibility, but the fact that she remained weak after the drug was discontinued makes this an unlikely diagnosis. An endocrine myopathy, such as those caused by hyperparathyroidism, and particularly hypothyroidism, need to be considered due to her elevated cholesterol and CK.

WHAT SHOULD BE DONE NEXT?

Thyroid-stimulating hormone was 211 mIU/L (normal, 0.35–5.50 mIU/L). Thyroxine was below 0.5 µg/dL (normal, 4.5–13 µg/dL). A complete blood count was normal, except for a hematocrit of 30.4% with mean corpuscular volume of 106.0 fL (normal, 80–100 fL), mean corpuscular hemoglobin, 35 pg/cell (normal, 27–33 pg/cell), and mean corpuscular hemoglobin concentration, 33.3 g/dL (normal, 33–36 g/dL). Rheumatoid factor was negative. B_{12} was 1020 pg/mL (normal, >200 pg/mL).

She was diagnosed as having a hypothyroid myopathy and treated with thyroid supplement.

DISCUSSION

This patient manifested with muscle weakness and pain and had elevated serum CK; she was initially thought to have a statin-induced myopathy,[1] but in patients on these drugs with elevated CK, one always should be aware of other possible causes.[2,3] Her symptoms persisted after discontinuation of atorvastatin calcium, and she was found to have hypothyroidism. This case emphasizes that serum CK levels and liver enzymes should always be measured in patients with hyperlipidemia *prior* to starting statins, and if these levels are elevated, the patient should have thyroid function tests, as an elevated CK and hyperlipidemia are seen in hypothyroidism.

The thyroid hormone is important for neuromuscular function. It is bound to intracellular receptors such as the adrenergic receptors, regulating glycogenolysis and mitochondrial oxidation. It also regulates the activity of calcium ATPase.[4] The hormone participates in the mobilization of mucopolysaccharides, and hypothyroidism results in deposits of mucopolysaccharides in tissues and can cause carpal tunnel syndrome.

The symptoms of hypothyroidism include thickening of facial features and limb skin, lethargy, cold intolerance, constipation, hair loss, fatigue, muscle stiffness, and paresthesias. Clinical findings could include weakness, myoedema, and slow relaxation of ankle reflexes. Myoedema consists of clinically silent muscle contractures produced by percussion of muscles.

The neuromuscular manifestations of thyroid disease are multiple and include, for example, ophthalmopathy that could mimic or be associated with myasthenia gravis; in hyperthyroidism, this could also cause a myopathy or be associated with hypokalemic periodic paralysis.[5]

Patients with hypothyroidism may develop polyneuropathy with numbness and paresthesias. Pathologically, there are deposits of mucinous material in nerves, with glycogen aggregates in Schwann cells and capillaries. There are also mitochondrial aggregates with axonal degeneration and demyelination. The pathology also involves the small unmyelinated axons.[6,7]

Cranial nerve dysfunction can also occur in this disorder, including hoarseness, anosmia, hearing loss, and, rarely, diaphragmatic paralysis. Entrapment neuropathies are not uncommon, particularly carpal tunnel syndrome and tarsal tunnel syndrome. Patients might manifest with an asymptomatic CK elevation or a myopathy that might be mild[8] or severe[9] with rhabdomyolysis.[10–12] Most often they have myalgias, weakness, and pain; muscle biopsy findings include fiber atrophy with internalized nuclei; and some necrosis could also be seen. Mitochondrial swellings with inclusions, myofibrillary disorganization, and accumulation of glycogen and lipids are seen on electromicroscopy.[13]

Electrophysiologic studies in patients with hypothyroidism could be normal or show fibrillation potentials and, rarely, myotonia; the motor unit action potentials could be normal or small. Those with a peripheral neuropathy have low-amplitude SNAPs and CMAPs with mild conduction slowing.

The disease could also manifest with the Hoffman syndrome, a condition that consists of muscle hypertrophy and pain with prominent myoedema.[14,15] In children, this could manifest with muscle swelling but without pain and with dysmorphic features; this is called Kocher–Debré–Sémélaigne syndrome.[16]

The exact cause of elevated CK in patients without a myopathy is not clear. It is possible that there is necrosis in muscles that are not biopsied. It has also been suspected that this could be caused by a decreased clearance of the enzyme from plasma.[17,18]

The treatment of hypothyroidism consists of thyroid replacement; its associated entrapment syndromes might require decompression surgery.[19]

SUMMARY

This woman had muscle weakness with pain, particularly in the legs. She had hyperlipidemia and was on atorvastatin calcium that was initially assumed to be the cause of weakness.

The patient also had an elevated CK that was also thought to be related to her statin drug, but the symptoms remained when the drug was discontinued. She was later found to be hypothyroid.

IMPORTANT POINTS

- Hypothyroidism should be considered in the differential diagnosis of patients with hyperlipidemia and a high serum CK, prior to exposing the patient to expensive and painful diagnostic tests.
- Serum CK and liver enzymes should be tested *prior* to starting statins.
- Symptoms of hypothyroidism include weight gain, low-temperature intolerance, constipation, depression, and muscle weakness. There might be a mild neuropathy.
- Patients could develop proximal lower extremity weakness, myalgias, cramps, and muscle hypertrophy. There are rare reports of rhabdomyolysis.
- Other neurologic complications include polyneuropathy, carpal tunnel syndrome, and, rarely, other mononeuropathies. The syndrome of hypothyroidism with severe muscle stiffness, hypertrophy, and pain in adults is called the Hoffman syndrome and in children it is called Kocher–Debré–Sémélaigne syndrome. The latter is also accompanied by dysmorphic features; patients do not have pain.
- Characteristic clinical findings of hypothyroid myopathy include myoedema (focal electrically silent contractures of muscle after percussion) and a delayed relaxation of the ankle reflexes.
- Electromyography might show a mild peripheral neuropathy with scattered rare denervation potentials with small or large motor units.
- The histopathology of hypothyroid myopathy reveals the atrophy of type I and type II fibers, scattered hypertrophy of fibers, and increased internalized nuclei. There could also be mitochondrial swelling and inclusions; rarely, there could be severe necrosis.
- The exact pathogenesis of hypothyroid myopathy is not known. Decreased thyroid hormone level impairs the metabolism of carbohydrates and fatty acids, leading to decreased adenosine triphosphate production.

REFERENCES

1. Thompson PD, Clarkson P, Karas RH. Statin-associated myopathy. *JAMA*. 2003;289(13):1681–1690.
2. Rando LP, Cording SA, Newnham HH. Successful reintroduction of statin therapy after myositis: was there another cause? *Med J Aust*. 2004;180(9):472–473.
3. Vladutiu GD, Simmons Z, Isackson PJ, et al. Genetic risk factors associated with lipid-lowering drug-induced myopathies. *Muscle Nerve*. 2006;34(2):153–162.
4. Crum BA, Bolton CF. Peripheral neuropathy in systemic disease. In: Brown WF, Bolton CF, Aminoff MJ, eds. *Neuromuscular Function and Disease*. Philadelphia, PA: WB Saunders; 2002: 1081–1108.
5. Al-Shekhlee A, Kamaniski HJ, Ruff RL. Endocrine myopathies and muscle disorders related to electrolyte disturbance. In: Katirji B, Kaminski HJ, Preston DC, Ruff RL, Shapiro BE, eds. *Neuromuscular Disorders in Clinical Practice*. Boston, MA: Butterworth-Heinemann; 2002:1187–1204.
6. Dyck PJ, Lambert EH. Polyneuropathy associated with hypothyroidism. *J Neuropathol Exp Neurol*. 1970;29:631–658.
7. Shirabe T, Tawara S, Terao A, Araki S. Myxedematous polyneuropathy: a light and electron microscopic study of the peripheral nerve and muscle. *J Neurol Neurosurg Psychiatry*. 1975; 38:241–247.
8. Tornero Estébanez C. Myopathy in hypothyroidism [in Spanish]. *An Med Interna*. 2001;18(6):345–346.
9. Scott KR, Simmons Z, Boyer PJ. Hypothyroid myopathy with a strikingly elevated serum creatine kinase level. *Muscle Nerve*. 2002;26(1):141–144.
10. Kar PM, Hirani A, Allen MJ. Acute renal failure in a hypothyroid patient with rhabdomyolysis. *Clin Nephrol*. 2003;60(6):428–429.
11. Kisakol G, Tunc R, Kaya A. Rhabdomyolysis in a patient with hypothyroidism. *Endocr J*. 2003;50(2):221–223.
12. Barahona MJ, Mauri A, Sucunza N, et al. Hypothyroidism as a cause of rhabdomyolysis. *Endocr J*. 2002;49(6):621–623.
13. Cakir M, Samanci N, Balci N, Balci MK. Musculoskeletal manifestations in patients with thyroid disease. *Clin Endocrin (Oxf)*. 2002;59:162–167.
14. Benito-Leon J, Martin E, Mendez M, et al. Muscle pseudohypertrophy associated with hypothyroidism (Hoffman's syndrome). *Rev Neurol*. 2001;32(10):998–999.
15. Mastropasqua M, Spagna G, Baldini V, et al. Hoffman's syndrome: muscle stiffness, pseudohypertrophy and hypothyroidism. *Horm Res*. 2003;59(2):105–108.
16. Tullu MS, Udgirkar VS, Muranjan MN, et al. Kocher-Debré-Sémélaigne syndrome: hypothyroidism with muscle pseudohypertrophy. *Indian J Pediatr*. 2003;70(8):671–673.
17. Asami T, Uchiyama M. Elevated serum creatinine levels in infants with congenital hypothyroidism: reflection of decreased renal function? *Acta Paediatr*. 2000;89(12):1431–1434.
18. Karlsberg RD, Roberts R. Effect of altered thyroid function on plasma creatine kinase clearance in the dog. *Am J Physiol*. 1978;235:E614–E618.
19. Bassam B, Bertorini TE. Neuromuscular manifestations of acquired metabolic endocrine, and nutritional disorders Chapter 21. In: Bertorini TE, ed. *Neuromuscular Disorders: Treatment and Management*. Amsterdam, Netherlands: Elsevier; 2022. 2nd ed.

An Older Woman With Leg Weakness and Atrophic Muscle Fibers on Biopsy

A 72-year-old woman presented with a 1-year history of lower extremity weakness and pain with difficulty going upstairs. She denied numbness or tingling paresthesias.

Previous workup by the referring neurologist included an EMG that showed "mild peripheral neuropathy" with many polyphasic motor unit action potentials. A muscle biopsy showed only mild type II muscle fiber smallness.

Past medical history was significant for gout, which was well controlled with allopurinol. She did not smoke or drink.

Examination revealed normal mentation and cranial nerves. She could not rise from a chair without using her hands, could not sit on a stool without assistance, and had difficulty sitting from a supine position, but gait was normal. Manual muscle testing revealed mild weakness only of the hip flexor abductors and extensors. Reflexes were normal without delayed relaxation of the ankle reflex or myoedema. Sensory and cerebellar examinations were normal. She had no pathologic reflexes.

WHAT IS THE DIFFERENTIAL DIAGNOSIS?

The differential diagnosis in an older person with slowly progressive lower extremity weakness and pain includes peripheral neuropathy secondary to diabetes or several other causes such as pernicious anemia, toxins, and an alcoholic or paraneoplastic neuropathy. She did not have the characteristic glove-and-stocking sensory loss associated with a neuropathy. Spinal stenosis causes weakness with leg and back pain. The lack of dry mouth, pupillary abnormalities, and normal reflexes is against Eaton–Lambert syndrome.

The lower extremity proximal weakness could be from an inflammatory myopathy such as polymyositis or inclusion body myositis (IBM). The lack of neck flexor or proximal arm weakness was against polymyositis; the lack of significant quadriceps and distal muscle involvement was against IBM, and her muscle biopsy apparently ruled out both possibilities. The possibility of a late-onset muscular dystrophy was not supported by the biopsy. Endocrine myopathies such as hypothyroidism (see Case 87) and hyperparathyroidism can cause predominant leg weakness, and the muscle biopsy may show type II muscle fiber atrophy. Polymyalgia rheumatica, in addition to disuse atrophy due to muscle pain, should be considered, but polymyalgia rheumatica does not cause weakness.

WHAT OTHER TESTS SHOULD BE DONE?

Blood chemistry profile was normal, except for glucose of 115 mg/dL (normal, 74–113 mg/dL), blood urea nitrogen, 21 mg/dL (normal, 5–20 mg/dL), calcium, 11.4 mg/dL (normal, 8.6–10.4 mg/dL), and alkaline phosphatase, 197 IU/L (normal, 39–134 IU/L). Thyroxine and thyroid-stimulating hormone were normal. Erythrocyte sedimentation rate was normal. Glycosylated hemoglobin was 6.26 g/dL (normal, 4.40–6.40 g/dL). Serum creatine kinase (CK) was 150 IU/L (normal, 50–200 IU/L).

AN EMG TEST WAS PERFORMED

Motor Nerve Studies

Nerve and Site	Latency (ms)	Amplitude (mV)	Conduction Velocity (m/s)
Peroneal Nerve R.	**Normal ≤ 5.7**	**Normal ≥ 3**	**Normal ≥ 40**
Ankle	3.7	3	–
Fibular head	10.3	3	51
Knee	11.7	3	52
Before exercise	–	3	–
Posttetanic	–	3	–
Tibial Nerve L.	**Normal ≤ 5.3**	**Normal ≥ 4**	**Normal ≥ 40**
Ankle	4.7	4	–
Pop. fossa	12.7	3	51

Nerve and Site	Latency (ms)	Amplitude (mV)	Conduction Velocity (m/s)
Ulnar Nerve R.	**Normal ≤ 3.6**	**Normal ≥ 8**	**Normal ≥ 50**
Wrist	2.9	15	–
Elbow	6.7	14	61

F-Wave and Tibial H-Reflex Studies

Nerve	Latency (ms)	Normal Latency ≤ (ms)
Peroneal nerve R.	53.5	54
Tibial nerve L.	53.0	54
Ulnar nerve R.	29.9	30
H-reflex R.	34.0	34
H-reflex L.	34.0	34

Sensory Nerve Studies

Nerve	Onset Latency (ms)	Normal Onset Latency ≤ (ms)	Peak Latency (ms)	Normal Peak Latency ≤ (ms)	Amp (μV)	Normal Amp ≥ (μV)	Conduction Velocity (m/s)	Normal Conduction Velocity ≥ (m/s)
Sural nerve R.	3.1	3.5	3.6	4.0	13	11	45	40
Superficial peroneal nerve R.	2.8	3.5	3.3	4.0	12	8–10	50	40
Ulnar nerve R.	2.5	2.6	3.0	3.1	15	13	50	50

EMG Data

Muscle	Insrt Activity	Fibs	Pos Waves	Fasc	Amp	Dur	Poly	Pattern
Deltoid R.	Norm	None	None	None	**Dec**	**Brief**	**Few**	Full
Biceps brachii R.	Norm	None	None	None	Norm	Norm	None	Full
Brachioradialis R.	Norm	None	None	None	Norm	Norm	None	Full
Flexor carpi radialis R.	Norm	None	None	None	Norm	Norm	None	Full
Flexor carpi ulnaris R.	Norm	None	None	None	Norm	Norm	None	Full
First dorsal interosseous R.	Norm	None	None	None	Norm	Norm	None	Full
Tensor fasciae latae R.	Norm	None	None	None	Norm	Norm	**Few**	Full
Vastus lateralis R.	Norm	None	None	None	Norm	Norm	**Few**	Full
Tibialis anterior R.	Norm	None	None	None	Norm	Norm	None	Full
Peroneus longus R.	Norm	None	None	None	Norm	Norm	None	Full
Gastrocnemius R.	Norm	None	None	None	Norm	Norm	None	Full

WHAT WERE THE EMG FINDINGS?

This test showed normal nerve conduction velocities and CMAP and SNAP amplitudes and latencies. There was no posttetanic facilitation. There were scattered small polyphasic motor unit action potentials in the proximal leg and arm muscles with normal recruitment and without denervation potentials. This study suggested that she had a mild myopathy.

The muscle biopsy that was reviewed showed some scattered small fibers, mainly type II of both subtypes; there were no esterase-positive atrophic fibers, fiber grouping, or other abnormalities (Fig. 97-1).

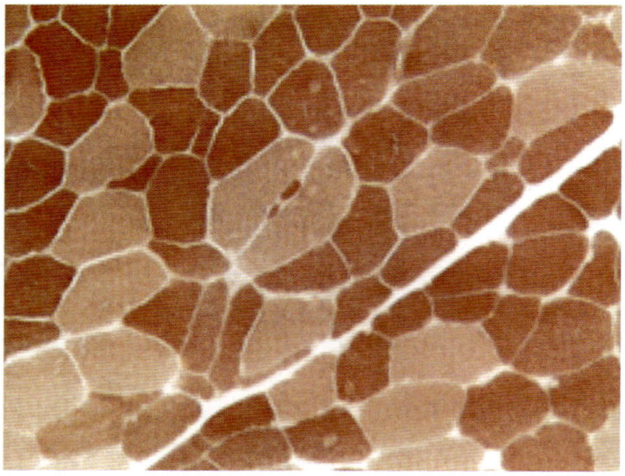

FIG. 97-1 Muscle biopsy showing scattered small muscle fibers, mainly type II (ATPase, pH 9.4, ×200).

WHAT DO THESE TESTS SUGGEST?

The normal CK test and the findings on biopsy are against muscular dystrophy or an inflammatory myopathy. The normal sedimentation rate argued against polymyalgia rheumatica. She had a normal thyroid profile and a borderline high blood sugar level, but her glycosylated hemoglobin was normal. The normal nerve conduction tests did not demonstrate a peripheral neuropathy. The normal CMAP amplitude and lack of posttetanic facilitation were against Eaton–Lambert syndrome. The lack of denervation or large motor units in the legs was against spinal stenosis. Thyroid studies were normal, but the mildly elevated calcium level raises the possibility of hyperparathyroidism. Another consideration is multiple myeloma or metastatic bone disease causing the elevated calcium level.

WHAT OTHER TESTS NEED TO BE DONE?

Ionized calcium level was 5.7 mg/dL (normal, 4.6–5.4 mg/dL). Phosphate was 3.3 mg/dL (normal, 1.0–1.5 mg/dL). Magnesium was 1.7 mg/dL (normal, 1.5–2.5 mg/dL); intact parathyroid hormone was 128 pg/mL (normal, 11–64 pg/mL), and alkaline phosphatase was 125.3 IU/L (normal, 8.6–10.6 IU/L). These tests were diagnostic of hyperparathyroidism.[1] B_{12} was normal.

Thyroid ultrasound showed a small node in the left lobe of the thyroid which was consistent with a parathyroid adenoma. The adenoma was removed, and there was a moderate postsurgical improvement of symptoms.

One month later, the patient had recurrent weakness and pains, and repeat calcium remained high at 11.1 mg/dL (normal, 4.6–5.4 mg/dL). No recurrent adenoma was found and she declined exploratory surgery. She was treated with pamidronate but developed an allergic reaction. There was some improvement with Miacalcin nasal spray.

DISCUSSION

This patient presented with muscle weakness. She had a normal serum CK and type II muscle fiber atrophy on muscle biopsy. She was found to have elevated calcium and parathyroid hormone levels and was diagnosed as having primary hyperparathyroidism. Her symptoms improved following the removal of a parathyroid adenoma. The recurrence of symptoms indicated that there was residual functional adenoma.

Primary hyperparathyroidism manifests as fatigability with proximal muscle weakness in the lower extremities, and, rarely, with pain.[2–5] The weakness ranges from mild to severe, and patients may develop dysphagia and dysarthria[4] with wasting and atrophy, sometimes, mimicking amyotrophic lateral stenosis. The muscle stretch reflexes are normal to increased. Diplopia, myotonia, or severe hypotonia can also occur, but rarely.[4] A necrotizing myopathy secondary to hyperparathyroidism has been reported.[5] A significant peripheral neuropathy is not seen in hyperparathyroidism, in spite of patients' complaints of paresthesias and dysesthesias.

Electromyography in hyperparathyroid myopathy usually shows short-duration polyphasic motor unit potentials, suggestive of a primary myopathy, and the muscle biopsy reveals type II muscle fiber atrophy, as in this patient. Scattered atrophic esterase-positive fibers, indicating denervation and calcium deposits in the endomysial vessels, can also be seen.[6]

The mechanism by which primary hyperparathyroidism leads to neuromuscular disease is unclear, but elevated parathyroid hormone, hypercalcemia, hypophosphatemia, and hypomagnesemia might impair muscle function. The degree of hypercalcemia or hypophosphatemia does not correlate with the severity of weakness.

Proximal weakness also occurs in vitamin D deficiency and osteomalacia, suggesting a link between abnormal vitamin D metabolism and neuromuscular disease in both primary and secondary hyperparathyroidism, which have similar clinical manifestations.[7]

Increased parathyroid hormone promotes bone resorption increasing renal calcium and phosphate reabsorption and promotes increased dihydroxy calciferol and 1,25-vitamin D levels. Parathyroid hormone activates sarcoplasmic reticulum calcium channels by cyclic adenosine monophosphate secondary messenger in muscle.[8] Excessive parathyroid hormone increases muscle proteolysis and impairs energy production and utilization,[9] in part by mitochondrial calcium overload.[10] Abnormalities of neuromuscular transmission can occur, as demonstrated by increased jitter on single-fiber EMG.[3,11]

Parathyroid adenomas are diagnosed by ultrasound and neck MRI and treated by surgical excision.[12,13] Secondary hyperparathyroidism in renal failure is treated with vitamin D supplementation and, additionally, in severe cases, by intravenous calcitriol.[7,14] In those cases, renal transplantation can improve muscle strength. The clinical and laboratory characteristics of hyperthyroidism and other endocrinopathies that manifest with muscle weakness are outlined in Table 97-1.

TABLE 97-1 Myopathies in Endocrine Disorders

Acromegaly
- Proximal weakness, carpal tunnel syndrome, and neuropathy could be seen
- Muscle atrophy
- Normal CK, but could be mildly elevated, elevated growth hormone and IgF-1 levels, TSH levels
- EMG: normal or myopathic
- Biopsy: nonspecific, some fiber necrosis could be seen
- Treatment: removal of the tumor

Hypopituitarism
- Weakness could be severe
- Muscle fatigue
- Normal CK
- Multiple hormone deficiencies
- EMG, biopsy: not defined
- Treatment: hormone replacement

Adrenal Insufficiency—Addison Disease
- Proximal weakness
- Cramps
- Fatigue
- Elevated potassium, reduced cortisol levels, abnormally high ACTH, and normal CK
- EMG: normal
- Biopsy: nonspecific findings
- Treatment: hormone replacement

Hyperadrenalism—Cushing Disease (Primary or Drug-Induced)
- Proximal weakness
- Myalgias
- Truncal adipose tissue accumulation, moon face, and other manifestations of Cushing syndrome
- Normal CK, low potassium, elevated plasma cortisol
- EMG: could show myopathic motor units
- Biopsy: atrophy of type II fibers, mainly IIb
- Treatment: reduction of steroids, removal of tumor

Hyperthyroid or Thyrotoxic Myopathy
- Proximal weakness with little atrophy, more common in women
- In 20% weakness is distal, some with bulbar involvement; Graves ophthalmopathy can occur
- Fasciculations and myokymia can be seen
- Normal CK, high T_4, T_3, reduced TSH levels
- Myopathy on EMG with fibrillations and fasciculations sometimes
- Biopsy: normal or nonspecific findings
- Treatment: beta-blockers, surgery, and radioactive iodine

Thyrotoxic periodic paralysis
- Occurs mainly in Asians, but also in other races, more common in men
- Sporadic or an autosomal-dominant predisposition

(continued)

TABLE 97-1 Myopathies in Endocrine Disorders—cont'd

Attacks of weakness with hypokalemia, usually after high-carbohydrate meals
Elevated CK during attacks
Biopsy: nonspecific, could show vacuolated fibers
EMG: normal except for decreased CMAPs during attacks or after exercise
Treatment: beta-blockers, potassium supplement, PTU, surgery
Hypothyroidism (Adults: Hoffmann Syndrome; Children: Kocher–Debré–Sémélaigne Syndrome)
Proximal weakness
Muscle spasms, and pain (adults)
Myoedema, delayed relaxation of reflexes
Elevated CK, elevated TSH, low T_4
EMG: nonspecific
Biopsy: nonspecific
Treatment: thyroid replacement
Diabetes
Myopathies are unusual
Muscle infarcts occur, causing unilateral weakness, swelling, and high CK
Proximal muscle weakness seen in diabetics, caused by disuse or from neuropathies (as in diabetic amyotrophy and mononeuritis multiplex)
Hyperparathyroidism
Primary, or secondary from renal disease
Proximal weakness and atrophy, muscle cramps; some have hypotonia
Elevated calcium levels usually low phosphate and high alkaline phosphatase, normal or mildly elevated CK
Elevated PTH and vitamin D levels (in secondary hyperparathyroidism, vitamin D levels are low)
EMG: small polyphasic motor units
Biopsy: type II fiber atrophy, angular atrophic fibers, increased calcium in capillaries
Treatment: removal of the adenoma, vitamin D supplementation (for secondary hyperparathyroidism)
Hypoparathyroidism
Hypocalcemia-induced tetany (Chvostek, Trousseau signs)
Cramps
Mildly elevated CK, hypocalcemia, hypomagnesemia
Multiplex discharges on EMG
Treatment: calcium and vitamin D

CK, Creatine kinase; *PTH*, parathyroid hormone; *PTU*, propylthiouracil; *TSH*, thyroid-stimulating hormone.

SUMMARY

This elderly woman presented with proximal muscle weakness and mild type II muscle fiber atrophy on biopsy.

Her elevated serum calcium level prompted investigations leading to the diagnosis of hyperparathyroidism.

IMPORTANT POINTS

- Primary hyperparathyroidism is caused by parathyroid adenomas; secondary hyperparathyroidism occurs in patients with renal failure and osteomalacia.
- Patients with primary hyperparathyroidism have high levels of calcium, parathyroid hormone, and 1,25-hydroxy-vitamin D levels; serum phosphate is usually low. In secondary hyperparathyroidism, vitamin D levels are low.
- Neuromuscular complications in hyperparathyroidism include fatigue and lower extremity weakness. Hoarseness, dysarthria, and diplopia have been reported. There are rare patients who present with a syndrome resembling amyotrophic lateral sclerosis; others might have severe hypotonia or a necrotizing myopathy.
- An elevated serum calcium level should be a clue for the diagnosis of hyperparathyroidism.
- The histopathology of hyperparathyroidism includes type II muscle fiber atrophy and mild neurogenic atrophy. The routine EMG findings are usually nonspecific.
- Parathyroid hormone increases muscle proteolysis and impairs energy production and utilization.
- The treatment of primary hyperparathyroidism is surgical removal of the adenoma.

REFERENCES

1. Younes NA, Shafagoj Y, Khatib F, Ababneh M. Laboratory screening for hyperparathyroidism. *Clin Chim Acta*. 2005;353(1–2):1–12.
2. Patten BM, Bilezikian JP, Mallette LE, et al. Neuromuscular disease in primary hyperparathyroidism. *Ann Intern Med*. 1974;80:182–193.
3. Ljunghall S, Akerstrom G, Johansson G, et al. Neuromuscular involvement in primary hyperparathyroidism. *J Neurol*. 1984;231:263–265.
4. McElduff S. Posen: hyperparathyroidism: a clinical review. In: Massry SG, Fujita T, eds. *New Actions of Parathyroid Hormone*. New York, NY: Plenum Press; 1989:379–386.
5. Al-Shekhlee A, Kawish HJ, Ruff RL. Endocrine myopathies and muscle diseases related to electrolyte disturbance. In: Katirji B, Kaminski HJ, Preston DC, Ruff RL, Shapiro BE, eds. *Neuromuscular Disorders in Clinical Practice*. Boston, MA: Butterworth-Heinemann; 2002:1187–1204.
6. Bertorini TE. Histologic studies in muscle of hyperparathyroidism. In: Massry SG, Fujita T, eds. *New Actions of Parathyroid Hormone*. New York, NY: Plenum Press; 1989:173–182.
7. Mallette LE, Patten BM, Engel WK. Neuromuscular disease in secondary hyperparathyroidism. *Ann Intern Med*. 1975;82:474–483.
8. Garber AJ. Effects of parathyroid hormone on skeletal muscle protein and amino acid metabolism in the rat. *J Clin Invest*. 1983;71(6):1806–1821.
9. Baczynski R, Massry SG, Magott M, et al. Effect of parathyroid hormone on energy metabolism of skeletal muscle. *Kidney Int*. 1985;28(5):722–727.
10. Wrogemann K, Pena SD. Mitochondrial calcium overload: a general mechanism for cell-necrosis in muscle disease. *Lancet*. 1976;1:672–674.
11. Kaplan PE, Hines JR, Leestma JE, Ruder HJ. Neuromuscular junction transmission deficit in a patient with primary hyperparathyroidism. *Electromyograph Clin Neurophysiol*. 1980;20:359–367.

12. Wersall-Robertson E, Hamberger B, Ehren H, et al. Increase in muscular strength following surgery for primary hyperparathyroidism. *Acta Med Scand*. 1986;220:233–235.
13. Delbridge L, Marshman D, Reeve T, et al. Neuromuscular symptoms in elderly patients with hyperparathyroidism: improvement with parathyroid surgery. *Med J Austral*. 1988;149:74–76.
14. Bassan B, Bertorini TE. Neuromuscular manifestations of acquired metabolic, endocrine, and nutritional disorders Chapter 21. In: Bertorini TE, ed. *Neuromuscular Disorders: Treatment and Management*. Amsterdam, Netherlands: Elsevier; 2022:528–558. 2nd ed.

98A CASE

A Woman With Muscle Weakness and a Skin Rash

A 30-year-old White woman presented with a 7-month history of muscle weakness, pain and stiffness, mild nocturnal fever, and leg swelling. She developed an erythematous rash on the face and knuckles 2 months prior to our evaluation and had difficulty swallowing, climbing stairs, and rising from the toilet.

Past medical history included a Bell palsy and partial hysterectomy 4 years previously for uterine cancer.

Physical examination was unremarkable, except for erythema in the hands, face, elbows, and knuckles, and capillary proliferation in the periungual areas of the fingers (Fig. 98A-1). There were no subcutaneous calcifications. Muscle strength was 4−/5 in neck flexors, 4/5 in deltoids, biceps, triceps, hip flexors, extensors, and abductors, and normal elsewhere. Her gait was normal but she had difficulty rising from a chair and sitting up from a supine position. Reflexes, sensory, and cerebellar examinations were normal. Her vital capacity was 2.04 L, 66% of predicted for her age and size. The examination was otherwise normal.

WHAT IS THE DIFFERENTIAL DIAGNOSIS?

The patient had proximal muscle weakness of recent onset with an otherwise normal neurologic examination. This is consistent with an acquired myopathy. The characteristic skin rash is typical for dermatomyositis. The history of cancer raised the possibility of a paraneoplastic dermatomyositis, but in those patients, the association is usually with other cancers such as lung, ovary, and breast.[1,2] The history of recurrent Bell palsy suggests sarcoidosis, but her rash was not typical of this disease. Another possibility was dermatomyositis associated with a connective tissue disorder such as lupus.

WHAT SHOULD BE DONE NEXT?

Laboratory studies revealed normal complete blood count and metabolic profile; erythrocyte sedimentation rate was 39 mm/h (normal, <30 mm/h), serum creatine kinase level was 461 IU/L (normal, 41–186 IU/L), and aspartate transaminase, 57 IU/L (normal, <29 IU/L).

AN EMG TEST WAS PERFORMED

Motor Nerve Responses

Nerve and Site	Latency (ms)	Amplitude (mV)	Conduction Velocity (m/s)
Peroneal Nerve R.	**Normal ≤ 5.7**	**Normal ≥ 3**	**Normal ≥ 40**
Ankle	3.5	11	–
Fibular head	11.7	11	41
Knee	13.4	9	44

Nerve and Site	Latency (ms)	Amplitude (mV)	Conduction Velocity (m/s)
Ulnar Nerve R.	**Normal ≤ 3.6**	**Normal ≥ 8**	**Normal ≥ 50**
Wrist	3.0	12	–
Below elbow	7.1	12	57
Above elbow	9.2	12	57

F-Wave Studies

Nerve	Latency (ms)	Normal Latency ≤ (ms)
Peroneal nerve R.	51.4	54
Ulnar nerve R.	27.2	30

Sensory Nerve Studies

Nerve	Onset Latency (ms)	Normal Onset Latency ≤ (ms)	Peak Latency (ms)	Normal Peak Latency ≤ (ms)	Amp (μV)	Normal Amp ≥ (μV)	Conduction Velocity (m/s)	Normal Conduction Velocity ≥ (m/s)
Sural nerve R.	3.2	3.5	3.7	4.0	16	11	44	40
Ulnar nerve R.	2.4	2.6	2.9	3.1	18	13	50	50

EMG Data

Muscle	Insrt Activity	Fibs	Pos Waves	Fasc	Amp	Dur	Poly	Pattern
Deltoid R.[a]	Norm	None	None	None	**Dec**	**Brief**	**Many**	Full[a]
Biceps brachii R.	Norm	None	None	None	**Dec**	**Brief**	**Many**	Full[a]
Triceps R.	Norm	None	None	None	**Dec**	**Brief**	**Few**	Full

EMG Data—cont'd

Muscle	Insrt Activity	Fibs	Pos Waves	Fasc	Amp	Dur	Poly	Pattern
First dorsal interosseous R.	Norm	None	None	None	Norm	Norm	None	Full
Vastus lateralis R.	Norm	None	None	None	Norm	Norm	None	Full
Tensor fasciae latae R.	Norm	None	None	None	**Dec**	**Brief**	**Few**	Full[a]
Iliopsoas R.	Norm	None	None	None	**Dec**	**Brief**	**Few**	Full[a]
Tibialis anterior R.	Norm	None	None	None	Norm	Norm	None	Full

[a]Rapid recruitment of motor unit action potentials.

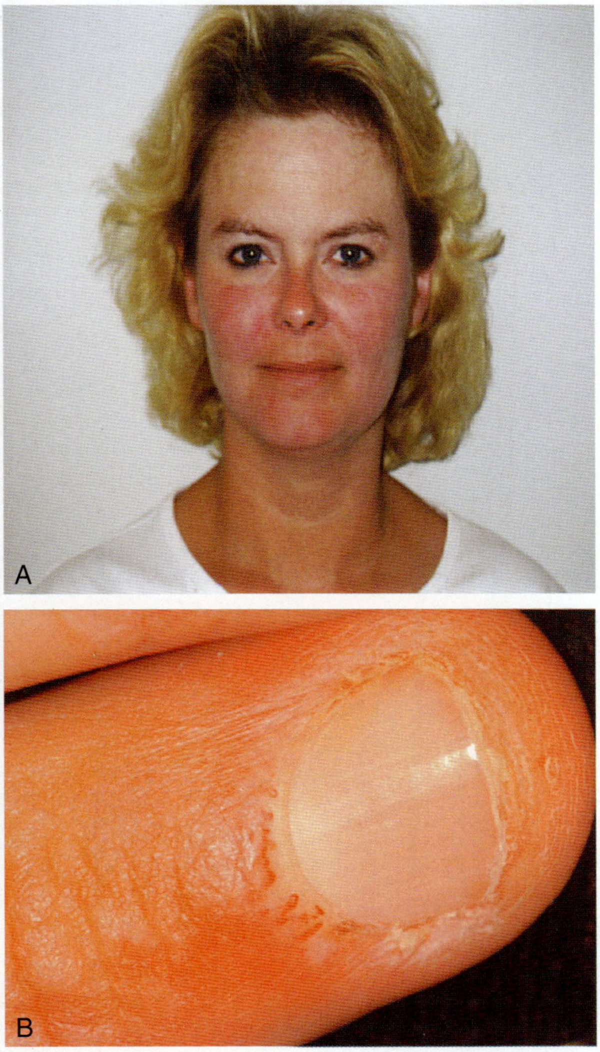

FIG. 98A-1 **A**, Erythematous rash on the face of the patient in Case 98A. **B**, Capillary dilatation and proliferation in the base of fingernails and thickening of the fingertips.

WHAT WERE THE EMG FINDINGS?

Nerve conduction tests were normal, but the needle test showed small polyphasic motor unit action potentials with fast recruitment for the level of effort, characteristic of a myopathy. Increased insertional activity and fibrillation potentials, often seen in inflammatory myopathies,[3] were not present.

WHAT SHOULD BE DONE NEXT?

Although she appeared to have dermatomyositis, it is always important to have a tissue diagnosis. A deltoid muscle biopsy was done. This showed mild evidence of necrosis with phagocytosis, some in the perifascicular area, but there was no prominent perifascicular atrophy. There were, however, inflammatory cell infiltrates in the interstitial and perivascular areas (Fig. 98B-2A–C).

A skin biopsy showed foci of lymphocytic infiltrates (Fig. 98B-2D).

She was initially treated with prednisone 60 mg/day with marked improvement, but she developed mild Cushingoid features and increasing weakness while tapering prednisone. Methotrexate 7.5 mg/week was started with marked improvement.

For further discussion, important points, and references, see Case 98B.

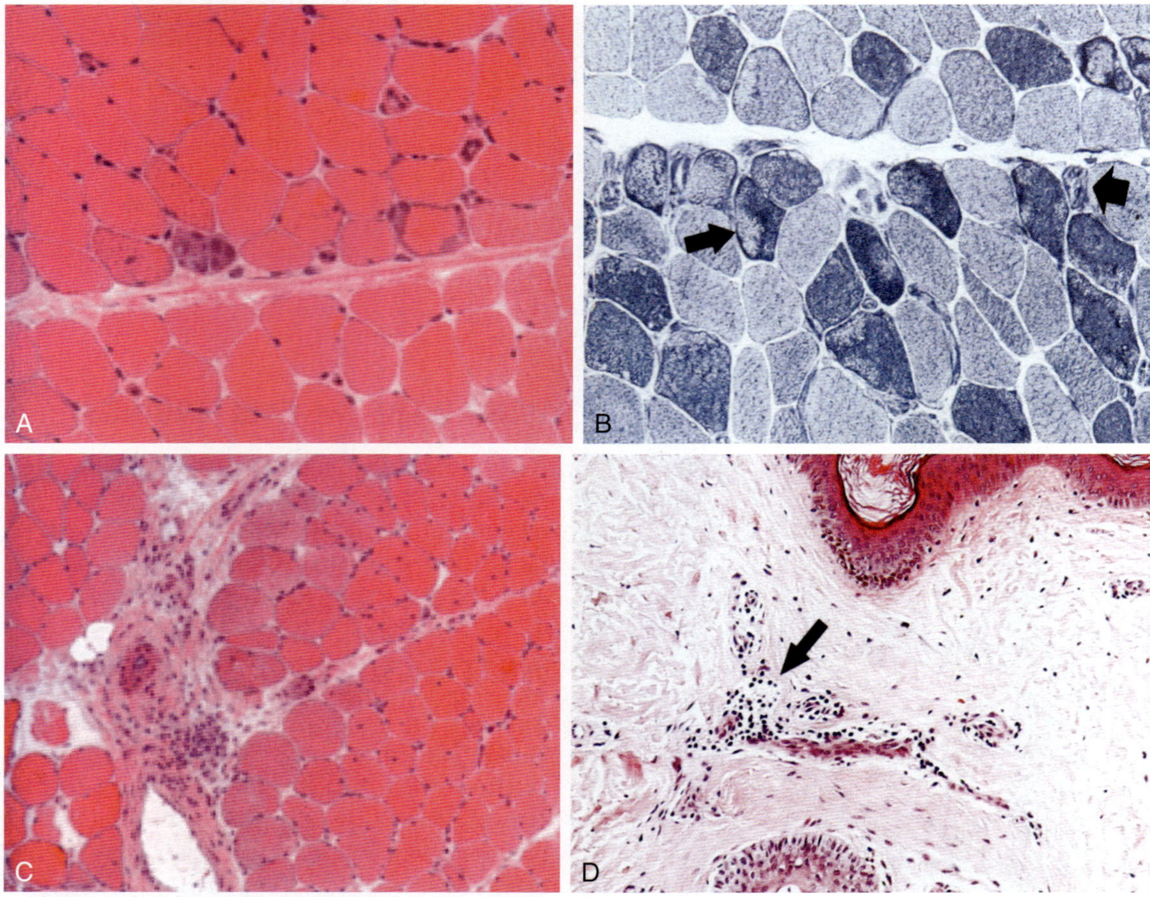

FIG. 98A-2 **A**, Necrotic fibers, some in the perifascicular area (H&E stain, ×200). **B**, Notice pale centers (NADH-TR stain, ×200). **C**, Perivascular inflammatory infiltrates and internalized nuclei close to the perivascular area (H&E stain, ×100). **D**, Skin biopsy; notice lymphocytic infiltrates in the dermis (*arrow*).

A Child With Muscle Weakness and a Skin Rash

A 5-year-old boy (son of the patient in Case 98A) presented with muscle stiffness, finger swelling, diffuse erythema, pain in the wrist joints, and difficulty climbing stairs which started 3 months after his mother. On further questioning, his mother was diagnosed recognized that the erythema had been present for the past year.

Past medical history was negative.

His examination was unremarkable, except for a positive Gowers sign, although examination was limited due to poor cooperation, and manual muscle testing was difficult to do; gait was normal. He had erythema on the face, fingers, and knees[1] (Fig. 98B-1).

Laboratory studies revealed a creatine kinase of 35 IU/L (normal, 4–88 IU/L); erythrocyte sedimentation rate was 32 mm/h (normal, <20 mm/h); antinuclear antibodies were elevated with a 1/1280 titer. C3 was 92 mg/dL (normal, 89–173 mg/dL), and C4 was 21 mg/dL (normal, 17–42 mg/dL). Test for extractable nuclear antigens was normal. Human leukocyte antigen typing for DQA1, 01, and 02 was negative.

AN EMG TEST WAS PERFORMED

Motor Nerve Studies

Nerve and Site	Latency (ms)	Amplitude (mV)	Conduction Velocity (m/s)
Median Nerve R.	**Normal ≤ 4.2**	**Normal ≥ 6**	**Normal ≥ 50**
Wrist	3.4	18	–
Elbow	8.0	18	55
Peroneal Nerve R.	**Normal ≤ 5.7**	**Normal ≥ 3**	**Normal ≥ 40**
Ankle	3.1	8	–
Fibular head	11.5	8	42
Knee	13.0	8	43

F-Wave Studies

Nerve	Latency (ms)	Normal Latency ≤ (ms)
Median nerve R.	26.8	30
Peroneal nerve R.	46.2	54

Sensory Nerve Studies

Nerve	Onset Latency (ms)	Normal Onset Latency ≤ (ms)	Peak Latency (ms)	Normal Peak Latency ≤ (ms)	Amp (μV)	Normal Amp ≥ (μV)	Conduction Velocity (m/s)	Normal Conduction Velocity ≥ (m/s)
Median nerve R.	2.1	2.6	2.6	3.1	40	20	62	50
Sural nerve R.	3.3	3.5	3.8	4.0	25	11	42	40

EMG Data

Muscle	Insrt Activity	Fibs	Pos Waves	Fasc	Amp	Dur	Poly	Pattern
Deltoid R.	None	None	None	None	**Dec**	**Brief**	**Many**	Full
Biceps brachii R.	None	None	None	None	**Dec**	**Brief**	**Many**	Full
Triceps R.	None	None	None	None	**Dec**	**Brief**	**Few**	Full
First dorsal interosseous R.	None	None	None	None	Norm	Norm	**None**	Full
Iliopsoas R.	None	None	None	None	**Dec**	**Brief**	**Few**	Full
Vastus lateralis R.	None	None	None	None	**Dec**	**Brief**	**Few**	Full

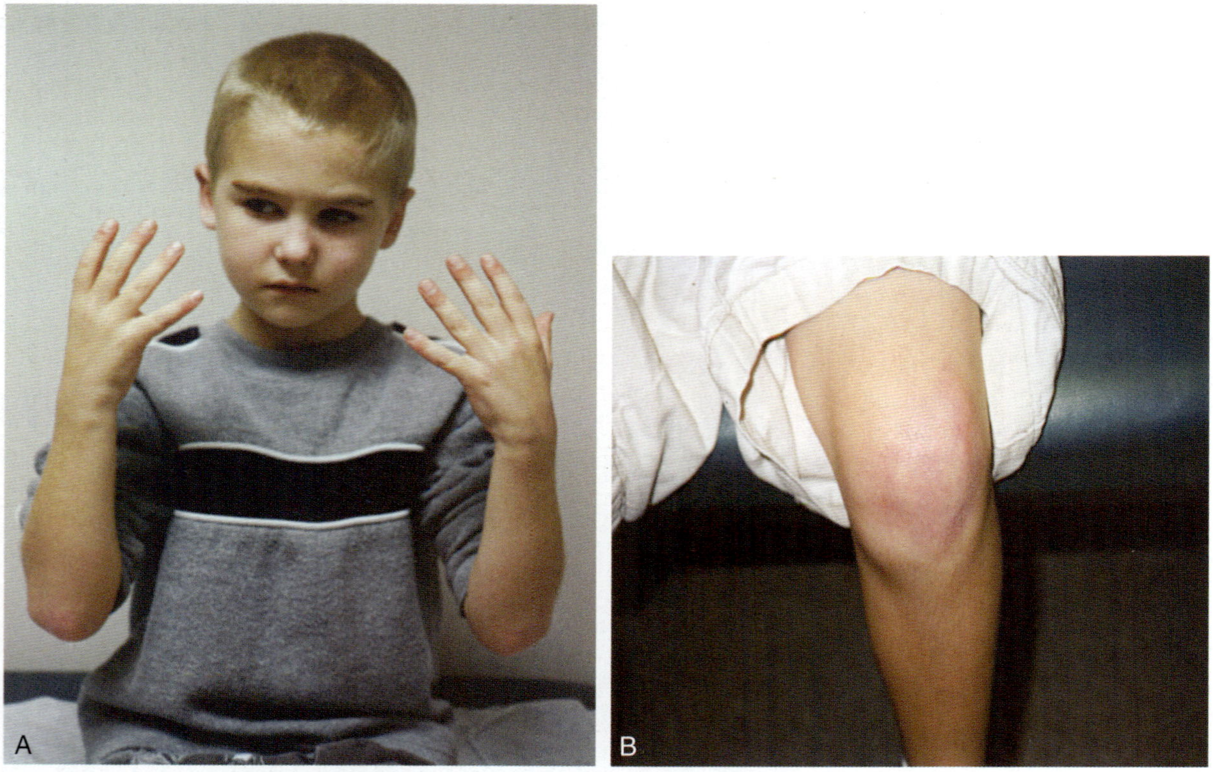

FIG. 98B-1 **A**, Patient in Case 98B showing erythema in the knuckles. **B**, The same patient showing erythema in the knees.

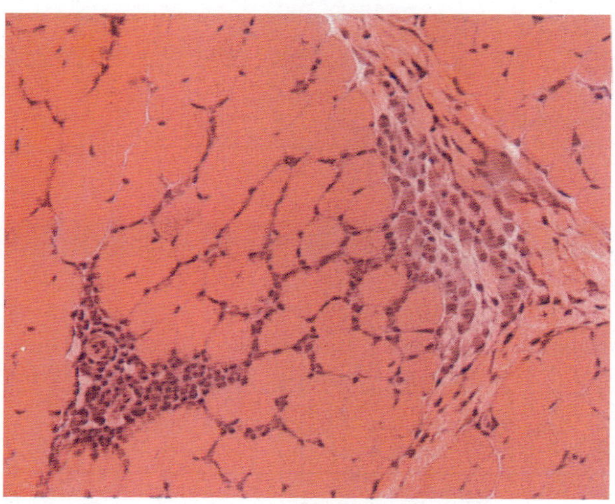

FIG. 98B-2 Muscle biopsy of patient in Case 98B showing inflammatory infiltrates in the interstitial and perivascular area (H&E stain, ×200).

WHAT WERE THE EMG FINDINGS?

Nerve conduction studies were normal, and the needle test showed many small polyphasic motor unit action potentials in proximal muscles.

A muscle biopsy showed inflammatory infiltrates (Fig. 98B-2) with necrosis and atrophy in the perifascicular area which was characteristic of dermatomyositis,[4] and although he had positive lupus serology, he had no systemic manifestations of lupus erythematosus.

He showed significant improvement with prednisone 30 mg/day, which was later tapered.

WHAT IS THE MOST LIKELY DIFFERENTIAL DIAGNOSIS?

Weakness presenting in a mother and child suggests either an autosomal-dominant or X-linked recessive disease, such as in muscular dystrophy. However, the rash in these two cases was very characteristic of dermatomyositis, an acquired autoimmune disorder, and thus indicates an unusual familial dermatomyositis.

Both patients improved with corticosteroids. However, the mother became Cushingoid, and she was changed to methotrexate with marked improvement.

DISCUSSION (CASES 98A AND 98B)

These patients' symptoms and clinical presentations were characteristic of dermatomyositis, and they responded well to immunosuppressant therapy.

Autoimmune diseases, such as dermatomyositis, are usually sporadic, but some occur in families, including among siblings. A genetic predisposition appears to play an important role in inflammatory myopathies and other autoimmune disorders.[5–11] Dermatomyositis and lupus have been reported in twins.[12,13] There is also an increased incidence of dermatomyositis and other autoimmune diseases in first-degree relatives.[14–16] Some human leukocyte antigen types are associated with inflammatory myopathy, particularly DRB1 "0301 and DQA1" 0501.[17–19] JO-1 antibodies are strongly associated with Dr3 M5–2 types; dermatomyositis is associated with Dr7/Dr53/DQA1*0201.[19,20] These human leukocyte antigen types were not present in the child or his mother.

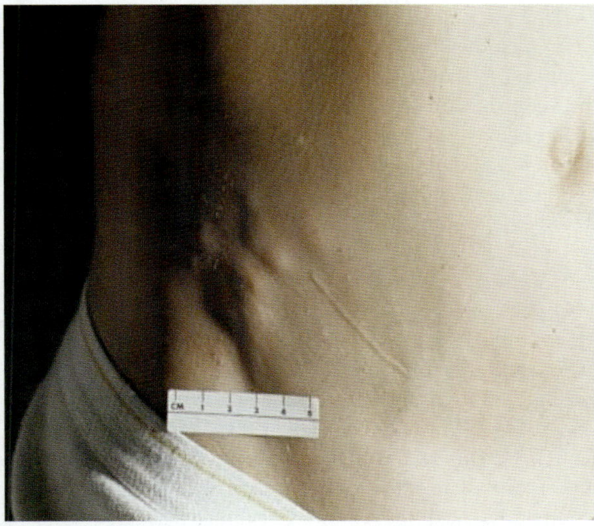

FIG. 98B-3 Subcutaneous calcifications seen in another patient with dermatomyositis.

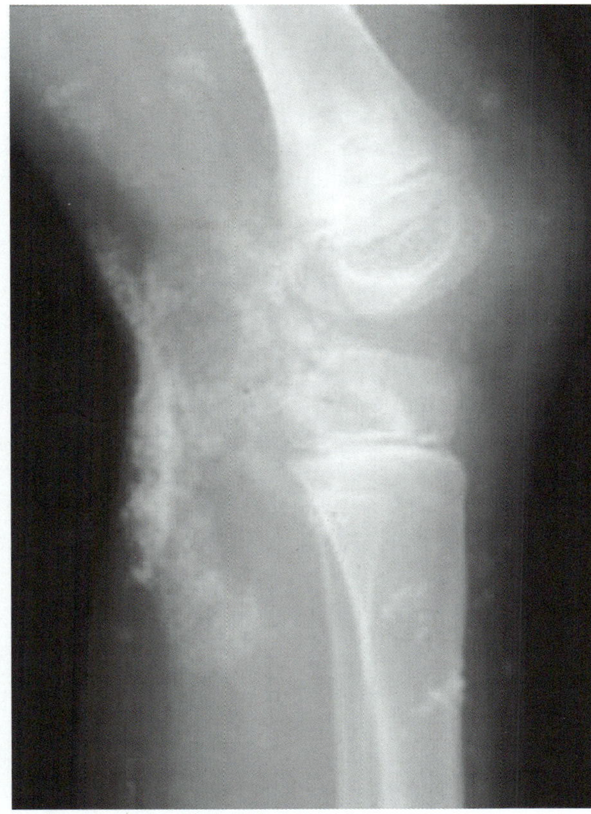

FIG. 98B-4 Calcifications seen on the x-ray of a patient with dermatomyositis.

Dermatomyositis is an autoimmune myopathy similar to polymyositis but is characterized not only by muscle weakness but also by a skin rash,[21] which consists of the classic heliotrope or erythema on the eyelids, rash over the knuckles (Gottron's sign), and some patients have a rash without weakness or an amyopathic dermatomyositis,[25] and there are cases without clear changes in muscle biopsy characteristic of the disease. Other skin changes are erythema of the shoulders (shawl sign), scaling of the dorsal surface of joints, proliferation of capillaries in the periungual area of the fingers, and the characteristic carpenter's fingers with thickening of skin in the digits. Patients with dermatomyositis may develop subcutaneous calcifications[1] (Figs. 98B-3 and 98B-4).

Laboratory studies reveal an elevated erythrocyte sedimentation rate; creatine kinase and other muscle enzymes, however, could be normal in some patients, particularly children.

EMG shows myopathic features, frequently accompanied by increased insertional activity and fibrillation potentials, while the muscle biopsy demonstrates the characteristic inflammation, necrosis, and perifascicular fiber atrophy.

MRI of muscles could also show increased signal in T2-weighted images; contrast MRI could help.

Dermatomyositis can be associated with other connective tissue disorders, and in persons over 50 years of age there could be an association with carcinoma. Dermatomyositis can also be caused by drugs such as penicillamine[22] and by retroviral infections.[20]

Systemic involvement in inflammatory myopathies includes interstitial lung fibrosis, particularly in those with elevated JO-1 antisynthetase antibodies.[23] Arthralgias, gastrointestinal angiopathy, and myocarditis can occur. There are several other myositis-specific antibodies that can occur in some cases,[24,25] while patients could also have antibodies associated with connective tissue disorders.

As discussed earlier, infections, environmental factors, and genetic predisposition likely play a role in the pathogenesis. For example, patients with dermatomyositis and other connective tissue disorders, such as scleroderma or Raynaud's phenomenon, have PM-CL antinuclear antibodies and the human leukocyte antigen DQA1*0501 and DRB1*0301 allelic markers.[20]

In dermatomyositis there is evidence of a humoral-mediated immune response against the vascular endothelium with deposits of C5b-9 membrane attack complexes of complement and IgG in the capillaries, which causes capillary depletion and ischemic muscle fiber injury.[26,27] In polymyositis and inclusion body myositis there is evidence of a close interaction between CD8 cells and nonnecrotic muscle fibers[28]; this appears to destroy them and, thus, in those there appears to be primarily a cell-mediated immune response.

In these inflammatory myopathies, T cells express cytokines, which contribute to the local inflammatory response and myofiber degeneration, and thus perpetuation of the autoimmune process.[29] This process includes T-cell activation, recruitment of mononuclear cells, and increased expression of major histocompatibility complex molecules on damaged fibers, which could be demonstrated by immunohistochemistry. Also, chemotactic and inflammatory chemokines are found in muscles of patients with these disorders. Cytokine expression causes the upregulation of cell-surface antigens that promote T-cell migration into muscle, followed by adherence and activation.[20] In addition, there is expression of adhesion molecules, such as intercellular adhesion molecule-1 on endothelial cells and muscle fibers[30–32]; this promotes T-cell homing. Cytokines that inhibit inflammation can also be expressed.

Dermatomyositis is treated with corticosteroids in doses of 1–2 mg/kg daily, switching to alternating days after 1 or 2 months if the patient improves.[1] Pulse intravenous steroids appear to yield a higher remission rate.[33] Azathioprine, methotrexate, and other immunosuppressants[34] are also helpful in refractory cases and are used in patients who experience significant side effects from corticosteroids. Immunoglobulin infusions are also beneficial, particularly in dermatomyositis.[35] Rituximab is used in refractory cases.[25]

For a more detailed discussion on immunotherapy, see Chapter 3.

SUMMARY

A mother and her son presented with classic dermatomyositis. These cases emphasize the fact that autoimmune disorders might have a genetic predisposition, while environmental factors and infections may also play a role. The close-time association of their presentations suggests an unidentified environmental factor that was not obvious.

IMPORTANT POINTS

- Dermatomyositis can occur in families, indicating a genetic predisposition, as in other autoimmune disorders.
- Characteristics of dermatomyositis include proximal muscle weakness, heliotrope and erythematous rash, scaling, Gottron's sign, shawl erythema, carpenter's fingers, capillary proliferation of the periungual areas of the fingers, and subcutaneous calcifications.
- Systemic manifestations of dermatomyositis include, among others, vasculitis of the gastrointestinal tract, myocarditis, pulmonary fibrosis, subcutaneous calcifications, and arthralgias.
- EMG in inflammatory myopathies frequently shows increased insertional activity, denervation potentials, and small polyphasic units with normal or increased recruitment.
- Muscle biopsy in dermatomyositis shows inflammation, necrosis, and perifascicular muscle fiber atrophy.
- Dermatomyositis can be associated with malignancies, other autoimmune disorders, retroviral infections, and drugs such as penicillamine.
- The treatment of dermatomyositis consists of corticosteroids or immunosuppressants; IgG infusions can also be beneficial.

This case was studied with Dr. Masanori Igarashi.

REFERENCES

1. Bertorini TE. Inflammatory myopathies (polymyositis, dermatomyositis, inclusion body myositis). *Compr Ther.* 1998;24(10):494–502.
2. Buchbinder R, Hill CL. Malignancy in patients with inflammatory myopathy. *Curr Rheumatol Rep.* 2002;4(5):415–426.
3. Bertorini TE. EMG in polymyositis and dermatomyositis. In: Dalakas MC, ed. *Polymyositis and Dermatomyositis.* Woburn, MA: Butterworth; 1988:217–234.
4. Bertorini TE. Histopathology of the inflammatory myopathies. In: Dalakas MC, ed. *Polymyositis and Dermatomyositis.* Woburn, MA: Butterworth; 1988:157–194.
5. Garlepp MJ. Genetics of idiopathic inflammatory myopathies. *Curr Opin Rheumatol.* 1996;8:514–520.
6. Shamim EA, Rider LG, Miller FW. Update on the genetics of the idiopathic inflammatory myopathies. *Curr Opin Rheumatol.* 2000;12:482–491.
7. Arnett FC, Shulman LE. Studies in familial systemic lupus erythematosus. *Medicine (Baltimore).* 1976;55:313–322.
8. Reveille JD, Wilson RW, Provost TT, et al. Primary Sjögren's syndrome and other autoimmune diseases in families: prevalence and immunogenetic studies in six kindreds. *Ann Intern Med.* 1984;101:748–756.
9. Maddison PJ, Stephens C, Briggs D, et al. Connective tissue disease and autoantibodies in the kindreds of 63 patients with systemic sclerosis. The United Kingdom Systemic Sclerosis Study Group. *Medicine (Baltimore).* 1993;72:103–112.
10. Lambie JA, Duff IF. Familial occurrence of dermatomyositis: case reports and a family survey. *Ann Intern Med.* 1963;59:839–847.
11. Andrews A, Hickling P, Hutton C. Familial dermatomyositis. *Br J Rheumatol.* 1998;37:231–232.
12. Harati Y, Niakan E, Bergman EW. Childhood dermatomyositis in monozygotic twins. *Neurology.* 1986;36:721–723.
13. Ginn LR, Lin JP, Plotz PH, et al. Familial autoimmunity in pedigrees of idiopathic inflammatory myopathy patients suggests common genetic risk factors for many autoimmune diseases. *Arthritis Rheum.* 1998;41:400–405.
14. Lewkonia RM, Buxton PH. Myositis in father and daughter. *J Neurol Neurosurg Psychiatry.* 1973;36:820–825.
15. Mbauya A, Plotz PH, Wilder RL, Miller FW. Increased prevalence of autoimmune disease in first-degree relatives of patients with idiopathic inflammatory myopathy [abstract]. *Arthritis Rheum.* 1993;36(Suppl 9):S255.
16. Plamondon S, Dent PB, Reed AM. Familial dermatomyositis. *J Rheumatol.* 1999;26:2691–2692.
17. Reed AM, Stirling JD. Association of the HLA-DQA1*0501 allele in multiple racial groups with juvenile dermatomyositis. *Hum Immunol.* 1995;44:131–135.
18. Garlepp MJ, Mastaglia FL. Autoantibodies in inflammatory myopathies. *Am J Med Sci.* 2000;319:227–233.
19. Hollingsworth PN, Garlepp MJ, Dawkins RL. Autoimmune diseases of muscle. In: Rose NR, Mackay I, eds. *The Autoimmune Diseases.* 3rd ed. San Diego, CA: Academic Press; 1998:663–686.
20. Mastaglia FL, Garlepp MJ, Phillips BA, Zilko PJ. Inflammatory myopathies: clinical, diagnostic and therapeutic aspects. *Muscle Nerve.* 2003;27(4):407–425.
21. Okogbaa J, Batiste L. Dermatomyositis: an acute flare and current treatments. June 18, 2019. Clin Med Insights Case Report. https://doi.org/10.1177/1179547619855370.
22. Carroll GJ, Will RK, Peter JB, et al. Penicillamine induced polymyositis and dermatomyositis. *J Rheumatol.* 1987;14:995–1001.
23. Fathi M, Dastmalchi M, Rasmussen E, et al. Interstitial lung disease, a common manifestation of newly diagnosed polymyositis and dermatomyositis. *Ann Rheum Dis.* 2004;63(3):297–301.
24. Dalakas MC. Inflammatory myopathies: update on diagnosis, pathogenesis and therapies, and COVID-19-related implications. *Acta Myol.* 2020;39(4):289–301.
25. Dalakas MC. Treatment and management of autoimmune myopathies Chapter 22. In: Bertorini TE, ed. *Neuromuscular Disorders: Treatment and Management.* Amsterdam, Netherlands: Elsevier; 2022:554–571. 2nd ed.
26. Emslie-Smith AM, Engel AG. Microvascular changes in early and advanced dermatomyositis: a quantitative study. *Ann Neurol.* 1990;27:343–356.

27. Mendell JR, Garcha TS, Kissel JT. The immunopathogenic role of complement in human muscle disease. *Curr Opin Neurol.* 1996;9:226–234.
28. Arahata K, Engel AG. Monoclonal antibody analysis of mononuclear cells in myopathies, III: immunoelectron microscopy aspects of cell-mediated muscle fiber injury. *Ann Neurol.* 1986;19:112–125.
29. Lepidi H, Frances V, Figarella-Branger D, et al. Local expression of cytokines in idiopathic inflammatory myopathies. *Neuropathol Appl Neurobiol.* 1998;24:73–79.
30. De Blecker JL, Engel AG. Expression of cell adhesion molecules in inflammatory myopathies and Duchenne dystrophy. *J Neuropathol Exp Neurol.* 1994;53:369–376.
31. Sallum AM, Marie SK, Wakamatsu A, et al. Immunohistochemical analysis of adhesion molecule expression on muscle biopsy specimens from patients with juvenile dermatomyositis. *J Rheumatol.* 2004;31(4):801–807.
32. Hohlfeld R, Engel AG, Goebels N, Behrens L. Cellular immune mechanisms in inflammatory myopathies. *Curr Opin Rheumatol.* 1997;9:520–526.
33. Matsubara S, Sawa Y, Takamori M, et al. Pulsed intravenous methylprednisolone combined with oral steroids as the initial treatment of inflammatory myopathies. *J Neurol Neurosurg Psychiatry*. 1994;57:1008.
34. Bromberg M. Advances in diagnosis and management of inflammatory myopathies. *J Clin Neuromuscul Dis.* 2005;6:167–179.
35. Dalakas MC. High-dose intravenous immunoglobulin in inflammatory myopathies: experience based on controlled clinical trials. *Neurol Sci.* 2003;24(Suppl 4):S256–S259.

99 CASE

A Man With Muscle Pains

A 55-year-old man was referred for evaluation of muscle pains at rest, mainly in the thighs and calves and occasionally in the arms, and an elevated serum creatine kinase (CK). The muscle pains were present for 8 months, while the patient was on atorvastatin calcium for hyperlipidemia but persisted when the medication was discontinued. He denied weakness.

Past medical history was unremarkable. He did not smoke or drink. Family history was negative for neurologic disorders.

Examination revealed normal mentation and cranial nerves. There was normal muscle bulk and muscle strength. Reflexes were normal, and there were no pathologic reflexes. No myotonia, myoedema, or fasciculations were detected. Sensation, coordination, and gait were normal. There were no skin lesions, and the examination was otherwise unremarkable.

WHAT IS THE DIFFERENTIAL DIAGNOSIS?

Hypothyroidism is an important consideration in patients with hyperlipidemia and muscle pains. It is unlikely that atorvastatin was the cause of his symptoms as they persisted after discontinuation of the drug.

Metabolic myopathies usually cause pain during or after exercise.

An inflammatory myopathy is also a possibility as such patients have muscle pains and elevated serum CK, but they usually also have muscle weakness. Fasciitis and polymyalgia rheumatica could cause muscle pains, but in these the CK levels are usually normal.

AN EMG TEST WAS PERFORMED

Motor Nerve Studies

Nerve and Site	Latency (ms)	Amplitude (mV)	Conduction Velocity (m/s)
Peroneal Nerve R.	**Normal ≤ 5.7**	**Normal ≥ 3**	**Normal ≥ 40**
Ankle	5.3	9	–
Fibular head	12.2	8	45
Knee	14.2	8	48
Ulnar Nerve R.	**Normal ≤ 3.6**	**Normal ≥ 8**	**Normal ≥ 50**
Wrist	3.1	8	–
Below elbow	7.1	8	54
Above elbow	9.4	8	55

F-Wave and Tibial H-Reflex Studies

Nerve	Latency (ms)	Normal Latency ≤ (ms)
Peroneal nerve R.	51.1	54
Ulnar nerve R.	29.7	30
H-reflex R.	30.2	34
H-reflex L.	31.6	34

Sensory Nerve Studies

Nerve	Onset Latency (ms)	Normal Onset Latency ≤ (ms)	Peak Latency (ms)	Normal Peak Latency ≤ (ms)	Amp (μV)	Normal Amp ≥ (μV)	Conduction Velocity (m/s)	Normal Conduction Velocity ≥ (m/s)
Sural nerve R.	3.4	3.5	3.9	4.0	16	11	41	40
Superficial peroneal nerve R.	3.2	3.5	3.7	4.0	19	8–10	44	40
Ulnar nerve R.	2.2	2.6	2.7	3.1	17	13	55	50

EMG Data

Muscle	Insrt Activity	Fibs	Pos Waves	Fasc	Amp	Dur	Poly	Pattern
Deltoid R.	Norm	None	None	None	Norm	Norm	None	Full
Biceps brachii R.	Norm	None	None	None	Norm	**Brief**	**Few**	Full[a]
Extensor digitorum com. R.	Norm	None	None	None	Norm	**Brief**	**Few**	Full[a]
First dorsal interosseous R.	Norm	None	None	None	Norm	Norm	None	Full
Vastus lateralis R.	Norm	None	None	None	Norm	**Brief**	**Few**	Full[a]
Tibialis anterior R.	Norm	None	None	None	Norm	**Brief**	**Few**	Full
Gastrocnemius R.	Norm	None	None	None	Norm	Norm	None	Full

[a]Rapid recruitment of motor unit action potentials.

WHAT WERE THE EMG FINDINGS?

This study showed normal nerve conduction velocities and CMAP and SNAP amplitudes and latencies. There were scattered small polyphasic motor unit action potentials and no evidence of denervation or fasciculations. The findings were suggestive of a mild myopathy.

WHAT SHOULD BE DONE NEXT?

Serum CK was 8682 IU/L (normal, <200 IU/L); FANA, protein electrophoresis, erythrocyte sedimentation rate, thyroid-stimulating hormone, and HIV titers were normal.

A quadriceps muscle biopsy showed rare, scattered necrotic fibers undergoing phagocytosis. There was mild interstitial inflammation (Fig. 99-1). Histochemical stains showed the absence of myoadenylate deaminase (MAD) (Fig. 99-2).

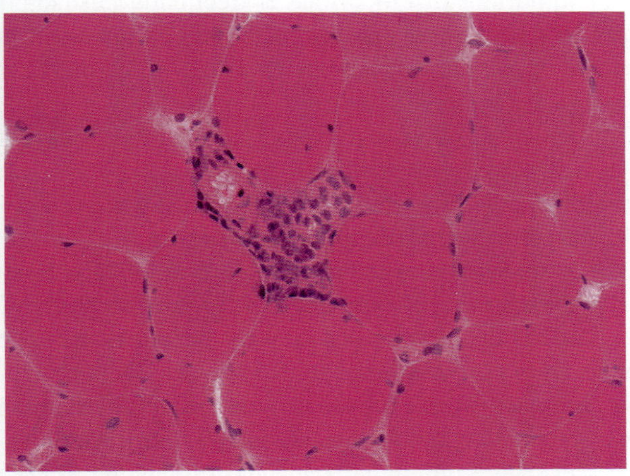

FIG. 99-1 Muscle biopsy showing necrotic fibers and mild inflammation (H&E stain, ×400).

WHAT IS THE MOST LIKELY DIAGNOSIS?

This patient with muscle pains and elevated CK was diagnosed with a necrotizing myopathy with inflammation and deaminase deficiency. Immunotherapy was considered, but he opted against this.

Eighteen months later, he presented with increasing muscle pain and fatigue.

Examination revealed the weakness of 4/5 in neck flexors and shoulder muscles and 4−/5 in the iliopsoas and glutei. Other muscles were normal. Forced vital capacity was 3.22 L, 70% of predicted for his age and size. Serum CK was again elevated at 4750 IU/L.

A Second EMG Test Was Performed

Motor Nerve Studies

Nerve and Site	Latency (ms)	Amplitude (mV)	Conduction Velocity (m/s)
Peroneal Nerve R.	**Normal ≤ 5.7**	**Normal ≥ 3**	**Normal ≥ 40**
Ankle	4.3	8	–
Fibular head	11.3	8	46
Knee	13.3	7	48
Ulnar Nerve R.	**Normal ≤ 3.6**	**Normal ≥ 8**	**Normal ≥ 50**
Wrist	2.9	9	–
Below elbow	6.6	9	62
Above elbow	8.6	9	60

F-Wave Studies

Nerve	Latency (ms)	Normal Latency ≤ (ms)
Peroneal nerve R.	51.4	54
Ulnar nerve R.	26.8	30

Sensory Nerve Studies

Nerve	Onset Latency (ms)	Normal Onset Latency ≤ (ms)	Peak Latency (ms)	Normal Peak Latency ≤ (ms)	Amp (μV)	Normal Amp ≥ (μV)	Conduction Velocity (m/s)	Normal Conduction Velocity ≥ (m/s)
Sural nerve R.	2.8	3.5	3.3	4.0	18	11	50	40
Ulnar nerve R.	2.1	2.6	2.6	3.1	20	13	57	50

EMG Data

Muscle	Insrt Activity	Fibs	Pos Waves	Fasc	Amp	Dur	Poly	Pattern
Deltoid R.	Norm	None	None	None	**Dec**	**Brief**	**Many**	Full[a]
Biceps brachii R.	Norm	None	None	None	**Dec**	**Brief**	**Many**	Full[a]
First dorsal interosseous R.	Norm	None	None	None	Norm	Norm	None	Full
Tensor fasciae latae R.	Norm	None	None	None	**Dec**	**Brief**	**Many**	Full
Vastus lateralis R.	Norm	None	None	None	Norm	Norm	None	Full
Tibialis anterior R.	Norm	None	None	None	Norm	Norm	None	Full

[a]Rapid recruitment of motor unit action potentials.

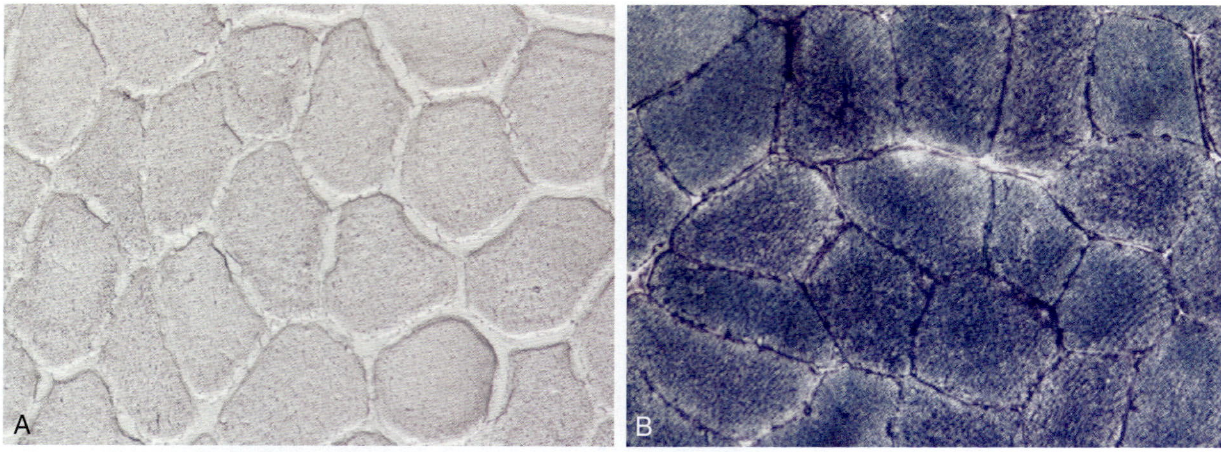

FIG. 99-2 Muscle biopsy showing absence of deaminase staining (**A**) compared with normal control (**B**) (myoadenylate deaminase stain, ×400).

WHAT WERE THE FINDINGS OF THE SECOND TEST?

This study showed normal nerve conduction tests but abnormal needle EMG with frequent small polyphasic motor unit action potentials; no spontaneous potentials were seen, again compatible with a myopathy.

He was treated with prednisone 1 mg/kg. He did not improve after 3 months and became Cushingoid. Methotrexate 7.5 mg/week was started and increased to 10 mg and later to 17.5 mg/week; with this, he showed only minimal improvement after 3 months, and his white cell count was borderline low.

WHAT SHOULD BE DONE NEXT?

The use of higher doses of methotrexate parenterally was considered, but he was then given gamma globulin infusions 2 g/kg with remarkable improvement. His serum CK went down to 800 IU/L. Prednisone was discontinued; he continued taking methotrexate 12.5 mg weekly and has been stable for 4 years. Myositis antibodies were not elevated.

DISCUSSION

This patient presented initially with myalgias and elevated serum CK. His muscle biopsy showed MAD with mild necrosis and inflammation. He did not receive treatment during the initial presentation but later developed progressive weakness. He did not respond initially to prednisone and methotrexate, but he did respond when methotrexate was increased, in addition to IV IG infusions.

He was diagnosed as having polymyositis (PM), an autoimmune myopathy caused by cell-mediated activation of cytotoxic lymphocytes with necrosis and inflammation. (See discussion of Cases 98A and 98B.) PM can be idiopathic: it is sometimes associated with other connective tissue disorders and with cancer, and it is also seen in HIV-infected patients.[1] The response to immunotherapy in this case was slow and required a combination of drugs, demonstrating that immunotherapy may take longer to work. The dosages, especially of methotrexate, should be increased if there is no response prior to assuming a wrong diagnosis, particularly if there are no significant side effects or significant leukopenia. This is very important in PM, which is frequently misdiagnosed in patients with other conditions,[2,3] such as inclusion body myositis, or even limb-girdle dystrophies, which might show inflammation on muscle biopsies.

This patient also had MAD deficiency, but it is unlikely that this played a role in his weakness. This disease could be associated with muscle pain, but the pain in this case was likely caused by PM, as it improved with immunotherapy.

MAD deficiency was initially reported in 1978 by Fishbein et al., who described patients with muscle dysfunction after exercise.[4] MAD is the enzyme that converts adenosine monophosphate to inosine monophosphate with a release of ammonia. It plays an important role in muscle function as it participates in energy production by the generation of intermediators of the citric acid cycle from amino acids and stimulation of glycolysis. Most patients with MAD deficiency are asymptomatic, and their deficiency is found only incidentally in muscle biopsies and could be diagnostic of other conditions.[5,6] Some have myalgias that worsen with exercise. In this disease the ischemic exercise test shows a lack of rise of serum ammonia, while there is a normal rise of lactate.[7] It seems unusual that most MAD-deficient cases do not have more significant muscular symptoms, as MAD is an important enzyme. Myoglobinuria, however, has been reported, rarely, in patients with homozygous mutations of the *AMPD1* gene.[8]

The diagnosis of MAD deficiency is based on muscle biopsy demonstrating the absence of the enzyme, and this can be confirmed by biochemistry.

The disease is considered to have two forms. The "primary" form is autosomal-recessive, and a single mutant allele, harboring a nonsense mutation that results in a truncated peptide, is responsible for all cases. The "secondary" form, as in this case, includes those patients in which the deficiency is associated with other conditions.[9]

Most individuals with inherited MAD have a single mutant allele of the *AMPD1* gene that is located in the short arm of chromosome 1. Common mutations include nucleotide substitutions or small deletions, duplications, or rearrangements.[10,11] There is no treatment for MAD.

It is unlikely that in this patient the PM and the MAD deficiency had a synergistic effect, as it occurs rarely in some patients who have two combined metabolic defects impairing energy production,[12] sometimes called "double-trouble." It appears that the cause of this patient's symptoms was PM, because of the improvement with therapy.

SUMMARY

This patient presented with muscle pain and later developed weakness. He was found to have MAD deficiency and a necrotizing inflammatory myopathy. He was diagnosed as having PM and responded to immunotherapy. MAD deficiency might have been an incidental finding on muscle biopsy.

IMPORTANT POINTS

- MAD deficiency can manifest with muscle pains but might be an incidental finding in patients with other conditions.
- In patients with MAD deficiency there is a lack of rise in ammonia, but a normal rise of lactic acid during ischemic exercise test.
- This disorder may, rarely, cause myoglobinuria.
- Patients with PM can also present with muscle pains and weakness, and they should be treated aggressively if there is no response to conventional immunotherapy.

REFERENCES

1. Bertorini TE. Inflammatory myopathies (polymyositis, dermatomyositis, inclusion body myositis). *Comp Ther*. 1998;24:494–502.
2. van der Meulen MF, Bronner IM, Hoogendijk JE, et al. Polymyositis: an overdiagnosed entity. *Neurology*. 2003;61(3):316–321.
3. Amato AA, Griggs RC. Unicorns, dragons, polymyositis and other mythological beasts. *Neurology*. 2003;61(3):288–289.
4. Fishbein WN, Armbrustmacher VW, Griffin JL. Myoadenylate deaminase deficiency: a new disease of muscle. *Science*. 1978;200:545–548.
5. Kar NC, Pearson CM. Muscle adenylate deaminase deficiency: report of six new cases. *Arch Neurol*. 1981;38:279–281.
6. Mercelis R, Martin JJ, de Barsy T, Van den Berghe G. Myoadenylate deaminase deficiency: absence of correlation with exercise intolerance in 452 muscle biopsies. *J Neurol*. 1987;234:385–389.
7. Bertorini TE. Clinical evaluation and clinical laboratory tests. In: Bertorini TE, ed. *Clinical Evaluation and Diagnostic Tests for Neuromuscular Disorders*. Boston, MA: Butterworth-Heinemann; 2002:15–98.
8. Baumeister FA, Gross M, Wagner DR, et al. Myoadenylate deaminase deficiency with severe rhabdomyolysis. *Eur J Ped*. 1993;152(6):513–515.
9. Yiomaz EY, Pourmand R. Evaluation of a patient presenting with muscle cramps and calf hypertrophy. *J Clin Neuromuscul Dis*. 2002;3:29–35.
10. Gross M. Clinical heterogeneity and molecular mechanisms in inborn muscle AMP deaminase deficiency. *J Inherit Metab Dis*. 1997;20:186–192.
11. Sabina RL. Myoadenylate deaminase deficiency: a common inherited defect with heterogeneous clinical presentation. *Neurol Clin*. 2000;18:185–194.
12. Rubio JC, Martin MA, Bautista J, et al. Association of genetically proven deficiencies of myophosphorylase and AMP deaminase: a second case of "double trouble". *Neuromuscul Disord*. 1997;7:387–389.

100A CASE

An Older Woman With Progressive Muscle Weakness

A 62-year-old woman presented with progressive muscle weakness for more than 6 years. She had been previously diagnosed with polymyositis; she was treated with corticosteroids without benefit and subsequently referred to us. The patient complained of difficulty going up and down stairs and in turning door knobs but denied any problems swallowing, muscle pains, or sensory complaints.

Past medical history was unremarkable; she did not smoke or drink alcohol.

General examination, mentation, and cranial nerves were normal; in particular, there was no evidence of facial weakness, tongue atrophy, or fasciculations.

There was moderate symmetrical atrophy of the biceps, triceps, and quadriceps muscles (Fig. 100A-1). Manual muscle testing demonstrated MRC scoring in neck flexors of 5−/5, extensors, 5/5; shoulder muscles, 4+/5; biceps, 3+/5; triceps, 3/5; wrist extensors, 4/5; wrist flexors, 3+/5; finger extensors, 3−/5; flexors, 3−/5; and intrinsic hand muscles, 3+/5. In the lower extremities the iliopsoas muscles were 4/5; quadriceps, 3−/5; adductors, glutei, and hamstrings, 4/5; foot dorsiflexors and evertors, 4/5; and flexors, 5/5. Reflexes were 1+ all over, except for trace at the knees. Vibration, pinprick, and touch sensations were normal. No fasciculations were detected. There was no percussion or grip myotonia. The examination was otherwise unremarkable.

Blood tests revealed normal complete blood count; the serum creatine kinase (CK) was 360 IU/L (normal, <200 IU/L); comprehensive metabolic panel, thyroid function tests, FANA, and erythrocyte sedimentation rate were all normal.

WHAT IS THE DIFFERENTIAL DIAGNOSIS?

This older woman presented with progressive weakness and mildly elevated serum CK. The differential diagnosis includes a motor neuron disorder, such as progressive spinal muscular atrophy, which could have a similar presentation, and mildly elevated CK, but the slow progression and lack of fasciculations are somewhat against that diagnosis. The long history of nonfluctuating weakness and atrophy, lack of cranial nerve abnormalities, and mildly elevated CK are also against a disorder of neuromuscular transmission, and she had no sensory deficits to suggest a polyneuropathy.

This patient appeared to have a progressive myopathy. The differential diagnosis of this is extensive and includes limb-girdle dystrophy, an endocrine or metabolic myopathy, and proximal myotonic myopathy (PROMM), even if there is no clinical myotonia. Inflammatory myopathies, such as polymyositis and inclusion body myositis (IBM), are also important considerations; the distribution of weakness, age, and the lack of response to steroids suggest the latter.

AN EMG TEST WAS PERFORMED

Motor Nerve Responses

Nerve and Site	Latency (ms)	Amplitude (mV)	Conduction Velocity (m/s)
Peroneal Nerve R.	**Normal ≤ 5.7**	**Normal ≥ 3**	**Normal ≥ 40**
Ankle	3.8	5	–
Fibular head	11.8	5	48
Median Nerve R.	**Normal ≤ 4.2**	**Normal ≥ 6**	**Normal ≥ 50**
Wrist	3.2	8	–
Elbow	8.6	8	57
Ulnar Nerve R.	**Normal ≤ 3.6**	**Normal ≥ 8**	**Normal ≥ 50**
Wrist	2.8	10	–
Below elbow	3.7	10	55
Median Nerve L.	**Normal ≤ 4.2**	**Normal ≥ 6**	**Normal ≥ 50**
Wrist	3.8	9	–
Elbow	8.0	9	57

F-Wave Studies

Nerve	Latency (ms)	Normal Latency ≤ (ms)
Peroneal nerve R.	51.6	54
Median nerve R.	28.2	30
Ulnar nerve R.	27.6	30
Median nerve L.	28.8	30

Sensory Nerve Studies

Nerve	Onset Latency (ms)	Normal Onset Latency ≤ (ms)	Peak Latency (ms)	Normal Peak Latency ≤ (ms)	Amp (μV)	Normal Amp ≥ (μV)	Conduction Velocity (m/s)	Normal Conduction Velocity ≥ (m/s)
Median nerve R.	2.4	2.6	2.9	3.1	23	20	54	50
Ulnar nerve R.	2.2	2.6	2.7	3.1	15	13	55	50

EMG Data

Muscle	Insrt Activity	Fibs	Pos Waves	Fasc	Amp	Dur	Poly	Pattern
Deltoid R.	Norm	None	None	None	**Red**	**Brief**	**Few**	Full
Biceps brachii R.	Norm	None	None	None	**Red**	**Brief**	**Many**	Full
Tensor fasciae latae R.	Norm	None	None	None	Norm	Norm	**Many**	Full
Gluteus medius R.	Norm	None	None	None	Norm	Norm	**Few**	Full
Vastus lateralis R.	**Inc**	**1+**	None	None	**Lg**	**Inc**	**Few**	**Red**
Gastrocnemius R.	Norm	None	None	None	Norm	Norm	None	Full
Deltoid L.	Norm	None	None	None	**Red**	**Brief**	**Few**	Full
Biceps brachii L.	Norm	None	None	None	**Red**	**Brief**	**Few**	Full
Brachioradialis L.	Norm	None	None	None	Norm	Norm	None	Full

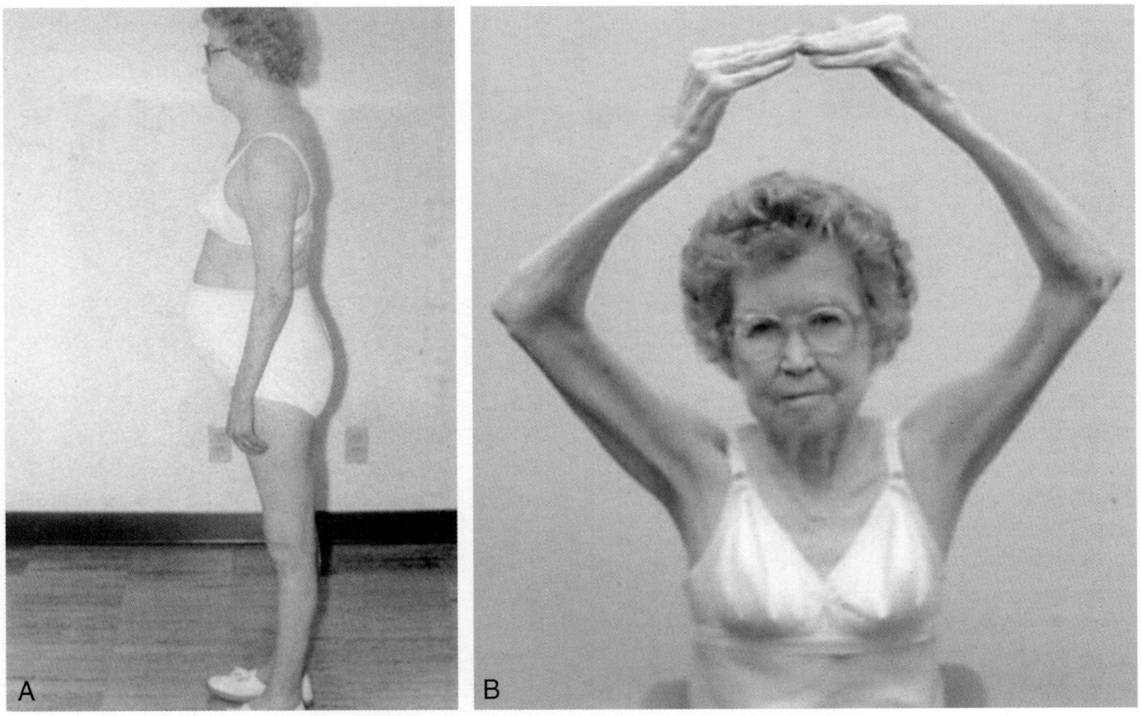

FIG. 100A-1 A, Case 100A during initial presentation; note the quadriceps wasting, overextended knee. **B**, Four years later, she was wheelchair-bound; notice wasting of the forearms.

WHAT WERE THE EMG FINDINGS?

This test showed normal nerve conduction velocities and CMAP and SNAP latencies and amplitudes. There were no denervation potentials, except for some fibrillations in the vastus lateralis muscle. Scattered, small polyphasic motor unit action potentials (MUAPs) were seen in most muscles, suggestive of a primary myopathy. There were some large MUAPs with reduced interference patterns, only in the quadriceps. No myotonia or fasciculations were seen.

WHAT IS THE DIFFERENTIAL DIAGNOSIS GIVEN THESE EMG FINDINGS?

The lack of fasciculations, diffuse denervation, and small motor units ruled out a motor neuron disorder. The absence of myotonia is against acid maltase deficiency or PROMM. Normal CMAP amplitudes and elevated CK are against Eaton–Lambert syndrome; similarly, there was no cranial nerve involvement, and the atrophy and elevated CK are against myasthenia gravis. A repetitive stimulation test was not done.

It was concluded that this patient has a primary myopathy. The lack of fibrillation potentials, except in the quadriceps muscle, is somewhat against an inflammatory myopathy, but the combination of small motor units with large units in some muscles can be seen in IBM,[1,2] a disease in which there is a prominent forearm and quadriceps muscle weakness, as in this case.

WHAT SHOULD BE DONE NEXT?

A left vastus lateralis muscle biopsy showed scattered necrotic fibers and interstitial inflammation. There were also rimmed vacuoles with deposits of congophilic material, as well as myeloid bodies and filamentous inclusions on electromicroscopy (Fig. 100A-2).

Rimmed vacuoles without inclusion bodies can also be seen in other conditions, such as Welander and Nonaka distal muscular dystrophies, some types of limb-girdle muscular dystrophies, and Emery–Dreyfuss dystrophy. They are also seen in oculopharyngeal muscular dystrophy, in some cases chronic partial denervation with reinnervation, and toxic myopathies such as those caused by chloroquine. Rimmed vacuoles with inclusion bodies can be seen in the autosomal-recessive familial-inclusion body myopathy or quadriceps-sparing distal muscular dystrophy.[3] The presentations of these disorders are different from those in this case, and the muscle biopsies do not show evidence of inflammation.

DISCUSSION

Based on the clinical presentation, the mildly elevated CK, and the presence of rimmed vacuoles, inclusion bodies, and inflammation, it was concluded that this patient had IBM.

IBM is the most common inflammatory myopathy among older people, occurring more frequently in men but also seen in women. This disease can be misdiagnosed as amyotrophic lateral sclerosis, other myopathies, and polymyositis; and this case reinforces the importance of a muscle biopsy prior to making a diagnosis or prior to the use of corticosteroids in cases with this presentation.

Historically, Adams et al. initially reported a myopathy with cellular inclusions in 1965,[4] and Chou reported in 1967[5] a patient

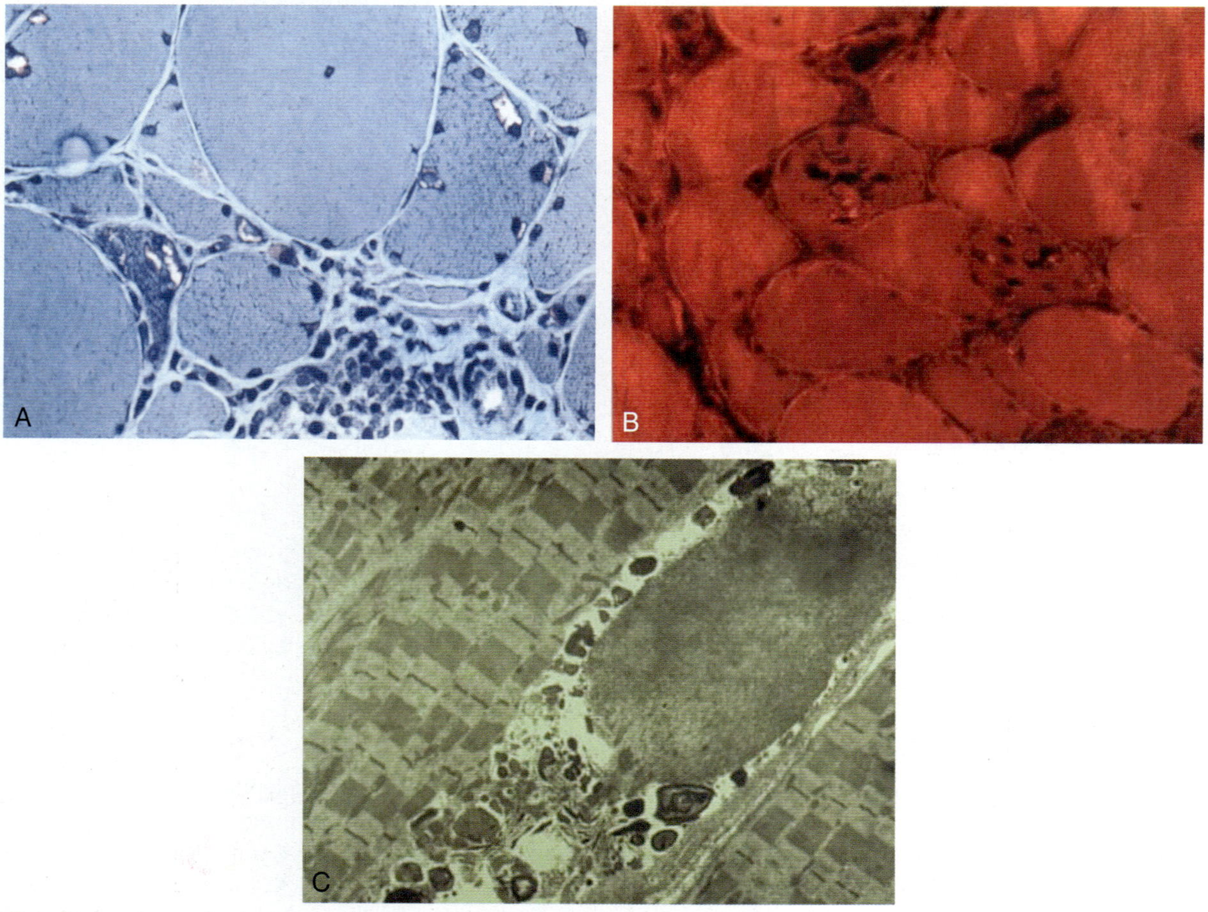

FIG. 100A-2 A, Rimmed vacuoles in muscle fibers, also fiber atrophy (trichrome stain, ×400). **B**, Congo red stain showing fluorescent inclusion viewed using a confocal laser scanning microscope (×200). **C**, Inclusion body and myeloid bodies on electromicroscopy (×7000).

with polymyositis and myxovirus-like inclusion and suggested a viral etiology for the disease. It is likely that patient had IBM, but as discussed later on in this case, these inclusions are not viral, but rather are deposits of a β-amyloid. In 1971 Yunis and Samaha coined the name *inclusion body myositis*.[6]

Since then, IBM has been recognized as a separate entity with a characteristic pattern of weakness, with prominent involvement of the quadriceps, the forearms, the wrist and finger flexors, and the foot dorsiflexor muscles. Later, patients also develop dysphagia that could cause aspiration.[7–10]

Unlike polymyositis and dermatomyositis, IBM is not associated with myocarditis, interstitial lung disease, or malignancy, although about 15%–20% might have an associated autoimmune disorder.

The diagnosis of IBM should be considered based on the clinical presentation in older patients with quadriceps and distal weakness. The biopsy could be misdiagnosed as polymyositis if the rimmed vacuoles and inclusion bodies are not conspicuous, and if the examiner does not look carefully for their presence, or particularly if the biopsy is studied on paraffin sections.

It is not clear if IBM is an autoimmune disorder or a degenerative disease with secondary inflammation. The disease is strongly associated with the HLDA-Dr3, Dr52, and B8 types,[11,12] and patients do not have the apparent protective HLA-Dr53 antigen.[12] IBM has been reported in HIV-infected patients at an age younger than those with the classic disease.[13] (See Case 101.) Patients with IbM could have antibodies against. 5'-nucleotidase, but this test is not very sensitive for diagnosis.[14]

As in polymyositis, the endomysial inflammatory infiltrates are dominated by CD8+ T lymphocytes. The cytoplasm of vacuolated fibers has an accumulation of β-amyloid positive filaments, myelin-like bodies, and lysosomal debris; ragged red fibers are also frequently seen. On EM the inclusions consist of paired helical filaments of 15–21 nm diameters and are seen in the nucleus, cytoplasm, or both. They contain phosphorylated tau protein and resemble the filaments of Alzheimer disease. Other molecules that accumulate that accumulate in IBM muscle include presenilin-1 apolipoprotein E, α-synuclein, ubiquitin, α I antichymotrypsin, and TDP-43[15] basic fibroblast growth factor, and cellular prion protein. This protein is different from that found in the human brain of patients with prion diseases[7] and is also expressed in other inflammatory myopathies.[15] Up to about 20% of the normal muscle fibers overexpress alpha B crystallin.[16]

An accumulation of mutant ubiquitin UBB+1 in muscle fibers could be pathogenic by inhibiting the ubiquitin-proteosome system, which is the main degrading pathway for proteins, leading to the accumulation of misfolded proteins.[17–19] The exact trigger, however, is unknown. IBM is usually an acquired disorder; there are, however, cases of familial IBM occurring in siblings or with an autosomal-dominant inheritance.[19] There is controversy over whether IBM is autoimmune or a degenerative disease.[20,21]

The treatment of IBM remains conservative. The finger tendon transplantation has been recommended to improve hand function,[22,23] percutaneous endoscopic gastronomy tube placement is sometimes necessary for feeding, and knee bracing is used to ameliorate ambulation from severe quadriceps weakness.[23] Patients do not respond to immunotherapy, and although some benefit was observed with immunoglobulin infusion,[24] this has not been confirmed in controlled studies.[25,26] A trial using alemtuzumab, a monoclonal antibody that blocks transduction molecules such as CD52 and causes lymphocytic depletion, is currently underway at the National Institutes of Health.[27] Antithymocyte globulin, which is a potent polyclonal antibody against T cells, is another promising drug for IBM.[28]

SUMMARY

This woman presented with weakness, predominantly in the quadriceps and distal upper extremity muscles. She was initially diagnosed to have polymyositis but did not improve with steroid therapy and was later found to have IBM.

IMPORTANT POINTS

- IBM is an inflammatory myopathy of older persons which manifests with weakness, predominantly in the quadriceps femoris, forearm muscles, and ankle dorsiflexors.
- The EMG in IBM shows small polyphasic motor units, but there could also be large motor units.
- The cause of IBM is unknown, and it is not clear if this is a primary inflammatory disorder or if the inflammation is secondary.
- The characteristic muscle biopsy findings in IBM are the presence of necrosis, inflammation, and rimmed vacuoles with congophilic inclusions; ragged red fibers are also seen. Electromicroscopy demonstrates myeloid debris and the characteristic inclusions formed by filamentous proteins that contain phosphorylated tau protein. Rimmed vacuoles seen in IBM are also seen in other disorders, such as familial inclusion body myopathy, some distal muscular dystrophies, oculopharyngeal dystrophy, and some toxic myopathies, and in cases of chronic partial denervation.
- There is no cure for IBM, and its response to immunosuppressant therapy is disappointing.
- A muscle biopsy should always be done in a patient with myopathy, particularly prior to initiating immunotherapy.

REFERENCES

1. Bertorini TE. Inflammatory myopathies (polymyositis, dermatomyositis, inclusion body myositis). *Comp Ther.* 1998;24:494–502.
2. Bertorini TE. EMG in polymyositis and dermatomyositis. In: Dalakas MC, ed. *Polymyositis and Dermatomyositis.* Woburn, MA: Butterworth; 1998:157–196.
3. Bertorini TE, Horner LH. Histology and histochemistry of muscle and nerve. In: Bertorini TE, ed. *Clinical Evaluation and Diagnostic Tests for Neuromuscular Disorders.* Boston, MA: Butterworth-Heinemann; 2002:595–691.
4. Adams RD, Kakulas BA, Samaha FA. A myopathy with cellular inclusions. *Trans Am Neurol Assoc.* 1965;90:213–216.
5. Chou SM. Myxovirus-like structures in a case of human chronic polymyositis. *Science.* 1967;158(807):1453–1455.

6. Yunis EJ, Samaha FJ. Inclusion body myositis. *Lab Invest.* 1971;25(3):240–248.
7. Askanas V, Engel WK, Mirabella M. Idiopathic inflammatory myopathies: inclusion-body myositis, polymyositis, and dermatomyositis. *Curr Opin Neurol.* 1994;7:448–456.
8. Carpenter S. Inclusion body myositis: a review. *J Neuropathol Exp Neurol.* 1996;55:1105–1114.
9. Garlepp MJ, Mastaglia FL. Inclusion body myositis. *J Neurol Neurosurg Psychiatry.* 1996;60:251–255.
10. Griggs RC, Askanas V, DiMauro S, et al. Inclusion body myositis and myopathies. *Ann Neurol.* 1995;38:705–713.
11. Garlepp MJ, Laing B, Zilko PJ, et al. HLA associations with inclusion body myositis. *Clin Exp Immunol.* 1994;98:40–45.
12. Badrising UA, Schreuder GM, Giphart MJ, et al. Associations with autoimmune disorders in HLA class I and II antigens in inclusion body myositis. *Neurology.* 2004;63:2396–2398.
13. Cuper EJ, Leon-Monzon M, Miller J, et al. Inclusion body myositis in HIV-1 and HTLV-1 infected patients. *Brain.* 1996;119(Pt 6): 1887–1893.
14. Lilleker JB, Rietveld A, Pye SR, Mariampillai K, et al. Cytosolic 5′-nucleotidase 1A autoantibody profile and clinical characteristics in inclusion body myositis. *Ann Rheum Dis.* 2017;76(5):862–868. https://doi.org/10.1136/annrheumdis-2016-210282.
15. Weihl CC, Temiz P, Miller SE, Watts G, et al. TDP-43 accumulation in inclusion body myopathy muscle suggests a common pathogenic mechanism with frontotemporal dementia. *J Neurol Neurosurg Psychiatry.* 2008;79(10):1186–1189.
16. Askanas V, Engel WK. Inclusion-body myositis: newest concepts of pathogenesis and relation to aging and Alzheimer disease. *J Neuropathol Exp Neurol.* 2001;60:1–14.
17. Banwell BL, Engel AG. αB-Crystallin immunolocalization yields new insights into inclusion body myositis. *Neurology.* 2000;54:1033–1041.
18. Fratta P, Engel WK, Van Leeuwen FW, et al. Mutant ubiquitin UBB+1 is accumulated in sporadic inclusion body myositis muscle fibers. *Neurology.* 2004;63(6):1114–1117.
19. Fratta P, Engel WK, McFerrin J, et al. Proteasome inhibition and aggresome formation in sporadic inclusion body myositis and in amyloid-beta precursor protein-overexpression cultured human muscle fibers. *Am J Pathol.* 2005;167(2):517–526.
20. Needham M, Mastaglia FL, Garlepp MJ. Genetics of inclusion-body myositis. *Muscle Nerve.* 2007;35:549–561.
21. Mammen AL. Inclusion body myositis: autoimmune or myodegenerative disease? *Neurology.* 2022;98(13):521–522. doi: 10.1212/WNL.0000000000200188. Epub 2022 Feb 7.
22. Waclawick AJ, Rao VK. Effective treatment of severe finger flexion weakness inclusion-body myositis using tendon transfers. *J Clin Neuromuscul Dis.* 2002;4:31–32.
23. Loyd T. *Management of Inclusion Body Myositis.* Waltham, MA: UpToDate; 2021.
24. Soueidan SA, Dalakas MC. Treatment of inclusion body myositis with high-dose intravenous immunoglobulin. *Neurology.* 1993;43(5):876–879.
25. Amato AA, Barohn RJ, Jackson CE, et al. Inclusion body myositis: treatment with intravenous immunoglobulin. *Neurology.* 1994;44(8):1516–1518.
26. Dalakas MC, Koffman B, Fujii M, et al. A controlled study of intravenous immunoglobulin combined with prednisone in the treatment of IBM. *Neurology.* 2001;56(3):323–327.
27. Lindberg C, Trysberg E, Tarkowski A, Oldfors A. Anti-T-lymphocyte globulin treatment in inclusion body myositis: a randomized pilot study. *Neurology.* 2003;61(2):260–262.
28. Dalakas MC. Treatment and management of autoimmune myopathies Chapter 22. In: Bertorini TE, ed. *Neuromuscular Disorders: Treatment and Management.* 2nd ed. Amsterdam, Netherlands: Elsevier; 2022:554–571.

An Elderly Man With Weakness Diagnosed as Having a Myopathy and a Neuropathy

This 79-year-old patient developed cramps in the legs that had been present for about 4 years. Two years prior to evaluation, he developed weakness in his feet which became progressively worse, particularly in the foot dorsiflexors. Previous EMG showed evidence of peripheral neuropathy with denervation in the distal and proximal muscles. He had a normal MRI of the back and neck.

The family history was negative.

Workup revealed normal MRI of the back and neck.

Examination revealed normal mentation and cranial nerves. There was weakness in both biceps, triceps, interossei, and grip, particularly with weakness in the finger flexors. In the lower extremities, there was mild weakness of the hip flexors, moderate weakness of the feet dorsiflexors and evertors, and severe weakness of the toe dorsiflexors. Reflexes were normal, except for absence at the ankles, and there was absence vibration sense in the toes and decreased in the ankles and knees and there was decreased pinprick to the middle of the feet. Position sense was normal. Gait showed some steppage gait and difficulty walking on the heels.

AN EMG TEST WAS PERFORMED

Motor Nerve Conduction

Nerve and Site	Latency (ms)	Amplitude (mV)	Segment	Conduction Velocity (m/s)
Peroneal R.				
Ankle	4.3	0.1	Extensor digitorum brevis–ankle	
Fibular (head)	15.8	0.1	Ankle–fibula (head)	30
Popliteal fossa	18.9	0.1	Fibula (head)–popliteal fossa	29
Tibial L.				
Ankle	5.7	0.5	Abductor hallucis–ankle	
Popliteal fossa	19.2	0.5	Ankle–popliteal fossa	33
Ulnar R.				
Wrist	45	1.9	Abductor digiti minimi (manus)–wrist	
Below elbow	11.1	1.5	Wrist–below elbow	39
Above elbow	13.4	1.2	Below elbow–above elbow	52

F-Wave Studies

Nerve	M-Latency (ms)	F-Latency (ms)
Peroneal R.	Absent	Absent
Tibial L.	5.7	64.8
Ulnar R.	4.5	37.9

Sensory Nerve Conduction

Nerve and Site	Onset Latency	Peak Latency	Amplitude	Segment	Latency Difference	Distance	Conduction Velocity
Sural R.: lower leg	NR	NR	NRµV	Ankle–lower leg	ms	mm	m/s
Superficial peroneal R.: ankle	NRs	NR	NRµV	Dorsum of foot–ankle	ms	mm	m/s
Ulnar R.: wrist	NRs	NR	NRµV	Digit V (little finger)–wrist	ms	mm	m/s

H-Wave Studies

Nerve	Latency	Amplitude (max)
Tibial R.		
M-wave	4.9 ms	0.6 mV
H-wave	Absent	Absent
Tibial L.		
M-wave	6.8 ms	0.7 mV
H-wave	Absent	Absent

Needle EMG Examination

	Insertional	Spontaneous Activity			Volitional MUAPs				
Muscle	Insertional	Fibs	+Wave	Fasc	Duration	Amplitude	Poly	Config	Recruitment
Vastus lateralis R.	Normal	None	None	None	Normal	Normal	None	Normal	Normal
Tibialis anterior R.	Normal	None	None	None	Normal	Normal	Few	Normal	Reduced
Gastrocnemius R.	Normal	None	None	None	Sl. Incr.	Sl. Incr.	None	Normal	Normal
Deltoid R.	Normal	None	None	None	Normal	Normal	None	Normal	Normal
Biceps brachii R.	CRD	None	1+	None	Decr.	Decr.	Few	Normal	Normal
First dorsal interosseous R.	Normal	None	None	Few	Sl. Incr.	Sl. Incr.	None	Normal	Normal
Vastus lateralis L.	Increased	1+	1+	None	Decr.	Decr.	Few	Normal	Normal

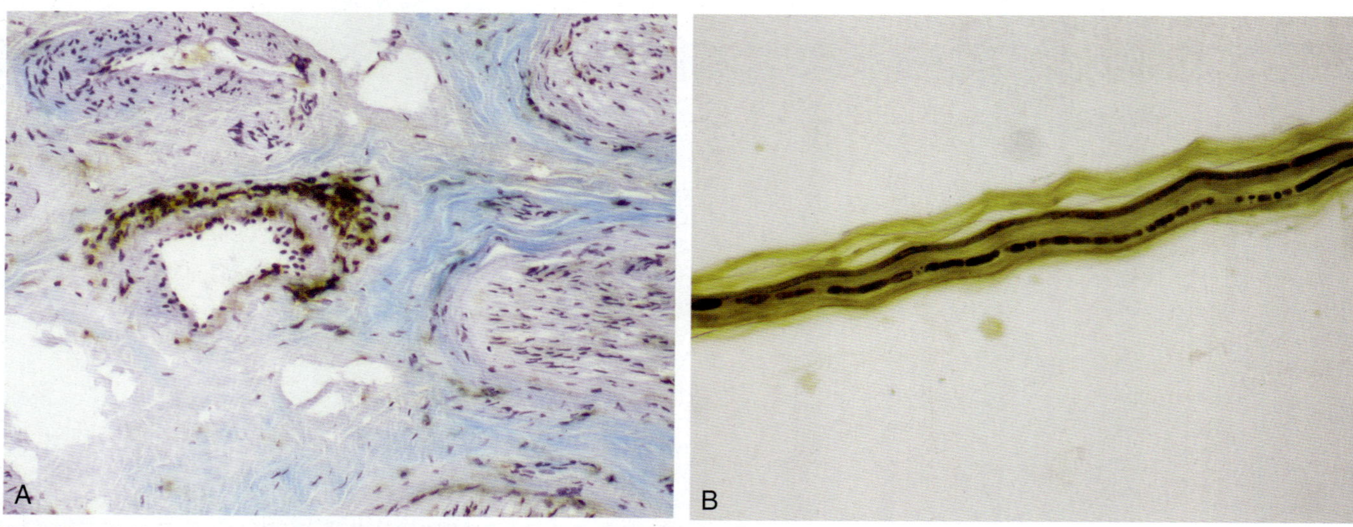

FIG. 100B-1 **A**, Nerve biopsy, CD45 shows inflammatory infiltrates (×100). **B**, Teased nerve preparation showing evidence of axonal degeneration (×100).

WHAT IS THE DIFFERENTIAL DIAGNOSIS?

This patient has an acquired peripheral neuropathy, and the possibilities are multiple including diabetes, autoimmune neuropathy, nutritional and metabolic, or B_{12} deficiency, but the patient's weakness also suggests that he has a feature of a myopathy, and suggested that he could have inclusion body myositis (IBM), particularly with finger flexor weakness. The association of a proximal and distal weakness is unusual in a neuropathy.

WHAT TO DO NEXT?

Serum creatine kinase was 320 IU/L (normal, <200 IU/L). FANA, B_{12}, T4, TSH, and hemoglobin A1C were normal. Rheumatoid factor and ANA were normal. Angiotensin-converting enzyme test was normal.

WHAT TESTS NEED TO BE DONE?

This EMG showed evidence of a predominantly sensorimotor neuropathy with mild demyelination and evidence of myopathic features with irritability in the proximal muscles and small polyphasic motor units and action potentials.

A biceps muscle biopsy and sural nerve were ordered.

The biceps muscle biopsy showed no muscle tissue, only fat, and nerve biopsy showed evidence of inflammation and axonal degeneration (Fig. 100B-1).

Two years later, the patient developed hip pain and underwent hip replacement and during that time a muscle biopsy was

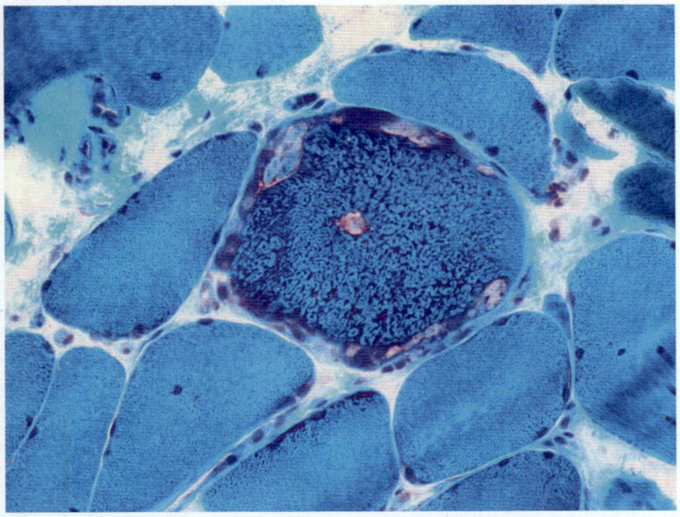

FIG. 100B-2 Muscle biopsy showing rimmed vacuoles on modified trichrome stain. There is also variation in fiber size and internalized nuclei (×200).

done. The muscle biopsy showed inflammation, mild proliferation of connective tissue, and evidence of rimmed vacuoles (Fig. 100B-2).

The patient was treated with methotrexate 10 mg a week, and he stabilized.

DISCUSSION

This patient had Inclusion Body Myositis in addition to a peripheral neuropathy could occur in older persons due to multiple causes, none of this was evident; he was not diabetic, did not have a vitamin deficiency, and did not drink alcohol.[1] Although rimmed vacuoles were seen on biopsy due to chronic denervation, in his muscle biopsy there was also evidence of inflammation; the patient had features of IBM with prominent finger flexor weakness.

There has always been a debate about where neuropathy occurs in IBM. In a study of electromicroscopy of 14 cases of IBM, they all had abnormalities that were nonspecific, but none of them had inflammation.

In an electrophysiological study of 50 cases of IBM, 36% had evidence of a peripheral neuropathy and 6% had Sjögren syndrome.[2] In an electrophysiological study, 35% of patients had abnormalities in conduction velocities and 50% had abnormalities on thermal threshold.[3] Barkaus et al.[4] used quantitative EMG in the biceps muscle, but this could be secondary to sampling. It is conceivable that the inflammatory neuropathy was a coincidental finding; however, it is also possible that they are associated.[5–7]

There is also a debate about whether IBM is a degenerative disease because of the presence of beta-amyloid and other abnormal proteins in muscles, while others believe that this is autoimmune and the amyloid deposits are secondary.[8,9] Evidence of an autoimmune etiology in IBM is the association with autoimmune diseases as well as HIV (see Case 101) and HTLV-1 with upregulation of the MHC and the presence of T cells in nonnecrotic fibers.[9] There is also a proliferation of cytotoxic T cells.[10] There is also the possibility that the abnormal filaments trigger an autoimmune response.[11]

This controversy, however, remains if IBM is primarily degenerative or primarily an autoimmune disease. This case had an inflammatory polyneuropathy and myopathy with features of IBM suggesting that both have an autoimmune etiology; however, this could just be a coincidental association.

IMPORTANT POINTS

- IBM could be associated with an inflammatory neuropathy.
- IBM disorder affects proximal-distal muscles, although peripheral neuropathy is not frequent.
- In patients with a prominent neuropathy and IBM, a nerve biopsy could be necessary to document the presence of inflammation.

REFERENCES

1. Hermanns B, Molnar M, Schröder JM, et al. Peripheral neuropathy associated with hereditary and sporadic inclusion body myositis: confirmation by electron microscopy and morphometry. *J Neurol Sci.* 2000;179:92–102.
2. Naddaf E, Shelly S, Mandrekar J, Chamberlain AM, et al. Survival and associated comorbidities in inclusion body myositis. *Rheumatology.* 2022;61(5):2016–2024. https://doi.org/10.1093/rheumatology/keab716.
3. Lee JH, Boland Freitas R, Liang C, et al. Neuropathy in sporadic inclusion body myositis: a multi-modality neurophysiological study. *Clin Neurophysiol.* 2020;131(11):2777.
4. Barkaus PE, Periquet MI, Nandedkar SD. Quantitative electrophysiological studies in sporadic inclusion body myositis. *Muscle Nerve.* 1999;22(4):480–487.
5. Askanas V, Engel WK. Sporadic inclusion-body myositis and hereditary inclusion-body myopathies: current concepts of diagnosis and pathogenesis. *Curr Opin Rheumatol.* 1998;10: 530–542.
6. Askanas V, Engel WK, Nogalska A. Sporadic inclusion-body myositis: a degenerative muscle disease associated with aging, impaired muscle protein homeostasis and abnormal mitophagy. *Biochim Biophys Acta.* 2015;1852:633–643.
7. Weihl CC, Temiz P, Miller SE, Watts G, et al. TDP-43 accumulation in inclusion body myopathy muscle suggests a common pathogenic mechanism with frontotemporal dementia. *J Neurol Neurosurg Psychiatry.* 2008;79(10):1186–1189. https://doi.org/10.1136/jnnp.2007.131334.
8. Dalakas MC. Interplay between inflammation and degeneration: using inclusion body myositis to study "neuroinflammation". *Ann Neurol.* 2008;64(1):1–3.
9. Badrising UA, Schreuder GM, Giphart MJ, et al. Associations with auto immune disorders and HLA class I and II antigens in inclusion body myositis. *Neurology.* 2004;63(12):2396–2398.
10. Greenberg SA. Inclusion body myositis: clinical features and pathogenesis. *Nat Rev Rheumatol.* 2019;15(5):257–272.
11. Dalakas MC. Treatment and management of autoimmune myopathies. Chapter 22. In: Bertorini TE, ed. *Neuromuscular Disorders: Treatment and Management.* Amsterdam, Netherlands: Elsevier; 2022. 2nd ed.

101 CASE

An HIV-Infected Man With Muscle Weakness and Spasms

A 41-year-old man was referred for complaints of muscle weakness, stiffness, and chronic back pain for 10 months. The patient stated that, when he stretched his legs, they would not relax, and he could not put them down because of thigh stiffness. He was found to be HIV-positive 10 years previously and had chronic back pain related to a car accident 3 years prior to presentation. He had also had a previous lumbar laminectomy.

He complained of some neck and back stiffness. MRI of the neck showed a bulging disk, and MRI of the back was essentially normal except for postoperative changes.

The patient had been on lamivudine and abacavir for his HIV. Because of the weakness and an elevated serum creatine kinase (CK) of 3700 IU/L (normal, 60–210 IU/L), he underwent a muscle biopsy elsewhere, and this showed "inflammation and mitochondrial changes." He had had an EMG that showed scattered denervation potentials and normal nerve conduction tests.

Viral load was low and lymphocyte counts had been stable.

Past medical history and family history were noncontributory, except for a brother who died of leukemia. He stated that he had lost over 20 lb. He smoked and drank alcohol only occasionally.

Examination revealed normal mentation and cranial nerves. His gait had a mild waddle. Manual muscle testing revealed neck flexors and extensors to be 5/5; shoulder abduction and extension, 5−/5; biceps and triceps, 4+/5; wrist extensors, flexors, hand muscles, and finger extensors and flexors, 5−/5. Iliopsoas strength was 5−/5 and the glutei were 5−/5. Quadriceps were 4/5; adductors, 5−/5; and hamstrings, 5−/5. Distal lower extremity strength was normal. Reflexes in the upper extremities were 2+. He only had trace reflexes in the knees and ankles. Sensation to vibration and pinprick were normal in the legs and arms. There were no fasciculations or myotonia present. Straight leg raising test was negative. While the patient was seated, his knee was extended; he had slow relaxation, but there were no contractures and the knee could be flexed completely on passive range-of-motion testing. The rest of the examination was unremarkable.

Forced vital capacity was 3.88 L, which is 79% of predicted.

AN EMG TEST WAS PERFORMED

Motor Nerve Studies

Nerve and Site	Latency (ms)	Amplitude (mV)	Conduction Velocity (m/s)
Peroneal Nerve R.	**Normal ≤ 5.7**	**Normal ≥ 3**	**Normal ≥ 40**
Ankle	4.7	3	–
Fibular head	12.6	3	40
Knee	14.4	3	44
Tibial Nerve L.	**Normal ≤ 5.3**	**Normal ≥ 4**	**Normal ≥ 40**
Ankle	4.1	4	–
Pop. fossa	14.4	4	41

Nerve and Site	Latency (ms)	Amplitude (mV)	Conduction Velocity (m/s)
Ulnar Nerve R.	**Normal ≤ 3.6**	**Normal ≥ 8**	**Normal ≥ 50**
Wrist	3.6	9	–
Below elbow	8.0	9	55
Above elbow	10.0	8	60

F-Wave and Tibial H-Reflex Studies

Nerve	Latency (ms)	Normal Latency ≤ (ms)
Peroneal nerve R.	52.6	54
Tibial nerve L.	53.4	54
Ulnar nerve R.	29.8	30
H-reflex R.	34.0	34
H-reflex L.	33.8	34

Sensory Nerve Studies

Nerve	Onset Latency (ms)	Normal Onset Latency ≤ (ms)	Peak Latency (ms)	Normal Peak Latency ≤ (ms)	Amp (μV)	Normal Amp ≥ (μV)	Conduction Velocity (m/s)	Normal Conduction Velocity ≥ (m/s)
Sural nerve R.	3.2	3.5	3.7	4.0	12	11	44	40
Ulnar nerve R.	2.3	2.6	2.8	3.1	14	13	52	50

EMG Data

Muscle	Insrt Activity	Fibs	Pos Waves	Fasc	Amp	Dur	Poly	Pattern
Deltoid R.	**CRD**	None	None	None	Norm	Norm	None	Full
Biceps brachii R.	**CRD**	None	None	None	Norm	Norm	None	Full
Triceps R.	Norm	None	None	None	Norm	Norm	None	Full
Brachioradialis R.	Norm	None	None	None	Norm	Norm	None	Full
Flexor carpi ulnaris R.	Norm	None	None	None	Norm	Norm	None	Full
First dorsal interosseous R.	Norm	None	None	None	Norm	Norm	None	Full
Tensor fasciae latae R.	**CRD**	None	None	None	Norm	**Brief**	**Few**	Full
Rectus femoris R.	**CRD**	None	None	None	Norm	**Brief**	**Many**	Full
Tibialis anterior R.	Norm	None	None	None	Norm	Norm	None	Full
Gastrocnemius R.	Norm	None	None	None	Norm	Norm	None	Full
Gastrocnemius L.	**CRD**	None	None	None	Norm	Norm	None	Full

WHAT WERE THE EMG FINDINGS?

This test showed normal nerve conduction studies. On the needle examination there were scattered, brief polyphasic motor unit action potentials, and frequent complex repetitive discharges (CRDs), particularly in the quadriceps, suggesting an inflammatory myopathy.

WHAT IS THE DIFFERENTIAL DIAGNOSIS?

This patient had weakness and spasms mainly in the thigh muscles. He had progressive muscle weakness, elevated CK, and abnormal EMG, suggesting an inflammatory myopathy associated with HIV. He was not taking zidovudine, which can be associated with mitochondrial myopathy and weakness.

His stiffness suggests a disorder of motor unit hyperexcitability, causing frequent spasms as in Isaacs syndrome, but his EMG was not consistent with this. Stiff-person syndrome also causes muscle stiffness, but this was only evident in the patient's thighs and was not generalized, and the EMG ruled that disorder out. It is also possible that his back problem caused the spasms and EMG abnormalities, but these were diffuse, including the upper extremities. It was concluded that the findings were secondary to the inflammatory myopathy.

This patient's muscle biopsy was reviewed and did show severe necrosis and inflammation with scattered rimmed vacuoles (Figs. 101-1 and 101-2) and ragged red fibers (Fig. 101-3). There were eosinophilic inclusions (Fig. 101-4). The Congo red stain revealed deposits of congophilic material (Fig. 101-5). No electromicroscopy was done.

The patient was treated with oxcarbazepine with marked improvement of muscle spasms. After 3 months, because of progressive weakness, he was started on prednisone 30 mg/day, with careful monitoring of his lymphocyte counts, and IgG infusions monthly with marked improvement.

DISCUSSION

This patient has HIV and a necrotizing myopathy with inflammation and rimmed vacuoles. HIV patients manifest with several myopathies,[1–3] including typical polymyositis, a myopathy

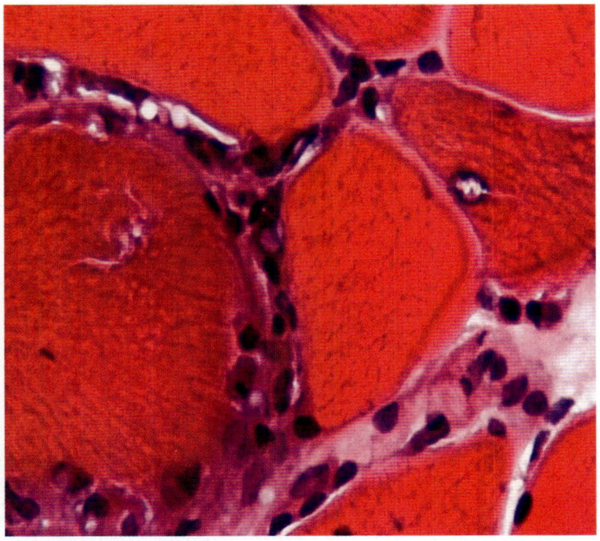

FIG. 101-1 Rimmed vacuoles and small lymphocytic inflammatory infiltrate (H&E stain, ×400).

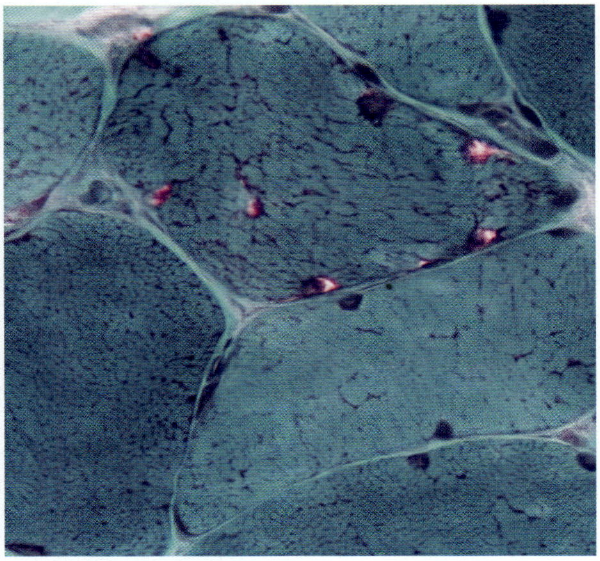

FIG. 101-2 Muscle fibers showing multiple rimmed vacuoles (modified trichrome stain, ×400).

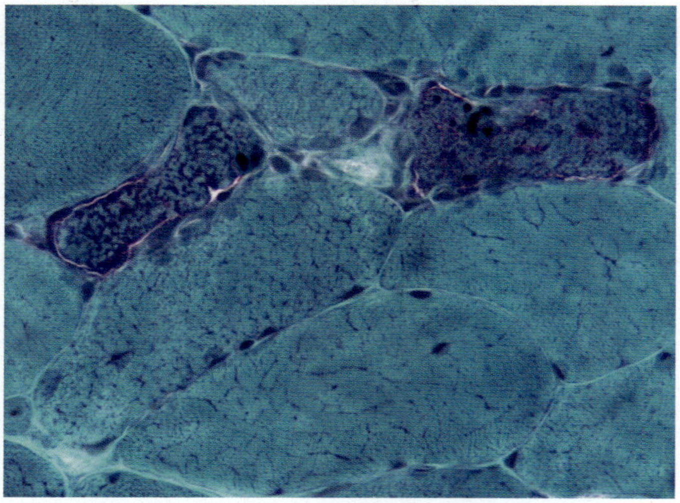

FIG. 101-3 Ragged red fibers (modified trichrome stain, ×200).

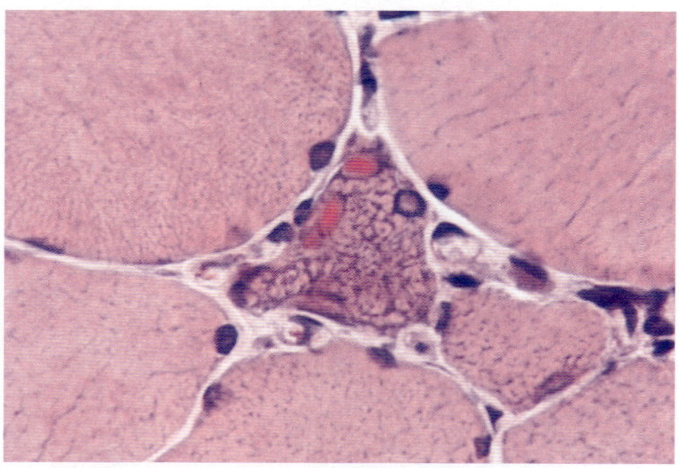

FIG. 101-4 Muscle fiber showing an eosinophilic inclusion (H&E stain, ×200).

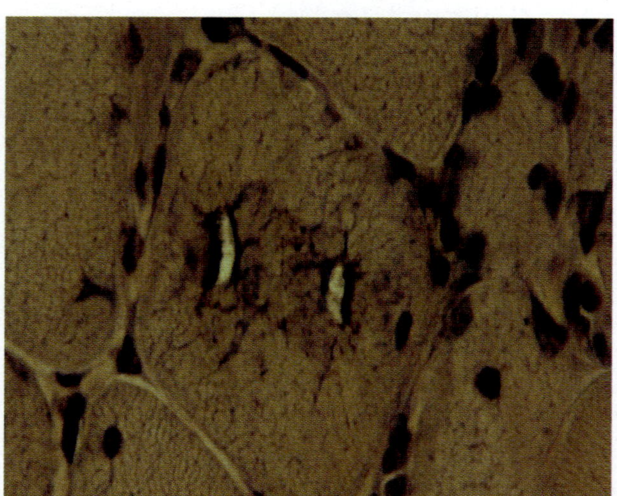

FIG. 101-5 Congo red stain viewed under polarized light; notice birefringent congophilic material (×400).

with rod bodies with or without inflammation, pyomyositis, and inclusion body myositis (IBM). Occasional cases have myoglobinuria. They could also develop type II muscle fiber atrophy as a manifestation of a cachetic syndrome.[4–6] HIV-infected patients could also develop a myopathy caused by drugs, particularly zidovudine, which is associated with cytoplasmic bodies, nemaline rods, and ragged red fibers, secondary to drug-induced mitochondrial DNA depletion.[7] (See Case 40 for another HIV patient who presented with an acute neuropathy.)

The distribution of weakness and the muscle biopsy were diagnostic of IBM, and the muscle spasms and difficulty in relaxing the thighs were likely secondary to neuromuscular irritability, manifesting as frequent CRDs.

This case demonstrates that sodium channel blockers can help patients with increased neuromuscular irritability, not only those with myotonia but also in cases with muscle spasms.

IBM has been reported in HIV-infected patients with a clinical phenotype very similar to sporadic IBM, but usually in younger individuals.[8] Muscle biopsies show endomysial inflammation[9] with rimmed vacuoles and inclusion bodies similar to sporadic IBM. The inflammatory cells consist of CD8 lymphocytes bearing the TCR Vβ5.1 and Vβ13 chains around nonnecrotic muscle fibers.[8] Viral antigens are found in macrophages around, but not within, fibers.[8]

Patients infected with human T-lymphotropic virus 1 can also be associated with an inflammatory myopathy.[10-12] In these patients, there is evidence of viral messenger ribonucleic acid in inflammatory cells.[10]

The treatment of HIV-associated myositis is similar to that of polymyositis, consisting of corticosteroids, immunosuppressants, and IgG infusions. While the immunotherapy of sporadic IBM is not rewarding, this case demonstrates that HIV-associated IBM might respond to immunotherapy.

SUMMARY

This HIV-positive patient developed weakness and muscle stiffness. His EMG demonstrated many CRDs, particularly in the quadriceps muscle. The stiffness improved with oxcarbazepine. His biopsy showed an inflammatory myopathy with rimmed vacuoles and congophilic inclusions. He was then treated with low doses of prednisone and IgG infusions, and this produced significant improvement.

IMPORTANT POINTS

- HIV can manifest in several neuromuscular disorders and particularly myopathies, such as polymyositis, IBM, a cachetic syndrome with type II muscle fiber atrophy, and, rarely, myoglobinuria. Zidovudine can cause a mitochondrial myopathy.
- The presentation of IBM in HIV-positive patients is similar to that of the sporadic disease in non-HIV patients.
- Patients with neuromuscular irritability causing spasms should be treated with sodium channel blockers.

- Patients with HIV-associated myositis should be treated carefully with immunosuppressant therapy, and HIV-associated IBM may respond to this form of therapy.

REFERENCES

1. Dalakas MC, Pezeshkpour GH, Gravell M, Sever JL. Polymyositis associated with AIDS retrovirus. *JAMA*. 1980;256:2381–2383.
2. Dalakas MC, Pezeshkpour GH. Neuromuscular disease associated with human immunodeficiency virus infection. *Ann Neurol*. 1988; 23(Suppl):S38–S48.
3. Dalakas MC, Wichman A, Sever JL. AIDS and the nervous system. *JAMA*. 1989;261:2396.
4. Dalakas MC. Virus-related muscle disorders. In: Engel AG, Franzini-Armstrong C, eds. *Myology*. 3rd ed. New York, NY: McGraw-Hill; 2004:1389–1417.
5. Simpson DM, Bender AN. Human immunodeficiency virus-associated myopathy: analysis of 11 patients. *Ann Neurol*. 1988; 24:79–84.
6. Lange DJ, Britton CB, Younger DS, Hays AP. The neuromuscular manifestations of human immunodeficiency virus infections. *Arch Neurol*. 1988;45:1084–1088.
7. Cupler EJ, Danon MJ, Jay C, et al. Early features of zidovudine-associated myopathy: histopathological finding and clinical correlations. *Acta Neuropath (Berl)*. 1995;90:1–6.
8. Cupler EJ, Leon-Monzon M, Miller J, et al. Inclusion body myositis in HIV-1 and HTLV-1 infected patients. *Brain*. 1996;119:1887–1893.
9. Dalakas MC. Myopathies and neuropathies in HIV-infected adults and children. In: Pizzo PA, Wilfert CM, eds. *Pediatric AIDS*. 3rd ed. Baltimore, MD: Williams & Wilkins; 1998: 403–415.
10. Ozden S, Gessain A, Gout O, Mikol J. Sporadic inclusion body myositis in a patient with human T cell leukemia virus type-1 associated myelopathy. *Clin Infect Dis*. 2001;32:510–514.
11. Khan RB, Bertorini TE, Levin MC. HTLV-1 and its neurological complications. *Neurologist*. 2001;7:271–278.
12. Neike C, Kleefeld F, Preusse C, Ruck T, Stenzel W. Inclusion body myositis and associated diseases: an argument for shared immune pathologies. *Acta Neuropathol Commun*. 2022;10(1):84.

102 CASE

A Patient With Rapidly Progressive Muscle Weakness and Rather Elevated Creatine Kinase

A 44-year-old man presented with a progressive proximal weakness for 2 months and an elevated serum creatine kinase (CK) of 17,209 U/L (normal, <22–269 U/L). Physical examination revealed symmetrical Medical Research Council 2/5 proximal strength of the upper and lower limb girdle. The remainder of the examination including motor reflex testing, cranial nerve and sensory testing, and dermatological examinations were within normal limits.

Computed tomography scan of the chest, abdomen, and pelvis showed no evidence for malignancy. Lab workup includes HIV, thyroid-stimulating hormone, T4, Jo-I antibody, anti-Smith antibody, and anti-RNP antibody. Hepatitis A, B, and C panels were all negative. Chest radiograph did not show abnormalities.

WHAT IS THE DIFFERENTIAL DIAGNOSIS?

This patient appeared to have a rapidly progressive myopathy with rather elevated CK. Polymyositis is a possibility, although this is very unusual in patients who do not have connective tissue disease. Dermatomyositis is even less likely, because there is no skin rash. Adult-onset Pompe disease is a possibility, although the rapidly progressive weakness is somewhat against this. Another possibility is limb-girdle muscular dystrophy, for which the rapid progression is unlikely. He is too young to have inclusion body myositis.

Other conditions include carnitine deficiency or another metabolic myopathy. A necrotizing myopathy is seen in those who have been on statins and have the HMG-CR antibody. Some patients with signal recognition particle (SRP) antibodies can also have a necrotizing myopathy.

WHAT TO DO NEXT?

An EMG showed evidence of many fibrillation potentials and brief polyphasic motor units, suggestive of a necrotizing or an inflammatory myopathy, although this can also occur in other conditions such as some limb-girdle muscular dystrophies, toxic myopathies, and Pompe disease and other metabolic myopathies.

WHAT SHOULD BE DONE NEXT?

The patient had an elevation of signal recognition antibodies.

A muscle biopsy revealed an active necrotizing myopathy with fiber atrophy, necrosis, phagocytosis, and some regenerating fibers with minimal inflammation (Fig. 102-1A and B) with only rare scattered CD45-positive lymphocytes in the interstitium or vessels. There were CD4 lymphocytes in muscle fibers (Fig. 102-1C and D).

WHAT TO DO NEXT?

We treated the patient with prednisone 1 g/kg and he remained weak, so he received IVIG therapy with significant improvement, but CK remained elevated. He first received azathioprine and then methotrexate as a steroid-sparing agent to taper the prednisone. He improved some, but 2 years later, he got weaker with a CK of 6566. He received IVIG for 6 months and is maintained on monthly IVIG therapy.

DISCUSSION

Rapidly progressive muscle weakness in this person suggests an inflammatory myopathy such as polymyositis, which is rare but has been reported in patients with 3-hydroxy-3-methylglutaryl-coenzyme A reductase (HMGR) antibodies, even if not taking statins,[1,2] and the muscle biopsy shows evidence of a necrotizing myopathy. This is also seen in patients with SRP antibodies as in this case. The SRP is a ubiquitous cytosolic RNA protein that mediates the translation of newly synthesized protein across the endoplasmic reticulum. Antibodies against the SRP have been reported as causing a necrotizing myopathy.[1]

Necrotizing myopathy is not an uncommon autoimmune muscle disease that has been recently recognized.[3–5] Patients present with moderate-to-severe muscle weakness, elevated CK, and there are minimal or no inflammatory cells present, but there is active necrosis. This has also been associated in patients who have received checkpoint inhibitors,[6] and recently, some patients infected with COVID-19 developed a necrotizing myopathy.[7]

SRP antibody–mediated myositis has a somewhat heterogenous presentation,[8] and its response to treatment with immunosuppressants such as gamma globulin and the response to first-line therapy, as in this case, is not ideal, and patients may require additional treatment with immunosuppressants and gamma globulin infusion.[7,9] There could be an association with pulmonary disease, and the myopathy and lung disease respond to rituximab.[10]

SUMMARY

In conclusion, this patient has a necrotizing myopathy associated with SRP antibodies; he did not respond well to prednisone and immunosuppressant and required IVIG therapy.

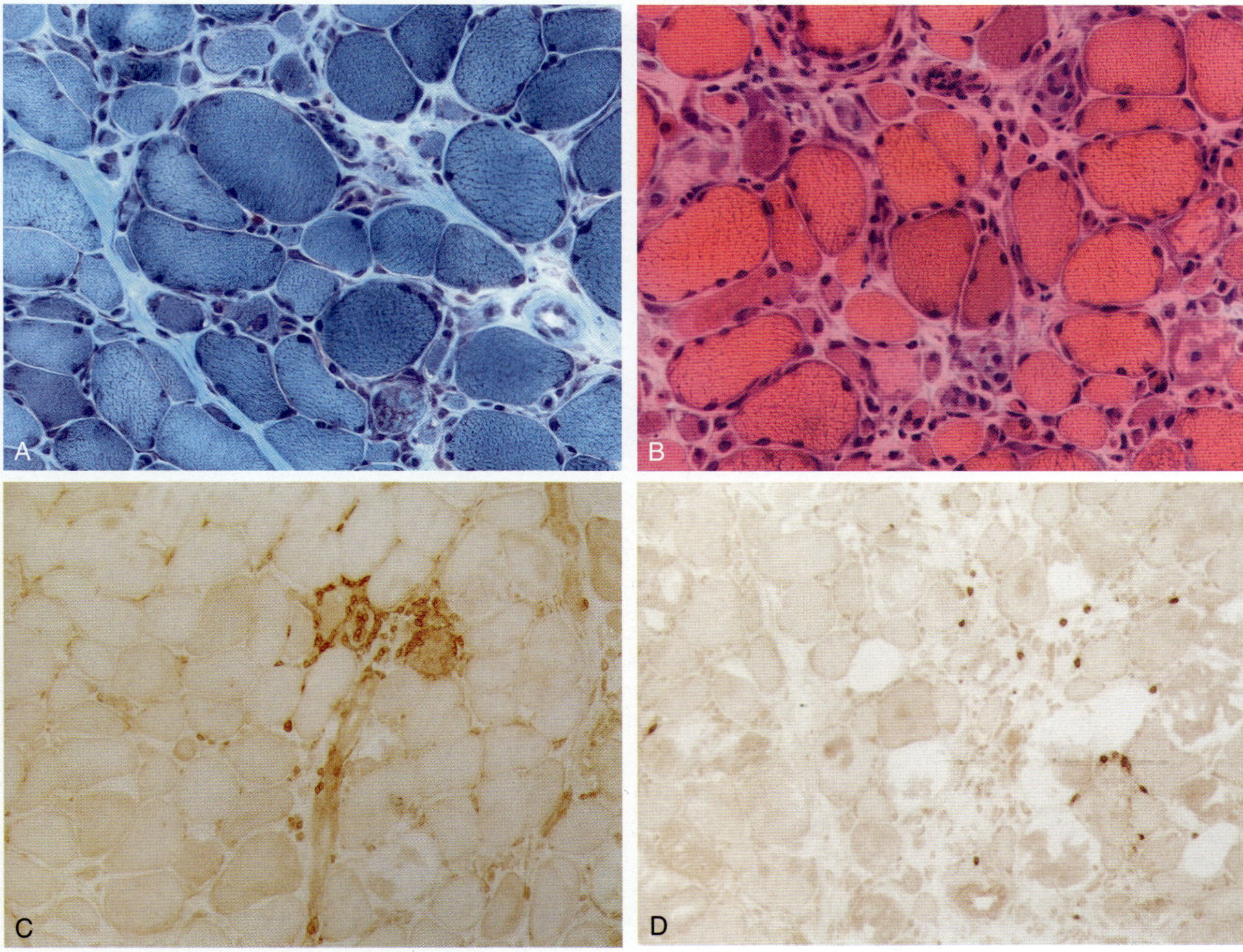

FIG. 102-1 **A**, Modified trichrome stain showing variation in fiber size, scattered necrotic fibers, and some undergoing phagocytosis. There is a mild increase in the endomysial connective tissue (×100). **B**, H&E stain showing frequent necrotic fibers undergoing phagocytosis, but no interstitial inflammation. There is mild variation in fiber size (×100). **C**, Immunohistochemistry stain for CD4 showing positive lymphocytes invading muscle fibers (×100). **D**, Immunohistochemistry for CD8 showing no positive staining of CD8 lymphocytes (×100).

IMPORTANT POINTS

- A rapidly progressive myopathy with rather elevated CK could be caused by a necrotizing myopathy.
- Necrotizing myopathy occurs in patients with HMGR antibodies and SRP antibodies and has also been reported after COVID-19 infections and in patients who received checkpoint inhibitors.
- These patients do not respond to first-line therapy and may require immunotherapy and gamma globulin infusions.

This case was reported as Garcia-Rosell M, Moore S, Pattanaik D, et al. Signal recognition antibody-positive myopathy and response to intravenous immunoglobulin G (IVIG). J Clin Rheumatol. 2013:19(4): 214–217.

REFERENCES

1. Watanabe Y, Uruha A, Suzuki S, et al. Clinical features and prognosis in anti-SRP and anti-HMGCR necrotizing myopathy. *J Neurol Neurosurg Psychiatry*. 2016;87(10):1038–1044. https://doi.org/10.1136/jnnp-2016-313166.
2. Dalakas M. Myositis: are autoantibodies pathogenic in necrotizing myopathy? *Nat Rev Rheumatol*. 2018;14(5):251–252. https://doi.org/10.1038/nrrheum.2018.54.
3. Turgoff IN, Johnson AE, Miller FW. Antibody to signal recognition particle in polymyositis. *Arthritis Rheum*. 1990;33:1361–1370.
4. Kaib AH, Lacomis D, Lucas M, et al. Anti-signal recognition particle autoantibody in patients with and patients without idiopathic inflammatory myopathy. *Arthritis Rheum*. 2004;50:209–215.
5. Henextman CJD, ter Laak HJ, Vree Egberts WTM, et al. Anti-signal recognition particle autoantibodies: marker of a necrotising myopathy. *Ann Rheum Dis*. 2006;65:1635–1638.
6. Dalakas MC. Neurological complications of immune checkpoint inhibitors: what happens when you 'take the brakes off' the immune system. *Ther Adv Neurol Disord*. 2018; Sep 14;11:1756286418799864.
7. Dalakas MC. Inflammatory myopathies: update on diagnosis, pathogenesis and therapies, and COVID-19-related implications. *Acta Myol*. 2020;39:289–301.
8. Suzuki S, Nishikawa A, Kuwana M, Nishimura H, et al. Inflammatory myopathy with anti-signal recognition particle

antibodies: case series of 100 patients. *Orphanet J Rare Dis.* 2015;10:61. https://doi.org/10.1186/s13023-015-0277-y.
9. Miller T, Al-Lozi MT, Lopate G, Pestronk A. Myopathy with antibodies to the signal recognition particle: clinical and pathological features. *J Neurol Neurosurg Psychiatry.* 2002;73(4):420–428.
10. Mazeda C, Cunha R, Ferreira PG, Barcelos A, Aguiar R. Myopathy associated with anti-signal recognition particle antibodies with pulmonary involvement and response to rituximab. *Rheumatol Int.* 2022;42(7):1265–1269. https://doi.org/10.1007/s00296-021-04904-5.

A Woman With Painful and Swollen Legs

A 46-year-old woman presented with a 2-month history of progressive fatigue, generalized edema, myalgia, and proximal muscle weakness. She had a 30-lb weight gain, diffuse large joint arthralgias, and morning stiffness; she also had an erythematous rash over her upper extremities, trunk, and back. She denied recent infections other than chronic sinusitis and had no fever, lymphadenopathy, dysphagia, or changes in bowel habits.

Examination revealed prominent limb edema and induration. There was a splotchy maculopapular rash on her proximal upper extremities, chest, and back. She had discomfort on range-of-motion testing but no warmth, inflammation, or joint infusions. Neurologic examination revealed tenderness on muscle palpation and a very mild proximal muscle weakness in the lower extremities, likely due to poor effort from pain. The examination was otherwise unremarkable.

Pertinent laboratory tests included a serum creatine kinase (CK) of 84 IU/L (normal, <200 IU/L); white blood count, 16 thou/mm^3 (normal, 5–10 thou/mm^3) with a differential significant for elevated eosinophils of 35%; hematocrit, 36% (normal, 37%–47%); and platelets, 436 mm^3 (normal, 150–400 mm^3). Alanine transaminase was 38 IU/L (normal, 0–30 IU/L); aspartate transaminase, 21 IU/L (normal, 0–30 mm^3); albumin, 2.3 g/dL; blood urea nitrogen, 33 mg/dL (normal, 6–20 mg/dL); the chemistry profile was otherwise normal, and the antinuclear antibody titer of 1:160 with a speckled pattern. Hepatitis B and C, HIV, antineutrophil cytoplasmic antibodies, and antichromatin antibodies were all negative.

WHAT IS THE MOST LIKELY DIAGNOSIS?

Stiffness, erythema, and edema with eosinophilia are suggestive of an eosinophilic fasciitis. The absence of significant weakness and normal CK are against an inflammatory myopathy, which sometimes presents with subcutaneous edema. Amyloidosis and cysticercosis could also manifest with muscle swelling, but not with the skin changes seen in this case. It is also unlikely that she had myopathy with muscle enlargement, such as in the myotonias, as the swelling was not in the muscles and appeared to be subcutaneous. The absence of joint deformities argues against rheumatoid arthritis, although she did have joint pains. There were no systemic manifestations of lupus erythematosus. The prominent edema and the absence of sclerodactyly or systemic involvement argue against systemic sclerosis. However, systemic sclerosis and fasciitis may require biopsy and observation of therapeutic response to differentiate. Finally, fasciitis can occur secondary to toxic oil syndrome and in the eosinophilic syndrome secondary to contaminated tryptophan ingestion. This patient denied exposure to tryptophan. Systemic histiocytosis can sometimes manifest by fasciitis, but she had no evidence of a systemic disease.

WHAT SHOULD BE DONE NEXT?

A deltoid muscle and fascia biopsy were performed. This demonstrated normal muscle fibers without atrophy or necrosis. There were abundant mononuclear cells infiltrating the fascia and extending into the perimysium (Fig. 103-1) but not into the endomysium (Fig. 103-2). This infiltrate consisted mainly of macrophages and lymphocytes with very rare eosinophils. The macrophages stained very intensely with nonspecific esterase (Fig. 103-3) and some with acid phosphatase (Fig. 103-4) and NCL-MACRO 68 Ab. Most cells were CD45 positive. There were numerous CD8+ (Fig. 103-5) and only a few CD4+ lymphocytes.

WHAT IS THE TREATMENT?

She was treated with steroids which resulted in decreased arthralgia, myalgia, and edema, and she returned to her normal weight.

DISCUSSION

This patient had diffuse fasciitis and polymyositis with eosinophilia (Shulman syndrome), a condition first described in 1984,[1] which is characterized by diffuse fasciitis, peripheral edema, skin induration, and blood eosinophilia. Other clinical features include joint stiffness and contractures, skin rippling, visible separation of muscle fascicles (groove sign), and myositis.[2–5] It is interesting to note that most cases are preceded by an episode of strenuous physical exertion. The presentation varies depending on the degree of systemic involvement and the extent of muscle and fascial inflammation. Some patients have skin hardening as in scleroderma. The diagnosis is clinical and confirmed by muscle and fascial biopsy. Contrast MRI has demonstrated isolated fascial enhancement in one patient whose muscle biopsy confirmed the diagnosis of Shulman syndrome[6] and may have increased utility in the future for noninvasive diagnosis.

In a study of 24 muscle biopsies of suspected eosinophilic fasciitis the classic findings of inflammatory cell infiltrates were seen in 15; these were composed mainly of macrophages and lymphocytes involving the fascia and perimysium, with eosinophils present in only five cases.[7] Another study found

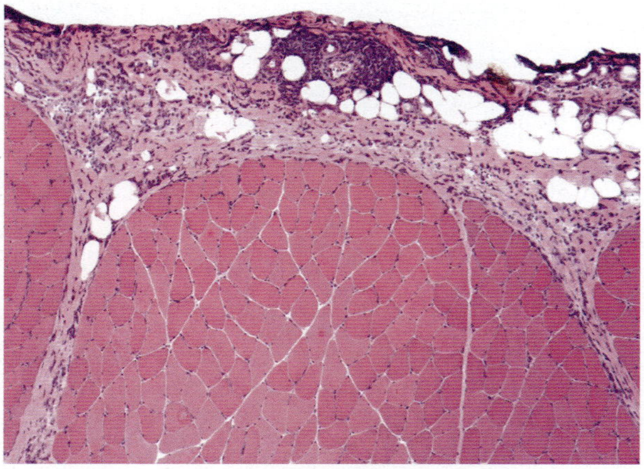

FIG. 103-1 Muscle and fascia biopsy showing an inflammatory infiltrate of mononuclear cells in the fascia and perimysium, but normal muscle fibers (hematoxylin and eosin stain, ×100).

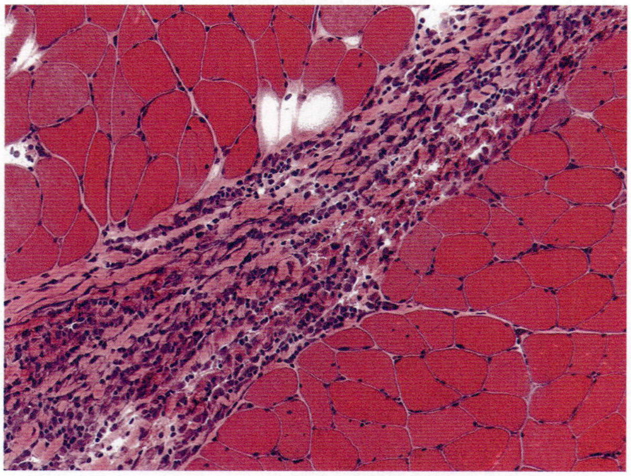

FIG. 103-2 Large population of mononuclear cells in the perimysial area, again with normal muscle fibers (hematoxylin and eosin stain, ×200).

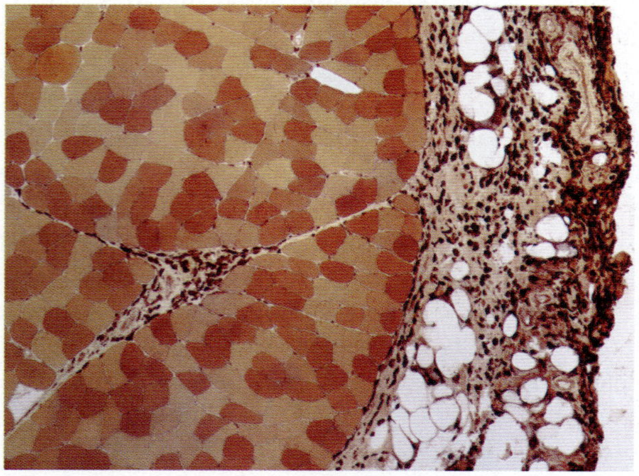

FIG. 103-3 Abundant macrophages in the fascia and perimysium (nonspecific esterase stain, ×100).

predominantly CD8+ lymphocytes with granzyme-B expression, which suggests that this syndrome is triggered by either infectious or environmental factors.[8] It has been theorized that

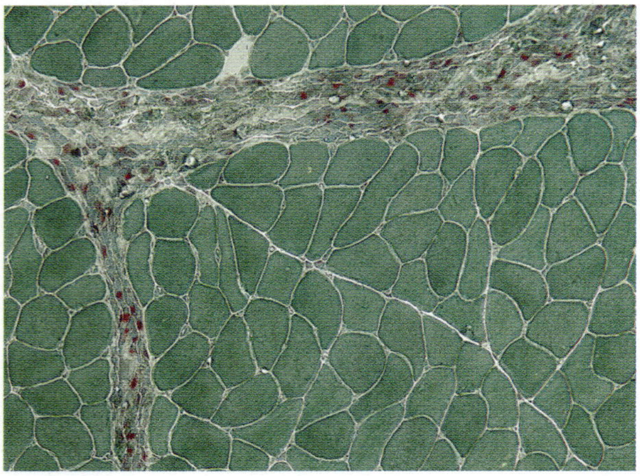

FIG. 103-4 Increased acid phosphatase activity in cells in the perimysial area (acid phosphatase stain, ×200).

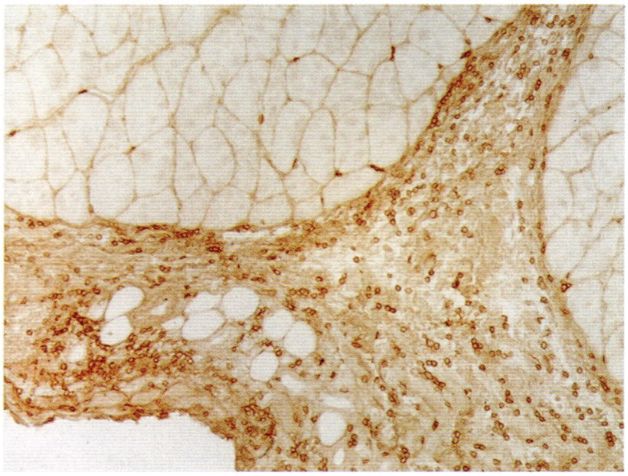

FIG. 103-5 CD8+ lymphocytes in the perimysium (immunoperoxidase stain, ×200).

Shulman syndrome is a variant of scleroderma.[9–11] However, unlike scleroderma, Shulman syndrome responds well to early treatment with steroids.[4,8] Clues to this diagnosis include the lack of weakness and a normal serum CK that differentiates this disease from other inflammatory myopathies. A muscle and fascia biopsy should always be done in patients with muscle pains and limb swelling, as failure to include fascial tissue with the muscle biopsy may lead to an incorrect diagnosis. These will often demonstrate an inflammatory infiltrate composed of macrophages and CD8+ lymphocytes confined to the fascia and perimysium without evidence of muscle atrophy, necrosis, or inflammation, as in this case.

Some cases of Shulman syndrome are associated with *Borrelia* infections,[12–14] while others occur during phenytoin therapy,[15] suggesting that in those, the eosinophilic syndrome represents an allergic reaction. Most cases are idiopathic. These occurred in patients who took L-tryptophan contaminated with an acetaldehyde/triptophan derivative.[16]

Eosinophilic fasciitis should be considered in the differential diagnosis of an inflammatory myopathy with peripheral blood eosinophilia.

SUMMARY

This patient had arthralgias, stiffness, erythema, and edema in the limbs with blood eosinophilia. Muscle and fascia biopsy showed fasciitis and perimyositis. The patient responded to oral steroid treatment.

IMPORTANT POINTS

- Eosinophilic fasciitis is a relatively benign condition characterized by limb edema, occasional erythema, and eosinophilia.
- Fasciitis should be considered in the differential diagnosis of patients presenting with myalgia. In such cases a muscle biopsy should also include fascia, which could help in the diagnosis.
- Fasciitis can occur in the eosinophilic syndrome and in connective tissue disorders, systemic histiocytosis, toxic oil syndrome, and tryptophan toxicity.
- The inflammatory cells in the fascia and muscle in eosinophilic fasciitis consist mainly of macrophages and lymphocytes.
- Eosinophilic syndrome responds to oral steroids and immunosuppressants.

This case was reported by Owens W, Bertorini T, Holt H Jr, Shadle M. Diffuse fasciitis with eosinophilia (Shulman syndrome). J Clin Neuromuscul Dis. 2004;6(2):99–101.

REFERENCES

1. Shulman LE. Diffuse fasciitis with hypergammaglobulinemia and eosinophilia: a new syndrome [Abstract]. *J Rheumatol.* 1984;11:569–570.
2. Mosconi S, Streit M, Bronimann M, Braathen LR. Eosinophilic fasciitis (Shulman syndrome). *Dermatology.* 2002;205:204–206.
3. Falanga V, Medsger TA Jr. Frequency, levels, and significance of blood eosinophilia in systemic sclerosis, localized scleroderma, and eosinophilic fasciitis. *J Am Acad Dermatol.* 1987;17:648–656.
4. Krauser RE, Tuthill RJ. Eosinophilic fasciitis. *Arch Dermatol.* 1977; 113:1092–1093.
5. Fitzpatrick TB, Eisen AZ, Wolff K, et al., eds. *Dermatology in General Medicine.* 4th ed, Vol. 1, Section 14. New York, NY: McGraw-Hill; 1993:1159–1160.
6. Imai T, Saitoh M, Matsumoto H. Eosinophilic fasciitis: MRI evaluation. *Neurology.* 2003;61(3):416.
7. Serratrice G, Pellissier JF, Roux H, Quilichini P. Fasciitis, perimyositis, myositis, polymyositis and eosinophilia. *Muscle Nerve.* 1990;13(5): 385–395.
8. Toquet C, Hamidou MA, Renaudin K, et al. In situ immunophenotype of the inflammatory infiltrate in eosinophilic fasciitis. *J Rheumatol.* 2003;30(8):1811–1815.
9. Torres VM, George WM. Diffuse eosinophilic fasciitis: a new syndrome or variant of scleroderma? *Arch Dermatol.* 1977;112: 1591–1593.
10. Rodnan GP, DiBartolomeo A, Medsger TA. Eosinophilic fasciitis: report of six cases of a new recognized scleroderma-like syndrome. *Arthritis Rheum.* 1975;18(51):525.
11. Urbano-Marquez A. Eosinophilic fasciitis evolving into scleroderma. *Ann Intern Med.* 1983;99:412.
12. Grahamann F, Schmidi J, Meier C. Shulman syndrome as a precursor of acrodermatitis chronica atrophicans Herxheimer: another manifestation of lyme borreliosis? *Zentralbl Bakteriol.* 1989;18:172–177.
13. Granter SR, Barnhill RL, Hewins ME, Duray PH. Identification of Borrelia burgdorferi in diffuse fasciitis with peripheral eosinophilia: borrelial fasciitis. *JAMA.* 1994;272:1283–1285.
14. Hashimoto Y, Takahashi H, Matsuo S, et al. Polymerase chain reaction of Borrelia burgdorferi flagellin gene in Shulman syndrome. *Dermatology.* 1996;192:136–139.
15. Buchanan RR, Gordon DA, Muckle TJ, et al. The eosinophilic fasciitis syndrome after phenytoin (Dilantin) therapy. *J Rheumatol.* 1980;7:733–736.
16. Dalakas MC. Treatment and management of autoimmune myopathies Chapter 21. In: Bertorini TE, ed. *Neuromuscular Disorders: Treatment and Management.* Amsterdam, Netherlands: Elsevier; 2022:554–571. 2nd ed.

104 CASE

A Man With a Bent Spine

A 65-year-old man developed a sudden onset of nonradiating, severe back pain, and he had to lie down on the floor for several hours. The next day he felt weak and had difficulty straightening out his back. The pain went away after 3 days, but he continued to have difficulty stretching and standing erect. He walked bent forward, his gait was unsteady, and he used a cane to prevent his trunk from bending. He was very uncomfortable when he walked and became tired after long walks. He also had difficulty raising his arms above his head due to lack of stability.

Past medical history included surgery for back pain in the remote past, inguinal hernia repair, hemorrhoidectomy, kidney stones, and prostatic hypertrophy. He was on a cholesterol-lowering drug but never took antipsychotics. His family history was noncontributory. He did not smoke and drank socially.

Examination revealed normal mentation and cranial nerves. He stood with a forward-bent posture (Fig. 104-1). Muscle strength testing showed mild weakness of the neck flexors but no weakness or atrophy in the upper or lower extremities, except for 4/5 weakness in the hip and thoracic extensors. He was able to rise up from a chair without using his hands and even squatted normally. His back was flattened. Reflexes were 2+ and symmetrical, except for trace at the ankles; no pathologic reflexes were detected. There was no rigidity, tremors, or dystonia. Sensory examination and coordination were normal. Straight leg raising was negative. The rest of the examination was unremarkable.

WHAT IS THE DIFFERENTIAL DIAGNOSIS?

This patient appears to have *bent spine syndrome*, or *camptocormia*, from the Greek *kamptos* (bent forward) and *kormos* (trunk). This syndrome might be secondary to neurogenic atrophy of the thoracic paraspinal muscles or a primary myopathy. Thus the term *isolated trunk extensor myopathy* is also used. The possibility of a dystonic process was considered, but there was no evidence of dystonia, as when the patient lay in a lateral position, there was no spontaneous bending of the trunk.

WHAT TESTS SHOULD BE DONE?

Complete blood profile and thyroid studies were normal. Serum creatine kinase was 66.1 IU/L (normal, <200 IU/L). Acetylcholine receptor antibodies, FANA, and erythrocyte sedimentation rate were normal. Bone density studies revealed evidence of mild osteopenia.

AN EMG TEST WAS PERFORMED

Motor Nerve Studies

Nerve and Site	Latency (ms)	Amplitude (mV)	Conduction Velocity (m/s)
Peroneal Nerve R.	**Normal ≤ 5.7**	**Normal ≥ 3**	**Normal ≥ 40**
Ankle	4.0	11	–
Fibular head	11.6	10	41
Knee	13.5	9	50

Nerve and Site	Latency (ms)	Amplitude (mV)	Conduction Velocity (m/s)
Tibial Nerve R.	**Normal ≤ 5.3**	**Normal ≥ 4**	**Normal ≥ 40**
Ankle	5.2	19	–
Pop. fossa	15.1	17	45

Nerve and Site	Latency (ms)	Amplitude (mV)	Conduction Velocity (m/s)
Ulnar Nerve R.	**Normal ≤ 3.7**	**Normal ≥ 8**	**Normal ≥ 50**
Wrist	3.6	14	–
Below elbow	7.8	13	56
Above elbow	10.1	13	52
Axilla	12.1	12	60

F-Wave and Tibial H-Reflex Studies

Nerve	Latency (ms)	Normal Latency ≤ (ms)
Peroneal nerve R.	52.7	54
Tibial nerve R.	53.4	54
Ulnar nerve R.	29.2	30
H-reflex R.	33.8	34
H-reflex L.	33.2	34

Sensory Nerve Studies

Nerve	Onset Latency (ms)	Normal Onset Latency ≤ (ms)	Peak Latency (ms)	Normal Peak Latency ≤ (ms)	Amp (μV)	Normal Amp ≥ (μV)	Conduction Velocity (m/s)	Normal Conduction Velocity ≥ (m/s)
Sural nerve R.	3.5	3.5	4.0	4.0	18	11	40	40
Superficial peroneal nerve R.	3.4	3.5	3.9	4.0	10	10	41	40
Ulnar nerve R.	2.8	2.6	3.3	3.1	15	13	43	50
Ulnar nerve L.	2.6	2.6	3.1	3.1	18	13	50	50

Repetitive stimulation of the right accessory nerve was normal.

EMG Data

Muscle	Insrt Activity	Fibs	Pos Waves	Fasc	Amp	Dur	Poly	Pattern
Lumbar paraspinals R.	**Inc**	**1+**	**1+**	None	Norm	Norm	None	Full
Thoracic paraspinals R.	**Inc**	**1+**	**1+**	None	Norm	Norm	**Few**	Full
Gluteus medius R.	Norm	None	None	None	Norm	Norm	None	Full
Gluteus maximus R.	Norm	None	None	None	Norm	Norm	None	Full
Tibialis anterior R.	Norm	None	None	None	Norm	Norm	None	Full
Vastus lateralis R.	Norm	None	None	None	**Lg**	**Inc**	None	Full
First dorsal interosseous R.	Norm	None	None	None	Norm	Norm	None	Full
Deltoid R.	Norm	None	None	None	Norm	Norm	None	Full

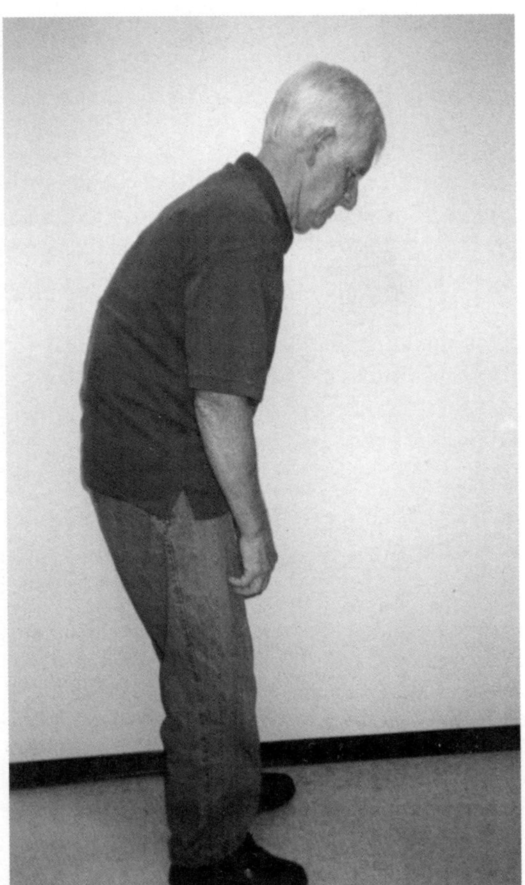

FIG.104-1 Lateral view of the patient showing the bent spine.

WHAT WERE THE EMG FINDINGS?

This test showed normal motor and sensory nerve conduction velocities and CMAP and SNAP amplitudes and latencies. A repetitive stimulation test was normal. There were scattered, large motor unit action potentials, particularly in the vastus lateralis muscle, and there were few fibrillation potentials present in the lumbar and thoracic paraspinal muscles. The findings were nonlocalizing and could have been related to previous radiculopathy and back surgery but could also suggest a chronic lumbosacral radiculopathy or spinal stenosis.

WHAT OTHER TESTS SHOULD BE DONE?

MRI of the spine showed atrophy of the thoracic and lumbar paraspinal muscles (Fig. 104-2) but no other abnormalities. A quadriceps muscle biopsy was normal, and a thoracic paraspinal muscle biopsy showed neurogenic atrophy (Fig. 104-3).

WHAT SHOULD BE DONE NEXT?

A trial of corticosteroids was given, despite the lack of inflammation on the biopsy, and this treatment was unsuccessful. Levodopa/carbidopa trial was also unsuccessful. Back exercises and physical therapy were not helpful.

DISCUSSION

Involuntary forward bending of the spine when standing, or bent spine syndrome, appears to be a condition similar to the head drop syndrome,[1,2] described in *Case 31*. Although a bent

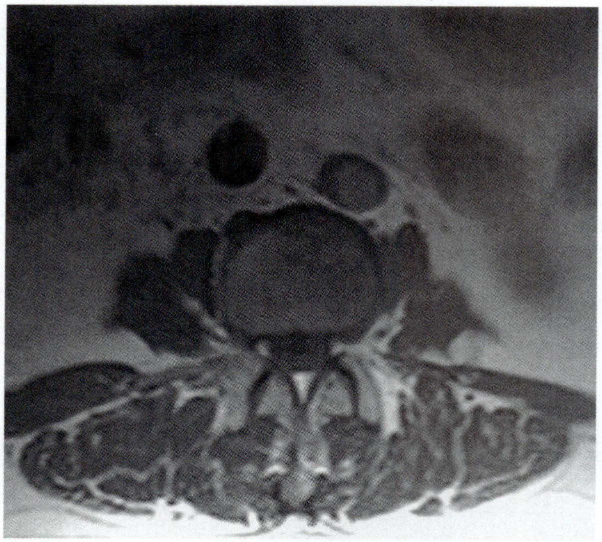

FIG. 104-2 Thoracic axial T1-weighted MRI image showing atrophy and partial replacement of paraspinal muscles by fat.

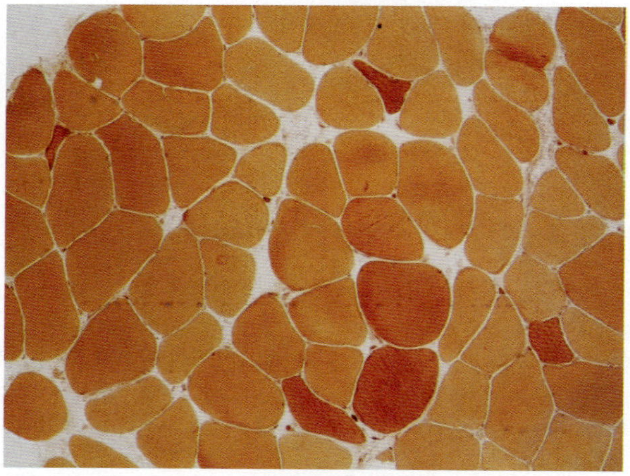

FIG. 104-3 Muscle biopsy of thoracic paraspinal muscles showing scattered, atrophic esterase-positive angular fibers (nonspecific esterase, ×200). (A quadriceps muscle biopsy was normal.)

spine can be caused from structural spinal abnormalities, the term is usually applied to patients who have a reducible and not fixed posture. This is sometimes seen in dystonia and Parkinson disease. The syndrome was initially described by Brodie in 1837,[1] and the term *camptocormia* was first used by Souques in 1915.[3] This refers to soldiers during World War I who had traumatic injury, and the possibility of a psychogenic illness cause was considered then.

This patient has camptocormia; however, the case is unusual, as the symptoms occurred suddenly and because he had previous spinal surgery. The denervation and atrophy in the paraspinal muscles support the hypothesis that idiopathic camptocormia is caused by weakness of these muscles from denervation,[4] but in this case it was only mild.

Like the head drop syndrome, bent spine syndrome can be a manifestation of various neuromuscular disorders causing weakness, including amyotrophic lateral sclerosis,[5,6] inclusion body myositis,[7] nemaline (rod) myopathy,[8] facioscapulohumeral dystrophy, and other myopathies.[9] Camptocormia has also been reported in idiopathic or postencephalitic Parkinson disease[10,11] and in patients with valproic acid toxicity,[12] dystonia, and other movement disorders.[13,14] Several conditions can manifest with neck or trunk extension weakness; these include polymyositis, dermatomyositis, myotonic dystrophy, mitochondrial myopathy, Cushing disease, hypothyroidism, chronic inflammatory demyelinating polyradiculoneuropathy, and a "truncal muscle extensor myopathy."[12] All these disorders should be considered in the differential diagnosis.[1,2]

Although head drop and camptocormia in neuromuscular disorders can be caused by muscle weakness, they are seen more often in the elderly with decreased tissue elasticity; chronic stretch injury could be a contributing factor.[13–16] As discussed, denervation could play a role,[4] but paraspinal muscle denervation in the elderly is a nonspecific finding.[17–19] It is more likely that several factors contribute to the development of the syndrome.[2]

The treatment of idiopathic camptocormia is conservative except in those cases with an identifiable primary disease that is treatable, such as Parkinson disease.

SUMMARY

This patient has bent spine syndrome and in his case it is not associated with a neuromuscular generalized disease. He had had previous back surgery; his MRI showed atrophy of the thoracic and lumbar paraspinal muscles. The muscle biopsy showed mild neurogenic atrophy that could have played a role in the pathogenesis.

IMPORTANT POINTS

- Camptocormia, from the Greek *kampto* (bent forward) and *kormos* (trunk), is a condition seen in the elderly and has multiple causes but frequently is idiopathic and associated with atrophy of the paraspinal muscles and hip extensor weakness.
- Other conditions should be ruled out, such as myositis, mitochondrial myopathy, amyotrophic lateral sclerosis, myasthenia gravis and muscular dystrophy, and a familial myopathy.
- The disease has similarities to head drop syndrome; it might be related to the influence of gravity, causing difficulty maintaining an erect posture because of trunk extensor muscle weakness.
- No specific treatment is available for idiopathic camptocormia.

REFERENCES

1. Katz JS, Barohn RJ. Paraspinous myopathies: dropped head and bent spine syndromes. In: Katirji BE, Kaminski HJ, Preston DC, Ruff RL, Shapiro BE, eds. *Neuromuscular Disorders in Clinical Practice*. Boston, MA: Butterworth-Heinemann; 2002:1181–1186.
2. Umapathi T, Chaudhry V, Cornblath D, et al. Head drop and camptocormia. *J Neurol Neurosurg Psychiatry*. 2002;73:1–7.
3. Souques A, Rosanoff-Saloff M. La camptocormia: incurvation du tronc, consecutive aux traumatisms du dos et des lombes; considerations morphologiques. *Rev Neurol (Paris)*. 1914–15;28: 937–939.
4. Serratrice G, Pouget J, Pellissier JF. Bent spine syndrome. *J Neurol Neurosurg Psychiatry*. 1996;60:51–54.

5. Kuncl RW, Cornblath DR, Griffin JW. Assessment of thoracic paraspinal muscles in the diagnosis of ALS. *Muscle Nerve*. 1988; 11:484–492.
6. Gowers W. A manual of diseases of the nervous system. *Classics of Neurology and Neurosurgery Library*. Birmingham, AL: Gryphon Editions; 1983:350–377.
7. Hund E, Heckl R, Goebel HH, Meinck HM. Inclusion body myositis presenting with isolated erector spinae paresis. *Neurology*. 1995;45(5):993–994.
8. Carpenter S, Karpati G, eds Adult onset nemaline myopathy. *Pathology of Skeletal Muscle*. New York, NY: Oxford University Press; 2001:474. 2nd ed.
9. Peng Y, Zhu M, Zheng J, Zhu Y, et al. Bent spine syndrome as an initial manifestation of late-onset multiple acyl-CoA dehydrogenase deficiency: a case report and literature review. *BMC Neurol*. 2015;15:114. https://doi.org/10.1186/s12883-015-0330-7.
10. Djaldetti R, Mosberg-Galili R, Sroka H, et al. Camptocormia (bent spine) in patients with Parkinson's disease: characterization and possible pathogenesis of an unusual phenomenon. *Mov Disord*. 1999;14:443–447.
11. Martin JP. Curvature of the spine in post-encephalitic Parkinsonism. *J Neurol Neurosurg Psychiatry*. 1965;28:395–400.
12. Long Man Y, Rose M, Coakley G. Failure to stand corrected: camptocormia, a rare cause of bent spine. *Rheumatol Adv Pract*. 2018(suppl 1). https://doi.org/10.1093/rap/rky033.108.
13. Kiuru S, Livanainen M. Camptocormia, a new side effect of sodium valproate. *Epilepsy Res*. 1987;1:254–257.
14. Azher SN, Jankovic J. Camptocormia: pathogenesis, classification, and response to therapy. *Neurology*. 2005;65:355–359.
15. Katz JS, Wolfe GI, Burns DK, et al. Isolated neck extensor myopathy: a common cause of dropped head syndrome. *Neurology*. 1996;46(4):917–921.
16. Laroche M, Delisle MB, Aziza R, et al. Is camptocormia a primary muscular disease? *Spine*. 1995;20:1011–1016.
17. Penisson-Besnier I, Menef P, Dubas F, et al. Histological demonstration of the process of paraspinal muscle denervation in a case of reducible lumbar kyphosis (camptocormia). *Rev Rhum Ed Fr*. 1994;61:868–870.
18. Wharton SB, Chan KK, Pickard JD, Anderson JR. Paravertebral muscles in disease of the cervical spine. *J Neurol Neurosurg Psychiatry*. 1996;61(5):461–465.
19. Lacomis D, Chad DA, Smith TW. Myopathy in the elderly: evaluation of the histopathological spectrum and the accuracy of clinical diagnosis. *Neurology*. 1993;43(4):825–828.

105 CASE

A Man With Muscle Stiffness and Later With Diplopia

A 31-year-old, right-handed man presented with left hip and low back spasms which eventually spread to all four limbs and the entire back bilaterally.

Neurologic examination showed normal mental status and cranial nerves. He had a well-developed musculature with pronounced lordosis (Fig. 105-1) and had firm muscles, particularly of the lower back. There were no muscle rippling, Chvostek, Trousseau, or Babinski signs. Strength was normal. He had mildly hyperactive reflexes and normal sensation. There was no myotonia. The examination was otherwise unremarkable.

WHAT IS THE DIFFERENTIAL DIAGNOSIS?

There are several diseases to be considered in the differential diagnosis of muscle stiffness (Table 105-1). Most importantly, there was no evidence of long tract signs to suggest a myelopathy, and the stiffness was more prominent in the trunk and not focal, as in dystonia. He did not have slow relaxation of muscles to suggest hypothyroid myopathy,[1] nor did he have clinical myotonia to suggest a myotonic syndrome, such as myotonia congenita.[2] There was no evidence of muscle rippling to suggest rippling disease, and the stiffness was persistent and not exercise-induced, as seen in metabolic myopathies. This was present all the time, not just during relaxation after exercise, to suggest Brody disease[3]; also, there was no evidence of muscle fibrosis to suggest drug-induced muscle stiffness.[4] Tetanus is another possibility, but the chronic presentation and lack of trismus are against this. Tetany might present with muscle stiffness, but such patients usually have positive Chvostek or Trousseau signs, which were not present in this patient.

Another possibility is neuromyotonia, or Isaacs syndrome; patients with this have stiffness with impaired relaxation, muscle aches, and cramps that are generalized and have difficulty relaxing the grip, but percussion myotonia is not frequent. Electromyographic studies show evidence of myokymia and other spontaneous discharges; the disease is caused by antibodies against voltage-gated potassium channels.[5]

Stiff-person syndrome (SPS) is an important consideration as it manifests with marked lordosis and difficulty in relaxing muscles, as in this case. Fig. 105-2 shows the steps for the evaluation of patients with muscle spasms.

AN EMG TEST WAS PERFORMED

Motor Nerve Studies

Nerve and Site	Latency (ms)	Amplitude (mV)	Conduction Velocity (m/s)
Ulnar Nerve R.	**Normal ≤ 3.6**	**Normal ≥ 8**	**Normal ≥ 50**
Wrist	2.8	11	–
Below elbow	6.7	11	54
Above elbow	8.7	10	60
Peroneal Nerve R.	**Normal ≤ 5.7**	**Normal ≥ 3**	**Normal ≥ 40**
Ankle	3.8	6	–
Fibular head	11.4	6	44
Knee	12.8	6	50

F-Wave and Tibial H-Reflex Studies

Nerve	Latency (ms)	Normal Latency ≤ (ms)
Ulnar nerve R.	28.8	30
Peroneal nerve R.	51.2	54
H-reflex R.	33.8	34
H-reflex L.	33.5	34

Sensory Nerve Studies

Nerve	Onset Latency (ms)	Normal Onset Latency ≤ (ms)	Peak Latency (ms)	Normal Peak Latency ≤ (ms)	Amp (μV)	Normal Amp ≥ (μV)	Conduction Velocity (m/s)	Normal Conduction Velocity ≥ (m/s)
Ulnar nerve R.	2.1	2.5	2.6	3.1	22	13	57	50
Sural nerve R.	3.2	3.5	3.7	4.0	15	11	44	40

EMG Data

Muscle	Insrt Activity	Fibs	Pos Waves	Fasc	Amp	Dur	Poly	Pattern
Deltoid R.	Norm	None	None	None	Norm	Norm	None	Full
Biceps brachii R.	Norm	None	None	None	Norm	Norm	None	Full

EMG Data—cont'd

Muscle	Insrt Activity	Fibs	Pos Waves	Fasc	Amp	Dur	Poly	Pattern
Triceps R.	Norm	None	None	None	Norm	Norm	None	Full
First dorsal interosseous R.	Norm	None	None	None	Norm	Norm	None	Full
Lumbar paraspinals R.	Norm	None	None	None	Norm	None	None	Full[a]
Tensor fasciae latae R.	Norm	None	None	None	Norm	Norm	None	Full[a]
Vastus lateralis R.	Norm	None	None	None	Norm	Norm	None	Full[a]
Tibialis anterior R.	Norm	None	None	None	Norm	Norm	None	Full
Vastus lateralis L.	Norm	None	None	None	Norm	Norm	None	Full
Gastrocnemius L.	Norm	None	None	None	Norm	Norm	None	Full[a]

[a]Continuous firing of normal-appearing motor units that disappeared with 10 mg of IV diazepam.

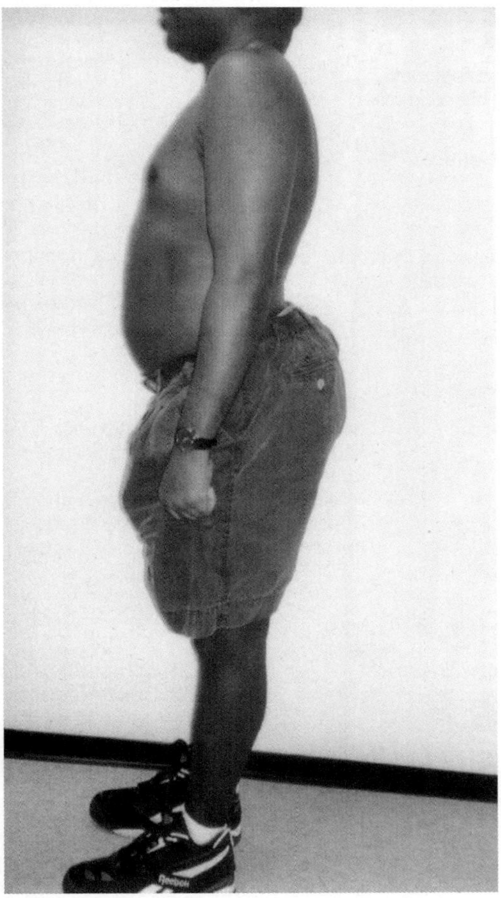

FIG. 105-1 Patient showing prominent lordosis.

WHAT WERE THE EMG FINDINGS?

The EMG showed essentially normal nerve conduction studies, and needle examination showed no myotonia or myokymia, which is against a diagnosis of Isaacs syndrome and myotonic syndromes. The needle test had normal motor unit potentials which appeared spontaneously and did not disappear upon relaxation. They did disappear with 10 mg of intravenous diazepam. This appeared diagnostic of SPS.

Other diagnostic tests included normal complete metabolic panel, thyroid profile, and FANA. He had an elevated glutamic acid decarboxylase (GAD) antibody count of 159 U/mL (normal, <1 U/mL).

TABLE 105-1 Differential Diagnosis of Muscle Stiffness/Spasms

- Central
  - Akinetic-rigid syndromes (i.e., Parkinson disease, progressive supranuclear palsy)
  - Stiff-person syndrome
  - Progressive encephalomyelitis with rigidity
  - Dystonias
  - Tetanus
  - Myelopathy
- Peripheral nerve
  - Neuromyotonia
  - Tetany
  - Benign cramps
- Muscle
  - Hypothyroid myopathy
- Myotonic syndromes
  - Myotonic dystrophy (DM1 and DM2)
  - Proximal myotonic myopathy
  - Myotonia congenital
  - Paramyotonia congenital
  - Schwartz–Jampel syndrome and
- Metabolic myopathies (with exercise-induced spasms)
  - Myophosphorylase deficiency (McArdle disease)
  - Phosphofructokinase deficiency (Tarui disease)
  - Phosphorylase b kinase deficiency
  - Phosphoglycerate mutase deficiency
  - Phosphoglycerate kinase deficiency
  - Lactate dehydrogenase deficiency
- Brody disease
- Rippling muscle disease
- Muscle fibrosis
  - Muscular dystrophies (i.e., Emery–Dreifuss type)
  - Drug-induced muscle fibrosis

Reprinted from Ahmed S, Bertorini T, Narayanaswami P, Senthilkumar K. Clinical approach to a patient presenting with muscle stiffness. *J Clin Neuromuscul Dis*. 2003;4(3):151.

WHAT IS THE MOST LIKELY DIAGNOSIS?

The clinical presentation and electromyographic findings are typical for SPS, and he also had elevated GAD antibodies. He was treated with oral baclofen 10 mg twice a day.

In this disease there is an insidious onset of muscular rigidity in the limbs and axial muscles, most prominent in the

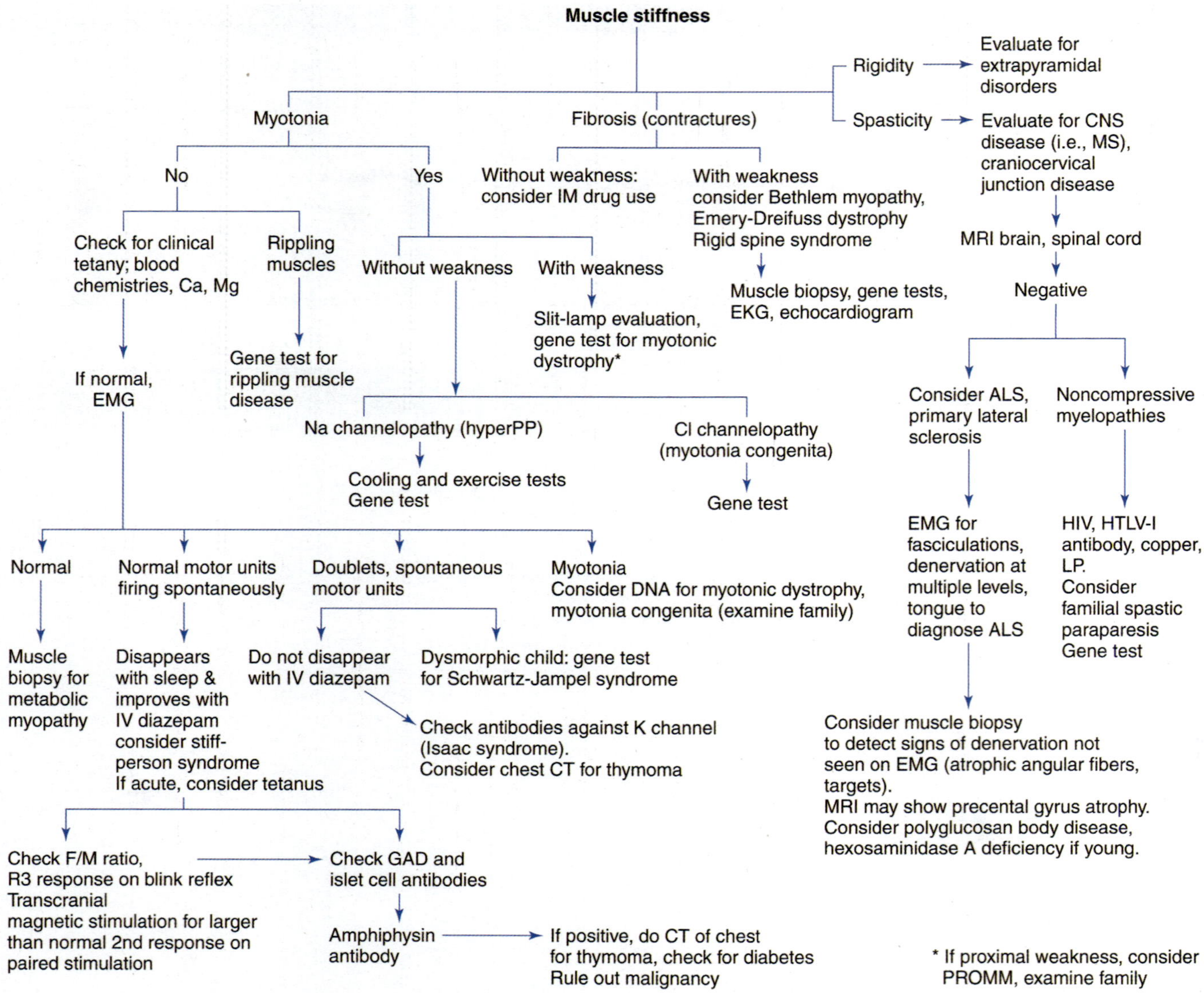

FIG. 105-2 Evaluation of a patient presenting with muscle stiffness. *ALS*, Amyotrophic lateral sclerosis; *Ca*, calcium; *Cl*, chloride; *CNS*, central nervous system; *CT*, computed tomography; *EKG*, electrocardiogram; *EMG*, electromyogram; *F/M ratio*, F-response to M-response amplitude ratio; *GAD*, glutamic acid decarboxylase; *HIV*, human immunodeficiency virus; *HTLV-1*, human T-lymphotropic virus-1; *IM*, intramuscular; *IV*, intravenous; *K*; potassium; *LP*, lumbar puncture; *Mg*, magnesium; *MRI*, magnetic resonance imaging; *Ms*, multiple sclerosis; *PP*, periodic paralysis; *PROMM*, myotonic dystrophy type 2 (DM2). Edited and reproduced with permission from Bertorini TE. Clinical Evaluation and Diagnostic Tests for Neuromuscular Disorders. Boston, MA: Butterworth-Heinemann; 2002. Fig. A10.7.

abdominal and thoracolumbar paraspinals, with difficulty in turning or bending. There is continuous cocontraction of agonist and antagonist muscles with the inability to relax, as confirmed clinically and electrophysiologically; there could be episodic spasms superimposed on the rigidity, precipitated by unexpected noises, tactile stimuli, or emotional upset. There are no signs of other neurologic diseases or chronic pain syndromes that can explain stiffness and spasms.[6,7]

FOLLOW-UP

The patient presented later with a 3-week history of a droopy right upper eyelid with intermittent diplopia which worsened through the day and improved with rest.

Examination showed normal cranial nerves except for ptosis on the right, and he used the frontalis muscles to elevate the eyelid (Fig. 105-3A). He had a limitation to adduction of the right eye and the left eye, with fatigue. Muscle strength testing revealed 4+/5 in proximal muscles and normal distal muscles without fatigue. Reflexes were normal. Plantar responses were flexor. He walked with marked lordosis. The examination was otherwise normal.

WHAT IS THE MOST LIKELY DIAGNOSIS?

The new onset of diplopia and droopy eyelid could suggest a central nervous disorder, such as multiple sclerosis or a brainstem tumor. The fluctuating symptoms without long tract signs

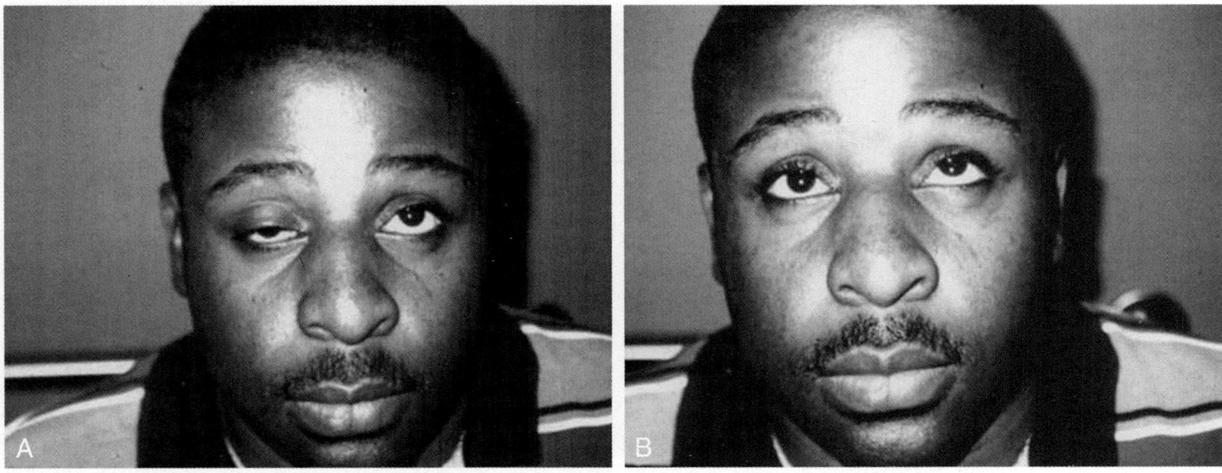

FIG. 105-3 A, The patient showing ptosis in the right eye. **B**, Improvement of ptosis after 6 mg of IV edrophonium.

are against these diagnoses. There was no evidence of exophthalmos to suggest thyroid ophthalmopathy; the eye findings fluctuated and were not symmetrical to suggest a mitochondrial disorder or other ocular myopathies. The presentation suggested myasthenia gravis.

A Second EMG Test Was Performed

Motor Nerve Studies

Nerve and Site	Latency (ms)	Amplitude (mV)	Conduction Velocity (m/s)
Ulnar Nerve R.	**Normal ≤ 3.7**	**Normal ≥ 8**	**Normal ≥ 50**
Wrist	2.7	8	–
Below elbow	6.2	8	64
Above elbow	8.0	8	66

F-Wave Studies

Nerve	Latency (ms)	Normal Latency ≤ (ms)
Ulnar nerve R.	29.6	30

Sensory Nerve Studies

Nerve	Latency (ms)	Normal Latency ≤ (ms)	Amp (μV)	Normal Amp ≥ (μV)
Ulnar nerve R.	2.9	3.1	14	13

Repetitive Stimulation

Ulnar nerve R.	Normal
Facial nerve R.	Normal

Accessory Nerve R.

Potential Number	Amp (mV)	Amp Decrement (%)	Area Decrement (%)
Before Exercise			
1	4.00	0	0
2	3.57	6	8
3	3.56	6	8
4	3.04	**10**	**11**
5	3.03	**10**	**14**
Posttetanic			
1	4.11	0	0
2	4.11	0	0
3	3.55	5	3
4	3.51	6	3
5	3.52	6	2
1 min Postexercise			
1	4.08	0	0
2	3.50	8	**10**
3	2.54	**10**	**10**
4	2.21	**10**	**11**
5	2.21	**10**	**11**
2 min Postexercise			
1	4.11	0	0
2	2.82	**15**	**11**
3	2.82	**15**	**13**
4	2.77	**16**	**13**
5	2.77	**16**	**13**
3 min Postexercise			
1	4.10	0	0
2	3.14	**11**	**14**
3	3.14	**11**	**14**
4	3.08	**13**	**16**
5	3.08	**13**	**16**

WHAT WERE THE FINDINGS OF THE SECOND EMG?

The repeat EMG demonstrated normal ulnar nerve conduction tests. There was a CMAP decrement on the repetitive stimulation test of the accessory nerve while recording on the trapezius muscle 2 minutes after exercise.

An edrophonium test showed improvement of ptosis (Fig. 105-3B). Acetylcholine receptor modulating antibody titers were 28 nmol/L (normal, 0–20 nmol/L); acetylcholine-binding antibodies were 0.50 nmol/L (normal, ≤0.02 nmol/L); acetylcholine receptor blocking antibodies were 0.0%.

A CT scan of the chest showed an enlarged thymus gland. The patient underwent a thymectomy that showed thymus hyperplasia. It was concluded that he had SPS with myasthenia gravis. As in this case, SPS has been reported with thymoma and myasthenia gravis with improvement after thymectomy.[7,8] He received pyridostigmine 60 mg four times a day and later was treated with prednisone, 60 mg daily, then tapering down. He is now stable and having some muscle stiffness and very mild ptosis.

DISCUSSION

This patient had SPS, a disorder initially described by Moersch and Woltman in 1956, who were the first to call it stiff-man syndrome.[6] This occurs equally in both sexes with the onset after age 40, and patients usually have progressive generalized muscle stiffness, prominent lordosis, painful spasms, and difficulty ambulating. They may develop swallowing difficulties and autonomic dysfunction, and there could be sudden death due to cardiac arrhythmias; seizures could also occur.[7–9] SPS can be associated with diabetes and other autoimmune disorders, such as Hashimoto's thyroiditis, pernicious anemia, and myasthenia gravis[10] (Table 105-2). There are variants of this disorder including partial SPS or stiff limb syndrome and progress with encephalomyelitis, rigidity, and myoclonus, and all of these are grouped in the stiff-person spectrum disorders.[11]

TABLE 105-2 Stiff-Person Syndrome Associations

Autoimmune Associations
Diabetes mellitus, type I
Hashimoto thyroiditis
Graves disease
Pernicious anemia
Vitiligo
Myasthenia gravis without thymoma
Premature ovarian failure
Premature gray hair
Autoimmune adrenal failure
Paraneoplastic Associations
Myasthenia gravis with thymoma
Breast adenocarcinoma
Colon Adenocarcinoma

Patients with SPS have antibodies to GAD.[12] Testing spinal fluid is helpful. However, GAD antibodies can be present in serum in people with other autoimmune disorders.[11] GAD is an enzyme that participates in the formation of the inhibitory neurotransmitter γ-aminobutyric acid, and thus there is a lack of inhibition with spontaneous firing of α-motor neurons.[13,14] GAD is present in nervous system neurons and also in the islet cells of the pancreas, and patients with SPS have GAD 65 or islet cell cytoplasmic antibodies and could develop insulin-dependent diabetes. In some cases SPS might be associated with a neoplasm and autoimmune diseases[15] and could have antibodies against amphiphysin, a nerve terminal protein that plays a role in endocytosis.[16] Antibodies against gephyrin, a cytosolic protein concentrated in the inhibitory synapses, have also been reported in SPS.[17,18] The other antibodies are those against the alpha units of the glycine receptor[19] and against the dipeptidyl peptide-like protein 6 and SABA receptor. Paraneoplastic SPS has been associated with anti-Ri neuronal nuclear antibody 2, or ANA2.[19]

The treatment of SPS consists of the use of muscle relaxants, such as diazepam or baclofen. Immunosuppressants, and particularly immunoglobulin infusions, are beneficial.[20,21] Rituximab, a drug that inhibits humoral-mediated autoimmunity, has also been found to be helpful.[22]

SPS in patients with thymoma and myasthenia gravis improve after thymectomy.[23–26] This patient improved later after corticosteroid therapy.

SUMMARY

This patient was diagnosed as having SPS and was treated symptomatically with baclofen. He later developed ptosis and diplopia and was diagnosed as also having myasthenia gravis. He had thymic hyperplasia but had no response to thymectomy. However, he later benefited from pyridostigmine and corticosteroids.

This case reinforces the fact that an autoimmune disease can manifest with another autoimmune disorder affecting different target organs.

IMPORTANT POINTS

- The differential diagnosis of a patient with muscle stiffness includes hypothyroidism, myotonia, Isaacs syndrome, SPS, chronic tetany, and muscle fibrosis from drugs. Tetanus is more acute. Metabolic myopathies present with stiffness only after exercise.
- Patients with SPS manifest with stiffness, autonomic hyperactivity, and lordosis and frequently have an elevation of GAD and antiislet cell antibodies.
- The syndrome is diagnosed by EMG demonstrating lack of myotonia or other spontaneous discharges; in addition, there are spontaneous-firing, normal-appearing motor unit action potentials that disappear after intravenous diazepam.
- The treatment for SPS includes muscle relaxants such as baclofen; immunotherapy including gamma globulin infusions is also beneficial.

- SPS patients might develop diabetes, seizures, and other autoimmune conditions such as myasthenia gravis.
- Patients with myasthenia gravis and SPS respond to immuno therapy.

REFERENCES

1. Ianuzzo D, Patel P, Chen V, et al. Thyroidal trophic influence on skeletal muscle myosin. *Nature*. 1977;270:74–76.
2. Surtees R. Inherited ion channel disorders. *Eur J Pediatr*. 2000; 159(Suppl 3):S199–S203.
3. Danon MJ, Karpati G, Charuk J, Holland P. Sarcoplasmic reticulum adenosine triphosphatase deficiency with probable autosomal dominant inheritance. *Neurology*. 1988;38:812–815.
4. Levin BE, Engel WK. Iatrogenic muscle fibrosis: arm levitation as an initial sign. *JAMA*. 1975;234:621–624.
5. Newsom-Davis J, Mills KR. Immunological associations of acquired neuromyotonia (Issacs' syndrome): report of five cases and literature review. *Brain*. 1993;116:453–469.
6. Moersch FP, Woltman HW. Progressive fluctuating muscular rigidity and spasm ("stiff-man" syndrome): report of a case and some observations in 13 other cases. *Proc Staff Meet Mayo Clin*. 1956;31:421–427.
7. Ahmed SN, Bertorini TE, Narayanaswami P, Senthilkumar K. Clinical approach to a patient presenting with muscle stiffness. *J Clin Neuromuscul Dis*. 2003;4(3):150–160.
8. Srinivassau J, Thoma D, Sabin I. Tetanus. In: Katirji B, Kaminski HJ, Preston DC, Ruff RL, Shapiro BE, eds. Neuromuscular Disorders in Clinical Practice. Boston, MA: Butterworth-Heinemann; 2002:1157–1269.
9. McEvoy K. Stiff man syndrome. In: Samuels MA, Feske S, eds. *Office Practice of Neurology*. New York, NY: Churchill Livingstone; 1996:691–695.
10. Piccolo G, Cosi V. Stiff-man syndrome, dysimmune disorder, and cancer. *Ann Neurol*. 1989;26(1):105.
11. El-Abassi R, Soliman MY, Vllemarette-Pittman N, England JD. SPS: understanding the complexity. *J Neurol Sci*. 2019;404:137–149. https://doi.org/10.1016/j.jns.2019.06.021. Epub 2019 Jul 17.
12. Dalakas MC, Fujii M, Li M, et al. The clinical spectrum of anti-GAD antibody-positive patients with stiff person syndrome. *Neurology*. 2000;55:1531–1535.
13. Solimena M, Folli F, Aparisi R, et al. Autoantibodies to GABA-ergic neurons and pancreatic beta cells in stiff-man syndrome. *N Engl J Med*. 1990;322:1555–1560.
14. Dalakas MC, Li M, Fujii M, et al. Stiff person syndrome quantification, specificity and intrathecal synthesis of GAD65 antibodies. *Neurology*. 2001;57:780–784.
15. Rakocevic G, Alexopoulos H, Dalakas MC. Quantitative clinical and autoimmune assessments in stiff person syndrome: evidence for a progressive disorder. *BMC Neurol*. 2019 Jan 3;19(1):1. https://doi.org/10.1186/s12883-018-1232-z.
16. Butler MH, Hayashi A, Ohkoshi N, et al. Autoimmunity to gephyrin in stiff-man syndrome. *Neuron*. 2000;26(2):307–312.
17. De Camilli P, Thomas A, Cofiell R, et al. The synaptic vesicle-associated protein amphiphysin is the 128-kD autoantigen of stiff-man syndrome with breast cancer. *J Exp Med*. 1993;178: 2219–2223.
18. Espay AT, Chen R. Rigidity and spasms from autoimmune encephalomyelopathies: stiff-person syndrome. *Muscle Nerve*. 2006;34:677–690.
19. Thumen A, Moser. An uncommon paraneoplastic Ri-positive opsoclonus-myoclonus-like syndrome and stiff-person syndrome with elevated glutamate/GABA ratio in the cerebrospinal fluid after breast cancer. *J Neurol*. 2010;257(7):1215–1217.
20. Martinez-Hernandez E, Arino H, McKeon A, Iizuka T, et al. Clinical and immunological investigations in patients with stiff-person spectrum disorder. *JAMA Neurol*. 2016;73(6):714–720.
21. Ortiz JF, Ghani MR, Cox AM, Tambo W. Stiff-person syndrome: a treatment update and new directions. *Cureus*. 2020;12(12):e11995. https://doi.org/10.7759/cureus.11995.
22. Baker MR, Das M, Isaacs J, et al. Treatment of stiff person syndrome with rituximab. *J Neurol Neurosurg Psychiatry*. 2005;76(7):999–1001.
23. Nicholas AP, Chatterjee A, Arnold MM, et al. Stiff-persons' syndrome associated with thymoma and subsequent myasthenia gravis. *Muscle Nerve*. 1997;20:493–498.
24. Piccolo G, Martino G, Moglia A, et al. Autoimmune myasthenia gravis with thymoma following the spontaneous remission of a stiff man syndrome. *Ital J Neurol Sci*. 1990;11(2):177–180.
25. Thomas S, Critchley P, Lawden M, et al. Stiff person syndrome with eye movement abnormality, myasthenia gravis, and thymoma. *J Neurol Neurosurg Psychiatry*. 2005;76:141–142.
26. Dalakas MC, Fujii M, Li M, et al. High-dose intravenous immune globulin for stiff-person syndrome. *N Engl J Med*. 2001;345(16):1870–1876.

106 CASE

A Woman With Muscle Cramps and Fasciculations

A 53-year-old woman complained of frequent muscle spasms, cramps, and mild fluctuating weakness in the arms and legs for 6 years. She initially had difficulty rising from a squat position and had pharynx and tongue spasms that occasionally caused dysphagia. Her symptoms improved recently with celecoxib and clonazepam. She denied difficulty breathing or constipation.

Past medical history was unremarkable. She had three healthy children. Her father was diagnosed with amyotrophic lateral sclerosis (ALS) and died after an 18-year history of progressive weakness, but there are no details of his clinical presentation. One sister had a history of muscle cramps, spasms, and an elevated serum creatine kinase (CK). Another sister had epilepsy and one died of leukemia. She also had three healthy siblings.

Examination revealed normal mentation and cranial nerves. There was no tongue atrophy or fasciculations, and the palate was intact (Fig. 106-1). She had mild hip extensor weakness, and mild hand tremor and fasciculations were seen after muscle activity, but there was no myotonia. Sensation was normal except for mildly decreased vibration sense in the toes. Gait was normal. There were no Babinski signs. The rest of the examination was normal.

Laboratory studies revealed a normal complete blood count, comprehensive metabolic panel, thyroxine and thyroid-stimulating hormone, alanine transaminase, aspartate aminotransferase, and L-lactate dehydrogenase. Serum immunoelectrophoresis was normal except for an IgG of 1840 mg/dL (normal, 700–1600 mg/dL); there were normal GM1 ganglioside antibodies and hexosaminidase A. Serum CK was 520 IU/L (normal, 60–218 IU/L). Spinal fluid was normal with a protein level of 31 mg/dL.

WHAT IS THE DIFFERENTIAL DIAGNOSIS?

Fasciculations are frequently seen in normal people,[1] although in some these might be more frequent, and these individuals are considered to have a syndrome of *benign fasciculations*.[2] When cramping is more severe, this is called the *cramp fasciculation syndrome*. These can be disabling and may be associated with mildly elevated CK.[3]

Muscle fasciculations can also be seen in various neurologic conditions, including particularly some neuropathies, like multifocal motor neuropathy, and motor neuron diseases, such as ALS, Kennedy syndrome, and spinal muscular atrophy (SMA).[4,5] These can be occasionally seen focally in radiculopathies, and also occur in debranching enzyme deficiency.[5]

The family history of her father having "slowly progressive ALS" and one sister with cramps and elevated CK suggests an autosomal-dominant inheritance and is against the autosomal-recessive chromosome 5–associated SMA of adult onset.[6] An autosomal-dominant SMA has also been reported.[7] Autosomal-dominant ALS, with prominent lower motor neuron signs and slow progression, is another possibility.

AN EMG TEST WAS PERFORMED

Motor Nerve Studies

Nerve and Site	Latency (ms)	Amplitude (mV)	Conduction Velocity (m/s)
Peroneal Nerve R.	**Normal ≤ 5.7**	**Normal ≥ 3**	**Normal ≥ 40**
Ankle	3.8	8	–
Fibular head	8.8	6	50
Knee	10.4	6	50

Nerve and Site	Latency (ms)	Amplitude (mV)	Conduction Velocity (m/s)
Tibial Nerve L.	**Normal ≤ 5.3**	**Normal ≥ 4**	**Normal ≥ 40**
Ankle	3.3	19	–
Pop. fossa	10.6	17	48

Nerve and Site	Latency (ms)	Amplitude (mV)	Conduction Velocity (m/s)
Median Nerve R.	**Normal ≤ 4.2**	**Normal ≥ 6**	**Normal ≥ 50**
Wrist	**4.5**	14	–
Elbow	7.8	14	58
Ulnar Nerve R.	**Normal ≤ 3.6**	**Normal ≥ 8**	**Normal ≥ 50**
Wrist	2.6	11	–
Below elbow	5.6	11	58
Above elbow	7.5	11	64

F-Wave and Tibial H-Reflex Studies

Nerve	Latency (ms)	Normal Latency ≤ (ms)
Peroneal nerve R.	40.5	54
Tibial nerve L.	45.0	54
Median nerve R.	24.3	30
Ulnar nerve R.	24.6	30
H-reflex R.	33.6	34
H-reflex L.	33.8	34

Sensory Nerve Studies

Nerve	Onset Latency (ms)	Normal Onset Latency ≤ (ms)	Peak Latency (ms)	Normal Peak Latency ≤ (ms)	Amp (μV)	Normal Amp ≥ (μV)	Conduction Velocity (m/s)	Normal Conduction Velocity ≥ (m/s)
Sural nerve R.	2.9	3.5	3.4	4.0	14	11	48	40
Superficial peroneal nerve R.	3.0	3.5	3.5	4.0	**5**	8–10	46	40
Sural nerve L.	2.8	3.5	3.3	4.0	**5**	11	50	40
Median nerve R.	2.6	2.6	3.1	3.1	**11**	20	50	50
Ulnar nerve R.	2.1	2.6	2.6	3.1	**3**	13	57	50
Radial nerve R.	2.0	2.6	2.5	3.1	**11**	30	50	50

EMG Data

Muscle	Insrt Activity	Fibs	Pos Waves	Fasc	Amp	Dur	Poly	Pattern
Tongue	Norm	None	None	**Few**	**Lg**	**Inc**	None	Full
Deltoid R.	**Myok**	None	None	None	**Lg**	**Inc**	None	Full
First dorsal interosseous R.	Norm	None	None	**Few**	**Lg**	**Inc**	None	**Red**
Vastus lateralis R.	**Inc**	None	**1+**	**Few**	**Lg**	**Inc**	None	**Red**
Vastus medialis R.	Norm	None	None	None	**Lg**	**Inc**	None	Full
Tibialis anterior R.	**Inc**	None	**2+**	**Few**	**Lg**	**Inc**	None	Full
Gastrocnemius R.	Norm	None	None	None	**Lg**	**Inc**	None	Full

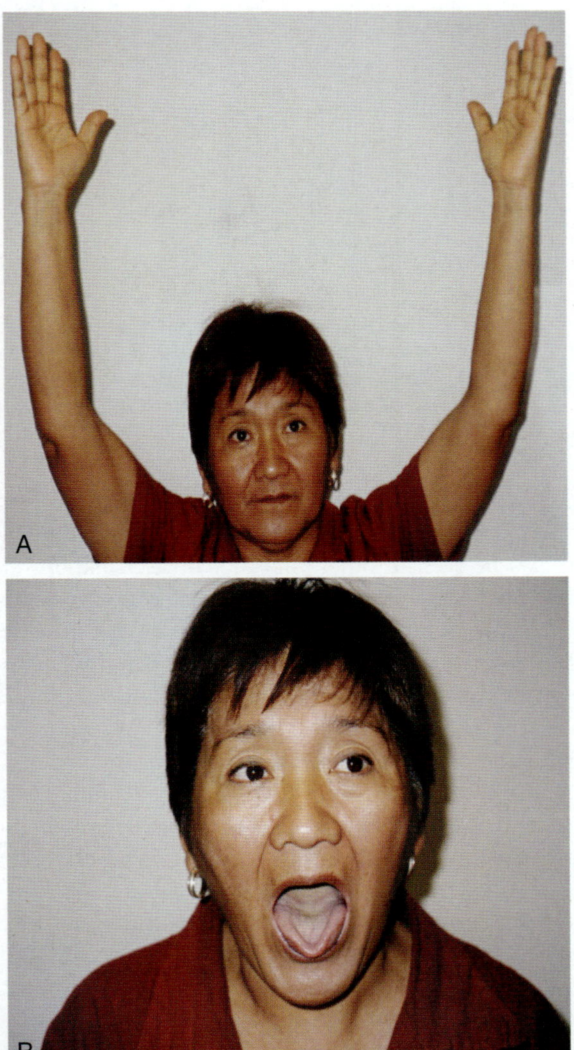

FIG. 106-1 **A**, The patient was able to raise her arms normally and had no atrophy. **B**, The patient showing no evidence of tongue wasting.

WHAT WERE THE EMG FINDINGS?

The EMG showed normal motor nerve conduction velocities and latencies and normal CMAP amplitudes; F-wave and tibial H-reflex were normal. Several SNAPs were of low amplitude. There was mild evidence of denervation in the vastus lateralis and tibialis anterior muscles. Frequent fasciculations and large, fast-firing spontaneous motor unit potentials were seen diffusely after activation, including in the tongue. She developed cramps after voluntary muscle contractions. There was also decreased recruitment of voluntary-activated motor unit action potentials, which were large (Fig. 106-2). Automatic motor unit interference "cloud" analysis confirmed a neurogenic disease with increased motor unit amplitudes and reduced number of turns.[8]

The large motor unit potentials indicate denervation with reinnervation. Their presence in the tongue indicates the involvement of bulbar motor neurons.

It was concluded that she had a motor neuron disorder. Low-amplitude SNAPs suggest that there was also the involvement of the sensory axons; thus she likely had a motor and sensory neuronopathy.

A left quadriceps muscle biopsy showed scattered necrotic fibers undergoing phagocytosis and frequent esterase-positive atrophic angular fibers and fiber-type grouping (Fig. 106-3). A sural nerve biopsy showed a decreased number of myelinated axons, rare axonal degeneration, and some segmental demyelination (Fig. 106-4).

The patient responded well to phenytoin treatment in addition to clonazepam.

WHAT OTHER TESTS SHOULD BE DONE?

DNA testing for Cu/Zn superoxide dismutase mutations and chromosome 5q deletions of SMA and androgen receptor gene

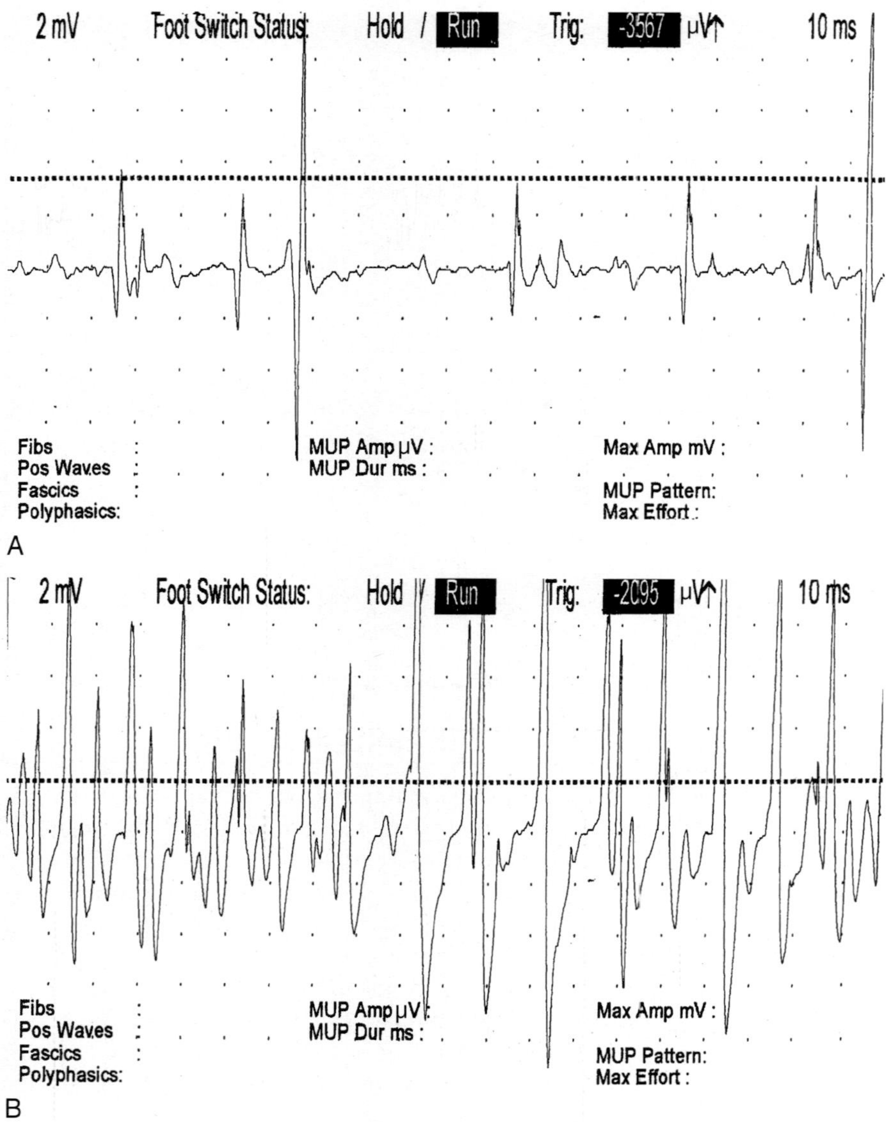

FIG. 106-2 A, Large motor unit action potentials, deltoid muscle (2 mV/10 ms). **B**, Large motor unit action potentials in the tongue; the patient developed a cramp during recording (2 mV/10 ms).

DNA test, for the remote possibility that the patient was a manifest carrier of Kennedy disease, were all normal.

DISCUSSION

This patient had a relatively benign lower motor neuron disorder, manifested mainly by muscle cramps, fasciculations, and mild and fluctuating muscle weakness.

The large motor unit action potentials on EMG, which correlated with the muscle biopsy, seemed to indicate that the patient and her family had an adult-onset autosomal-dominant SMA, but the sensory involvement indicates that she had a neuronopathy, and we presumed that her father was misdiagnosed as having ALS.

This patient also had elevated CK, which occurs in motor neuron disease.[9] This could be secondary to her motor unit excitability with fasciculations and cramps.

Fasciculations are caused by spontaneous depolarization of the whole or part of the motor unit which can occur in normal people; they are usually associated with disorders of the motor neurons.[5] Progressive motor neuron disorders, such as ALS or progressive muscular atrophy, must be considered when fasciculations are associated with weakness, although this could also be seen in other conditions. Fasciculations appear to originate in the axon, but their exact pathogenesis is not clear.[5] Electrophysiologic studies demonstrate that patients with the *cramp fasciculation syndrome* have active-discharges and develop cramps during repetitive nerve stimulation, indicating axonal hyperexcitability.[10]

The combination of muscle spasms, fasciculations, and cramps suggested that *cramp fasciculation syndrome*, which is often a benign condition, may rarely be an early presentation of a progressive motor neuron disorder.[11] Sometimes, the cramp fasciculation syndrome is hereditary; in other cases, it is sporadic. Some individuals with the sporadic form have antibodies against potassium channels in peripheral nerves, as in Isaacs syndrome—another disorder of increased motor unit excitability with which it could have some similarities. Patients could have peripheral and central hyperexcitability.[12]

The presentation, apparent inheritance, and DNA testing in this patient indicated that she did not have a chromosome

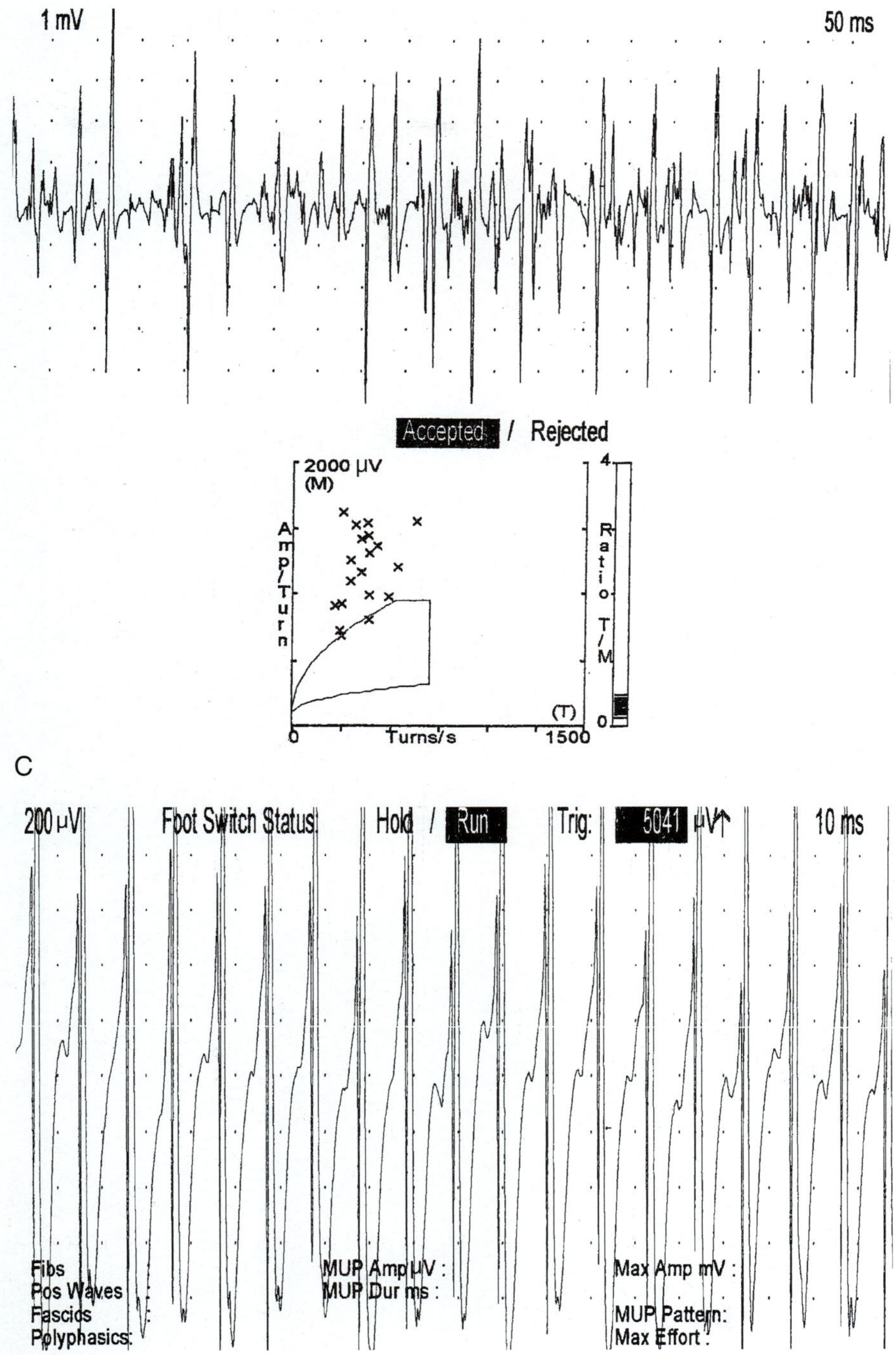

D

FIG. 106-2, cont'd **C**, Large motor unit action potentials, quadriceps muscle (1 mV/50 ms); the cloud analysis documented large units with decreased number of turns (2000 µV). **D**, Single motor unit firing at about 90 Hz, biceps muscle (200 µV/10 ms).

5–associated SMA. Adult-onset autosomal-dominant forms of SMA also occur. Patients usually have a relatively benign course. The genetic defect has not been documented in this form.[7]

This patient had a neuronopathy as in bulbospinal muscular atrophy (Kennedy syndrome), caused by mutations of the androgen receptor gene on the X-chromosome.[13] Autosomal-dominant forms have been rarely described.[14] She did not have a known Kennedy disease mutation, nor was there evidence that her father had clinical manifestations of Kennedy disease. There is a very similar autosomal-dominant syndrome reported in Japan characterized by slowly progressive muscle weakness and atrophy with fasciculations, areflexia, abnormal sensory conduction tests, and elevated serum CK. This is caused by mutations in chromosome 3.[15] The treatment is symptomatic with medication like carbamazepine or mexiletine.

One patient who had diabetes and thyroiditis responded to plasma exchange.[12]

SUMMARY

This woman has a history of muscle cramps, fasciculations, and mild weakness, her sister had similar symptoms, and her father apparently also had a slowly progressive motor neuron disease. The electrophysiologic findings indicate that she has a neuronopathy. Her cramps improved with phenytoin.

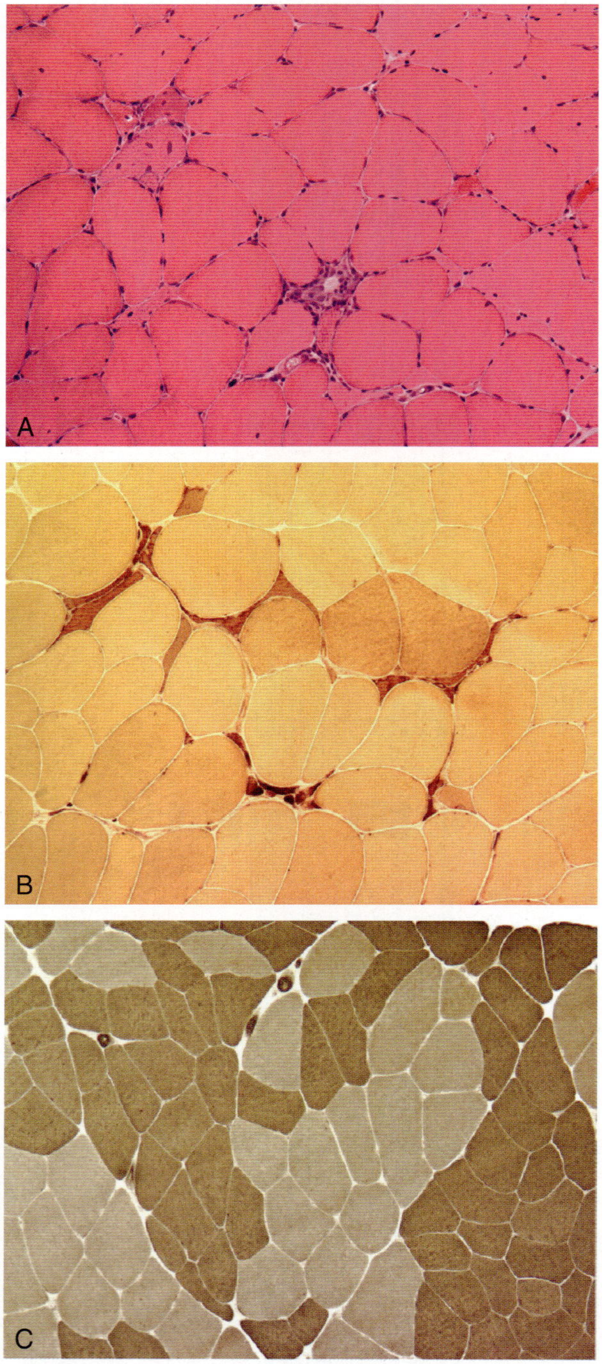

FIG. 106-3 **A**, Fiber necrosis with phagocytosis and atrophic muscle fibers (H&E stain, ×200). **B**, Esterase-positive atrophic fibers (nonspecific esterase stain, ×200). **C**, Fiber-type grouping (ATPase stain, pH 9.4, ×100).

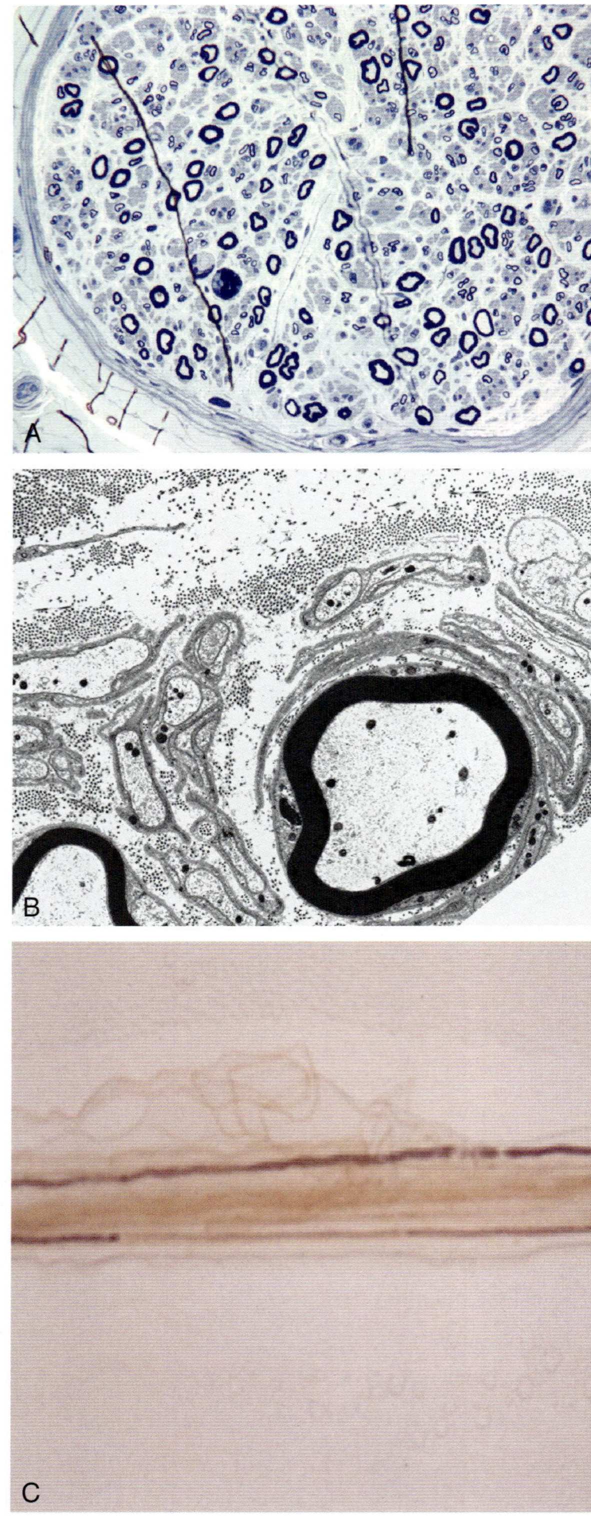

FIG. 106-4 **A**, Sural nerve biopsy showing a mildly decreased number of myelinated axons (osmicated plastic-embedded, toluidine blue stain, ×400). **B**, Early onion bulb formation on a large axon with thin myelin (EM, ×840,000). **C**, Teased nerve preparation showing small fibers, myelin ovoids indicating axonal degeneration, and some axons undergoing segmental demyelination (×100).

IMPORTANT POINTS

- Cramps and fasciculations can be benign but are frequently associated with lower motor neuron syndromes such as SMA.
- Mildly elevated CK occurs not only in myopathy but also in motor neuron disease.
- Large motor unit potentials with decreased recruitment are characteristic of chronic neurogenic disease with reinnervation.
- Not all familial motor neuron diseases have a defined genetic defect, nor are they all rapidly progressive.
- Cramp and fasciculations may respond to anticonvulsant therapy or sodium channel blockers.
- "Benign" fasciculations and cramp fasciculation syndrome might not always be benign.

REFERENCES

1. Reed DM, Kurland LT. Muscle fasciculations in a healthy population. *Arch Neurol.* 1963;9:363–367.
2. Blexrud MD, Windebank AJ, Daube JR. Long-term follow-up of 121 patients with benign fasciculations. *Ann Neurol.* 1993;34: 622–625.
3. Tahmoush AJ, Alonso RJ, Tahmoush GP, Heiman-Patterson TD. Cramp-fasciculation syndrome: a treatable hyperexcitable peripheral nerve disorder. *Neurology.* 1991;41:1021–1024.
4. Roth G. The origin of fasciculations. *Ann Neurol.* 1982;12:542–547.
5. Kimura J. Routine needle electromyography. In: Bertorini TE, ed. *Clinical Evaluation and Diagnostic Tests for Neuromuscular Disorders.* Boston, MA: Butterworth-Heinemann; 2002:331–364.
6. Meadows JC, Marsden CD, Harriman DG. Chronic spinal muscular atrophy in adults: 1. The Kugelberg-Welander syndrome. *J Neurol Sci.* 1969;9:527–550.
7. Rietschel M, Rudnik-Schoneborn S, Zerres K. Clinical variability of autosomal dominant spinal muscular atrophy. *J Neurol Sci.* 1992; 107:65–73.
8. Stalberg E, Chu J, Bril V, et al. Automatic analysis of the EMG interference pattern. *Electroencephalogr Clin Neurophysiol.* 1983; 56(6):672–681.
9. Rudnik-Schoneborn S, Lutzenrath S, Borkowska J, et al. Analysis of creatine kinase activity in 504 patients with proximal spinal muscular atrophy types I–III from the point of view of progression and severity. *Eur Neurol.* 1998;39(3):154–162.
10. Harrison TB, Benatar M. Accuracy of repetitive nerve stimulation for diagnosis of the cramp-fasciculation syndrome. *Muscle Nerve.* 2007;35(6):776–780.
11. de Carvalho M, Swash M. Cramps, muscle pain, and fasciculations: not always benign? *Neurology.* 2004;63:721–723.
12. Liewluck T, Klein CJ, Jones, LK. Jr. Cramp-fasciculation syndrome in patients with and without neural autoantibodies. *Muscle Nerve.* 2014;49(3):351–356.
13. Schiffer D, Brignolio F, Chio A, et al. Clinical-anatomic study of a family with bulbo-spinal muscular atrophy in adults. *J Neurol Sci.* 1986;73:11–22.
14. Ikezoe K, Yoshimura T, Taniwaki T, et al. Autosomal dominant familial spinal and bulbar muscular atrophy with gynecomastia. *Neurology.* 1999;53(9):2187–2189.
15. Takashima H, Nakagawa M, Nakahara K, Suehara M, et al. A new type of heredity motor and sensory neuropathy linked to chromosome 3. *Ann Neurol.* 1997;41(6):771–780.

107 CASE

A Young Man With Large and Stiff Muscles

An 18-year-old patient had complained of muscle stiffness since he was 2½ years old, impairing his ability to exercise. He felt less stiff after warming up, and cold made the symptoms worse. His past medical history was unremarkable, and a review of systems was negative. He denied weakness or other neurologic symptoms. Family history revealed that his mother had muscle stiffness with a well-developed musculature all her life.

On examination he had normal mentation and cranial nerves, except for delayed relaxation of the orbicularis oculi muscles after forceful contraction. He was well built with prominent muscles (Fig. 107-1) but had no weakness. There was delayed relaxation after a muscle contraction from gripping or percussion. Reflexes, coordination sensory tests, and the rest of the examination were normal.

WHAT IS THE MOST LIKELY DIAGNOSIS?

The differential diagnosis of muscle enlargement includes hereditary myopathies, such as Becker's dystrophy, and some limb-girdle dystrophies, myotonia congenita, amyloidosis, hypothyroidism, stiff-person syndrome, and parasitic infection, among others (Table 107-1). Myotonic dystrophy sometimes presents initially without prominent weakness or atrophy, but those patients do not have muscle hypertrophy. Schwartz–Jampel syndrome manifests with muscle hypertrophy and myotonia, but the patient did not have the short stature or skeletal anomalies seen in this disease.[1] The family history and early onset are against an acquired disorder of muscle irritability such as Isaacs syndrome.[2] He had no activity-exacerbated myotonia to suggest paramyotonia congenita.[3]

The most likely consideration in this case with hereditary muscle hypertrophy and myotonia is myotonia congenita, Thomsen type.

AN EMG TEST WAS PERFORMED

Motor Nerve Studies

Nerve and Site	Latency (ms)	Amplitude (mV)	Conduction Velocity (m/s)
Median Nerve R.	**Normal ≤ 4.2**	**Normal ≥ 6**	**Normal ≥ 50**
Wrist	3.2	15	–
Elbow	6.7	15	59
Peroneal Nerve R.	**Normal ≤ 5.7**	**Normal ≥ 3**	**Normal ≥ 40**
Ankle	4.7	8	–
Fibular head	12.7	7	42
Knee	14.1	7	46

F-Wave Studies

Nerve	Latency (ms)	Normal Latency ≤ (ms)
Median nerve R.	27.8	30
Peroneal nerve R.	48.0	54

Sensory Nerve Studies

Nerve	Onset Latency (ms)	Normal Onset Latency ≤ (ms)	Peak Latency (ms)	Normal Peak Latency ≤ (ms)	Amp (μV)	Normal Amp ≥ (μV)	Conduction Velocity (m/s)	Normal Conduction Velocity ≥ (m/s)
Median nerve R.	2.3	2.6	2.8	3.1	35	20	57	50
Sural nerve R.	3.1	3.5	3.6	4.0	20	11	45	40

EMG Data

Muscle	Insrt Activity	Fibs	Pos Waves	Fasc	Amp	Dur	Poly	Pattern
Deltoid R.	**Myot**	None	None	None	Norm	Norm	None	Full
Biceps brachii R.	**Myot**	None	None	None	Norm	Norm	None	Full
Flexor carpi radialis R.	**Myot**	None	None	None	Norm	Norm	None	Full
Extensor digitorum com. R.	**Myot**	None	None	None	Norm	Norm	None	Full
First dorsal interosseous R.	**Myot**	None	None	None	Norm	Norm	None	Full
Vastus lateralis R.	**Myot**	None	None	None	Norm	Norm	None	Full
Tibialis anterior R.	**Myot**	None	None	None	Norm	Norm	None	Full
Gastrocnemius R.	**Myot**	None	None	None	Norm	Norm	None	Full

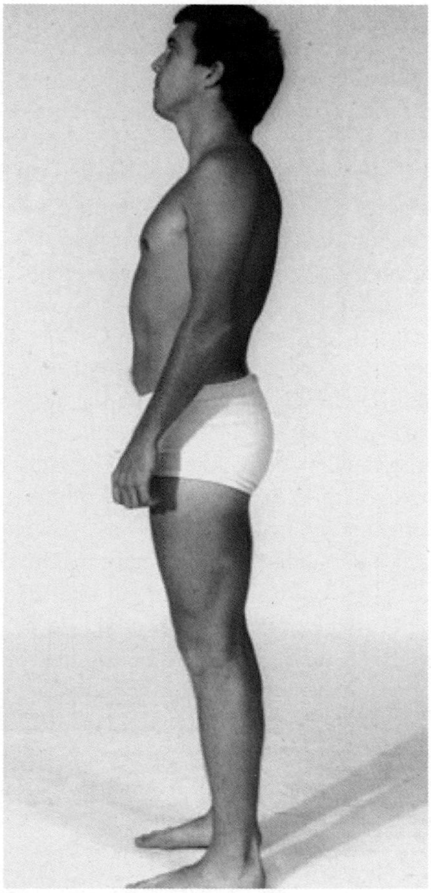

FIG. 107-1 Notice patient's prominent muscles.

TABLE 107-1 Neuromuscular Causes of Muscle Hypertrophy

Generalized hypertrophy
Juvenile spinal muscular atrophy (usually early, mainly calves)
Postpolio pseudohypertrophy
Acromegaly
Hypothyroid myopathy
Schwartz–Jampel syndrome
Isaacs syndrome
Myotonia congenita
Paramyotonia congenita
Duchenne muscular dystrophy (can be generalized but mainly in the calves)
Becker muscular dystrophy
Limb-girdle muscular dystrophy (mainly in the calves, but could be generalized in some)
Flier syndrome
Sarcoidosis (can be focal)
Parasites (cysticercosis, schistosomiasis, and trichinosis)
Amyloidosis
Focal hypertrophy
Sarcoidosis
Radiculopathy of other causes of partial denervation (e.g., tethered cord)
Tendon rupture

Adapted from Griggs R, Mendell JR, Miller RG, eds. Evaluation of the patient with myopathy. In: *Evaluation and Treatment of Myopathies*. Contemporary Neurology Series. Philadelphia, PA: FA Davis; 1995:26.

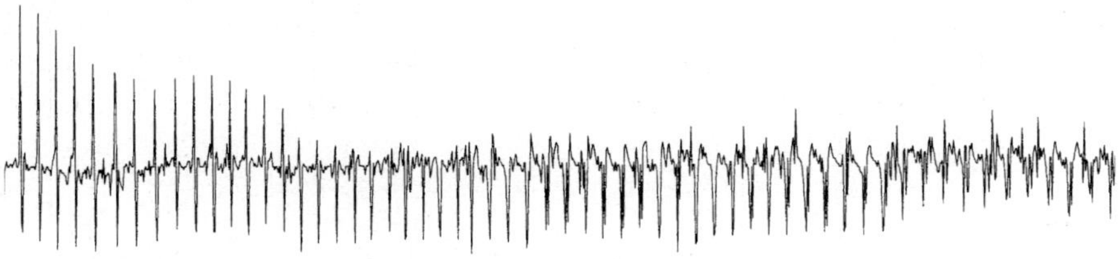

FIG. 107-2 Myotonic discharges in first dorsal interosseus muscle (200 μV/20 ms).

WHAT WERE THE EMG FINDINGS?

This study showed normal nerve conduction tests. The motor unit action potentials were normal, and there were characteristic waxing and waning myotonic discharges in the needle test, indicating a myotonic disorder, likely myotonia congenita (Fig. 107-2).

DISCUSSION

Myotonia, a term that comes from the Greek words *myo* (muscle) and *tonus* (tension), was initially used by Strumpell in 1891 (cited in Ref. 4) to describe muscle stiffness due to hyperexcitability of the muscle during voluntary contraction or percussion, causing delayed relaxation. Myotonia decreases during increased activity, or "warming up," unlike paradoxical myotonia in paramyotonia congenita in which the stiffness increases with activity.[3,4] Clinical myotonia can also be seen in myotonic dystrophy and, by a lesser degree, in hyperkalemic periodic paralysis.

Myotonia congenita is a hereditary disorder of the muscle chloride channel, caused by mutations of the *CLCN1* gene. It manifests with muscle enlargement and clinical myotonia. The abnormalities of the chloride channel cause repetitive depolarization of the muscle membrane, appearing on the EMG as repetitive discharges that wax and wane in amplitude. Myotonia congenita, or nondystrophic myotonia (to differentiate it from myotonic dystrophy), is thus a muscle chloride channelopathy.

Muscle channelopathies are disorders of ion channels. They also include malignant hyperthermia, which affects the calcium channel–ryanodine receptor; paramyotonia congenita and hyperkalemic periodic paralysis, which are caused by disorders of the voltage-gated muscle calcium channel; and hypokalemic paralysis, which could be a calcium or sodium channelopathy.

WHAT CAUSES MYOTONIA?

Normally when a nerve impulse arrives at a neuromuscular junction, the voltage-gated calcium channel opens, causing calcium influx that triggers the release of acetylcholine. Acetylcholine attaches to the muscle receptor, opening its ionic channel and triggering an endplate potential. When this endplate potential exceeds the depolarization threshold, the voltage-gated muscle sodium channels are open, leading to voltage changes that produce the muscle action potential. The depolarization travels through the tubular system and then triggers the opening of the calcium channels of the sarcoplasmic reticulum, initiating the mechanism of muscle contraction.

During generation of the muscle action potential, the voltage-gated muscle sodium channel allows extracellular sodium to enter the intercellular space, increasing the intracellular muscle resting potential from −80 to +20 or +30 mV, causing sarcoplasmic depolarization. Repolarization is initiated by closing the sodium channels and opening the voltage-gated potassium channels.

After depolarization, potassium ions accumulate in the tubular system until they are removed by the sodium-potassium ATPase pump. The prolonged presence of potassium in the extracellular space can cause repetitive depolarizations which are buffered by chloride that mobilizes due to the high conductance of the chloride channel.

In chloride channelopathies, chloride channels function poorly. Chloride ions cannot egress to neutralize the extracellular potassium causing excessive depolarization currents, which manifest as myotonia[5–8] (Fig. 107-3). In myotonia congenita the repetitive muscle depolarization causes muscle hypertrophy.

Similar mechanisms of a *loss of function* of the chloride channel occur in myotonic mice and goats, also called "fainting goats," which drop to the ground after becoming stiff from stimuli such as loud noise[7] (Fig. 107-4). Detailed studies of these animals have allowed a better understanding of the pathophysiology of myotonia in humans.

The myotonia in sodium channelopathies, such as hyperkalemic paralysis and paramyotonia congenita, is caused by a *gain of function* of the sodium channel. This allows an excessive influx of sodium into the intracellular space during depolarization. Thus the muscle fiber does not return to its resting state but remains depolarized. This prolonged depolarization produces repetitive discharges (myotonia), or inexcitability, causing weakness[9] (see Fig. 107-3B).

There are two major forms of myotonia congenita, autosomal-recessive (Becker's type) and autosomal-dominant (Thomsen's type), both caused by a mutation of the CLCN1 channel. The autosomal-recessive form starts in late childhood and tends to be much more severe (Fig. 107-5), while the autosomal-dominant type starts early but has a less severe phenotype.

Characteristically, patients complain of muscle stiffness, which improves with exercise (in paramyotonia congenita, a sodium channelopathy, myotonia worsens with exercise), and develop muscle enlargement. Occasionally, patients have reflexive stiffness, which could make them fall after hearing a loud noise. They are usually not weak but could develop weakness later, particularly in the recessive form. The neurologic examination is normal, except for muscle hypertrophy and clinical myotonia (Figs. 107-6 and 107-7).

The CIC1 channel is *homodimeric* and is encoded by the *CLCN1* gene in chromosome 7q35.[4] Splice mutations cause the recessive phenotype, while truncations and missense mutations of the gene can cause either the dominant or the recessive form.

The CIC1 channel has a double-barrel structure with two independent pores having fast and slow opening mechanisms. Both pores are affected by the recessive mutation. A slow-gated structure is affected by the dominant mutation.[10]

A less frequent third form of myotonia congenita is characterized by muscle stiffness but also by pain, which is not seen in the other two forms. This third form is caused by mutations of the sodium channel.[8,11]

In myotonia congenita the serum creatine kinase may be mildly elevated. Nerve conduction studies are normal, and

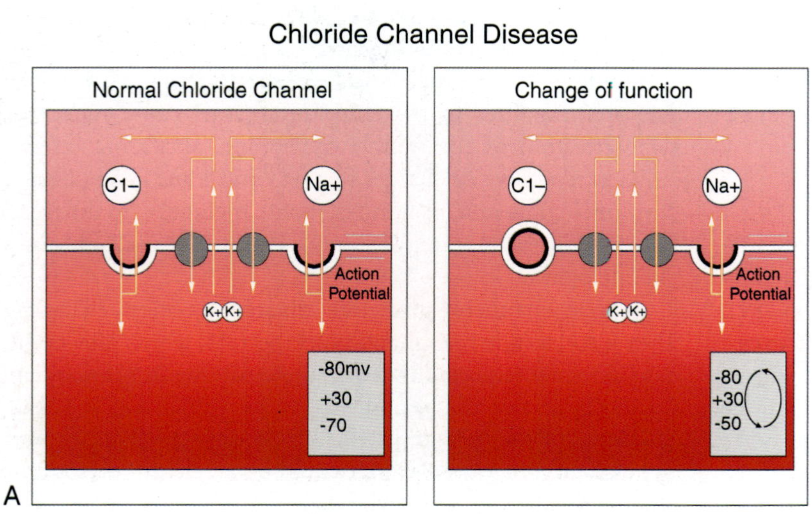

FIG. 107-3 A, Muscle membrane in the T tubular system, enlarged on the right, from a normal muscle (*upper representation*), and from a patient with myotonia congenita (*lower representation*). The circles are the channels. Notice in the normal muscle where, on generation of an action potential, there is increased entrance of sodium to the intracellular space from the tubular system, and the membrane depolarizes. This is counteracted by the exit of potassium. The membrane then returns to normal. In chloride channelopathy (*bottom*) the chloride channel does not function, and during depolarization there is an excess of potassium in the lumen of the tubular system. Chloride ions do not exit to neutralize this so that the membrane takes longer to achieve resting state and can have repeated depolarizations.

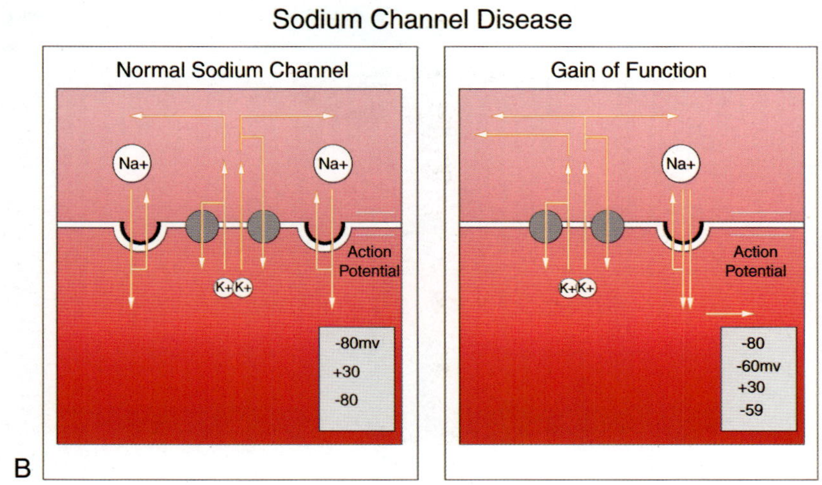

FIG. 107-3, cont'd B, Notice in a normal muscle (*upper representation*), sodium enters the cell and the membrane goes from −80 mV and becomes positive generating an action potential. In a patient with sodium channelopathy (*lower representation*), there is an excessive entrance of sodium so that the fiber does not return to resting membrane potential of −80 mV. Modified with permission from Hoffman E. Duchenne-Becker muscular dystrophy and the non-dystrophic myotonias: paradigms for loss of function and change of function of gene products. *Arch Neurol.* 1993;30(11):1227–1237.

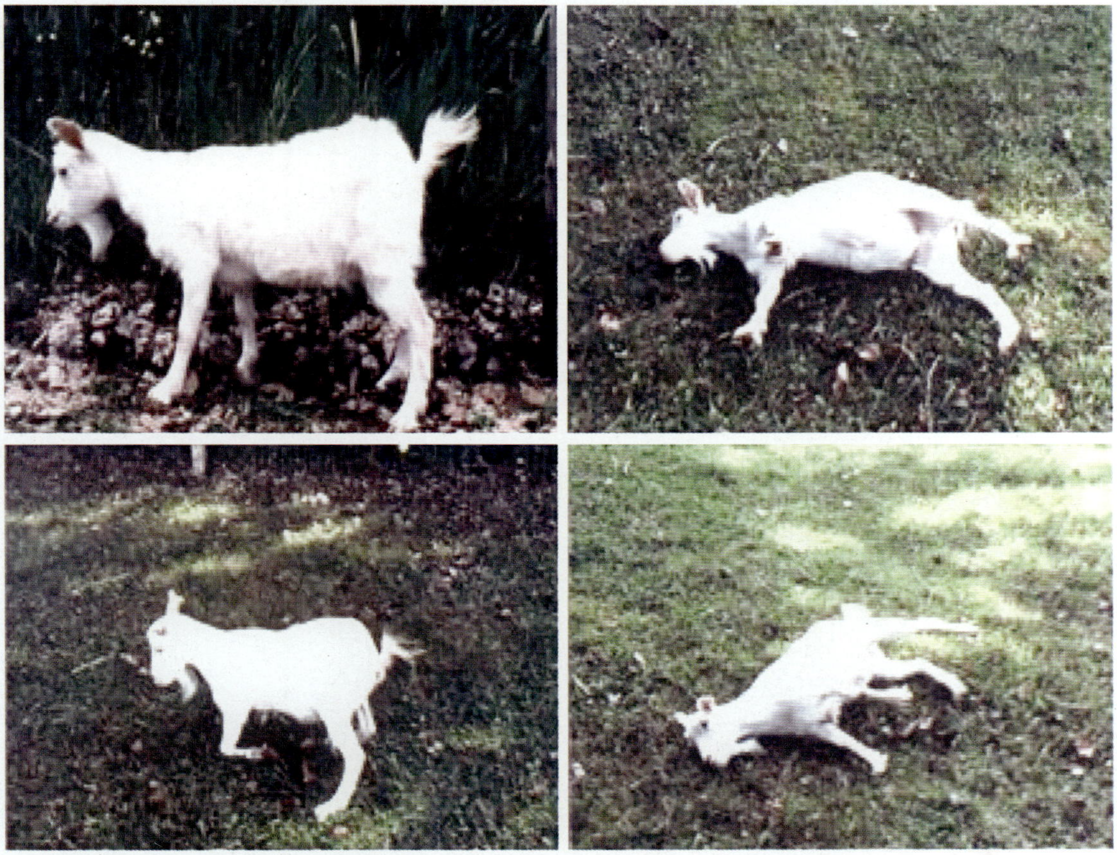

FIG. 107-4 Myotonic goat falling to the ground after hearing a loud noise. Courtesy Dr. Daniel Jacome.

needle electromyography shows normal- or short-duration motor unit action potentials and the characteristic waxing and waning myotonic discharges at rest or with needle movement. These increase with cooling. Repetitive nerve stimulation tests may show a decremental response of the CMAP, particularly in the recessive form of the disease.[11] In those patients there is an absence of type IIB muscle fibers on muscle biopsy.[12] The biopsy is otherwise normal or shows nonspecific findings.

The *short exercise test* is used in the electrophysiologic evaluation of channelopathies.[13] This consists of stimulating the ulnar nerve and recording the CMAP at the abductor digiti minimi muscle for 2–3 minutes to establish a baseline with single stimulation at 1-minute intervals. The patient then performs a tetanic muscle contraction for 5–10 seconds. The nerve is immediately stimulated after this, and every 10 seconds until the CMAP returns to the baseline, thereafter for 1–2 minutes. In

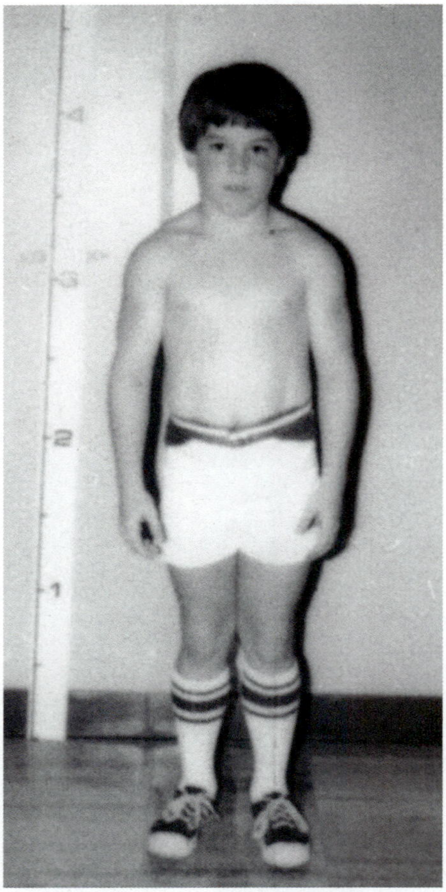

FIG. 107-5 A child with autosomal-recessive myotonia congenita.

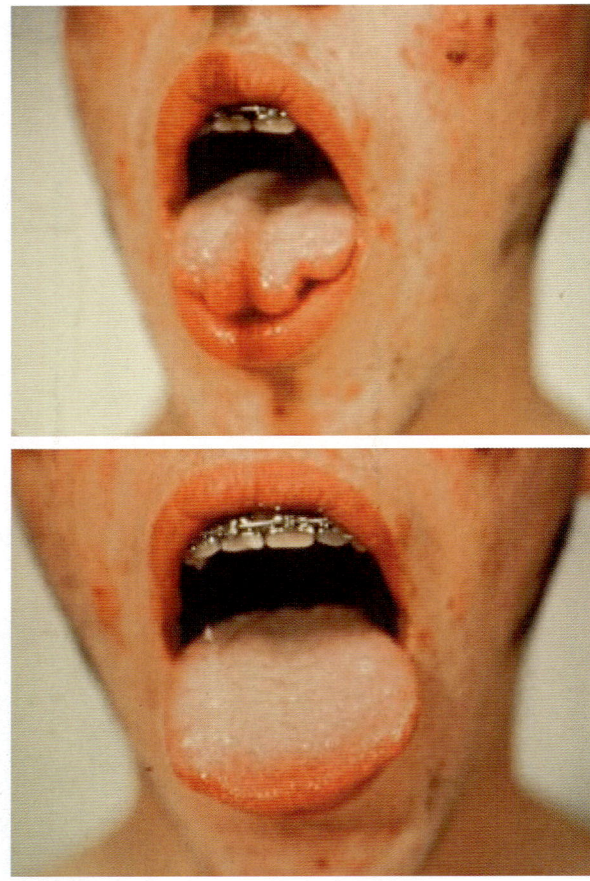

FIG. 107-7 A gentle tap of the tongue produces myotonic contractions (*top*) in another patient the tongue is seen at rest (*bottom*).

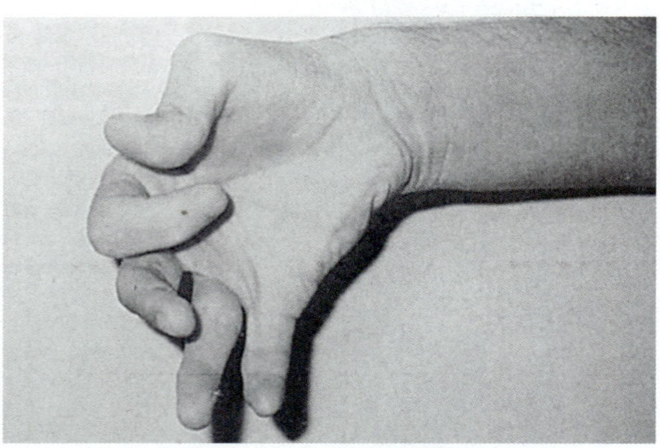

FIG. 107-6 Myotonia. Notice the patient's delay in opening the hand after grip.

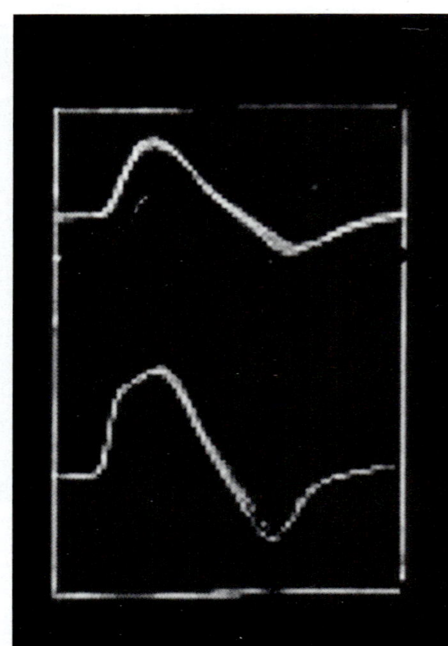

FIG. 107-8 CMAP of the abductor digiti minimi muscle stimulating the ulnar nerve before (*bottom*) and after (*top*) 10 s of tetanic contraction.

chloride channelopathy there is a lower amplitude of the CMAP immediately after the tetanic contraction (Fig. 107-8), and this recovers after 1–2 minutes.[14] The decreased amplitude is more pronounced in the recessive form. In paramyotonia congenita the CMAP might not recover to its normal size for several minutes.

The *prolonged exercise test* uses the same recording technique as the short exercise test, except in this, the patient is asked to contract the muscle for 15 seconds, then relaxing for 5 seconds, repeating this cycle for 3–5 minutes. The CMAP is recorded before and after the exercise. The nerve is then stimulated immediately and at every 1–2 minutes for 40–60 minutes. In periodic paralysis the CMAP does not change immediately after the exercise or could become only slightly larger, but there is a decline in the CMAP amplitude after 20–40 minutes. This test is usually normal in myotonia congenita[15] and is used in periodic paralysis.[14]

WHAT IS THE TREATMENT OF MYOTONIA CONGENITA?

There is no cure for myotonia congenita, and the treatment consists of the use of sodium channel blockers, such as carbamazepine, or antiarrhythmics, such as mexiletine.[16] Tocainide can also be used,[17,18] but it could produce toxic effects.

SUMMARY

This young patient presented with muscle hypertrophy and stiffness, and myotonia was present clinically and on EMG. These are consistent with myotonia congenita, a muscle chloride channelopathy.

IMPORTANT POINTS

- The differential diagnosis of muscle hypertrophy includes myotonia congenita, hypothyroidism, amyloidosis, Isaacs syndrome, some forms of limb-girdle muscular dystrophies, myotubular myopathy, dystrophinopathies such as Becker dystrophy, stiff-person syndrome, Schwartz–Jampel syndrome, and parasite infestations.
- Myotonia congenita manifests by muscle stiffness and enlargement without weakness. This condition is caused by the mutation of the *CLCN1* gene in chromosome 7q35. There is an autosomal-recessive form and an autosomal-dominant form. A third form is caused by the mutation of the sodium channel and is associated with muscle pain.
- In myotonia congenita the genetic defect causes loss of function of the chloride channel, which results in decreased chloride conductance and repeated muscle depolarizations.
- Myotonia is treated with sodium channel antagonists such as carbamazepine and mexiletine.

REFERENCES

1. Ishpekova B, Rasheva M, Moskov M. Schwartz-Jampel syndrome: clinical, electromyographic and genetic studies. *Electromyogr Clin Neurophysiol.* 1996;36(3):151–155.
2. Isaacs H. A syndrome of cutaneous muscle fiber activity. *J Neurol Neurosurg Psychiatry.* 1961;24:319–325.
3. Jurkat-Rott K, Muller-Hocker J, Pongratz D, Lehmann-Horn F. Chloride and sodium channel myotonias. In: Karpati G, ed. *Structural and Molecular Basis of Skeletal Muscle Diseases.* Basel, Switzerland: ISM Neuropath Press; 2002:90–94.
4. Jurkat-Rott K, Lehmann-Horn F, Rudel R. Chloride and sodium channel myotonias. In: Rose MR, Griggs RL, eds. *Channelopathies of the Nervous System.* Boston, MA: Butterworth-Heinemann; 2001:141–157.
5. Adrian RH, Bryant SH. On the repetitive discharge in myotonic muscle fibers. *J Physiol.* 1974;240:505–515.
6. Lehmann-Horn F, Jurkat-Rott K. Voltage-gated ion channels and hereditary disease. *Physiol Rev.* 1999;79:1317–1372.
7. Bryant SH. Cable properties of external intercostal muscle fibers from myotonic and nonmyotonic goats. *J Physiol.* 1969;204(3):539–550.
8. Koch MC, Steinmeyer K, Lorenz C, et al. The skeletal muscle chloride channel in dominant and recessive human myotonia. *Science.* 1992;257:797–800.
9. Lehmann-Horn F, Kuther G, Ricker K, et al. Adynamia episodica hereditaria with myotonia: a non-inactivating sodium current and the effect of extracellular pH. *Muscle Nerve.* 1987;10:363–374.
10. Saviane C, Conti F, Pusch M. The muscle chloride channel CIC-1 has double-barreled appearance that is differentially affected in dominant and recessive myotonia. *J Gen Physiol.* 1999;113:457–468.
11. McMannis P. Channelopathies. In: Brown W, Bolton CHF, Aminoff MJ, eds. *Neuromuscular Function and Disease.* Philadelphia, PA: WB Saunders; 2002:1459–1478.
12. Crews J, Kaiser KK, Brooke MH. Muscle pathology of myotonia congenita. *J Neurol Sci.* 1976;28(4):449–457.
13. Streib EW. AAEM minimonograph 27: differential diagnosis of myotonic syndromes. *Muscle Nerve.* 1987;10(7):603–615.
14. Kuntzer T, Flocard F, Vial C, et al. Exercise test in muscle channelopathies and other muscle disorders. *Muscle Nerve.* 2000; 23(7):1089–1094.
15. Boegle AK, Narayanswami P. Treatment and management of disorders of neuromuscular hyperexcitability and periodic paralysis Chapter 18. In: Bertorini TE, ed. *Neuromuscular Disorders: Treatment and Management.* 2nd ed. Amsterdam, Netherlands: Elsevier; 2022:414–445.
16. Leheup B, Himon F, Morali A, et al. Value of mexiletine in the treatment of Thomsen-Becker myotonia. *Arch Fr Pediatr.* 1986; 43(1):49–50.
17. Rudel R, Dengler R, Ricker K, et al. Improved therapy of myotonia with the lidocaine derivative tocainide. *J Neurol.* 1980;222(4): 275–278.
18. Puniani TS, Bertorini TE. Tocainide therapy in muscle cramps and spasms due to neuromuscular disease. *Muscle Nerve.* 1991; 14(3):280–285.

108 CASE

A Woman With Generalized Increased Insertional Activity on EMG

A 41-year-old woman with no past medical history was referred for an EMG because of right shoulder pain. She denies neck pain. There was no family history. She denies stiffness.

Physical examination was unremarkable, except for some tenderness to palpation of the shoulder joint. Muscle strength, reflex, and sensory exams were normal.

Laboratory studies included a normal creatine kinase (CK) level.

AN EMG TEST WAS PERFORMED

Motor Nerve Conduction

Nerve and Site	Muscle	Latency (ms)	Ref. (ms)	Amplitude (mV)	Ref. (mV)	Distance (mm)	Velocity (m/s)	Ref. (m/s)
R. Peroneal								
Ankle	EDB	4.69	≤6.50	3.4	≥2.0	90		
Fibula (head)	EDB	11.25		3.2		300	45.7	≥44.0
Popliteal fossa	EDB	12.71		3.1		80	54.9	≥44.0
R. Median								
Wrist	APB	3.69	≤4.40	6.5	≥4.0	70		
Elbow	APB	8.77		5.5		300	59.0	≥49.0
R. Ulnar								
Wrist	ADM	3.02	≤3.30	11.7	≥6.0	30		
Below elbow	ADM	7.19		10.5		220	52.8	≥49.0
Above elbow	ADM	9.06		11.1		120	64.0	≥49.0

F-Wave Studies

Nerve	F-Latency (ms)	Ref. (ms)	M-Latency (ms)
R. Peroneal—EDB	12.5	≤56.0	48.4
R. Median—APB	30.0	≤31.0	8.8
R. Ulnar—ADM	30.5	≤32.0	9.1

Sensory Nerve Conduction

Nerve and Site	Rec. Site	Peak Latency (ms)	Ref. (ms)	Amplitude (μV)	Ref. (μV)	Segments	Distance (mm)
R. Sural—Ankle (Calf)							
Calf	Ankle	3.2	≤4.4	12	≥6.0	Calf–ankle	140
R. Ulnar—Digit V (Antidromic)							
Wrist	Dig V	2.7	≤3.1	***22***	≥17.0	Wrist–Dig V	110
R. Median—Digit II (Antidromic)							
Wrist	Dig II	2.5	≤3.5	***42***	≥20.0	Wrist–Dig II	130
R. Median—Palmar (Orthodromic)							
Mid-palm	Wrist	1.8	≤2.2	***55***	≥50.0	Mid-palm–wrist	80

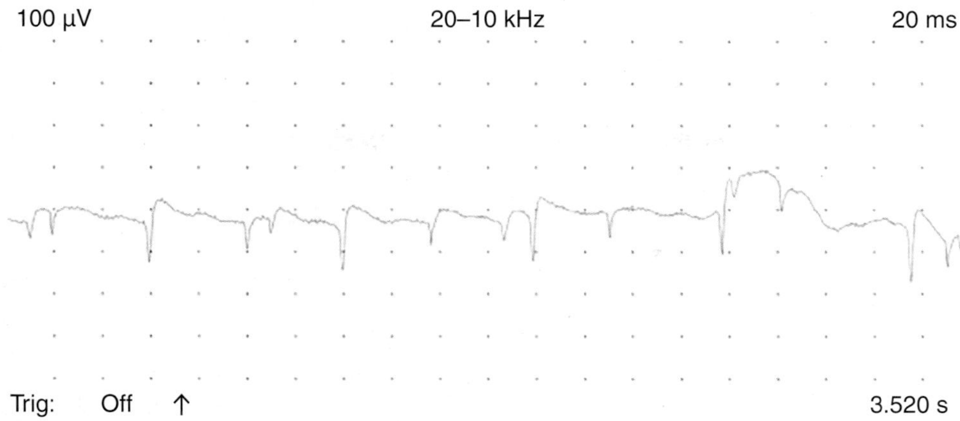

FIG. 108-1 Train of positive waves provoked by needle movement in electromyogram of the right vastus lateralis.

H-waves

Nerve	H-Lat (ms)		
	Left	Right	Ref
Tibial—Soleus	31.6	30.6	≤34

EMG Summary Table

			Spontaneous				MUAP			Recruitment	
Muscle	Nerve	Roots	IA	Fib	PSW	Fasc	Duration	Amplitude	PPP	Pattern	Effort
R. Deltoid	Axillary	C5–C6	Normal	1+[a]	1+	None	Decr.	Normal	Normal	Normal	Normal
R. Biceps brachii	Musculocutaneous	C5–C6	Incr.	1+[a]	1+[a]	None	Normal	Decr.	Normal	Normal	Normal
R. Iliopsoas	Femoral	L2–L3	Normal	None	None	None	Normal	Normal	Normal	Normal	Normal
R. Quadriceps	Femoral	L2–L4	Incr.	1+[a]	1+[a]	None	Decr.	Decr.	Normal	Normal	Normal
R. Tibialis anterior	Deep peroneal (fibular)	L4–L5	Normal	None	None	None	Normal	Normal	Normal	Normal	Normal
R. Gastrocnemius (medial head)	Tibial	S1–S2	Incr.	1+[a]	1+[a]	None	Normal	Normal	Normal	Normal	Normal
L. Tibialis anterior	Deep peroneal (fibular)	L4–L5	Incr.	1+[a]	1+[a]	None	Normal	Normal	Normal	Normal	Normal
L. Gastrocnemius (medial head)	Tibial	S1–S2	Incr.	1+[a]	1+[a]	None	Decr.	Normal	Normal	Normal	Normal

[a]Myotonia.

An EMG revealed increased insertional muscle activity in all muscles sampled (Fig. 108-1) proximally and distally. This appeared as short runs of positive, short waves. Nerve conductions were normal. Motor unit action potentials were normal.

WHAT SHOULD BE DONE NEXT?

This patient has increased insertional activity on EMG in various muscles and we considered that these findings represented myotonia. This could have many causes, but her normal CPK, lack of family history, lack of weakness, and normal motor unit action potentials suggest that this could be a chloride channelopathy or PROMMs. An MRI of the shoulder showed subacromial bursitis.

DNA sequencing was done, and the patient had evidence of *CLCNA1* gene mutation that revealed C2 to T transition at position 1649 resulting in threonine and methionine substitution in codon 550. There were no increased repeat expansions of the *DMPK* and *ZNF* genes.

DISCUSSION

Increased insertional activity, positive waves, and myotonia originate in muscle fibers when there is destabilization of the membrane potential.[1] Insertional activity results from tissue damage from the needle insertion by producing unstable membrane potential. This could be seen in a variety of conditions including some myopathies like Pompe disease, other metabolic and inflammatory myopathies, some muscular dystrophies, and toxic myopathies. Wiechers and Johnson reported increased insertional activity in asymptomatic people for which the cause is unknown,[2] and for this "EMG disease" has been quoted. This has also been considered a form of myotonia congenita. Because myotonia congenita has clinical variability in individuals and affected families the term "latent myotonia" was used.[3] Barkhaus and Nandedkar[4] demonstrated slow myotonic discharges in DM1, and they reported that this could be manifest by seeing fibrillations and positive waves.[4] We have also observed a similar phenomenon in a patient with DM2,[5] a condition in which the clinical findings may not be obvious.

The *CLCN1* gene expresses the major skeletal muscular chloride channel that contributes to stabilize the resting membrane potential. Mutations of the genes expressing this channel could cause myotonia.[6,7] The DNA mutation in this case has been reported in those with an autosomal-dominant inheritance,[8] but this patient did not have a positive family history of the disorder.

SUMMARY

This woman had shoulder pain from joint disease and no symptoms of muscle disease. She was found to have diffuse increased insertional activity on EMG; DNA testing revealed that she had a myotonia congenita mutation.

IMPORTANT POINTS

- Diffuse insertional activity on EMG could be a form of myotonia.
- Electrical myotonia can be seen in several conditions including myotonic dystrophy and chloride channelopathies, Pompe disease, carnitine deficiency, some dystrophies, and inflammatory and toxic myopathies. Patients with myotonia or increased insertional activity on EMG should be investigated for a channelopathy.
- There is no such thing as "EMG disease."

REFERENCES

1. Dumitru D. Single muscle fiber discharges (insertional activity, end-plate potentials, positive sharp waves and fibrillation potentials): a unifying proposal. *Muscle Nerve*. 1996;19: 216–226.
2. Wiechers DG, Johnson EW. Diffuse abnormal electromyographic insertional activity: a preliminary report. *Arch Phys Med Rehabil*. 1979;60:419–422.
3. Colding-Jorgensen E. Phenotypic variability in myotonia congenita. *Muscle Nerve*. 2005;32:19–34.
4. Barkhaus PE, Nandedkar SD. "Slow" myotonic discharges. *Muscle Nerve*. 2006;34:799–800.
5. Pendley C, Mansour S, Bertorini TE. Myotonic myopathy type 2 with electrical myotonia without weakness. In: *Presented at The AANEM Annual Meeting*. Orlando, FL; 2012.
6. George AL Jr, Sloan-Brown K, Fenichel GM, Mitchell GA, Spiegel R, Pascuzzi RM. Nonsense and missense mutations of the muscle chloride channel gene in patients with myotonia congenita. *Hum Mol Genet*. 1994;3:2071–2072.
7. Meyer-Klein C, Steinmeyer K, Ricker K, Jentsch TJ, Koch MC. Spectrum of mutations in the major human skeletal muscle chloride channel gene (CLCN1) leading to myotonia. *Am J Hum Genet*. 1995;57:1325–1334.
8. Wu FF, Ryan A, Devaney J, et al. Novel CLCN1 mutations with unique clinical and electrophysiological consequences. *Brain*. 2002;125:2392–2407.

A Boy With Short Stature, Small Jaw, Muscle Hypertrophy, and Stiffness

A 5-year-old boy was seen for muscle stiffness. He was the product of a normal pregnancy of a 27-year-old woman and had normal developmental milestones until he developed progressive limb spasms and difficulty opening and closing his mouth at age 2 years. He had marked muscle hypertrophy and short stature; he was treated with carbamazepine, which produced some improvement of the spasms. The patient had one healthy brother and two healthy sisters. Family history was otherwise negative.

Physical examination revealed a boy with short stature for his age at 92 cm, which is below the limits of normal for his age (normal, 100 cm) (Fig. 109-1), and a very small jaw, low-set ears, and prominent eyebrows. Neurologic examination was normal except for marked muscle hypertrophy, muscle stiffness, and percussion myotonia. The rest of the examination was unremarkable.

WHAT IS THE DIFFERENTIAL DIAGNOSIS?

The differential diagnosis of this patient with prominent muscles and stiffness is rather limited. It includes hypothyroidism, but the myotonia is against this diagnosis. Myotonia congenita is another consideration. The patient's facial deformities and prominent eyebrows, micrognathia, and short stature are consistent with Schwartz–Jampel syndrome.[1]

AN EMG TEST WAS PERFORMED

Motor Nerve Conduction

Nerve and Site	Latency (ms)	Amplitude (mV)	Conduction Velocity (m/s)
Ulnar Nerve R.	**Normal ≤ 3.6**	**Normal ≥ 8**	**Normal ≥ 50**
Wrist	2.4	13	–
Below elbow	4.8	13	63
Above elbow	6.8	12	60

Motor Nerve Conduction—cont'd

Nerve and Site	Latency (ms)	Amplitude (mV)	Conduction Velocity (m/s)
Ulnar Nerve R.	**Normal ≤ 3.6**	**Normal ≥ 8**	**Normal ≥ 50**
Peroneal Nerve R.	**Normal ≤ 5.7**	**Normal ≥ 3**	**Normal ≥ 40**
Ankle	2.3	6	–
Fibular head	5.5	6	53
Knee	7.5	6	50

F-Wave Studies

Nerve	Latency (ms)	Normal Latency ≤ (ms)
Ulnar nerve R.	23.1	30
Peroneal nerve R.	41.0	54

Sensory Nerve Studies

Nerve	Onset Latency (ms)	Normal Onset Latency ≤ (ms)	Amp (μV)	Normal Amp ≥ (μV)
Ulnar nerve R.	2.6	3.1	18	13
Sural nerve R.	3.2	4.0	20	11

EMG Data

Muscle	Insrt Activity	Fibs	Pos Waves	Fasc	Amp	Dur	Poly	Pattern
Deltoid R.	**Myot CRDs**	None	None	None	Norm	**Brief**	**Few**	Full
Biceps brachii R.	**Myot CRDs**	None	None	None	Norm	**Brief**	**Many**	Full
First dorsal interosseous R.	**Myot CRDs**	None	None	None	Norm	**Brief**	**Few**	Full
Vastus lateralis R.	**Myot**	None	None	None	Norm	**Brief**	**Many**	Full
Tibialis anterior R.	**Myot CRDs**	None	None	None	Norm	**Brief**	**Few**	Full
Gastrocnemius R.	**Myot**	None	None	None	Norm	**Brief**	**Few**	Full

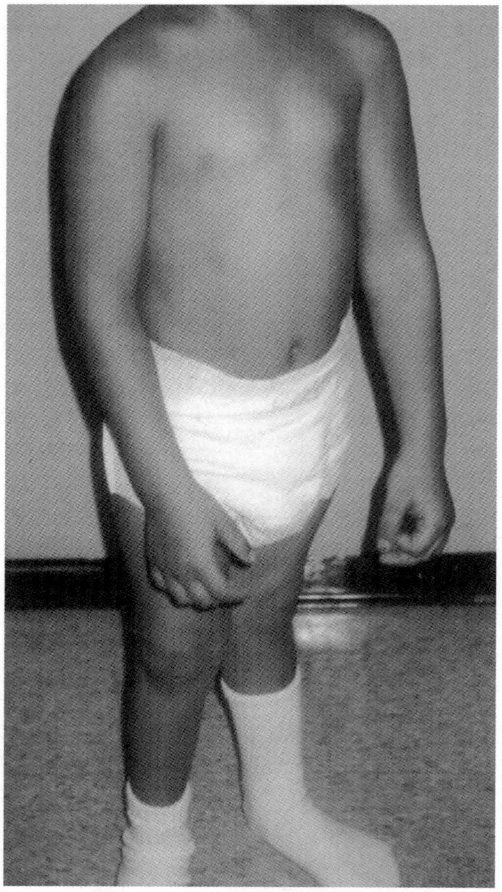

FIG. 109-1 Patient showing very prominent muscles. He had a small chin. The face is not shown at parent's request.

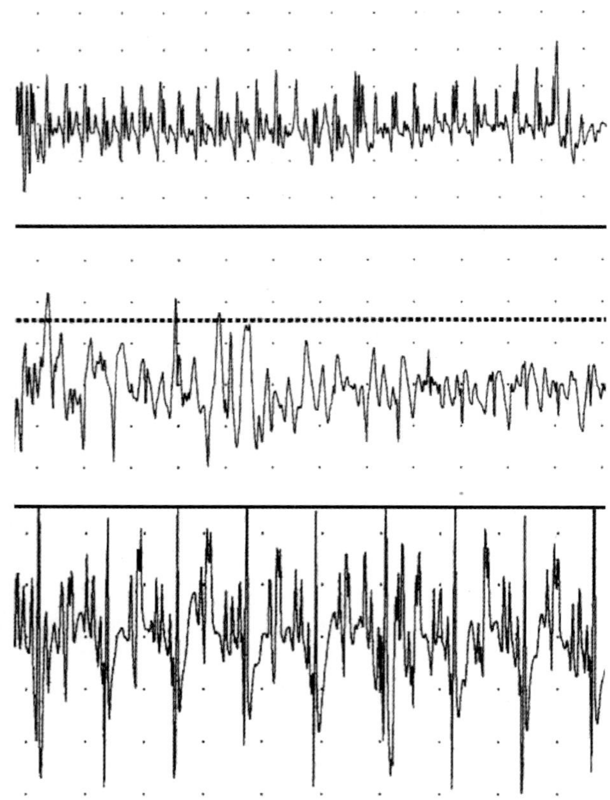

FIG. 109-2 Tracings of electromyography, quadriceps muscle, showing complex repetitive discharges (*top and bottom*) and myotonic discharges (*middle*) (100 μV/20 ms).

WHAT WERE THE EMG FINDINGS?

The EMG showed normal nerve conduction studies. The needle examination demonstrated prominent myotonia and complex repetitive discharges (CRDs) in all muscles tested (Fig. 109-2). The motor unit action potentials appeared small and polyphasic, but these were hard to evaluate because of poor cooperation.

Although there were only a few clinical skeletal anomalies, the patient was diagnosed as having Schwartz–Jampel syndrome.

Because of persistent jaw tightness, he received 5 units of botulinum toxin in each masseter muscle with significant relief.

WHAT IS SCHWARTZ–JAMPEL SYNDROME?

Schwartz–Jampel syndrome, or chondrodystrophic myotonia, is an autosomal-recessive disorder initially described in 1962.[1] It is characterized by short stature, skeletal and facial anomalies including small jaw, blepharophimosis, short neck, low-set ears, prominent eyebrows, hip dysplasia, pectus carinatum, pectus excavatum, myotonia, and muscle hypertrophy.[1,2] Other features include bowing or external rotation of the femur with coxa valga, talipes valgus or varus, hip dislocation, and arthrogryposis.

There are three forms of the disease.[2,3] Type 1A starts in childhood with moderate myotonia and dysmorphic features. Type 1B presents at birth with profound skeletal anomalies. Type 2 patients have contractures, bone deformities, and early death due to laryngeal spasms[4] or Stuve–Wiedemann syndrome which is really a different disorder.[5]

The syndrome is caused by mutations of chromosome 1p36.1–35 of the *perlecan* gene.[6–8] Although the exact pathophysiology of the myotonia is unclear, there is evidence of a persistent opening of the sodium channels causing spontaneous depolarization muscle contractions with secondary hypertrophy.[8] Patients could also have elevated serum creatine kinase levels.

Perlecan, or heparin sulfate proteoglycan, is a large multifunctional protein with homologies to laminin, low-density lipoprotein receptor neural cell adhesion molecules, and an epidermal growth factor. The protein contains domains that regulate fibroblast growth factor activity and release[9]; these have a role in clustering of acetylcholine receptors at the neuromuscular junctions.[10, 11] Perlecan interacts with integrins to connect the basal lamina with the plasma membrane. The mutation produces dysfunctional protein that disrupts the neuromuscular and cartilage–bone junctions.[8,11]

The treatment of Schwartz–Jampel syndrome includes sodium channel blockers, such as carbamazepine.[12] In this case we used local botulinum toxin injections, which relieved masseter spasms.

SUMMARY

This child has Schwartz–Jampel syndrome characterized by facial deformities, short stature, myotonia, and stiffness.

The treatment consists of carbamazepine, and, as in this case, botulinum toxin.

IMPORTANT POINTS

- Schwartz–Jampel syndrome is an autosomal-recessive disorder caused by a mutation of the *perlecan* gene at 1p36.1–35.
- The disease is associated with skeletal anomalies, facial deformities, myotonia, and short stature.
- Perlecan is a large multifunctional protein that participates in fibroblast growth factor release and activity.
- The treatment of this disease is symptomatic with sodium channel blockers, such as carbamazepine.

REFERENCES

1. Schwartz O, Jampel RS. Congenital blepharophimosis associated with a unique generalized myotonia. *Arch Ophthalmol.* 1962;68: 52–77.
2. Spaans F, Theunissen P, Reekers AD, et al. Schwartz-Jampel syndrome, I: clinical, electromyographic, and histologic studies. *Muscle Nerve.* 1990;13(6):516–527.
3. Giedion A, Boltshauser E, Briner J, et al. Heterogeneity in Schwartz-Jampel chondrodystrophic myotonia. *Eur J Pediatr.* 1997;156:214–223.
4. Spranger J, Hall BD, Hane B, et al. Spectrum of Schwartz-Jampel syndrome includes micromelic chondrodysplasia, kyphomelic dysplasia, and Burton disease. *Am J Med Genet.* 2000;94(4): 287–295.
5. Mallineni SK, You CKY, King NM. Schwartz-Jampel syndrome: a review of the literature and case report. *Spec Care Dentist.* 2012; 32(3):105–111.
6. Fontaine B, Nicole S, Topaloglu H, et al. Recessive Schwartz-Jampel syndrome (SJS): confirmation of linkage to chromosome 1p, evidence of genetic homogeneity and reduction of the SJS locus to a 3-cM interval. *Hum Genet.* 1996;98(3):380–385.
7. Kallunki PM, Eddy RL, Byers MG, et al. Cloning of human heparan sulfate proteoglycan core protein, assignment of the gene (HSPG2) to 1p36.1-p35 and identification of a BamHI restriction fragment length polymorphism. *Genomics.* 1991;11:389–396.
8. Hoffman EP, Pegoraro E. Heparin sulfate proteoglycan (perlecan) deficiency. Schwartz-Jampel syndrome. In: Karpati G, ed. *Structural and Molecular Basis of Skeletal Muscle Diseases.* Basel, Switzerland: ISN Neuropath Press; 2002:43–44.
9. Lehmann-Horn F, Iaizzo PA, Franke C, et al. Schwartz-Jampel syndrome, II: Na+ channel defect causes myotonia. *Muscle Nerve.* 1990;13(6):528–535.
10. Nugent MA, Nugent HM, Iozzo RV, et al. Perlecan is required to inhibit thrombosis after deep vascular injury and contributes to endothelial cell-mediated inhibition of intimal hyperplasia. *Proc Natl Acad Sci USA.* 2000;97:6722–6727.
11. Peng HB, Xie H, Rossi SG, Rotundo RL. Acetylcholinesterase clustering at the neuromuscular junction involves perlecan and dystroglycan. *J Cell Biol.* 1999;145:911–921.
12. Squires LA, Prangley J. Neonatal diagnosis of Schwartz-Jampel syndrome with dramatic response to carbamazepine. *Pediatr Neurol.* 1996;15(2):172–174.

110 CASE

An Elderly Woman With Muscle Spasms

An 81-year-old woman with a history of thyroidectomy for thyroid carcinoma presented 2 years later with recurrent muscle spasms, muscle pain, and weakness.

Her serum calcium levels were consistently in the range of 4.3–4.5 mEq/L (normal, 4.3–5.3 mEq/L), despite aggressive therapy with calcium (Os-Cal 1500 mg three times a day) and vitamin D (50,000 IU three times a week). She had carpopedal spasms that persisted, with weakness in the lower extremities, and she also developed difficulty swallowing.

Examination revealed a clinically ill-appearing woman. Cranial nerves and mentation were normal. She had mild leg weakness and stiffness. Reflexes were 2+ to 3+ symmetrical; there were no Babinski signs. Sensation was normal. There was no myotonia or fasciculations. She had positive Chvostek and Trousseau signs. The rest of the examination was normal.

WHAT IS THE DIFFERENTIAL DIAGNOSIS?

This woman had weakness and neuromuscular irritability of recent onset; for this the differential diagnosis is very limited. There was no history to suggest myotonia nor was this seen clinically. Muscle rigidity and spasms occur in hypothyroidism, but these are usually not accompanied by carpopedal spasms.[1] Acquired neuromyotonia, such as Isaacs syndrome, is a consideration and should be thought of in the differential diagnosis, but although generalized stiffness is seen in Isaacs syndrome, there are no carpopedal spasms.[2] The most likely possibility is tetany due to her hypocalcemia.[3]

It was determined that this patient developed hypoparathyroidism due to the removal of the parathyroid glands, which caused recurrent hypocalcemia and tetany.

AN EMG TEST WAS PERFORMED

Motor Nerve Studies

Nerve and Site	Latency (ms)	Amplitude (mV)	Conduction Velocity (m/s)
Peroneal Nerve R.	**Normal ≤ 5.7**	**Normal ≥ 3**	**Normal ≥ 40**
Ankle	5.3	4	–
Fibular head	8.6	4	51
Tibial Nerve L.	**Normal ≤ 5.3**	**Normal ≥ 4**	**Normal ≥ 40**
Ankle	4.8	4	–
Pop. fossa	11.6	4	54

This case was reported as Puniani TS, Bertorini TE. Tocainide therapy in muscle cramps and spasms due to neuromuscular disease. *Muscle Nerve*. 1991;14:382–385.

Motor Nerve Studies—cont'd

Nerve and Site	Latency (ms)	Amplitude (mV)	Conduction Velocity (m/s)
Ulnar Nerve R.	**Normal ≤ 3.6**	**Normal ≥ 8**	**Normal ≥ 50**
Wrist	3.2	9	–
Below elbow	6.7	9	51

F-Wave Studies

Nerve	Latency (ms)	Normal Latency ≤ (ms)
Peroneal nerve R.	52	54
Tibial nerve L.	53	54
Ulnar nerve R.	29	30

Sensory Nerve Studies

Nerve	Onset Latency (ms)	Normal Onset Latency ≤ (ms)	Peak Latency (ms)	Normal Peak Latency ≤ (ms)	Amp (μV)	Normal Amp ≥ (μV)	Conduction Velocity (m/s)	Normal Conduction Velocity ≥ (m/s)
Sural nerve R.	3.4	3.5	3.9	4.0	11	11	41	40
Ulnar nerve R.	2.5	2.6	3.0	3.1	13	13	50	50

EMG Data

Muscle	Insrt Activity	Fib	Pos Waves	Fasc	Amp	Config	Poly	Pattern
Thoracic paraspinals R.	**CRD**	None	None	None	Norm	Norm	None	Full
Vastus lateralis R.	Norm	None	None	None	Norm	**Multiplets**	None	Full
Biceps long head R.	Norm	None	None	None	Norm	**Multiplets**	None	Full

Continued

EMG Data—cont'd

Muscle	Insrt Activity	Fib	Pos Waves	Fasc	Amp	Config	Poly	Pattern
Tibialis anterior R.	Norm	None	None	None	Norm	**Multiplets**	None	Full
Gastrocnemius R.	Norm	None	None	None	Norm	Norm	None	Full
Deltoid R.	Norm	None	None	None	Norm	**Multiplets**	None	Full
Triceps R.	Norm	None	None	None	Norm	Norm	None	Full
Biceps brachii R.	Norm	None	None	None	Norm	Norm	None	Full
Extensor digitorum com. R.	Norm	None	None	None	Norm	Norm	None	Full
Flexor carpi ulnaris R.	Norm	None	None	None	Norm	Norm	None	Full
First dorsal interosseous R.	**CRD**	None	None	None	Norm	**Multiplets**	None	Full

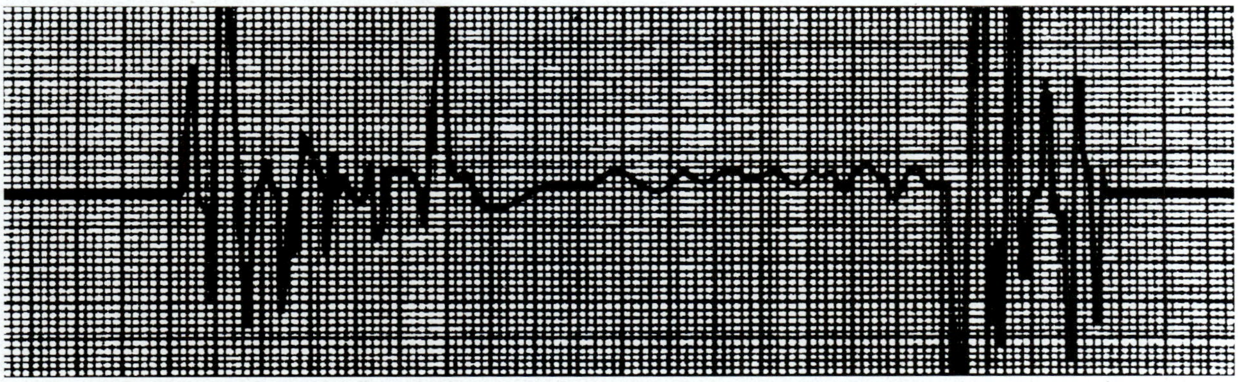

FIG. 110-1 EMG performed with a TECA TD20 machine, using sweep speed of 10 ms, gain of 200 mV, low-frequency filter of 20 Hz, and high-frequency filter of 10 kHz. Shows quadruplets muscle action potentials in left gastrocnemius muscle at rest.

WHAT WERE THE EMG FINDINGS?

The EMG revealed normal motor and sensory conduction results. The motor unit action potentials appeared normal, and she had no myotonia or denervation potentials. She had complex repetitive discharges and quadruplet potentials, in agreement with the diagnosis of tetany (Fig. 110-1).

WHAT SHOULD BE DONE NEXT?

She was treated appropriately with calcium supplement with minimal improvement; phenytoin 300 mg/day was added. This produced some symptomatic improvement, but tetany persisted with periodic worsening associated with fluctuations in serum calcium levels due to recurrent diarrhea, the cause of which was not apparent; this was treated symptomatically. Tocainide 200 mg twice a day abolished the symptoms after 4 days. Later, her diarrhea and hypocalcemia disappeared with oral calcium supplement and calcitriol.

DISCUSSION

This elderly woman, who had a previous thyroidectomy for thyroid carcinoma, developed resistant tetany, which was caused by hypocalcemia and is common in these patients.[3] This could also be caused by hypomagnesemia[4] causing neuromuscular irritability.[3,4] It is not known why her symptoms presented in spite of calcium-supplement therapy. The addition of calcitriol is more helpful, as regular vitamin D is inactive due to the lack of parathyroid hormone (PTH). Calcitriol is the active form of vitamin D_3 which stimulates intestinal calcium absorption and renal reabsorption, even though it actually suppresses PTH secretion and synthesis.

Most cases of acquired hypoparathyroidism are caused by the removal of the parathyroid gland during thyroidectomy. Hypoparathyroidism can produce several neurologic manifestations, such as chronic myopathy with increased serum creatine kinase levels,[5,6] and even myoglobinuria.[7] The most characteristic manifestations, however, are tetany, caused by hypocalcemia when plasma calcium levels are below 4.3 mg/dL, and hypomagnesemia, which is aggravated by alkalosis, making the axons hyperexcitable with spontaneous repetitive discharges. Symptoms of tetany include paresthesias and carpopedal spasms, which consist of extension and adduction of the fingers with flexion of the fingers at the carpophalangeal joints and cramps. Electrophysiologically, there are fast-firing motor unit action potentials with interdischarge intervals of 2–20 m/s that are spontaneous during contraction. They could fire two (doublets), three (triplets), or more than three (multiplets) times or may fire in large bursts.[8–10] Increased nerve irritability is triggered by the decreased calcium concentration, which shifts the resting potential toward its action potential,[11–13] thus less current is required to elicit an action potential.[13] Causes of tetany include complete thyroidectomy, excessive enema treatments, pancreatitis, alkalosis in dialysis patients, and hypomagnesemia. Normocalcemic tetany could also occur as a familial disorder.[14]

Treatment consists of intravenous calcium with vitamin D and, particularly, calcitriol. However, some patients do not respond to this form of treatment. The use of sodium channel blockers, such as tocainide, relieves cramps.[15] As this is toxic, other channel blockers could be used and are beneficial, useful, and also help patients with myotonia.[16]

SUMMARY

This elderly woman had hypocalcemia due to radical thyroidectomy. She had characteristic tetany with carpopedal spasms, with positive Chvostek and Trousseau signs. The patient had only a partial response with vitamin D and calcium supplementation. She was treated with tocainide with some improvement and she later improved with calcitriol.

IMPORTANT POINTS

- Tetany is caused by neuromuscular irritability from hypocalcemia, hypomagnesemia, or alkalosis. A normocalcemic tetany has also been reported to occur in families.
- The characteristic clinical findings in tetany include carpopedal spasms, with positive Chvostek sign, characterized by contractures of the facial muscles upon tapping the facial nerves, and the Trousseau sign, which consists of carpopedal spasms after ischemia.
- The characteristic EMG findings of tetany include a spontaneous discharge from motor units in the form of multiplet motor unit discharges, such as duplets, triplets, or quadruplets.
- The treatment of tetany includes calcium gluconate and calcitriol. Sodium channel blockers could also be beneficial.

REFERENCES

1. Duyff RF, Van den Bosch J, Laman DM, et al. Neuromuscular findings in thyroid dysfunction: a prospective clinical and electrodiagnostic study. *J Neurol Neurosurg Psychiatry*. 2000;68(6):750–755.
2. Isaacs H, Heffron JJ. The syndrome of continuous muscle-fibre activity cured: further studies. *J Neurol Neurosurg Psychiatry*. 1974;37(11):1231–1235.
3. Yamashita H, Murakami T, Noguchi S, et al. Postoperative tetany in Graves disease: important role of vitamin D metabolites. *Ann Surg*. 1999;229(2):237–245.
4. Flink EB. Magnesium deficiency: etiology and clinical spectrum. *Acta Med Scand*. 1981;647(Suppl):125–137.
5. Hower J, Struck H, Tackmann W, Stolecke H. CPK activity in hypoparathyroidism. *N Engl J Med*. 1972;287:1098.
6. Kruse K, Scheunemann W, Baier W, Schaub J. Hypocalcemia myopathy in idiopathic hypoparathyroidism. *Eur J Pediatr*. 1982;138:280–282.
7. Akmal M. Rhabdomyolysis in a patient with hypocalcemia due to hypoparathyroidism. *Am J Nephrol*. 1993;13:61–63.
8. Amato AA, Dumitru D. Acquired myopathies. In: Dumitru D, Amato AA, Zwarts MJ, eds. *Electrodiagnostic Medicine*. Philadelphia, PA: Hanley & Belfus; 2002:937–1041. 2nd ed.
9. Swash M, Schwartz MS. *Neuromuscular Diseases: A Practical Approach to Diagnosis and Management*. London, England: Springer-Verlag; 1988.
10. Partanen VS, Lang AH. An analysis of double discharges in the human electromyogram. *J Neurol Sci*. 1978;36:363–375.
11. Frankenhaeuser B, Hodgkin AL. The action of calcium on the electric properties of squid axons. *J Physiol*. 1957;137:218–244.
12. Frankenhaeuser B. The effect of calcium on the myelinated nerve fiber. *J Physiol*. 1957;137:245–260.
13. Brink F. The role of calcium ions in neural processes. *Pharmacol Rev*. 1954;6:243–298.
14. Day JW, Parry GJ. Normocalcemic tetany abolished by calcium infusion. *Ann Neurol*. 1990;27:438–440.
15. Puniani TS, Bertorini TE. Tocainide therapy in muscle cramps and spasms due to neuromuscular disease. *Muscle Nerve*. 1991;14:280–285.
16. Modoni A., D'Amico A., Primiano G., et al. Long-term safety and usefulness of mexiletine in a large cohort of patients affected by non-dystrophic myotonias. *Front Neurol*. 2020;11:300. doi: 10.3389/fneur.2020.00300. eCollection 2020.

A Woman With Proximal Muscle Weakness and Neuromuscular Irritability

A 67-year-old woman presented with a 6-year history of mild difficulty climbing stairs, rising from a chair, and lifting her grandchild. She denied difficulty swallowing, numbness, shortness of breath, fasciculations, or muscle stiffness. Forty years earlier, she developed mild, nonspecific cataracts. During a routine medical evaluation, she was found to have a serum creatine kinase (CK) of 1032 IU/L (normal, <200 IU/L) and was referred to a neurologist.

Her family history was positive for a grandfather diagnosed with "neuromotor ataxia," her father had "spinal muscular atrophy," and a brother had similar symptoms.

Her initial electrophysiologic testing (done elsewhere) demonstrated a "myopathic" EMG with polyphasic motor units and many positive sharp waves diffusely. She had an abnormal muscle biopsy that led to the diagnosis of limb-girdle dystrophy; she was then referred for evaluation at our center.

Neurologic examination revealed normal mentation and cranial nerves without ptosis, cataracts, or facial anomalies. She had more proximal than distal muscle weakness (Fig. 111-1). Neck flexors were 3−/5, extensors, 4−/5; shoulder muscles, 4/5; biceps, triceps, and distal muscles were 5−/5. Distal hand muscles were normal. In the lower extremities the iliopsoas and glutei were 4/5, while the quadriceps, adductors, and distal muscles were 5/5. Reflexes were 2− and symmetrical without pathologic reflexes. There were no fasciculations or atrophy, no grip or eyelid myotonia was evident, and mild percussion myotonia was present. Sensation and coordination were normal. The rest of the examination was unremarkable.

Blood chemistry profile included normal thyroid studies and a CK of 573 IU/L (normal, <200 IU/L). No other abnormalities were detected.

AN EMG TEST WAS PERFORMED

Motor Nerve Studies

Nerve and Site	Latency (ms)	Amplitude (mV)	Conduction Velocity (m/s)
Peroneal Nerve R.	**Normal ≤ 5.7**	**Normal ≥ 3**	**Normal ≥ 40**
Ankle	3.9	3	–
Fibular head	11.0	3	43
Median Nerve R.	**Normal ≤ 4.2**	**Normal ≥ 6**	**Normal ≥ 50**
Wrist	3.5	8	–
Elbow	8.7	7	50

F-Wave Studies

Nerve	Latency (ms)	Normal Latency ≤ (ms)
Peroneal nerve R.	53.6	54
Median nerve R.	28.9	30

Sensory Nerve Studies

Nerve	Onset Latency (ms)	Normal Onset Latency ≤ (ms)	Peak Latency (ms)	Normal Peak Latency ≤ (ms)	Amp (μV)	Normal Amp ≥ (μV)	Conduction Velocity (m/s)	Normal Conduction Velocity ≥ (m/s)
Sural nerve R.	3.3	3.5	3.8	4.0	13	13	42	40
Median nerve R.	2.6	2.6	3.1	3.1	25	20	50	50

EMG Data

Muscle	Insrt Activity	Fibs	Pos Waves	Fasc	Amp	Dur	Poly	Pattern
Deltoid R.	**Myot**	None	None	None	**Dec.**	**Brief**	**Few**	Full
Triceps R.	**Myot**	None	**2+**	None	**Norm**	Norm	**Few**	Full
Biceps brachii R.	**Mtot**	None	**1+**	None	**Dec.**	**Brief**	**Few**	Full
Pronator teres R.	**Myot**	None	**1+**	None	Norm	Norm	**Few**	Full
Extensor digitorum com. R.	**Myot**	None	**1+**	None	Norm	Norm	**Few**	Full
First dorsal interosseous R.	**Myot**	None	**1+**	None	Norm	Norm	**Few**	Full
Opponens pollicis R.	**Myot**	None	**1+**	None	Norm	Norm	**Few**	Full

WHAT WERE THE EMG FINDINGS?

Nerve conduction tests were normal. The needle examination showed abundant short runs of myotonic discharges (Fig. 111-2) in several muscles and frequent polyphasic motor unit action potentials (MUAPs); some were small.

Her muscle biopsy was reviewed and showed many internalized nuclei, some fiber splitting and variation in fiber size, and pale centers; type I fibers were smaller than type II fibers (Fig. 111-3).

Her brother, aged 60 years, was evaluated later and found to have a slightly elongated face, baldness, mild cataracts, proximal weakness, and percussion and mild grip myotonia.

WHAT IS THE MOST LIKELY DIAGNOSIS?

The differential diagnosis in this patient with proximal muscle weakness includes myopathies, such as limb-girdle dystrophy. Other diagnoses, such as spinal muscular atrophy, adult-onset rod myopathy, and an endocrine or mitochondrial myopathy, should also be considered. Acid maltase deficiency and an inflammatory myopathy are important considerations because of the presence of myotonia on EMG, but these diseases are not accompanied by clinical myotonia. The suggestion of an autosomal-dominant inheritance is unlikely for acid maltase deficiency or an acquired myopathy such as polymyositis.

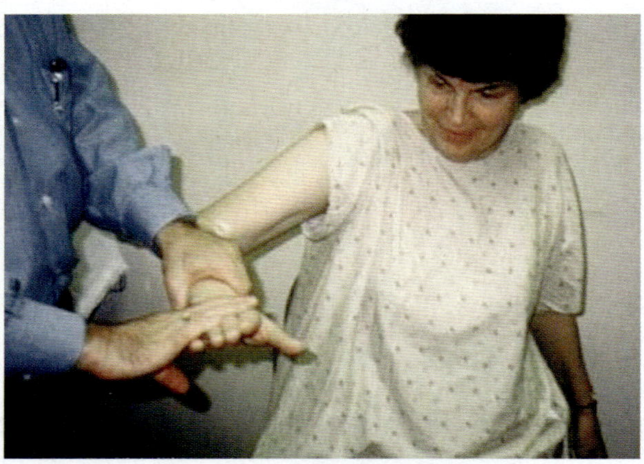

FIG. 111-1 Patient demonstrating normal facial features and more proximal than distal weakness.

The findings of small polyphasic MUAPs on EMG and the myotonia are against a motor neuron disorder and make limb muscular dystrophy, rod myopathy, endocrine disease, or mitochondria disorder unlikely.

The predominantly proximal weakness makes the diagnosis of classic myotonic dystrophy or dystrophic myotonia (DM) unlikely. The weakness and lack of prominent myotonia are against the diagnosis of myotonia congenita.

The autosomal-dominant inheritance and proximal weakness with electrical myotonia, and her brother having clinical myotonia, are suggestive of proximal myotonic myopathy, or PROMM.

WHAT SHOULD BE DONE NEXT?

DNA studies by PCR amplification and high-resolution electrophoresis showed 11,000 CCTG repeat expansions (normal, 10–30) in intron 1 of the zinc finger protein 9 (*ZNF9*) gene.

DISCUSSION

This patient had an autosomal-dominant disease characterized by proximal muscle weakness that was previously diagnosed as limb-girdle muscular dystrophy. Her father was diagnosed as having spinal muscular atrophy but likely had the same disease. She had mild percussion myotonia, and myotonia that was prominent on EMG, whereas her brother has more significant clinical myotonia. It is likely that her first EMG finding of "positive sharp waves" was actually short runs of myotonic discharges.

The association of muscle weakness and myotonia is characteristic of DM. In this disease the phenotype consists of facial, neck flexor, and *distal* limb weakness (Fig. 111-4), balding, and cataracts with other systemic manifestations such as cardiomyopathy.

Most DM patients have CTG repeat expansions of the *DMPK* gene in chromosome 19 and are now classified as DM1.[1] Patients with DM who lack this genetic defect are classified as DM2. In those the genetic defect is located in chromosome 3.[1] Patients with predominantly proximal weakness and myotonia are considered to have PROMM,[2–4] the diagnosis of this patient. The gene for PROMM is mapped to the same 3q locus as DM2 in many patients and thus is the same disease

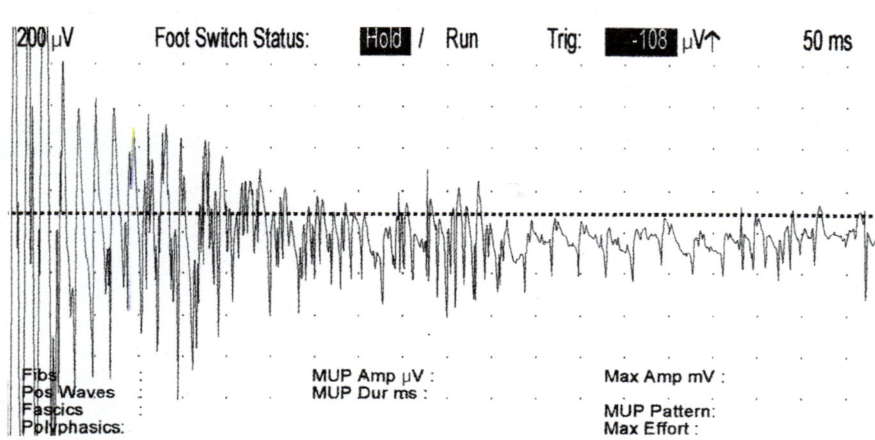

FIG. 111-2 Myotonic discharges in the deltoid muscle (200 μV/50 ms).

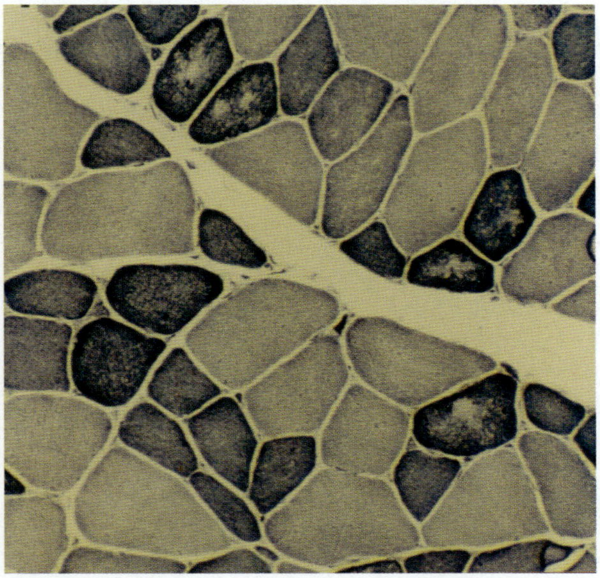

FIG. 111-3 Muscle biopsy showing type I muscle fiber smallness and pale centers (NADH-TR stain, ×200).

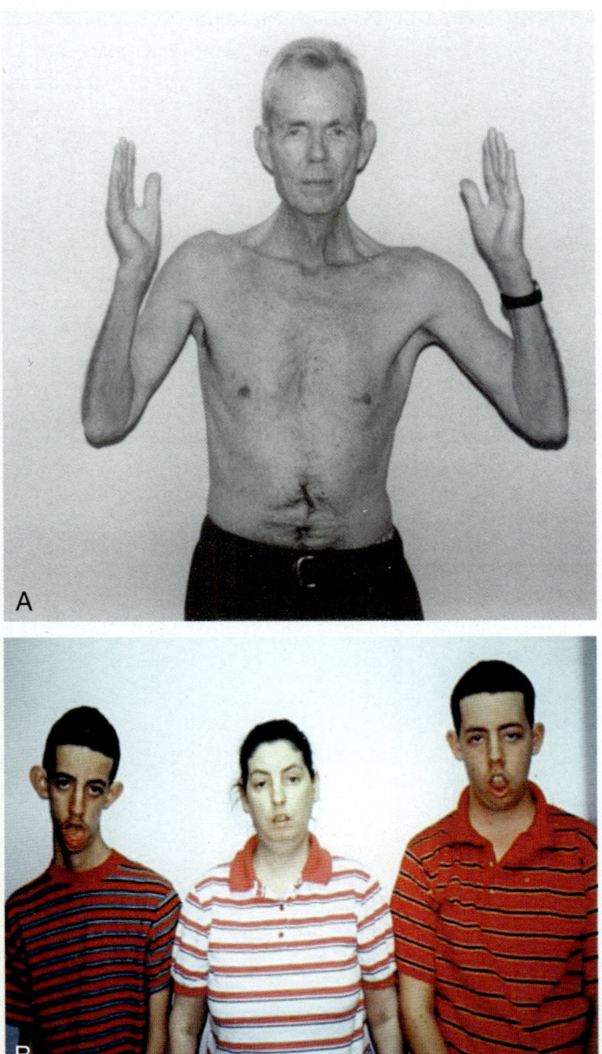

FIG. 111-4 **A**, A patient with classic myotonic dystrophy (DM1) showing elongated face and distal muscle wasting. **B**, A mother and her two sons with DM1; notice the elongated faces.

with some variations in the phenotype.[5,6] Anticipation is rare in PROMM. The genetic defect in PROMM/DM2 consists of a CCTG tetranucleotide repeat expansion in intron 1 of the *ZNF9/CNBP* gene.[6,7] Mutant transcripts aggregate as nuclei foci that sequester RNA-binding proteins resulting in a spliceopathy of effector genes. Other factors like changes in gene expression, translation, and micro-RNA metabolism occur.[8]

PROMM is characterized by proximal weakness and myotonia. Early cataracts can occur.[6] The clinical myotonia can fluctuate and might be missed during clinical examination. We actually diagnosed a case with myotonia only on EMG. There is one report with myotonia that was evident only during pregnancy.[8]

The diagnosis of PROMM should be made by careful clinical evaluation in patients with limb-girdle weakness and autosomal-dominant inheritance having myotonia clinically. DNA analysis demonstrates a lack of the CTG repeat expansion of DM on chromosome 19, and patients should be investigated for the CCTG repeat expansions in chromosome 3q.[9]

PROMM/DM2 is usually a more benign disease than DM1, although systemic manifestation, including cardiomyopathy, can occur.[4,6,7,10] A severe clinical presentation with mental retardation that can occur in DM1 is not seen in these patients.[1,7]

Muscle biopsies of DM2/PROMM typically do not show the characteristic type I fiber atrophy and ring fibers in DM1; instead, they show more prominent type II muscle fiber atrophy; frequent internalized nuclei and pyknotic nuclei are also common.[11,12] This case had smaller type I muscle fibers.

There is no cure for PROMM other than conservative management. Sodium channel blockers may help those with prominent myotonia.

SUMMARY

This patient has proximal weakness, mild percussion myotonia, and obvious myotonia on EMG. Her brother had a similar presentation resembling DM1. She was diagnosed as having PROMM, a disease characterized by proximal weakness and myotonia caused by a mutation in chromosome 3.

IMPORTANT POINTS

- PROMM is an autosomal-dominant disease characterized by proximal weakness and myotonia. Other features include cataracts, and cardiomyopathy might occur.
- Myotonic dystrophies have two recognized genetic loci. The one in chromosome 19 is characterized by increased CTG repeat expansion in the DMPK gene, and the other has mutations in chromosome 3q, which is a CCTG tetranucleotide repeat expansion in the *ZNF9* gene in chromosome 3q (DM2), as PROMM.
- The pathogenesis of the myotonia and weakness in these conditions is unclear.

REFERENCES

1. Moxley RT III. The myotonias: their diagnosis and treatment. *Comp Ther*. 1996;22:8–21.

2. Moxley RT III, Udd B, Ricker K. Proximal myotonic myopathy (PROMM) and other proximal myotonic syndromes. *Neuromuscul Disord.* 1998;8:519–520.
3. Ricker K, Koch MC, Lehmann-Horn F, et al. Proximal myotonic myopathy: a new dominant disorder with myotonia, muscle weakness, and cataracts. *Neurology.* 1994;44(8):1448–1452.
4. Ricker K, Koch MC, Lehmann-Horn F, et al. Proximal myotonic myopathy: clinical features of a multisystem disorder similar to myotonic dystrophy. *Arch Neurol.* 1995;52:25–31.
5. Liquori CL, Ricker K, Moseley ML, et al. Myotonic dystrophy type 2 caused by a CCTG expansion in intron 1 of ZNF9. *Science.* 2001;293(5531):864–867.
6. Day JW, Ricker K, Jacobsen JF, et al. Myotonic dystrophy type 2: molecular, diagnostic and clinical spectrum. *Neurology.* 2003; 60(4):657–664.
7. Machuca-Tzili L, Brook D, Hilton-Jones D, et al. Clinical and molecular aspects of the myotonic dystrophies: a review. *Muscle Nerve.* 2005;32:1–18.
8. Newman B, Meola G, O'Donovan DG, et al. Proximal myotonic myopathy (PROMM) presenting as myotonia during pregnancy. *Neuromuscul Disord.* 1999;9:144–149.
9. Moxley RT III, Udd B, Ricker K. Proximal myotonic myopathies, PROMM, and other proximal myotonic syndromes. *Neuromuscul Disord.* 1998;8:519–520.
10. Vihola A, Bassez G, Meola G, et al. Histopathological differences of myotonic dystrophy type 1 (DM1) and PROMM/DM2. *Neurology.* 2003;60(11):1854–1857.
11. Schoser BG, Schneider-Gold C, Kress W, et al. Muscle pathology in 57 patients with myotonic dystrophy type 2. *Muscle Nerve.* 2004;29:275–281.
12. Meola G, Cardani R. Myotonic dystrophies: an update on clinical aspects, genetic, pathology, and molecular pathomechanisms. *Biochim Biophys Acta.* 2015;1852(4):594–606.

A Woman With Focal Spontaneous Muscle Movements

A 42-year-old right-handed, Black woman came complaining that her leg muscles got tight and "moved on their own" for about 4–5 months prior to presentation and had gotten progressively worse. The symptoms were more prominent in the thighs and buttocks but occasionally involved the anterior abdominal wall and chest. She had spasms with swelling which produced discomfort and pain. She denied numbness, paresthesias, or other neurological complaints. Exercise might make the movements appear more often.

Past medical history was remarkable for "benign cysts" in the axilla and a Bartholin cyst. She had been on a muscle relaxer without benefit. She did not smoke, drink alcohol, or use recreational drugs. Family history was negative.

General physical examination was normal, but she was observed to have spontaneous waveform-like contractions in the thigh muscles (Fig. 112-1). She could reproduce these contractions by massaging and pressing the thighs. There was no rash. She had normal mentation and cranial nerves, without ptosis, fatigue, diplopia, or muscle weakness and wasting. Reflexes were slightly brisk but symmetrical, and plantar responses were flexor. Coordination and sensory examinations were normal. There was no grip or percussion myotonia, but there was mild myoedema. The rest of the examination was unremarkable.

WHAT IS THE DIFFERENTIAL DIAGNOSIS?

This patient appears to have a syndrome of neuromuscular irritability. There was no clinical myotonia to indicate a myotonic syndrome. The contractions were focal and not persistent or prominent in the trunk to suggest stiff-person syndrome. These appeared and disappeared spontaneously and rapidly and were not the characteristic contractions seen in the glycogenesis. The movements resembled cramps but there were no fasciculations present as in the cramp-fasciculation syndrome. Issacs syndrome is another consideration because of the spasms and focal contractions.

Comprehensive metabolic and thyroid-stimulating hormones were normal. HIV was nonreactive. FANA titers were elevated at 1:640 speckles, rheumatoid factor was 194 IU/mL (normal, <14 IU/mL). Serum creatine kinase was 1150 IU/L (normal, 0–165 IU/L). Erythrocyte sedimentation rate was 84 mm/h (normal, <30 mm/h). Complete blood count showed normal white blood cells, but her hematocrit was 22%–84%; hemoglobin was 6.6 g/dL.

A CAT scan of the chest was normal. Stool for occult guaiac was negative.

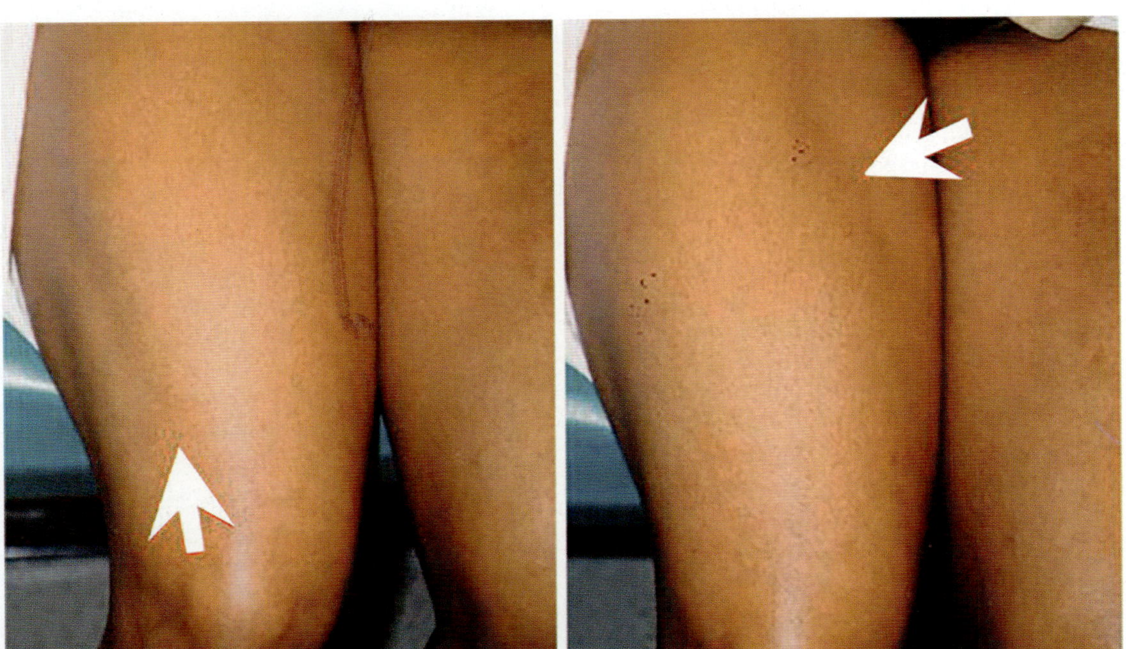

FIG. 112-1 Notice the spontaneous contractions in the thighs (*arrows*).

AN EMG TEST WAS PERFORMED

Nerve conduction studies were normal, and on EMG there was no evidence of myokymia, myotonia, or other abnormal electrical discharge at rest. The motor units were normal and did not fire spontaneously. The waveform contractions observed clinically were not associated with electrical action potentials.

It was concluded that she had rippling muscle disease (RMD).

A muscle biopsy showed some myofiber necrosis with phagocytosis and mild interstitial inflammatory infiltrates with patchy decreased staining for caveolin (Fig. 112-2).

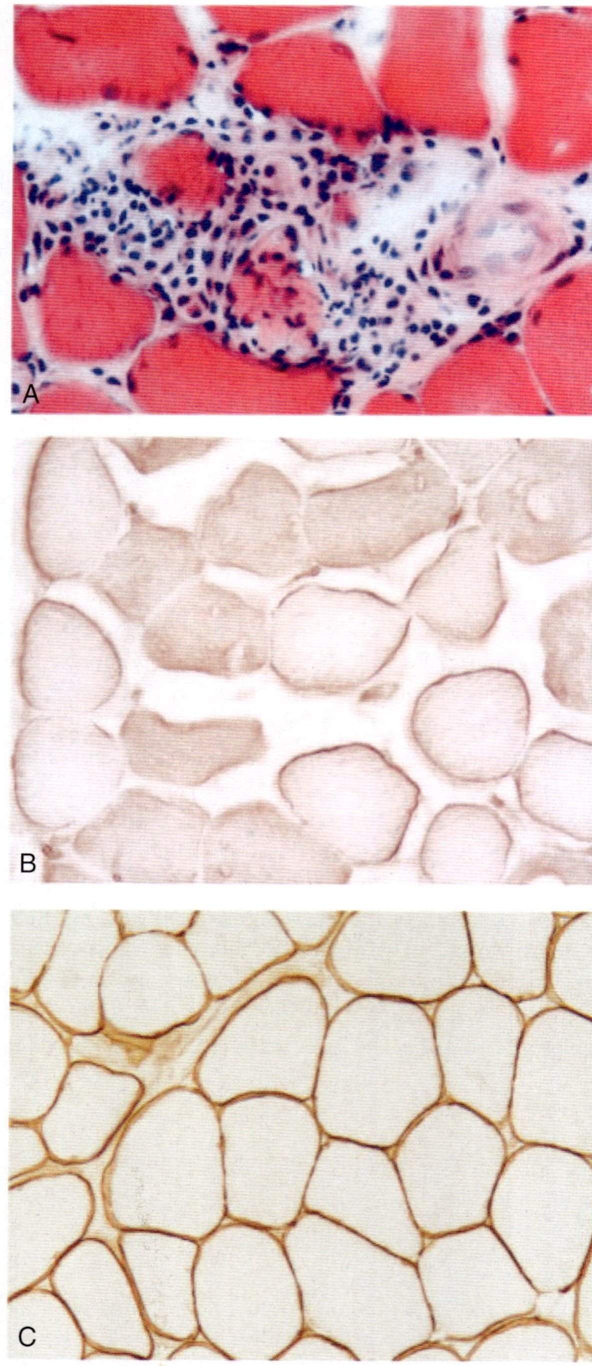

FIG. 112-2 A, Focal muscle necrosis and inflammatory cell infiltrates; there are also freezing artifacts (H&E stain, ×200). **B**, Scattered fibers without, or with patchy caveolin stain. Compare with normal in control. **C**, (immunoperoxidase, ×200).

DISCUSSION

This patient has RMD, a condition that manifests with electrically silent wave-like contractions, and although she had no clinical evidence of lupus erythematosus, her lupus tests were positive. The erythrocyte sedimentation rate was also elevated, but her anemia could have contributed to this.

She was treated with metaxalone with minimal improvement; the addition of dantrolene also helped, and later prednisone 30 mg/day caused marked improvement. She was also found to have iron-deficiency anemia, believed to be from heavy menses, and was treated with iron replacement.

RMD is characterized by muscle hyperexcitability with spasms and contractions which can be induced by muscle stitching, pressure, and percussion. The contractions are silent.[1,2]

RMD could be hereditary[3-7] or acquired.[6,8] The disease is named for the self-propagation, rippling, or rolling of muscle with a velocity of about 0.6 m/s. Additional clinical features are myoedema or localized mounding of the muscles after percussion. There is usually no associated weakness, although distal weakness can be seen rarely.

As in this patient, acquired RMD may be immune-mediated, and some patients have myasthenia gravis.[8-10] They could also have antibodies against striated muscle and potassium voltage-gated muscle channels.[11] There are cases with hypothyroidism.[12]

RMD was originally described by Torbergsen in 1975[13] and Ricker in 1989[14] who first used the descriptive name. The classic hereditary form is autosomal-dominant with variable presentations as associated with mutations of the caveolin gene linked to chromosome C1q41; some cases have cardiomyopathy.[15] This genetic defect has been excluded in some patients.[16,17] A caveolin-3 mutation on chromosome 3p25 has been associated with RMD and is allelic to limb-girdle dystrophy 1C.[4,7] A severe autosomal-recessive RMD has also been described.[16,17]

The exact cause of muscle rippling is unknown, but the region of the C1q42 contains important proteins that participate in excitation–contraction coupling, including α-actinin, α-actin troponin I, and cardiac ryanodine receptor. The pathogenesis in those with caveolin mutations may be explained by the important role of caveolin in the structural integrity of the sarcoplasm and signal translation.[17] To explain the mechanism of rippling, in vitro studies show after-contractions with increased sarcolemma excitability due to a delayed released of calcium by the sarcoplasmic reticulum.[4] Alterations of the tubular system have also been observed.[18] Recently, Lamb suggested that rippling is caused by action potential in the tubular system that does not excite the sarcolemma. Those are not detectable by electromyography and thus are considered to be "silent."[19]

A focal-decreased staining of caveolin has been demonstrated in acquired RMD, likely caused by antibodies against the sarcolemma.[20]

There is no cure for RMD, but some patients respond to muscle relaxants, and those with the acquired form might also respond to immunotherapy.

SUMMARY

This patient had wave-like muscle contractions that were electrically silent; she was diagnosed as having RMD. In her case, this was likely autoimmune and responded to dantrolene and steroids.

IMPORTANT POINTS

- Spontaneous, electrically silent muscle contractures that are persistent for minutes occur in metabolic myopathy. In RMD, they have wave-like characteristic but appear and disappear promptly.
- RMD can be hereditary from mutations of C1q41 and the *CAV 3* gene in chromosome 3p25 but can have an autoimmune etiology, sometimes associated with myasthenia gravis and hypothyroidism.
- The disease responds to dantrolene, and steroids in the acquired form.

REFERENCES

1. So YT, Zu L, Barraza C, et al. Rippling muscle disease: evidence for phenotypic and genetic heterogeneity. *Muscle Nerve*. 2001; 24(3):340–344.
2. Ansevin CF. Phenotypic variability in rippling muscle disease. *Neurology*. 2000;5(2):273–274.
3. Koul RL, Chand RP, Chacko A, et al. Severe autosomal recessive rippling muscle disease. *Muscle Nerve*. 2001;24(11):1542–1547.
4. Betz RC, Schoser BC, Kasper D, et al. Mutations in CAV 3 cause mechanical hyperirritability of skeletal muscle in rippling muscle disease. *Nat Genet*. 2001;28(3):218–219.
5. Stephan DA, Hoffman EP. Physical mapping of the rippling muscle disease locus. *Genomics*. 1999;55(3):268–274.
6. Torbergsen T. Rippling muscle disease: a review. *Muscle Nerve*. 2002;11:S103–S107.
7. Vorgerd M, Ricker K, Ziemssen F, et al. A sporadic case of rippling muscle disease caused by a de novo caveolin-3 mutation. *Neurology*. 2001;57:2273–2277.
8. Ansevin CF, Agamanolis DP. Rippling muscles and myasthenia gravis with rippling muscles. *Arch Neurol*. 1996;53(2):197–199.
9. Greenberg SA. Acquired rippling muscle disease with myasthenia gravis. *Muscle Nerve*. 2004;19:143–146.
10. Muller-Felber W, Ansevin CF, Ricker K, et al. Immunosuppressive treatment of rippling muscles in patients with myasthenia gravis. *Neuromuscul Disord*. 1999;9:604–607.
11. Walker GR, Watkins T, Ansevin CF. Identification of autoantibodies associated with rippling muscles and myasthenia gravis that recognize skeletal muscle proteins: possible relationship of antigens and stretch-activated ion channels. *Biochem Biophys Res Commun*. 1999;264:430–435.
12. Ducci RDP, Scola RH, Lorenzoni PJ, et al. Immune-mediated rippling muscle disease in a patient with treated hypothyroidism. *J Neurol Sci*. 2017;383:53–55.
13. Torbergsen T. A family with dominant hereditary myotonia, muscular hypertrophy and increased muscular irritability, distinct from myotonia congenita of Thomsen. *Acta Neurol Scand*. 1975;51:225–232.
14. Ricker K, Moxley RT, Rohkamm R, et al. Rippling muscle disease. *Arch Neurol*. 1989;46:405–408.
15. Stephan DA, Buist NR, Chittenden AB, et al. A rippling muscle disease gene is localized to 1q41: evidence for multiple genes. *Neurology*. 1994;44:1915–1920.
16. Vorgerd M, Bolz H, Patzold T, et al. Phenotypic variability in rippling muscle disease. *Neurology*. 2000;54:273–274.
17. Burns J, Bretag AH, Blumbergs PC, Harbord MG. Benign familial disease with muscle mounding and rippling. *J Neurol Neurosurg Psychiatry*. 1994;57:344–347.
18. Woodman SE, Sotgia F, Galbiati F, et al. Caveolinopathies: mutations in caveolin-3 cause four distinct autosomal dominant muscle disease. *Neurology*. 2004;62:538–543.
19. Lamb GD. Rippling muscle disease may be caused by "silent" action potentials in the tubular system of skeletal muscle fibers. *Muscle Nerve*. 2005;31:652–658.
20. Schulte-Mattler WJ, Kley RA, Rothenfusser-Korber E, et al. Immune-mediated rippling muscle disease. *Neurology*. 2005;64:364–367.

INDEX OF CASES BY DIAGNOSIS

INDEX

Note: Page numbers followed by f indicate figures; those followed by t indicate tables.

A

B

C

E

F

G

H

I

M

N

O

P

Q

R

S

T

U

V

W

X

Z